Essentials of Human Diseases and Conditions

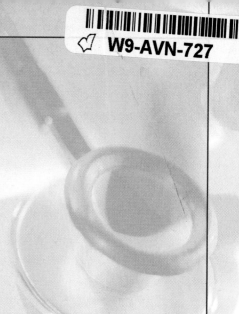

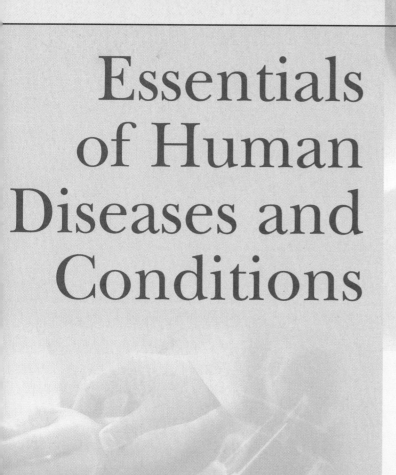

Essentials of Human Diseases and Conditions

third edition

Margaret Schell Frazier, RN, CMA, BS
Retired
Department Chair, Health and Human Services Division
Program Chair, Medical Assisting Program
Ivy Tech State College, Northeast
Fort Wayne, Indiana
Owner, Consultant
M&M Consulting
Hudson, Indiana

Jeanette Wist Drzymkowski, RN, BS
Formerly
Associate Faculty
Ivy Tech State College, Northeast
Fort Wayne, Indiana

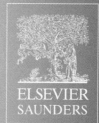

ELSEVIER
SAUNDERS

ELSEVIER
SAUNDERS

An Imprint of Elsevier

11830 Westline Industrial Drive
St. Louis, Missouri 63146

Essentials of Human Diseases and Conditions, Third Edition   0-7216-0256-8

DISCLAIMER
Every effort has been made to make this text complete and accurate, but no guarantee, warranty, or rep-
resentation is made for its accuracy or completeness.
W.B. Saunders Company, Margaret S. Frazier, and Jeanette W. Drzymkowski are not providing any legal
or professional service/advice in presenting these codes and bear no liability for how the codes are used.
THE PUBLISHER

NOTICE

Medical assisting is an ever-changing field. Standard safety precautions must be followed, but as new
research and clinical experience broaden our knowledge, changes in treatment and drug therapy
may become necessary or appropriate. Readers are advised to check the most current product information provided by the manufacturer of each drug to be administered to verify the recommended dose, the method and duration of administration, and contraindications. It is the responsibility of the licensed health-care provider, relying on experience and knowledge of the patient, to
determine dosages and the best treatment for each individual patient. Neither the publisher nor the
author assumes any liability for any injury and/or damage to persons or property arising from this
publication.

Previous editions copyrighted 2000, 1996

International Standard Book Number 0-7216-0256-8

Publishing Director: Andrew Allen
Executive Editor: Adrianne Rippinger
Senior Developmental Editor: Rae L. Robertson
Publishing Services Manager: Linda McKinley
Senior Project Manager: Julie Eddy
Senior Designer: Julia Dummitt

Printed in the United States of America

Last digit is the print number: 9   8   7   6   5   4   3   2   1

Third Edition Editorial Review Board

To Dave, always my strength and love, and to
Margaret Sarah Musser, the newest Margaret in the family, our joy and beloved granddaughter.

Love, Margie and Grandma

*Mere change is not growth. Growth is the synthesis of change and continuity,
and where there is no continuity there is no growth.*
Selected Literary Essays, *Hamlet: The Prince or the Poem* (1942)
From *The Quotable C.S. Lewis*

In addition to the work of research and the development of this text,
much of the creativity of this edition results from a synthesis
of life experiences, both professional and personal.
This edition therefore is gratefully and properly dedicated to my teachers
who endowed me with a solid foundation for growth;
to my students with whom I engaged in learning
and often was challenged with change;
to those who have been under my professional care
and have gifted me with their trust and appreciation;
to my colleagues, whose thoughtful contributions
ensure the quality of the manuscript;
and to my family and friends—*you know who you are*—who
in one way or another offered their talents and enduring support.

Jeanette Drzymkowski

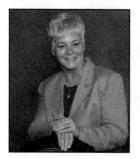
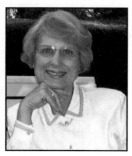

Recently, health care has experienced dramatic and far-reaching changes. The first edition of *Essentials of Human Diseases and Conditions* was visualized as an encyclopedic handbook. As the format progressed, however, a textbook with a systematic approach to pathophysiology evolved. While many disease entities and their concepts may remain constant, their diagnosis and treatment may experience changes. The second edition was updated to reflect many of these changes. Once again, review and revision are in order, and the authors have gathered data and sought experts to critique and assist in the writing of the third edition.

Essentials of Human Diseases and Conditions, Third Edition, is a user-friendly reference intended to serve as a stimulating and practical textbook for students as well as an invaluable tool as a handbook for healthcare providers in any type of health-care setting. Instructors of such classes as anatomy and physiology, disease conditions, medical coding, and medical transcription will likely appreciate the value of this edition as a required text. This encyclopedic but simplified handbook includes comprehensive information about hundreds of diseases and conditions. Supplementary facts highlighted throughout the text offer further clarification of information. The appendices offer valuable information about diagnostic testing, pharmacology, and resource agencies. A new concept in reference information has been added in the form of websites that have been specifically designed to help the student and/or health-care professional in researching supplementary sources of comprehensive information.

Distinctive Features of Our Approach

Because disease conditions are universally experienced, there is a natural curiosity about them and an interest in understanding them. Written by experienced nurses who are educators of medical paraprofessionals, this book condenses and simplifies current medical information on the more common clinical disorders encountered in the health field and physician's office. Students in the field of medical assisting, medical transcription, insurance coding, or other allied health programs *who have had a prior introduction to basic anatomy and physiology of the human body and medical terminology* will find this system of learning orderly, concise, and easy to comprehend. The sheer magnitude of the body of knowledge represented in this field would overwhelm any beginning student if it were not streamlined into a logical format.

Chapter 1 introduces the reader to general principles of pathophysiology. This is followed by a discussion of pediatric situations in Chapter 2. After these general discussions, the text progresses through body systems in a logical sequence. Chapter 14 is entirely devoted to discussion of mental disorders, including phobias, grief response, posttraumatic stress disorders, alcohol abuse, and other conditions covered by DSM-IV. This chapter also includes a comprehensive chart on drugs of abuse, their street names, and their effects on the abuser. The final chapter includes information about traumatic insults, both physical and emotional, that equips the health-care worker with practical knowledge when faced with a variety of traumatic injuries. This material includes lightning injuries; insect, animal, and snake bites; child abuse, psychological abuse, elder abuse, sexual abuse, and rape.

Text Features

A logical sequence for the progression of the information is followed. Each chapter is introduced with a brief review of the normal function of the specific body system discussed in the chapter, and this review is reinforced with clear illustrations.

Important pathologic mechanisms are explained and illustrated as well. Each disease entity is presented in a format that begins by describing and discussing the nature of the disease as seen in the symptoms experienced by the patient and signs detected by the physician. The format continues with sections devoted to etiologic factors, diagnosis, treatment options, prognosis, prevention, and patient teaching related to the disease entity. A diagnostic code is assigned to each disease entity. **(See important notes at the end of the preface.)** This format also follows the inherent progression of a patient's experience: (1) the individual reports symptoms to a health-care provider, usually in a clinical setting; (2) abnormal signs of a clinical disorder may be elicited during the physical examination and/or subsequent diagnostic testing; (3) an appropriate treatment option is initiated and monitored for results; (4) the patient is given appropriate teaching to encourage compliance to ensure an optimal outcome. The usual prognosis for the condition and possible preventive measures are discussed.

Boldfaced words found in the text are listed in the Key Terms at the beginning of each chapter, as well as in the Glossary at the back of the book. The Key Terms list provides pronunciations for important words related to chapter content. Italicized words found in the chapters are defined in the Glossary for purposes of review or clarification of meaning. The authors have kept in mind the advantages to the student and health-care worker in better understanding clinical disorders. These include (1) great professional gain when one comprehends the effects that a disease has on a person, (2) increased communication skills with the entire health-care team, and (3) personal education that has many practical applications.

Enrichment boxes are used to give the reader pertinent information that is not discussed in the typical 10-point format. Occasionally, relevant information does not lend itself to the usual format; this information is discussed as **Enrichments.** Likewise, essential warnings (cautions and precautions) that require discussion may require special treatment. This information is presented in the **Alert boxes** found throughout the book. To give the reader visual images of facts being addressed, more than 475 color illustrations are included. Several tables give the reader another visual medium to improve understanding. The glossary is a supplementary resource provided for your convenience. Boldfaced words throughout the chapters are defined in the glossary.

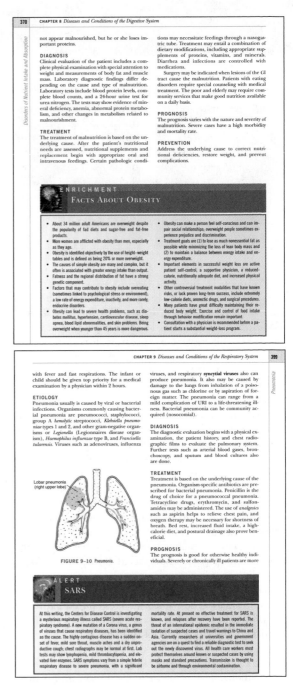

Three appendices are found in the back of the book. The Common Laboratory and Diagnostic Tests appendix discusses tests often ordered by the physician. Reference values are listed for laboratory tests, followed by possible causes of each variation above normal or below normal. Reference values or expected normal results are discussed for imaging and other studies. Again, causes of variations from normal are provided. It is imperative that the reader using this information recognize that reference values may vary according to the laboratory in which the test is performed and reported. Another appendix contains pharmacology information. Representative drugs are listed by group and include name of drug, usual intended therapeutic objective, possible side effects, and general comments. The presentation of this appendix follows the chapters in the text. Once again, the reader must recognize that drugs and drug substances may be continually changing and that any specific material must be confirmed by referencing a current PDR or pharmacology reference source. The final appendix contains listings of resource agencies. Most contain names of agencies, mailing addresses, telephone contact numbers, and website information. Resource agencies tend to change locations, telephone numbers, and websites; therefore the reader may view updates by using the Evolve site for this book.

The authors believe it is important to define the role of patient screening in each discussion. Therefore the discussion of each particular disease entity begins with a feature called *Patient Screening;* the remarks therein usually are tailored to the disease entity being discussed. Because the vast majority of patients first seek access to health-care services by telephone, many healthcare facilities have a written, standardized protocol for medical personnel who take incoming calls. The comments offered in the *Patient Screening* feature of this text are not intended to diagnose the caller's medical condition or give curative advice. The feature typically offers *general clues* to recognizing the urgency for an appointment, identifying emergencies, and discerning the kind of calls that require referral to the physician for response. This feature is not to be confused with the skill of medical triage, which state practice acts generally reserve for certain licensed professionals. Carefully listening to the patient who is calling often identifies information that helps the telephone screener select the appropriate action required by the caller. Ideally, the outcome of telephone communication between caller and screener will benefit the patient and avoid potential medical-legal problems. Maintaining a sensitivity to human suffering, keeping strict confidentiality, and upholding the priority of meeting the needs of patients cannot be overemphasized as skills necessary in a medical telephone screener.

In this regard, we also would like to add a list of serious and life-threatening conditions that require immediate assessment and intervention. These include but are not limited to:

- Sudden onset of unexplained shortness of breath
- Crushing pain across the center of the chest
- Difficult breathing occurring suddenly and rapidly worsening, often in the middle of the night
- Vomiting of blood that is bright red or with a very dark "coffee grounds" appearance
- Sudden onset of weakness and unsteadiness or severe dizziness
- Sudden loss of consciousness or paralysis
- Flashes of light in field of vision
- Sudden and progressively worsening abdominal, flank, or pelvic pain
- Sudden onset of blurred vision accompanied by severe throbbing in the eye

A report of any of these symptoms must be immediately relayed to the physician. The physician will then offer additional instructions to give to the individual calling for help.

Extensive Supplemental Resources
Student Workbook

This new workbook features comprehenisve additional review exercises and practice activities in a variety of formats to reinforce chapter topics.

- **Word Definitions** and **Glossary Terms** review important key terms covered in each chapter.
- **Short Answer** and **Fill-in-the-Blank** questions review key chapter concepts.
- An **Anatomical Structures** section in select chapters presents diagrams representing key body structures to be labeled by the student.
- A **Patient Screening** section guides students in the practice of appointment scheduling or specialist referral based on a patient's described signs and symptoms.
- A **Patient Teaching** section guides students in the practice of performing patient education for various diseases and disorders.
- **Essay** questions invite students to further investigate key chapter topics.
- A **Certification Exam Review** helps students prepare for the certification exam with questions focused on chapter content in multiple choice format.

Internet Resources

Students and health-care providers need a method of keeping current on developments, trends, changes, and news in the medical arena. The specially designed complimentary **Evolve** website offers an extensive list of pertinent links to information for over 500 diseases and disorders. It also provides periodic updates to information found in the text. The Evolve site gives students or heath-care professionals an avenue for accessing necessary information from the ever-changing field of medicine and health care. The vast amount of information provided by sources found on this Evolve website is available for access at http://evolve.elsevier.com/Frazier/essentials/.

Instructor's Curriculum Resource With CD-ROM

Included is the Instructor's Curriculum Resource in both print and CD-ROM formats. This resource contains pedagogy to aid the instructor in teaching a course in pathophysiology.

This supplementary material is readily available to the instructor to enhance the educational process. An introduction provides an insight into material contained in the ICR. This is followed by suggested course outlines for teaching in an 11-week quarter, a 16-week semester, two 11-week quarters, and two 16-week semesters. Generalized teaching strategies for the classroom are suggested. Specific important guidelines for students using the internet for assignments are included. It is highly recommended that students be given a copy of these guidelines before they attempt to research assignments on the Internet. The final aspect of generalized information includes disclaimers about the use of the book for insurance coding, patient teaching, and patient screening.

A chapter-by-chapter outline is as follows:
- Introduction to and overview of information available in that chapter
- Key terms
- Chapter learning objectives
- Suggested activities to promote learning
- Review-challenge questions and answers covering pertinent chapter material
- Summary of the information presented in each chapter
- Real-Life Challenge questions and answers
- Worksheets for students to complete

The ICR also includes:
- Test bank for each chapter available, with answers, in both printed and Exam-View format
- Student workbook answer key
- Glossary

All the above features are available to the instructor for easy download, allowing the instructor to apply his or her creativity; all of these features may be revised to accommodate any instructor's lesson plan.

The information presented in this book represents research into the mainstream of medical knowledge and its application in clinical practice. In the actual practice of the dynamic art and science of medicine, great variations and opposing views result in either more conservative or more aggressive concepts. The material presented in this text should not take the place of individualized consultation with medical experts.

Important Information

NOTE: Regarding the diagnostic codes included in this publication, it is *imperative* to consider the following:

Medical coding is an intricate and intense process requiring study and understanding to ensure maximum reimbursement from insurance companies, for participation in Medicare and Medicaid programs, and for statistical tabulation. A diagnostic code used in the health-care setting has been assigned to each disease entity in this publication *to help students and workers in the health-care setting to understand the ICD-9-CM coding process in reporting clinical information.* Diagnostic codes are subject to changes, revisions, and additions; therefore it is imperative that you always refer to a *current* listing of ICD-9-CM codes. The authors have kept in mind that financial reimbursement directly correlates with the reporting of current, valid codes, which may require modification to ensure greatest specificity found in the most current coding manual and guidelines. Therefore the authors recommend referral to a current edition of a coding manual.

Regarding *patient teaching*, the authors are mindful of legal parameters addressed in state acts governing the practice of medical assistants.

NOTE: *Readers, please consult your state code regarding licensing for the rules and regulations applying to medical assistant practice.* State practice laws vary; they identify the tasks the properly prepared medical assistant can perform. Regarding the responsibility issue, the medical assistant in a medical office must know whom his or her supervisor is; it may be the physician. Medical assistants should ask about a written office policy regarding any delegation of tasks by the physician or nurse.

The authors consider it important, and in the patient's best interest, that all health-care workers as members of a clinical team understand the principles, goals, and specifics of patient teaching. *Licensing regulations, and state practice acts generally permit only nurses and physicians to perform patient teaching and make triage judgments.*

As with the previous editions, research, revision, and consultation with health-care professionals were required. A systematic approach to the revision of preexisting material was implemented. Suggestions for additional diseases to be discussed were obtained and addressed.

Experts in the various fields were consulted, and some helped to rewrite or add to specific areas. Others reviewed and suggested important revisions and additions. We want to acknowledge the input from our field of experts and identify their area of expertise.

Carol O'Hear, BA—Areas pertaining to cancer

William Shiel, MD, FACP, FACR

Barbara Shang, MD—Areas pertaining to the eye

Margaret Ann Frazier, MS/LFMT

Pegi Frazier, BS/FMLT, Angola, IN, Private Practice—Mental wellness and illness

Marlise Fletter, MS, APRN.BC, Family Nurse Practitioner, Angola, IN—Dermatology and urinary tract disorders

Jeffery P. Shriver, RPh, BS, Practicing Pharmacist, Keltsch Pharmacy, Decatur, IN—Pharmacology as related to disease treatment

Robert Fulcher, BS, BSPh, RPh—Pharmacology appendix revision and consultation

Lauri Burnett, Bachelors of Ministry, Insurance Claim Reviewer—Identification and assignment of ICD-9-CM codes

In addition, the professional reviewers kept us on our toes with their astute reviews of every word and comment.

The Evolve website will give instructors extensive resources for teaching material. In addition to the website, instructors are offered the "slide show" of more than 750 slide images with legends to be selected for additional visuals and for specific lessons. This vast array of illustrations uses most of the printed illustrations from the book and about 300 additional images of supplementary material.

The test bank in the ExamView format gives instructors the option of evaluating students' retained knowledge by chapter in a comprehensive format. This tool is capable of assessing retention of essential information necessary for excellence in functioning in the workplace.

Students completing education in medical assisting will find this book an invaluable tool as they move into the professional arena. It has been designed to provide information relevant in the medical office environment and will remain a handy reference during employment. The website updates will offer a resource covering current changes in the health-care field to help keep the graduate current.

The established health-care provider, whether a medical assistant, nurse, transcriber, coder, respiratory therapist, massage therapist, receptionist, EMT, or other, will find this reference material a valuable resource in his or her work with the patient. Knowledge of the disease and its related factors is essential in the provision of quality care.

Margaret Schell Frazier, RN, CMA, BS
Jeanette Wist Drzymkowski, RN, BS

Acknowledgments

A great big thanks goes to Adrianne Rippinger, Executive Editor, whose vision and support helped us to keep sight of our goal. Her comprehensive view of the total project directed our efforts keeping us on task and we are grateful for her involvement. Reinforcing our editor's guidance, Rae Robertson, Senior Developmental Editor, was an important member of our Elsevier team, working with us on a daily basis as we brought the book to fruition. Thank you Rae.

In the revising of this edition, we sought out additional expertise in the form of contributing authors. These individuals worked with us, one on one, to bring a different perspective to specific areas. We are grateful to each one, and their names are listed in the Contributing Author's list on p. v. The expertise of the following professionals assures the readers that the information presented in this book was discussed and reviewed for its accuracy. We thank them for taking the time to critique the material and to offer us expert advise and insight. Special thanks to the following professionals who so patiently answered our numerous questions as we revised the manuscript: Dean D. Dauscher, MD; Mischelle Frazier Musser, RN, ASN; Eugenia M. Fulcher, RN, BSN, Med, EdD, CMA; David P. Schlueter, MD; Carolyn Steinbacher, ORT; Thomas Van Den Driessche, MD; Diana M. Wade, RN; and Kimberly Weaver, RN, ASN.

We would be remiss if we did not continue to remember the contribution made by Maverick Luther Musser and his family. Once again, we thank you for teaching us about the joy and value of life by displaying courage and strength during the 19 months Maverick blessed our lives. Also, we gratefully acknowledge your making us aware of the technology available to very premature neonates. The situations you faced enlightened us to the challenges and possible conditions resulting from premature birth as well as the courage and strength required of families thrust into similar situations.

Our gratitude also is extended to the members of our immediate families. Children, their respective spouses, and our wonderful grandchildren all had to be tolerant of Mom and Grandma when the book took priority. You are our immortality, and this book is your legacy. Thanks for your patience and understanding. And of course, we saved the best for almost last. To the other half of our partnerships, Dave and Frank, we thank you from the bottom of our hearts for everything, your patience, your technical support, your understanding and encouragement, and most of all your love.

Finally, to each other. Once again we have shared joys and sorrows, laughter and tears, and still accomplished this revision long distance thanks to air travel, hotels, and the Internet. Modern travel, technology, and friendships are wonderful.

Contents

Essentials of Human Diseases and Conditions

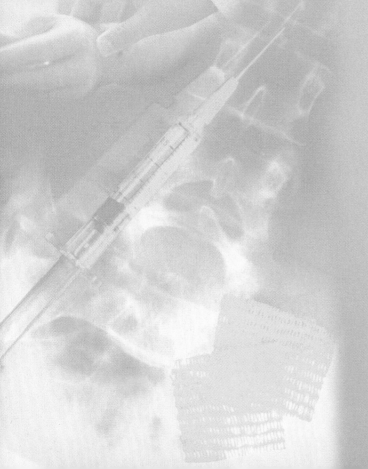
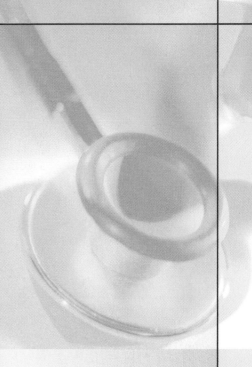

CHAPTER 1

Mechanisms of Disease, Diagnosis, and Treatment

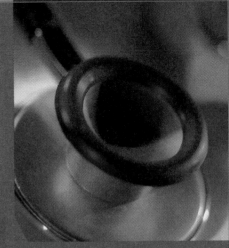

Chapter Outline

Learning Objectives

After studying Chapter 1, you should be able to:

1. Explain how a pathologic condition affects the homeostasis of the body.
2. Describe the difference between:
   Signs and symptoms of disease
   Acute and chronic disease
   Benign and malignant neoplasms
3. Identify the predisposing factors of disease.
4. Describe the ways in which pathogens may cause disease.
5. Track the essential steps in diagnosis of disease.
6. List the prevention guidelines for cancer.

7. Explain the inflammation response to disease.
8. Describe the hospice concept of care.
9. Name two ways an individual can practice positive health behavior.
10. Describe (a) the physiology of pain, (b) how pain may be treated, and (c) what is meant by referred pain.
11. Define the holistic approach to medical care.
12. Describe examples of alternative medical therapies.
13. Discuss the principals and goals of patient teaching.

Key Terms

allergen (**AL**-ler-jen)
anaphylaxis (**an**-ah-fih-**LAK**-sis)
antigen (**AN**-tih-jen)
asymptomatic (a-sim-toh-**MAH**-tik)
auscultation (**aws**-kel-**TAY**-shun)
cachexia (kah-**KEX**-e-ah)
carcinogenic (**kar**-sih-no-**JEN**-ik)
chromosome (**KRO**-mo-sohm)
genotype (**JEN**-o-type)
homeostasis (**ho**-me-o-**STA**-sis)

hospice (**HAUS**-pis)
ischemia (is-**KEY**-me-ah)
karyotype (**KARE**-ee-o-type)
metastasis (meh-**TAS**-tah-sis)
mutation (meu-**TAY**-shun)
nociceptor (**no**-see-**SEHP**-tor)
oncogene (**AHN**-ko-jeen)
pathogenesis (**path**-o-**JEN**-eh-sis)
phagocytic (**fag**-o-**SIT**-ik)
somatoform (so-**MAT**-o-form)

PATHOLOGY AT FIRST GLANCE

PATHOLOGY, THE SCIENTIFIC STUDY of disease, is the objective description of the traits, causes, and effects of abnormal conditions. Pathologic conditions involve measurable changes in normal structure and function that threaten the internal stability, or **homeostasis,** of the body.

In human disease, the negative characteristics, or departures from normal status, are described subjectively by patients as symptoms. Signs, or abnormal objective findings, are the evidence of disease found by physical examination and diagnostic testing. Signs of disease often correlate with the symptoms. In other instances, the signs of disease may be noted in an **asymptomatic** patient, as in the discovery of a painless tumor or the finding of an abnormal blood pressure reading in a person with undiagnosed essential hypertension. A defined collection of signs and symptoms that

characterize a disorder or condition is termed a *syndrome.*

The development of disease occurs in stages, described as the **pathogenesis.** In the course of infection, for instance, the pathogenesis may include an incubation period, a period of full-blown symptoms, and then remission or convalescence. The pathogenesis of a disease varies with the individual patient, the causative factors, and medical intervention.

Diseases often are described as acute or chronic. *Acute* refers to an abrupt onset of more or less severe symptoms that run a brief course (usually shorter than 6 months) and then resolve or, in some cases, result in death. When a disease develops slowly, or is intermittent, and lasts longer than 6 months, it is described as *chronic.*

Additionally, persons who have continuous pain as part of chronic syndromes often experience depression.

MECHANISMS OF DISEASE

HUMAN DISEASE, A UNIVERSAL occurrence, has varied manifestations, any of which threatens a person's ability to adapt to internal and external stressors and to maintain a state of well-being. Systemic health, or internal equilibrium, is preserved by numerous body organs and structures that work in concert to meet specific cellular needs. Any disruption of the body's equilibrium produces degenerative changes at the cellular level that may produce signs and symptoms of disease. Major disruptions in the body's cellular equilibrium that threaten homeostasis include fluid and electrolyte imbalance and excessive acidity (acidosis) or alkalinity (alkalosis).

Elements involved either directly or indirectly in pathogenesis include predisposing factors, access to preventive health care, genetic diseases, infection, inflammation and repair, neoplasms, physical trauma, chemical agents, malnutrition, immune disorders, aging, psychological factors, and mental disorders.

Predisposing Factors

Predisposing factors, also called *risk factors,* make a person or group more vulnerable to disease. Although the recognition of risk factors may be significant in prevention, diagnosis, and prognosis, it does not precisely predict the occurrence of disease, nor does the absence of predisposing factors necessarily protect against the development of disease. A person may be susceptible to one or more risk factors that overlap or occur in combination, to a greater or lesser degree. Predisposing factors include age, gender, lifestyle, environment, and heredity.

Age. From complications during pregnancy and the postpartum period to maladies associated with aging, some increased risks of diseases are simply intrinsic to one's stage in the human life cycle.

Gender. Certain diseases are more common in women (e.g., multiple sclerosis and osteoporosis) and other disorders are more common in men (e.g., gout and Parkinson's disease).

Lifestyle. Occupation, habits, or one's usual manner of living can have negative cumulative effects that can threaten a person's health. It is possible to alter some known risk factors associated with lifestyle, thereby promoting health instead of predisposing one to disease; examples include smoking, excessive drinking of alcohol, risky sexual behavior, poor nutrition, lack of exercise, and certain psychological stressors.

Environment. Air and water pollution is considered a major risk factor for illnesses such as cancer and pulmonary disease. Poor living conditions, excessive noise, chronic psychological stress, and a geographic location conducive to disease proliferation also are environmental risk factors.

Heredity. Genetic predisposition (inheritance) currently is considered a major risk factor. Family histories of coronary disease, cancer, certain arthritic conditions, and renal disease are known hereditary risk factors. Hereditary factors in disease that appear regularly in successive generations are likely to affect males and females equally. Hereditary or genetic diseases often develop as a result of the combined effects of inheritance and environmental factors. Examples are mental illness, cancer, hypertension, heart disease, and diabetes. Some evidence shows that smoking, a sedentary lifestyle, and a diet high in saturated fat, combined with a positive family history, compound a person's risk for heart disease and cancer. Schizophrenia may result from a combination of genetic predisposition and numerous psychological and sociocultural causes.

Preventive Health Care

Preventive health care places emphasis on strategies for preventing disease and injury. Current statistical evidence indicates that positive personal health behavior, in conjunction with prophylactic medical services, may reduce the mortality rate associated with certain diseases, such as cardiovascular disease. Identifying risk factors and employing specific screening tests to detect alterations give individuals information they can use to modify their lifestyles. Using available medical measures can help prevent the onset of disease or at least minimize complications.

Many injuries may be prevented by implementing (1) improved safety measures involving the operation of machinery and automobiles; (2) protective labeling and packaging of food, drugs, and toxic products; and (3) general public safety education. Family violence, another possible threat to one's health, is a serious and growing epidemic in the United States that results in both psychological stress and physical trauma. In many cases, early intervention may prevent such abuse. Involving legal, social, and medical authorities early on can serve to identify and protect those caught up in the cycle of domestic violence before serious medical consequences result.

Health-care institutions are challenged daily to uphold infection control measures that protect patients against hospital-acquired infections (known as *nosocomial infections*). Continuing education requirements fulfilled by physicians and other health care providers give them the skills to help diminish occasions of iatrogenic disorders, that is, those diseases or conditions that are a result of medical procedures or treatment.

Genetic Diseases

Every cell in the body is coded with genetic information arranged on 23 pairs of **chromosomes;** one chromosome from each pair is inherited from the father and the other from the mother. The X and Y chromosomes are known as the *sex chromosomes,* whereas the remaining 22 pairs are called *autosomes.* Each cell in an individual's body contains the same chromosomes and genetic code **(genotype).** A **karyotype** is an ordered arrangement of photographs of a full chromosome set (Fig. 1–1). Genes, the basic units of heredity, are small stretches of a DNA (deoxyribonucleic acid) molecule, situated at a particular site on a chromosome.

Genetic diseases are (1) produced by an abnormality in, or a mutation of, the genetic code in a single gene; (2) caused by several abnormal genes (producing so-called *polygenic* diseases); or (3) caused by the abnormal presence or absence of an entire chromosome or by alteration in the structure of chromosomes. Harmful genetic **mutations,** or changes in the genetic code, passed from one generation to the next may occur spontaneously or be caused by agents known to disrupt the normal

sequence of DNA units. Agents (called *mutagens*) that can damage DNA include certain chemicals, radiation, and viruses.

The main modes of inheritance for genetic diseases are as follows:

Autosomal dominant—the gene in question is located on an autosome and the mutant phenotype is seen even if a normal gene is present on the other chromosome in the pair. Examples include Marfan syndrome and Huntington disease.

Autosomal recessive—the gene is located on an autosome but is insufficient to produce the mutant phenotype in the presence of a normal gene on the paired chromosome. Both genes must be mutated for disease to occur. Examples include cystic fibrosis and phenylketonuria.

X-linked (sex-linked) recessive—the gene is located only on the X chromosome. Males are much more commonly affected by these diseases than are females. Examples include Duchenne muscular dystrophy and hemophilia A.

Individuals who have only one copy of a recessive gene and appear outwardly normal are known as carriers of the defective gene. The mutant gene may produce an abnormal protein that causes a disease, or it may fail to produce its normal cellular function. Hereditary diseases often are noted at birth, but they may not appear until later in life. Many genetic mutations are compatible with life, but some are not.

The following examples of genetic abnormalities are discussed in this book:

Huntington chorea
Down syndrome
Hemophilia
Klinefelter syndrome
Polycystic kidney
Dwarfism
Albinism
Hyperopia
Hemolytic anemia
Cystic fibrosis
Epilepsy
Hirschsprung disease
Phenylketonuria
Turner syndrome
Hemolytic disease of newborn
Cleft palate
Myopia

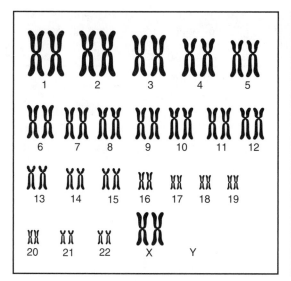

FIGURE 1–1 Examples of karyotypes. **A**, Normal female (46,XX). **B**, Normal male (46,XY). (From Damjanov I: *Pathology for the health-related professions,* Philadelphia, 1996, Saunders.)

Infection

Infectious diseases are caused by pathogens. The cardinal signs of local infection are redness, swelling, heat, pain, fever, pus, enlarged lymph glands, and red streaks. Symptoms of widespread infection are fever, headache, body aches, weakness, fatigue, loss of appetite, and delirium.

When disease-causing organisms find ideal conditions in which to grow and multiply in the body, they cause disease by (1) invasion and local destruction of living tissue and (2) intoxication or production of substances that are poisonous to the body. The end result is tissue damage that has the potential for producing systemic involvement.

The sources of infection can be endogenous (originating within the body) or exogenous (originating outside the body). Modes of transmission of pathogenic organisms are direct or indirect physical contact, inhalation or droplet nuclei, ingestion of contaminated food or water, or inoculation by an insect or animal. Pathogenic agents include bacteria, viruses, fungi, and protozoa (Table 1–1).

A communicable or contagious disease can be transmitted directly from one person to another. Carriers are asymptomatic persons or animals that harbor in their bodies pathogens that can be transferred to others.

The body's natural defense systems against infection include (1) natural mechanical and chemical barriers, such as the skin, the cilia, body pH, and normal body flora; (2) the inflammatory response; and (3) the immune response. When these mechanisms of defense fail to contain or eliminate infection, appropriate and prompt medical intervention is required to treat the host and to control transmission of the infectious disease. This is accomplished by first isolating and identifying the organism through laboratory testing. Subsequently, appropriate antimicrobial therapy using antibiotic (antibacterial), antifungal, antiparasitic, or antiviral agents can begin. Analgesics for pain and antipyretic agents for fever, as well as other comfort measures, are dispensed. Adequate fluid intake, infection control measures, and rest are important for management.

Fundamental to preventing the spread of certain infections are isolation of the infected individual when necessary, implementation of immunization programs, and rudimentary public health teaching. To facilitate early intervention and infection control measures, many infectious diseases such as encephalitis, syphilis, and tuberculosis must be reported to the local health department. The Centers for Disease Control and

TABLE 1–1
Common Pathogens and Some Infections or Diseases That They Produce

ORGANISM	RESERVOIR	INFECTION OR DISEASE
BACTERIA		
Escherichia coli (E. coli)	Colon, manure	Enteritis, mild to severe
Staphylococcus aureus	Skin, hair, anterior nares	Wound infection, pneumonia, food poisoning, cellulitis
Streptococcus (beta-hemolytic group A) organisms	Oropharynx, skin, perianal area	"Strep throat," rheumatic fever, scarlet fever, impetigo
Streptococcus (beta-hemolytic group B) organisms	Adult genitalia	Urinary tract infection, wound infection, endometritis
Mycobacterium tuberculosis	Lungs	Tuberculosis
Neisseria gonorrhoeae	Genitourinary tract, rectum, mouth, eye	Gonorrhea, pelvic inflammatory disease, infectious arthritis, conjunctivitis
Rickettsia rickettsii	Wood tick	Rocky Mountain spotted fever
Staphylococcus epidermidis	Skin	Wound infection, bacteremia
VIRUSES		
Hepatitis A virus	Feces, blood, urine	Hepatitis A (infectious hepatitis)
Hepatitis B virus	Feces, blood, all body fluids and excretions	Hepatitis B (serum hepatitis)
Herpes simplex virus	Lesions of mouth, skin, blood, excretions	Cold sores, aseptic meningitis, sexually transmitted disease
Human immunodeficiency virus (HIV)	Blood, semen, vaginal secretions (also isolated in saliva, tears, urine, breast milk, but not proven to be sources of transmission)	Acquired immunodeficiency syndrome (AIDS)
Hantavirus	Deer mouse urine, feces, and saliva	Upper respiratory infection (URI) to lower respiratory infection (LRI) to adult respiratory distress syndrome (ARDS)
West Nile virus	Mosquito-borne	Fever, rash, hepatitis, encephalitis
FUNGI		
Aspergillus organisms	Soil, dust	Aspergillosis
Candida albicans	Mouth, skin, colon, genital tract	Thrush, dermatitis
PROTOZOA		
Plasmodium falciparum	Mosquito	Malaria

Modified from Potter P, Perry A: *Fundamentals of nursing: concepts, process, and practice,* ed 5, St. Louis, 2001, Mosby.

Prevention (CDC) publishes notifiable diseases in the United States. In hospitals, the control of post-surgical bacterial wound infections relies on breaking the chain of transmission by killing the pathogen, isolating infected persons, and using precautions such as hand washing and sterilization to prevent cross-contamination.

Inflammation and Repair

Injury and disease impose stress on the body's equilibrium and disrupt or destroy cellular function. Acute inflammation, a normal protective physiologic response to tissue injury and disease, is accompanied by redness, heat, swelling, pain, and loss of function. Widespread inflammation is marked by systemic symptoms, such as fever, malaise, and loss of appetite. Blood testing may reveal an elevated white blood cell count or an elevated erythrocyte sedimentation rate (ESR). The intensity of inflammation depends on the cause, the area of the body involved, and the physical condition of the person. An inflammatory response is considered a nonspecific immune response. Infection with pathogens, the effects of toxins, physical trauma, **ischemia,** and *necrosis* are some conditions that induce the inflammatory response.

Acute inflammation, an exudative response, attempts to wall off, destroy, and digest bacteria and dead or foreign tissue. Vascular changes allow fluid to leak into the site; this fluid contains chemicals that permit **phagocytic** activity by white blood cells. The process prevents the spread of infection by way of antibody action and other chemicals released by cells with more specific immune activity. After the mechanisms of inflammation have contained the insult and "cleaned up" a damaged area, repair and replacement of tissue can begin (Fig. 1–2). A normal inflammatory response can be inhibited by immune disorders, chronic illness, or the use of certain medications, especially long-term steroid therapy.

When an inflammatory response is chronic or too intense, damage in the affected tissue can be the result, thereby inhibiting the healing process. Diseases with a chronic inflammation component include arthritis, asthma, and eczema.

Cancer

Cancer refers to a group of diseases characterized by uncontrolled cell proliferation. This abnormal growth leads to the development of tumors or *neoplasms,* a relentlessly growing mass of abnormal cells that proliferates at the expense of the healthy organism. Tumors are characterized as malignant or benign and according to the cell type and tissue of origin (Tables 1–2 and 1–3). Some of the main general types of cancer are carcinoma, cancer of epithelial cells; sarcoma, cancer of the supportive tissues of the body such as bone and muscle; lymphoma, cancer arising in the lymph nodes and tissues of the immune system; leukemia, cancer of blood cell precursors; and melanoma, cancer of the melanin-producing cells of the body.

Benign tumors develop slowly and can arise from any tissue. They tend to remain encapsulated and do not infiltrate surrounding tissue. When examined microscopically, benign tumor cells are well differentiated—they resemble the tissue of origin. Because tumors take up space, complications can result from compression of tissue by the lesion or obstruction of organs. Benign tumors rarely recur after surgical removal.

Malignant tumors can represent a serious threat to the life and well-being of a person. The tumors consist of invasive cells that multiply excessively and can infiltrate other tissues. They tend to bleed, ulcerate, and become infected. Cancer cells are variable in appearance and disorderly (anaplastic) with irreversible changes in structure. They are usually poorly differentiated and do not resemble the tissue of origin. Malignant tumors have the ability to invade the surrounding tissue. Often malignant cells enter the bloodstream or the lymphatic vessels and lead to tumor growth in other areas of the body. These secondary tumors are known as **metastases. Metastasis** makes the neoplasm more difficult to eradicate from the body.

Cancer is actually many different diseases with numerous causes. Cancer may be caused by both external exposure to *carcinogens* (chemicals, radiation, and viruses) and internal factors (hormones, immune conditions, and inherited mutations). Ten years or longer may pass between exposures or mutations and the onset of detectable cancer. Cancer can develop in anyone, but the frequency increases with age. Figure 1–3 shows the leading sites of cancer incidence and death.

Recommendations for decreasing the risk of cancer encompass guidelines and appropriate screening tests for early detection and treatment. Primary prevention guidelines include the following:

- Consumption of a low-fat, high-fiber diet rich in fruits and vegetables with vitamins A and E
- Elimination of active and passive exposure to cigarette smoke
- Limitation of skin exposure to sunlight
- Avoidance of heavy use of alcohol
- Avoidance of excessive exposure to radiation and radon
- Careful evaluation for estrogen replacement therapy (ERT)

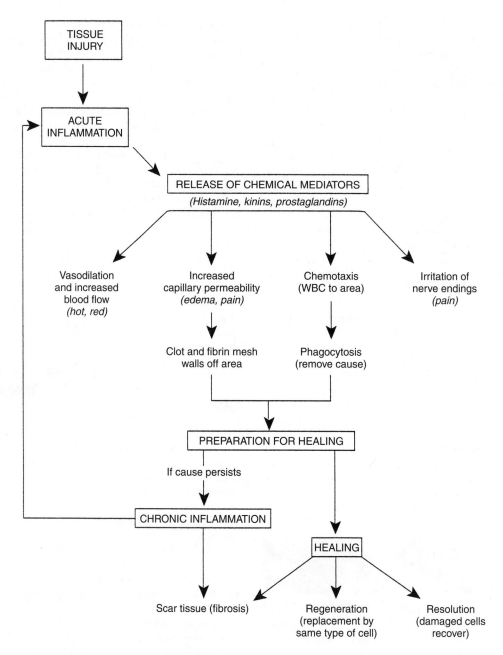

FIGURE 1–2 The course of inflammation and healing. (From Gould BE: *Pathophysiology for the health-related professions,* ed 2, Philadelphia, 2002, Saunders.)

TABLE 1-2
Comparison of Benign and Malignant Tumors

CHARACTERISTICS	BENIGN	MALIGNANT
Mode of growth	Relatively slow growth by expansion; encapsulated; cells adhere to each other	Rapid growth; invades surrounding tissue by infiltration
Cells under microscopic examination	Resemble tissue of origin; well differentiated; appear normal	Do not resemble tissue of origin; vary in size and shape; abnormal appearance and function
Spread	Remains localized	Metastasis; cancer cells carried by blood and lymphatics to one or more other locations; secondary tumors occur
Other properties	No tissue destruction; not prone to hemorrhage; may be smooth and freely movable	Ulceration and/or necrosis; prone to hemorrhage; irregular and less movable
Recurrence	Rare after excision	A common characteristic
Pathogenesis	Symptoms related to location with obstruction and/or compression of surrounding tissue or organs; usually not life threatening unless inaccessible	**Cachexia**; pain; fatal if not controlled

A 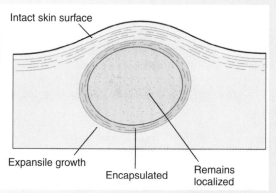 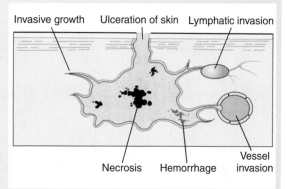 B

Gross appearance of benign **(A)** and malignant **(B)** tumors.

TABLE 1-3
Classification of Neoplasms by Tissue of Origin

TISSUE OF ORIGIN	BENIGN	MALIGNANT
Connective tissue		Sarcoma
Embryonic fibrous tissue	Myxoma	Myxosarcoma
Fibrous tissue	Fibroma	Fibrosarcoma
Adipose tissue	Lipoma	Liposarcoma
Cartilage	Chondroma	Chondrosarcoma
Bone	Osteoma	Osteogenic sarcoma

From Black JM, Matassarin-Jacobs E: *Medical-surgical nursing,* ed 6, Philadelphia, 2001, Saunders.   *Continued*

TABLE 1-3
Classification of Neoplasms by Tissue of Origin—cont'd

TISSUE OF ORIGIN	BENIGN	MALIGNANT
Epithelium		Carcinoma
Skin and mucous membrane	Papilloma	Squamous cell carcinoma
Glands		Basal cell carcinoma
		Transitional cell carcinoma
	Adenoma	Adenocarcinoma
	Cystadenoma	Cystadenocarcinoma
Pigmented cells (melanocytes)	Nevus	Malignant melanoma
Endothelium		Endothelioma
Blood vessels	Hemangioma	Hemangioendothelioma
		Hemangiosarcoma
		Kaposi sarcoma
Lymph vessels	Lymphangioma	Lymphangiosarcoma
		Lymphangioendothelioma
Bone marrow		Multiple myeloma
		Ewing sarcoma
		Leukemia
Lymphoid tissue		Malignant lymphoma
		Lymphosarcoma
		Reticulum cell sarcoma
Muscle tissue		
Smooth muscle	Leiomyoma	Leiomyosarcoma
Striated muscle	Rhabdomyoma	Rhabdomyosarcoma
Nerve tissue		
Nerve fibers and sheaths	Neuroma	Neurogenic sarcoma
	Neurinoma	
	(Neurilemoma)	
	Neurofibroma	(Neurofibrosarcoma)
Ganglion cells	Ganglioneuroma	Neuroblastoma
Glial cells	Glioma	Glioblastoma
Meninges	Meningioma	Malignant meningioma
Gonads	Dermoid cyst	Embryonal carcinoma
		Embryonal sarcoma
		Teratocarcinoma

From Black JM, Matassarin-Jacobs E: *Medical-surgical nursing*, ed 6, Philadelphia, 2001, Saunders.

- Avoidance of chemical agents known to be **carcinogenic**
- Increase in physical activity

The diagnosis of cancer is very prevalent in the U.S. society. Statistics from the American Cancer Society estimate that nearly 1.3 million Americans are diagnosed with invasive cancer and over 500,000 die of cancer per year. One out of every four deaths in the United States is cancer-related.

Cancer detection employs general and specific techniques of physical examination, medical history-taking, and laboratory screening tests. Screening examinations can detect cancers of the breast, rectum, colon, prostate, cervix, testis, tongue, mouth, and skin early, when treatment is more likely to succeed. These cancers account for approximately half of all new cancer cases.

Some tumor cells produce and secrete substances called *tumor markers*. Screening tests for elevation of

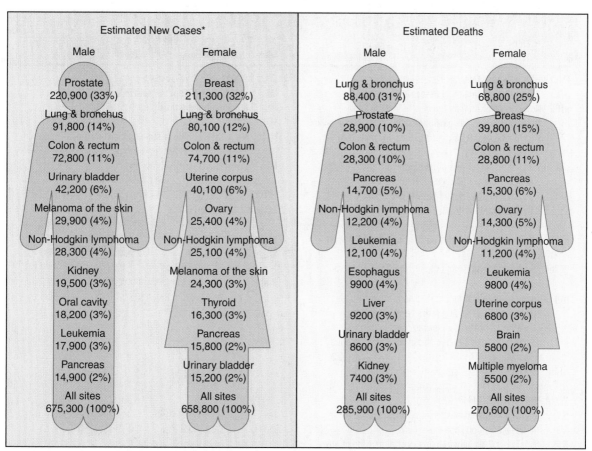

*Excludes basal and squamous cell skin cancers and in situ carcinoma except urinary bladder.
Percentages may not total 100% due to rounding.

FIGURE 1–3 Leading sites of new cancer cases and deaths—2003 estimates. (Reprinted with permission of the American Cancer Society, Inc., *Cancer Facts and Figures—2003.*)

blood serum levels of tumor markers, when considered with other diagnostic data, are shown to have clinical value in (1) helping determine the diagnosis of cancer and (2) evaluating response to therapy. For example, in primary and metastatic prostate cancer, elevated prostate-specific antigen (PSA) may be found.

If cancer is suspected, additional diagnostic investigation is achieved by using high-technology imaging techniques and, most decisively, by performing *biopsy* of the lesion.

After a cancer diagnosis has been confirmed, the patient undergoes an evaluation to determine the stage of the neoplasm. Stage reflects tu-

mor size and extent of tumor spread. It has important implications for determining choice of treatment options and prognosis. Staging is a method that institutions can use to communicate patient information, so the procedures and staging systems used for staging must be standardized worldwide. Types of cancer that are more prevalent in less-developed countries, such as cervical cancer, are often staged clinically and without use of technologies such as magnetic resonance imaging (MRI) and computed tomography (CT) scans. For some types of cancer, such as endometrial neoplasms, complete staging requires surgical removal of the affected organ and

TABLE 1–4
Melanoma Staging System of the American Joint Committee on Cancer (25)

PRIMARY TUMOR (PT)

pTX   Primary tumor cannot be assessed.

pT0   No evidence of primary tumor

pTis   Melanoma in situ (atypical melanotic hyperplasia, severe melanotic dysplasia), not an invasive lesion (Clark's Level I)

pT1   Tumor 0.75 mm or less in thickness and invades the papillary dermis (Clark's Level III)

pT3   Tumor more than 1.5 mm but not more than 4 mm in thickness and/or invades the reticular dermis (Clark's Level IV)

pT3a   Tumor more than 1.5 mm but not more than 3 mm in thickness

pT3b   Tumor more than 3 mm but not more than 4 mm in thickness

pT4   Tumor more than 4 mm in thickness and/or invades the subcutaneous tissue (Clark's Level V) and/or satellite(s) within 2 cm of the primary tumor

pT4a   Tumor more than 4 mm in thickness and/or invades the subcutaneous tissue

pT4b   Satellite(s) within 2 cm of primary tumor

LYMPH NODE (N)

NX   Regional lymph nodes cannot be assessed.

N0   No regional lymph node metastasis

N1   Metastasis 3 cm or less in greatest dimension in any regional lymph nodes

N2   Metastasis more than 3 cm in greatest dimension in any regional lymph node(s) and/or in-transit metastasis

N2a   Metastasis more than 3 cm in greatest dimension in any regional lymph node(s)

N2b   In-transit metastasis

N2c   Both (N2a and N2b)

DISTANT METASTASIS (M)

MX   Presence of distant metastasis cannot be assessed.

M0   No distant metastasis

M1   Distant metastasis

M1a   Metastasis in skin or subcutaneous tissue of lymph node(s) beyond the regional lymph nodes

M1b   Visceral metastasis

STAGE GROUPING

Stage	pT	N	M
Stage I	pT1	N0	M0
	pT2	N0	M0
Stage II	pT3	N0	M0
Stage III	pT4	N0	M0
	Any pT	N1, N2	M0
Stage IV	Any pT	Any N	M1

examination of the specimen by an experienced pathologist.

Although a number of different staging systems exist, the majority of cancers use a TNM system. TNM staging assesses the neoplasm in three different areas: the size or extent of the primary tumor (T), the extent of regional lymph node involvement by the tumor (N), and the number of distant metastases (M). Once all three parameters are defined, they are combined to assign a stage number of I, II, III, or IV to the cancer. I is an early stage tu-

mor and carries the best prognosis, whereas IV is the most advanced stage. Within each stage, subcategories are defined (Ia, Ib, etc.) to further aid in treatment planning and facilitation of communication between institutions and physicians. See Table 1–4 for an example of staging.

Stage usually offers the best indicator of prognosis. Prognosis reflects the estimation of the likelihood of cancer recurrence and death, independent of the treatment given. In general, the diagnosis of cancer in an early stage offers a greater chance for cure. Prognosis is usually reported statistically as the percentage of patients with that cancer who are still alive after a certain period of time. The patient may be cured of the disease, in remission, or still undergoing treatment. The most often–reported time period for survival is 5 years. It can be reported as "overall 5-year survival," which takes into account all the people, regardless of stage, with that cancer, or it can reflect the 5-year survival for people in the various stages of cancer. For example, the overall 5-year survival rate for all types of cancer combined is 62% (i.e., for every 100 people diagnosed with cancer, 62 will be alive 5 years later), but the 5-year survival for stage IV colorectal cancer is 8%. It is important to note, however, that the current 5-year survival rates actually represent data from patients diagnosed with cancer at least 8 years ago and do not reflect more recent advances in treatment.

Depending on the type of neoplasm, other factors can impact prognosis. Examples include age of the patient, serum concentration of any tumor markers, time between diagnosis and treatment, and grade of the tumor. Tumor grade is determined through microscopic evaluation of the tumor or a biopsy specimen. Grade is assigned based on the degree of differentiation of the tumor cells. *Well-differentiated,* low grade tumor cells still retain features of the tissue cells from which they derived. *Poorly differentiated,* high grade tumor cells are more abnormal in appearance and do not resemble the tissue from which they derived. High grade tumor cells usually have a greater number of mitoses (divide more rapidly) and are associated with poorer survival.

One type of cancer in which grade is a very important indicator of prognosis is prostate cancer. The grading system is known as the Gleason grade, and it was designed with the knowledge that prostate cancer has different patterns of growth and that multiple patterns coexist in the prostate. Analysis of prostate tumor histology is done and the two predominant patterns are recorded and scored from one to five (one represents a well-differentiated histology; five is the most poorly differentiated). Both scores are summed to give a Gleason score from two to ten. The Gleason grade correlates with extent of disease throughout the body and with prognosis.

The goal of cancer treatment is to eradicate every cancer cell in the body. Treatment options involve localized therapy such as surgery and radiation, as well as systemic modalities such as chemotherapy, hormonal therapy, and immunotherapy. Surgery alone is curative only for early stage tumors. Usually, more than one treatment option is employed. Neoadjuvant therapy may be administered preoperatively to shrink the tumor to facilitate surgical removal.

Surgery is important for the treatment of solid cancers and is often used in the staging evaluation as well. As a treatment modality, the goal is either cure or palliative symptom control. When surgery is employed as a curative measure, surgeons try to achieve negative margins around the tumor, meaning that the surgeon will remove a certain amount of normal tissue along with the tumor to ensure the entire tumor has been removed. If negative margins are not achieved, surgery must be performed again or another type of treatment must be tried. At the time of surgery, the regional lymph nodes may be evaluated to determine whether the cancer cells have entered the lymphatic system and invaded the nodes. Affected nodes are generally removed. Palliative surgery is performed to relieve troublesome symptoms such as obstruction. Relief can be achieved by tumor resection, bypass, stenting, or laser ablation.

Chemotherapy involves the use of chemical agents to destroy cancer cells. Most of the drugs affect cell replication so chemotherapy is most effective against rapidly dividing cells, such as cancer cells. Normally occurring cells in other parts of the body that are known to divide rapidly also are destroyed, and this accounts for many of the classic side effects of chemotherapy. These cell populations (and the related side effects) include hair cells (alopecia), gastrointestinal (GI) mucosal cells (anorexia, vomiting, diarrhea), hematopoietic cells (anemia, bruising), and reproductive organs (infertility). Often drugs are administered in combination with other drugs that affect different steps in cell replication (combination chemotherapy). Chemotherapy usually is given in cycles that include a treatment period followed by a recovery period and is performed in the outpatient setting. Although cancer cells may be initially responsive to the drugs, cells tend to develop resistance to the drugs over time, and new drugs or different treatment modalities must be employed then.

The use of hormone therapy and immunotherapy in the treatment of cancer is continually evolving. Hormone therapy can be effective in hormone-

Cancer

dependent cancers such as breast cancer and prostate cancer. It may involve the administration of drugs that suppress hormone synthesis such as luteinizing hormone-releasing hormone (LHRH) antagonists or aromatase inhibitors that are used to treat prostate cancer, drugs that block the action of hormones such as the estrogen receptor modulator tamoxifen used to treat breast cancer, or surgical removal of hormone-producing glands such as *oophorectomy* and *orchiectomy*. The use of corticosteroids may be useful in some lymphomas and leukemias.

Immunotherapy, on the other hand, involves the use of monoclonal antibodies that are designed to target certain products of cancer cells that are not found in normal cells. Some of the antibodies currently approved for use include trastuzumab (Hercieptin), used in breast cancers that overexpress the HER2/neu protein, and rituximab (Rituxan), directed against a CD-20 molecule found in lymphoma.

In many cases of metastatic disease, cure is not possible, but these same treatment modalities may be useful in prolonging life or improving the quality of life for the patient. Even after the patient has achieved remission, he or she must be followed closely for several years. Micrometastases may exist at the time of diagnosis that can lead to eventual recurrence of the cancer if they are not eradicated by systemic therapy.

Advances in radiation and chemotherapy have diminished the need for radical surgery. Both radiation and most useful anticancer drugs have significant side effects that require constant surveillance and management. Pain management at every stage is a major concern for patients and includes generous use of various analgesics and noninvasive techniques that promote relaxation and distraction. Terminally ill persons can be referred to **hospice** care for compassionate, holistic case management. (See the Enrichment box describing hospice care.)

One aspect of cancer treatment that is becoming more important as a greater number of patients are being cured of their cancer is the consequence of therapy. Chemotherapy and radiation therapy are very toxic, not only to cancer cells but also to the body in general. Some of the effects of this toxicity are not seen until many years after therapy. Patients are predisposed to develop other malignancies, especially lymphomas and

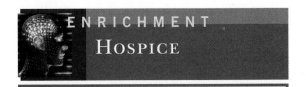
leukemias. The effect of cancer therapy is even more dramatic in many children. Growth retardation and cognitive impairment may result. Still, cancer therapies are constantly evolving and methods are being developed that may not have such long-term side effects.

Research into cancer therapy points to useful information about new approaches to cancer treatment that show promise. One theory is based on starving a tumor by inhibiting its blood supply. Experimental studies have shown that inhibiting the growth of new blood vessels (angiogenesis), which feed the tumor, causes the tumor to shrink. Since 1994, two angiogenesis inhibitors, angiostatin and endostatin, have had positive results in mice. Humans are beginning to receive experimental treatments with angiogenesis inhibitors.

Certain forms of cancer are inherited; thus much of the current research is focused on cancer at its genetic roots. Scientists are investigating genetic switches that cause healthy cells to become disorderly. It has been observed that broken genes can send cells into spirals of cancerous growth. Such **oncogenes** and tumor suppressor genes are proposed targets for therapy. One drug currently targeting an oncogene is imatinib mesylate (Gleevec), which inhibits the *bcr-abl* tyrosine kinase in chronic myelogenous leukemia.

Specific types of cancer are discussed in subsequent chapters of this book.

Physical Trauma and Chemical Agents

Physical trauma is the major cause of death in children and young adults. Common mechanisms of acute injury are falls; motor vehicle accidents, including those involving pedestrians; physical abuse; penetrating injuries; drowning; and burns. Emergency management begins with triage to determine the priorities of care. Persons who sustain trauma require precise assessment and management to prevent infection, to minimize the insult to the body tissues, to combat shock and hemorrhage, and to restore homeostasis.

Chemical agents or irritants that are potentially injurious include pollutants, poisons, drugs, preservatives, cosmetics, and dyes. Extreme heat or cold, radiation, electrical shock, and insect and snake bites are other instruments of injury to the body.

See Chapter 15 for a discussion of specific types of trauma.

Malnutrition

Disorders of nutrition, as discussed in Chapter 8, may be the result of a deficient diet or of disease conditions that do not allow the body to break down, absorb, or use food. An example of a severe deficiency disease is protein-calorie malnutrition (kwashiorkor), the starvation associated with famine. Other nutritional disorders include iron deficiency, anemia, obesity, and hypervitaminoses.

Immune Disorders

The immune system is a complex network of specialized cells and organs that has evolved to defend the body against attacks by foreign organisms. Immune disorders are the result of a breakdown in the body's defense system that may generate (1) hypersensitivity (allergy), (2) autoimmune diseases, or (3) immunodeficiency disorders.

Allergic disease is a hypersensitivity of the body to a substance (**allergen**) ordinarily considered harmless. Common allergens include inhalants (dust, molds, and fungi), foods, drugs, chemicals, and physical agents (heat, cold, and radiation). Initial exposure to an allergen, which acts as an **antigen** (a substance that causes the allergic response), stimulates the production of immunoglobulin E (IgE) antibodies, and the person thus is sensitized. Subsequent exposures trigger the allergic response, which is an antigen-antibody reaction causing the release of histamine and other chemicals (Fig. 1–4). The chemicals cause a variety of persistent and bothersome symptoms, including nasal congestion, sneezing, coughing, wheezing, itching, burning, swelling, and diarrhea. Common allergic conditions include seasonal allergic rhinitis (hay fever), allergic sinusitis, bronchial asthma, urticaria (hives), eczema, and food, drug, or venom allergy. These conditions may range from mild and self-limiting to severe and life threatening.

When the offending allergens can be identified, they are eliminated from the diet or the environment. Symptomatic treatment includes the use of antihistamines, bronchial dilators, and corticosteroids. Desensitization with a series of injections may be recommended to build immunity to some antigens. Severe systemic manifestations of allergic responses include **anaphylaxis,** serum sickness, arthralgia, and *status asthmaticus.* For example, anaphylactic shock, the result of a severe systemic allergic reaction, calls for emergency lifesaving intervention.

Autoimmune diseases represent a large group of disorders marked by an inappropriate or excessive response of the body's defense system that allows the immune system to become self-destructive. Normally, the immune system is able to distinguish self-antigens, which are harmless, from foreign antigens, which present a threat to the body. In autoimmune diseases, antibodies are formed

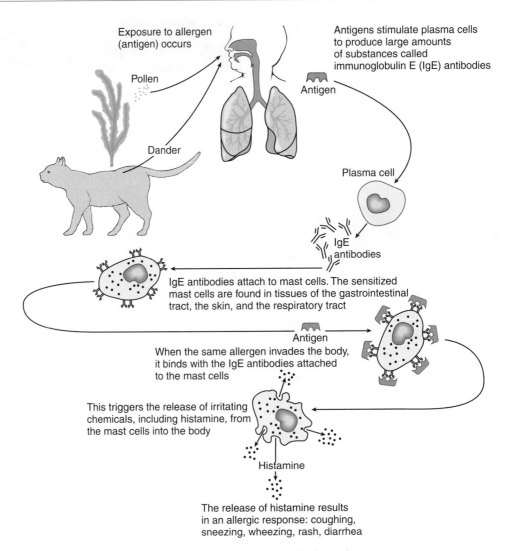

Exposure to allergen (antigen) occurs

Pollen

Dander

Antigens stimulate plasma cells to produce large amounts of substances called immunoglobulin E (IgE) antibodies

Antigen

Plasma cell

IgE antibodies

IgE antibodies attach to mast cells. The sensitized mast cells are found in tissues of the gastrointestinal tract, the skin, and the respiratory tract

Antigen

When the same allergen invades the body, it binds with the IgE antibodies attached to the mast cells

This triggers the release of irritating chemicals, including histamine, from the mast cells into the body

Histamine

The release of histamine results in an allergic response: coughing, sneezing, wheezing, rash, diarrhea

FIGURE 1–4 Mechanisms of allergic reaction.

against self-antigens mistakenly identified as foreign. Why the body becomes confused or what triggers an autoimmune response remains a mystery. Many serious diseases appear to have a strong autoimmune component. Examples are glomerulonephritis (see Chapter 11), Hashimoto disease (see Chapter 4), and rheumatoid arthritis (see Chapter 3).

Immunodeficiency disorders result from a depressed or absent immune response. Causative factors can be primary, manifested by a characteristic decrease in the number of T cells and B cells, leaving the body unable to adequately defend itself against infection and tumors. Immunodeficiency also may be secondary to disease or infection or may be the result of damage to the immune system caused by drugs, radiation, or surgery. Acquired immunodeficiency syndrome (AIDS), a prominent example of an immunodeficiency state, is caused by infection with a virus.

Chapter 3 discusses specific diseases of the immune system.

Aging

Because of the gradual diminishment of body functions, the aging process, although not considered a disease in itself, is a risk factor for the onset of many health problems. For this reason, a yearly physical examination with specific screening tests is recommended after age 50 years. Screening examinations include determination of blood cholesterol levels for *hyperlipidemia, electrocardiogram* (ECG) for heart disease, rectal examination for bowel cancer and prostate enlargement, blood pressure check for hypertension, Pap (Papanicolaou) smear for cervical cancer, mammogram for breast cancer, and urinalysis for possible diabetes and renal disease.

Knowing the special needs of older persons is becoming a more critical component of health care because the percentage of Americans over the age of 65 is growing dramatically. Currently, 13% of the population is over age 65, and they account for over one third of all health expenditures. It is predicted that this percentage will double over the next 15 years as the "baby boomers" approach late adulthood. Attention must be paid to the functional status and to the health issues of elderly patients. Common concerns are substance abuse, overmedication, loss of mental acuity, depression, and nutritional problems. Regular exercise three to five times a week, proper nutrition, and creating a hazard-free environment to prevent falls all should be emphasized. Older adults can have many significant life stresses such as financial hardships, relocation, loss of normal roles in life, and death of loved ones. Such added stress in a person's life may be a contributing factor in disease development or progression. Drug therapy is another major issue because many older adults take a number of different prescribed medications, in addition to nonprescription drugs that the health care professionals providing care might not know about. These older persons are at high risk for adverse drug reactions and may have to be hospitalized for such problems. Older adults also may not be able to tolerate the standard dose of medications because of metabolic and other changes in body composition (increased adipose tissue, decreased total body water, etc.) that occur with aging.

Psychological Factors

The constant interaction between mind and body can potentially affect a person's state of wellness or illness. When a person seeks medical attention, assessment of mental status is intertwined with physical evaluation. Psychological evaluation encompasses the observation of behavior, appearance, mood, communication, judgment, and thought processes. Because people react differently to disease, or the threat of illness, treatment plans must be tailored to meet their psychological needs as well. Preservation of self-esteem is of great importance.

Illness can disrupt daily activities; it can significantly change a patient's life and also the lives of involved family. In the face of disease, the person experiences an altered body image and emotional and social changes that are best understood in terms of past personal experience and perception. For example, when the patient was a child, did illness elicit empathy and a "chicken soup" approach or was illness met with aversion and a "tough it out" attitude?

Chronic disease is a stressor that can affect a person's self-esteem and behavior. Fear, helplessness, and lack of control are typical feelings. Patients pass through stages of anxiety, shock, denial, anger, withdrawal, and depression as they adjust to the presence of disease. If these stages are sustained and the person fails to accept the reality of the disease, the patient may develop psychological disturbances in addition to physical alterations.

Pain

All of us experience pain at some time in our lives. What is pain, how do we describe pain, how do we interpret pain, what are the types of pain, why are tolerance levels different for different people, and why do we have pain at all? Knowing the answers to these questions is a necessary component of developing an understanding of pain and how the health-care provider can facilitate relief of pain for patients.

Describing Pain

Pain is subjective and individualized and perceived only by the individual experiencing it. It can be physiologic or psychological. The vocabulary people use to express their sensations of pain varies widely; pain may be described as an uncomfortable sensation, an unpleasant experience, distress, strong discomfort, suffering, agony, or simply hurting. Dull and aching are words used often to describe pain resulting from overuse of the musculoskeletal system. Pain along a nerve route that is described as "burning" is often an indication of peripheral nerve insult. Patients use the term *cramping* to characterize an abdominal–visceral type of pain. Head pain or pain felt along a blood vessel commonly is described as *throbbing*. Other descriptive terms include shooting, stabbing, and stinging and in reference to thermal injury, pain may be described as a burning sensation. When expressing concern about how pain is affecting them, patients may use terms such as frightening, sickening, tiring, discomforting, intense, unbearable, mild, excruciating, and vicious to categorize the pain.

Because pain interpretation is subjective, the intensity with which it is felt depends on many factors. An individual's perception of pain and response to pain may be based on cultural values, past experiences, religious beliefs, emotional support or the lack thereof, anxiety, level of education, and the specific situation in which pain is being felt. Pain perception may be absent when a person is in the midst of a life-threatening situation and returns only when the person has escaped the danger. A variety of pain rating scales, using numbers and figures, are sometimes used to help measure an individual's perception of pain intensity and quality (Fig. 1–5).

Physiology of Pain

Pain is a necessary entity in life. The physiology of pain involves the stimulation of specialized nerve endings called **nociceptors.** These pain receptors are found on free sensory nerve endings in the superficial portions of the skin, in some tissues of internal or visceral organs, in joint capsules, in the periosteum of bones, surrounding the walls of blood vessels, and in certain deep tissue. Pain often is a signal of injury or tissue damage and as such is a protective mechanism that makes people aware of tissue insult.

Pain is the result of tissue insult from noxious (harmful) stimuli, including heat and cold, pressure, chemicals, electrical shock, and trauma. Pain receptors respond to three types of stimuli: (1) temperature extremes; (2) mechanical damage; and

(3) dissolved chemicals, including potassium, acids, histamines, acetylcholine, bradykinin, and prostaglandins. A very strong stimulus may excite all three types, creating a burning-type sensation. Additional causes of painful stimuli include hypoxia and ischemia to the tissues and muscle spasms.

Pain impulses travel from the nerve ending through the spinal cord to the thalamus, and then proceed to the sensory cortex. Adaptation to painful stimuli does not occur because the receptors continue to respond as long as the stimulus remains, stopping only when the tissue damage has ended.

Pain is a signal that helps locate and eliminate or reduce the source of tissue damage. Pain may be a part of the normal healing process too—a reaction to the inflammatory process. It is also possible for pain to occur in the absence of physical injury (this is referred to as psychological pain). Stress can alter both perception and response to pain. The cerebral cortex is responsible for the interpretation of pain and therefore must be functioning at normal capacity for interpretation to occur.

Pain is not always reported accurately. Many of the internal organs are poorly supplied with nociceptors, and therefore the tissue insults in these organs are not always reported as such. The free nerve endings have large receptive fields, consequently making it difficult to determine the true source of the pain stimuli. Additionally, neurons from certain organs may travel a parallel pathway along the spinal cord to the brain, resulting in *referred pain.* Generally, the referred pain follows a *dermatome* that is supplied by the same spinal nerve as the nerve that has been stimulated by the insult, causing the pain to be projected to the body surface. For example, the patient experiencing myocardial ischemia or angina describes the pain as chest pain radiating to the left arm. Likewise, the nervous tissue of the brain has no pain receptors; nevertheless, headaches are commonly reported. Often the pain is caused by pressure on the blood vessel walls or pressure on the meninges. Tissue insult or inflammation to the gallbladder often results in pain referred to the right scapular region (Fig. 1–6).

Pain Classification

Pain may be classified as acute, chronic, transient, or intractable. Acute pain usually has a sudden onset and is severe in intensity. It also usually is of short duration. Individuals with acute pain have a

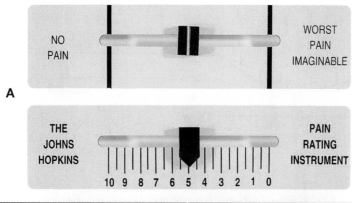

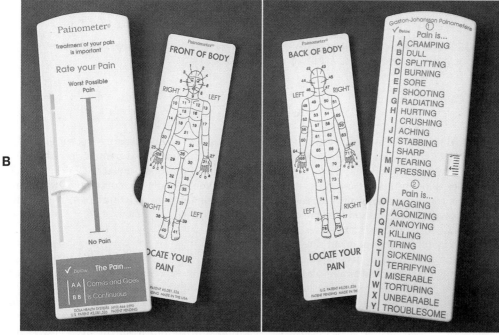

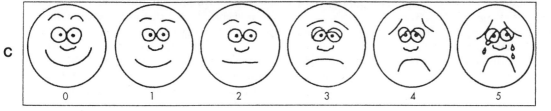

FIGURE 1–5 Pain rating scales and instruments. **A,** Self-contained, portable, pain-rating instrument that can provide an immediate assessment of pain. **B,** The painometer. **C,** The Wong/Baker Faces Rating Scale. (**A** from Grossman SA et al: A comparison of the Hopkins Pain Rating Instrument with standard visual analogue and verbal descriptor scales in patients with cancer pain, *Pain Symptom Manag* 7: 196-203, 1992; **B** courtesy of Dr. Fannie Gaston-Johansson, School of Nursing, The Johns Hopkins University; **C** from Wong DL, et al: *Wong's Essentials of Pediatric Nursing,* ed 6, St. Louis, 2001, p. 1301. Copyrighted by Mosby, Inc. Reprinted by permission.

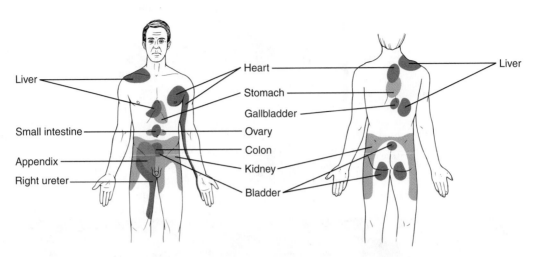

FIGURE 1–6 Referred pain, anterior and posterior views. (From Miller-Keane: *Encyclopedia and dictionary of medicine, nursing, & allied health,* ed 7, Philadelphia, 2003, Saunders.)

tendency to guard the painful area; may exhibit distractive behavior, such as crying or moaning; are restless, anxious, or listless; and may have altered thought processes. Blood pressure and pulse often increase, whereas respiratory rates may increase or decrease. Occasionally, sudden onset of very severe pain may cause vascular collapse and a resulting state of shock. Facial movements may indicate a grimace, and the skin may become *diaphoretic*. Acute pain, such as the pain experienced as a result of myocardial infarction, postoperative pain after surgical intervention, pain resulting from severe trauma, and pain felt during terminal illness, can be treated with narcotics or opioid-related drugs. Chronic pain is usually less severe and has a duration of longer than 6 months. Pain from inflammatory conditions such as arthritis and bursitis is considered chronic. Patients with chronic pain often exhibit weight loss or gain, insomnia or altered sleep patterns, anorexia, inability to continue normal activities, and guarded movements. Psychosocial relationships may be altered. Chronic pain often is treated with acetaminophen, antiprostaglandins, steroids, or antiinflammatory agents such as nonsteroidal antiinflammatory drugs (NSAIDs). Chronic intractable pain, usually generated by nerve damage, is debilitating and can cause depression. Transient pain comes and goes, usually has a brief duration, and often is not significant.

Pain also can be classified as superficial, deep, or visceral. Superficial pain is described as being located on the body surface. Deep pain refers to pain that usually is correlated with muscles, joints, or tendons. Visceral pain is attributed to internal organs.

Pain Relief

As previously mentioned, pain relief can be achieved by the use of analgesic drugs including narcotics and non-narcotic agents. Other methods include massage of the painful area to increase the blood flow to and from the area and to increase the flow of lymph from the area. Acupuncture, an ancient therapeutic treatment, is thought to elicit pain relief by way of the needles used to stimulate nerves deep in the tissue, thus arousing the pituitary gland and other parts of the brain to cause release of endorphins, the brain's own natural opioids. Endorphins reduce the perception of pain while the stimulus remains. Transcutaneous electrical nerve stimulation (TENS) sends electrical impulses to the nerve endings with the intention of blocking nerve transmission to the brain. (Some insurance companies consider TENS and electrical stimulation for pain relief to be experimental and will not provide reimbursement for this procedure.)

Function of Pain

Pain is necessary for survival. It is a warning signal that tissue damage is occurring. Without pain, an individual would have no idea that something was going wrong in the body. An example of this is a person who inadvertently develops a fracture in a leg bone as a result of disease such as osteoporosis; without pain the person would continue to walk until the broken bone protruded through the skin, finally creating awareness of the fracture. At that point the damage would be much more severe, and the person would also be exposed to microbial infection. Another example is a person whose coronary vessels are narrowing because of plaque build-up. If no anginal pain was felt with increased activity, he or she would continue the activity, unaware of the ischemia and permanent damage being done. The vessels could become completely occluded, and death would be the outcome. Yet another example is a woman with an ectopic pregnancy. Without pain, she would not be cognizant that the pregnancy growing inside the fallopian tube had caused the tube to rupture until she experienced vaginal bleeding. At that point, immediate surgical intervention would be needed to save her life. Even when an injury is external, pain is a necessary defense mechanism. A child who touches an object that is hot will withdraw his or her hand because of the pain it causes, thus preventing additional tissue damage. Although pain is most often thought to be an unpleasant experience, it is nevertheless an essential part of human existence.

Psychological Pain

Psychological or emotional pain is as real as pain with a physical cause to the person experiencing it. This type of pain also can be acute, chronic, transient, or intractable.

Acute psychological pain often is triggered by a catastrophic event, such as the death of a loved one, severe trauma, an extreme loss, witnessing brutal or cruel incidents, and being subjected to abusive situations. Coping or defense mechanisms usually are instinctively initiated but are not always effective in helping people deal with the extreme stress they feel. A person's reaction to an acute stressor may be immediate or it may be delayed. Psychological pain may be described as feelings of despair, anger, helplessness, rage, depression, and/or hopelessness. Thought processes and sleep patterns may be disrupted. An individual may cry or may exhibit signs of withdrawal. Often, those experiencing psychological pain become nonfunctional in a normal environment, or they may be able to function but are unaware of their surroundings as they go through the motions. Diagnoses for these conditions include major depression, posttraumatic stress disorder, and a variety of anxiety disorders. If an individual is noted to have these manifestations, intervention is indicated in the form of counseling, drug therapy, or both.

Chronic psychological pain usually has a more subtle and insidious onset. Often individuals are unaware of the personality changes and alterations in functioning that are taking place. The gradual onset of symptoms, the adaptive behavior they display, and the defense or coping mechanisms they employ assist them in continuing to live in a fairly normal fashion. Over a period of time, however, family, friends, coworkers, and even the individuals themselves will begin to notice the personality and functional changes. As with acute emotional pain, thought processes and sleep patterns are altered as are eating habits. Individuals may experience anorexia or overeating, with corresponding weight loss or gain. A change in appearance may take place as attention to personal hygiene and dress become less important. Posture begins to slump and energy diminishes. Sadness is expressed often with tears and crying, and laughter and a sense of humor are experienced less often. Depression, a delayed reaction to posttraumatic stress, seasonal affective disorder, situational involvement or lack of involvement, loss, and the grieving process are all components of chronic emotional pain. Intervention in the form of counseling and drug therapy is helpful in relieving this pain.

Transient emotional pain, like transient physical pain, is of very short duration and often resolves itself as the precipitating situation modifies.

Intractable psychological pain is a true emergency. An individual experiencing this feels him- or herself to be in a hopeless situation and has very few coping mechanisms on which to rely. When intractable psychological pain is brought to the attention of the health-care provider, immediate intervention should be initiated. If left to their own resources, these individuals may react to the hopelessness of the situation either with violent behavior or with attempted, and many times successful, suicide.

Health-care providers must understand the importance of having an awareness of the depth and significance of psychological pain. Such understanding is essential if they are to provide the best and most appropriate care possible to patients. By acknowledging the significance of this pain, they can help make the community more aware of the incidence of mental disorders and can help mitigate the stigma of mental illness.

Mental Disorders

Generally, mental disorders are described as being clinically significant behavioral or psychological syndromes that are associated with psychic pain or distress or impairment of function. Although sometimes cloaked in mystery, their common occurrence and their potential for causing disability dictate that the same ardent handling is needed for mental disorders as it is for any other sickness. Chapter 14 discusses mental disorders in more detail, including grief response, dementia, mood disorders, and **somatoform** disorders.

Diagnosis of Disease

When a person seeks medical attention and exhibits symptoms and/or signs of disease, the clinician begins an orderly series of steps to investigate the cause and make a diagnosis (Fig. 1–7). Establishing a diagnosis is a decision-making process in which data collected from the medical history, physical examination, and diagnostic tests are analyzed, integrated, and interpreted. A diagnosis provides a logical basis for determining treatment and prognosis.

The importance of the patient's medical history cannot be overstated; as the primary source of data, it provides vital clues and background information that helps direct the remainder of the assessment. During the patient interview, medical information such as predisposing factors or preexisting conditions, drug allergies, and current therapies is carefully noted. This can provide the foundation for an individualized treatment plan. And finally, the clinician focuses questions on the onset and nature of the present illness.

Next, a methodical physical examination of the patient from head to toe (a systems review) is per-

formed to detect the physical signs of disease. Assessment skills used to evaluate health status are inspection (observation and measurement, including vital signs), **auscultation** (trained listening), palpation (investigation by sense of touch), and percussion (tapping that produces vibration and sound). The information gathered is then measured against norms or standards.

The final source of assessment data is that which can be obtained by conducting a wide variety of appropriate diagnostic studies and laboratory tests. These include microscopic examination of cells and tissues and chemical analysis. Although diagnostic testing is considered to be an important scientific measure of function, these laboratory data are not interpreted apart from other clinical data gathered from the history and physical examination. In the process of deciding or confirming the identification of a disease, the results of diagnostic studies are integrated with the medical history and physical examination findings. In fact, physicians now have computer systems that can analyze large numbers of patient records to quantify probabilities and to devise an orderly approach to diagnosis (a decision tree). As a result, the physician is reminded of a full range of possible diagnoses for a given set of symptoms and signs; in other words, the physician is aided in making a *differential diagnosis,* especially when two or more diseases resemble one another in respect to signs and symptoms.

Laboratory tests, particularly biochemical profiles obtained by testing blood and urine, are used routinely to screen for imbalances or to detect early signs of disease. They also are used to monitor the effectiveness of therapeutic medications and other medical treatment (Box 1–1).

Treatment of Disease

After the initial assessment is completed and a diagnosis is established, appropriate medical intervention is implemented. The plan of treatment is directly related to an identified expected outcome. The goal may be specifically to cure, to control symptoms, or to be supportive, or it may be a combination of these. Therapeutic elements of a conventional medical care plan may be used conservatively or aggressively and include one or more of the following: preventive measures, therapeutic procedures, administration of medications, surgery,

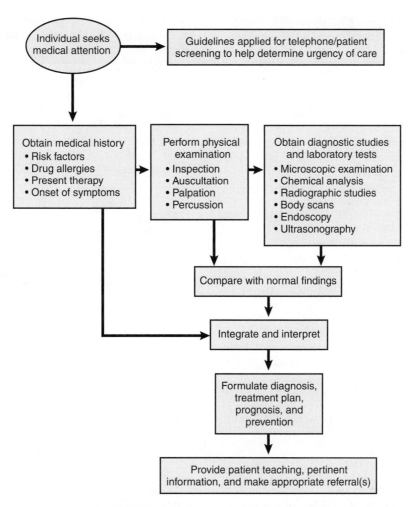

FIGURE 1–7 Essential steps in diagnosis.

physical therapy, diet modification, psychotherapy, patient education, and follow-up care.

After a medical treatment plan is implemented, it is evaluated and modified as needed. The current trend is to involve patients directly in the choices of treatment and to emphasize their responsibility to make choices that promote their recovery. A team approach to medical treatment, involving the patient, medical personnel, family, and community support systems, is optimum for complicated cases.

The concept of holistic medicine is comprehensive care that focuses on the needs of the whole person (Fig. 1–8). The physical and psychological well-being of the individual are dependent on each other. It is this established mind-and-body interac-

tion that compels the holistic health-care provider to consider the patient as a whole person. Rather than narrowly defining a disease only in terms of physical pathologic changes, the clinician also considers the patient's social, emotional, intellectual, and spiritual components. Individualizing care is important; the personality, environment, and lifestyle of the patient all need to be factored into the care plan. The holistic practitioner acknowledges the uniqueness of the patient in regard to his or her needs, aspirations, perception, comprehension, and insight. The illness or health-altering event is considered to be a dysfunction of the entire, or whole, person and not just an isolated dimension.

Encouraging the patient's active participation in the recovery process is essential to this system of

BOX 1-1
Common Laboratory and Diagnostic Tests

BLOOD ANALYSIS

Complete blood count (CBC): Evaluation of cellular components of the blood. Includes red blood cell count, red blood cell indices, white blood cell count, white blood cell differential, hemoglobin, hematocrit, and platelet count. Sometimes referred to as hemogram. Often the differential must be ordered specifically as CBC with differential.

Hemoglobin (Hgb): Measurement of the oxygen-carrying pigment of the red blood cells.

Hematocrit (HCT): Measurement of the percentage of red blood cells in a volume of whole blood.

Chemistries: Normal chemistry profiles may contain blood serum levels for albumin, alkaline phosphatase, aspartate aminotransferase, bilirubin, calcium, creatinine, lactate dehydrogenase, phosphorus, total protein, urea nitrogen, and uric acid.

Thyroid function tests: Thyroid thyroxine (T4), triiodothyronine (T3), and thyroid-stimulating hormone (TSH).

Lipid profile: Total cholesterol, triglycerides, high-density lipoprotein (HDL) cholesterol, low-density lipoprotein (LDL) cholesterol.

Electrolytes (lytes): Blood serum test for chloride, potassium, sodium, and carbon dioxide.

Clotting and coagulation studies: Partial thromboplastin time (PTT), prothrombin time (PT), platelet (thrombocyte) count, bleeding times.

Erythrocyte sedimentation rate (ESR): The rate at which red blood cells (erythrocytes) fall out of well-mixed whole blood to the bottom of the test tube.

Glucose tolerance test (GTT): Fasting blood glucose (FBG) levels.

Toxicology studies, drug screens.

Drug levels: Digoxin, digitoxin, theophylline, lidocaine, lithium, and various drugs for therapeutic and/or toxic levels.

Arterial blood gas (ABG) analysis: Measurement of dissolved oxygen and carbon dioxide in arterial blood. Also measures pH and O_2 saturation of the arterial blood.

Cardiac enzymes: Creatine kinase (CK), CK isoenzymes, lactate dehydrogenase (LD), lactate dehydrogenase isoenzymes, aspartate aminotransferase (AST, SGOT), alanine aminotransferase (ALT, SGPT)

URINE STUDIES

Urinalysis (UA): A screening test using a urine specimen that gives a picture of the patient's overall state of health and the state of the urinary tract. Measurements include pH and specific gravity of the urine, presence of ketones, protein, sugars, bilirubin, urobilinogen. Color and odor are noted, as is the presence of abnormal blood cells, casts, bacteria, other cells, and crystals.

Culture and sensitivity (C & S) of urine: *Culture:* Sample of urine specimen is placed in/on culture medium to see whether microbial growth occurs. If growth occurs, identification of the pathogenic microbe is determined. *Sensitivity:* A portion of the specimen is placed on a sensitivity disk (which has been impregnated with specific antibiotics) to determine which antibiotic the pathogen is resistant to or to which it will be responsive.

CARDIOLOGY TESTS

Electrocardiogram (ECG, EKG): A record of the electrical activity of the myocardium used to diagnose ischemia, arrhythmias, conduction difficulties, activity of cardiac medications.

Echocardiogram: An ultrasound examination of the cardiac structure to define the size, shape, thickness, position, and movements of the cardiac structures, including valves, walls, and chambers.

Holter monitor: A miniature electrocardiograph that records the electrical activity of the heart for an extended period of time, usually 24 to 48 hours. The patient records all activities during the time period for the examiner to correlate activity with cardiac abnormalities.

Thallium scan: A scan to indicate myocardial profusion and the location and extent of myocardial ischemia and/or infarction and to predict the possible prognosis of the cardiac condition.

MUGA scan: A scan that assesses the function of the left ventricle and identifies abnormalities of the myocardial walls.

Stress testing, treadmill, exercise tolerance testing: An assessment of cardiac function during moderate exercise after a 12-lead electrocardiogram.

Pulse oximeter: An instrument (spectrophotometer) that provides a noninvasive measurement of the O_2 saturation of the arterial blood.

Cardiac catheterization: Fluoroscopic visualization of right or left side of heart by passing a catheter into right or left chamber and injecting dye. Angiograms consist of the catheter being passed into the coronary vessels where the dye is injected and fluoroscopic images are recorded.

IMAGING STUDIES

Radiographs: Visualization of internal organs and structures by electromagnetic radiation. Radiographs of bone; the ab-

BOX 1–1
Common Laboratory and Diagnostic Tests—cont'd

domen; the chest; paranasal sinuses; and kidneys, ureters, and bladder (KUB) and mammograms do not require contrast medium. Contrast medium is used to distinguish soft tissue and some organs such as the gallbladder, esophagus, stomach, and small and large intestines.

Magnetic resonance imaging (MRI): Uses a magnetic field instead of radiation to visualize internal tissues. It is possible to view tissue and organs in a three-dimensional manner with MRI. Helpful in determining blood flow to tissues and organs, in studying condition of blood vessels, in detecting tumors, in differentiating healthy and diseased tissues, and in detecting sites of infection. The patient is not exposed to ionizing radiation during MRI.

Computed tomography (CT) scans: A radiographic technique using a scanner system that can provide images of the internal structure of tissue and organs both geographically and characteristically.

Fluoroscopy: A real-time imaging process that provides continuous visualization of the area undergoing radiography. Still films and video recordings are made of the process for more extensive examination. Used in procedures and to study the functioning of tissues and organs.

Sonograms, ultrasound, echogram: A beam of sound waves is projected into target tissues or organs, resulting in a bouncing back of the wave off the target structure. An outline of the structure is produced and recorded on film or videotape for examination.

Myelogram: An imaging examination of the spinal cord and spinal nerve roots. Contrast medium (dye) and/or air are injected into the subarachnoid space and recorded on radiographic film and videotape. Fluoroscopy generally is used in this procedure.

STOOL ANALYSIS
Guaiac tests: For occult blood.
Ova and parasite tests

SPUTUM ANALYSIS
Sputum studies: Microscopic studies of sputum, including culture and sensitivity, acid-fast bacteria culture and stain, Gram stain, and cytology studies.

ENDOSCOPY TESTS
Endoscopy: Visual inspection of internal organs and/or cavities of the body using appropriate scope.
Gastroscopy: Visualization of the stomach by a gastroscope.

Colonoscopy: Visualization of the colon with a colonoscope.
Sigmoidoscopy: Visualization of the sigmoid portion of the colon and the rectum with a sigmoidoscope.
Proctoscopy: Visualization of the rectum with a proctoscope.
Cystoscopy: Visualization of the structures of the urinary tract with a cystoscope.
Colposcopy: Visualization of the cervical epithelium, vagina, and vulvar epithelium with a colposcope.
Bronchoscopy: Visualization of the trachea and bronchi with a bronchoscope.

PULMONARY FUNCTION STUDIES
Peak flow: The patient blows into a flowmeter to determine the volume of an expiratory effort.
Spirometry: A measurement of lung capacity, volume, and flow rates by a spirometer.
Methacholine challenge: A test for asthma in which measurement of lung volumes is taken before and after the inhalation of methacholine, a bronchial constrictor.
Pulmonary function
Tidal volume, expiratory reserve volume, residual volume, inspiratory reserve volume

MISCELLANEOUS TESTS
Culture and sensitivity (C & S): *Culture:* Sample of specimen is placed in/on culture medium to see whether microbial growth occurs. If growth occurs, identification of the pathogenic microbe is determined. *Sensitivity:* A portion of the specimen is placed on a sensitivity disk (which has been impregnated with specific antibiotics) to determine which antibiotic the pathogen is resistant to or to which it will be responsive. The specimen could be blood, stool, urine, sputum, any discharge fluid, or from a wound.
Bone marrow studies: Aspiration of bone marrow by needle from the sternum, posterior or superior iliac spine, or the anterior iliac crest for diagnosis of neoplasms, metastasis, and blood disorders.
Immune and immunoglobulin studies: Studies of the functioning or nonfunctioning of the patient's immune system.
Serologic testing: Analysis of blood specimens for antigen–antibody reactions. Used to detect bacterial infections, including syphilis, Lyme disease, chlamydia, and streptococcal infections; antibodies from viral sources including infectious mononucleosis, rubella, hepatitis, rabies, HIV, herpes, and cytomegalovirus; antibodies from fungal

Continued

BOX 1-1
Common Laboratory and Diagnostic Tests—cont'd

sources such as histoplasmosis and *Candida;* and antibodies from the parasitic source, toxoplasmosis.

Biopsies: The excision of tissue from the living body, followed by microscopic examination, for purpose of exact diagnosis.

Lumbar punctures (LP): A surgical procedure to withdraw spinal fluid for analysis.

Electroencephalogram (EEG): A recording of the electrical activity of the cerebral cortex of the brain.

Electromyelogram (EMG): An electrodiagnostics assessment and recording of the activity of the skeletal muscles.

Gastric analysis: Used in the diagnosis of pernicious anemia and peptic ulcers.

Pregnancy tests: Human chorionic gonadotropin (HCG–UCG). Used in diagnosis of pregnancy, abortion, ectopic pregnancy, and uterine pathology.

Gram stain: Used to identify gram-positive or gram-negative microorganism of infectious process.

SCREENING

Hepatic screening: Liver function tests–Liver profile: Usually includes alanine aminotransferase, alkaline phosphatase, aspartate aminotransferase, bilirubin, and gamma-glutamyl transpeptidase.

Tuberculosis (TB) screening: *Mantoux:* An intradermal injection of tuberculin is done usually on the inner aspect of the lower arm. Localized thickening of the skin in the area,

along with redness, indicates the presence of active or dormant tuberculosis. Positive reaction requires further investigation, usually including a chest radiograph.

Prostatic-specific antigen (PSA): A serum blood test to determine the level of PSA. Increased levels may indicate benign prostatic hypertrophy, prostate cancer, inflammatory conditions of the prostate. This is a screening test that should be followed by a digital rectal examination of the prostate gland to determine any abnormalities. Often additional diagnostic studies are indicated.

Pap (Papanicolaou) smear: A cytologic examination of cells that have been scraped or aspirated from the cervix and cervical os. A screen test is done annually, especially before any female hormones are prescribed.

Mammograms: A radiographic examination of the breast tissue. A screen test is done on an annual basis for women older than 40 years of age to detect the presence of breast disease. This screening also should be accompanied by a manual examination of the breast tissue by a physician. Monthly breast self-examinations are recommended.

These are many of the common diagnostic procedures that may be ordered and performed. Many more diagnostic procedures may be used in the process of arriving at the patient's diagnosis and prognosis. More diagnostic tests and procedures are discussed, along with the corresponding disease or condition, in subsequent chapters.

Refer to Appendix I for additional information regarding normal and abnormal values and indications for tests.

care. Feelings of love, humor, hope, and enthusiasm are part of the healing process, whereas feelings of hostility, fear, anger, grief, rage, shame, and greed fuel the illness process.

The absence of illness does not necessarily indicate optimal health. Holistic care encourages the patient to consciously pursue the highest possible expressions of being, including those of spirit, mind, emotion, environment, socialization, and physical being. Although integrating all the needs of a patient is compatible with the comprehensive treatment plans of traditional medicine, holistic medicine also may incorporate a variety of nontraditional methods of treatment, which may be empirical or experimental.

Cultural Diversity

One important aspect of holistic medicine is recognition of the cultural diversity of patients. The United States continues to grow more culturally diverse. According to the U.S. Census Bureau, the number of foreign-born U.S. residents increased from 19 million to over 28 million between 1990 and 2000. Health-care providers must be aware of the challenges of caring for such a diverse population, challenges such as differences in language, religious beliefs, views about health issues, and life experiences.

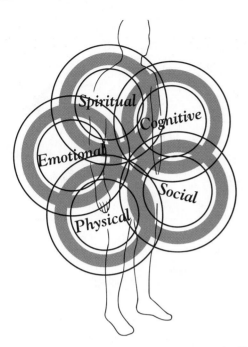

FIGURE 1-8 Human beings from a holistic viewpoint. The expanding and receding circles represent the dynamic interaction of the physical, social, emotional, spiritual, and cognitive needs that constitute humanness. (From Luckmann J, Sorensen K: *Medical–surgical nursing: a pathophysiologic approach,* Philadelphia, 1987, Saunders.)

Overcoming the challenges that cultural diversity presents begins with a willingness on the part of the health-care provider to learn about cultural issues, to overcome language barriers, and to take the time necessary to understand what the patient is trying to convey. Many hospitals and clinics have interpreters available to facilitate communication with more prominent minority groups in their communities. Even so, it takes time, patience, and flexibility to acquire knowledge of different cultures and their ways of explaining, understanding, and treating health problems.

Alternative Medicine

Many patients and practitioners now accept safe alternative medicine as an adjunct to traditional medicine. Some of the therapies are osteopathy, chiropractic, massage, reflexology, aromatherapy, herbs, diet and nutrition, acupuncture, acupressure, shiatsu, magnetic therapy, hypnosis, relaxation, Reiki, energy movement, and music therapy.

Osteopathy is probably the most widely accepted form of alternative medicine. In the United States, osteopathic physicians (Doctors of Osteopathy [DOs]) are trained medical doctors who emphasize stimulation of the body's natural processes as a means to promote healing and well-being. In addition to traditional medical and surgical concepts, osteopathic physicians use manipulation techniques to realign body structure, thereby restoring balance and promoting healing.

Chiropractic medicine is based on the concept that the body's nervous system is the foundation of health and that undue pressure on or an insult to the nervous system may result in pain and disease. Correct alignment of the spinal vertebrae is emphasized; therefore many chiropractic adjustments involve manipulation of the spine.

Massage, although not a new concept, is just now being recognized by the U.S. medical community as a valid alternative therapy or type of medicine. According to the Eastern philosophy and also the Swedish concepts, massage encourages drainage of the lymphatic system and increases circulation to the tissues.

Reflexology, a form of massage, directs its efforts primarily toward massage of the feet and sometimes of the hands. The theory is that the body is divided into zones and that these zones are reflected in specific areas of the feet or hands. Manipulation of these areas is expected to cause a therapeutic effect on the organ or system represented in that zone.

Aromatherapy uses essential oils to promote wellness and healing and to relieve stress. Although this therapy mainly involves inhalation and the olfactory system (Fig. 1–9), the oils used are absorbed through the skin and transported to the various body tissues and systems by the circulatory system as well. The essential oils are diluted and then massaged into the skin or placed in a steam inhaler for inspiration. Some of the more common essential oils used in aromatherapy are chamomile, clary sage, clove, eucalyptus, geranium, ginger, lavender, orange, peppermint, rosemary, sage, tea tree, and ylang ylang. Often aroma therapists mix the oils to meet the specific needs of their patients.

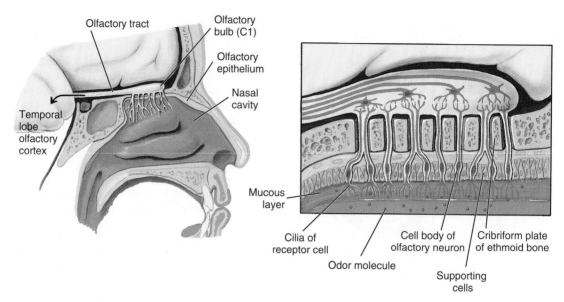

FIGURE 1–9 Structure of the olfactory receptors. (From Applegate EJ: *The anatomy and physiology learning system,* ed 2, Philadelphia, 2000, Saunders.)

Herbs have been used as medicines for many centuries, with ancient Egyptians being the first culture known to record lists of herbs. Sometimes called natural medicines, herbs now are being substituted for pharmaceutical products by some. Common herbal products include *Ginkgo biloba,* garlic, saw palmetto, ginseng, passion flower, angelica, chamomile, fennel, lavender, peppermint, rosemary, sage, Saint John's wort, valerian, and yarrow. Herbs may be purchased in a pharmacy or herbal drug store, or by mail. Herbal remedies are professed to treat allergies, arthritis, gastrointestinal (GI) problems, headaches, hypertension or hypotension, insomnia, urinary problems, menstrual or menopausal symptoms, and skin diseases. Many of these products do not have FDA approval and may damage health if taken unwarily or in conjunction with prescription drugs. Lack of FDA regulation also means that the ingredients stated on the outside of the bottle may not necessarily be inside the bottle or may not be present in the amounts indicated.

Diet and nutrition therapy certainly is not a new concept; however, many are following special diets and addressing nutritional needs, hoping to eliminate toxins from the body and allow it to function at optimum level. Diet therapy may include fat-free, low saturated fat, low-sugar, high-protein, low-carbohydrate, vegetarian, no or low-caffeine, and seafood diets. Vitamin and mineral supplements often are added to the daily routine, but should be done so with caution because megadoses may be toxic. Patients should check with a physician or pharmacist before starting any nutritional supplement regimen.

Acupuncture, an Asian therapy that uses meridians, attempts to adjust the body's energy (chi [chee]) flow by inserting needles into acupuncture points. After insertion, the needles are manipulated by twirling or by a gentle pumping action. Recent advances in techniques use electrical or laser stimulation. Only professionals trained in the art should attempt acupuncture.

Acupressure, similar to acupuncture, involves the manipulation of acupoints by means of finger pressure. The intent is to balance the flow of energy along the meridians to promote healthy functioning of internal organs. Acupressure often is incorporated into massage as a method of muscle relaxation and stress reduction.

Shiatsu (she-AT-sue), a form of therapy from Japan that is similar to acupressure, usually is performed on a mat on the floor. The patient remains clothed, and the therapist applies pressure to the acupoints and along the meridians using the fingertips, knuckles, elbows, knees, or even the feet.

Magnetic therapy, a relatively new concept in the United States, has not been approved by the FDA.

However, it is being used extensively in veterinary medicine, especially in equine veterinary medicine. In Europe and the United Kingdom, magnetic therapy has been accepted for use in humans as well. Although the theory has not been proved according to FDA standards, it is believed that magnets increase circulation to the area being treated, thereby increasing the available amount of oxygen (O_2) and nutrients while at the same time transporting away the waste products of metabolism and the inflammatory process. It also is postulated that the magnetic field interferes with the conduction of the sensory nerves by preventing movement of the sodium (Na) and potassium (K) ions in and out of the nerve cell; this reduces the conduction capability of the sensory nerve. Advocates of this therapy state that magnets are useful in relieving muscle and nerve pain, reducing inflammation, and mitigating migraines.

Hypnosis and hypnotherapy have been accepted means of psychological therapy only for approximately the past 40 years. The therapist places the patient in a trance-like state, often resembling sleep. While in this trance, the subject follows acceptable suggestions. Often relaxation and pain relief can be achieved using this therapy. Only a qualified practitioner who is trained specifically in the art of hypnosis should attempt this therapy.

Relaxation can be thought of as a form of self-hypnosis. Many techniques for achieving relaxation are available to the individual. Physical relaxation usually is the starting point for the subject, with psychological relaxation often being the next step. Relaxation is used to treat stress-related physical and emotional problems, pain, anxiety, asthma, arthritis, depression, panic attacks, and hypertension. Many forms of relaxation include repetition of an action, images, or sounds that then passively erase everyday thoughts from the mind.

Reiki (ray-KEE) is a transference of healing energy from the practitioner to the patient. Usually the practitioner starts the ritual at the patient's head and either touches the head or moves the hands close to the head within the patient's aura. The practitioner's hands then touch other parts of the patient's body, or the hands move into the aura space outlining the body. Healing energy then is transferred to the patient. The intention of this therapy is the promotion of physical, emotional, and spiritual well-being.

The practitioner using energy movement perceives shortages in the energy field of the patient and attempts to balance the energies with interaction. Energy from a "higher power" is transferred through the practitioner to the patient, thus not exhausting the practitioner's own energy supply. This noninvasive approach uses energy balancing to effect significant changes in the physical, emotional, and spiritual well-being of the patient.

Music therapy recognizes the involvement of vibrations, rhythms, and sound in the well-being of individuals. Listening to music by composers of the Baroque period, such as Mozart, can help achieve relaxation. Music along with anesthesia or pain medication is used to elevate mood, to create a calming effect, and to lessen muscle tension and to alleviate feelings of fear and anxiety by manifesting a state of relaxation. Trained and qualified music therapists design the therapy to fit the particular patient's needs.

Homeopathy, polarity therapy, rolfing, tai chi (tie-CHEE), iridology, naturopathy, hydrotherapy, and Ayurveda are some additional forms of alternative medicine. Although any of these therapies may be considered as a form of alternative medicine, the patient and practitioner should check with the physician before attempting to include these therapies in the course of treatment. When used, they should be considered as adjunct treatment and not necessarily proven medical treatment. Health-care providers should inquire routinely about a patient's use of alternative therapies because a large percentage of the population does use them, and many do not think to report this use to their physicians.

Genetic Counseling

For many genetic diseases, the responsible gene or chromosomal abnormality has been identified, and it is possible to test for the presence of the mutation in an individual. The discovery of a genetic disease in a family member often raises the questions of whether other family members are affected, whether others are carriers of the disease, and whether future offspring will be affected by it. Genetic counseling is a communication process that is centered on the occurrence or risk of occurrence of a genetic disorder in a family. Such counseling should be offered to all families affected by the diagnosis of a genetic disease in one or more members.

Genetic counseling is more than simply reproductive counseling concerning inherited disorders; it helps to bridge the gap between complicated medical and scientific concepts and the emotional aspects of being diagnosed with a certain condition. Counselors help the family understand the diagnosis, course of disease, and available treatment options. They talk about heredity and risk of occurrence in other family members and future offspring. If genetic testing is available for the disorder, the counselors first explain the test and the benefits of taking/not taking the test. They help prepare the family for any outcome of the genetic test. Common feelings experienced after receiving a diagnosis of a genetic disorder are a sense of being "labeled," guilt that other family members may be affected, worry about insurance discrimination, or a sense of hopelessness if the disease has no cure. Even if the patient receives the "good" news that he or she is not affected, there may be a feeling of "survivor guilt." With the increase in availability of genetic testing for many conditions, genetic counselors are usually available at most major hospitals.

Gene Therapy

Gene therapy refers to the experimental intervention of adding, repairing, or blocking the expression of specific genes to treat a disease, whether in-herited or acquired. A therapeutic gene is delivered using a vector (a chaperone molecule that accompanies and aids in the safe delivery of the DNA). Protocols may be done *ex vivo* (outside the body) or *in vivo* (inside the body). In *ex vivo* protocols, the cells to be modified are removed from the body, modified, and returned to the patient. *In vivo* therapies treat the patient with a gene delivery vehicle that will target the desired cells for the gene modification. Gene therapy aims to treat autosomal or X-linked recessive diseases by addition of a functional copy of the defective gene. The goal for autosomal dominant disease is to inhibit or repair the defective gene. Most of the vectors used for DNA delivery to date involve viruses, but nonviral methods, such as liposomes (small, spherical, artificial particles consisting of a lipid bilayer that encloses, in this case, the gene to be delivered), are being investigated as well. Experimental gene therapy protocols have been designed to treat diseases such as cystic fibrosis, sickle cell anemia, hemophilia B, and various forms of cancer. Although many studies have been done to determine the feasibility of gene therapy, few, if any, of these trials demonstrated clinical benefit to those who had been treated. Still, much research is underway and hopefully one day it will be possible to surmount the technical difficulties that currently prohibit the use of gene therapy in the treatment of a wide variety of illnesses.

PATIENT TEACHING

NOTE: *Please consult your state code regarding licensing regulations for an explanation of the rules and regulations governing medical assistant practice in your location.* Practice laws address what tasks the properly prepared medical assistant can perform; these laws differ from state to state. It is important that medical assistants know who their legally responsible supervisor is in a medical office; it may be the physician. Medical assistants should ask to see the written office policy regarding any delegation of tasks by the physician or nurse.

The authors consider it important, and in the patient's best interest, that all health-care workers, as members of a clinical team, understand the principles, goals, and specifics of patient teaching. *Licensing regulations and state practice acts gen-erally permit only nurses and physicians to actually do patient teaching and make triage judgments.*

General Principles of Patient Teaching

- The concept of patient teaching is based on patient-centered care, with the patient being a partner in the process of learning skills, solving problems, and preventing complications.
- The education process is ongoing, interactive, and directed toward achieving the patient's plan of care.
- Patient teaching is a course of action that involves assessment, critical thinking, and

compromise directed towards successful compliance.

- Effective patient teaching policies indicate who has primary legal responsibility for patient teaching and documentation (outlined in nurse state practice acts).

Goals of Patient Teaching

- Encourage the patient to comply with the personalized medical treatment plan to assure recovery.*
- Offer guidance, support, and clear instruction to both the patient who requires medical attention and to the family or caregiver.
- Develop a trusting relationship with patients through empathy, effective communication, and knowledge about the subject matter being taught.
- Give an individual the confidence needed to take responsibility for his or her health or recovery.

Reasons for Patient Teaching

- Ease anxiety
- Answer questions
- Instill confidence through individualized education
- Evaluate the patient's perception of the treatment plan, and make any necessary adjustments
- Reinforce the physician's instructions
- Highlight reasonable goals for recovery
- Encourage the individual to take responsibility for his or her health care
- Help build the esteem that creates a sense of self-sufficiency and control
- Educate the primary caregiver or family about specific aspects of the care plan
- Improve patient/family coping

---

*NOTE: According to the American Medical Association – Report 2 of the Council on Scientific Affairs, 1998, between 30% and 50% of all patients fail to follow their prescribed therapy.

- Provide an opportunity to practice skills associated with care
- Reduce clinic visits and hospitalization
- Supply the patient and caregiver with educational materials (booklets, websites, community resources)
- Suggest participation in appropriate social support groups
- Supply a list of phone numbers to call for answers to questions or medical concerns during recovery
- Stress the importance of keeping future appointments for follow-up care

The Specifics of Patient Teaching: Addressing the Patient's Concerns

"What's wrong with me?"

Answering this question provides an opportunity to reinforce or explain *only what has been expressed to the patient by the medical professional with primary responsibility for care.* It is not appropriate to "second guess" or give false or unsubstantiated information to a patient.

"What are these tests for?"

Again your response will depend on guidelines given by the medical professional ordering the tests.

- Explain any special preparation and the purpose for the test.
- In plain words, explain the procedure and what to expect during and after the procedure.
- Make sure the patient understands warning signs of complications that may occur, if any.
- Tell the patient when to expect the test results, and advise when to call or wait to be called for those results.
- Be prepared to discuss the cost to the patient or insurance company, if asked.

"What is this disease?"

Again, you should review and explain the diagnosis made by the physician. When possible, use illustrations and plain language to explain the pathophysiology of the disease. Try to point to the history of symptoms that may relate to the disease. This will help the patient monitor changes in symptoms during his or her recovery.

"What causes this disease?"

Review the physician's explanation of the cause(s) and contributing factors. This could include the source of infection, genetic influences, lifestyle, age, diet, trauma, or epidemic factors. Understanding prevention measures is helpful in some cases.

"Why do I need this medication?"

Explain the purpose and expected results. Review the dosage schedule and route of administration. Discuss the common side effects, as well as what side effects to report to the physician. Give special instructions such as how to handle skipped doses, and explain why some medications must not be stopped abruptly without the advice of the doctor. Be sure to mention over-the-counter drugs to avoid.

"When should I call the doctor?"

Review warning signs of possible complications from the disease or any medical intervention that require notification of the nurse or physician: sudden increase in pain, signs of infection or bleeding, neurologic changes, muscle pain or weakness, etc. Advise the patient on how to obtain refills for medications.

"How long do I have to do this therapy?"

Explain the goal(s) of treatment or therapy: physical therapy, therapeutic topical applications of heat or ice, eye drops, wound care, extra rest, or avoidance of certain activity. Demonstrate and give the patient time to practice a prescribed treatment or evaluation such as glucose monitoring, or the use of an inhaler.

"Would you explain this diet?"

Instruct the patient on the relationship of diet and his or her recovery and health. Warn the patient about the possible interactions between specific herbs and certain medications. List the signs of dehydration. Refer to a dietitian as needed.

"The doctor says I need an operation."

Preoperative Care

- Offer reasonable assurance because preoperative anxiety is universal.
- Review the preoperative instructions given by the physician.
- Ask the patient if he or she understands what to expect from the operation and offer as much information as possible to the family or caregiver.
- Arrange for any preoperative blood work, radiology or scans. Answer related questions. Give laboratory phone numbers and hours of service.
- Give the patient complete directions and parking instructions.

Postoperative Care

- After surgery, make sure the patient understands the medical plan: wound care, how to take medications, and when to resume activity and return to work.
- The patient needs reassurance about pain control, and what to expect during the recovery process.
- Explain warning signs of complications: fever, bleeding, infection, shock, dehydration, and emotional depression.
- The patient and caregiver should be given written instructions and the phone numbers of the nurse or physician to call for answers to questions.
- Make appropriate referrals to support groups.

"When do I have to be seen again?"

Make a follow-up appointment for the patient. Explain the importance of ongoing care during the recovery process. Encourage the patient to ask questions about any aspect of his or her medical care. Long-term treatment and medical concerns are addressed on an ongoing basis.

Special Considerations for the Patient With Cancer or Life-Threatening Disease

When the clinician interrelates with patients and families faced with life-shortening illness, he or she has many opportunities to offer important responses and guidance. Seriously ill patients benefit from an interdisciplinary approach to the clinical management of their disease. Clinicians can expect to address many special needs of the person diagnosed with the disease itself and also with side effects of therapeutic interventions. The issues to be addressed are many and varied.

- Keep patients and families from feeling abandoned by providing support based on their personal needs and goals.
- Give verbal and written instructions.
- Welcome feedback on all aspects of the care plan.
- Encourage discussion about side effects of medications, especially chemotherapy, radiation, or any therapeutic procedures.
- Review warning signs to report to the physician (i.e., weight loss, dehydration, or pain that is not controlled by prescription medication).
- Address the physical, psychological, social, and spiritual aspects of care.

- Bear in mind the two main fears of those with life-threatening illness: being in pain and becoming a burden to others.
- Make appropriate and timely referrals to support groups or comprehensive programs of end-of-life care, such as hospice.
- Reinforce the concept of palliative care being prescribed when curative treatment offers no hope.
- Address the caregiver's concerns including adjusting to role changes, providing physical care, and ethical issues and dilemmas.

CONCLUSION

Human pathologic processes involve complex mechanisms that can be weighed separately as elements of the disease process but that ultimately converge into the total picture of how and why an individual is sick and what is required as a remedy.

It is worth the effort to strive to understand the nature and impact of human disease on the person and on humankind. One can expect to find great personal and professional satisfaction in knowing the nature, signs, symptoms, causes, and treatment of the pathologic conditions that alter or seriously threaten health. This knowledge also fosters insight into the scenario imposed by diseases and fosters compassion for the people affected by them.

REVIEW CHALLENGE

Answer the following questions:

1. How may the following predisposing factors make a person more vulnerable to disease?
   Age
   Gender
   Lifestyle
   Environment
   Heredity
2. Describe three ways that genetic diseases are caused.
3. Name three of the body's natural defense mechanisms.
4. How does acute inflammation protect against infection?
5. Discuss the behavioral characteristics of malignant neoplasms.
6. What is the goal of cancer treatment and what therapeutic measures may be used?
7. What is allergic disease? What are the symptoms and how may they be treated?
8. List the normal sequence of steps in formulating diagnosis.
9. What is the difference between benign and malignant tumors?
10. What is the emphasis in preventive health care?
11. Explain the importance of knowing the types of pain, the possible causes, and how it may be described by the patient.
12. List some of the stresses and special needs of older persons.
13. What are the components of the holistic concept of medical care?
14. Discuss osteopathy as a form of alternative medicine.
15. How does genetic counseling help families?
16. How does good patient teaching affect the positive outcome of disease?

INTERNET ASSIGNMENTS

1. Explore the plethora of information available for information and research from the National Cancer Institute. Report on your personal points of interest on this subject.
2. Navigate the website for the Centers for Disease Control and Prevention, available in English or Spanish, and explore such material as the Health Topics A-Z page.
3. Explore the Genetic Alliance for resources available regarding any particular genetic disease.
4. Access the American Academy of Allergy and Immunology website and explore such pages as the NAB report on pollen and mold.

CHAPTER 2

Developmental, Congenital, and Childhood Diseases and Disorders

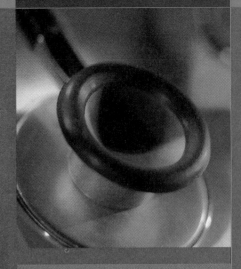

Chapter Outline—Cont'd

Learning Objectives

After studying Chapter 2, you should be able to:

1. List the possible causes of congenital anomalies.
2. Discuss the purpose and procedure of amniocentesis.
3. Trace fetal circulation.
4. Describe the condition of prematurity and associated disorders: the causes and the treatment.
5. Distinguish between muscular dystrophy and cerebral palsy.
6. Describe patent ductus arteriosus.
7. Name and describe the most common congenital cyanotic cardiac defect.
8. List the major clinical manifestations of cystic fibrosis.
9. Distinguish between Klinefelter syndrome and Turner syndrome.
10. Describe the clinical condition of congenital rubella syndrome.
11. Discuss the treatment of asthma.
12. List the symptoms and signs of anemia; describe the pathology of leukemia.
13. Explain the etiology of erythroblastosis fetalis.
14. Name some warning signs of lead poisoning.
15. Describe the infant born with fetal alcohol syndrome.

Key Terms

acetabulum (**ass**-eh-**TAB**-u-lum)
acyanotic (a-**sigh**-ah-**NOT**-ik)
adenosarcoma (**ad**-eh-no-sar-**KO**-mah)
amniocentesis (**am**-nee-o-sen-**TEE**-sis)
anencephalic (**an**-en-seh-**FAL**-ik)
ataxic (ah-**TACH**-sik)
azoospermia (azo-**SPIR**-me-a)

bicornate (bye-**KOR**-nate)
contracture (kon-**TRACK**-chur)
dysplasia (dis-**PLAY**-zee-ah)
dystrophy (**DIS**-troe-fee)
electromyography (e-**LECK**-tro-my-**og**-ra-fee)
foramen ovale (for-**A**-men o-**VAL**-a)
meconium (meh-**KOH**-nee-um)

Key Terms—Cont'd

meninges (men-**IN**-jeez)
neonates (**NEE**-o-nates)
pyelography (**pye**-eh-**LOH**-grah-fee)
pylorus (pye-**LOR**-us)

stenosis (ste-**NO**-sis)
syncope (**SIN**-koh-pee)
tachypnea (**tack**-ip-**NEE**-ah)
trisomy (**TRY**-so-me)

DEVELOPMENTAL AND CONGENITAL DISORDERS

DEVELOPMENTAL CHARACTERISTICS AND CONGENITAL ANOMALIES

Developmental Characteristics

The developmental process begins with conception and progresses as a gradual modification of the structure and characteristics of the individual (Fig. 2–1). The first 2 months of the gestational period is considered the embryonic period, after which the developing human being is considered a fetus. At any point in this prenatal development, during the birth process (perinatal period), or during the neonatal and postnatal periods, the development may diverge from normal, generating a developmental dilemma. Causes of these dilemmas can be many or even unknown. Pregnant women are encouraged to abstain from smoking, consuming alcohol, and taking any form of medication or drugs without their physician's knowledge and consent and to avoid any situation that may expose the developing fetus to toxic substances. Table 2–1 describes the specific stages of development during this important period of life.

Congenital Anomalies

Congenital anomalies can be mental or physical and can vary widely in severity, from trivial to fatal. They are present at birth but might not be detected until later in infancy or childhood. The limbs or organs may be malformed, duplicated, or entirely absent. Organs sometimes fail to move to their proper location or fail to open or close at the right time. Anomalies are seldom isolated and are likely to occur in multiple.

The cause of congenital defects may be genetic, nongenetic, or a combination of both. Nongenetic causes include infection in the mother, drugs taken by the mother, the age of the mother, radiographic examination made early in pregnancy, or injury to the pregnant woman or the fetus. The cause often is unknown. However, prenatal care and advanced surgical techniques have greatly improved the management of anomalies that are compatible with life.

Parents of a special-needs child face emotional and physical challenges and deserve medical attention. A team approach is ideal, including medical assessment by physicians and appropriate therapy for the child, and family involvement and participation in a support group for the parents.

Methods of Prenatal Diagnosis

One can diagnose congenital anomalies in a fetus by taking a fluid sample from the amniotic sac between the 15th and 18th weeks of pregnancy. This procedure, known as **amniocentesis,** allows amniotic fluid to be tested and cells to be microscopically examined for abnormal substances or chromosomal abnormalities. An example of an abnormal substance is an elevated alpha-fetoprotein (AFP) level. Amniocentesis is not without risk to mother and baby.

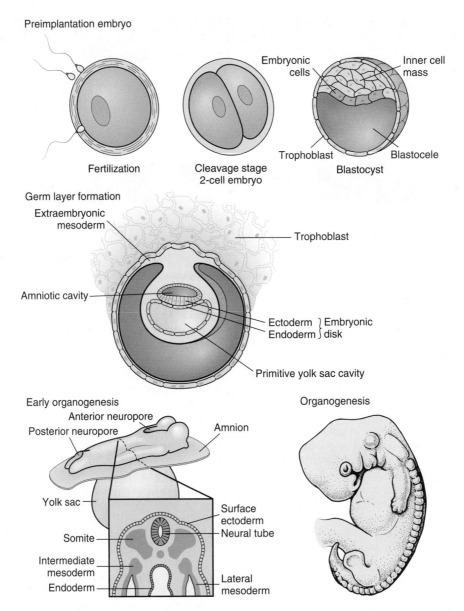

FIGURE 2–1 Normal prenatal development can be divided into several stages. (From Damjanov I: *Pathology for the health-related professions,* ed 2, Philadelphia, 2000, Saunders.)

Abnormalities of the spine and skull may be discovered during ultrasound studies of the fetus. An alternative procedure called chorionic villus biopsy (CVB) can be performed in the second month of pregnancy. The gynecologist, guided by ultrasound, directs an instrument toward the placenta in the womb and obtains a tissue sample. The safety of this procedure has not been proved, and some data link this test to limb abnormalities.

Many, but not all, congenital disorders can be detected (Fig. 2–2).

TABLE 2–1
Monthly Changes During Prenatal Development

END OF MONTH*	SIZE OF EMBRYO OR FETUS	DEVELOPMENTS DURING THE MONTH
1	6 mm	Arm and leg buds form; heart forms and starts beating; body systems begin to form
2	23-30 mm, 1 g	Head nearly as large as body; major brain regions present; ossification begins; arms and legs distinct; blood vessels form and cardiovascular system fully functional; liver large
3	75 mm, 10-45 g	Facial features present; nails develop on fingers and toes; can swallow and digest amniotic fluid; urine starts to form; fetus starts to move; heartbeat detected; external genitalia develop
4	140 mm, 60-200 g	Facial features well formed; hair appears on head; joints begin to form
5	190 mm, 250-450 g	Mother feels fetal movement; fetus covered with fine hair called lanugo hair; eyebrows visible; skin coated with vernix caseosa, a cheesy mixture of sebum and dead epidermal cells
6	220 mm, 500-800 g	Skin reddish because blood in the capillaries is visible; skin wrinkled because it lacks adipose in the subcutaneous tissue
7	260 mm, 900-1300 g	Eyes open; capable of survival but the mortality rate is high; scrotum develops; testes begin their descent
8	280-300 mm, 1400-2100 g	Testes descend into the scrotum; sense of taste is present
9	310-340 mm, 2200-2900 g	Reddish skin fades to pink; nails reach tips of fingers and toes or beyond
10	350-360 mm, 3000-3400 g	Skin smooth and plump because of adipose in subcutaneous tissue; lanugo hair shed; fetus usually turns to a head-down position; full term

*These are 4-week (28-day) months.
From Applegate EJ: *The anatomy and physiology learning system: Textbook*, Philadelphia, 2000, Saunders.

Prematurity

DESCRIPTION
Preterm birth or prematurity is the result of birth before the 37th gestational week of pregnancy. The condition of prematurity describes the birth of a low-weight, underdeveloped, and short-gestational infant and is considered the leading cause of death during the neonatal period. These high-risk infants are born with incomplete development of organ systems.

■ ICD-9-CM Code **765.00** *(Extreme immaturity)*
Usually implies a birth weight of less than 1000 grams. This code requires the additional code for weeks of gestation (765.20-765.29).

■ ICD-9-CM Code **765.10** *(Other preterm infants)*
Usually implies birth weight of 1000–2499 grams. This code requires the additional code for weeks of gestation (765.20-765.29).

Weeks of Gestation:
765.20 *(Unspecified weeks of gestation)*
765.21 *(Less than 24 completed weeks of gestation)*
765.22 *(24 completed weeks of gestation)*
765.23 *(25-26 completed weeks of gestation)*
765.24 *(27-28 completed weeks of gestation)*

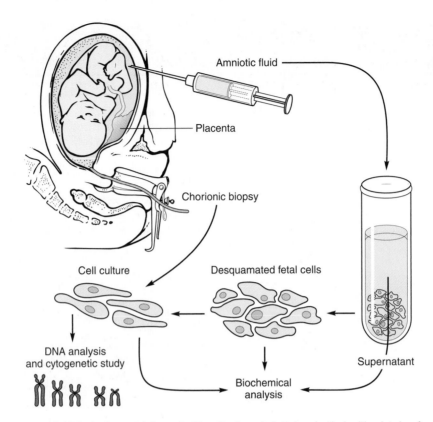

FIGURE 2–2 Methods of prenatal diagnosis. (From Damjanov I: *Pathology for the health-related professions,* ed 2, Philadelphia, 2000, Saunders.)

765.25 *(29-30 completed weeks of gestation)*
765.26 *(31-32 completed weeks of gestation)*
765.27 *(33-34 completed weeks of gestation)*
765.28 *(35-36 completed weeks of gestation)*
765.29 *(37 or more completed weeks of gestation)*

SYMPTOMS AND SIGNS

Premature babies may range in weight from 12 ounces to 5 pounds, 8 ounces. Their physical development is at various stages depending on the length of gestational time. The smaller of these infants has little subcutaneous fat, palms and soles with few creases, possible undescended testes in the male, and a prominent clitoris in the female.

Many of these very tiny and immature babies lack the ability to suck or swallow or have weakened sucking or swallowing reflexes. The lungs are often underdeveloped, leading to respiratory dangers. An immature immune system makes the risk of infection high.

PATIENT SCREENING

Pregnant patients who contact the physician to say they may be in labor require prompt attention. The pregnant patient who is more than three weeks before her due date and thinks she is in labor must be assessed as quickly as possible. Many physicians prefer that these patients go directly to the hospital at which they plan to deliver. Others prefer to see the patient in the office as soon as possible. When the patient arrives at the office, she should be placed in the examination room and the physician notified that she is in the office.

ENRICHMENT
CONJOINED TWINS

URING THE CONCEPTION PROCESS, the fertilized egg, the embryo, may divide, creating identical twins. Conjoined twins result when the separation process of identical twins fails to complete before the 13th day after fertilization (Fig. 2–3). As with identical twins, the embryo originates from a single fertilized ovum and occupies one placenta. For an unidentifiable reason, however, the normal separation of the embryo into twins stops before completion, resulting in a partially separated embryo that continues to mature into conjoined fetuses. Conjoined twins occur more often in female embryos than in male embryos and result in two fetuses who are joined at some point on their bodies. More of these children are being born alive as a result of specific prenatal diagnosis and surgical intervention to facilitate the delivery.

These children may be joined at different locations of the body and may share various organs. The attachment to each other may involve a small portion of tissue or may be as extensive as fusion at the head or sharing of an organ or body part. Common types or variations usually are categorized by the location and involvement of the junction through the term *pagus*, meaning fastened, included in the classification terminology.

Twins with a cranial union are considered to be craniopagus. Those with anterior junction at the chest, often sharing the heart and vital portions of the chest wall and internal organs, are called thoracopagus conjoined twins. The term *pygopagus* describes those twins who are joined posteriorly at the rump. Another posterior junction occurring at the sacrum and coccyx is termed *ischiopagus*. When the connection proceeds from the breastbone to the waist, the term *omphalopagus* describes the junction. A very rare form, dicephalus, is the condition in which the individual has one body and two separate heads and necks.

Modern technology and medical advances have recently helped physicians and surgical teams to successfully separate some of these twins. In some separation procedures, one or both of the children have died during or shortly after the surgery. The children and their families require emotional support and education about the possible outcomes of the condition.

ETIOLOGY

There are many reasons that these infants enter the world before reaching the traditionally accepted gestational age of 40 weeks and have very low birth weights. Causes of premature labor resulting in a premature infant are an *incompetent cervix,* **bicornate** uterus, toxic conditions, maternal infection, trauma, premature rupture of the amniotic membranes, multiple gestation, intrauterine fetal growth retardation, and other physical conditions of the mother, such as pregnancy-induced or chronic hypertension.

DIAGNOSIS

Diagnostic criteria include a gestational age of less than 37 weeks and a weight of less than 5 pounds, 8 ounces. **Neonates** diagnosed as small for gestational age (SGA) are not premature but are low-weight infants.

TREATMENT

Treatment varies depending on the gestational age, weight, present or subsequent conditions, anomalies,

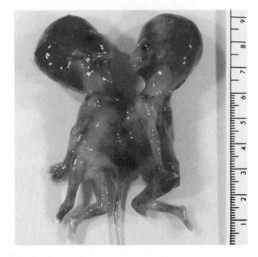

FIGURE 2–3 Conjoined twins at 12 weeks of development. (From Moore KL, Persaud TVN, Shiota K: *Color atlas of clinical embryology,* ed 2, Philadelphia, 2000, Saunders; courtesy Dr. DK Kalousek, Department of Pathology, University of British Columbia, Children's Hospital, Vancouver, British Columbia, Canada.)

Prematurity

and nutritional status. Intravenous (IV) fluids and *hyperalimentation* are necessary to encourage growth and development of the premature infant. Airway management and pulmonary functioning are monitored very closely. Many of the smallest babies are intubated endotracheally, and respiration is maintained by mechanical ventilation. Pulse oximeters constantly monitor oxygen (O_2) saturation levels and heart rate. Body temperature is monitored closely and maintained at normal levels (Fig. 2–4).

PROGNOSIS

Advances in technology have made survival of low-weight and short-gestation infants possible. The prognosis for these children varies depending on gestational age, weight, and the occurrence of anomalies and developmental deficits. There are documented cases of 12-ounce and/or 22-gestational-week babies surviving. They fall into the 1% of those born at that weight and gestational age. Being born before the normal prenatal development is complete, these children often have many problems to overcome (Fig. 2–5).

A primary risk is a cerebral bleed, which may occur during the labor and delivery process or may result from handling after delivery. The cerebral bleed may cause the development of cerebral palsy or mental functioning deficiencies.

Another major concern is underdevelopment of the pulmonary system, including the lung tissue and the airway. Some pulmonary conditions these infants experience are infant respiratory distress syndrome (IRDS), bronchopulmonary **dysplasia** (BPD), laryngomalacia, tracheomalacia, and bronchomalacia. Lack of body fat can affect the maintenance of body temperature. Underdevelopment of the central nervous system (CNS) and the circulatory system may result in hydrocephalus. Any stress or increased or high supplemental O_2 flow may be responsible for retinopathy of prematurity (ROP) and possible blindness. Necrotizing enterocolitis (NEC) is a danger in the digestive system because of the reduced tolerance of the alimentary tract. Atrial septal defect (ASD) and patent ductus arteriosus (PDA) often are present because the fetal circulatory system has failed to mature.

About 1% of those with extreme prematurity survive the birth process and the perinatal period. Improvements in technology are making it possible for more and more of these tiniest infants to survive (Fig. 2–6).

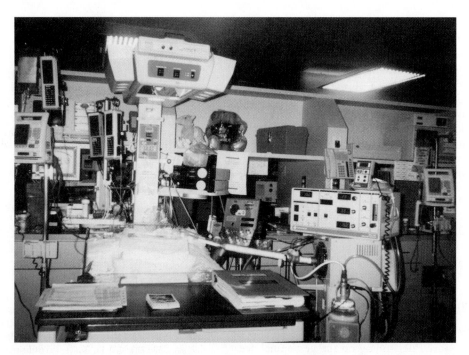

FIGURE 2–4 Technology in a neonatal intensive care unit. (Courtesy David L. Frazier, 1999.)

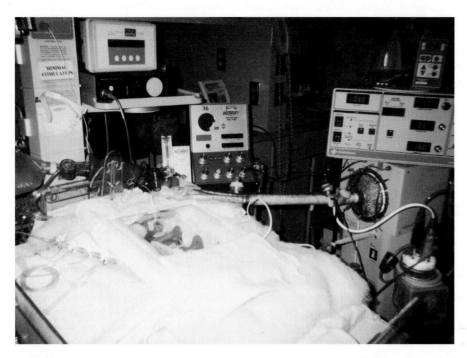

FIGURE 2–5 Four-day-old premature infant. Weight is 14.6 oz, and gestational age is 22 weeks. (Courtesy David L. Frazier, 1999.)

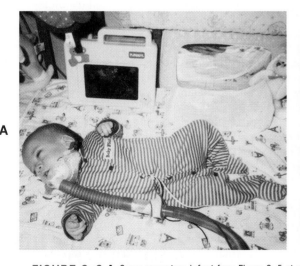

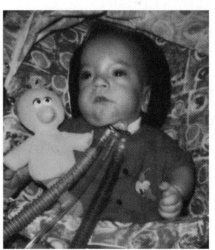

A

B

FIGURE 2–6 A, Same premature infant from Figure 2–5 at age 9 months, weight 11 lbs, 8 oz. **B,** Same infant at age 10 months, weight 13 lbs. (Courtesy David L. Frazier, 1999.)

PREVENTION

Preventing prematurity requires good prenatal care, adequate nutrition, and assessment of the pregnant patient's risk factors for premature labor. Abstaining from alcohol and cigarettes helps to reduce the risk of premature birth. Additionally, bed rest of the expectant mother may delay the onset of premature labor and create more time for the fetus to develop. Drug therapy may be used in an attempt to stop premature labor that results in premature birth. (Refer to Chapter 12, Premature Labor.)

PATIENT TEACHING

Encouraging pregnant women to obtain prenatal care and to follow guidelines is important. Pregnant women should be instructed to contact their physician at the first sign of labor, especially labor before the 37th week of gestation. Parents of premature infants will need emotional support and should be educated in the possibility of complications resulting from prematurity.

Infant Respiratory Distress Syndrome
DESCRIPTION

IRDS or hyaline membrane disease is similar to adult respiratory distress syndrome in that the patient suffers acute hypoxemia caused by infiltrates within the alveoli.

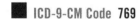 **ICD-9-CM Code 769**

SYMPTOMS AND SIGNS

Shortly after birth, the neonate exhibits signs of respiratory distress, including nasal flaring, grunting respirations, and sternal retractions. Blood gas studies indicate reduced oxygen tension and ineffective gas exchange. The infant becomes *cyanotic*, with mottled skin.

PATIENT SCREENING

The infant will be hospitalized, usually in a neonatal intensive care unit (NICU). The NICU staff observes the infant for signs of respiratory distress, and immediate intervention is instituted at the first signs of distress.

ETIOLOGY

The lungs of the neonate lack the *surfactant* needed to allow the alveoli to expand. The surfactant normally is produced relatively late in fetal life; consequently, premature infants are at risk. The outcome of this inability of the lungs to expand is inadequate surface area for proper gas exchange and a potentially fatal lack of oxygen in the blood.

DIAGNOSIS

The first indications of IRDS are increased respiratory efforts of the newborn and a history of prematurity. Blood gas studies demonstrate the reduced potential for adequate gas exchange. Radiographic chest films indicate the presence of the infiltrate or hyaline membrane.

TREATMENT

Treatment consists of the administration of carefully titrated supplemental oxygen, usually administered by mechanical ventilation and positive end-expiratory pressure (PEEP), and is of primary importance. Drug therapy, including the aerosol infusion of an exogenous surfactant such as beractant (Survanta) or colfosceril palmitate (Exosurf) into the pulmonary tree by an endotracheal tube as soon as possible after birth, helps to provide an artificial surfactant, allowing the alveoli to expand. This treatment should begin within the first 48 hours of life and continue until the alveoli are expanded.

PROGNOSIS

The prognosis for these infants' survival has improved greatly because of a better understanding of the condition and advanced technology in drug and respiratory therapy.

PREVENTION

Prevention is the best treatment; therefore, if time permits, the mother is injected with a corticosteroid (betamethasone [Celestone Soluspan]) 12 hours before delivery in an attempt to mature the surfactant-synthesizing system.

PATIENT TEACHING

Give the parents printed information about the disease. Parents will need emotional support and understanding. They should be referred to community support groups.

Unfortunately, the occurrence of IRDS, along with its treatment modalities, often predisposes premature infants to the development of bronchopulmonary dysplasia (BPD).

ENRICHMENT

LARYNGOMALACIA, TRACHEOMALACIA, AND BRONCHOMALACIA

LARYNGOMALACIA, TRACHEOMALACIA, AND bronchomalacia all are forms of airway obstructive conditions. They can evolve as separate entities or can develop in a combination of two or even all three conditions. Although most often observed in the infant or young child, these conditions may be found in adults. The primary cause in all conditions is softened or underdeveloped cartilage (malacia), allowing the airway structure or structures to partially or completely collapse and compromise the airway.

The infant with laryngomalacia exhibits respiratory stridor that is louder on inspiration. The infant with tracheomalacia also exhibits respiratory stridor; however, the stridor is more pronounced on expiration. All these congenital conditions cause infants to experience dyspnea and possibly episodes of cyanosis. Oxygen saturation levels decrease, and infants may experience bradycardia. Infants occasionally experience feeding difficulties. Diagnostic studies include chest radiographs, computed tomography (CT), and magnetic resonance imaging (MRI) scan; bronchoscopy; angiography; and echocardiography. Treatment is based on the underlying cause after it has been determined. Most of these children outgrow the disorders.

Bronchopulmonary Dysplasia

DESCRIPTION

BPD, a chronic lung disease, results after an insult to the neonate's lungs. This may be a sequela to IRDS, a lung infection, or extreme prematurity. The lungs are stiff, obstructed, and hard to ventilate.

 ICD-9-CM Code 770.7

SYMPTOMS AND SIGNS

The infant experiences periods of dyspnea, including **tachypnea,** wheezing, cyanosis, nasal flaring, and sternal retractions. O_2 saturation rates decrease, as does the heart rate. The infant may experience coughing and difficulty feeding. These babies appear to be working very hard to breathe. Wet or crackling sounds are heard on auscultation of the lungs with a stethoscope.

PATIENT SCREENING

The infant will be hospitalized, usually in an NICU. The NICU staff observes the infant for signs of respiratory distress, and immediate intervention is instituted at the first signs of distress.

ETIOLOGY

BPD occurs in many premature infants after IRDS, mechanical ventilation with supplemental oxygen, and infection or pneumonia. The pressure and oxygen needed to maintain life-sustaining oxygen levels can damage soft and fragile lung tissue, causing overinflation or scarring.

DIAGNOSIS

Observation of the infant reveals early respiratory distress. Radiographs of the chest are abnormal, indicating alveolar damage, either scarring or overinflation, sometimes described as a "ground glass" appearance. Arterial blood gases (ABGs) indicate a problem. Oxygen levels in the lungs may be low and carbon dioxide (CO_2) levels high.

TREATMENT

The goal of treatment is replacement of the damaged alveoli. Children grow new alveoli until about 8 years of age. Infants who have BPD need to grow new alveoli to replace those damaged by scarring. As this replacement occurs, the severity of the condition lessens. Supportive treatment includes supplemental oxygen and adequate nutritional support. The types of medications used include diuretics and bronchodilators, including beta$_2$-agonists, anticholinergic drugs, and theophylline. Antiinflammatory drugs such as steroids also may help.

Supplemental O_2 therapy may be needed for several weeks, occasionally for more than 1 year. This therapy usually is by nasal canula; however, if the infant has a tracheostomy, it may be delivered by a tracheostomy collar or by *continuous positive airway pressure (CPAP)*. O_2 saturation levels must be monitored with a pulse oximeter so they can be maintained at 90% or greater. The pulse oximeter also monitors heart rate. As the infant grows and matures, blood oxygen saturation levels may be maintained on room air, usually by the age of 1 year.

Diuretics help to reduce fluid accumulation in the lungs and reduce the incidence of pulmonary hypertension and right-sided heart failure. Bronchodilators are administered to reverse the narrowing of the bronchi resulting from inflammation or bronchospasm, thus allowing more oxygen to reach the lung tissue. These drugs may be administered orally as syrups or by aerosol inhalation. The antiinflammatory drugs help to prevent the inflammatory process from becoming severe.

Adequate nutrition is needed for the infant's growth and to meet the increased caloric demand resulting from difficult breathing. High-calorie formulas are fed to the infant. The infant must be held with the head raised slightly and the formula given frequently in small amounts to prevent gastroesophageal reflux disease (GERD). Some infants are given medications to prevent GERD and medications such as antacids or histamine-2 blockers to reduce gastric acid.

PROGNOSIS

Prognosis is good with early and aggressive intervention, prudent monitoring, and maintenance of adequate oxygen saturation levels and heart rate. Resolution of the condition is slow, and improvement is gradual. Complications include pulmonary edema and hypertension, right-sided heart failure (cor pulmonale), respiratory infections, apnea, tracheomalacia, asthma, and gastrointestinal (GI) reflux and aspiration. These children are particularly susceptible to respiratory infections such as pneumonias, including respiratory syncytial virus (RSV), and they may experience poor growth or delayed development. Many of these children outgrow the condition, but others may be susceptible to respiratory distress for life. Apneic periods and low oxygen saturation levels for an extended period of time may cause hypoxia to the brain, which may result in developmental deficits. Some infants may not survive.

PREVENTION

There is currently no way to prevent BPD; however, early weaning from mechanical respiratory support may reduce its incidence. Early and aggressive intervention and treatment may prevent complications and permanent conditions, even death.

PATIENT TEACHING

Help parents find community support groups and agencies to assist with emotional and financial stressors. The parents should receive emotional support because this condition usually requires prolonged or frequent hospitalizations. Encouraging parents to become as involved as possible in the care of their infant helps them to become familiar with the infant's health-care needs and bond with the infant.

Retinopathy of Prematurity

DESCRIPTION

ROP, or retrolental fibroplasia, is an abnormal growth of the blood vessels in the retinas of the infant's eyes. The condition occurs in the eyes of premature infants.

 ICD-9-CM Code 362.21

SYMPTOMS AND SIGNS

ROP occurs in infants born before 28 weeks of gestation. There are no visible symptoms. Screening examinations are performed routinely on premature infants weighing less than 1500 g with a gestational age of less than 31 weeks. The entire retina is visualized to determine the stages of development of the blood vessels supplying it. These examinations first are performed when the infant is 4 to 6 weeks old (Fig. 2-7).

PATIENT SCREENING

The infant will be hospitalized, usually in an NICU. An ophthalmologist performs routine examinations of the retina. If the infant has been dismissed from the hospital and later exhibits signs of complications, an immediate appointment or examination should be arranged.

ETIOLOGY

The vascularization of the retina begins at the back central part of the eye, as vessels grow out toward the edges. The blood vessels to the retina do not begin development until about the 28th week of gestation. In premature infants, this vascularization

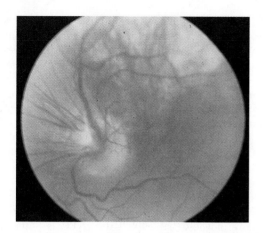

FIGURE 2-7 Retrolental fibroplasias. (From Zitelli BJ, Davis HW: *Atlas of pediatric physical diagnosis,* ed 4, St. Louis, 2002, Mosby.)

is incomplete. Regardless of gestational age at birth, most ROP originates at 34 to 40 weeks after conception.

No specific risk factors for the development of ROP have been identified. However, there is a group of risk factors that contribute to it. The more premature and the lower the birth weight of the infant, the greater is the risk of developing ROP. High supplemental oxygen concentrations are responsible for many incidents of ROP. However, close monitoring of oxygen saturation levels and appropriate adjustment and titration of oxygen concentration levels to the infant reduces the risk. Certain drugs, such as surfactant and indomethacin, administered to the neonate for treatment of immature lungs and PDA may increase the risk for the premature infant. Recently, intense artificial lighting in the nursery or crib has been considered a risk factor. Other risk factors cited include seizures, mechanical ventilation, anemia, blood transfusions, and multiple spells of apnea and bradycardia.

DIAGNOSIS

Diagnosis is made by an ophthalmologist using an indirect ophthalmoscope and scleral depression to visualize the retina. The lens and iris also are examined at this time.

TREATMENT

Most mild forms of ROP resolve without treatment. Laser treatment to the area anterior to the vascular shunt eliminates abnormal vessels before they deposit enough scar tissue to cause retinal detachment. Severe cases may require other procedures. Occasionally, the damage is so severe that blindness results.

PROGNOSIS

As previously mentioned, mild forms of this condition may resolve by themselves. Laser surgery may be required in more serious cases. Blindness may result from serious damage. ROP that has resolved can have later complications. These include crossed or wandering eyes (strabismus), "lazy eye" (amblyopia), nearsightedness (myopia), glaucoma, and late-onset retinal detachment. Many of these children may require corrective glasses.

PREVENTION

There is no way to prevent ROP in the premature infant. Close monitoring and titration of oxygen concentrations have reduced the incidence of the condition. NICUs now protect premature infants' eyes from excessive exposure to artificial lighting. Attempts are made to avoid exposing premature infants to stress factors. Screening examinations, staging (determining extent of vascular damage), and appropriate intervention help to reduce the severity of the condition and prevent blindness.

PATIENT TEACHING

Parents should be told of the risk for this condition in the premature infant. Give them printed material about the condition and help them to contact support groups in the community.

Necrotizing Enterocolitis

DESCRIPTION

Necrotizing enterocolitis (NEC) is an acute inflammatory process caused by ischemic necrosis of the mucosal lining of the small intestine, large intestine, or both. It is a condition of premature infants or sick neonates that develops after birth, when the fragile intestinal tract of the premature or compromised newborn becomes active.

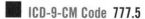 **ICD-9-CM Code 777.5**

SYMPTOMS AND SIGNS

Feeding intolerance, abdominal distention, bile-colored emesis, diarrhea, blood in the stool, decreased or absent bowels sounds, lethargy, and body temperature instability a few days after birth are some of the initial symptoms exhibited by the preterm or low-weight infant. The state of well-being degrades as these infants experience respiratory problems to brief apneic periods, reduced urine output, hyperbilirubinemia, and erythema. The abdomen is tender to palpation.

PATIENT SCREENING

The infant will be hospitalized, usually in an NICU. The NICU staff observes the infant for signs of NEC, and the neonatologist is notified and immediate intervention are instituted at first signs of distress.

ETIOLOGY

The etiology of NEC is unknown; however, it is thought to be a breakdown in normal defense systems of the GI tract, allowing the *normal flora* of the GI tract to invade the intestinal mucosa. This can happen when blood is shunted away from the GI tract, resulting in convulsive vasoconstriction of the mesenteric vessels and diminished blood supply, interfering with the normal production of protective mucus.

In addition to prematurity, factors that may predispose infants to NEC include hypovolemia, sepsis, umbilical catheters, exchange transfusions, and IRDS. Another factor is oral feeding of high-calorie concentrated formula.

DIAGNOSIS

Observation of changes in the infant's feeding patterns or activity level, impaired body temperature maintenance, and respiratory difficulties, along with abdominal distention and tenderness, calls for further investigation. Complete blood count (CBC) indicates an elevated *white blood cell (WBC) count,* and guaiac test results of stool specimens for occult blood are positive. Blood and stool cultures are performed and may confirm the presence of bacteria. Radiographs of the intestine confirm the condition.

TREATMENT

Aggressive and immediate intervention is necessary if the infant is to survive. Feedings are stopped, making the infant's status NPO (nothing by mouth). A small tube is inserted into the stomach by way of the nose or mouth for decompression. Fluids are administered intravenously, as are antibiotics. Respiratory status and pH are monitored by

ABGs. The infant's weight, intake, and output are monitored closely, and fluid and electrolyte balance is maintained. Abdominal distention is monitored through frequent measurements of the abdomen by a tape measure. Radiographic monitoring of the intestinal tract also is performed. Complications of intestinal perforation or peritonitis require surgical intervention with removal of the necrotic tissue. When necrosis is extensive, ileostomy or colostomy may be necessary until the infant grows, and closure with *anastomosis* can be performed.

PROGNOSIS

Without immediate and aggressive intervention, many of these babies will die. NEC is a serious complication of prematurity, and some babies die even with aggressive treatment. Resection of a portion of the bowel can lead to an obstruction of the bowel or to malabsorption syndrome. Perforation can lead to sepsis and death.

PREVENTION

Most of these babies are still in the hospital when NEC develops. Prudent nursing observations and reporting of any symptoms of NEC are essential. Because the infection can be spread from infant to infant, meticulous hand-washing techniques must be followed. Breast milk appears to offer some immunity to this condition. An awareness of the high-risk infant is fundamental in the prevention and early intervention of this disease.

PATIENT TEACHING

Parents will require emotional support along with information about the condition. Meticulous hand-washing techniques should be reviewed, and the dangers of infection should be explained.

Diseases of the Nervous System

Cerebral Palsy

DESCRIPTION

Cerebral palsy (CP), the most common crippler of children, is a congenital, bilateral, nonprogressive paralysis that results from damage to the central nervous system (CNS).

■ **ICD-9-CM Code 343.9** *(Infantile cerebral palsy, unspecified)*
Infantile CP is coded by type. Refer to the physician's diagnosis and then to the current edition of the ICD-9-CM coding manual to ensure the greatest specificity of pathology and any appropriate modifiers.

SYMPTOMS AND SIGNS

This syndrome affects primarily motor performance and might be noticed shortly after birth, when the infant has difficulty with sucking or swallowing. The muscles may be floppy or stiff, with reduced voluntary movement. When the infant is lifted from behind, the legs may be difficult to separate and the infant may cross his or her legs. There are three major types of CP:

Spastic cerebral palsy is characterized by hyperactive reflexes or rapid muscle contractions. The older child manifests the scissor gait by walking on the toes and crossing one foot over the other. Approximately 70% of patients with CP fall into this category.

Athetoid cerebral palsy is characterized by involuntary muscle movements, especially during times of stress, and reduced muscle tone. The child has difficulty with speech. About 20% of cases of CP fall into this category.

Ataxic cerebral palsy is characterized by lack of control over voluntary movements, poor balance, and a wide gait.

A patient may exhibit signs of all three types in varying degrees from mild to severe. The symptoms tend to be more exaggerated as the child grows; however, they may be static (i.e., they neither get worse nor improve). Some patients have other related complications, including visual and auditory deficits, seizure activity, and mental retardation.

PATIENT SCREENING

Most times CP is suspected during routine well-baby or well-child visits. However, when a parent calls the office about previously mentioned symptoms, the child should be scheduled for an evaluation as soon as possible. The condition usually is not life-threatening; nevertheless, the parent's anxiety is high, and it may appear as an emergency to the parent.

ETIOLOGY

CP usually stems from inadequate blood or oxygen supply to the brain during fetal development, during the birth process, or in early childhood until about 9 years of age. The syndrome is more common in premature infants and in male babies. Most insults to the brain result from an interruption in the circulation of blood to the brain during labor and delivery or from infection or head trauma during the first month of life. It often is impossible to determine the exact cause of CP.

DIAGNOSIS

Diagnosis is made from the clinical picture and neurologic examination findings. The child is examined to determine the degree of physical and mental impairment.

TREATMENT

There is no cure for CP. In mild or severe cases, the goal of treatment is to minimize the handicap by providing every possible therapeutic measure to help the child reach his or her potential. This takes a team effort involving the family or caretaker and various medical specialists. Physical therapy, speech therapy, and special education may be required. Orthopedic intervention with casts, braces, and traction or surgery may be indicated. If the child experiences seizure activity, anticonvulsant agents are prescribed. Muscle relaxants help to reduce spastic muscle activity.

PROGNOSIS

The brain damage cannot be reversed; therefore there is no cure for cerebral palsy. Supportive treatment is important and is intended to provide the child with the best quality of life obtainable.

PREVENTION

Measures to prevent oxygen deprivation in the developing brain during the prenatal, perinatal, and neonatal periods are essential. Additional steps to prevent head injury or brain infection during these periods of cerebral development are important.

PATIENT TEACHING

Encourage and help parents to contact community support groups. Reinforce the fact that there is no cure for CP and that parents should take advantage of support services available in the community. When possible, assist parents by giving them the names of agencies that provide services to children with CP and their families.

Muscular Dystrophy

DESCRIPTION

Muscular **dystrophy** (MD) is a progressive degeneration and weakening of the skeletal muscles. There are several types of the disease, but all are rare. The most common and best-known type is Duchenne MD, which begins soon after birth or during early childhood, usually before the age of 5 years.

■ **ICD-9-CM Code 359.1** *(Hereditary progressive muscular dystrophy)*
MD is coded by type. Refer to the physician's diagnosis and then to the current edition of the ICD-9-CM coding manual to ensure the greatest specificity of pathology and any appropriate modifiers.

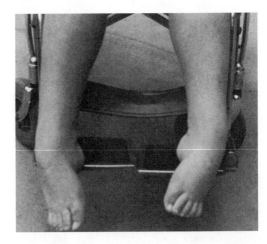

FIGURE 2–8 Contracture of the feet in a patient with muscular dystrophy. (From Jahss MH: *Disorders of the foot and ankle,* vol 1, ed 2, Philadelphia, 1991, Saunders.)

SYMPTOMS AND SIGNS

MD initially affects the muscles of the shoulders, the hips, and the thighs and calves of the legs, causing the characteristic waddling gait and toe walking. Affected muscles sometimes look larger than normal because fat replaces atrophied muscle. The child also may have lordosis or other spinal deformities. In addition, the child has difficulty climbing stairs and running, tends to fall easily, and has difficulty getting up. As the disease progresses, it involves all the muscles, causing crippling and immobility (Fig. 2–8). **Contractures** typically develop, and the child becomes increasingly susceptible to serious pulmonary infections such as pneumonia. Children with Duchenne MD also often are impaired mentally.

PATIENT SCREENING

MD usually is first suspected during routine well-baby or well-child visits. However, when a parent calls the office about previously mentioned symptoms, the child should be scheduled for an evaluation as soon as possible. The condition usually is not life-threatening; nevertheless, the parent's anxiety is high, and it may appear as an emergency to the parent.

ETIOLOGY

Duchenne MD is the result of a genetic defect. As is the case for hemophilia and color blindness, the disease affects only males and generally is inherited through female carriers. In one third to one half of cases, there is no family history of MD. This means that the disease may be caused by a newly acquired mutation.

DIAGNOSIS

Characteristic symptoms along with family history of MD suggest the diagnosis. Muscle biopsy and **electromyography (EMG)** confirm the diagnosis. Also, an elevated serum creatine kinase (CK) level is evident in the blood.

TREATMENT

There is no known successful treatment for Duchenne MD. Physical therapy, exercise, surgery, and the use of orthopedic appliances can minimize deformities and preserve mobility.

PROGNOSIS

The prognosis for a child with Duchenne MD is poor. The child usually is confined to a wheelchair by the age of 9 to 12 years. Death usually results from cardiac or respiratory complications within 10 to 15 years of the onset of the disease.

PREVENTION

MD is genetic, and therefore prevention is unlikely.

PATIENT TEACHING

With no cure for MD at present, parents will need emotional support. Help them contact support

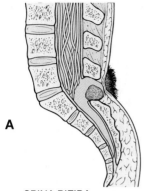
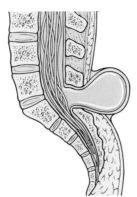
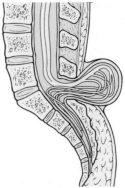

SPINA BIFIDA
Posterior vertebral arches have not fused; there is no herniation of the spinal cord or meninges

MENINGOCELE
External protruding sac contains meninges and CSF

MYELOMENINGOCELE
External sac contains meninges, CSF, and the spinal cord

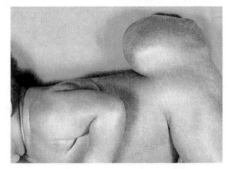

FIGURE 2–9 A, Congenital spinal cord defects. **B,** Myelomeningocele. *CSF,* Cerebrospinal fluid. (**B** from Zitelli BJ, Davis HW: *Atlas of pediatric physical diagnosis,* ed 2, St. Louis, 1992, Mosby.)

groups and services for MD patients and their families. Offer families educational material on the supportive treatment and care of the child with MD.

Spina Bifida

DESCRIPTION

Spina bifida is a group of malformations of the spine in which the posterior portion of the bony canal containing the spinal cord (usually in the lumbar region) is completely or partially absent (Fig. 2–9, *A*). Also called neural tube deficits, the three different levels of the condition originate during early weeks of gestation as the spinal cord and bony canal develop. During this developmental stage, there is a failure of the posterior spinal processes to close, usually in the lumbar region. This failure of complete closure allows the **meninges** and, in severe cases, the spinal cord to herniate. Depending on the extent of the herniation and the amount of the neural tube that has herniated, various degrees of

neural deficits or impairment occur. The three types of spina bifida are spinal bifida occulta, meningocele, and myelomeningocele.

Spina Bifida Occulta

DESCRIPTION

In the defect called spinal bifida occulta, the posterior arches of the vertebrae, commonly in the lumbosacral area, fail to fuse, but there is no herniation of meninges or spinal cord. Usually there is no spinal cord or spinal nerve involvement.

■ **ICD-9-CM Code** **756.17** *(Spina bifida occulta)*
741.90 *(Spina bifida without mention of hydrocephalus)*
Spina bifida is coded according to involvement of hydrocephalus and region affected. Refer to the physician's diagnosis and then to the current edition of the ICD-9-CM coding manual to ensure the greatest specificity of pathology and any appropriate modifiers.

SYMPTOMS AND SIGNS

When this malformation occurs without displacement of the cord or the meninges, spina bifida occulta is asymptomatic. At other times, the only evidence of the neural tube defect is a dimpling, a tuft of hair, or a hemangioma over the site where the vertebrae have not completely fused.

PATIENT SCREENING

Most cases are discovered during the newborn examination. Parents requesting an appointment to discuss the condition should be scheduled as soon as possible. It is important to remember the amount of anxiety the parents may experience.

ETIOLOGY

The etiology of this congenital anomaly is unknown, but it has been associated with exposure to ionizing radiation during early uterine life. A recent theory considers the possibility of a metabolic abnormality in which reduced levels of vitamin A and folic acid may contribute to the incidence of spina bifida. The condition occurs when the neural tube fails to close in the early stages of fetal development, possibly as a result of such a metabolic imbalance.

DIAGNOSIS

Maternal blood levels of AFP may be measured to detect possible neural tube defects. Diagnosis is made by prenatal ultrasonography or by postnatal physical examination, detection of neurologic symptoms, visual inspection of the spine, and radiographic studies. If the infant is asymptomatic, the condition may not be discovered unless it is sought.

TREATMENT

Spina bifida occulta usually requires no intervention other than prudent observation throughout the child's growth and development. Treatment depends on the degree of neurologic involvement. If the child becomes symptomatic with neurologic problems, surgical intervention to repair the deficit is necessary.

PROGNOSIS

The prognosis is good for children with spina bifida occulta.

PREVENTION

Because the etiology of this condition is unknown, methods of prevention are also unknown. However, avoiding exposure to ionizing radiation during pregnancy is a wise precaution and significant in the prevention of this disorder. Increased intake of folic acid is encouraged in females planning to become pregnant and during early stages of pregnancy. Because many pregnancies are unplanned, all females of child-bearing age capable of becoming pregnant are encouraged to take the recommended amount of folic acid each day.

PATIENT TEACHING

The value of regular observation during the growth and development period should be emphasized to both the child and the parent. In addition, the parents and child should be urged to watch for neurologic symptoms and report symptoms.

Meningocele

DESCRIPTION

The second level of failure of the spinal column to fuse during the developmental stage is meningocele. The meninges protrude through an opening in the spinal column, thus forming a sac that becomes filled with cerebrospinal fluid (CSF) (see Fig. 2–9, *B*).

 ICD-9-CM Code 741.90 *(Meningocele without mention of hydrocephalus)*
Meningocele is coded according to the region affected. Refer to the physician's diagnosis and then to the current edition of the ICD-9-CM coding manual to ensure the greatest specificity of pathology and any appropriate modifiers.

SYMPTOMS AND SIGNS

There is no nerve involvement; therefore the infant usually has no neurologic problems. The sac formed over the deficit will permit the passage of light during transillumination, indicating no spinal cord or neurologic involvement. The skin over the area may be fragile, and rupture of the sac is a potential problem.

PATIENT SCREENING

Most cases are discovered during the newborn examination. Parents requesting an appointment to discuss the condition should be scheduled as soon as possible. It is important to remember the anxiety parents may be experiencing. As the child grows and matures, the parents may detect the onset of neurologic symptoms. When this happens, the child requires immediate assessment.

ETIOLOGY

As in spina bifida occulta, the posterior portion of the neural tube fails to close. The exact cause is not known. However, genetic and environmental factors may play a role. Recent postulation considers the possibility of a metabolic abnormality in which reduced levels of vitamin A and folic acid may contribute to the incidence of spina bifida.

DIAGNOSIS

Diagnosis is made by visual examination of the spinal area and verification of the presence of a sac. Radiographic studies of the spine confirm the clinical findings. The infant is assessed for hydrocephalus, which often is associated with neural tube defects.

TREATMENT

Treatment usually consists of surgical intervention to correct the deficit in the first 24 to 48 hours of life. Because the spinal cord is not involved, paralysis usually does not occur. These children require prudent follow-up and usually develop normally.

PROGNOSIS

With early surgical intervention, the outlook for these children is good.

PREVENTION

Because the etiology of this condition is unknown, methods of prevention are also unknown. However, avoiding exposure to ionizing radiation during pregnancy is a wise precaution and significant in the prevention of this disorder. Increased intake of folic acid is encouraged for females planning to become pregnant and during early stages of pregnancy. Because many pregnancies are unplanned, all females of child-bearing age capable of becoming pregnant are encouraged to take the recommended amount of folic acid each day.

PATIENT TEACHING

The value of regular observation during the growth and development period should be emphasized to both the child and the parents. In addition, the parents and child should be urged to watch for neurologic symptoms and report symptoms.

Myelomeningocele
DESCRIPTION

Myelomeningocele (also known as spina bifida cystica) is a protrusion of a portion of the spinal cord

and the meninges through a defect in the spinal column, usually in the lumbar region (see Fig. 2–9, *A* and *B*).

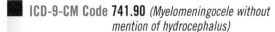

ICD-9-CM Code 741.90 *(Myelomeningocele without mention of hydrocephalus)*
Myelomeningocele is coded according to the region affected. Refer to the physician's diagnosis and then to the current edition of the ICD-9-CM coding manual to ensure the greatest specificity of pathology and any appropriate modifiers.

SYMPTOMS AND SIGNS

Myelomeningocele is the most severe form of spina bifida. Because spinal nerves or the spinal cord are present in this herniation, the infant exhibits neurologic symptoms. The infant may have musculoskeletal malformation, immobile joints, or paralysis of the lower extremities. Depending on the level of the anomaly, bowel or bladder control may be affected.

PATIENT SCREENING

This condition will be apparent during the newborn examination. Parents requesting an appointment to discuss the condition should be scheduled as soon as possible. It is important to remember the amount of anxiety the parents may be experiencing. As the child grows and matures, the parents may detect the onset of increased neurologic symptoms. When this happens, the child requires immediate assessment.

ETIOLOGY

As in spina bifida occulta and meningocele, the neural tube fails to close during fetal development. This allows the meninges, spinal nerves, and spinal cord to herniate through the opening of the posterior aspect of the spinal column. The etiology may include genetic factors; spinal cord defects are more common when prior offspring of the mother have had a similar defect.

DIAGNOSIS

Diagnosis is made by physical examination and imaging. Electromyography is used to determine the extent of neurologic involvement. Surgical exploration verifies the severity of the disorder.

TREATMENT

Treatment is surgical intervention, usually within the first 24 hours of life, to prevent further deterioration of the involved nerves, infection, and rupture of the herniation. As the child grows, additional procedures may be required to correct evolving problems. Children with myelomeningocele may have other anomalies, including hydrocephalus. Many of these children have no bowel or bladder control and may never be able to walk. A large number of these children die before the age of 2 years.

PROGNOSIS
Nerve damage is irreversible. Surgical intervention in early life may halt the progression of any paralysis. Physical therapy, including leg braces, crutches, and ambulation training, help to increase the child's mobility. Bladder and bowel problems will not improve, and the child and family must be trained to deal with them.

PREVENTION
As with other spina bifida conditions, the etiology of this condition is unknown, as are methods of prevention. However, avoiding exposure to ionizing radiation during pregnancy is a wise precaution and significant in the possible prevention of this disorder. Increased intake of folic acid is encouraged for females planning to become pregnant and during early stages of pregnancy. Because many pregnancies are unplanned, all females of child-bearing age capable of becoming pregnant are encouraged to take the recommended amount of folic acid each day.

PATIENT TEACHING
Parents are told that nerve damage is irreversible. Parents should be given information about spina bifida along with help in locating and contacting support groups. Females of child-bearing age who are capable of becoming pregnant are advised to take the daily recommendation of folic acid.

The value of regular observation during the growth and development period should be emphasized to both the child and the parents. In addition, the parents and child should be urged to watch for neurologic symptoms and report symptoms.

Hydrocephalus

DESCRIPTION
In hydrocephalus, the amount of CSF is increased greatly or its circulation is blocked, resulting in an abnormal enlargement of the head and characteristic pressure changes in the brain.

> ■ **ICD-9-CM Code** **741.0** *(With spina bifida only)*
> **331.3** *(Communicating)*
> **331.4** *(Obstructive)*

SYMPTOMS AND SIGNS
The fontanelles begin to bulge, the sutures of the skull separate, and scalp veins become distended. The infant has a high-pitched cry, is irritable, and may have episodes of projectile vomiting. Eventually, there is a downward displacement of the eyes. Neurologic signs include abnormal muscle tone of the legs.

PATIENT SCREENING
Many cases of hydrocephalus are apparent during the newborn examination, while others may be detected during well-baby examinations. Parents requesting an appointment to discuss the condition will have great anxiety and should be scheduled as soon as possible. When a parent contacts the office with concern about the child's head appearing to be unusually large, the child requires prompt assessment. The same policy should apply to parents contacting the office with concerns about possible neurologic signs.

ETIOLOGY
In hydrocephalus, a large amount of CSF accumulates in the skull, causing increased intracranial pressure. An impairment of the circulation of the CSF in the ventricular circulation (obstructive hydrocephalus) may be caused by a lesion within the system or by a congenital structural defect. An impairment of the flow of the CSF in the subarachnoid space (communicating hydrocephalus) prevents the CSF from reaching the areas where it normally would be reabsorbed by the arachnoid villi. This may be the result of intracranial hemorrhage resulting from head trauma, a blood clot, prematurity, or infection (meningitis) (Figs. 2–10 and 2–11).

DIAGNOSIS
Diagnosis is made through the clinical picture, physical examination, and radiographic skull studies. CT and MRI scans demonstrate the condition.

TREATMENT
Treatment consists of surgical intervention to place a shunt in the ventricular or subarachnoid spaces

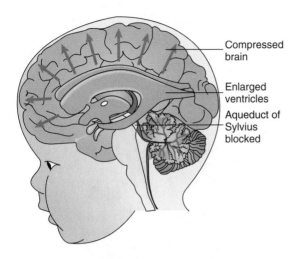

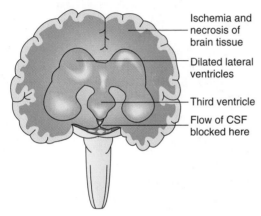

- Compressed brain
- Enlarged ventricles
- Aqueduct of Sylvius blocked

- Ischemia and necrosis of brain tissue
- Dilated lateral ventricles
- Third ventricle
- Flow of CSF blocked here

FIGURE 2–10 Hydrocephalus. (From Gould BE: *Pathophysiology for the health professions,* ed 2, Philadelphia, 2002, Saunders.)

to drain off the excessive CSF. Some catheters empty into the peritoneal cavity, and other shunt catheters empty into the right atrium of the heart (Fig. 2–12). One-way valves help to shunt the excessive CSF away from the cerebrospinal canal and to maintain a normal pressure. If left untreated, the increasing intracranial pressure of hydrocephalus causes mental retardation and eventually death (see Fig. 2–10).

PROGNOSIS

The prognosis for these children varies depending on the extent of the condition as well as the success of corrective interventions. Most children can function normally in society. Parents and the child must

watch for the onset of neurologic symptoms and seek medical assessment and treatment.

PREVENTION

There is no known prevention for the congenital form of this disorder. Good prenatal care along with prudent observation and assistance during labor and delivery help to prevent damage to the brain. Preventing infections and injury to the head during childhood, although challenging, may prevent some incidences.

PATIENT TEACHING

Parents and the child should be taught to recognize signs of malfunctioning shunts. In addition, they should be told the importance of promptly reporting any neurologic signs or symptoms to the physician.

Anencephaly

DESCRIPTION

This most severe form of neural tube deficit occurs early in gestation with failure of the cephalic aspect of the neural tube to close.

■ **ICD-9-CM Code 740.0**

SYMPTOMS AND SIGNS

The **anencephalic** fetus or neonate has no cranial vault and little cerebral tissue. Bones of the base of the skull and the orbits are present (Fig. 2–13). The microcephalic fetus or neonate has very small amounts of cerebral tissue and may survive a few hours or days. Although most of these infants die before birth or during the birth process, a few survive for a short time.

PATIENT SCREENING

This anomaly may be found during prenatal ultrasound. The mother or parents should be scheduled for an office visit at which the physician discusses the findings of the ultrasound. When the anomaly is not apparent until birth, the infant usually is stillborn or dies shortly after birth. This event produces great anxiety, and parents may request an appointment for additional information. An appointment should be scheduled promptly.

ETIOLOGY

The etiology is essentially unknown, but this anomaly is characterized by failure of the neural tube at the cephalic (cranial) end to close completely during

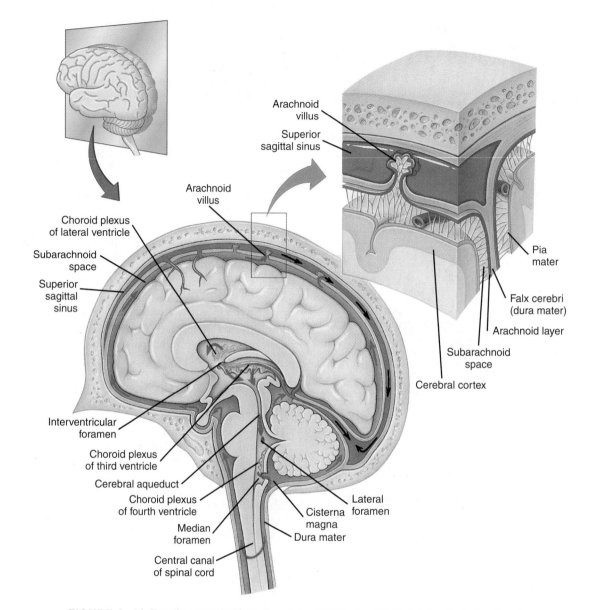

Arachnoid
villus

Superior
sagittal sinus

Arachnoid
villus

Choroid plexus
of lateral ventricle

Subarachnoid
space

Superior
sagittal
sinus

Pia
mater

Falx cerebri
(dura mater)

Arachnoid layer

Subarachnoid
space

Cerebral cortex

Interventricular
foramen

Choroid plexus
of third ventricle

Cerebral aqueduct

Choroid plexus
of fourth ventricle

Lateral
foramen

Cisterna
magna

Dura mater

Median
foramen

Central canal
of spinal cord

FIGURE 2–11 Flow of cerebrospinal fluid. (From Patton KT, Thibodeau GA: *Mosby's handbook of anatomy & physiology*, St. Louis, 2000, Mosby.)

the second or third week of prenatal development. The occurrence of this defect tends to be familial; females are affected more often than males.

DIAGNOSIS
Diagnosis is made by ultrasonographic examination of the fetal head when blood tests of the mother indicate an elevated AFP level. The ultra-sonogram shows symmetric absence of normal cranial bone structure and brain tissue.

TREATMENT
There is no effective treatment of this anomaly. Infants who survive the birth process die shortly afterward because many have several other neural tube anomalies incompatible with life.

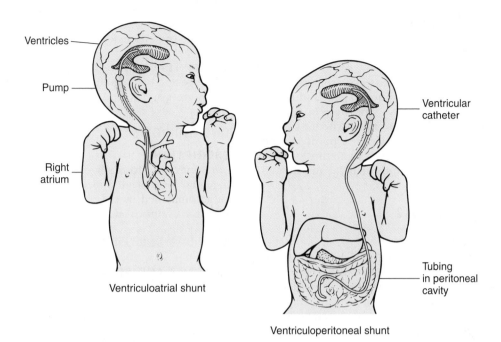

Ventricles

Pump

Right atrium

Ventriculoatrial shunt

Ventricular catheter

Tubing in peritoneal cavity

Ventriculoperitoneal shunt

FIGURE 2–12 Shunting procedures for hydrocephalus. Ventriculoperitoneal shunt is the preferred procedure.

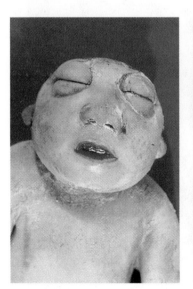 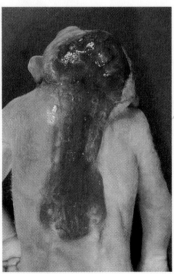

FIGURE 2–13 Anencephaly. (From Damjanov I: *Pathology for the health-related professions,* ed 2, Philadelphia, 2000, Saunders.)

PROGNOSIS

These fetuses or neonates lack sufficient cerebral tissue to sustain life.

PREVENTION

As with other neural tube deficits, the etiology is unclear. All females of child-bearing age and capability are urged to avoid radiation exposure and take the recommended amount of folic acid daily.

PATIENT TEACHING

Patient teaching includes answering the parents' questions. Encourage and help parents to learn about appropriate community resources.

Cri-du-Chat Syndrome (Cat's Cry Syndrome)

DESCRIPTION

The deletion of genetic material from chromosome 5 results in the condition called cri-du-chat. A rare disorder, "cat's cry" syndrome usually results in stillborn children or those who die shortly after birth. Those who survive the perinatal and neonatal periods may progress to maturity. These individuals will have various medical and mental problems.

■ **ICD-9-CM Code** **758.3**

SYMPTOMS AND SIGNS

Infants with cri-du-chat syndrome have an abnormally small head (microcephaly), with a deficiency of cerebral brain tissue, and mental retardation. Those who are born alive have a weak, mewing, catlike cry. The orbits of the eyes are spaced far apart. Surviving children will experience slow growth patterns, a small head, and poor muscle tone. Motor and language skills development may be delayed. Mental development may be slow and retarded, and behavioral problems may develop.

ETIOLOGY

Cri-du-chat syndrome, a hereditary condition, is the result of a chromosomal aberration caused by deletion of part of the short arm of chromosome 5 of the B group.

DIAGNOSIS

Diagnosis is made by the clinical picture of microcephaly and the characteristic catlike cry of the infant. The diagnosis is confirmed by a genetic study indicating the chromosomal defect.

TREATMENT

There is no cure, so treatment supports body functions until the infant dies. Many fetuses with this chromosomal aberration die in utero. Those infants who survive and progress into childhood will need special schooling and supportive care. These individuals can possibly experience a normal life span.

PROGNOSIS

There is no cure for this condition. With supportive treatment and special schooling, surviving individuals may possibly experience a normal life span.

PREVENTION

There is no prevention for this hereditary condition.

PATIENT TEACHING

Encourage and help parents to contact community support groups.

Down Syndrome

DESCRIPTION

Down syndrome (formerly called mongolism) is a congenital form of mild to severe mental retardation accompanied by characteristic facial features and distinctive physical abnormalities.

■ **ICD-9-CM Code** **758.0**

SYMPTOMS AND SIGNS

Down syndrome, in addition to mild to severe mental retardation, is associated with heart defects and other congenital abnormalities. The infant has

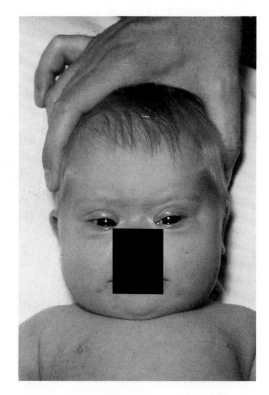

FIGURE 2–14 Typical face seen in a child with Down syndrome. (From Zitelli BJ, Davis HW: *Atlas of pediatric physical diagnosis*, ed 4, St. Louis, Mosby, 2002.)

a small head with a flat back skull, a typical slant to the eyes, a flat nasal bridge, low-set ears, a protruding tongue, and small weak muscles (Figs. 2–14 and 2–15). The hands are short with stubby fingers and a deep horizontal crease across the palm (simian line). There is an exaggerated space between the big and little toes.

PATIENT SCREENING

Down syndrome usually is diagnosed during the neonatal period and followed through normal infant and childhood office visits. When the parent of a Down child calls requesting an appointment, assessment will depend on the complaint. Consider the anxiety level of the parent, and schedule an appointment at the next available time.

ETIOLOGY

Infants with Down syndrome have an extra chromosome on number 21 (**trisomy** 21). It occurs in 1 in 650 live births and more often in infants born to women more than 35 years of age (Fig. 2–16).

DIAGNOSIS

Infants with severe Down syndrome usually are identified at birth; milder forms are diagnosed later. The physical characteristics may be blatantly obvious. Findings on examination of the eyes may include the presence of small white dots on the iris. A *karyotype* showing the chromosomal abnormality can confirm the diagnosis.

TREATMENT

Care of the child with Down syndrome depends on the severity of the physical defects and the degree of mental impairment. There is no known cure. The treatment plan is individual and includes a multidimensional approach to maximize the development of motor and mental skills. Life expectancy has

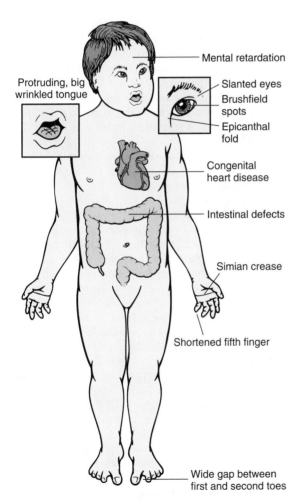

FIGURE 2–15 Typical features of Down syndrome. (From Damjanov I: *Pathology for the health-related professions,* ed 2, Philadelphia, 2000, Saunders.)

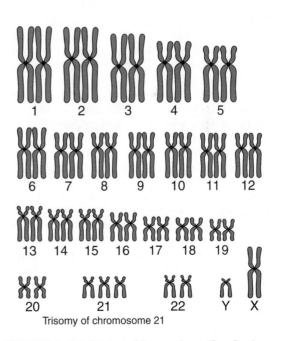

Trisomy of chromosome 21

FIGURE 2–16 Karyotype of Down syndrome. (From Damjanov I: *Pathology for the health-related professions,* ed 2, Philadelphia, 2000, Saunders.)

been improved through surgical correction of cardiac defects and antibiotic therapy for susceptibility to pulmonary disease. Some individuals may receive care in the home; others require residency at long-term care centers. Those who live longer are known for their affectionate and placid personalities.

PROGNOSIS

There is no known cure for Down syndrome; however, some of these individuals may be educable.

PREVENTION

There is no prevention for this condition.

PATIENT TEACHING

Help parents find and contact local support groups. Be available to answer parents' questions.

Congenital Cardiac Defects

Fetal Circulation

Oxygen and nutrients are supplied by the mother's blood to the developing fetus. The maternal blood supply also carries away waste products. The exchange takes place in the placental tissue. The umbilical vessels, two arteries and one vein, transport the blood between the placenta and the fetus (Fig. 2–17).

The umbilical vein transports oxygen-rich blood and nutrients to the fetus. The umbilical vein enters the fetal body by passing through the umbilical ring and then goes on to the liver. Fifty percent of this blood passes into the liver, and the other 50% bypasses the liver by way of the ductus venosus. The ductus venosus soon joins the inferior vena cava, allowing the oxygenated placental blood to mix with the deoxygenated blood coming from the lower fetal body. This blood then travels to the right atrium through the vena cava.

Because the fetal lungs are not functioning, this blood mostly bypasses the lungs. Most of the blood entering the right atrium by the inferior vena cava is shunted directly into the left atrium through the **foramen ovale**. There is a small valve on the left side of the atrial septum called the septum primum. This valve keeps blood from going back into the right atrium. The remaining fetal blood that has entered the right atrium contains a large

amount of oxygen-poor blood from the superior vena cava and travels to the right ventricle and into the pulmonary trunk. The pulmonary blood vessels have a high resistance to blood flow because of the collapsed state of the lungs, thus allowing only a small amount of blood to enter the pulmonary circulation. This small amount is enough to nourish the pulmonary tissue.

The blood that has been shunted away from the pulmonary circulation bypasses the lungs through the fetal vessel, the ductus arteriosus. This vessel connects the pulmonary trunk to the descending area of the aortic arch. The ductus arteriosus allows the blood with low oxygen concentration to bypass the lungs and also prevents it from entering the arteries leading to the brain.

The blood that has a high oxygen concentration and that has been shunted to the left atrium by way of the foramen ovale mixes with the small amount of blood returning from the pulmonary circulation by way of the pulmonary veins. This blood flows into the left ventricle and then into the aorta. From the aorta, some travels to the coronary and the carotid arteries. A portion travels on through the descending aorta to other parts of the fetal tissue. The remaining blood travels into the umbilical arteries and back to the placenta for exchange of gases, nutrients, and waste.

After the birth process, the infant's respiratory effort, and the initial inflation of the lungs, the circulatory system undergoes important changes. The resistance to blood flow through the lungs is reduced by the inflation of the tissue, allowing an increased blood flow from the pulmonary arteries. An increased volume of blood now flows from the right atrium into the right ventricle and the pulmonary arteries. In addition, the volume of blood flowing through the foramen ovale into the left atrium is reduced. The volume of blood returning by way of the pulmonary veins from the lungs to the left atrium is increased, causing an increase in the pressure in the left atrium. Blood is forced against the septum primum by decreased right atrial pressure and increased left atrial pressure, and the foramen ovale closes. If this does not occur, the infant has an atrial septal defect (ASD) (discussed subsequently under congenital anomalies). In most cases, however, the heart now is a two-sided pump.

With the lungs expanded and taking over the function of gas exchange, the infant no longer needs the ductus arteriosus to shunt blood from the pulmonary trunk to the descending aorta.

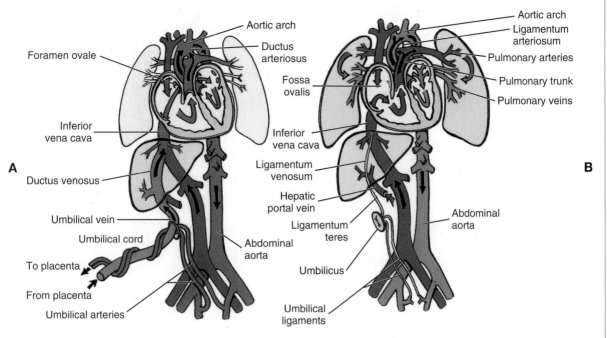

FIGURE 2-17 Circulation patterns before and after birth. **A,** Fetal circulation. **B,** Circulation after birth. (From Applegate EJ: *The anatomy and physiology learning system,* ed 2, Philadelphia, 2000, Saunders.)

Normally, the ductus arteriosus closes in the first few days after birth. If it does not close, it is termed *patent.* The patent ductus arteriosus (PDA) is a congenital birth defect (discussed subsequently).

SYMPTOMS AND SIGNS

Congenital cardiac defects are developmental anomalies of the heart or the great vessels of the heart. They are present at birth, and the defects cause mild to fatal stress of the cardiac muscle. Signs and symptoms vary according to the nature of the anomaly, the severity of the defect, and its effect on the heart and the circulatory system. More than one defect can be present, or a combination of defects can complicate the case. The common defects generally are categorized as follows: **acyanotic,** in which deoxygenated and oxygenated blood does not mix, and cyanotic, in which oxygenated and deoxygenated blood mixes.

Acyanotic Defects

DESCRIPTION

In this condition, oxygenated blood does not mix with deoxygenated blood and the infant usually maintains a fairly normal pink skin color. Cyanosis is not prevalent.

PATIENT SCREENING

Most cases will be discovered during the newborn examination. Parents requesting an appointment to discuss the condition should be scheduled as soon as possible. The parents may be experiencing great anxiety. Those cases not detected during the neonatal period of hospitalization may develop symptoms after dismissal from the hospital. When parents contact the office to relay concerns and symptoms, the infant requires prompt assessment.

Ventricular Septal Defect

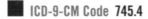 **ICD-9-CM Code 745.4**

The most common congenital cardiac disorder, ventricular septal defect, is an abnormal opening between the right and the left ventricles (Fig. 2-18). When the defect is small, there is little functional disease; when it is large, the results are serious. In this condition, blood is shunted from the left to the right side of the heart by higher pressure

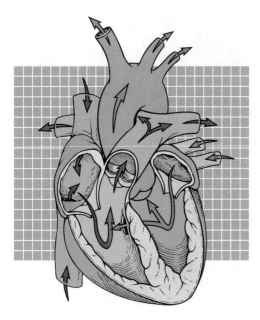

FIGURE 2–18 Ventricular septal defect. (Used with permission of Ross Products Division, Abbott Laboratories, from *Congenital heart abnormalities* [Clinical Education Aid no 7], 1992.)

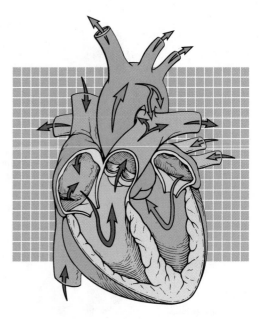

FIGURE 2–19 Patent ductus arteriosus. (Used with permission of Ross Products Division, Abbott Laboratories, from *Congenital heart abnormalities* [Clinical Education Aid no 7], 1992.)

in the left ventricle. A loud systolic *murmur* is heard during auscultation. Clinical features include failure to gain weight, restlessness, irritability, and increased heart rate and respirations. This condition may go undetected until later in childhood, adolescence, or adulthood.

Patent Ductus Arteriosus

■ **ICD-9-CM Code** **747.0**

PDA results when the ductus fails to functionally close. During normal fetal circulation, the patent ductus short-circuits shunting the circulation from the lungs and directs blood from the pulmonary trunk to the aorta. If PDA continues after birth, circulation of oxygen is compromised because this abnormal opening is a shunt that allows oxygenated blood to recirculate through the lungs (Fig. 2–19). PDA is detected during a physical examination when a classic "machinery" murmur is heard on auscultation and palpitation reveals a thrill. The infant's growth and development may be slowed, and various signs of heart failure may be present.

Closure may be attempted by drug therapy using an antiprostaglandin. The other option is surgical closure of the ductus.

This condition is fairly common in premature infants and often is accompanied by ASD with failure of the foramen ovale to close.

The prognosis for these infants depends on the presence of other anomalies. Closure by either drug therapy or surgical intervention establishes a normal postnatal circulation path and gives the infant the opportunity to grow and thrive. Currently no prevention is known.

Coarctation of the Aorta

■ **ICD-9-CM Code** **747.10**

This defect is characterized by a narrowed aortic lumen, causing a partial obstruction of the flow of blood through the aorta (Fig. 2–20). The result is increased left ventricular pressure and workload, with decreased blood pressure distal to the narrowing. Signs and symptoms can be evident shortly after birth or may not surface until adolescence.

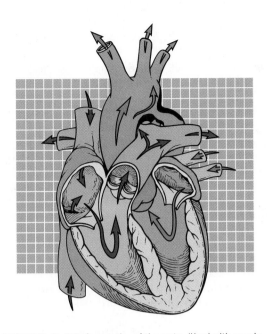

FIGURE 2–20 Coarctation of the aorta. (Used with permission of Ross Products Division, Abbott Laboratories, from *Congenital heart abnormalities* [Clinical Education Aid no 7], 1992.)

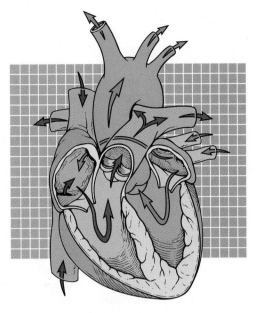

FIGURE 2–21 Atrial septal defect. (Used with permission of Ross Products Division, Abbott Laboratories, from *Congenital heart abnormalities* [Clinical Education Aid no 7], 1992.)

They include signs of left ventricular failure with pulmonary edema. The patient is pale and *cyanotic* with weakness, *dyspnea,* and *tachycardia.* Systemic blood pressure is elevated when measured in the arms, yet no pulse is felt in the leg vessels because pressure in them may be decreased.

Atrial Septal Defect

■ **ICD-9-CM Code 745.5**

ASD is an abnormal opening between the right and left atria (Fig. 2–21). Although the defect can vary in size and location, blood generally shunts from left to right in all atrial septal defects. Small defects may be undetected or cause symptoms such as fatigue, shortness of breath, and frequent respiratory tract infections. A large defect causes pronounced *cyanosis,* dyspnea, and **syncope.** A classic systolic cardiac murmur can be heard with a stethoscope. This condition often is associated with prematurity and PDA, and closure is achieved with surgical repair.

Cyanotic Defects

DESCRIPTION
Central cyanosis is a sign that the atrial blood is not fully oxygenated. The infant will appear cyanotic with a blue tinge to the skin.

PATIENT SCREENING
Most cases will be discovered during the newborn examination. Parents requesting an appointment to discuss the condition should be scheduled as soon as possible. One must remember the great anxiety the parents may be feeling. Those cases not detected during the neonatal period of hospitalization may develop symptoms after dismissal from the hospital. When parents contact the office to relay concerns and symptoms, the infant requires prompt assessment.

Tetralogy of Fallot

■ **ICD-9-CM Code** **745.2**

The most common cyanotic cardiac defect is a combination of four congenital heart defects: (1) ventricular septal defect, an abnormal opening in the ventricular septum; (2) pulmonary **stenosis,** a tightening of the pulmonary valve or vessel; (3) dextroposition (displacement to the right) of the aorta, which overrides (receiving circulation from both ventricles) the ventricular septal defect; and (4) right ventricular *hypertrophy,* caused by increased pressure in the ventricle (Fig. 2–22).

Affected infants are born as blue babies. In severe defects, deoxygenated blood enters the aorta, causing the symptoms of *hypoxia:* tachycardia, **tachypnea,** dyspnea, and seizures. Bone marrow hypoxia causes polycythemia, increased total red blood cell mass. Physical examination may reveal delayed physical growth and development along with clubbing of the fingers and toes. Cardiac murmurs can be heard. Older children assume a squatting position after exercise to relieve breathlessness caused by hypoxia.

Transposition of the Great Arteries

■ **ICD-9-CM Code** **745.10** *(Complete transposition of the great vessels)*

In this defect, the aorta and the pulmonary artery are reversed: the aorta originates from the right ventricle, and the pulmonary artery originates from the left ventricle. The result is two closed-loop circulatory systems: one between the heart and the lungs, and the other between the heart and systemic circulation (Fig. 2–23). Within a few hours of birth, neonates with this defect exhibit cyanosis and tachypnea, followed by signs of heart failure.

Immediate surgical intervention is indicated. Prostaglandins are administered to the infant in an effort to keep the ductus arteriosus patent and the foramen ovale from closing. As soon as surgery is possible, the blood flow is redirected by correction of the defect.

The prognosis for these infants is poor unless a pediatric surgical unit is readily available and transportation to it is swift. Another factor in the survival of the infant with this condition is the infant's response to the drug therapy to maintain the fetal

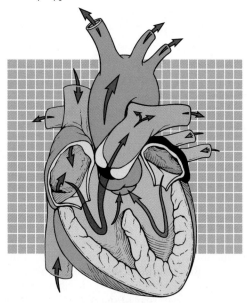

FIGURE 2–22 Tetralogy of Fallot. (Used with permission of Ross Products Division, Abbott Laboratories, from *Congenital heart abnormalities* [Clinical Education Aid no 7], 1992.)

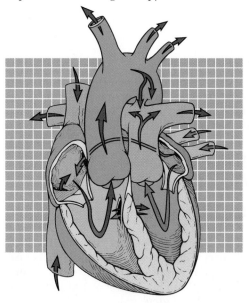

FIGURE 2–23 Transposition of the great arteries. (Used with permission of Ross Products Division, Abbott Laboratories, from *Congenital heart abnormalities* [Clinical Education Aid no 7], 1992.)

circulation and prevent the change to the normal postbirth circulatory system.

Methods of preventing this condition are unknown.

ETIOLOGY

The cause of congenital cardiac defects remains unknown. They may result from several factors, including chromosomal abnormalities and environmental conditions such as maternal infections and the mother's use of certain drugs during gestation. Several congenital disorders result from the failure of the circulatory system to shift from the fetal route of blood flow at the time of birth.

DIAGNOSIS

Physical examination and patient history are essential. The physician palpates the neck vessels and auscultates for blood pressure and murmurs. Diagnostic procedures depend on the initial findings and may include radiographic chest films, blood tests, cardiac catheterization, echocardiogram, and electrocardiogram. The diagnostic investigation determines the presence and severity of any structural or functional abnormality or defect.

TREATMENT

The medical management of congenital cardiac defects is determined by the type of defect, the degree of symptoms and signs, and the presence of life-threatening complications. Advances in surgical techniques enable surgeons to close septal defects, to reconstruct or replace a valve, and to repair or join blood vessels. These procedures make it possible to save, improve, and extend the lives of individuals born with congenital cardiac defects. Medications are available to strengthen and regulate the heartbeat. Supportive measures include prophylactic antibiotic administration to ward off infection.

PROGNOSIS

Prognosis varies and depends on the severity, the number of defects, and the gestational age of the infant or child. Most defects can be surgically repaired.

PREVENTION

There is no known prevention for these defects. Good prenatal care accompanied by good nutrition is always wise during any pregnancy.

PATIENT TEACHING

Parents and caretakers need understanding, encouragement, and teaching to cope with changes in individual and family lifestyle imposed by these conditions. Help and encourage parents to find and contact support groups in the community.

Musculoskeletal Diseases

Clubfoot (Talipes Equinovarus)

DESCRIPTION

Clubfoot is an obvious, nontraumatic deformity of the foot of the newborn in which the anterior half of the foot is adducted and inverted.

 ICD-9-CM Code 754.51 *(Talipes, unspecified)*

SYMPTOMS AND SIGNS

Besides the previously mentioned description, the heel is drawn up, with the lateral side of the foot being convex and the medial aspect being concave (Fig. 2–24, *A*). A true clubfoot cannot be manipulated to the proper position, while distortions that are caused by intrauterine position usually can be.

PATIENT SCREENING

Most cases will be discovered during the newborn examination. Parents requesting an appointment to discuss the condition should be scheduled as soon as possible. Remember the great anxiety the parents may be feeling. As treatment progresses, routine examinations are scheduled.

ETIOLOGY

Some sources suggest that fetal position is the cause, and other studies implicate genetic factors because of an abnormal development of the germ plasma during the embryonic stage.

DIAGNOSIS

The deformity is obvious at birth, with a resistance of the foot to return to a neutral position during manipulation. In addition, the Achilles tendon is shortened.

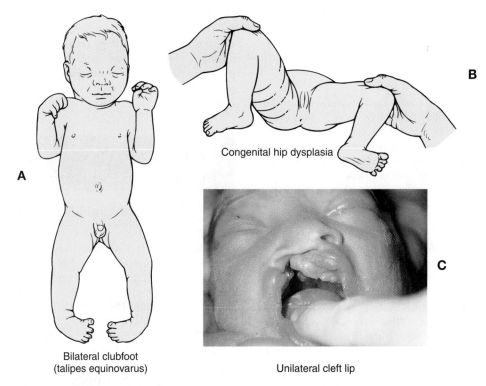

Congenital hip dysplasia

Bilateral clubfoot
(talipes equinovarus)

Unilateral cleft lip

FIGURE 2–24 Congenital musculoskeletal diseases. (From Behrman RE, Kliegman RM, Arvin AM: Slide set for *Nelson textbook of pediatrics,* ed 15, Philadelphia, 1996, Saunders.)

TREATMENT

Treatment consists of either cast application or the use of splints. Treatment must start early in the neonatal period. Casts are reapplied at frequent intervals as the correction increases and the infant grows. Splints include a bar affixed to shoes; the infant is placed in the shoes, which hold the feet and legs in position. Many physicians employ a combination of manipulative methods, with cast application followed by the use of splints as the child matures. The child must be observed throughout childhood for reversal of the improvement. If casting and splinting are unsuccessful, surgery may be indicated to correct the condition.

PROGNOSIS

Prognosis is good for these children when casting is performed or splints can be used early in life. When these modes of treatment do not completely resolve the condition, surgical intervention usually corrects the deformity.

PREVENTION

No prevention of this deformity is known or accepted.

PATIENT TEACHING

Parents will be extremely anxious and need information about this condition. Instruction in cast and skin care is important. The importance of observing continuously for any reversal of correction is stressed.

Congenital Hip Dysplasia

DESCRIPTION

•Congenital hip dysplasia (CHD) is an abnormal development of the hip joint that ranges from an unstable joint to dislocation of the femoral head from the **acetabulum.**

■ **ICD-9-CM Code 755.63** *(Other congenital deformity of hip [joint], Congenital anteversion of femur [neck])*

754.3 *(Congenital dislocation of hip)*
Refer to the physician's diagnosis and then to the current edition of the ICD-9-CM coding manual to ensure the greatest specificity of pathology and any appropriate modifiers.

SYMPTOMS AND SIGNS

Physical examination reveals asymmetric folds of the thigh of the newborn with a limited abduction of the affected hip. A shortening of the femur is noted when the knees and hips are flexed at right angles (see Fig. 2–24, *B*).

PATIENT SCREENING

This dysplasia will be apparent during the newborn examination. Parents requesting an appointment to discuss the condition should be scheduled as soon as possible. Remember the great anxiety the parents may be feeling. As treatment progresses, routine examinations are scheduled.

ETIOLOGY

The exact cause is unknown. Typical CHD occurs shortly before, during, or shortly after birth, possibly as a result of softening of the ligaments caused by the maternal hormone relaxin. CHD may result from a breech presentation and is more common in female infants.

DIAGNOSIS

Abnormal signs, including a positive *Ortolani sign,* may be detected at birth. Diagnosis is made during the physical examination and is confirmed by radiographic studies.

TREATMENT

Treatment includes the use of various devices to reduce the congenital hip dislocation. After the femoral head is returned to its proper position in the acetabulum, the legs are held in place by a Pavlik harness, a splint, or a cast, allowing stable maintenance of the hip in a position of flexion and abduction. Early treatment offers the best results and may avoid the necessity of surgical intervention.

PROGNOSIS

The prognosis for this deformity is good when therapy is instituted early in the neonatal period. If this therapy is unsuccessful, surgical intervention may be required.

PREVENTION

No prevention for this condition is known.

PATIENT TEACHING

Parents should be taught to care for the skin and the correctional device. In addition, the need for compliance in the treatment should be stressed. After the condition appears to have been corrected, parents should be told of the importance of follow-up assessments of the child.

Cleft Lip and Palate

DESCRIPTION

Cleft lip (harelip) is a congenital birth defect consisting of one or more clefts in the upper lip (see Fig. 2–24, *C*). Cleft palate is a birth defect in which there is a hole in the middle of the roof of the mouth (palate).

ICD-9-CM Code 749.20 *(Cleft palate with cleft lip, unspecified)*
Cleft palate and lip are coded by type. Refer to the physician's diagnosis and then to the current edition of the ICD-9-CM coding manual to ensure the greatest specificity of pathology and any appropriate modifiers.

SYMPTOMS AND SIGNS

The cleft may extend completely through the hard and soft palates into the nasal area. The defects appear singularly or may be linked and vary in severity. Some infants have difficulty with nasal regurgitation and feeding because of air leaks around the cleft. A major problem is the infant's appearance.

PATIENT SCREENING

These birth defects will be apparent during newborn examination. Parents may want an appointment to discuss the condition and treatment with the physician. Because of the great anxiety the parents may be feeling, a prompt appointment should be scheduled. As the repair and correction of conditions progress, the parents may contact the office about problems the child is having, especially in feeding. Prompt response to their requests is required.

ETIOLOGY

The cause is a failure in the embryonic development of the fetus. It is considered a multifactorial genetic disorder and occurs in about 1 in 10,000 births.

DIAGNOSIS

Cleft abnormalities are obvious during clinical inspection at birth.

TREATMENT

Cleft deformities usually are repaired surgically as soon as possible. Extensive deformities require a second repair. Special feeding devices can be tried. The child often requires speech therapy.

PROGNOSIS

Prognosis is good for this disorder with surgical repair. Advances in plastic surgery have made the repair look as natural as possible.

PREVENTION

No prevention of this disorder is known.

PATIENT TEACHING

Parents will need instruction on care of the surgical repair and on feeding of the infant. Help and encourage them to find and contact support groups in the community.

Genitourinary Diseases

Cryptorchidism (Undescended Testes)

DESCRIPTION

• Cryptorchidism is failure of one or both of the testicles to descend from the abdominal cavity into the scrotum.

ICD-9-CM Code 752.51

SYMPTOMS AND SIGNS

Cryptorchidism, or failure of the testicles to descend from the abdominal cavity into the scrotum, is detected at birth or shortly thereafter (Fig. 2–25). The condition may be unilateral or bilateral. During infancy and early childhood, there are no symptoms, just the absence of the testes. The condition is more common in premature infants.

PATIENT SCREENING

This condition is palpable and observed during the newborn examination. Parents may request an appointment to discuss the condition and possible treatment. The anxiety of the parents calls for an appointment at the earliest convenience of the parents and the physician.

ETIOLOGY

The cause of failure of the testes to descend during the final fetal development is not clearly understood. Some experts suspect that hormones play a role.

DIAGNOSIS

Diagnosis is by visual inspection and by palpation, starting above the inguinal ring and pushing downward on the inguinal canal toward the scrotum. The examination reveals no evidence of one or both testes in the scrotal sac. When the condition is bilateral, the scrotum appears underdeveloped.

TREATMENT

• The testes often descend spontaneously during the first year of life. If this does not happen by 4 years of age, the treatment is to place the undescended testes into the scrotum by either surgical manipulation (orchiopexy) or hormonal drug therapy. Treatment is important because untreated cryptorchidism may lead to sterility in the adult male. There is an increased risk of testicular cancer in untreated cryptorchidism.

PROGNOSIS

Prognosis is good when surgical intervention can move the testicles down into the scrotum and secure them. This procedure is necessary in early childhood to prevent sterility and possible cancer later in life.

PREVENTION

There is no accepted form of prevention.

PATIENT TEACHING

Parents need to be told the dangers of not employing suggested surgical intervention. After the procedure, they will need instructions in caring for the incisions.

Wilms' Tumor

DESCRIPTION

• Wilms' tumor, or nephroblastoma, is a highly malignant neoplasm of the kidney that affects children younger than 5 years. It is the most common kidney tumor of childhood.

ICD-9-CM Code 189.0

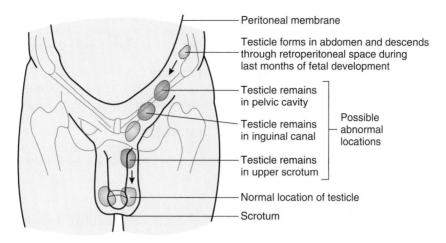

FIGURE 2–25 Cryptorchidism and possible positions of the undescended testis. (From Gould BE: *Pathophysiology for the health professions,* ed 2, Philadelphia, 2002, Saunders.)

SYMPTOMS AND SIGNS

The most common presentation is a mass in the kidney region, which is often discovered by a parent or examining physician. The mass is firm, nontender, and usually confined to one side of the body. The patient may experience other symptoms resulting from compression caused by the tumor mass, metabolic alterations due to the tumor, or metastasis. These include *hematuria,* pain in the abdomen or chest, hypertension, anemia, vomiting, intestinal obstruction, weight loss, and fever.

PATIENT SCREENING

A child experiencing hematuria, pain, and vomiting and who has a noticeable mass in the kidney region requires prompt assessment.

ETIOLOGY

Wilms' tumor is an **adenosarcoma** arising from abnormal fetal kidney tissue that is left behind during early embryonic life (Fig. 2–26). The tissue begins unrestrained cancerous growth after the child is born. About 20% of cases of Wilms' tumor are hereditary; however, there is no method to identify gene carriers. Wilms' tumor is associated with several congenital anomalies such as aniridia (absence of the iris) and genitourinary anomalies (such as cryptorchidism and ambiguous genitalia), and is a part of some familial cancer syndromes. Most tumors are unilateral, but 10% are bilateral or multicentric.

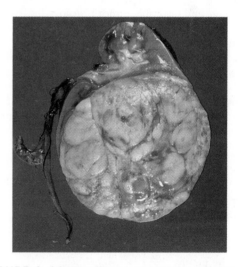

FIGURE 2–26 Wilms' tumor in the lower pole of the kidney with the characteristic tan-to-gray color and well-circumscribed margins. (From Kumar V, Cotran R, Robbins S: *Basic pathology,* ed 7, Philadelphia, 2002, Saunders.)

DIAGNOSIS

A child suspected of having Wilms' tumor often undergoes physical examination to palpate the kidney mass, to seek associated congenital anomalies, and to look for signs of malignancy (e.g., increased size of liver and spleen, lymphadenopathy, and anemia). Specific tests that help determine the extent of disease include abdominal ultrasound, CT scan, and urinalysis. Intravenous **pyelography** shows displacement and distortion of the pelvis of the kidney. Surgery is necessary for complete staging of the tumor. Staging is based on the degree the tumor extends beyond the kidney capsule, the presence of metastasis, and whether there is bilateral kidney involvement.

TREATMENT
Prompt recognition and treatment are imperative because the tumor is locally invasive and tends to metastasize. Surgical removal of the tumor and accessible metastatic sites is followed by chemotherapy with or without radiation therapy. The specific treatment choice is guided by tumor stage and histology.

PROGNOSIS
Wilms' tumor has one of the highest survival rates of all childhood cancers. The prognosis is largely based on stage and tumor histology. Patients with a low stage and favorable tumor histology have a 90% cure rate. For those with high stage or unfavorable histology, the cure rate drops to 60% to 70%. However, with the increased cure rate achieved through modern treatment methods, an increased risk of second primary tumors has been noted in these patients. This is likely either a result of the therapies used or a manifestation of the cancer syndromes with which Wilms' tumor is associated.

PREVENTION
No prevention is known.

PATIENT TEACHING
Help and encourage parents to find and contact support groups in the community as well as community resources that provide services to the child and the family.

Phimosis

DESCRIPTION
Phimosis is stenosis, or narrowing, of the opening of the foreskin in the male.

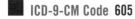 **ICD-9-CM Code 605**

SYMPTOMS AND SIGNS
Phimosis is stenosis, or narrowing, of the opening of the foreskin in the male infant. He may experience difficulty with urination, or the parents may have difficulty with cleaning the area under the prepuce of the glans penis, resulting in an accumulation of secretions. These symptoms may develop later in uncircumcised males.

ETIOLOGY
Many male infants are born with phimosis; the cause is unknown.

DIAGNOSIS
Diagnosis is made by visual examination and the inability to slide the prepuce back over the glans penis.

TREATMENT
Treatment is circumcision, the surgical removal of the prepuce. This procedure, which used to be routine for male newborns, is usually performed in the first few days of life.

PROGNOSIS
The prognosis is good.

PREVENTION
No prevention is known for this condition.

PATIENT TEACHING
Parents will require instruction in caring for the incised area.

Diseases of the Digestive System

Congenital Pyloric Stenosis

DESCRIPTION
Pyloric stenosis is a gastric obstruction associated with narrowing of the pyloric sphincter at the exit of the stomach. This condition may also be called congenital hypertrophic pyloric stenosis.

ICD-9-CM Code 750.5

SYMPTOMS AND SIGNS
The infant has episodes of projectile vomiting after feedings (Fig. 2–27) and fails to gain weight. Symptoms usually begin at 2 to 3 weeks of age. The infant appears hungry, continues to feed, and yet fails to gain weight. If left untreated, the infant becomes dehydrated and experiences electrolyte imbalances. A small olive-shaped hard mass may be palpated in the region of the pyloric sphincter, and

left to right peristalsis may be noted, followed by reverse peristalsis. The emesis contains no bile.

PATIENT SCREENING

The infant with sudden onset of projectile vomiting requires prompt assessment.

ETIOLOGY

There is a slight hereditary tendency, but the exact cause is unknown. It occurs four times more often in male than in female infants.

DIAGNOSIS

The condition is diagnosed from the history and the patient's physical condition. Diagnostic studies include upper gastrointestinal radiographic studies and ultrasonographic study of the **pylorus.**

TREATMENT

Treatment consists of surgical intervention in which the constricted pylorus is incised and sutured to relieve the obstruction.

PROGNOSIS

The prognosis is good with prompt surgical intervention.

PREVENTION

No prevention is known.

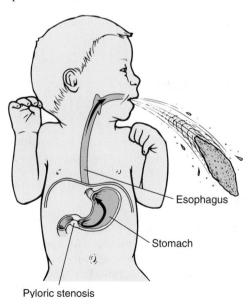

Esophagus

Stomach

Pyloric stenosis

FIGURE 2–27 Congenital pyloric stenosis. The abnormal narrowing of the opening of the pylorus causes episodes of projectile vomiting.

PATIENT TEACHING

Parents will need instruction in care of the incision. Reinforce the importance of postoperative visits.

Hirschsprung Disease (Congenital Aganglionic Megacolon)

DESCRIPTION

Hirschsprung disease is an impairment of intestinal motility that causes obstruction of the distal colon.

 ICD-9-CM Code 751.3 *(Unspecified, NOS)*

SYMPTOMS AND SIGNS

The symptoms and signs differ slightly depending on the age of the child experiencing an exacerbation of the condition. In the neonatal period, the newborn fails to pass **meconium** within 48 hours after birth. The infant may have bile-stained or fecal vomitus and does not want to feed. The abdomen becomes distended.

After the neonatal period, the symptoms and signs include a failure to thrive, with obstinate constipation, vomiting, and abdominal distention. When the condition worsens, the infant may become feverish and may have explosive, watery diarrhea.

The older child exhibits more chronic symptoms such as constipation, abdominal distention, ribbon-like stools that are foul smelling, easily palpable fecal masses, and visible peristalsis. The child appears malnourished and anemic.

PATIENT SCREENING

Infants or children with GI symptoms of bile-stained or fecal vomitus require prompt assessment, as do those children with obstinate constipation, especially when combined with vomiting and abdominal distension. Any child experiencing ribbon-like stools also should have prompt assessment.

ETIOLOGY

The defect lies in the abnormal innervation of the **intrinsic** musculature of the bowel wall. In Hirschsprung disease, the parasympathetic nerve ganglion cells are absent in a segment of the colon, usually in the rectosigmoid area. This deficiency of innervation results in lack of peristalsis in the affected portion of the colon and the succeeding backup of fecal material. The proximal portion of the colon becomes grossly distended, and intestinal obstruction results.

Statistics indicate that males are more likely than females to have a megacolon and that the risk is increased in children with Down syndrome. It is believed to be a familial congenital disease.

DIAGNOSIS

Diagnosis is based on family history, the clinical picture, radiographic studies of the bowel, and finally, biopsy that confirms the absence of the ganglionic cells.

TREATMENT

Treatment consists of relief of the obstruction by surgical intervention; the affected bowel is excised, and the normal colon is joined to the anus. A temporary colostomy is performed proximal to the aganglionic section of the colon. Electrolyte and fluid balance must be maintained. After the colon recovers function (6 months to 1 year), the colostomy is closed.

PROGNOSIS

The prognosis varies depending on the extent of colon involvement and the success of surgical intervention. Ideally, the colon will heal and the colostomy can be closed within a year.

PREVENTION

No prevention is known for this apparently familial congenital disease.

PATIENT TEACHING

Parents and the child will require training on caring for the stoma as well as dealing with the colostomy bags and drainage. Help and encourage families to find and contact support groups as well as other community resources. The parents, family, and child may require counseling. Provide nutritional and dietary information.

Metabolic Disorders

Cystic Fibrosis

DESCRIPTION

- Cystic fibrosis (CF) is a chronic dysfunction of the exocrine glands (glands that secrete through ducts) affecting multiple body systems; it is the most common fatal genetic disease.

 ICD-9-CM Code 277.0 *(Cystic fibrosis)*
Cystic fibrosis is coded according to the region involved. Refer to the physician's diagnosis and then to the current edition of the ICD-9-CM coding manual to ensure the greatest specificity of pathology and any appropriate modifiers.

SYMPTOMS AND SIGNS

Symptoms may become apparent soon after birth or may develop in childhood. The disease primarily attacks the lungs and the digestive system, producing copious thick and sticky mucus that accumulates and blocks glandular ducts. The clinical effects of CF can be immense, including a dry paroxysmal cough, exercise intolerance, pneumonia, bulky diarrhea, vomiting, and bowel obstruction. Pancreatic changes occur, with fat and fiber replacing normal tissue. Involvement of sweat glands causes increased concentrations of salt in sweat. Normal growth and ability to thrive are reduced (Fig. 2–28).

PATIENT SCREENING

Many of these children will become suspect for the disease during the neonatal period while still in the newborn nursery. The condition may become apparent during routine well-baby examinations. When parents report that the child has developed a cough producing thick, sticky mucus, prompt assessment of the child is indicated.

ETIOLOGY

- CF is an inherited disorder and is transmitted as an autosomal recessive trait.

DIAGNOSIS

The diagnostic workup includes a family history, a pulmonary function test, radiographic chest film, and stool studies. A sweat test reveals elevated levels of sodium and chloride and confirms the diagnosis.

TREATMENT

CF is considered a fatal disease. However, early diagnosis and treatment have greatly increased life expectancy during the past few decades. The treatment is supportive measures that help the child to lead as normal a life as possible and that prevent pulmonary infections. These measures include the use of a high-calorie, high–sodium-

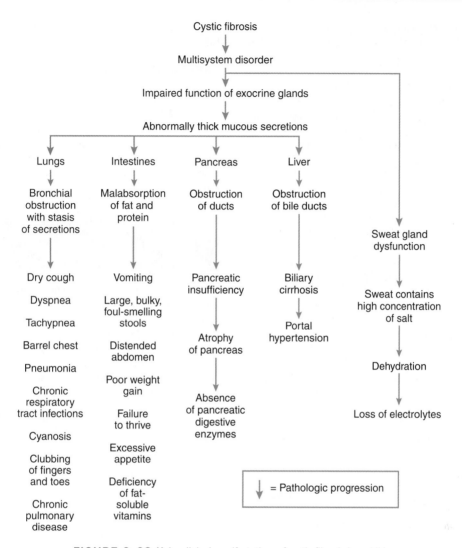

FIGURE 2–28 Major clinical manifestations of cystic fibrosis in a child.

chloride diet, chest physiotherapy, and pancreatic enzyme supplementation to aid in digestion. Broad-spectrum antibiotics are used aggressively to treat infection, and drugs that thin the mucus are given. Oxygen therapy may be required.

PROGNOSIS

Because CF is considered a fatal disease, the long-term prognosis is not favorable. Early diagnosis and compliance with treatment have improved the pos-

sibility for these children to have as near normal a life as possible and an increased life expectancy.

PREVENTION

CF is genetic, and no prevention is known.

PATIENT TEACHING

The family needs emotional support and teaching about the disease; referral to genetic counseling is helpful. Help and encourage the family to find and contact support groups and other resources in the community.

Phenylketonuria

DESCRIPTION

Phenylketonuria (PKU) is an inborn error in the metabolism of amino acids that causes brain damage and mental retardation when not corrected.

■ **ICD-9-CM Code 270.1**

SYMPTOMS AND SIGNS

In this defect, an enzyme needed to change an amino acid (phenylalanine) in the body into another substance (tyrosine) is lacking. As a result, phenylalanine accumulates in the blood and urine and is *toxic* to the brain. Symptoms may not begin until the infant is 4 months old, when a characteristic musty odor of the child's perspiration and urine is noted. Other signs include rashes, irritability, hyperactivity, personality disorders, and evidence of arrested brain development.

PATIENT SCREENING

Screening of all newborns is mandatory in all states, and a positive screen indicates immediate dietary intervention. When a parent or caregiver reports that the infant has a musty smell, especially in the urine, prompt assessment is indicated.

ETIOLOGY

PKU is inherited as an autosomal recessive trait and causes defective enzymatic conversion in protein metabolism, resulting in the accumulation of phenylalanine in the blood.

DIAGNOSIS

PKU is detected by mandatory screening of the newborn blood. A positive *Guthrie test* result indicates the presence of phenylalanine in the blood. The urine is tested for phenylalanine derivatives.

TREATMENT

The treatment is to place the infant on a phenylalanine-free diet. Because natural proteins contain phenylalanine, the patient must remain on a protein-restricted diet.

PROGNOSIS

The prognosis is excellent when the infant is placed on a phenylalanine-free diet soon after birth. Late dietary intervention does not reverse brain damage.

PREVENTION

No prevention is known.

PATIENT TEACHING

Close follow-up with testing for phenylalanine levels in the blood may allow some modification of the difficult dietary restrictions. Emotional support is important for the child and the parent. Genetic counseling is advised.

Endocrine Diseases

Klinefelter syndrome and Turner syndrome are examples of genetic, chromosomal diseases that are not inherited. They result from nondisjunction, or the failure of a chromosome pair to separate, during *gamete* production (Fig. 2–29).

Humans normally have 46 chromosomes, 22 pairs of *autosomes* and 2 sex chromosomes. The technical notation for a human female is 46,XX

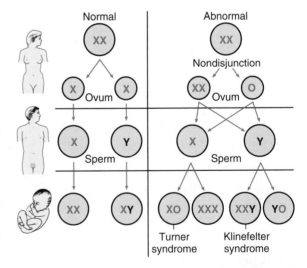

FIGURE 2–29 Pathogenesis of sex chromosome abnormalities (Turner and Klinefelter). (From Damjanov I: *Pathology for the health-related professions,* ed 2, Philadelphia, 2000, Saunders.)

and for a male, 46,XY. In a fertilized ovum, one chromosome from each pair of autosomes originates from the mother's ovum, and the other from the father's sperm. Each ovum normally contains a single X chromosome. Sperm cells may contain either an X or a Y chromosome. If a sperm bearing the X chromosome fertilizes the ovum, the fetus develops into a female. A sperm carrying the Y chromosome produces a male fetus. Sometimes, through what may be described as an accident of nature, extra chromosomes or the absence of chromosomes in the fertilized ovum cause congenital syndromes with a variety of physical and mental developmental effects.

Klinefelter Syndrome

DESCRIPTION

Klinefelter syndrome is male hypogonadism, appearing in males after puberty with at least two X chromosomes and one or more Y chromosomes (typically the 47,XXY pattern).

ICD-9-CM Code 758.7

SYMPTOMS AND SIGNS

The presence of two X chromosomes in affected males causes abnormal development of the testes and reduced levels of the male hormone testosterone. Puberty begins at the usual time and usually results in a normal-size penis, but the testes are small and body hair is scant. In general, the person appears normal, except for exceptionally long legs, above average height, and reduced muscle development. The most significant problem associated with Klinefelter syndrome is infertility resulting from *azoospermia*. Only rarely are patients fertile; these individuals have the mosaic form that carries the extra X chromosome in only one cell line. Other alterations include a mild delay in language acquisition and increased risk of behavioral and learning disabilities. Some affected individuals have mild to more significant intellectual impairment. The mammary glands may be enlarged in about half of the cases. Possible complications include osteoporosis and chronic pulmonary disease.

PATIENT SCREENING

The male infant appears normal at birth, and symptoms are usually not noted until puberty. The condition may be discovered during a routine sports or pre-camp physical. In other situations, the parent may call to discuss the delay in sexual maturation of the young male. Considering the anxiety that the family may be experiencing, an assessment should be performed promptly.

ETIOLOGY

Klinefelter syndrome results from the presence of at least two X chromosomes, typically the 47,XXY pattern. The extra X chromosome may be of either maternal or paternal origin. Other variants include XXYY, XXXY, and XXXXY. The disease is not inherited but results from a nondisjunction during gamete formation. This disorder affects an estimated 1 in 500 to 600 liveborn males.

DIAGNOSIS

The diagnostic workup includes a physical examination, serum and urine gonadotropin level determination, and semen analysis. A chromosomal smear analysis confirms the diagnosis and differentiates between the mosaic and true form of Klinefelter syndrome.

TREATMENT

At the time of normal puberty, long-term hormone replacement with testosterone by injection or a transdermal patch is given, usually under the supervision of an endocrinologist. Testosterone is necessary for the maintenance of normal sexual function and normal muscle and bone mass. However, fertility cannot be restored. Many patients report an improvement in energy and emotional stability with hormone therapy. Supplemental calcium intake is prescribed to help prevent osteoporosis.

PROGNOSIS

There is no cure for the syndrome, and natural fatherhood probably will never be achieved. Alteration of intelligence correlates with the number of extra X chromosomes. Many of these males achieve in their chosen profession and are productive members of society.

PREVENTION

Because Klinefelter syndrome is a chromosomal disorder, no prevention is known.

PATIENT TEACHING

Inform the patient and family of the importance of follow-up appointments to monitor hormone replacement and identify the target dosage. Explain the importance of adhering to the prescribed dosage schedule of medication to maintain proper blood levels. Describe the possible adverse effects of testosterone therapy, such as insomnia, anxiety, tremors, and dizziness; tell the patient to report these or other symptoms to the attending physician. Refer the patient and family to Klinefelter Syndrome and Associates for support, meetings, and conventions.

Turner Syndrome

DESCRIPTION

Turner syndrome is a chromosomal disease that occurs in females with a single sex chromosome, 45,XO.

 ICD-9-CM Code 758.6

SYMPTOMS AND SIGNS

Turner syndrome is the most common disorder of gonadal dysgenesis in females. At birth, the ovaries are immature or absent, and the female infant appears short, with swollen hands and feet and possible webbing of the neck. As these children grow, they experience lack of sexual maturation along with amenorrhea, sterility, dwarfism, and cardiac and kidney defects. If ovaries were present at birth, they slowly begin to disappear, leaving only small amounts of tissue. If the ovaries do not disappear, they typically contain no eggs, eliminating the possibility of pregnancy. Most of these female children may experience delayed speech and ambulation; however, they usually are of normal intelligence.

PATIENT SCREENING

Well-baby examinations may reveal signs of the disorder. The baby is referred for chromosome studies to confirm the diagnosis. As the child matures, appointments may be needed to assess possible cardiac or renal disorders.

ETIOLOGY

Turner syndrome results from a loss of the second X chromosome caused by nondisjunction during gamete formation. The anomaly is seen in about 1 in 1000 live female births.

DIAGNOSIS

Chromosomal smear studies show only one X chromosome instead of the normal 46,XX chromosomal pattern.

TREATMENT

Symptoms can be reduced by estrogen and growth hormone therapy. Surgical correction may be indicated for certain anomalies, such as webbing of the neck. Emotional support for the patient and the family helps them to develop strategies for coping with low self-esteem, body image disturbance, and potential cardiac or renal disorders that may develop.

PROGNOSIS

There is no cure for this genetic disorder; however, the prognosis is good if the patient has no other complicating conditions, including cardiac or kidney disorders. Moderate degrees of learning disorders are common. These females will never be able to conceive their own child, as they have no ovaries to produce eggs.

PREVENTION

As Turner syndrome is a chromosomal disorder, there is no prevention. These individuals will be sterile; therefore, they will have no offspring who could inherit the disorder.

PATIENT TEACHING

Help the child and parents to find and contact support groups and community resources. Encourage the family to help the girl build self-esteem and confidence. Make referrals for genetic counseling if requested.

CHILDHOOD DISEASES

Nothing causes more anxiety than a seriously ill child. Pathologic processes in children pose special threats because children are constantly changing physically and functionally. The journey through childhood normally results in maturation and expansion of the body's natural immune defense mechanisms. In addition, rapid advances in treatment and preventive medicine enable us to control many infectious diseases that formerly caused serious illness and disabling complications, even death. However, many infections and disease syndromes can interrupt the normal growth and development of any child. The following section describes the common diseases that affect children.

Infectious Diseases

Although the infant acquires limited natural immunity from the mother, the growing child is vulnerable to many infectious diseases and the disabilities that they cause. Many of these communicable diseases can be prevented. Dramatic results have been achieved in pediatric medicine through routine prophylactic immunization with vaccines that build specific and prolonged protection. To prevent epidemics of contagious diseases, all states in the United States require that children have inoculations before entering school (Table 2–2). (See the discussion of immunity in Chapter 3.)

Chickenpox (Varicella)

DESCRIPTION

Chickenpox is a highly contagious, acute viral infection that is common in children and young adults.

■ **ICD-9-CM Code** **052.9**

SYMPTOMS AND SIGNS

Chickenpox is a systemic disease with superficial cutaneous lesions that begin as red macules that progress to *papules* and then finally become *vesicles* that form crusts. The lesions first are seen on the

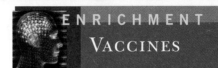

ENRICHMENT
VACCINES

A VACCINE IS A SUSPENSION of dead or attenuated organisms given to stimulate an active immune response that produces more or less permanent resistance to pathogenic organisms and viruses. Booster doses are smaller amounts of the original vaccine given at specified intervals to maintain serum antibody levels. Vaccines are controlled for potency and stability and are tested for safety and effectiveness. Some vaccines are grown in bird eggs or in animal organs or are weakened with chemicals. The patient is screened for certain allergies or previous reactions to vaccines. Local responses of soreness, redness, and swelling at the site of injection are common. Untoward responses include high fever, generalized swelling, difficulty in breathing, severe headache, arthralgia, and seizures. Any of these symptoms should be reported immediately to the physician.

Toxoids use an altered form of a bacterial toxin to stimulate antibody production and thereby impart protection against toxins.

face or the trunk and then spread over the extremities; they can be distributed everywhere on the body and even have been found internally. A day or two before the rash appears, the patient may experience fever, malaise, and anorexia. The lesions can continue to erupt for 3 to 4 days and cause intense itching. Recovery is usually complete within 2 weeks, leaving the person with lifetime immunity. Some possible complications include secondary bacterial infection, viral pneumonia, conjunctival ulcers, and Reye syndrome (Fig. 2–30).

PATIENT SCREENING

Contagious diseases present a challenge in the patient-screening process. Many physicians prefer not to have the contagious patient in the regular reception area. Many pediatricians have a "sick child" waiting room as well as a regular waiting room. At

TABLE 2–2
Typical Immunization Schedule for Normal Children

NAME OF VACCINE	NAME OF DISEASE	NUMBER OF DOSES	AGE GIVEN
Diphtheria and tetanus toxoids and pertussis vaccine (DTP)	Diphtheria, tetanus, pertussis	5	2 mo 4 mo 6 mo 15-18 mo 4-6 yr
Oral poliomyelitis vaccine (OPV)	Poliomyelitis	4	2 mo 4 mo 15 mo 4-6 yr
Measles, mumps, and rubella virus vaccine (MMR)	Measles, mumps, rubella	2	15 mo 4-6 yr, or before starting kindergarten or first grade
Haemophilus b conjugate vaccine (HibCV)	Meningitis	3	2, 4, 6 mo
Diphtheria and tetanus toxoids (Td)	Diphtheria	1	14-16 yr
Varicella virus vaccine	Chickenpox (varicella)	1	1-12 yr
Hepatitis B vaccine	Hepatitis B	3	Birth–2 mo 1–4 mo 6–18 mo

Special schedules are recommended for older children, adults, and people at special risk. The chronically ill, immigrants, foreign travelers, or those with lifestyle risks may need additional immunizations.
The American Academy of Pediatrics recommends routine hepatitis B vaccination of infants.
See text for additional information on varicella vaccine.

offices that have no "sick child" waiting area, the child is immediately placed in an examination room and the physician is notified. Some physicians prefer to have a telephone staff person obtain symptoms, body temperature information, and other pertinent information over the telephone, along with a telephone number where the parent can be reached. The physician reviews the information and calls the parent back to discus the situation.

ETIOLOGY
The causative organism is the varicella-zoster virus (VZV), a member of the herpes virus group. The virus is transmitted by direct or indirect droplet nuclei spread from the respiratory tract of the infected person or a carrier. Fluid from the cutaneous lesions is also infectious, but dried crusty lesions are not contagious. The patient is considered contagious for 1 to 2 days before the erup-

tions until about 6 days after the eruptions. The incubation period is 2 to 3 weeks.

DIAGNOSIS
Chickenpox usually is diagnosed via the history of exposure and the presence of characteristic cutaneous eruptions. Although laboratory testing is not usually necessary, the VZV can be visualized when a culture of vesicular fluid is examined microscopically. After the infection, antibodies are found in the serum.

TREATMENT
• Palliative treatment to alleviate *pruritus* includes cool bicarbonate of soda baths followed by a cornstarch dusting or the application of calamine lotion. This helps to control scratching that can lead to secondary infection and scarring. Other comfort measures include the administration of aceta-

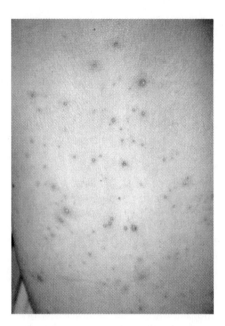

FIGURE 2–30 Chickenpox (varicella). (From Hill MJ: *Skin disorders—Mosby's clinical nursing series,* St. Louis, 1994, Mosby.)

minophen for fever and pain. ***Caution:*** Aspirin is *not* given to children with chickenpox because of the risk of Reye syndrome. The patient must be isolated until all lesions have crusted.

PROGNOSIS

Prognosis is good for recovery from chicken pox. The patient may have scarring from eruptions. Individuals who have had chickenpox are at risk of developing herpes zoster (shingles) later in life.

PREVENTION

A varicella virus vaccine (Varivax) is available for protection against chickenpox. For children, a single injection of the vaccine at 1 to 12 years of age is recommended. For adolescents and adults, a second dose is administered 4 to 8 weeks after the first dose. The need for booster doses has not been defined because the duration of protection of varicella vaccine currently is unknown.

Patients who are immunocompromised or otherwise at high risk can be given the varicella-zoster immune globulin within 4 days of exposure.

PATIENT TEACHING

Reinforce the need for good hand washing along with the use of tissues during coughing or sneezing episodes and the proper handling and disposal of soiled tissues. Encourage parents to minimize contact these children may have with others during the contagious period, which is 1 to 2 days before the eruptions until about 6 days after the eruptions.

Diphtheria

DESCRIPTION

Diphtheria is an acute communicable disease that causes necrosis of the mucous membrane in the respiratory tract.

ICD-9-CM Code 032.9 *(Unspecified)*
Refer to the physician's diagnosis and then to the current edition of the ICD-9-CM coding manual to ensure the greatest specificity of pathology and any appropriate modifiers.

SYMPTOMS AND SIGNS

The patient, most often a child, has sore throat, *dysphagia,* a cough, hoarseness, and chills. Fever, swollen regional lymph nodes, and foul breath can be noted. As the bacteria invade the nasopharynx, they multiply and produce a powerful *exotoxin* that travels in the blood throughout the body. Locally, the infection and inflammation cause grayish patches of thick mucous membrane to appear along the respiratory tract known as pseudomembrane, or false membrane. The membrane, which can be extensive, is composed of bacteria, inflammatory cells, dead tissue, and *fibrin;* it is surrounded by inflammation and swelling that can interfere with the airway, impairing swallowing and speech. As the toxin is absorbed, it affects other vital organ systems, with many possible complications, including otitis media, pneumonia, myocarditis, and paralysis.

Carriers, although infected, remain asymptomatic and do not contract active infection themselves.

PATIENT SCREENING

Children with fever, chills, and respiratory difficulties require prompt assessment. When a parent reports a child with respiratory difficulties, most protocol recommends the child be seen in an emergency facility.

Infectious Diseases

ETIOLOGY

The causative bacteria, *Corynebacterium diphtheriae*, is present in the nasopharynx of infected people or carriers and is transmitted by airborne respiratory droplets. The incubation period is 2 to 5 days. The patient is contagious for 2 to 4 weeks if untreated or for 1 to 2 days after initiating antibiotic treatment. Carriers of the disease remain asymptomatic but can infect the inadequately immunized individual.

DIAGNOSIS

The presence of the characteristic membrane adhering to the throat is diagnostic. Culture of the throat and laboratory stains are positive for *C. diphtheriae,* and antibodies are found in the serum. Immunity or susceptibility can be determined by the *Schick test.*

TREATMENT

Diphtheria antitoxin is given as soon as possible. The administration of antibiotics, such as penicillin and erythromycin, is indicated to kill the organism. The patient is isolated, restricted to bed rest, and given a diet as tolerated. The patient is observed for the possible complications related to systemic involvement. Carriers are given antibiotics to eliminate the organisms from their respiratory tract.

PROGNOSIS

With prompt intervention and completion of antibiotic drug therapy, the prognosis is good.

PREVENTION

Diphtheria, once common in North America and Europe, can be prevented by the administration of diphtheria toxoid to produce active immunity. Inoculation begins at 2 to 3 months, with booster doses given at appropriate intervals during childhood.

PATIENT TEACHING

Reinforce the need for good hand washing and the use of tissues during coughing or sneezing episodes. Instruct on the handling and disposal of soiled tissues. Encourage parents to minimize contact these children may have with others during the contagious period, which continues for 1 to 2 days after starting antibiotic therapy. Emphasize the importance of routine immunizations for children.

Mumps (Epidemic Parotitis)

DESCRIPTION

Mumps is an acute communicable disease causing inflammation and swelling of one or both parotid glands.

 ICD-9-CM Code 072.9 *(Without mention of complications)*
Refer to the physician's diagnosis and then to the current edition of the ICD-9-CM coding manual to ensure the greatest specificity of pathology and any appropriate modifiers.

SYMPTOMS AND SIGNS

The patient, usually a child, has tenderness in the neck in front of and below the ears in the region of the parotid glands and pain on swallowing (Fig. 2–31). Patients also may experience a headache and a low-grade fever, with loss of appetite and an earache that is aggravated by chewing. A common complication of the disease in the adult male is mumps *orchitis,* which may lead to sterility. Often, the infection is a subclinical illness without noticeable symptoms.

PATIENT SCREENING

Contagious diseases present a challenge in the patient-screening process. Many physicians prefer not to have the contagious patient in the reception area. When the parents feel an office visit is warranted,

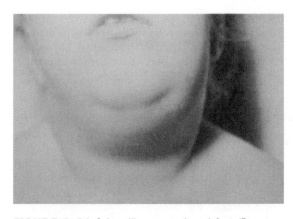

FIGURE 2–31 Submaxillary mumps in an infant. (From Grimes D: *Infectious diseases—Mosby's clinical nursing series,* St. Louis, 1991, Mosby.)

the child is immediately placed in an examination room, and the physician is notified. Some physicians prefer to have a telephone staff person obtain symptoms, body temperature information, and other pertinent information over the telephone, along with a telephone number where the parent can be reached. The physician reviews the information and either calls the parent back or has the telephone staff person call the parent back with instructions for care.

ETIOLOGY

The causative agent of mumps is an airborne virus that is spread by droplet nuclei from the respiratory tract. The incubation period is long, usually 14 to 21 days. The patient is contagious for 1 to 7 days before the swelling of the parotid glands and up to 9 days thereafter. Lifelong immunity develops after a clinical or subclinical infection; active immunization with the mumps vaccine also affords prolonged immunity.

DIAGNOSIS

Diagnosis is made from a history of exposure and a clinical picture that includes swelling of the parotid glands. The male patient is assessed for tenderness of the testes.

TREATMENT

Acetaminophen is given, and warm or cold compresses are applied for pain. A soft or liquid diet can help to minimize discomfort when eating. The male patient who is experiencing testicular tenderness and swelling may need scrotal support.

PROGNOSIS

Most children recover from mumps; however, meningitis and encephalitis are possible complications of mumps.

PREVENTION

Childhood immunization is the best prevention. An unimmunized person should be referred to a physician for active immunization within 48 hours of contact to prevent or alter the severity of the disease. Good hand washing and proper handling of soiled tissue helps prevent the spread of the disease among family members and other contacts.

PATIENT TEACHING

Reinforce the need for good hand washing and proper handling and disposal of soiled tissues.

Discuss the airborne viruses responsible for mumps and discuss the means of preventing the spread of the disease. Emphasize the importance of routine immunizations for children.

Pertussis (Whooping Cough)

DESCRIPTION

Whooping cough is a highly contagious bacterial infection of the respiratory tract.

 ICD-9-CM Code 033.9 *(Unspecified organism)*

SYMPTOMS AND SIGNS

The disease has three stages: (1) the highly contagious catarrhal stage, when the child seems to have a common cold; (2) the paroxysmal stage, when the cough becomes violent, ending in a high-pitched inspiratory whoop, often followed by vomiting of thick mucus; and (3) a convalescent period, when the cough gradually diminishes.

PATIENT SCREENING

A child exhibiting symptoms of violent coughing with high-pitched inspiratory whoop and vomiting of thick mucus requires prompt attention.

ETIOLOGY

The pertussis bacillus *Bordetella pertussis* reproduces in the respiratory tract, where it releases a toxin that leads to *necrosis* of the mucosa with a thick exudate. It is transmitted by droplet nuclei spread via direct or indirect contact with nasopharyngeal secretions of the contagious patient.

DIAGNOSIS

Bacterial studies of nasopharyngeal mucus are positive for the pertussis bacillus. The patient's white blood cell (WBC) count usually is elevated.

TREATMENT

Erythromycin is the antibiotic of choice for treatment. Fluid intake is encouraged to prevent dehydration. A nutritious diet is important to prevent weight loss. Quiet and rest are required because the episodes of prolonged coughing cause exhaustion and weakness. The patient should be observed closely for respiratory distress. Bronchopneumonia, convulsions, or hemorrhages are possible complications of severe disease.

PROGNOSIS

With prompt intervention, hydration monitoring and maintenance, and antibiotic therapy, the prognosis is good. However, when untreated, pertussis can be fatal.

PREVENTION

Pertussis can be prevented by immunization with the pertussis vaccine. Childhood immunization is the best prevention. Good hand washing and proper handling of soiled tissue helps prevent the spread of the disease among family members and other contacts. Emphasize the importance of routine immunizations for children.

PATIENT TEACHING

Reinforce the necessity of good hand washing and proper handling and disposal of soiled tissues. Discuss the airborne microbe responsible for pertussis, and discuss methods of preventing airborne spread of the disease. Emphasize the importance of routine immunizations for children.

Measles (Rubeola)

DESCRIPTION

Measles is an acute, highly contagious viral disease occurring in children who have not been vaccinated.

 ICD-9-CM Code 055.9 *(Without mention of complications)*

SYMPTOMS AND SIGNS

Early symptoms include coldlike symptoms, tracheobronchitis, conjunctivitis, and *photophobia*. The child has a fever, followed in 3 to 7 days by a red blotchy rash. The rash starts behind the ears, hairline, and forehead and then progresses down the body (Fig. 2–32). Before the eruption of the rash, Koplik spots can be detected on the oral mucosa as tiny white spots on a red background (Fig. 2–33).

PATIENT SCREENING

Contagious diseases present a challenge in the patient-screening process. Many physicians prefer not to have the contagious patient in the reception area. When the parents feel an office visit is warranted, the child is immediately placed in an examination room and the physician is notified. Some physicians prefer to have a telephone staff

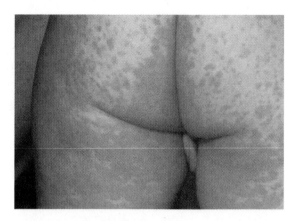

FIGURE 2–32 Rubeola (measles) rash on the third day. (From Grimes D: *Infectious diseases—Mosby's clinical nursing series,* St. Louis, 1991, Mosby.)

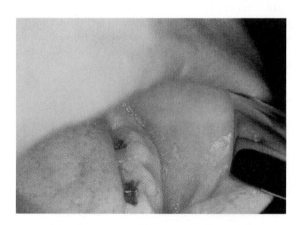

FIGURE 2–33 Koplik spots on the buccal mucosa 3 days before eruption of rubeola (measles) rash. (From Grimes D: *Infectious diseases—Mosby's clinical nursing series,* St. Louis, 1991, Mosby.)

person obtain symptoms, body temperature information, other pertinent information, and a telephone number over the telephone. The physician reviews the information and either calls the parent back or has the telephone staff person call the parent back with instructions for care.

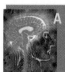

ALERT

SUBACUTE SCLEROSING PANENCEPHALITIS

Parents are encouraged to have their children immunized against measles.

Subacute sclerosing panencephalitis (SSPE), an infectious condition of the CNS, is considered a rare disorder and, as such, is listed in the National Organization for Rare Disorders, Inc (NORD). SSPE, one of three forms of encephalitis occurring secondary to measles virus, evolves after the dormant measles virus is reactivated. Symptoms of this progressive neurologic disorder emerge with an insidious onset and are identified by progressive motor and mental or intellectual deterioration, including personality changes, and neurologic deterioration subsequently resulting in severe dementia. Seizures, blindness, and fever are additional symptoms. Motor involvement leads to periodic involuntary movements and eventual decerebrate rigidity. The patient usually is 5 to 20 years of age and has experienced an attack of measles in the prior 2 to 10 years. The onset of this inappropriate immune response occasionally follows measles immunization.

The reactivation of the latent measles virus causes a cerebral infection. This infectious process causes atrophy of the cortical areas of the brain, demyelination of the nerves, or ventricular dilation. The brain tissue is diffusely inflamed.

SSPE is diagnosed from symptoms and a history of previous occurrence of measles or recent measles immunization. CSF shows elevated gamma globulin levels. The antibody titer is elevated indicating presence of measles virus antibodies.

There is no effective therapy or cure for SSPE. The treatment includes supportive measures, including drug therapy for seizure control. The duration of this disorder is several years, with progressive deterioration of the CNS. The patient usually is nonresponsive and unable to care for him- or herself for a period of time before ultimate death.

The mother of a young English singer who was afflicted by this rare disorder at the age of 18 years urges all parents to have their children immunized against measles, in the hope of preventing the condition that left her daughter blind and unable to speak. The daughter died 14 years after the onset of SSPE.

ETIOLOGY

The causative agent of measles is the measles virus. The infection is airborne, spread by direct contact with secretions from the nose or throat. The patient is contagious from about 4 days before the onset of the rash until about 4 days after the onset. The incubation period is 8 to 12 days after exposure.

DIAGNOSIS

Diagnosis is based on a history of exposure and the clinical picture, which includes the rash and the presence of Koplik spots on the oral mucosa.

TREATMENT

Uncomplicated measles runs its course in 7 to 10 days. Acetaminophen is given to treat the fever. If the fever is persistently high, tepid sponge baths may be given. The eyes may be protected from bright light as a comfort measure. If secondary infection occurs, antibiotics are prescribed to treat the infection. Pneumonia, otitis media, conjunctivitis, and encephalitis are complications of measles.

PROGNOSIS

The prognosis for uncomplicated measles is good. The complications of measles include pneumonia, otitis media, conjunctivitis, and encephalitis.

PREVENTION

Inoculation with the live measles vaccine is given during childhood to protect the individual and prevent epidemics of the disease. Measles immune globulin given 5 days after exposure to the disease creates passive immunity in unimmunized individuals at high risk. An attack of the disease usually creates immunity for life.

PATIENT TEACHING

Reinforce the necessity of good hand washing and proper handling and disposal of soiled tissues. Discuss the airborne microbe responsible for measles, and discuss methods of preventing airborne spread of the disease. Emphasize the importance of routine immunizations for children.

Infectious Diseases

Rubella (German Measles, Three-Day Measles)

DESCRIPTION
Rubella, a highly contagious viral disease, resembles measles clinically, but it has a shorter course and fewer complications.

■ **ICD-9-CM Code** **056.9** *(Without mention of complications)*

SYMPTOMS AND SIGNS
In this viral disease, the child has a rose-colored, slightly elevated rash that appears first on the face and head and then progresses downward on the body (Fig. 2–34). In addition, the child has a low-grade fever and can have tenderness and enlargement of the lymph nodes. Complications include a transient arthritis, myocarditis, and hemorrhagic manifestations.

Rubella causes great danger to the unborn children of pregnant women who contract the disease.

PATIENT SCREENING
Contagious diseases present a challenge in the patient-screening process. Many physicians prefer not to have the contagious patient in the reception area. When the parents feel an office visit is warranted, the child is immediately placed in an examination room and the physician is notified.

ETIOLOGY
The causative agent is the rubella virus, which is spread by direct contact with nasal or oral secretions. The incubation period after exposure is 14 to 21 days. The patient is contagious from 1 week before eruption of the rash until 1 week after the onset of rash. Although rubella is preventable through immunization, sporadic epidemics still arise, often on college campuses.

DIAGNOSIS
Diagnosis is made from a history of exposure and the clinical picture, including the rash. Because rubella resembles other diseases, a definitive diag-

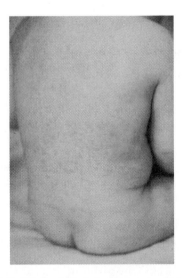

FIGURE 2-34 Acquired rubella (German measles) in 11-month-old infant. (From Grimes D: *Infectious diseases—Mosby's clinical nursing series,* St. Louis, 1991, Mosby.)

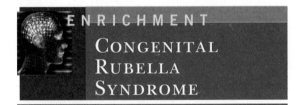

ENRICHMENT

CONGENITAL RUBELLA SYNDROME

WOMEN OF CHILDBEARING AGE who have not been immunized against rubella or who have not had the disease can transmit rubella to their infant if they become infected during pregnancy. When the virus is transferred to the fetus during the first trimester of pregnancy, a variety of congenital deformities, known as congenital rubella syndrome, occur in about 25% of births. The risk is lower if infection occurs later in pregnancy. Anomalies caused by congenital rubella syndrome include congenital cardiac disease, blindness, deafness, and mental retardation.

Pregnant women should be isolated from individuals infected with rubella to prevent perinatal infection; in addition, pregnant women must not be given the rubella vaccine. The best protection against congenital rubella syndrome is universal routine immunization with live rubella vaccine during infancy or as soon as possible in adulthood (Fig. 2–35).

Rubella causes great danger to the unborn children of pregnant women who contract the disease.

nosis includes a throat culture for the rubella virus and serologic studies to detect antibodies.

TREATMENT

Treatment consists of supportive measures, including the administration of a mild analgesic for fever and joint pain. The patient is isolated until the rash disappears.

PROGNOSIS

The prognosis is good. (Refer to the Enrichment box on Congenital Rubella Syndrome.)

PREVENTION

Active immunity conferred by the rubella vaccine in a patient older than 12 months prevents the disease.

PATIENT TEACHING

Reinforce the need for good hand washing and proper handling and disposal of soiled tissues. Discuss the microbe responsible for rubella, and discuss methods of preventing the spread of the disease via nasal and mucous routes. Emphasize the importance of routine immunizations for children.

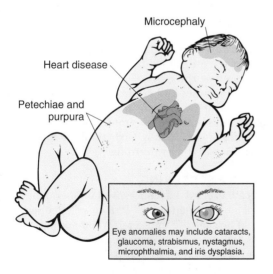

Microcephaly

Heart disease

Petechiae and purpura

Eye anomalies may include cataracts, glaucoma, strabismus, nystagmus, microphthalmia, and iris dysplasia.

FIGURE 2–35 Congenital rubella syndrome. (From Damjanov I: *Pathology for the health-related professions,* ed 2, Philadelphia, 2000, Saunders.)

Tetanus

DESCRIPTION

Tetanus is an acute, potentially deadly, systemic infection characterized by painful involuntary contraction of skeletal muscles.

 ICD-9-CM Code 037

SYMPTOMS AND SIGNS

The patient is extremely febrile (temperature greater than 101° F), is irritable, and sweats profusely. He or she has a stiff neck, a tight jaw (lockjaw), spasms of the facial muscles, and difficulty in swallowing. As the infection progresses, the muscles of the back and abdomen become rigid, with generalized convulsive muscle spasm (opisthotonos). These tonic spasms may cause death from asphyxiation.

PATIENT SCREENING

Patients who have experienced a soft-tissue wound, including animal bites, punctures from nails, burns, and abrasions, should be assessed for tetanus prophylaxis and instructed about the importance of receiving the "tetanus shot." Patients experiencing high fever, irritability, and profuse perspiration accompanied by stiff neck, a tight jaw (lockjaw), spasms of the facial muscles, and difficulty in swallowing require immediate assessment and intervention.

ETIOLOGY

The bacillus *Clostridium tetani* is found in contaminated soil and animal excreta and enters the skin through a puncture wound, laceration, abrasion, burn, or other injury. Puncture wounds are excellent breeding grounds for the bacillus because they lack a good oxygen supply and the bacillus thrives in dead tissue, producing a powerful exotoxin that attacks the nervous system. The incubation period is 3 to 21 days, with the onset commonly occurring at about 8 days. Tetanus antitoxin immunizations followed by booster doses every 10 years create immunity.

DIAGNOSIS

The patient's history may indicate inadequate immunization. The patient is fiercely ill as described previously. Laboratory test results do not always produce conclusive data for diagnosis.

Respiratory Diseases

TREATMENT

The medical management is chiefly supportive, with the administration of sedatives and muscle relaxants to relieve spasms and seizures; a quiet, dark environment promotes rest. If the patient suffers convulsions, respiratory integrity must be preserved.

The unimmunized patient at risk is given human tetanus immune globulin (TIG) within 72 hours of injury for temporary immunity. A booster injection of tetanus toxoid is needed if the injured person has not had tetanus immunization within 5 years.

PROGNOSIS

Tetanus carries a 35% mortality rate, so prevention is important.

PREVENTION

The best course is childhood immunizations, timely booster doses, and prompt cleaning of wounds with hydrogen peroxide.

PATIENT TEACHING

Encourage and stress the importance of tetanus booster immunizations. Cleansing of soft-tissue injuries also should be stressed.

Influenza

Influenza is an acute, highly contagious viral infection of the respiratory tract. Its highest incidence is in school children, and it is more severe in young children. Influenza occurs sporadically or as an epidemic and is transmitted by droplet nuclei or direct contact with moist secretions. Children tend to have high fevers with influenza and are susceptible to pulmonary complications and Reye syndrome. Because of the latter, acetaminophen, and *not* aspirin, is given to children and adolescents for fever and pain. A full description of influenza can be found in Chapter 9.

Common Cold

Young children have several colds a year, and most colds are self-limiting and run their course in 4 to 5 days. In infants, the nasal congestion can cause difficulty with eating and breathing. Supportive treatment consists of rest, increased fluid intake, and diet as tolerated. The possibility of secondary bacterial infection or extension of the infection into the lower respiratory tract or into the middle ear is potentially dangerous for the child. These complications warrant antibiotic therapy. For a complete discussion of the common cold, see Chapter 9.

Respiratory Diseases

Sudden Infant Death Syndrome

DESCRIPTION

Sudden infant death syndrome is the sudden and unpredicted death of an infant under the age of 1 year.

 ICD-9-CM Code   **798.0**

SYMPTOMS AND SIGNS

Sudden infant death syndrome (SIDS), formerly called crib death, is defined officially as the sudden death of an infant under the age of 1 year for which a cause cannot be established. It is the number-one cause of death among infants from 1 to 12 months of age; 1 in 500 infants dies mysteriously during the first year of life. Death occurs within seconds during sleep and without sound or struggle, and the baby does not suffer. Most SIDS infants appeared healthy before death. When found, the dead infant may have a mottled complexion and cyanotic lips and fingertips. There is often a trace of blood-tinged fluid coming from the mouth or the nose.

Known causes and contributing factors for the sudden death of an infant are ruled out. These may include an immature respiratory control system, a susceptibility to deadly arrhythmias, congenital heart disease, and myocarditis.

PATIENT SCREENING

Any call received that concerns an infant not breathing is an emergency, and 911 emergency services should be called to the scene. When an infant dies, the situation usually becomes a coroner's case and an autopsy is ordered. The parent desiring an appointment for a near-miss SIDS infant should be seen as soon as possible. Adequate information should be obtained to determine whether the situation is an emergency and whether the child needs to be entered into the emergency care system or can be seen in the office. If the parent of a child who has died of diagnosed SIDS calls for an appointment, remember the magnitude of the situation and schedule as soon as possible. During the entire process, remaining nonjudgmental is important.

ETIOLOGY

Although there are many theories and much misinformation about SIDS, the exact cause is uncertain. Research studies and autopsies point to certain pathologic findings in some SIDS infants that suggest more than one cause. Many maternal and infant risk factors are known: mother's age less than 20 years, poor prenatal care, smoking and drug abuse during pregnancy, prematurity, recent upper respiratory tract infection in the infant, and a sibling with apnea. The incidence is higher in males and during the winter months.

DIAGNOSIS

A complete postmortem investigation, including autopsy, a review of the child's medical history, and examination of the scene of death, fails to identify the cause of death.

TREATMENT

Resuscitation attempts fail. At this time, SIDS is not predictable or preventable. The American Academy of Pediatrics has added sleeping in the prone position to the list of risk factors. To reduce that risk, the academy recommends placing babies in bed on their sides or their backs instead of on their stomachs. A home apnea machine and cardiac monitor may be recommended during the age of peak vulnerability.

PROGNOSIS

Infants with near-miss SIDS are at risk for additional episodes and are placed on apnea monitors, usually until the age of 2 years. Parents who have had an infant die from SIDS are at higher risk of having another infant die of SIDS than those who have not. Subsequent children are placed on apnea monitors.

PREVENTION

Recent studies have isolated risk factors for SIDS. Although these risk factors may play a role in SIDS, parents must understand that by themselves these factors do not cause SIDS.

As previously mentioned, a supine sleeping position carries the lowest risk for SIDS. Exposure to cigarette smoke should be avoided. Firm bedding materials in a safety-approved crib are prudent. Research shows that overheating an infant by dressing in excessive clothing, especially during illness, is to be avoided. Other important factors include good prenatal care and breastfeeding. Breastfeeding is a source of immunity to the newborn infant.

PATIENT TEACHING

Survivors of SIDS should be offered sensitive interventions to help them to deal with the grief and possible feelings of guilt and anger. The Sudden Infant Death Syndrome Alliance is a national voluntary organization in the United States dedicated to eliminating SIDS through medical research. Help families find and contact SIDS support groups.

Croup

DESCRIPTION

Croup is an acute, severe inflammation and obstruction of the respiratory tract.

 ICD-9-CM Code 464.4

SYMPTOMS AND SIGNS

It usually is preceded by an upper-respiratory-tract infection. The symptoms include hoarseness, fever, a harsh, high-pitched cough, and **stridor** during inspiration caused by narrowing of the upper airways. The child may be anxious and frightened by the respiratory distress.

PATIENT SCREENING

Children experiencing signs and symptoms of respiratory distress, including hoarseness, fever, a harsh, high-pitched cough, and stridor during inspiration, require prompt, if not immediate, assessment and intervention.

ETIOLOGY

Croup is usually a viral disease that involves the larynx, trachea, and bronchi. The clinical manifestations are caused by edema and spasm of the vocal cords, creating varying degrees of obstruction (Fig. 2–36, *B*).

DIAGNOSIS

Croup must be distinguished from epiglottitis. If necessary, blood or throat cultures may be performed

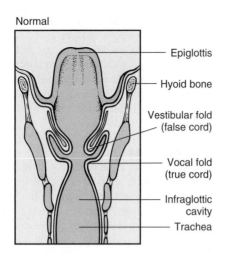

Normal
- Epiglottis
- Hyoid bone
- Vestibular fold (false cord)
- Vocal fold (true cord)
- Infraglottic cavity
- Trachea

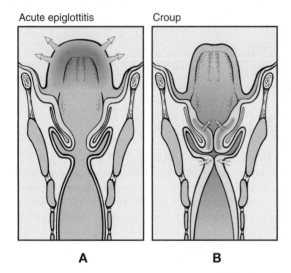

Acute epiglottitis   Croup

A   **B**

FIGURE 2–36 Acute inflammation of the larynx. **A,** Inflammation localized to the epiglottis (so-called acute epiglottitis). **B,** Inflammation of the entire larynx, causing diffuse laryngeal swelling and laryngospasm (croup). (From Damjanov I: *Pathology for the health-related professions,* ed 2, Philadelphia, 2000, Saunders.)

to identify certain bacterial causes. Laryngoscopy may be performed.

TREATMENT

The patient is treated symptomatically, with the administration of *antipyretic* agents, rest, increased fluid intake, cool humidification of air, and, if the cause is bacterial, antibiotic therapy. In severe cases, the patient is hospitalized for endotracheal intubation and oxygen therapy until the respiratory crisis passes. In most instances, the illness subsides in 3 to 4 days.

PROGNOSIS

The prognosis is good with prompt intervention. The child is likely to experience recurrences of the condition.

PREVENTION

Because croup is a viral disease, the only prevention is through avoidance of contact with respiratory viruses. Replace toothbrushes regularly and after any infectious process.

PATIENT TEACHING

Instruct the parents *not* to place anything in the child's mouth until the child is assessed by a health-care professional and the condition is determined not to be epiglottitis. Additional teaching includes instruction on handling and disposal of soiled tissues and the importance of good handwashing.

Epiglottitis

DESCRIPTION

Epiglottitis is an inflammation of the epiglottis, the thin, leaf-shaped structure that covers the entrance of the larynx during swallowing.

■ ICD-9-CM Code **464.30** *(Acute)*
              464.31 *(With obstruction)*
              476.1 *(Chronic)*

SYMPTOMS AND SIGNS

Epiglottitis typically strikes children between ages 3 and 7 years. The symptoms include a sore throat, croupy cough, fever, and respiratory distress caused by laryngeal obstruction. Visual inspection reveals a red and swollen epiglottis. Rapidly increasing dyspnea and drooling are the most significant signs of a critical respiratory emergency (see Fig. 2–36, *A*).

PATIENT SCREENING

Children experiencing any form of respiratory distress require immediate assessment and intervention. Instruct the parents *not* to place anything in the child's mouth until the child is assessed by a health-care professional.

ETIOLOGY

Epiglottitis may follow an upper-respiratory-tract infection. The most common cause is *Haemophilus influenzae* type B bacteria.

DIAGNOSIS

Radiographic films of the neck may reveal the enlarged epiglottis. If the obstruction is not significant, the throat is examined to inspect the epiglottis. Nothing is placed in the child's mouth until a health-care professional with the capability, equipment, and supplies needed to perform endotracheal intubation and tracheostomy is present.

TREATMENT

If the airway is obstructed, the child is hospitalized and given intensive care. The airway is established with tracheostomy or endotracheal intubation. Antibiotics, usually ampicillin, are given parenterally, and the patient is closely monitored.

PROGNOSIS

Prompt treatment affords a good prognosis.

PREVENTION

The American Academy of Pediatrics recommends that all children receive the *Haemophilus* B conjugate vaccine. Replace toothbrushes regularly and after any infectious processes.

PATIENT TEACHING

Instruct the parents *not* to place anything in the child's mouth until the child is assessed by a health-care professional. Additional teaching includes instruction in the handling and disposal of soiled tissues and the importance of good handwashing. Reinforce the recommendation for immunization with the *Haemophilus* B conjugate vaccine.

Acute Tonsillitis

DESCRIPTION

Acute tonsillitis is a painful inflammatory and infectious process affecting the tonsils.

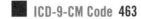 ICD-9-CM Code **463**

SYMPTOMS AND SIGNS

Tonsillitis, or inflammation of the tonsils, usually has a sudden onset. The patient has a mild to severe sore throat, chills, fever, headache, malaise, *anorexia,* and muscle and joint pain. The tonsils

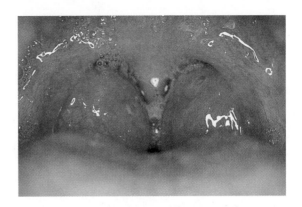

FIGURE 2–37 Acute tonsillitis. The tonsils are swollen and acutely inflamed, almost meeting in the middle. (From Stevens A, Lowe J: *Pathology: illustrated review in color,* ed 2, London, 2000, Mosby.)

appear inflamed and swollen, with yellowish exudate projecting from crypts. Lymph glands in the submandibular area are tender and enlarged (Fig. 2–37).

PATIENT SCREENING

The individual with pain, fever, and sore throat of sudden onset requires prompt assessment, with a culture and sensitivity test of the exudate obtained to determine the causative agent.

ETIOLOGY

Tonsillitis is caused by many organisms, with group A beta-hemolytic streptococci the most common cause.

DIAGNOSIS

The throat is examined, and a throat culture is performed to identify the causative organism. The WBC count may be elevated in response to the infection.

TREATMENT

When the throat culture is positive for streptococci, a full 10-day course of penicillin is given. This strict regimen is necessary to prevent rheumatic fever, rheumatic heart disease, and kidney complications. The child is placed on bed rest, is given a liquid diet, and is given saline throat irrigations. Tonsillectomy may be recommended for chronic tonsillitis or peritonsillar abscess.

PROGNOSIS

The prognosis is good with drug therapy. Surgery may be the option for chronic tonsillitis or peritonsillar abscess. Recovery from the surgical procedure usually is uneventful.

PREVENTION

As with any infectious process, good hand washing and proper handling and disposal of tissue helps to prevent exposure to microbes. Replace toothbrushes at least every 3 months or after any infectious processes.

PATIENT TEACHING

Teach the patient and family about the importance of hydration during illness. In addition, emphasize the importance of completing the entire recommended regimen of antibiotic therapy. Sharing of drinking glasses and eating utensils should be discouraged, and old toothbrushes should be replaced.

Adenoid Hyperplasia

DESCRIPTION

Adenoid hyperplasia is an abnormal enlargement of the lymphoid tissue located in the space above the soft palate of the mouth, causing partial breathing blockage, especially in children.

> ■ **ICD-9-CM Code** **474.12** *(Requires an extra digit modifier)*
> *Refer to the physician's diagnosis and then to the current edition of the ICD-9-CM coding manual to ensure the greatest specificity of pathology and any appropriate modifiers.*

SYMPTOMS AND SIGNS

Adenoids (and tonsils) are present at birth and play a role in the formation of immunoglobulins. After puberty, they normally atrophy.

Adenoid hyperplasia can contribute to recurrent otitis media and conductive hearing loss resulting from obstruction of the eustachian tube. The child is usually a mouth breather and snores during sleep. The child's speech has a nasal quality.

PATIENT SCREENING

Mouth breathing children who snore should be evaluated for adenoid enlargement. Schedule for an assessment.

ETIOLOGY

The cause of adenoid hyperplasia is unknown. Contributing factors include repeated infection, chronic allergies, and heredity.

DIAGNOSIS

The abnormal enlargement may be visualized on lateral pharyngeal radiographic films or with nasopharyngoscopic examination.

TREATMENT

Adenoidectomy is indicated for obstructive adenoids with recurrent otitis media or chronic serous otitis media with conductive hearing loss.

PROGNOSIS

Surgical removal of the adenoids usually corrects the condition.

PREVENTION

No prevention is known.

PATIENT TEACHING

Instruct the patient and family about the importance of hydration during illness. Teach comfort measures and routine postoperative care when adenoids have been removed.

Asthma

DESCRIPTION

Asthma is a chronic disease caused by increased reactivity of the tracheobronchial tree to various stimuli. It is a leading cause of chronic illness and school absenteeism in children.

> ■ **ICD-9-CM Code** **493.90**
> **493.20** *(Chronic asthma)*
> *Refer to the physician's diagnosis and then to the current edition of the ICD-9-CM coding manual to ensure the greatest specificity of pathology and any appropriate modifiers. Coding is done by extent of inflammation and type.*

SYMPTOMS AND SIGNS

The child presents with an incessant productive or nonproductive cough, a pronounced expiratory wheeze, and rapid shallow respirations. The labored breathing results in a rapid pulse, pallor, profuse perspiration, and an inability to speak more than a few words without halting to breathe. The patient often is anxious, is exhausted, and reports a "tight chest." The examining physician hears diminished breath sounds with wheezes and rhonchi in the lungs. The bronchial spasms trap air and thick mucus in the lungs. An asthmatic episode (Fig. 2–38) can be mild to severe, can last minutes or days, and may become a medical emergency. The attack may or may not have been preceded by a respiratory infection (Fig. 2–39).

PATIENT SCREENING

Asthmatic patients present an alarming situation. A possible respiratory compromise requires prompt assessment and intervention.

ETIOLOGY

A hereditary factor is strongly associated with the disease. Asthma is the result of "twitchy," or hyperactive and hypersensitive, bronchial tubes. The bronchial spasms of asthma can be triggered by many extrinsic (allergic) or intrinsic (nonallergic) factors, including stress, heavy exercise, infection, and inhalation of allergens or other substances. Allergens may include pollen, cockroaches and their excrement, molds, household dust mites, and pet dander. Additional "triggers" include air pollutants and irritants (perfumes, colognes, and aftershaves), smoke and second-hand smoke, cold air, emotional upsets, and exercise.

DIAGNOSIS

The best tool available to reveal the degree of airway obstruction is the pulmonary function test. However, this test may be normal between attacks. Radiographic chest films may show hyperinflation and changes in the lungs associated with mucous plugging. Specialists may order intradermal skin testing to identify inhalant and food allergies. Blood tests include a complete blood

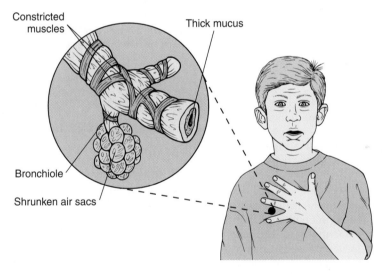

Constricted muscles — Thick mucus — Bronchiole — Shrunken air sacs

Symptoms
• Shortness of breath
• Wheezing
• Difficult breathing
• Cough
• Anxiety

Physical findings
• Rapid, shallow respirations
• Rapid pulse
• Pallor or cyanosis
• Diminished breath sounds
• Generalized retractions
• Frequent pausing to catch the breath when talking
• Hyperexpansion of the chest

FIGURE 2–38 An asthma attack with respiratory distress.

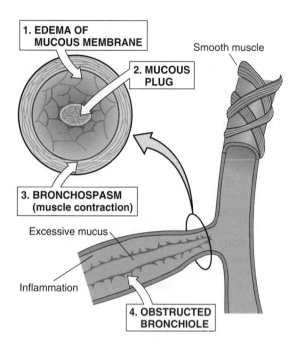

1. EDEMA OF MUCOUS MEMBRANE

Smooth muscle

2. MUCOUS PLUG

3. BRONCHOSPASM (muscle contraction)

Excessive mucus

Inflammation

4. OBSTRUCTED BRONCHIOLE

FIGURE 2-39 Asthma—acute episode. (From Gould BE: *Pathophysiology for the health professions,* ed 2, Philadelphia, 2002, Saunders.)

count (CBC) with differential leukocyte count, which may show an increased eosinophil count and elevated serum immunoglobulin E (IgE) levels.

TREATMENT

Many individuals with chronic asthma require medical management under the care of an expert. Strict compliance with a regimen of medications to relax and widen the bronchi and to release excessive mucus is important. Some of the drugs used are cromolyn sodium, albuterol, theophylline, and aerosol corticosteroids. Allergy evaluation and skin testing may indicate immunotherapy by desensitization injections, commonly called allergy shots. Avoiding infection, known allergens, and other triggers is strongly advised.

Severe acute asthma attacks are treated with injections of epinephrine and inhalation therapy. In a severe attack unresponsive to drug therapy, a condition called status asthmaticus may lead to fatal respiratory failure. The patient requires hospitalization for aggressive medical treatment and follow-up.

PROGNOSIS

The prognosis varies depending on the extent of the asthmatic attack as well as the causative factor. The use of prophylactic medications helps. Medication inhalers should be kept readily available at all times. Allergy testing may reveal the irritant, and allergy serum injections may help to alleviate or reduce the severity of the attack. As previously mentioned, unresponsive asthma, status asthmaticus, may result in death.

Prompt medical intervention is necessary when an attack cannot be resolved by usual and available methods.

PREVENTION

Avoiding the stimulating allergens may help to reduce the incidence and severity of the attacks. Injections of appropriate serum also may help prevent attacks.

PATIENT TEACHING

Encourage patients to use prophylactic medications and to avoid known triggering allergens. Teach caretakers the importance of seeking medical help when an attack does not resolve quickly with normal intervention.

Gastrointestinal Disorders

Infantile Colic

DESCRIPTION

Colic is intermittent abdominal distress in the newborn or during early infancy.

ICD-9-CM Code **789.00** *(Requires extra digits for greatest specificity)*
Refer to the physician's diagnosis and then to the current edition of the ICD-9-CM coding manual to ensure the greatest specificity of pathology and any appropriate modifiers.

SYMPTOMS AND SIGNS

The infant intermittently draws up the legs, clenches the fists, and cries as if in pain. During the episode, the infant may pass gas by mouth and rectum. The episodes of colic are likely to occur in the late afternoon and evening. These babies usually thrive, gain weight, and appear to tolerate the formula or mother's milk.

PATIENT SCREENING

Although not life-threatening, infantile colic is a very disruptive state in the life of the family with an infant. This child requires prompt assessment and should be scheduled as soon as convenient for all.

ETIOLOGY

The etiology of colic is unknown, although several theories have been advanced. One hypothesis suggests that improper feeding techniques may be responsible, and another theory blames overeating or the swallowing of excessive air. Sensitivity to cow's milk may be the causative factor, even for the nursing infant. In this case, the nursing mother is urged to eliminate cow's milk from her own diet. Another sensitivity may be to iron, requiring that supplemental iron be eliminated from either the infant's formula or the lactating mother's diet. Regardless of the cause, the infant is extremely uncomfortable and cries a great deal, with sleep pattern disturbance.

DIAGNOSIS

Diagnosis is made by the symptoms and a physical examination to rule out other causes of the apparent abdominal spasms.

TREATMENT

Investigation into possible causes is the first step in treatment. Eliminating any of the possible causative factors may help to lessen the symptoms. The infant usually outgrows the condition at about 3 months of age. Occasionally, in severe cases, an anticholinergic or antispasmodic drug may be given.

PROGNOSIS

The prognosis is good for the child to outgrow colic-type symptoms. Parents can become exhausted both physically and emotionally with the colicky, constantly crying baby. Intervention by another family member or support person may be advised to prevent abuse of the baby.

PREVENTION

With the etiology unknown, prevention is also undetermined.

PATIENT TEACHING

Encourage the use of support persons so parents can get needed rest. Many theories of treatment have been proposed; encourage parents to discuss these with the physician.

Helminth (Worm) Infestation

DESCRIPTION

Roundworms, pinworms, hookworms, and tapeworms all can take up residence in the GI tract. All of these worms are classified as helminthes, and helminth infestation describes the condition of these parasites occurring in the intestinal tract.

 ICD-9-CM Code 128.9 *(Unspecified)*

SYMPTOMS AND SIGNS

Worm infestations in children occur as children introduce eggs into their mouths from contaminated hands. After pinworm *(Enterobius vermicularis)* eggs are swallowed, they hatch in the intestine. The female worms migrate to the perianal area at night, where they lay their eggs. This process causes mild to intense itching and irritation in the area. The itching and scratching contaminates the fingers with the eggs and allows reingestion by the host.

PATIENT SCREENING

Children exhibiting behavior that suggests the presence of intestinal worms require prompt assessment and intervention.

ETIOLOGY

E. vermicularis (pinworm) is one of many possible parasitic worms. It is the most common cause of helminth infestation in the United States, and most patients are preschool or school-age children and the mothers of infected children. Pinworms are transmitted directly or indirectly from human to human (Figs. 2–40 and 2–41).

DIAGNOSIS

The diagnosis is made by detection of eggs or worms in the anal opening by the placing of transparent adhesive tape in the perianal area. A stool specimen examined microscopically may be positive.

TREATMENT

A complete course of anthelmintic agents is given; some physicians treat the entire family. Frequent showering and hand washing are advised. The worms and eggs also can be destroyed by the process of laundering clothing and linens in hot water with bleach.

PROGNOSIS

The prognosis is good when the entire family is treated.

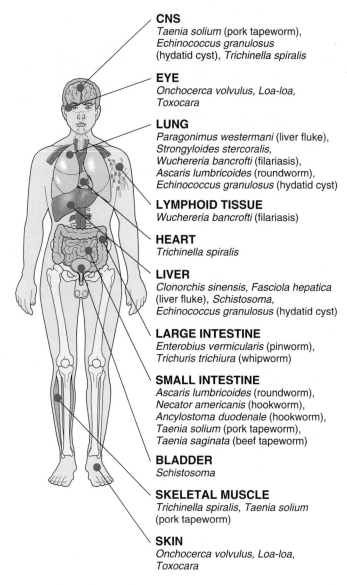

CNS
Taenia solium (pork tapeworm),
Echinococcus granulosus
(hydatid cyst), *Trichinella spiralis*

EYE
Onchocerca volvulus, Loa-loa,
Toxocara

LUNG
Paragonimus westermani (liver fluke),
Strongyloides stercoralis,
Wuchereria bancrofti (filariasis),
Ascaris lumbricoides (roundworm),
Echinococcus granulosus (hydatid cyst)

LYMPHOID TISSUE
Wuchereria bancrofti (filariasis)

HEART
Trichinella spiralis

LIVER
Clonorchis sinensis, Fasciola hepatica
(liver fluke), *Schistosoma,*
Echinococcus granulosus (hydatid cyst)

LARGE INTESTINE
Enterobius vermicularis (pinworm),
Trichuris trichiura (whipworm)

SMALL INTESTINE
Ascaris lumbricoides (roundworm),
Necator americanis (hookworm),
Ancylostoma duodenale (hookworm),
Taenia solium (pork tapeworm),
Taenia saginata (beef tapeworm)

BLADDER
Schistosoma

SKELETAL MUSCLE
Trichinella spiralis, Taenia solium
(pork tapeworm)

SKIN
Onchocerca volvulus, Loa-loa,
Toxocara

FIGURE 2–40 Helminthic infestations. (From Stevens A, Lowe J: *Pathology: illustrated review in color,* ed 2, London, 2000, Mosby.)

PREVENTION
Good hand washing and frequent showering help prevent infestation. Children should be encouraged not to touch or scratch the anus and not to put their hands in their mouths.

PATIENT TEACHING
Stress the importance of good hand washing and other cleanliness. Point out to parents the importance of teaching children good hygiene habits, especially in the toileting process.

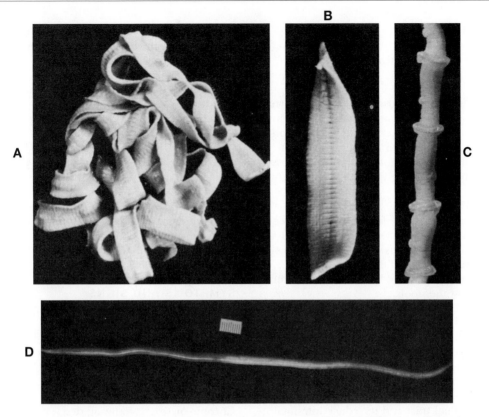

FIGURE 2–41 Intestinal worms. **A,** Tapeworms. Part of the tapeworm *Diphyllobothrium latum.* The total length of the worm is greater than 30 feet. The head is about 1 mm in diameter, and the immature segments (proglottides) are much smaller than are the segments shown (x 1.5). **B,** Part of the worm shown in A. It is made up of many segments, each of which is wider than it is long. **C,** Part of the tapeworm *Taenia saginata.* Each segment is longer than it is wide. **D,** *Ascaris lumbricoides.* This worm is the largest roundworm parasite of humans and superficially resembles an earthworm (from the Latin *lumbricus,* an "earthworm"). It ranges in length from 15 to 35 cm. The specimen was approximately 20 cm (8 inches) in length. Other common roundworms are considerably smaller: *Trichuris trichiura,* 3 to 5 cm; *Enterobius vermicularis,* 8 to 13 mm; and *Ancylostoma duodenale,* up to 1 cm. (The scale above the roundworm shown is 1 cm.) (From Walter JB: *An introduction to the principles of disease,* ed 3, Philadelphia, 1992, Saunders.)

Diarrhea

DESCRIPTION

◦ Diarrhea is rapid passage of stool through the intestinal tract, with a noticeable change in the frequency, fluid content, appearance, and consistency.

◼ ICD-9-CM Code 787.91 *(NOS)*
   Refer to the physician's diagnosis and then to the current edition of the ICD-9-CM coding manual to ensure the greatest specificity of pathology and any appropriate modifiers.

SYMPTOMS AND SIGNS

Diarrhea may be mild or severe, acute or chronic. In the infant or child, diarrhea can rapidly cause dehydration and electrolyte imbalance when fluid loss is profuse. Severe or prolonged diarrhea can produce metabolic *acidosis;* the patient may be lethargic and may hyperventilate. Depending on the cause, the symptoms could include intestinal cramping, weakness, nausea, irritability, and fever. Stool passage may become painful as a result of excoriation of the anus or skin in the diaper area.

PATIENT SCREENING

Children with diarrhea can dehydrate rapidly. Prompt assessment is indicated.

ETIOLOGY

Diarrhea has multiple causes: infection (viral, bacterial, or parasitic), medications, allergic reactions, emotions, anatomic abnormalities, malabsorption syndromes, mechanical or chemical irritation resulting from the diet, and toxicity. The cause may be unknown.

DIAGNOSIS

The clinician attempts to determine the degree of diarrheal disease, the underlying cause, and the fluid and electrolyte status of the patient. This requires a specific history of the onset and severity of symptoms, laboratory blood testing, stool cultures, and analysis of the stools.

TREATMENT

The treatment of diarrhea is directed at the cause, if known. Blood components are monitored for fluid and electrolyte balances. The frequency, color, consistency, and general composition of the stool are observed. Oral intake may be restricted to rest the intestinal tract and to reduce intestinal irritability. When infection is the cause, appropriate antibiotics may be given. Ignoring prolonged diarrhea in the infant or small child is dangerous. The patient may require hospitalization for intravenous (IV) fluid and electrolyte therapy.

PROGNOSIS

The prognosis is good with prompt intervention. Dehydration and electrolyte imbalance are factors in the outcome of the condition. Hospitalization may be necessary to maintain hydration, stable electrolytes, and nutrition.

PREVENTION

Prevention is many faceted because of the cause. Good hand washing is important in preventing microbial infections. Avoiding known allergens, certain medications, and dietary factors helps. Mechanical and chemical irritations in the diet may be eliminated. When the cause is anatomic abnormalities or malabsorption syndromes, preventive steps probably are few.

PATIENT TEACHING

Emphasize the importance of hydration to the parents. Care of the anal area may be required as a result of the irritation caused by the loose and irritating stools. Good hand washing is necessary after handling soiled diapers or any other clothing that may contain stool. Teach parents to observe urinary output for volume and color. When the child is in diapers, have parents count the number of soiled or wet diapers within a set time and report this to the office.

Vomiting

DESCRIPTION

Vomiting, or ejection through the mouth of stomach contents, is a common symptom in infants and children.

 ICD-9-CM Code 787.03

SYMPTOMS AND SIGNS

Vomiting can range from a mild regurgitation to projectile expulsion. The infant has a distended abdomen, is irritable, and often has a fever. Aspiration of vomitus into the lungs can result in pneumonia.

PATIENT SCREENING

Chronic or severe vomiting deserves special attention as a warning sign of disease or possible dehydration. Assessment is essential. Projectile vomiting requires prompt assessment.

ETIOLOGY

Vomiting, which is more common in infants than in children, usually results from trivial or temporary factors. However, it has a host of possible causes, including overfeeding, food allergy, gastric irritation, infection, drug poisoning, intracranial pressure, genetic defects such as pyloric stenosis, and habitual voluntary vomiting.

DIAGNOSIS

Vomiting in the infant or child always must be evaluated in the context of the child's total state of health. One assesses causative factors by performing a physical examination, taking the history, and monitoring the patient's vital signs, weight, nutritional status, and fluid and electrolyte balance. Radiographic studies of the intestinal tract may be indicated.

TREATMENT

Most vomiting can be expected to abate spontaneously. Food may be withheld for a time to rest the upper GI tract and to reduce gastric irritation. When treatment is indicated, it depends on the cause, severity, and nature of the vomiting. Infant feeding problems require changes in technique or intake. Other more serious causes, such as infection, poisoning, and congenital anomalies of the GI tract, may require direct medical or surgical intervention.

PROGNOSIS

The prognosis varies depending on the cause. Most vomiting subsides in a few hours. Longer periods of vomiting requiring medical or surgical intervention may or may not be corrected. Hydration, nutrition, and electrolyte balance are important factors in the resolution of the condition.

PREVENTION

Prevention varies depending on causative factors. Avoiding overfeeding, known food allergens, and substances that cause gastric irritation often is all that is necessary to prevent recurrence. Infection, drug poisoning, intracranial pressure, genetic defects such as pyloric stenosis, and habitual voluntary vomiting may not be preventable.

PATIENT TEACHING

Emphasize the importance of hydration and nutrition along with the use of good hand-washing technique after handling emesis.

Blood Disorders

Anemia

DESCRIPTION

Anemia is an abnormal reduction in the concentration of red blood cells (RBCs) or in the hemoglobin content of circulating blood. It is not a disease, but a symptom of various diseases. The manifestations of anemia are the result of tissue hypoxia. (See Chapter 10 for additional information on anemias.)

■ **ICD-9-CM Code 285.9** *(Unspecified)*
Refer to the physician's diagnosis and then to the current edition of the ICD-9-CM coding manual to ensure the greatest specificity of pathology and any appropriate modifiers.

SYMPTOMS AND SIGNS

Pallor, weakness, fatigability, and listlessness are noted initially in the anemic child or infant. Palpitation, tachycardia, cardiac enlargement, jaundice, and mental sluggishness are symptoms of severe anemia.

Laboratory signs indicating anemia vary with the underlying cause or type of anemia. Signs may include abnormal hemoglobin concentrations in the blood and a reduced hematocrit level.

PATIENT SCREENING

Children whose parents report that the child appears pale, weak, easily fatigued, and listless require prompt assessment.

ETIOLOGY

Iron deficiency is the most common cause of anemia in children. Other causes include acute or chronic blood loss, decreased blood formation, nutritional deficiency disorders, hemolytic diseases, inhibition or loss of bone marrow, and sickle-cell disease.

DIAGNOSIS

Diagnosis is based on physical examination and laboratory testing for signs and symptoms of anemia. Diagnostic tests include determination of hemoglobin concentration, hematocrit levels, serum iron levels, RBC count, mean corpuscular hemoglobin levels, and bone marrow studies. Abnormal RBCs may be seen microscopically.

TREATMENT

The first priority of treatment is to determine the cause of anemia. For iron deficiency anemia, iron-rich foods and oral preparations of ferrous iron are administered. When blood loss is the cause, blood volume is restored by transfusion. Replacement therapy is indicated in deficiency states (e.g., vitamin B_{12}, folic acid, and ascorbic acid deficiency). Specific hemolytic blood disorders are treated when the anemia is caused by excessive blood cell destruction. A planned program of activity balanced with rest is recommended during treatment.

PROGNOSIS

The prognosis varies depending on the cause. When diet modification can be recommended and followed, the prognosis is good. When the problem is bleeding and the source of the bleed can be determined and corrected, the prognosis is good with blood replacement and dietary supplement.

Hemolytic disorders have a fair prognosis with aggressive treatment.

PREVENTION

Diets meeting the daily requirement of iron and other vitamins and minerals help to prevent iron deficiency anemia. Prompt exploration of any unexplained type of bleeding helps to reveal underlying conditions and allows prompt treatment.

PATIENT TEACHING

Encourage parents to provide children with nutritious diets and recommended nutritional supplements and pediatric vitamins and minerals. Emphasize the importance of follow-up appointments for these children.

Leukemia

DESCRIPTION

Leukemia, a cancer of blood-forming tissues, is the most common childhood malignancy. It is characterized by an abnormal increase in the number of immature WBCs or undifferentiated blastocytes.

■ **ICD-9-CM Code 208.90** *(Unspecified)*
Refer to the physician's diagnosis and then to the current edition of the ICD-9-CM coding manual to ensure the greatest specificity of pathology and any appropriate modifiers.

SYMPTOMS AND SIGNS

Bone marrow infiltration by leukemic cells leads to anemia resulting from decreased RBCs, susceptibility to infection resulting from neutropenia, and prolonged bleeding time resulting from the reduction in the amount of platelets. Common signs and symptoms include fever, easy bruising, pallor, weakness, weight loss, bone and joint pain, and frequent or persistent infections. The abnormal cells invade various organs of the body, causing pressure symptoms in those areas. Lymph nodes and the spleen may become enlarged.

PATIENT SCREENING

A child whose parents report that the child has a fever, frequent infections, easy bruising, pallor, and weakness requires prompt assessment.

ETIOLOGY

Two general types of leukemia are found in children, acute lymphoid leukemia (ALL) and acute myelogenous leukemia (AML). These main types are further divided into subtypes based on the specific aberrations of WBCs. About 80% of childhood leukemias are ALL. The etiology is unknown. Predisposing factors include congenital disorders such as Down syndrome and radiation exposure. The peak age of incidence is between 2 years and 6 years. See Chapter 10 for additional discussion of leukemia.

DIAGNOSIS

A peripheral blood smear shows immature forms of WBCs. The complete blood cells often are reduced. Microscopic examination of bone marrow aspiration is necessary for definitive diagnosis. Chromosome analysis of the leukemic cells is performed because the presence of different characteristic abnormalities has prognostic value. A lumbar puncture is often performed to determine whether the central nervous system is involved.

TREATMENT

The disease is treated through systemic chemotherapy to eradicate leukemic cells and to induce remission. Chemotherapy is administered intrathecally as prophylaxis against central nervous system invasion. Bone marrow transplantation is a possible alternative for children with ALL during their second remission (after the first relapse) or for children with AML during the first remission (because AML carries a poorer prognosis than ALL when treated solely with chemotherapy). Psychological support for the child and the family must be provided.

PROGNOSIS

The best prognostic indicators in determining long-term survival are the patient's age at diagnosis, WBC count at diagnosis, cytogenetics, and sex of the child. For ALL, having a WBC count of $50,000/\mu L$, being over 10 years old, being male, and having certain cytogenic abnormalities such as Philadelphia chromosome (a translocation between chromosomes 9 and 22) are associated with a poorer prognosis. For AML, a WBC count greater than $100,000/\mu L$ and certain chromosomal abnormalities such as monosomy of chromosome 7 carry a poorer prognosis. In addition, failure to achieve remission by day 28 of therapy is associated with poor prognosis. Still, most children with leukemia survive the disease. Of those treated solely with chemotherapy, 80% achieve long-term, disease-free survival. Long-term survival for those undergoing bone marrow transplantation (BMT) ranges from 25% to 50%.

PREVENTION
There is no known prevention.

PATIENT TEACHING
Work with parents to contact support groups.

Erythroblastosis Fetalis (Hemolytic Disease of the Newborn)

DESCRIPTION
Erythroblastosis fetalis stems from an incompatibility of fetal and maternal blood, resulting in excessive rates of RBC destruction.

■ ICD-9-CM Code 773.2

SYMPTOMS AND SIGNS
Erythroblastosis fetalis is characterized by anemia, jaundice, *kernicterus,* and enlargement of the liver and spleen. In the most severe form, called hydrops fetalis, the fetus or infant is in great jeopardy because of extreme *hemolysis.* If the infant survives, the condition is marked by heart failure, edema, pulmonary congestion, lethargy, seizures, and mental retardation.

PATIENT SCREENING
Physicians caring for expectant mothers who have had prenatal care should understand the possibility of Rh incompatibility. New patients aware of possible Rh incompatibility because they know their Rh factor is negative should be scheduled to discuss the matter with the physician as soon as convenient for all parties. Newborn infants with hemolytic disease of the newborn will be identified during the newborn examination if not before birth, and treatment will be instituted as soon as possible.

ETIOLOGY
The cause is Rh factor incompatibility. Rh factor is the antigen found on RBCs of the Rh-positive individual. The mother, through a prior pregnancy, has become sensitized to the Rh factor (Rh isoimmunization) of the fetal RBCs. When sensitized ma-

ternal blood finds its way into fetal circulation, particularly during delivery, the antibodies in the mother's blood destroy the RBCs of the fetus (Figs. 2–42 and 2–43).

If an Rh-negative woman has children with an Rh-positive man, some or all of the infants will be Rh positive. During pregnancy, blood from the Rh-positive fetus may move from fetal circulation into the mother's bloodstream, where it can stimulate the mother's body to form antibodies against the Rh factor. When sufficient quantities of the antibodies pass back into the infant's circulation, the antibodies can clump and destroy Rh-positive cells, causing the symptoms of erythroblastosis fetalis.

DIAGNOSIS
Blood typing of the mother and father is essential. The maternal history includes pregnancy, elective and spontaneous abortions, and blood transfusions. A direct Coombs' test of umbilical cord blood measures Rh-positive antibodies in the newborn; a bilirubin test for *bilirubinemia* and hematocrit determination also are performed on the infant's blood. The amniotic fluid may be analyzed for hemolysis.

TREATMENT
The treatment is dictated by the degree of erythroblastosis fetalis and its effect on the fetus or newborn. Intrauterine transfusions may be indicated when the fetus shows signs of distress. When necessary, the delivery of the infant is planned 2 to 4 weeks before term. Exchange transfusion gives the infant fresh group-O, Rh-negative blood. *Phototherapy* and albumin infusion are used to reduce the amount of circulating bilirubin in the newborn.

PROGNOSIS
The prognosis is good when the disease is discovered early in pregnancy and closely monitored. Early delivery with immediate transfusion usually treats this condition successfully. Mothers with Rh-negative blood factor need to continue Rho-GAM injections for protection in subsequent pregnancies.

PREVENTION
Protection is now available for Rh-negative mothers who have never been sensitized, preventing the possibility of harm to an Rh-positive baby.

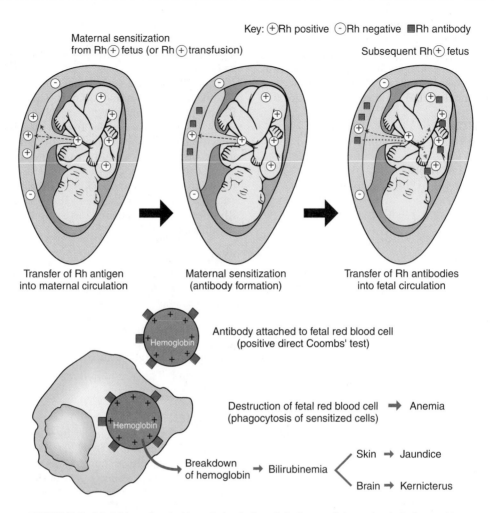

Maternal sensitization
from Rh⊕ fetus (or Rh⊕ transfusion)

Key: ⊕Rh positive ⊖Rh negative ■Rh antibody

Subsequent Rh⊕ fetus

Transfer of Rh antigen
into maternal circulation

Maternal sensitization
(antibody formation)

Transfer of Rh antibodies
into fetal circulation

Hemoglobin

Antibody attached to fetal red blood cell
(positive direct Coombs' test)

Hemoglobin

Destruction of fetal red blood cell ➡ Anemia
(phagocytosis of sensitized cells)

Breakdown
of hemoglobin ➡ Bilirubinemia ⟨ Skin ➡ Jaundice
Brain ➡ Kernicterus

FIGURE 2–42 Etiology of erythroblastosis fetalis (hemolytic disease of the newborn). (Redrawn with permission of Ross Products Division, Abbott Laboratories, from *Congenital heart abnormalities* [Clinical Education Aid no 7], 1992.)

Rho(D) immune globulin is given as soon as possible to the woman at risk after each exposure to Rh-positive blood (most often by giving birth to an Rh-positive infant) to prevent maternal Rh isoimmunization and complications in subsequent pregnancies.

PATIENT TEACHING

Emphasize the importance of Rh screening to all pregnant females. Those who are Rh negative require information about Rh-negative mothers with Rh-positive babies. Help with finding and contacting community support groups.

Lead Poisoning

DESCRIPTION

Lead poisoning is an environmentally caused blood toxicity resulting from ingestion or inspiration of lead dust or particles.

■ **ICD-9-CM Code 984.9** *(Unspecified)*
Refer to the physician's diagnosis and then to the current edition of the ICD-9-CM coding manual to ensure the greatest specificity of pathology and any appropriate modifiers.

Rh FACTOR INCOMPATIBILITY OF MATERNAL–FETAL BLOOD

(ERYTHROBLASTOSIS FETALIS, OR HEMOLYTIC DISEASE OF THE NEWBORN)

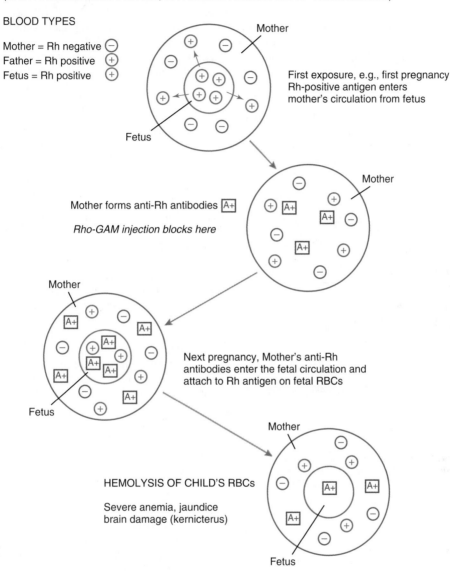

FIGURE 2–43 Rh incompatibility of maternal and fetal blood. RBCs, red blood cells. (From Gould BE: *Pathophysiology for the health professions,* ed 2, Philadelphia, 2002, Saunders.)

SYMPTOMS AND SIGNS

Children exposed to toxic levels of lead, a poisonous metallic element, exhibit signs of lead poisoning. Some warning signs are loss of appetite, vomiting, irritability, and **ataxic** gait. Chronic symptoms include anemia, weakness, colic, and peripheral neuritis. Evidence of mental retardation resulting from brain damage is possible. A child with acute lead intoxication presents as a medical emergency. The child has symptoms of encephalopathy with vomiting, headache, stupor, convulsions, and coma resulting from cerebral edema (Fig. 2–44).

PATIENT SCREENING

Children exhibiting fatigue, headaches, irritability, stomachaches, cramps, muscle and joint pain, and changes in behavior require prompt assessment.

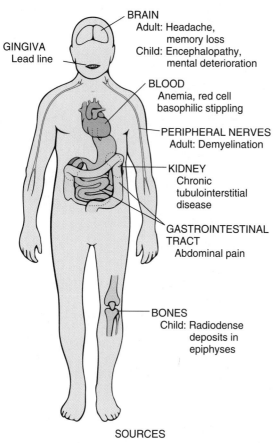

FIGURE 2–44 Clinical and pathological features of lead poisoning. (From Kumar V, Cotran R, Robbins S: *Basic pathology*, ed 7, Philadelphia, 2002, Saunders.)

ETIOLOGY

Any lead in the blood is abnormal. Exposure results from breathing or swallowing substances containing lead. The condition has developed in children who eat flakes of peeling lead paint, drink water from lead pipes, or ingest lead salts in certain foods. Lead dust may remain in soil contaminated by exhaust from previous use of leaded gasoline. Lead taken into the body is stored in many tissues; it is released into the blood and excreted in the urine.

DIAGNOSIS

The history of lead exposure and the presence of symptoms previously listed suggest the diagnosis. Blood tests reveal anemia and a blood lead level greater than 5 μg/dl. Lead excretion through the urine is increased. Characteristic changes in the ends of growing bones are noted on radiographic films.

TREATMENT

The source of poisoning first must be eliminated. The next goal of treatment is to remove the lead from the body. One attempts this by giving substances, known as chelating agents, that tie up the lead in a chemically inactive form in the bloodstream while it is transported to the kidneys for elimination. Antiemetics help to control nausea and vomiting, and sedation is given for convulsions. After acute therapy, penicillamine (a chelating agent for lead) is given orally for 3 to 6 months.

PROGNOSIS

The prognosis varies depending on the extent of damage and promptness in discovering the toxicity. Aggressive intervention and removal of the child from the contaminated environment help to prevent additional damage.

PREVENTION

An awareness of the environmental sources of lead, such as lead paint, lead plumbing, and other sources of lead dust is prudent. An act, Title X, or the Lead-Based Paint Hazard Act of 1992, helps prevent exposure to lead in homes built before 1978 by requiring disclosure of lead-based paint hazards in the home. Dust on vinyl mini-blinds may contain lead deposits.

PATIENT TEACHING

Teaching the parents about the hazards of lead poisoning and means of recognizing toxic sources is essential.

Miscellaneous Diseases

Reye Syndrome

DESCRIPTION

Reye syndrome is a combination of brain disease and fatty invasion of the inner organs, especially the liver.

 ICD-9-CM Code 331.81
Refer to the physician's diagnosis and then to the current edition of the ICD-9-CM coding manual to ensure the greatest specificity of pathology and any appropriate modifiers.

SYMPTOMS AND SIGNS

This rare syndrome is an acute and often fatal illness that may affect children through 15 years of age. The pathogenesis includes a disruption in the urea cycle that causes swelling of the brain, resulting in increased intracranial pressure. The symptoms of Reye syndrome progress through five stages: (1) lethargy, vomiting, and hepatic dysfunction; (2) hyperventilation, hyperactive reflexes, hepatic dysfunction, and delirium; (3) organ changes and coma; (4) deeper coma and loss of cerebral functions; and (5) seizures, loss of deep tendon reflexes, and respiratory arrest.

PATIENT SCREENING

Children who begin vomiting 3 to 6 days after viral illness such as chickenpox are possible candidates for Reye syndrome and require immediate assessment and intervention.

ETIOLOGY

The cause of Reye syndrome is unknown. However, it typically follows infection with influenza A or B viruses or chickenpox. It has been linked to the use of aspirin during these infections.

DIAGNOSIS

The medical history and the patient's clinical features suggest the disease. Laboratory blood studies show elevated serum ammonia levels. Liver function tests show elevated enzyme levels. Other tests include liver biopsy and CSF analysis.

TREATMENT

The early recognition and treatment of Reye syndrome has cut the mortality rate from 90% to 20%.

Hospitalization is required to stabilize the patient, to control cerebral edema, to monitor blood chemistries, to manage seizures, and to provide mechanical ventilation if needed. Recovery can be complete.

PROGNOSIS

The prognosis is good with prompt intervention and aggressive treatment.

PREVENTION

For prevention, the use of nonsalicylate analgesics and antipyretics, such as acetaminophen, is recommended instead of aspirin.

PATIENT TEACHING

Caution all parents or caretakers that children should not be given aspirin during possible viral infections.

Fetal Alcohol Syndrome

DESCRIPTION

Fetal alcohol syndrome (FAS) describes birth defects and other associated problems in infants born to alcoholic mothers who consume alcohol during the gestational period.

ICD-9-CM Code 760.71

SYMPTOMS AND SIGNS

Intrauterine exposure to sufficient levels of alcohol has been associated with fetal growth retardation, in which the infants are short and below average in weight. Facial characteristics of FAS include smaller eye openings with eyes spaced widely apart and a thin upper lip. FAS also is associated with mental retardation. The infant may exhibit signs of alcohol withdrawal shortly after birth.

PATIENT SCREENING

Maternal history and newborn examination usually reveal the condition. Parents seeking medical attention for the child at any stage of development should be scheduled for the earliest possible appointment.

ETIOLOGY

FAS is caused when alcohol enters the fetal blood as a result of chronic, excessive use of alcohol during gestation.

DIAGNOSIS
Typical clinical features present in the newborn and a maternal history of chronic alcoholism determine the diagnosis (Fig. 2–45).

TREATMENT
The treatment depends on the defects in the newborn. Much of the treatment is supportive because neurologic damage cannot be reversed. Proper nu-

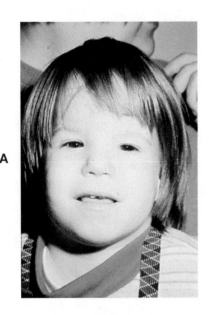

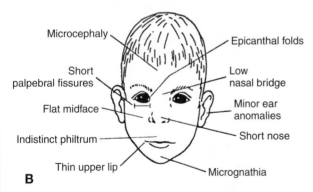

FIGURE 2–45 A, Fetal alcohol syndrome (FAS). **B,** Affected children typically have features that, when accompanied by mental retardation, are diagnostic of FAS. The features on the left are those most often seen in patients with FAS, whereas those on the right are features that are seen with increased frequency in this population compared with the general population. (From Jones KL, Smith DW, Ulleland CN, et al: Pattern of malformation in offspring of chronic alcoholic mothers. *Lancet* 1:1267, 1973.)

trition is vital. Because the baby may have poor sucking reflex, special adaptation may be necessary to ensure proper intake. The psychosocial needs of the infant and the mother must be addressed.

PROGNOSIS
As previously mentioned, neurologic damage cannot be reversed; therefore the prognosis varies depending on the amount of neurologic damage sustained.

PREVENTION
Preventive measures include prenatal care and education. Because experts do not agree on a safe maximum amount of alcohol intake during pregnancy, women generally are advised not to drink during gestation.

PATIENT TEACHING
Females should be advised not to drink during the gestational period. In addition, good prenatal care should be emphasized.

Diaper Rash

DESCRIPTION
Diaper rash, considered a contact dermatitis, is evident in the diaper area as an irritation or rash.

■ **ICD-9-CM Code** **691.0**

SYMPTOMS AND SIGNS
Diaper rash can vary from mild to severe and can be self-limiting or a chronic source of discomfort to the infant and dismay to the parent or caretaker. Diaper rash takes multiple forms from a mild excoriation, or *maculopapular* rash, to blisters and ulceration.

PATIENT SCREENING
Infants and toddlers with diaper rash that will not clear require prompt assessment.

ETIOLOGY
Infants with sensitive skin seem to have a hereditary predisposition to diaper rash, or irritant dermatitis. Diaper rash may be triggered by friction or prolonged exposure to moisture, feces, or the ammonia produced by bacterial action on urine. Poorly washed or rinsed diapers or the use of occlusive plastic pants over the diapers may contribute. Poor

hygiene or overzealous cleaning could irritate the diaper area.

DIAGNOSIS

One may need to differentiate diaper rash from seborrheic dermatitis, eczema, and secondary skin infection.

TREATMENT

In addition to frequent diaper changing and proper cleaning and drying of the diaper area, a bland protective agent such as zinc oxide or topical hydrocortisone may promote healing. Careful application of dry heat, as directed by the physician, may improve the condition. Topical antimicrobial agents are used for secondary skin infection. Cloth diapers should be rinsed of irritating residue.

PROGNOSIS

The prognosis is good.

PREVENTION

Frequent changing of diapers accompanied by thorough cleansing of the diaper area helps to prevent the rash. Leaving the area exposed to air for short periods often will allow the area to dry and help to prevent the rash from returning.

PATIENT TEACHING

Stress the importance of changing the infant's or toddler's diaper on a regular schedule and not leaving the child in a soiled diaper for extended periods. If necessary, demonstrate the method of cleansing the diaper area.

REVIEW
CHALLENGE

Answer the following questions:

1. List the possible causes of congenital anomalies.
2. What is the purpose of amniocentesis? Describe the procedure.
3. Trace fetal circulation.
4. Describe the condition of prematurity and list its causes. List the associated disorders, identifying their causes, and discuss the treatment options.
5. Explain the differences between muscular dystrophy and cerebral palsy.
6. Describe patent ductus arteriosus and its treatment.
7. Name and describe the most common congenital cyanotic cardiac defect.
8. List the major clinical manifestations of cystic fibrosis.
9. Explain the differences between Klinefelter syndrome and Turner syndrome.
10. Describe the clinical condition of congenital rubella syndrome.
11. Discuss the incidence, etiology, and treatment of asthma.
12. List the symptoms and signs of anemia; describe the pathology of leukemia.
13. Explain the etiology of erythroblastosis fetalis.
14. Name some warning signs of lead poisoning.
15. Describe the infant born with fetal alcohol syndrome.
16. Discuss the importance of childhood immunizations and list the schedule for the first year of life.

REAL-LIFE CHALLENGE

Asthma

A 6-year-old male presents coughing with audible expiratory wheezes and dyspnea. The child is pale, skin is moist and cool, and he has difficulty speaking more than a few words before stopping to catch his breath. His parents state the difficult breathing had a rapid onset approximately 1 hour earlier when he was playing with the neighbor's dog. The child has a history of previous asthma attacks, primarily after visiting his aunt's home where there are cats.

Assessment of the child shows T 98.6, P 120, R 40 and labored. Bilateral rales are heard on auscultation, louder on expiration but also present on inspiration. Cromolyn sodium had been prescribed prophylactically prior to visits to aunt's home. Child also has an Alupent inhaler to be used PRN. The use of the inhaler brought no relief.

QUESTIONS

1. Which diagnostic procedures would be ordered to reveal the degree of airway obstruction?
2. What changes in vital signs would be expected with the use of an Alupent inhaler?
3. Which immediate intervention may be ordered to relieve symptoms and provide comfort to the child?
4. What future testing may be ordered?
5. What is the cause of the dyspnea?
6. List allergens commonly responsible for asthma attacks.
7. Explain why asthma attacks are considered as medical emergencies and what steps should be taken on arrival of a patient in the midst of an asthma attack.

REAL-LIFE CHALLENGE

Patent Ductus Arteriosus

A premature infant weighing 1 pound, 10 ounces and 1 week old begins exhibiting reduced oxygen saturation levels, bradycardia, and cyanosis. The infant's respirations are being maintained with mechanical ventilation. Increased oxygen concentration is required to maintain oxygen saturation levels at 90%. The chest radiograph reveals IRDS as resolving. The echocardiogram indicates a PDA.

QUESTIONS

1. Explain the two treatment options, drug therapy, or a surgical procedure used to close the PDA.
2. Explain the complication that could occur due to high-concentration levels of oxygen.
3. What is the prognosis for the cardiac status of this child once closure has been achieved?
4. Which other congenital cardiac defect may be present?
5. Trace fetal circulation and explain the role of the ductus arteriosus prior to birth.

INTERNET ASSIGNMENTS

1. Go to the Asthma and Allergy Foundation of America website to ascertain and report on recent treatment options.

2. Go to the Cystic Fibrosis Foundation website to research new treatment options and support systems for patients and their family.

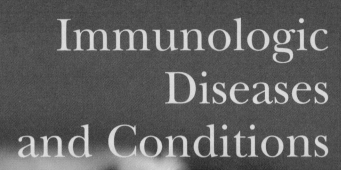

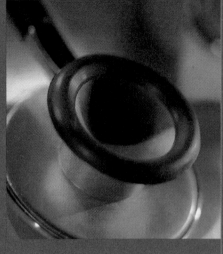

CHAPTER 3

Immunologic Diseases and Conditions

Chapter Outline—Cont'd

Learning Objectives

After studying Chapter 3, you should be able to:

1. Name the functional components of the immune system.
2. Characterize the three major functions of the immune system.
3. List examples of inappropriate responses of the immune system.
4. Explain the difference between natural and acquired immunity.
5. Trace the formation of T cells and B cells from stem cells.
6. Explain how T cells and B cells specifically protect the body against disease.
7. List the five immunoglobulins and explain complement fixation.
8. Explain the ways that human immunodeficiency virus (HIV) is transmitted.
9. List the guidelines for universal precautions and infection control.
10. Describe the primary absent or inadequate response of the immune system in the following diseases:
    - Common variable immunodeficiency
    - Selective immunoglobulin A deficiency
    - Severe combined immunodeficiency disease
11. Explain the destructive mechanisms in autoimmune diseases.
12. Describe the symptoms and signs of pernicious anemia. Name the primary treatment.
13. Recite the systemic features of systemic lupus erythematosus (SLE). Recall the diagnostic criteria.
14. Detail the pathology of rheumatoid arthritis.
15. Specify the primary objectives of the treatment for rheumatoid arthritis.
16. Compare the pathology of multiple sclerosis with that of myasthenia gravis.
17. List the distinguishing diagnostic features of ankylosing spondylitis.
18. Describe the pathology of vasculitis in general terms.

Key Terms

anticholinesterase (**an**–tee–koh–lyn–**ES**–ter–ase)
autoimmune (**aw**–toh–im–**YOON**)
candidiasis (**kan**–dih–**DIE**–ah–sis)
collagen (**KOLL**–ah–jen)
hematopoietic (**hem**–ah–toh–poy–**ET**–ik)
hypogammaglobulinemia
             (**hye**–poh–**gam**–a–**glob**–you–lyn–**EE**–me–ah)
immunocompetence (**im**–you–no–**KOM**–peh–tens)
immunodeficiency (**im**–you–no–deh–**FISH**–en–see)
immunoelectrophoresis (im–**you**–no–ee–**lek**–troh–foh–**REE**–sis)
immunogen (**IM**–you–no–jen)
immunoglobulin (**im**–you–no–**GLAHB**–you–lyn)
immunosuppressive (**im**–you–no–sup–**PRESS**–iv)
keratoconjunctivitis (**ker**–ah–toh–kon–**junk**–tih–**VIE**–tis)
lymph (**limf**)
lymphadenopathy (lim–**fad**–eh–**NOP**–ah–thee)
lymphocyte (**LIM**–foh–sight)
macrophage (**MACK**–roh–fayj)
phagocytes (**FAG**–oh–sights)
phagocytosis (**fag**–oh–sigh–**TOH**–sis)

ORDERLY FUNCTION OF THE IMMUNE SYSTEM

THE IMMUNE SYSTEM, a major defense mechanism, is responsible for a complex response to the invasion of the body by foreign substances. The concept of the immune system arose from an observation that a person who recovers from a specific infection does not get sick from that infection again. The person is thereafter "immune" to that particular infectious agent. Immunity is very specific in that a person who has developed immunity to a certain virus, such as the rubella virus, is still susceptible to infection by other similar viruses, such as the measles virus.

The immune response assists the body in maintaining its functional integrity, and it battles infection by bacteria, viruses, fungi, and parasites. The immune system involves lymphoid tissues classified as primary (thymus and bone marrow) or secondary (tonsils, adenoids, spleen, Peyer patches, appendix, etc.) (Fig. 3–1).

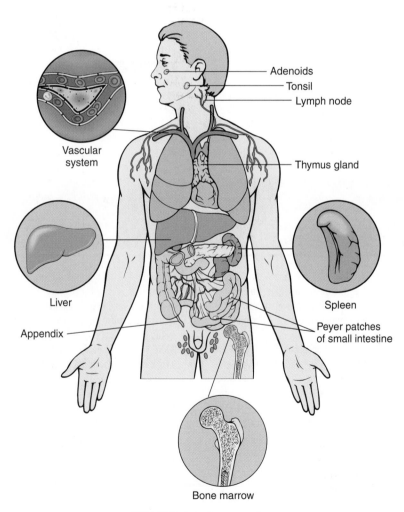

FIGURE 3–1 Immune system.

When the immune system reacts appropriately to an antigen and homeostasis is maintained, the process called **immunocompetence** is functioning well. If the immune system's response is inappropriate, either too weak or too strong, disruption of homeostasis results, which causes a malfunction in the system, or immuno*in*competence. Disruption of homeostasis is the cause of many diseases. Inappropriate responses or malfunctioning of the immune system are classified as follows:

- Hyperactive responses (e.g., allergies), in which the immune response is excessive
- **Immunodeficiency** disorders (e.g., acquired immunodeficiency syndrome [AIDS]), in which the immune response is inadequate
- **Autoimmune** disorders (e.g., systemic lupus erythematosus [SLE]), in which the immune response is misdirected
- Attacks on beneficial foreign tissue (e.g., reaction to blood transfusions or transplanted organ rejection). (See Enrichment box on Transplant Rejection.)

The immune response normally is activated whenever foreign substances, or antigens, enter the body by evading its first line of defense—the skin and mucous membranes. The body recognizes the antigen or **immunogen,** usually a protein, as foreign, or nonself, and produces *antibodies* in response to that specific antigen. It is crucial that the immune system be able to differenciate between self and foreign molecules. When this is not the case, autoimmune disease, conditions under which the body recognizes its own molecules as foreign and then attacks them, is the result.

The human body is protected by two types of immunity: innate immunity and acquired immunity. Innate immunity involves preformed and fully activated components that launch a nonspecific attack on a foreign organism as soon as it is detected. The main cells involved in innate immunity include the following:

- Natural killer (NK) cells that kill virus-infected cells and tumor cells by secreting certain toxins
- **Macrophages** that phagocytose bacteria, viruses, and other foreign substances
- Polymorphonuclear neutrophils (PMNs or simply neutrophils) that also phagocytose bacteria.

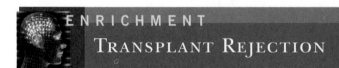

ENRICHMENT

TRANSPLANT REJECTION

KIDNEY, LIVER, HEART, LUNG, pancreas and corneal tissue all can be replaced with transplants. Skin transplants are used for the treatment of burns. Bone marrow transplantation is used to treat bone marrow failure, leukemia, and aplastic anemia.

To help prevent transplant rejection, donor and recipient are carefully matched for blood type and immunologic characteristics. The recipient is given antirejection (immunosuppressive) drugs, along with steroids to suppress the production of antibodies to the foreign tissue proteins. All homografts (a graft of tissue between two genetically dissimilar individuals of the same species) invariably evoke some transplant rejection, which is mediated by antibodies and a delayed cellular immune reaction.

Clinically distinct forms of transplant rejection are recognized:
- Hyperacute reaction—occurs during the operation. Such transplants must be removed immediately to prevent inevitable complications.
- Acute rejection—occurs most often within the first few weeks of transplantation, or later when antirejection drugs become ineffectual.
- Chronic rejection—evolves slowly over a period of months or years. Vascular injury and inflammation of the tissues and cells of the organ contributes to the ultimate deterioration of the transplanted organ (Fig. 3–2.)

Modified from Damjanov I: *Pathology for the health-related professions,* ed 2, Philadelphia, 2000, Saunders.

Acquired (or adaptive) immunity, on the other hand, takes days to become fully functional. It involves a specific response to a particular antigen, which becomes more efficient each time the body is exposed to that antigen. The development of the components required for adaptive immunity begins early in fetal life when the fetal liver produces stem cells, which in turn produce all cells of the **hematopoietic** system. Bone marrow assumes this role after birth (Fig. 3–3). Some of the stem cells migrate to the thymus gland, where they become

T cells (T **lymphocytes**), which multiply and develop the capacity to combine with specific foreign antigens derived from viruses, fungi, tumors, or transplanted tissue (Fig. 3–4). Those T cells coded to recognize self-antigens are destroyed. The remaining T cells are coded to seek out foreign invaders. The body produces several types of T cells; each has a different function:
• Cytotoxic T cells directly destroy virus-infected cells, tumor cells, and *allograft* cells by releasing certain toxins or by inducing *apoptosis.* These

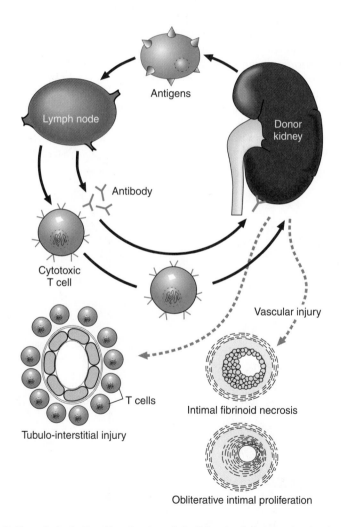

FIGURE 3–2 Transplant rejection. (From Damjanov I: *Pathology for the health-related professions,* ed 2, Philadelphia, 2000, Saunders.)

cells also may be referred to as CD8 cells because they carry the CD8 glycoprotein on their surface.

- Helper T cells stimulate the B cells to differentiate into plasma cells and to produce more antibodies. They also activate cytotoxic T cells and macrophages. Helper T cells carry the CD4 glycoprotein on their surface.
- Suppressor T cells inhibit both B and T cell activities and moderate the immune response.
- Memory T cells remain dormant until they are reactivated by the original antigen, allowing a rapid and more potent response years after the original exposure.

T cells are the major component of the type of acquired immunity known as *cell-mediated immunity*. The mononuclear phagocytic system, which used to be termed the *reticuloendothelial* system, initiates this immune response. Macrophages, which develop from monocytes, are found in the tissue of the liver, lungs, and **lymph** nodes. These large cells intercept and engulf the foreign invader antigens, then process and present them to the T cells. Cell-mediated immunity defends the body against viral and fungal attacks, mediates graft rejection and tumor cell destruction, and helps or suppresses an antibody-mediated response to infection.

The remaining stem cells develop into B cells (B lymphocytes) to produce the antibody-mediated (humoral) immunity that protects the body against bacterial and viral infections and reinfections (see Fig. 3–4). Once activated by exposure to an antigen, B cells are stimulated to proliferate and form a clone of cells that respond to that specific antigen. Some B cells become antibody-secreting plasma cells, whereas others become memory B cells, ready for a quick response if the target anti-

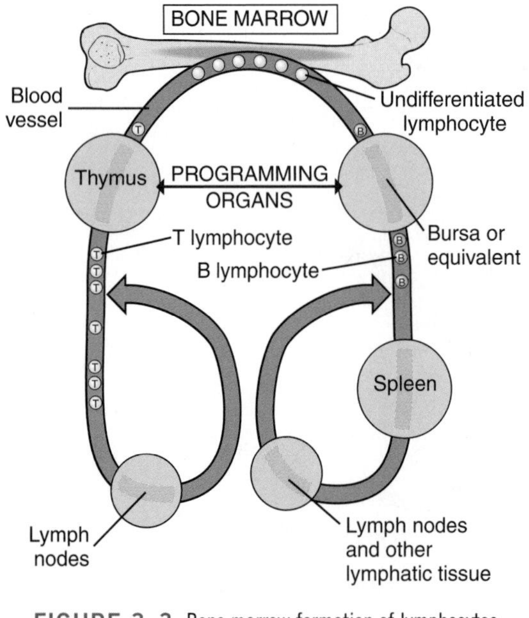

FIGURE 3–3 Bone marrow formation of lymphocytes.

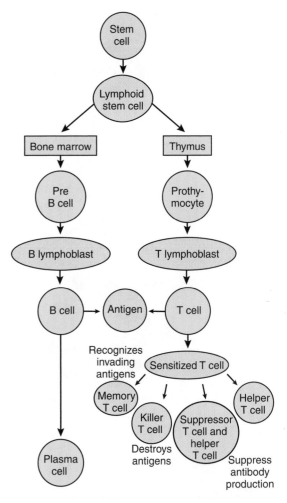

FIGURE 3–4 T cell and B cell formation.

gen presents itself again. The plasma cells are responsible for producing antibodies that attach to invading foreign antigens, thus marking the antigens for destruction by other cells of the immune system.

B cells are coated with **immunoglobulins,** giving them the ability to recognize foreign protein, and stimulate an antigen–antibody reaction. The five classes of immunoglobulins or antibodies are IgM, IgG, IgA, IgD, and IgE (Table 3–1). These immunoglobulins are usually all present during an antigenic response, although in varying amounts, depending on the stimulant and the health of the patient. Actions of the antigen–antibody complex include the following:

- Inactivation of the pathogen or its toxin through direct binding
- Stimulation of **phagocytosis** through opsonization, the process by which an antibody targets an infected cell for destruction by binding to the cell surface (Phagocytic cells recognize the antibody marker and engulf the infected cell.)

Activation of the complement system (complement fixation) involves several proteins found in plasma or body fluids. The antigen–antibody reaction initiates a series or cascade of reactions that activate the complement system, fixing the complement and consequently permitting the destruction of pathogens by the process of phagocytosis or lysis of the pathogen's cell membrane. This activation occurs during an immune reaction mediated by IgG or IgM.

Acquired immunity can be active or passive. *Active* immunity results when a person has had previous exposure to a disease or pathogen, for which the person was possibly asymptomatic and therefore the exposure was unrecognized, or when a person receives *immunizations* against a disease to stimulate the production of a specific antibody. Active immunity affords the person acquired permanent protection. *Passive* immunity bypasses the body's immune response to afford the benefit of immediate antibody availability. A person gains passive immunity by being given immune substances created outside that person's body for temporary immunity, such as when breast milk is fed to a child or immune globulin, an antibody-containing preparation made from the plasma of healthy donors, is given to help a person combat disease (Fig. 3–5).

Orderly Function of the Immune System

TABLE 3–1
Classes of Antibodies

CLASS	PERCENT OF TOTAL	LOCATION	FUNCTION
IgG	75–85	Blood plasma	Major antibody in primary and secondary immune responses; inactivates antigen; neutralizes toxins; crosses placenta to provide immunity for newborn; responsible for Rh reactions
IgA	5–15	Saliva, mucus, tears, breast milk	Protects mucous membranes on body surfaces; provides immunity for newborn
IgM	5–10	Attached to B cells; released into plasma during immune response	Causes antigens to clump together; responsible for transfusion reactions in the ABO blood typing system
IgD	0.2	Attached to B cells	Receptor sites for antigens on B cells; binding with antigen results in B cell activation
IgE	0.5	Produced by plasma cells in mucous membranes and tonsils	Binds to mast cells and basophils, causing release of histamine; responsible for allergic reactions

From Applegate EJ: *The anatomy and physiology learning system,* ed 2, Philadelphia, 2000, Saunders.

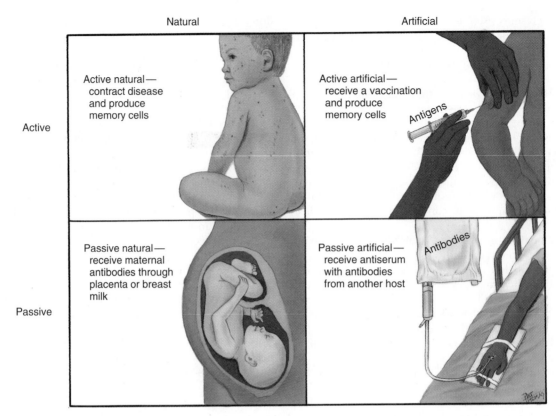

FIGURE 3–5 Acquired immunity. (From Applegate EJ: *The anatomy and physiology learning system,* ed 2, Philadelphia, 2000, Saunders.)

IMMUNODEFICIENCY DISEASES

AN ABSENT OR INADEQUATE RESPONSE of the immune system results in immunodeficiency conditions and increased susceptibility to other diseases and *opportunistic infections.* Immunodeficiency can occur in any of the following major components of the immune system: B cells, T cells, complement, or **phagocytes.** Although the deficiency may be in either the humoral or the cell-mediated responses, the consequences are similar: the individual does not have the capability to dispose of foreign and harmful substances. In general, an increased susceptibility to bacterial infections results from a B cell deficiency, whereas recurrent viral, fungal, and protozoan infections are usually due to decreased T cell function. Some of the conditions are genetic and present at birth, whereas other defects are not manifested until later in life or are acquired. Acquired immunoincompetence may result from a bacterial or viral insult to the body, malnutrition, or exposure to radiation or certain drugs. The severity of the immunodeficiency disease depends on the type of cell or cells that is affected. It can range from annoying chronic infections to severe life-threatening or fatal conditions.

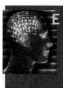

MALIGNANCIES AND COMMON OPPORTUNISTIC INFECTIONS AND CONDITIONS IN PATIENTS WITH AIDS

- Kaposi sarcoma is an aggressive malignancy of the blood vessels that appears as purple or blue patches on the skin, in the mouth, or anywhere else on the body (Fig. 3–6).
- Lymphomas are cancerous lesions of lymphoid tissues.
- *Pneumocystis carinii* pneumonia (PCP) is a lung infection that can progress to be life threatening. It is the most common lung disease in persons with AIDS.
- Tuberculosis is a tuberculous infection of the lungs or other organs.
- Herpes simplex consists of painful blister-like lesions of the mouth, genitalia, or anus caused by the herpes virus (Fig. 3–7).
- Herpes zoster (shingles) is characterized by clusters of red blister-like skin lesions that follow an inflamed nerve path.
- *Candida albicans* causes a fungal infection of the mucous membrane of the mouth, genitalia, or skin.
- Toxoplasmosis is an infection caused by a protozoan intracellular parasite. A rash and lymphadenopathy can be present, and the central nervous system, heart, or lungs can become involved.
- Neurologic complications include inflammation of nerves, neuropathy, neoplasms, and AIDS dementia complex.
- Diarrhea is a symptom of a host of bacterial and viral infections of the gastrointestinal tract, liver, or gallbladder.
- Epstein-Barr virus causes hairy leukoplakia that is characterized by white plaque visible on the tongue. This is associated with HIV-infected persons (Fig. 3–8).

Acquired Immunodeficiency Syndrome

DESCRIPTION
Acquired immunodeficiency syndrome (AIDS) is a progressive impairment of the immune system caused by the human immunodeficiency virus (HIV). This gradual destruction of the immune system affects many organ systems and has ultimately fatal consequences for the person infected.

ICD-9-CM Code 042

SYMPTOMS AND SIGNS
Initially it is not possible to tell whether people are infected with HIV by simply observing them. They may remain healthy for years during the latent period and may therefore unknowingly transmit the virus to other people. Within 1 to 2 weeks after exposure, the patient may experience a sore throat with fever and body aches. Lymphadenopathy, weight loss, fatigue, diarrhea, and night sweats are common as the clinical course progresses. The body's resistance becomes lower, and this leads to frequent infections, especially opportunistic infections; pneumonia; fever; and malignancies (see the Enrichment box for Malignancies and Common Opportunistic Infections and Conditions in Patients with AIDS). Often, in the later stages, en-

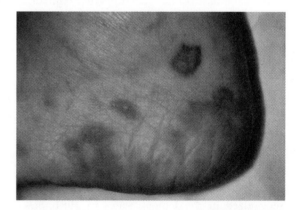

FIGURE 3–6 Kaposi sarcoma of distal heel and lateral foot. (Courtesy The Centers for Disease Control and Prevention, 1992. From Mudge-Grout C: *Immunologic disorders—Mosby's clinical nursing series,* St. Louis, 1992, Mosby.)

cephalopathy and malignancy lead to dementia and death (Fig. 3–9).

PATIENT SCREENING
An individual who complains of weight loss, fatigue, swollen glands, night sweats, and/or a persistent flulike syndrome needs an appointment with a physician for a medical evaluation as soon as possible. When an individual reports a known HIV

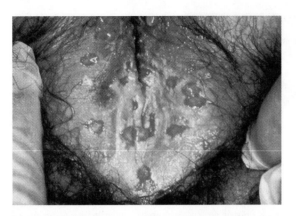

FIGURE 3–7 Primary perineal herpes with methylene blue stain. (Courtesy The Centers for Disease Control and Prevention, 1992. From Mudge-Grout C: *Immunologic disorders—Mosby's clinical nursing series,* St. Louis, 1992, Mosby.)

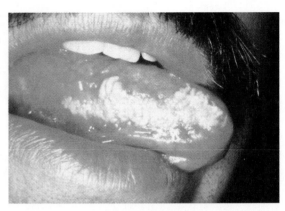

FIGURE 3–8 Hairy leukoplakia on the tongue of a patient with AIDS. (Courtesy J.S. Greenspan, DDS, University of California–San Francisco; courtesy The Centers for Disease Control and Prevention, 1992. From Mudge-Grout C: *Immunologic disorders—Mosby's clinical nursing series,* St. Louis, 1992, Mosby.)

exposure through unprotected sexual contact or puncture with a contaminated needle, immediate medical care should be arranged.

ETIOLOGY

AIDS is caused by HIV, type 1 or 2 (HIV-1 is found worldwide, HIV-2 is mainly in West Africa), *retroviruses* that contain *RNA;* they cannot survive apart from human cells. HIV attacks helper T lymphocytes (CD4 cells), the body's safeguard against tumors, viruses, and parasites. The destruction of T cells and the proliferation of HIV leave the body defenseless against infection and malignancy by reducing cell-mediated immunity. The virus also directly damages the nervous system. AIDS first was recognized in the United States in 1981. Since then, it has become a top killer of young men and a worldwide threat to humankind. It is estimated that more than 33 million people are currently infected with the AIDS virus. The time from infection with HIV to death is approximately 10 years. To date, neither a cure nor an effective vaccine has been found for this disease.

HIV is spread most readily by direct contact with the blood or semen of an infected person. It is not transmitted by casual contact such as touching, handshaking, and hugging. Sexual contact is the primary means of transmission. Although AIDS initially was associated with homosexual activity, more recent statistics show an increase in the number of women infected through heterosexual transmission. AIDS also can be transmitted through blood and blood products. Infants of infected mothers can contract the disease in utero, through the placenta, during the birth process and postpartum, and from breast milk. Sharing of needles by intravenous drug users also leads to infection. The risk of transmission of HIV to and from health-care workers and patients is minimized by strict adherence to the universal precautions for infection control.

DIAGNOSIS

The most common laboratory screening test used to detect the presence of HIV antibodies in the blood is the *enzyme-linked immunosorbent assay (ELISA)*. If the findings are positive, the test is repeated, and the result is then confirmed by using a *Western blot test*. A positive p24 antigen test indicates circulating HIV antigen. The lymphocyte count is monitored for the evaluation of immunocompetence—as the disease progresses, the T cell count decreases. Other tests can detect impairment of the immune system and monitor the total health status of the HIV-infected person. ELISA tests are often negative during the first month of infection, although a p24 antigen test or polychromase chain reaction (PCR) assay may be positive. Transmission of HIV is possible during all stages of infection, even early on, before it can be detected by laboratory tests.

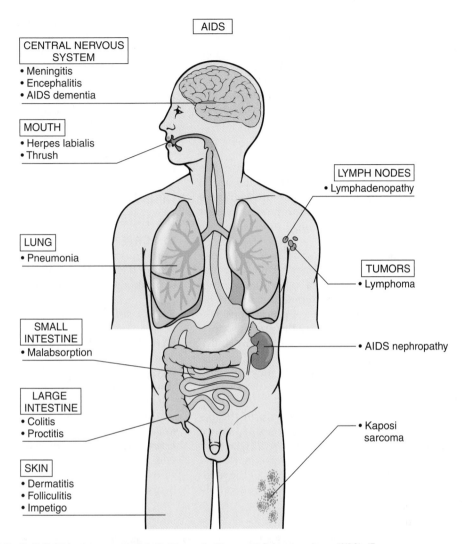

FIGURE 3–9 Pathologic changes associated with acquired immunodeficiency syndrome (AIDS). (From Damjanov I: *Pathology for the health-related professions,* ed 2, Philadelphia, 2000, Saunders.)

TREATMENT

Currently, no cure exists for AIDS. The goal of medical management is to maintain the best possible immune status by using immunizations and antiinfective therapy. The current treatment of choice involves the use of two nucleoside inhibitors, lamivudine and zidovudine (AZT), and a protease inhibitor called indinavir. This combination is referred to as HAART (highly active antiretroviral therapy).

Although these drugs have been effective at prolonging life and maintaining the quality of life for patients, they are associated with a number of toxicities and serious side effects. Surgery for the removal of *neoplasms* may be suggested to prolong life and to provide some comfort. Individualized supportive treatment plans vary with the body systems affected and the needs of each patient. Addressing the psychological needs of the patient with AIDS is essential.

Health-care practitioners who are involved in various forms of patient care with exposure to body fluids and blood should follow the principles of infection control and universal precautions (see the Alert box for Infection Control and Universal Precautions). All body fluids and blood from any patient should be handled with extreme care, as if the patient were known to be infected with HIV.

PROGNOSIS

Although AIDS is ultimately a fatal disease, the number of Americans dying of AIDS each year has dropped. Better access to care and more aggressive use of newer drugs are thought to be reasons that people with AIDS are living longer now.

PREVENTION

Because HIV is transmitted directly from human to human, prevention measures relate to avoiding risk factors for sexually transmitted diseases and infection control by using universal precautions. Use of condoms and not sharing needles are highly recommended. The drugs used in highly active antiviral therapy (HAART) can be administered as postexposure prophylaxis after a needle-stick injury.

PATIENT TEACHING

Describe the diagnostic tests and inform the patient concerning when to expect test results. Assure the patient of medical confidentiality. Make sure the HIV-positive individual knows how the disease is transmitted. Stress important aspects of the medication regimen and the dangers of noncompli-

ance. Explain side effects of the therapeutic drugs, and encourage him or her to contact the health-care worker with questions or concerns. Other teaching points will include how to minimize infections, the need for lifelong therapies, and the responsibility to inform healthcare providers about the HIV diagnosis. The psychological, social, and financial ramifications of having HIV require referrals for community support. Eventually referrals will be required to meet a variety of home care needs.

Common Variable Immunodeficiency (Acquired Hypogammaglobulinemia)

DESCRIPTION

Common variable immunodeficiency (CVID) is an acquired B cell deficiency that results in an absence of antibody production and/or function.

 ICD-9-CM Code 279.06

SYMPTOMS AND SIGNS

The person with CVID has a history of chronic infections. The *sinopulmonary* symptoms include sinus tenderness, cough, fever, runny nose, abnormal sputum, and *dyspnea.* Gastrointestinal symptoms include diarrhea, abdominal pain, and weight loss. **Lymphadenopathy,** *splenomegaly,* and *hepatomegaly* often are observed. Recurrent *otitis media* is experienced as well. When CVID is associated with *autoimmune* disorders, rashes, bleeding, bruising, fatigue, arthralgia (painful joints),

---

ALERT

INFECTION CONTROL AND UNIVERSAL PRECAUTIONS

Guidelines: Treat blood and body fluids as if infected and remember to use the following precautions:

1. Practice frequent and thorough handwashing.
2. Report any accidental needle-sticks.
3. Wear personal protective equipment, including mask, gown, gloves, and goggles.
4. Use caution with laboratory specimens.
5. Dispose of contaminated sharps in designated biohazard containers. *Caution:* Do not recap or break needles.

6. Use proper linen disposal containers.
7. Use clean mouthpieces and resuscitation bags.
8. Obtain hepatitis B vaccination to protect against occupational exposure to blood.
9. Use proper decontamination techniques.
10. Absorb blood spills with paper towels, then clean the area with soap and water, followed by disinfection of the area with a 1:10 solution of household bleach.

muscle weakness, and pain may be noted. As the disease progresses and T cell involvement occurs, susceptibility to opportunistic and viral infections and malignancies escalates.

PATIENT SCREENING

When a child or young teenager is seemingly susceptible to frequent infection, it is recommended that an appointment to discuss options be made with the health care provider or that office policy regarding referral to a pediatrician be followed. When the individual, particularly a younger adult, experiences frequent bacterial infections, an appointment for an in-depth medical investigation is indicated.

ETIOLOGY

CVID has two peaks of incidence: one between the ages of 25 and 45 years, and a smaller peak from ages 5 to 15 years. Although the exact cause of acquired **hypogammaglobulinemia** is not known, it is thought to be a result of defective T cell signaling. The number of circulating B cells is often normal, but the ability of the B cells to produce all types of immunoglobulins is reduced. Cell-mediated immunity usually remains intact.

DIAGNOSIS

A history of repeated and chronic infections along with the clinical findings should lead to further investigation of immunoglobulin levels, B cell titers, and B cell and T cell quantities. Evaluations of sinopulmonary status include cultures, radiographic studies, and pulmonary function tests. Abnormal findings in any of these studies necessitate a *biopsy* of lymph tissue. Decreased plasma cell presence is indicative of the disease.

TREATMENT

Treatment is aimed at preventing infections and implementing early treatment with appropriate antibiotic administration when infections occur. Proper nutrition and adequate rest are encouraged. Immune globulin replacement on a regular basis is helpful, and fever is treated with acetaminophen. Sinus and ear infections may be treated surgically to ensure proper drainage. *People known to have CVID must never be immunized with live virus vaccines.*

PROGNOSIS

Although the use of immune globulin and prophylactic antibodies has improved prognosis, patients eventually succumb to chronic lung disease, liver failure due to viral hepatitis, or malignancies. Males often have a higher mortality rate than do females.

PREVENTION

No methods of prevention are known.

PATIENT TEACHING

Teaching points include steps to take to avoid infection and to ensure good nutrition, adequate rest, and regular follow-up care.

Selective Immunoglobulin A Deficiency

DESCRIPTION

Patients with selective immunoglobulin A (IgA) deficiency fail to produce the normal levels of IgA. Selective deficiencies of IgM or IgG have been reported but are rare.

 ICD-9-CM Code 279.01

SYMPTOMS AND SIGNS

The majority of patients with IgA deficiency are asymptomatic, perhaps because of a compensatory increase in IgM production in these patients. Those who do experience symptoms have chronic sinopulmonary infections with subsequent respiratory allergy. Food allergies are also common. Celiac disease, ulcerative colitis, regional enteritis, and other autoimmune diseases often are associated with this condition. Children with selective IgA deficiency typically exhibit recurrent otitis media and respiratory tract disease. Spontaneous production of IgA may occur and if so, the ear and respiratory tract problems usually subside as a result.

ETIOLOGY

Failure to produce adequate levels of IgA is relatively common in the general population. Autosomal dominant or recessive inheritance appears to play a role in the etiology of this condition, in which B cells are apparently not secreting IgA. The cause may be a failure of heavy chain gene switching, the process that allows the production of different classes of immunoglobulins that have a specificity for the same antigen that elicited the immune response. It is thought that some patients with the disease will progress to common variable immunodeficiency (CVID).

DIAGNOSIS

Immunologic studies indicate below-normal levels of circulating IgA along with an absence of IgA in saliva and nasal, bronchial, and intestinal secretions. Other immunoglobulin levels are normal. Circulating B cells have a normal appearance.

TREATMENT

No cure for this condition is known, although some patients may spontaneously begin to produce IgA. Treatment is geared toward the prevention and management of infection. Prophylactic antibiotics are given. *Immune globulin must never be administered to these patients because sensitization can lead to anaphylaxis if blood products are administered later.*

PROGNOSIS

In most cases no significant medical problems are to be expected and prognosis is good. Some children may show a slow, spontaneous resolution of the condition.

PREVENTION

No method of prevention is known.

PATIENT TEACHING

Teaching points include steps to take to avoid infection and to ensure good nutrition, adequate rest, and regular follow-up care. Explain the purpose of prophylactic antibiotic therapy, as prescribed.

⁃ X-Linked Agammaglobulinemia

DESCRIPTION

X-linked agammaglobulinemia (Bruton agammaglobulinemia) is a condition of severe B cell deficiency.

 ICD-9-CM Code 279.04

SYMPTOMS AND SIGNS

The infant with X-linked agammaglobulinemia has recurrent severe gram-positive infections, including bacterial otitis media, bronchitis, pneumonia, and meningitis. These usually occur after 4 to 6 months of age, when the natural transplacental immunity from the mother has been depleted. Additional symptoms may include conjunctivitis *(purulent)*, dental caries, and rheumatoid arthritis–type symptoms. Lymphadenopathy and splenomegaly are noticeably absent.

PATIENT SCREENING

Recurrent severe bacterial infections in an infant signal the need for in-depth medical investigation to determine a possible underlying cause(s). Follow office policy for referral to a pediatrician, when appropriate.

ETIOLOGY

This congenital X-linked disorder affects only males. It is due to a defect in the Bruton tyrosine kinase, which is normally expressed in B cells during all stages of development. This kinase is also present in myeloid and erythroid cells. All five immunoglobulin classes are usually absent, along with the absence of circulating B cells and the presence of normal numbers of circulating T cells. Parents of these children are encouraged to seek genetic counseling regarding future pregnancies. Atypical forms of the disease have been documented in which low numbers of B cells and the usual symptoms occur later in life.

DIAGNOSIS

The clinical findings, along with a thorough history including age at onset and family history of relatives who died of severe infections, will suggest X-linked agammaglobulinemia. **Immunoelectrophoresis** indicates decreased levels of serum IgM, IgA, and IgG; however, relying on this method of diagnosis is not valid before the infant is 6 to 8 months of age. Other findings suggestive of this disease are normal T cell numbers along with low or absent B cell numbers.

TREATMENT

Treatment is directed at improving the child's immune defenses, controlling infections, and relieving rheumatoid arthritis–like symptoms. Intravenous infusions of immune globulin every 2 to 4 weeks, occasional infusions of fresh frozen plasma, and appropriate antibiotics are administered. *These children must never be immunized with live virus vaccines, nor should corticosteroids or immunosuppressive drugs be administered.*

PROGNOSIS

Although this condition cannot be cured, regular infusions of immune globulin may provide the child with an almost normal lifestyle.

PREVENTION

No methods of prevention are known.

PATIENT TEACHING

Discuss the importance of avoiding infections. Explain the procedure for immune globulin infusions. Caution the parents about the contraindication for live virus vaccines, and **immunosuppressive** drugs.

– Severe Combined Immunodeficiency

DESCRIPTION

Severe combined immunodeficiency (SCID) is a group of disorders that result from a disturbance in the development and function of both T cells and B cells. This leads to an absence of both cell-mediated (T cell) and antibody-mediated (B cell) immunity.

 ICD-9-CM Code 279.2

SYMPTOMS AND SIGNS

SCID manifests as severe, recurrent infections with bacteria, viruses, fungi, and protozoa. This occurs by the age of 3 to 6 months, when the natural maternal placental immunity begins to deplete. The most common infections are *Pneumocystis* pneumonia and mucocutaneous **candidiasis.** In addition, the infant fails to thrive and experiences chronic otitis media and diarrhea. The infant usually has a low-grade fever until the natural maternal acquired immunity is depleted, and then severe infections erupt. Discernible lymphoid tissue (enlarged tonsils, palpable lymph nodes, etc.) may be absent. Abnormal laboratory findings often include hypogammaglobulinemia and abnormal lymphocyte populations.

PATIENT SCREENING

The history of pneumonia in the first weeks of life, followed by frequent, severe infections in the young infant are indicative of underlying conditions that need a complete medical evaluation. These infections are potentially life threatening in the infant and immediate medical care is required. Follow office policy for referral to a pediatrician.

ETIOLOGY

Two types of SCID are known: X-linked and autosomal recessive. Both are due to a defect in stem cell differentiation into B cells and T cells. The X-linked type is due to a mutation in a cytokine receptor gene. This leads to the blockage of several cytokine pathways that are necessary for lymphocyte development. Autosomal recessive SCID stems from a mutation in either a gene encoding a tyrosine kinase (Jak-3) or a gene encoding a recombinase enzyme. Both defects result in a disruption in lymphocyte development.

DIAGNOSIS

If the clinical findings indicate suspicion of SCID, many laboratory tests are performed. These include measurement of immunoglobulin levels, antibody titers, and numbers of T cells and B cells. T cell proliferation should be measured *in vitro* if the lab findings are abnormal. Western blots of lymphocyte lysates showing the absence of the Jak-3 tyrosine kinase is diagnostic for one type of autosomal recessive SCID.

TREATMENT

Bone marrow transplantation is the only curative treatment for all types of SCID at present, although the role of gene therapy is being investigated. Preventing exposure to infection and assisting the immune response through bone marrow transplantation are the goals of treatment. Compatible bone marrow donors are usually siblings. Children with SCID are placed in completely sterile environments (usually a plastic "bubble") to prevent exposure to infectious agents.

PROGNOSIS

Not being able to detect defective antibody-mediated immunity in a child before the age of 6 months to 1 year compromises timely diagnosis of the condition. Consequently, many of these children die of overwhelming infection before the age of 1 year.

PREVENTION

No methods of prevention are known.

PATIENT TEACHING

Explain the medical and surgical interventions used to protect against infection and restore immune response. Refer parents to available community support organizations that can help with the psychological, physical, and financial burdens precipitated by the infant's prognosis of severe illness and early death. During hospitalizations, encourage the parents to visit and interact with the infant as much as possible. Refer the parents to a genetic counselor.

DiGeorge Anomaly (Thymic Hypoplasia or Aplasia)

DESCRIPTION
DiGeorge anomaly is a congenital condition of immunodeficiency that results from a small or absent thymus (thymic hypoplasia or aplasia). In some coding manuals, this disease may be listed as DiGeorge syndrome.

ICD-9-CM Code 279.11

SYMPTOMS AND SIGNS
DiGeorge anomaly is identified in young children by confirming a set of structural anomalies. These anomalies include abnormally wide-set, downward slanting eyes; low-set ears with notched pinnas; a small mouth (Fig. 3–10); and cardiovascular defects, possibly tetralogy of Fallot. The thymus and parathyroid glands are absent or underdeveloped. The infant exhibits signs of *tetany* due to hypocalcemia caused by hypoparathyroidism. Some degree of cognitive impairment often is present. The patient is susceptible to severe viral, fungal, and protozoan infections. The most common of these are pneumonia and thrush in infants.

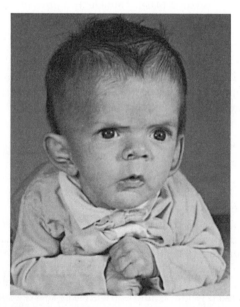

FIGURE 3–10 Infant with thymic hypoplasia (DiGeorge anomaly). (Courtesy Dr. Russell W. Steele, Washington, DC. From Stiehm RS: *Immunologic disorders in infants & children*, ed 4, Philadelphia, 1996, Saunders.)

PATIENT SCREENING
Infants or children with DiGeorge anomaly need prompt medical treatment when signs of infection occur.

ETIOLOGY
DiGeorge anomaly is the result of abnormal development of the third and fourth pharyngeal pouches during the 12th week of gestation. This causes the thymus gland to be underdeveloped or absent. If the thymus gland is underdeveloped, it is abnormally located (ectopic). The disease has two forms: complete and partial. In the complete form, the thymus is absent or weighs less than 1 gram. T cell number is very low or absent, B cells are present, but little antibody is produced. Partial forms have variable T cell number and function, depending on the amount of ectopic thymus tissue. Antibody production is usually normal. Most patients with DiGeorge anomaly have a microdeletion on one copy of chromosome 22.

DIAGNOSIS
A definitive diagnosis requires a reduced number of T cells and two of the following three features: cardiovascular defects, hypocalcemia of over 3 weeks' duration, and a microdeletion involving chromosome 22 (detected by fluorescence in situ hybridization). Absence, hypoplasia, or abnormal placement of the thymus gland can be detected radiographically. *Hypoparathyroidism* is diagnosed by low serum calcium levels, elevated serum phosphorus levels, and lack of parathyroid hormone.

TREATMENT
Aggressive treatment of the hypocalcemia with intravenous infusion to replace calcium is essential to restore the electrolyte balance and to reduce the risk of seizures. Vitamin D and parathyroid hormone replacement therapy are also necessary. Repair of cardiac anomalies may be attempted. Intravenous immune globulin may be helpful. Limited data suggest that a human fetal thymus transplantation may reconstitute immune function in some patients. Parents are taught to control exposure of the infant to prevent infections.

PROGNOSIS
Complete DiGeorge anomaly is usually fatal in early childhood because of cardiac dysfunction, hypocalcemia, and/or infection. For some patients

with partial DiGeorge anomaly, immune function may improve with age.

PREVENTION
No methods of prevention are known.

PATIENT TEACHING
Congenital structural anomalies, the complications thereof, and the child's susceptibility to infections determine what information is most helpful to parents and caregivers. Procedures such as intravenous infusions of immune globulin or those given to treat hypocalcemia are explained.

Chronic Mucocutaneous Candidiasis

DESCRIPTION
Chronic mucocutaneous candidiasis (CMC) is a chronic syndrome of persistent and recurrent candidal (fungal) infections of the skin, nails, and mucous membranes.

◼ ICD-9-CM Code 112
Refer to the physician's diagnosis and then to the current edition of the ICD-9-CM coding manual to ensure the greatest specificity of pathology and any appropriate modifiers.

SYMPTOMS AND SIGNS
Symptoms usually develop during the first 2 or 3 years of life or, if late-onset CMC, in young adulthood. Large circular lesions appear on the skin, mucous membranes, nails, or vagina. Sores in the mouth make eating difficult (Fig. 3–11). Recurrent thrush or diaper rash is often the first symptom of the disease in infants. Older children exhibit lesions, often beginning on the scalp and also involving the nails. Patients in late stages of the disease experience recurring respiratory tract infections. Other infections with bacteria, viruses, and other fungi are also more common in these individuals.

Glands can become involved (endocrinopathies), and the particular symptoms of hypofunction, such as hypocalcemia, hypoparathyroidism, and pernicious anemia, are related to the specific glands or organs affected. Some patients experience severe viral infections before the onset of the endocrinopathies.

Syndromes of CMC are chronic oral candidiasis (disease affecting the mucosa of the lips, tongue, and buccal cavity), chronic mucocutaneous candidiasis with endocrinopathy (hypoadrenalism, hy-

pothyroidism, hypoparathyroidism, and ovarian failure in females), chronic localized candidiasis (cutaneous lesions with hyperkeratosis), chronic diffuse candidiasis (widespread infection of the skin, nails, and mucous membranes) (Fig. 3–12), and candidiasis with thymoma (candidiasis accompanied by hypogammaglobulinemia, neutropenia, aplastic anemia, or myasthenia gravis).

PATIENT SCREENING
Frequent, persistent fungal infections of the mouth, skin, or nails in the young child necessitate a prompt appointment with the physician for medical evaluation and to begin treatment.

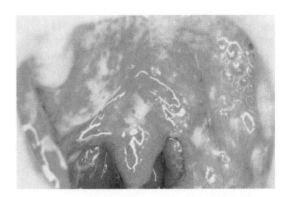

FIGURE 3–11 Candidiasis. (From Sigler B: *Ear, nose, and throat disorders—Mosby's clinical nursing series,* St. Louis, 1994, Mosby.)

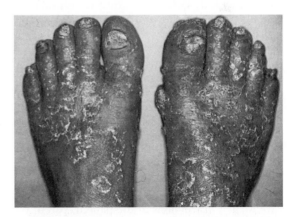

FIGURE 3–12 Chronic mucotaneous candidiasis of the feet. (From Stiehm RS: *Immunologic disorders in infants & children,* ed 4, Philadelphia, 1996, Saunders.)

ETIOLOGY

In the immunocompetent individual, *Candida albicans* is a nonpathogenic normal flora. Patients with CMC have a T cell deficit specific to *Candida* that makes them susceptible to infection. Other T cell and B cell functions are normal. An inherited defect in the T cell–mediated immune system that permits autoantibodies to develop against target organs appears to be a factor in this syndrome. This is associated with the endocrinopathies.

DIAGNOSIS

Blood studies indicate normal T cell circulation and normal antibody response to all organisms except *Candida*. Patients have normal immunoglobulin levels, normal lymphocyte numbers, and normal response to non-*Candida* antigens. Other immunodeficiency diseases need to be ruled out, and all endocrine functions should be evaluated. Any other abnormalities are evaluated according to the organs involved.

TREATMENT

Treatment is directed at eliminating the infections along with correcting the immunologic defects. The drug of choice for initial therapy is nystatin (Mycostatin) because of the lack of significant side effects with this drug. Other systemic antifungal agents are usually successful in cases not responding to nystatin. Topical treatment with antifungal agents appears to improve skin and nail lesions. Symptoms arising from other organs and glands are addressed according to the organ or gland involved. Treatment of the immunologic defect includes thymus transplantation, lymphocyte infusions, or bone marrow transplantation.

PROGNOSIS

Treatment with antifungals has good results, but most patients will relapse after cessation of these agents. Treatments aimed at correcting the immunologic defect may result in a cure.

PREVENTION

No method of prevention is known.

PATIENT TEACHING

Give written instructions to the patient/parent on the medication regimen. Teach comfort measures for mouth lesions such as a soft diet and the use of a mild mouthwash and a soft toothbrush. Instruct the patient/parent not to delay medical attention for any infections or signs of relapse. Address questions regarding any endocrine involvement as appropriate to the diagnosis. Give preoperative/postoperative information and instructions if thymus transplantation or bone marrow transplant is scheduled.

Wiskott-Aldrich Syndrome

DESCRIPTION

Wiskott-Aldrich syndrome is a congenital disorder that is characterized by inadequate B and T cell function.

 ICD-9-CM Code 279.12

SYMPTOMS AND SIGNS

The child with Wiskott-Aldrich syndrome experiences eczema and **thrombocytopenia** with severe bleeding. These childen also display an increased susceptibility to bacterial, viral, and fungal infections. Bleeding manifestations include *petechiae, purpura,* hematemesis, epistaxis, and hematuria, as well as the more serious gastrointestinal (GI) and intracranial bleeding. By the age of 1 year, the bleeding subsides somewhat and eczema develops. These children are predisposed to the development of autoimmune disorders (hemolytic anemia, vasculitis, etc.), leukemia, and lymphoma.

PATIENT SCREENING

Severe bleeding manifestations call for immediate assessment and medical care. If the child is being treated for Wiskott-Aldrich syndrome and signs of infection are reported, prompt medical attention is indicated.

ETIOLOGY

This rare immunodeficiency disorder is inherited as an X-linked trait affecting only males. It arises from mutations in the gene encoding the Wiskott-Aldrich syndrome protein (WASP), which is expressed in hematopoietic cells. The thymus gland is normal at birth but decreases in size as the child becomes older, resulting in decreased B and T cell functions. This compromises the child's immunity and increases the risk of infection. Additionally, metabolic defects in platelet synthesis that cause platelets to be short lived and phagocytes to be incompetent are both present. The average age at diagnosis is 21 months.

DIAGNOSIS

Diagnosis is suspected in a boy with thrombocytopenia and small platelet size, especially when accompanied by eczema and frequent infections. The diagnosis is supported by finding a mutation in WASP. The numbers of T cells and B cells may be low.

TREATMENT

Bone marrow transplantation (BMT) is the only curative therapy. A high success rate can be expected when the donor is an HLA-matched sibling. If BMT is not feasible, then splenectomy may result in an increase in platelet number and size. Additional treatment consists of intravenous immune globulin and/or appropriate antibiotic therapy for infections.

PROGNOSIS

Long-term survival is good for patients who receive a BMT before the age of 5 years. Patients who have a splenectomy without a BMT have a median survival of 25 years, whereas those who receive neither therapy often die before the age of 5 years. Bleeding is the main cause of death.

PREVENTION

No methods of prevention are known.

PATIENT TEACHING

Encourage the parent/caregiver to express concerns about episodes of bleeding. Discuss the signs of bleeding that require emergency care, such as signs of shock. Explain the importance of timely and aggressive treatment for infections. If bone marrow transplant is scheduled, discuss the procedure and reinforce the surgeon's explanation of expected results. If the child is experiencing symptoms of eczema, demonstrate the topical application of medication as prescribed.

AUTOIMMUNE DISEASES

AUTOIMMUNE DISEASES OCCUR when autoantibodies develop and begin to destroy the body's own cells. Tolerance to self-antigens is believed to commence during fetal life. As the body ages or experiences various disease processes, the immune system misidentifies body cells and develops antibodies against its own cells and tissues, resulting in self-destruction. Present theories consider *autoimmunity* to be acquired, not congenital; however, certain genetic markers identify patients at increased risk for many autoimmune diseases. Currently, the specific gene products involved are mostly undetermined.

Autoimmune diseases can occur in many body systems when lymphocytes and antibodies are sensitized to develop against self. The production of the autoantibodies may occur by means of several mechanisms including disease, injury, metabolic change, and a mutation of immunologically competent cells. Additionally, viral infection, trauma, and certain drugs or chemicals may alter specific body proteins, thereby thwarting recognition and terminating in their rejection as being foreign. Systems or body tissue particularly affected by autoimmunity and some of the resulting disease entities are listed in Table 3–2.

Hematopoietic Disorders

– Autoimmune Hemolytic Anemia

DESCRIPTION

Autoimmune hemolytic anemia is an autoimmune condition in which red blood cells (RBCs) are destroyed by antibodies.

 ICD-9-CM Code 283.0

SYMPTOMS AND SIGNS

Autoimmune hemolytic anemia causes the patient to experience fatigue, weakness, chills, fever, dyspnea, and itching. The skin is pale and *jaundiced* and bruises easily. Additionally, the patient may be hypotensive.

PATIENT SCREENING

Schedule a "same day" appointment for the patient experiencing the symptoms listed above. Patients with mild or fewer symptoms may be scheduled with less urgency.

Hematopoietic Disorders

TABLE 3-2
Autoimmune Diseases

BODY SYSTEM OR TISSUE	DISEASE
Hematopoietic system	Autoimmune hemolytic anemia
	Pernicious anemia
	Idiopathic thrombocytopenic purpura
	Idiopathic neutropenia
Kidney	Goodpasture syndrome
	Immune complex glomerulonephritis
Rheumatoid and collagen	Systemic lupus erythematosus
	Progressive scleroderma (systemic sclerosis)
	Sjögren syndrome
	Rheumatoid arthritis
	Juvenile rheumatoid arthritis
Endocrine system*	Graves disease
	Hashimoto disease (chronic thyroiditis)
	Type I diabetes
Neurologic system	Multiple sclerosis
	Myasthenia gravis
Vascular system	Small vessel vasculitis
	Systemic necrotizing vasculitis

*See Chapter 4.

ETIOLOGY

Because of failure of the immune response, B cell–produced antibodies are not able to identify RBCs as self, resulting in an attack on and destruction of the red corpuscles. The two types of hemolytic anemia are warm antibody (agglutinin) anemia and cold antibody (agglutinin) anemia. Warm antibody anemia is associated with an excess of IgG antibodies that react with protein antigens on the RBC surface at body temperature. Although most cases are *idiopathic,* some may be stimulated by certain drugs (e.g., penicillins), autoimmune diseases (e.g., systemic lupus erythematosus), or malignancies (especially chronic lymphocytic leukemia). Cold antibody anemia results from fixation of complement proteins on IgM that occurs at colder temperatures (best around 30° C). This type is regularly seen in conjunction with infectious mononucleosis or *Mycoplasma* pneumonia.

DIAGNOSIS

A direct Coombs test indicates antibody-coated RBCs that agglutinate when antiglobulin is added to the medium. Some RBCs are spherical; serum bilirubin levels are elevated; and RBC count, platelet count, hemoglobin concentration, and *hematocrit* usually are all decreased. The reticulocyte count is usually elevated. Examination of a peripheral blood smear for agglutination of RBCs and flow cytometry may be performed. In mild or sporadic disease, these previously mentioned results might not be evident when the patient is tested.

TREATMENT

Treatment should first address any underlying disease or drug use that could be causing the hemolytic anemia. Warm and cold antibody anemias are treated differently. In warm antibody anemia, corticosteroids and cytotoxic drugs are administered to reduce antibody production. Splenectomy or immune globulin administration may be done to reduce antibody effectiveness. Red cell transfusions may be attempted. The most useful therapy in the treatment of cold antibody anemia is avoidance of the cold—dressing warmly even in the summer, wearing gloves and warm hats, spending the colder months in warmer climates. *Plasmapheresis* may be helpful in reducing hemolysis.

PROGNOSIS

Anemia resulting from infection or drug use will usually abate after the infection resolves or the drug is discontinued. Anemia resulting from other causes is often chronic and poorly responsive to therapy. Warm antibody anemia is generally self-limiting in children, disappearing within 1 to 3 months.

PREVENTION

No methods of prevention are known.

PATIENT TEACHING

Explain the diagnostic tests and tell the patient when to expect results. If the cause has been determined, explain how the RBCs are being destroyed and how the treatment regimen is expected to help. Discuss expected results from immune globulin administration or, if indicated, the removal of the spleen.

Pernicious Anemia

DESCRIPTION

Pernicious anemia is caused by decreased gastric production of hydrochloric acid and the resulting shortage of intrinsic factor, which lead to impaired vitamin B_{12} absorption.

ICD-9-CM Code 281.0

SYMPTOMS AND SIGNS

The patient with pernicious anemia has a sore tongue, weakness, and tingling and numbness in the extremities. The lips, tongue, and gums appear pale, whereas the sclera and skin appear slightly jaundiced (Fig. 3–13). Because of the decreased hydrochloric acid production and atrophy of the gastric mucosa, the patient experiences disturbances in digestion such as *anorexia,* nausea, vomiting, diarrhea, constipation, flatulence, and weight loss. In this condition the individual is more vulnerable to infections. Vitamin B_{12} deficiency causes demyelination of the peripheral nerves and eventually the spinal cord. This leads to neuritis, peripheral weakness, numbness, and *paresthesia.* Ataxia (muscular incoordination), lightheadedness, altered vision, *tinnitus,* and optic muscle *atrophy* are additional symptoms that may occur as the anemia progresses. Central nervous system changes may cause headaches, irritability, and depression. Reduced hemoglobin levels are responsible for decreased oxygen-carrying capacity, leading to fatigue, weakness, and lightheadedness. The patient may experience palpitations, dyspnea, *tachycardia,* premature ventricular contractions, and even congestive heart failure.

PATIENT SCREENING

Initially the patient may present with insidious and vague symptoms; unless the symptoms are severe, the patient is scheduled for a medical evaluation at as soon as convenient. Patients complaining of weakness or cardiovascular symptoms (e.g., a rapid heart rate) require prompt medical care. A "same day" appointment is scheduled for the patient being treated for pernicious anemia if physical or psychological complications develop.

ETIOLOGY

Over 90% of patients with pernicious anemia have antiparietal cell antibodies, which can be cytotoxic to the *parietal* cells. A majority of patients also have antiintrinsic factor antibodies. Intrinsic factor must be present in the gastric mucosa for vitamin B_{12} absorption to occur. Vitamin B_{12} is necessary for RBC formation, and a deficiency causes RBCs to be deformed and reduced in number. Pernicious anemia is often associated with other autoimmune diseases such as Graves disease or Hashimoto thyroiditis. It is particularly common in people of Northern European descent between the ages of 40 and 70, but it can be seen in any ethnic group.

DIAGNOSIS

Diagnosis is confirmed by the clinical findings and laboratory tests. The Schilling test and/or an evaluation for the presence of antiparietal cell or antiintrinsic factor antibodies is performed. Blood tests reveal decreased hemoglobin (Hb) level, decreased RBC count, and increased mean cell volume (MCV). The RBCs and the platelets are large and malformed. Bone marrow studies indicate abnormal RBC production and other changes typical of vitamin B_{12} deficiency. Reduced amounts or absence of gastric acid is found on gastric analysis. Vitamin B_{12} is also necessary for proper *myelin* formation; a myelin deficiency can cause damage to the nerves.

TREATMENT

Monthly intramuscular injections of vitamin B_{12} are the primary treatment of this type of anemia, and they must be continued for life. Blood replacement may be indicated in severe cases. Supportive measures include adequate rest, gentle nonirritating mouth care, a well-balanced diet high in vitamin B_{12}, and the use of tranquilizers for behavioral problems.

PROGNOSIS

No cure for pernicious anemia is known, but early detection and treatment with vitamin B_{12} maintains a normal hemogram and neurologic function in most patients.

PREVENTION

No method of prevention for the primary condition is known. Patients who have had extensive gastric surgery benefit from vitamin B_{12} replacement.

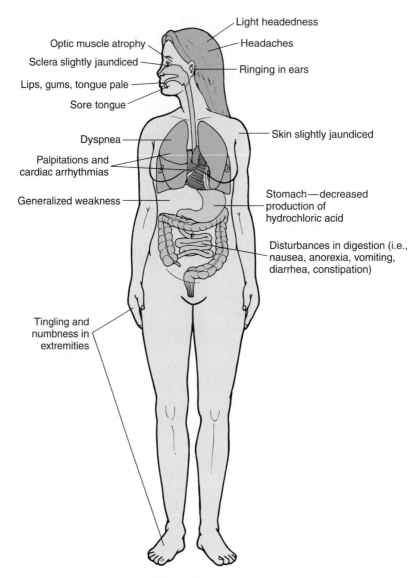

Light headedness

Headaches

Ringing in ears

Optic muscle atrophy

Sclera slightly jaundiced

Lips, gums, tongue pale

Sore tongue

Dyspnea

Palpitations and cardiac arrhythmias

Generalized weakness

Skin slightly jaundiced

Stomach—decreased production of hydrochloric acid

Disturbances in digestion (i.e., nausea, anorexia, vomiting, diarrhea, constipation)

Tingling and numbness in extremities

FIGURE 3–13 Symptoms and signs of pernicious anemia.

PATIENT TEACHING

During the diagnostic phase, give careful instructions about the 24-hour urine collections needed for an accurate Schilling test. If bone marrow studies are ordered, explain the procedure. Once diagnosed, inform the patient that improvement is likely within weeks of treatment and good compliance with the treatment regimen. To promote compliance, explain the importance of lifelong vitamin B_{12} replacement therapy; demonstrate injection technique to the patient or caregiver if required.

Review signs of any complications that should be reported to the physician.

Idiopathic Thrombocytopenic Purpura

DESCRIPTION

Idiopathic thrombocytopenic purpura (ITP) is an acquired disorder that results from an isolated deficiency of platelets (i.e., other blood counts are normal).

ICD-9-CM Code 287.3

SYMPTOMS AND SIGNS

Symptoms are related to an inability of the blood to clot and include spontaneous hemorrhages in the skin, mucous membranes, or internal organs. Petechiae, small spiderlike hemorrhages under the surface of the skin, and ecchymoses, larger hemorrhagic areas, are apparent. The patient may experience *epistaxis* (nosebleeds), gastrointestinal bleeding, *menorrhagia, hematuria,* and easy bruising. The clinical symptoms vary with patient age, with older patients exhibiting more severe bleeding symptoms.

PATIENT SCREENING

Multiple bruising of unknown cause in a child or an adult requires prompt medical attention. (NOTE: An event of spontaneous bruising in a child can cause a parent to become extremely alarmed and also precipitates a natural concern by medical personnel in regard to the child's welfare. Care must be taken by medical personnel to avoid judgmental attitudes toward parents until a sound reason to suspect child abuse has been established.)

ETIOLOGY

Thrombocytopenic purpura often is considered idiopathic (unknown cause), although antibodies that reduce the life of platelets have been found in most cases. Some cases may occur after a viral infection, especially rubella or mumps. Additionally, the spleen may be destroying the damaged platelets.

DIAGNOSIS

The diagnosis of ITP is often one of exclusion; therefore other causes of thrombocytopenia must be ruled out first. A complete blood count (CBC) analysis and a peripheral blood smear are performed. The clinical symptoms, along with prolonged bleeding time and reduced platelet count, suggest the diagnosis. The size and shape of the platelets may be abnormal. Circulating platelet time is reduced to hours instead of the normal days. HIV testing is often performed to rule out HIV infection as a cause of the thrombocytopenia.

TREATMENT

Corticosteroid administration increases capillary integrity for a short time. Intravenous immune globulin may be administered to increase the platelet count. Anemia needs to be corrected with blood transfusion, and vitamin K administration improves clotting mechanism. Therapeutic plasma exchange occasionally is attempted. Splenectomy is a last resort; however, this treatment is effective. Platelet numbers will increase after the procedure. Children are often just given supportive therapy and short-term steroid treatment because ITP in children is usually self-limited.

PROGNOSIS

Children often have a spontaneous remission of the disease, many times occurring within 2 to 8 weeks of diagnosis. The adult forms are rarely self-limited. With appropriate treatment, which may be long-term, only about 1% of patients will die from their disease.

PREVENTION

No methods of prevention are known.

PATIENT TEACHING

Explain the purpose and procedure of prescribed infusion therapy. The parents of a young child will benefit from reassurance that complete remission is likely. Adults with chronic ITP, who fail to respond to initial treatment with corticosteroids, may require preoperative instructions for splenectomy.

Immune Neutropenia

DESCRIPTION

The term *immune neutropenia* is used to describe neutropenia, a decreased number of circulating neutrophils, which is usually caused by the production of antineutrophil antibodies.

ICD-9-CM Code 288.0

SYMPTOMS AND SIGNS

The patient with immune neutropenia experiences malaise, fatigue, weakness, fever, and *stomatitis*. Recurrent infections are common, especially upper respiratory infections and otitis media in infants.

PATIENT SCREENING

Schedule an infant with a respiratory infection for a prompt medical evaluation. Subsequently, follow office policy for a referral to a pediatrician. The adult patient complaining of the above symptoms needs a medical evaluation at the first available opportunity.

ETIOLOGY

Immune-mediated neutropenia is most often due to accelerated turnover of neutrophils—production is increased, but an even greater increase in destruction mediated by the antineutrophil antibodies occurs. The number is diminished to almost complete absence of neutrophils in the blood. The neutropenia may be associated with infection, drug exposure, ITP, autoimmune hemolytic anemia, collagen vascular disease, or acute rheumatoid arthritis. A type of immune neutropenia, isoimmune neutropenia, is a rare disorder caused by the transplacental transfer of maternal IgG that reacts with fetal neutrophils. This type of neutropenia usually resolves in 12 to 15 weeks.

DIAGNOSIS

Neutropenia is confirmed by the significantly reduced numbers of neutrophils displayed in a white blood cell (WBC) count. Detection of antineutrophil antibodies is possible in many patients using assays such as immunofluorescence, agglutination tests, and antiglobulin analysis.

TREATMENT

Infants with idiopathic neutropenia usually require no specific treatment because their disease typically resolves spontaneously. Children, adults, and infants with severe disease may be treated with corticosteroids, immune globulin, or G-CSF (granulocyte-colony stimulating factor, a hematopoietic growth factor). Appropriate antibiotics are administered to treat bacterial infections. Transfusions of WBC concentrates may be indicated. Care must be taken to avoid exposure to any type of infection.

PROGNOSIS

Disease in infants usually resolves spontaneously. Neutropenia in children and adults often follows a benign course, especially with appropriate treatment.

PREVENTION

No methods of prevention are known.

PATIENT TEACHING

The parents of infants with immune neutropenia can benefit from understanding the relationship between frequent infections and the condition. When treatment is required, explain the effect of immune therapy, transfusion, or the need for antibiotics as prescribed.

Renal Disorders

Goodpasture Syndrome

DESCRIPTION

Goodpasture syndrome (also known as anti-GBM antibody disease) is an autoimmune kidney disease characterized by the presence of antibodies directed against an antigen in the glomerular basement membrane (GBM).

ICD-9-CM Code 446.21
In some coding manuals this disease may be spelled "Goodpasture's syndrome."

SYMPTOMS AND SIGNS

The patient with Goodpasture syndrome experiences acute glomerulonephritis, relatively acute renal failure with *proteinuria,* anemia, hemoptysis, and hematuria. Systemic complaints may include weight loss, fatigue, and fever.

PATIENT SCREENING

Symptoms of acute renal failure, such as scanty urine, blood in urine, and systemic complaints, signal critical illness that requires immediate medical care.

ETIOLOGY

The cause of this rare disease is obscure. Antibodies cause complement-mediated tissue damage in the glomerular and alveolar basement membranes, resulting in glomerulonephritis and pulmonary hemorrhage. Progression of the disease may lead to end-stage renal failure.

DIAGNOSIS

The diagnosis is suspected in any patient with acute glomerulonephritis, especially if accompanied by pulmonary hemorrhage and acute renal failure. Detection of anti-GBM antibodies in the serum or the kidney is necessary for definitive diagnosis. This can be done by performing ELISA, immunofluorescence, or renal biopsy. Urinalysis indicates the presence of protein and blood in the urine.

TREATMENT

The treatment of choice is plasmapheresis (to remove anti-GBM antibody) combined with immunosuppressive agents (corticosteroids and cyclophosphamide). The treatment is usually administered for 6 to 12 months. Hemodialysis and kidney transplants are last resorts for severely compromised patients.

PROGNOSIS

Goodpasture syndrome is often self-limited, and those who survive for a year after the initial diagnosis and maintain intact renal function usually do well. Patient survival during that time correlates with the degree of renal impairment at presentation and the amount of pulmonary involvement. Relapses can occur.

PREVENTION

No methods of prevention are known.

PATIENT TEACHING

Explain the purpose and procedure for the diagnostic studies. After the diagnosis has been made, discuss the effects of renal impairment on body systems, as appropriate to the patient's symptoms. Explain the purpose of plasmapheresis and the expected results from the medical regimen. Refer the patient to a dietician for instruction on how best to maintain optimal nutritional status. Teach the patient how to monitor weight, intake and output of fluids, and warning signs of complications. Encourage questions regarding treatment options as presented by the physician to the severely compromised patient.

Collagen Diseases

The main component of connective tissue, the essential part of all structures in the body, is a fibrous, insoluble protein called **collagen.** Collagen constitutes 30% of the total body protein.

Collagen diseases are known as *autoimmune disorders*. In autoimmune disorders, the immune system malfunctions and works against itself. In these collagen diseases, the immune system attacks and destroys the collagen, resulting in damage to some of the body's connective tissue. The reason for the malfunction of the immune system is unknown, but genetic factors do play some role. The immune system incorrectly identifies the body's own tissues as foreign and attacks them.

No cures for collagen diseases are known; treatment is directed at inhibiting the overactive immune system. In some patients, serious damage to the heart, lungs, or kidneys occurs.

Two well-known examples of the many collagen diseases are systemic lupus erythematosus and rheumatoid arthritis.

Systemic Lupus Erythematosus

DESCRIPTION

Lupus is a chronic, inflammatory autoimmune disease characterized by unusual antibodies in the blood that target tissues of the body.

 ICD-9-CM Code 710.0

SYMPTOMS AND SIGNS

Systemic lupus erythematosus (SLE), also called *lupus*, can inflame and damage connective tissue anywhere in the body. SLE most commonly produces inflammation of the skin, joints, nervous system, kidneys, lungs, and other organs. A characteristic butterfly rash, or erythema, may be present on the face, spreading from one cheek, across the nose, to the other cheek (Fig. 3–14, *A.*). Similar rashes may appear on other exposed areas of the body. Exposure to the sun can aggravate the rash. SLE may begin acutely with fever, fatigue, joint pain, and malaise, or may develop slowly over a period of years, with intermittent fever, malaise, joint deformities, and weight loss. Raynaud phenomenon and hair loss are common in SLE. This disease occurs most often in young women in their 30s or 40s.

PATIENT SCREENING

The manifestation of an unexplained cluster of symptoms, as mentioned above, requires the need for a complete medical evaluation. After the initial diagnostic evaluation, follow office policy for referral to a rheumatologist.

ETIOLOGY

The cause of SLE is unknown; however, it is thought to be an autoimmune disorder. Genetic, environmental, and hormonal factors may

Collagen Diseases

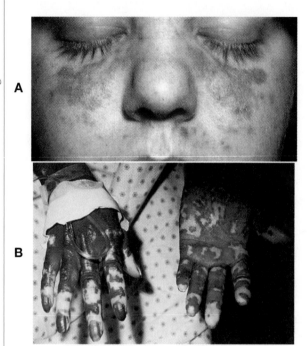

A

B

FIGURE 3–14 A, Typical butterfly rash of systemic lupus erythematosus. **B,** Systemic lupus erythematosus in black skin. (**A** from Goldstein BJ and Goldstein AO: *Practical dermatology,* ed 2, St Louis, 1997, Mosby; Courtesy the Department of Dermatology, University of North Carolina at Chapel Hill. **B** from Hill MJ: *Skin disorders—Mosby's clinical nursing series,* St. Louis, 1994, Mosby.)

predispose a person to this disease. Events that can precipitate SLE include stress, immunization reactions, pregnancy, and overexposure to ultraviolet light.

DIAGNOSIS

Patients with symptoms of SLE are evaluated for other rheumatic diseases (including rheumatoid arthritis, dermatomyositis, scleroderma, and Sjögren disease), other autoimmune diseases (including autoimmune hemolytic anemia, thyroiditis, and pernicious anemia), and diseases that are not autoimmune (e.g., cancer and infections).

The diagnosis of SLE can be made if four or more of the following symptoms or positive laboratory tests are present either at the same time or sequentially: a butterfly rash on the face, a *discoid* skin lesion (Fig. 3–14, *B*), photosensitivity, nasopharyngeal ulceration, polyarthritis without de-

formity, seizures or psychosis, chronic pleuritis or pericarditis, a false-positive serologic test result for syphilis or DNA or Sm (Smith, an uncharacterized nuclear antigen) antibodies in the blood, more than 0.5 g of protein in the urine in a 24-hour period, the presence of cellular casts in the urine, hemolytic anemia, thrombocytopenia, the presence of abnormal antibodies in the bloodstream, and the characteristic leukocytes (WBCs) called *LE cells,* which are not found in the circulation but are created in the laboratory as part of the testing. Diagnostic tests include a CBC with differential leukocyte count, platelet count, *erythrocyte sedimentation rate (ESR),* antinuclear antibody determination, and anti-DNA test. The anti-DNA test is the most specific test for SLE, but it is reliably positive only with active disease.

TREATMENT

In mild cases, antiinflammatory drugs, including aspirin, may be all that is needed to relieve the fever and joint pain. Sometimes antimalarial medications are added. For severe cases, corticosteroids are indicated. Immunosuppressive medications are useful when life-threatening or severe crippling disease is present. Immunosuppressive agents are also helpful when the patient fails to respond to conventional therapy or when intolerable side effects develop.

The prognosis for SLE is guarded. It improves slightly with early detection and treatment, but remains poor for persons with renal, cardiovascular, or neurologic complications. Morbidity and mortality increases with serious bacterial infection.

PROGNOSIS

The outlook for patients with systemic lupus continues to improve each decade with the development of more accurate monitoring tests and treatments. The prognosis depends on internal organ involvement. Patients with lupus are at a somewhat increased risk for developing cancer. The cancer risk is most dramatic for blood cancers, such as leukemia and lymphoma, but is also increased for breast cancer.

PREVENTION

It is essential that patients are diligent in adhering to their medication regimens. Flare-ups of disease can be prevented by not missing doses of prescribed medications and avoiding unnecessary sunlight exposure.

PATIENT TEACHING

Teaching the patient and family about the elements of the disease and laboratory testing can beneficially impact the health of lupus patients.

 # Scleroderma (Systemic Sclerosis)

DESCRIPTION

Scleroderma is a chronic, progressive disease characterized mostly by sclerosis (hardening) of the skin; scarring of certain internal organs can occur as well.

■ **ICD-9-CM Code 710.1**

SYMPTOMS AND SIGNS

Scleroderma is characterized by sclerosis (hardening) and shrinking of the skin and certain internal organs, including the gastrointestinal tract, heart, lungs, and kidneys. Involved skin becomes taut, firm, and edematous and is firmly attached to the subcutaneous tissue (Fig. 3–15). The skin feels tough and leathery, it may itch, and pigmented patches may occur. Raynaud phenomenon (see Raynaud disease in Chapter 10) is often the first symptom of scleroderma. This is followed by swelling, stiffness, and pain in the joints.

PATIENT SCREENING

Arrange an appointment for a consultation and medical evaluation to determine options for a person describing unexplained skin changes.

ETIOLOGY

The cause of scleroderma is unknown, but it appears to be an autoimmune disease. It occurs four times as often in women, especially those between 30 and 50 years of age, as in men.

DIAGNOSIS

A complete history and physical examination are all that is necessary for a diagnosis to made. Laboratory testing including Scl-70 and centromere antibodies can be supportive of the diagnosis. A skin biopsy is performed only rarely. Blood tests and urinalysis are performed to rule out complications or accompanying conditions. Patients with scleroderma are also evaluated for signs of systemic lupus erythematosus, polymyositis, Sjögren disease, and hypothyroidism. Lung function testing is helpful to detect pulmonary disease, and an

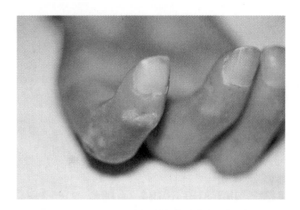

FIGURE 3–15 Crest syndrome of scleroderma. (From Hill MJ: *Skin disorders—Mosby's clinical nursing series,* St. Louis, 1994, Mosby.)

echocardiogram can be helpful to detect pulmonary hypertension.

TREATMENT

No specific treatment for scleroderma is known. A large number of drugs have been tried, including corticosteroids, vasodilators, and immunosuppressive agents, but their effects are merely *palliative.* Physical therapy helps patients maintain muscle strength but does not change the course of joint disease.

PROGNOSIS

The prognosis for patients with scleroderma depends on which organs are affected and the severity of the organ involvement. Patients with pulmonary hypertension and those with uncontrolled blood pressure have a higher risk of mortality.

PREVENTION

How to prevent scleroderma is not known. Preventing its complications, such as those from Raynaud phenomenon and esophageal reflux, can require medications and lifestyle changes.

PATIENT TEACHING

Teaching the patient and family about the elements of the disease and laboratory testing can beneficially impact the health of patients with scleroderma. Offer referrals to support groups for individuals coping with chronic disease.

— Sjögren Syndrome

DESCRIPTION

Sjögren syndrome is an autoimmune disease that features inflammation in various glands of the body.

■ **ICD-9-CM Code 710.2**
In some coding books this disease may be spelled "Sjogren's syndrome."

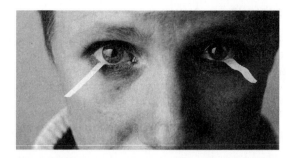

FIGURE 3–16 Schirmer tear test. (From Mudge-Grout C: *Immunologic Disorders—Mosby's clinical nursing series,* St. Louis, 1992, Mosby.)

SYMPTOMS AND SIGNS

Sjögren syndrome symptoms include rheumatoid arthritis, *xerostomia,* and **keratoconjunctivitis sicca.** This dryness of the nasal, oral, and laryngeal pharynx causes difficulty with talking, chewing, and swallowing. The patient may experience sores on or in the mouth and nose and dental decay may occur. Sjögren syndrome can follow the onset of rheumatoid arthritis.

PATIENT SCREENING

The onset of symptoms may be insidious or present with much discomfort due to dryness in the eyes or oral cavity; in the latter case offer the patient the first available appointment for medical evaluation.

ETIOLOGY

The exact cause of Sjögren syndrome is not known. Genetic (inherited) factors seem to play a role in predisposing a person to developing Sjögren syndrome. It is found more commonly in families that have members with other autoimmune illnesses. Most Sjögren syndrome patients are female.

DIAGNOSIS

Patients with symptoms of Sjögren syndrome are screened for medication side effects, thyroid disease, rheumatoid arthritis, systemic lupus erythematosus, sarcoidosis, and scleroderma associated with Sjögren syndrome. Dry eyes can be defined by abnormal Schirmer testing for dryness (Fig. 3–16). Enlarged salivary glands may prompt further investigation, including a lower lip biopsy, which may indicate a characteristic infiltration of lymphocytes. The blood studies will demonstrate anemia, decreased WBC count, and elevated ESR. Additional studies will show autoantibodies, called *Sjögren syndrome antibodies* (SSA and SSB antibodies), and high *rheumatoid factor* titers.

TREATMENT

Treatment is directed toward relieving symptoms, especially for the dryness in the oral cavity and eyes. Increasing fluid intake, chewing sugarless gum, and using oral sprays help to relieve oral dryness. Artificial tears are used in the eyes, and wearing sunglasses is recommended. Sometimes ophthalmologists will block the tear ducts with silicone to maintain adequate eye moisture. Occasionally, prednisone and/or antimalarial medications such as hydroxychloroquine are used to lessen the immune inflammation.

PROGNOSIS

Prognosis depends on what complications the patient develops, such as infections in the respiratory tract. A rare complication of Sjögren syndrome is cancer of the lymph glands (lymphoma).

PREVENTION

Prevention focuses on avoiding irritation of tissues caused by dryness, monitoring for the development of cancer, and the early management of infections.

PATIENT TEACHING

Patients with Sjögren syndrome can benefit by learning about the immune system and precisely how their bodies are affected by the condition. An awareness of the early warning signs of infection can prevent many serious complications.

Rheumatoid Arthritis

DESCRIPTION

Rheumatoid arthritis (RA) is a chronic, inflammatory, systemic disease that affects the joints (Fig. 3–17). It is one of the most severe forms of arthritis, commonly causing deformity and disability. RA affects 2.1 million Americans, women 3 times more often than men. RA may begin at any age, but it most commonly strikes individuals in their 30s and 40s.

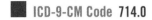 **ICD-9-CM Code 714.0**

SYMPTOMS AND SIGNS

RA causes inflammation and edema of the synovial membranes surrounding a joint. Eventually, this inflammation spreads to other parts of the affected joint and, if left untreated, has the capacity to destroy cartilage, deform joints, and destroy adjacent bone (Fig. 3–18). Most commonly many joints, on both sides of the body, are affected (polyarthritis) by RA. Occasionally, only one or two joints may be affected. When the neck is involved, the spinal cord can be at risk for damage, potentially leading to paralysis or death. RA is called a systemic disease because it can affect the entire body. It can cause generalized inflammation in the cardiac muscle, in blood vessels, and within the layers of the skin.

RA may begin without any obvious symptoms in the joints. The person may have unexplained weight loss, fatigue, a persistent low-grade fever,

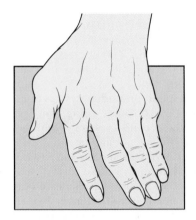

FIGURE 3–17 Joints affected by rheumatoid arthritis.

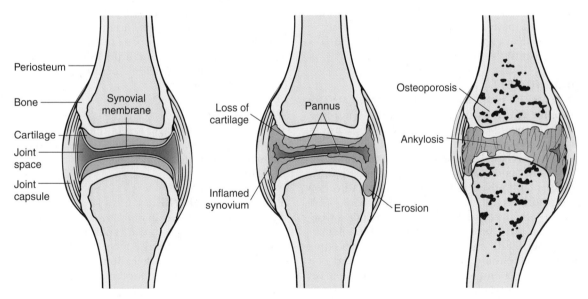

FIGURE 3–18 Schematic presentation of the pathologic changes in rheumatoid arthritis. The inflammation (synovitis) leads to pannus formation, obliteration of the articular space, and, finally, to ankylosis. The periarticular bone shows diffuse atrophy in the form of osteoporosis. (From Damjanov I: *Pathology for the health-related professions,* ed 2, Philadelphia, 2000, Saunders.)

and general malaise. This may accompany or precede joint stiffness, which is noticed especially on wakening and during periods of inactivity. Edema, pain, tenderness, erythema, and warmth in one or more joints occurring in a symmetric pattern gradually emerge as the principal symptoms. Joints generally affected are those of the fingers, wrists, knees, ankles, and toes. RA occurs less often in the spine or the hips, which are more susceptible to osteoarthritis (see Osteoarthritis in Chapter 7).

In some patients, the joint symptoms appear suddenly without any precursor symptoms. In other cases, joint symptoms are accompanied by bursitis or anemia. Some persons may have only one mild attack, whereas others may have several episodes that may leave them increasingly disabled.

PATIENT SCREENING

RA may have an insidious onset with vague systemic symptoms and joint pain, but occasionally the onset is abrupt. Initially the patient should be seen for diagnostic evaluation. Subsequently, follow office policy for referral to a rheumatologist.

ETIOLOGY

The exact cause of RA is unknown, although it is thought to be an autoimmune disorder. Heredity may predispose some persons to the disease; in other patients, a viral infection may trigger the disease process.

DIAGNOSIS

Patients with symptoms of RA are first evaluated for systemic lupus erythematosus, Sjögren syndrome, scleroderma, polymyositis, hormone disorders, cancer, and other possible causes of polyarthritis. Diagnosis is based on a review of the symptoms, patient and family history, physical examination, radiographic studies, and blood tests that will show elevated levels of rheumatoid factor in most patients. Other useful laboratory tests include a CBC, synovial fluid analysis, serum protein electrophoresis, ESR, and antinuclear antibody titer. Occasionally, the diagnosis of RA is achieved only after observation of the disease progression for several weeks or months.

TREATMENT

The primary objectives of treatment are the reduction of inflammation and pain, the preservation of joint function, and the prevention of joint deformity. These require a combination of medication, rest, special exercises, and joint protection. Antiinflammatory medications, including high doses of aspirin, are among the first choices to ease pain and stiffness, to reduce edema, and to control inflammation. Nonsteroidal antiinflammatory drugs (NSAIDs) are prescribed as an alternative to aspirin. Corticosteroids, by mouth or by local injection, often are given to control acute flare-ups. Even more potent disease-modifying antirheumatic drugs (DMARDs), such as gold compounds, penicillamine, immunosuppressive agents, and newer biologic response modifiers, may slow the disease process or even stop its progression.

Special splints and other devices to make dressing, bathing, cooking, eating, and performing other daily activities easier often are recommended to prevent, or at least reduce, deformities. Surgery is not often required, but it may be used to correct a deformity, relieve severe pain, and improve range of motion in persons with severe disease. For patients who no longer have adequately functioning joints, replacement with artificial joints may be recommended.

PROGNOSIS

The outlook for patients with RA depends on the adequacy of treatment, which must involve a close interaction between the patient and a physician skilled in the management of the disease. Without treatment, joint destruction, deformity, and disability are common.

PREVENTION

To prevent joint damage, loss of function, and disability, aggressive early medical intervention is mandatory. This generally means the early use of DMARDs.

PATIENT TEACHING

Patients with RA can benefit by learning about the immune system, joint anatomy, and the pathophysiology of the rheumatoid joint. An understanding of their medications and how their potential side effects are monitored can help ensure compliance and minimize complications. Referral to a physical therapist is helpful for individualized therapeutic exercises. Other supportive measures include splinting of inflamed joints and plenty of sleep each night. Give the patient information about the Arthritis Foundation and its support programs.

Juvenile Rheumatoid Arthritis

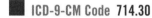

DESCRIPTION

Juvenile rheumatoid arthritis (JRA) is a form of RA that affects children (less than 16 years of age) and begins most commonly between the ages of 2 and 5 years.

■ **ICD-9-CM Code 714.30**

SYMPTOMS AND SIGNS

The various forms of JRA include pauciarticular (only a few joints affected), polyarticular (many joints affected), and systemic onset JRA with high fevers and a rash (also known as *Still disease*). JRA usually involves the large joints; the attacks last for several weeks and tend to lessen in severity with time, usually disappearing completely by puberty.

The child with systemic onset of JRA may have the following symptoms: a temperature fluctuating from normal in the morning to about 103° F in the evening; poor appetite, with resulting weight loss; a blotchy, salmon-colored rash over the limbs and trunk of the body; anemia; and swollen, stiff, and painful joints, most commonly involving the neck, elbows, knees, and ankles. Other possible symptoms include red, painful eyes; swollen cervical or axillary lymph glands; irritability; and acute pericarditis. Skeletal development may be impaired if the epiphyseal, or growth, plates of the long bones are damaged because of the inflammation around the joints.

Sites of JRA development vary considerably from child to child, and girls are affected four times as often as boys. The inflammation usually develops gradually but can be abrupt. In a few cases, the inflammation in the joints leads to partial or crippling deformity as a result of the recurring attacks. Unlike adult RA, complete remission of JRA occurs in approximately 75% of affected children.

PATIENT SCREENING

A young child with fever, rash, and/or swelling and stiffness in the joints should be seen for medical evaluation as soon as possible.

ETIOLOGY

The specific cause of JRA is unknown, but it generally is believed that the pathologic changes in the joints are related to an autoimmune disorder. Heredity may play a role in some children, particularly those with spondylitis.

DIAGNOSIS

Diagnosis is based on history and physical examination and the results of blood tests for the rheumatoid factor. Examination may show a lack of growth or delayed physical growth that would be appropriate for the age of the child. Other forms of arthritis that can affect children include spondylitis, the arthritis of inflammatory bowel disease, psoriatic arthritis, and sarcoidosis.

TREATMENT

Treatment of children with JRA is often similar to that of an adult with RA (see Rheumatoid Arthritis). Medication dosages are based on the child's weight. Parents should encourage the child's independence. Participation in school and social activities that do not increase joint pain or cause undue fatigue are also important for the child. A well-balanced diet with plenty of protein is essential. Physical therapy exercises are crucial for minimizing the pain and reducing the crippling effects of arthritis. Braces or splints may be needed to correct growth disturbances and joint contracture.

PROGNOSIS

With proper therapy, children with all forms of arthritis will usually get better over time. Indeed, the vast majority of children with arthritis grow up to lead normal lives with no significant physical limitations.

PREVENTION

To prevent joint damage, loss of function, and disability, aggressive early medical intervention is mandatory. This generally means the early use of DMARDs under the guidance of a qualified physician. A physical therapist can play a central role in helping the child maintain optimal function.

PATIENT TEACHING

Patients and families must have as good an understanding of the disease and its management as is possible. Stress the importance of follow-up care and regular eye examinations. The child should be encouraged to be as independent as possible.

Ankylosing Spondylitis

DESCRIPTION

Ankylosing spondylitis is a systemic, usually progressive, inflammatory disease affecting primarily the spinal column.

 ICD-9-CM Code 720.0

SYMPTOMS AND SIGNS

Ankylosing spondylitis (AS) commonly affects young men. It is several times more common in men than in women. Typically it first affects the sacroiliac area of the spine and adjacent soft tissue structures. The patient may present with recurring morning low back pain and stiffness that improves with activity. Constitutional symptoms such as fatigue, weight loss, fever, and/or diarrhea also may be present at the onset, as well as eye pain and photophobia due to uveitis. Pain and tenderness may be noted over the site of inflammation. The history may include heel pain, inflammatory bowel disease, or family incidence of arthritic conditions. Less often patients present with cervical or thoracic axial pain and stiffness and with paraspinal muscular spasm. Peripheral large joints can be involved, particularly in women. Women often have a more mild form of the disease.

As the disease progresses, perhaps over a period of 20 years, the physical examination can reveal limited range of motion in affected joints due to fusion (ankylosis). The inflammation and ossification can progress up the spine, greatly inhibiting the activities of daily life. Eventually, the spinal vertebrae become fused, inflexible and rigid; the patient's posture exhibits the typical forward flexion of the spine.

PATIENT SCREENING

Schedule the patient presenting with back pain and stiffness for a medical evaluation. Subsequently, follow office policy for a referral to a rheumatologist.

DIAGNOSIS

AS shares a number of diagnostic features with other arthritic diseases; thus early clinical diagnosis is often missed, especially in women. The clinical evaluation includes back pain and stiffness, joint pain with limitation of motion, and positive family history. Laboratory results reveal a negative rheumatoid factor and confirm the inflammatory nature of the disease with a mildly elevated erythrocyte sedimentation rate (ESR) or C reactive protein. The HLA-B27 tissue antigen is present in nearly 90% of individuals with AS. Characteristic x-ray findings are noted years after the onset and include bilateral sacroiliitis, "squaring" of the vertebrae, fusion of joints, and generalized osteoporosis. These changes produce the classic appearance of a "bamboo spine."

ETIOLOGY

The exact cause of AS is not known. Studies support a genetic basis and an association with the antigen HLA-B27. This immunogenic factor may predispose one to the development of an immune response directed at joint tissue after having succumbed to the effects of particular infectious agents, which have yet to be clearly defined.

TREATMENT

No cure for AS is known. The goal of treatment is to relieve pain and swelling with antiinflammatory medication and analgesics. Patients benefit from physical therapy and moderate exercise to maintain good posture and maximize mobility. Surgical procedures are rarely indicated.

PROGNOSIS

The course of AS is variable with periods of remission and episodes of exacerbation. A poorer prognosis is associated with early onset of the disease and male gender. Occasionally the disease takes a severe and rapid course, resulting in systemic complications and severe deformity.

PREVENTION

No preventive measures for AS are known, but its complications can be prevented or at least lessened with adequate exercise and medications. Because AS is occasionally associated with lung scarring, patients with AS must not smoke.

PATIENT TEACHING

Discuss the importance of maintaining prescribed medication and keeping follow-up appointments.

Counsel the patient on individual comfort measures and positional modification in the work environment, as indicated. Stress the importance of moderate, low-impact exercise, such as swimming, to maintain range of motion and good posture. Discuss the progressive nature of the disease and encourage the patient to contact the local Arthritis Foundation chapter for group support.

Polymyositis

DESCRIPTION

Polymyositis is a disease of muscle that features inflammation of the muscle fibers. The muscles affected are mostly those closest to the trunk or torso. This results in weakness that can be severe. It is a chronic illness with periods of increased symptoms, called *flares* or *relapses,* and decreased symptoms, known as *remissions.*

 ICD-9-CM Code 710.4

SYMPTOMS AND SIGNS

Muscle weakness is the most common symptom of polymyositis, usually involving the muscles closest to the trunk of the body. The onset can be gradual or rapid. This results in varying degrees of loss of muscle power and atrophy. The loss of strength can be noted as difficulty in getting up from chairs, climbing stairs, or lifting above the shoulders. Trouble with swallowing and weakness in lifting the head from the pillow can occur. Occasionally, the muscles ache and are tender to the touch. This disease may be accompanied by skin inflammation, in which case it is referred to as dermatomyositis. In such cases, a rash may appear and spread over the face, shoulders, arms, and bony prominences (e.g., knuckles, elbows, and knees). Nearly two thirds of patients with this disease are women. The person with polymyositis may feel generally fatigued and unwell.

PATIENT SCREENING

The patient will present with diffuse muscle weakness. Schedule the first available appointment for medical evaluation.

ETIOLOGY

The cause of polymyositis is unknown; however, it is thought to be an autoimmune disorder. Polymyositis occurs when white blood cells, the immune cells of inflammation, spontaneously invade muscles.

Neurologic Disorders

DIAGNOSIS

The history and physical examination should include a thorough search for muscle conditions, such as muscular dystrophy, drug toxicity (such as that caused by cholesterol drugs), thyroid disorder, sarcoidosis, and infections (e.g., HIV and parasites). Moreover, because polymyositis can sometimes accompany cancers, an intense screening for cancer is crucial. A medical history and physical examination document weakness. Blood analysis is used to detect elevated levels of muscle enzymes (CPK or creatinine phosphokinase, aldolase, serum glutamate oxaloacetate transaminase [SGOT], serum glutamate pyruvate transaminase [SGPT], and lactate dehydrogenase [LDH]). An electromyography (EMG) demonstrates a typical abnormal pattern of electrical activity in the inflamed muscle, and muscle biopsy confirms the diagnosis.

TREATMENT

Treatment of polymyositis is directed toward stopping the inflammation and inhibiting the overactive immune system. High doses of steroids usually are prescribed to suppress the inflammation. Immunosuppressive agents, such as cyclophosphamide and methotrexate, also are used. Gradually, exercise therapy is added to rebuild strength and prevent muscle atrophy.

PROGNOSIS

Patients ultimately can recover well from the effects, especially with early medical treatment of the disease and disease flares. The disease often becomes inactive. Rehabilitation of atrophied muscle can be accomplished with long-term physical therapy.

PREVENTION

It is essential that patients are diligent in taking their medications and that they closely monitor their muscle symptoms. Optimal outcomes are achieved with intervention at the earliest sign of activation of muscle inflammation.

PATIENT TEACHING

Patients should be instructed clearly about the purpose and importance of regular medications. Physical therapy and occupational therapy instructions play major roles in the recovery process.

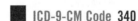

Neurologic Disorders

Multiple Sclerosis

DESCRIPTION

Multiple sclerosis (MS) is an inflammatory disease of the central nervous system. It attacks the myelin sheath, a fatty substance covering most of the nerves in the brain and spinal cord, and ultimately causes scarring (sclerosis) that debilitates the nerves (Fig. 3–19).

■ **ICD-9-CM Code 340**

SYMPTOMS AND SIGNS

The sclerosis prevents the transmission of stimuli to the brain and spinal cord and causes the following sensory and motor abnormalities:

- Weakness or numbness in one or more limbs
- Optic neuritis
- Loss of vision in one eye
- *Diplopia*
- Unsteady gait
- Vertigo

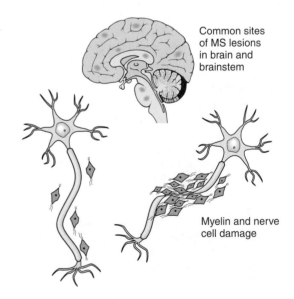

Common sites of MS lesions in brain and brainstem

Myelin and nerve cell damage

FIGURE 3–19 Myelin degeneration in multiple sclerosis (MS).

- Difficulty with urinating, leading to increased urinary tract infections
- Facial numbness or pain
- Speech problems
- *Dysphagia*
- Hearing loss
- Impotence in men
- Fatigue
- Emotional disturbances, including depression, irritability, and short-temperedness (Fig. 3–20)

ETIOLOGY

The cause of MS is unknown. It is thought that the immune system is involved in some way; an inher- ited trait that increases one's susceptibility to the disease may be a factor as well. A common theory holds that an unknown virus triggers the immune system to turn against the body and attack the myelin, which eventually results in MS. No virus has been conclusively implicated, however. The inci- dence of MS varies geographically, with the risk in- creasing as one moves from south to north in lati- tude. The risk is also greater in the white populations. MS is rare in children; in about two thirds of cases, it develops in people between the ages of 20 and 40 years; and it occurs rarely in peo- ple older than 60 years. MS occurs more often in women than in men.

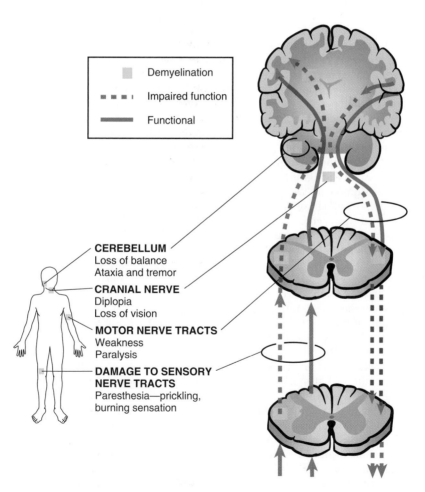

Demyelination

Impaired function

Functional

CEREBELLUM
Loss of balance
Ataxia and tremor

CRANIAL NERVE
Diplopia
Loss of vision

MOTOR NERVE TRACTS
Weakness
Paralysis

DAMAGE TO SENSORY NERVE TRACTS
Paresthesia—prickling, burning sensation

FIGURE 3–20 Multiple sclerosis—distribution of lesions. (From Gould B: *Pathophysiology for the health professions,* ed 2, Philadelphia, 2002, Saunders.)

Neurologic Disorders

The most common characteristic of MS is relapse, the onset of clinical dysfunction, followed by a remission during which the symptoms resolve for a period of time. MS can be defined as one of several types:

- Relapsing-remitting—relapses followed by recovery with no progression of neurologic dysfunction between relapses
- Primary-progressive—disease progression with no remissions
- Secondary-progressive—disease begins as relapsing-remitting, but later becomes progressive with few remissions
- Progressive-relapsing—progressive disease from the onset, with relapses and disease progression during the period between relapses

DIAGNOSIS

MS is difficult to diagnose because the symptoms are so variable and sporadic. A physical examination done in the early stages may elicit completely normal findings. Often, the diagnosis is determined by eliminating other possible causes of the symptoms. Usually, the patient has had two or more distinct episodes of CNS dysfunction with resolution of symptoms between episodes. The diagnosis is made clinically and supported by other test findings. Magnetic resonance imaging (MRI) is the modality of choice for supporting the diagnosis. A characteristic cerebral or spinal plaque is often found. Examination of the cerebrospinal fluid (CSF) often results in normal findings, although it may reveal an elevated immunoglobulin level.

TREATMENT

Acute attacks are treated with corticosteroids. Those with diagnosed relapsing-remitting disease may be started on one of the five medications approved by the United States Food and Drug Administration (USFDA) for treatment of this form of MS (interferon beta-1a [Avonex], interferon beta-1b [Betaseron], glatiramer [Copaxone], Rebif, and mitoxantrone [Novantrone]). Immunosuppressive therapies may be useful in the treatment of progressive disease (radiation, steroids, immune globulin, cytotoxic drugs). Otherwise, the disease is treated symptomatically. This may include taking muscle relaxants; taking vitamin supplements to prevent a vitamin B deficiency, which might contribute to nerve damage; undergoing physical therapy to help preserve as much muscle function as possible; wearing braces; and using a cane, walker, or wheelchair. Adequate rest and a well-balanced diet are also important.

PROGNOSIS

No cure for MS is known, and the duration of the disease is variable. Some patients die within a few months after onset of the disease; the average duration is 30 years or longer. Several prognostic indicators are known. A more favorable prognosis is seen in females, early age onset, relapsing disease (rather than progressive), and in patients with impairment of sensory pathways as an initial symptom.

PREVENTION

No method of prevention is known.

PATIENT TEACHING

Describe diagnostic procedures as prescribed, because many will be ordered before the definitive diagnosis is made. Discuss the many possible treatments that address varied symptoms (e.g., speech therapy, assistive devices, bladder training, and physical therapy). Explaining the possibility of remission and exacerbations is helpful. Discuss the medications that are prescribed, and how they will be monitored for side effects. Make referrals to community support groups such as the National Multiple Sclerosis Society.

Myasthenia Gravis

DESCRIPTION

Myasthenia gravis is a chronic, progressive neuromuscular disease that is thought to stem from the presence of autoantibodies to the acetylcholine receptor.

 ICD-9-CM Code 358.0

SYMPTOMS AND SIGNS

Myasthenia gravis is characterized by extreme muscular weakness (without atrophy) and progressive fatigue. The onset, although usually gradual, may be sudden, with symptoms of muscular weakness generally appearing first and most noticeably in the face. Drooping eyelids, diplopia, and difficulty with talking, chewing, and swallowing may be the first signs that something is wrong. The degree of weakness varies considerably from hour to hour, day to day, and year to year. Muscle weakness typically occurs late in the day or after strenuous exercise. Short periods of rest characteristically restore muscle function. Muscle weakness is progressive in myasthenia gravis, and eventually paralysis occurs. A myasthenic crisis (sudden inability to swallow and respiratory distress) may be so severe that mechanical ventilation becomes necessary. Prolonged exposure to sunlight, cold, infections, and emotional stress exacerbate the symptoms.

PATIENT SCREENING
The abrupt onset of symptoms as listed above can be disconcerting to the patient and might be confused with symptoms of stroke. Thus the patient should receive prompt medical attention.

ETIOLOGY
The disease mainly affects women between the ages of 20 and 40 years and men over the age of 60. It is thought to be caused by an autoimmune mechanism in which a faulty transmission of nerve impulses to and from the central nervous system occurs, especially at the neuromuscular junction. Autoantibodies against the acetylcholine receptor are found in 80% to 90% of patients. A majority of patients have either thymus hyperplasia or thymoma, and this may play a role in the development of the disease.

DIAGNOSIS
When myasthenia gravis is suspected, a physical examination is done that aims to test for fatigability of different muscle groups. The Tensilon test, intravenous administration of a short-acting acetylcholinesterase inhibitor, is performed to see whether the administration improves muscle strength. Tests are done to check for the presence of antibodies against the acetylcholine receptor. *Electromyography* also may be performed.

TREATMENT
The treatment of myasthenia gravis is *symptomatic* and supportive. Treatment choice is largely based on the patient's age and pregnancy status. Restricted activity, complete bed rest for severe cases, and a soft or liquid diet may be necessary. **Anticholinesterase** drugs are effective initial treatment for the fatigue and muscle weakness, but they become less effective as the condition worsens. Pyridostigmine bromide (Mestinon) is the drug of choice for treatment. If a thymus gland tumor (thymoma) is present, a thymectomy is needed. Corticosteroids are effective in patients who have not been aided by the thymectomy. A useful adjunct to alternate-day therapy with corticosteroids is immunosuppression. Myasthenic crisis is treated by intubation and withdrawal of anticholinesterase medications, followed by reintroduction of the drugs and plasmapheresis.

PROGNOSIS
Unexplained, spontaneous remissions can occur; however, the disease is usually a lifelong condition characterized by remissions and exacerbations. The prognosis for patients who experience myasthenic crisis has improved over the years, but such an event can still leave many patients who had been independent before the crisis functionally dependent afterward.

PREVENTION
No methods of prevention are known.

PATIENT TEACHING
Give the patient information about the diagnostic tests prescribed. Explain the medical management of symptoms and what side effects to report. Encourage the patient to take initiative in deciding on his or her own supportive care. List the warning signs of impending myasthenic or cholinergic crisis.

Vasculitis

Vasculitis is an inflammation in the walls of blood vessels. The affected vessel becomes necrotic when it is obstructed by a thrombus, and an *infarct* is the outcome. Biopsies of an involved vessel can demonstrate the presence of immunoglobulins and cells of inflammation in the blood vessel wall. Any blood vessel can be involved, and the many forms of vasculitis are characterized by which vessels are involved. Vasculitis can be classified into two main types, small vessel vasculitis and systemic necrotizing vasculitis. Each of these types have many sub-types.

Small Vessel Vasculitis

DESCRIPTION
Small vessel vasculitis is the category of vasculitis that primarily affects the capillaries, arterioles, and venules.

ICD-9-CM Code 447.9 *(Unspecified disorders of arteries and arterioles)*

SYMPTOMS AND SIGNS

Inflammation of the small vessels causes petechiae (nonblanching), purpura, erythema, ulcerations, and edema; these are found most often on the skin of the lower extremities. Pain and a burning sensation can accompany these lesions. Additionally, depending on the type of small vessel syndrome that the patient experiences, symptoms can include ocular lesions, genital or oral ulcerations, abdominal pain, arthralgia, and weakness.

PATIENT SCREENING

The patient describing a syndrome as listed above will need prompt medical evaluation. Subsequently, follow office policy regarding referral to a specialist for immune disorders.

ETIOLOGY

Although the exact cause is unknown, vasculitis often accompanies other immune disorders. Exposure to certain chemicals, foreign proteins, drugs, foods, and infections have been suggested as possible etiologic factors.

DIAGNOSIS

Diagnosis is confirmed by the histology and often immunofluorescence studies of biopsied tissue. The presence of the immunoglobulins and complement in the blood vessels, as well as the pattern of vascular involvement and the cell types present, can help define the subtype of small vessel vasculitis. Bleeding disorders, anticoagulant medication, and even aspirin can cause skin findings that mimic small vessel vasculitis.

TREATMENT

Treatment consists of identifying and avoiding exposure to the causative agent or managing the underlying disease. Corticosteroid therapy may afford relief; analgesics are given and rest is encouraged.

PROGNOSIS

The outlook for patients with small vessel vasculitis is generally very good. The condition tends to readily respond to treatment.

PREVENTION

For those patients who have developed small vessel vasculitis as a result of reaction to certain medications, avoidance of those medications in the future is the key to prevention.

PATIENT TEACHING

The importance of regular medical follow-up and adherence to the medication regimen cannot be overemphasized.

Systemic Necrotizing Vasculitis

DESCRIPTION

Systemic necrotizing vasculitis tends to primarily affect medium and large arteries.

 ICD-9-CM Code 447.8 *(Other specified disorders of arteries and arterioles)*

SYMPTOMS AND SIGNS

Systemic necrotizing vasculitis occurs in numerous cutaneous and systemic conditions. Symptoms differ depending on the body system involved; they can include headaches, fever, weakness, fatigue, *malaise,* anorexia, and weight loss. Patients also may experience muscle and joint pain, *angina,* dyspnea, hypertension, and visual disturbances. Impaired tissue perfusion causes *ischemic* pain in the system or tissues involved. Ulceration of the skin can result. Paralysis of an affected nerve can lead to weakness or numbness.

PATIENT SCREENING

Rapid evaluation by a qualified physician experienced in the evaluation and management of vasculitis is crucial.

ETIOLOGY

It is not clear how the inflammation and necrosis of blood vessels develop. Each subtype of systemic necrotizing vasculitis has specific clinical features with several probable mechanisms involved. Autoimmune responses constitute the causes and are mediated by antibodies, T cells, or IgA. Some forms have been clearly related to amphetamine use as well as the development of hepatitis B and C.

DIAGNOSIS

A complete history and a thorough physical examination are important. Comprehensive blood studies, including CBC, ESR, RA factor determination, and serum tests for immunoglobulins are done. The CBC indicates anemia and usually elevated WBC and platelet counts. The ESR is elevated during the acute stage. When the pulmonary system is involved, radiographic chest films show pulmonary infiltrates. Hematuria and proteinuria are present with renal involvement. Aneurysms and myocardial ischemia are indicators of cardiac involvement. Biopsy specimens of involved vessels ultimately confirm the diagnosis by demonstrating the invasion of leukocytes in the blood vessel wall. An alternative to biopsy, in some cases, can be an x-ray test of the blood vessels called an *angiogram.*

TREATMENT

Treatment focuses on decreasing the inflammation of the arteries and improving the function of affected organs. Treatment addresses the underlying causative factors and the systemic involvement. Corticosteroids and analgesics afford relief of the effects of inflammation. Immune suppressing medications and plasmapheresis are also used to lessen the immune activation. Hypertension is treated with antihypertensive drugs, usually *angiotensin-converting enzyme (ACE)* inhibitors. Ocular problems should be closely monitored.

PROGNOSIS

The outlook for patients with systemic necrotizing vasculitis is guarded until the condition is controlled with medications to suppress inflammation and immune activity. This category of vasculitis can permanently damage organs.

PREVENTION

No method of prevention for systemic necrotizing vasculitis is known.

PATIENT TEACHING

The importance of regular medical follow-up, monitoring for signs of activation of disease, and adherence to the medication regimen cannot be overemphasized. Patients with skin damage should be taught good skin care and those who smoke should be encouraged to stop.

REVIEW CHALLENGE

Answer the following questions:

1. Name the functional components of the immune system.
2. Describe the three major functions of the immune system.
3. List examples of inappropriate responses of the immune system.
4. Explain the difference between natural and acquired immunity and give examples of each.
5. Trace the formation of T cells and B cells from stem cells.
6. Explain how T cells and B cells specifically protect the body against disease.
7. List the five immunoglobulins.
8. Explain complement fixation and its importance in the immune system.
9. Describe the invasion of human immunodeficiency virus (HIV) into the T helper cells.
10. Explain the ways that HIV is transmitted.
11. List the guidelines for universal precautions and infection control.
12. Describe the primary absent or inadequate response of the immune system in the following diseases:
    - Common variable immunodeficiency
    - Selective immunoglobulin A deficiency
    - Severe combined immunodeficiency disease
13. Explain the destructive mechanisms in autoimmune diseases.
14. Describe the symptoms and signs of pernicious anemia. Name the primary treatment.
15. Describe the systemic features of SLE. Recall the diagnostic criteria.
16. Detail the pathology of rheumatoid arthritis (RA).
17. Specify the primary objectives of the treatment for RA.
18. Compare the pathology of multiple sclerosis to that of myasthenia gravis.
19. Explain the cause of the typical forward flexion of the spine in the patient with advanced ankylosing spondylitis.
20. Discuss the treatment and prognosis for patients with polymyositis.

REAL-LIFE CHALLENGE

Pernicious Anemia

A 46-year-old female patient reports fatigue, loss of appetite with occasional nausea and vomiting, a sore tongue, and weight loss. She also mentions weakness and numbness and loss of feeling in her hands, lower arms, feet, and lower legs. She has recently experienced lightheadedness, visual disturbances, ringing in the ears, shortness of breath, rapid pulse, and palpitations. In addition, she mentions experiencing headaches, irritability, and depression. Examination shows pale-appearing lips, tongue, and gums. Her skin and sclera appear jaundiced.

Hematology tests reveal reduced hemoglobin, RBC, WBC, and platelets and increased MCV. The RBCs and platelets appear large and malformed. Studies of bone marrow are indicative of abnormal RBC production. Gastric acid is either reduced or absent.

QUESTIONS

1. What is meant by megaloblastic anemia?
2. What is the importance of the intrinsic factor?
3. Why would the patient experience gastrointestinal-type symptoms?
4. What is the cause of the neurologic symptoms?
5. Why would the patient experience lightheadedness, fatigue, and weakness?
6. How long must the patient continue treatment after the symptoms abate?
7. Why is the patient unable to take the vitamin B_{12} orally?
8. At the present time, what is the cure for pernicious anemia?

REAL-LIFE CHALLENGE

Rheumatoid Arthritis

A 33-year-old woman reports the recent onset of pain in the joints of her fingers and hands. She recently has experienced weight loss, fatigue, and a persistent low-grade fever. On examination, the joints of the hands and fingers display tenderness, redness, warmth, and swelling. Blood tests indicate an elevated level of the rheumatoid factor. Further observation over a period of a few months shows a continuation of the symptoms with involvement of additional joints. The patient is diagnosed with rheumatoid arthritis.

QUESTIONS

1. Compare the incidence of rheumatoid arthritis in males and females.
2. Compare the symptoms and signs of rheumatoid arthritis and osteoarthritis. (See Chapter 7 for osteoarthritis.)
3. Describe the projected course of rheumatoid arthritis that is left untreated.
4. What is the cause of rheumatoid arthritis?
5. Which diagnostic tests usually are ordered when rheumatoid arthritis is suspected?
6. With the primary treatment being to reduce inflammation and pain, preserve joint function, and prevent deformities, what is the usual prescribed treatment?
7. Explain the side effects the patient may experience with NSAID therapy.

INTERNET ASSIGNMENTS

1. Explore the American Lupus Society website for breaking news. Learn how to use the website to locate the chapter of the Lupus Foundation nearest to you.
2. Explore the National AIDS Hotline and report on such information as the latest U.S. AIDS trends, or discuss findings at the linked site on STD resources for teens.

3. Go to the National Multiple Sclerosis Society to identify promising areas of disease research and list some current clinical trials.

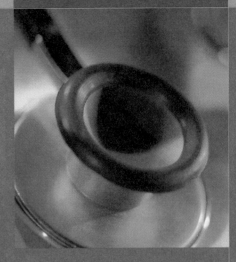

CHAPTER 4

Diseases
and Conditions
of the Endocrine
System

Learning Objectives

After studying Chapter 4, you should be able to:

1. List the major glands of the endocrine system.
2. Describe the importance of hormones and explain some of the critical body functions that they control.
3. Explain the importance of normal pituitary function.
4. Compare gigantism to acromegaly.
5. Describe the condition of dwarfism and its etiology.
6. Explain the cause of diabetes insipidus.
7. Explain the treatment of a simple goiter.
8. List the signs and symptoms of Graves' disease.
9. Distinguish between cretinism and myxedema.
10. Explain the pathogenesis of diabetes mellitus.
11. Identify the two major types of diabetes mellitus.
12. Distinguish between diabetic coma and insulin shock.
13. Explain the medical management of all three types of diabetes mellitus.
14. Explain why hypoglycemia can be a serious medical condition.
15. Compare the signs and symptoms of thyroid hypofunction with those of thyroid hyperfunction.
16. Describe the signs and symptoms of thyroid malignancy. Discuss the most important prognostic factor.

Key Terms

acidosis (**ass**–ih–**DOE**–sis)
corticotropin (**kor**–tih–ko–**TRO**–pin)
epiphyseal (**eh**–pih–**FEEZ**–e–al)
gonadotropin (**go**–nad–oh–**TRO**–pin)
hyperglycemia (**hye**–per–gli–**SEE**–me–ah)
hyperkalemia (**hye**–per–ka–**LEE**–me–ah)
hypocalcemia (**hye**–poh–kal–**SEE**–me–ah)
hypothalamus (**hye**–poh–**THAL**–ah–mus)
panhypopituitarism (pan–**high**–poh–pih–**TOO**–ih–tair–ism)
polydipsia (**pahl**–ee–**DIP**–see–ah)

polyphagia (**pahl**–ee–**FAY**–jee–ah)
polyuria (**pahl**–ee–**U**–ree–ah)
pruritus (pruh–**RI**–tus)
radioimmunoassay (**ray**–dee–oh–**IM**–u–no–**ass**–a)
somatotropin (**soh**–mat–oh–**TROH**–pin)
thyrotoxicosis (**thye**–roh–tox–ih–**KOH**–sis)
thyrotropin (thye–**ROT**–roe–pin)
thyroxine (thye–**ROKS**–in)
triiodothyronine (**try**–eye–oh–doh–**THYE**–row–neen)
vasopressin (**vaz**–oh–**PRES**–in)

ORDERLY FUNCTION
OF THE ENDOCRINE SYSTEM

BODY ACTIVITIES, HOMEOSTASIS, and the response to stress are controlled by two distinct but interacting systems: the nervous system and the endocrine system. The systems interact as one system starts, ends, or extends the activity of the other. The nervous system (discussed in Chapter 13) creates an immediate but short-lived response, operating on the principles of electricity, through impulse conduction. The endocrine system has a slightly slower onset and a longer duration of action, and uses highly specific and powerful hormones to control its response chemically. Hormones are chemical messengers classified as either amino acids (proteins) or steroids.

The endocrine system is composed of many glands scattered throughout the body; these glands secrete unique and potent chemicals called hormones directly into the bloodstream (Fig. 4–1). Most hormones direct their action to target glands or tissues at distant receptor sites, thereby regulating critical body functions such as urinary output, cellular metabolic rate, and growth and development. Hormonal secretions typically are regulated by negative feedback; information about the hormone level or its effect is fed back to the gland, which then responds accordingly (Fig. 4–2).

Certain endocrine glands are stimulated to secrete hormones in response to other hormones.

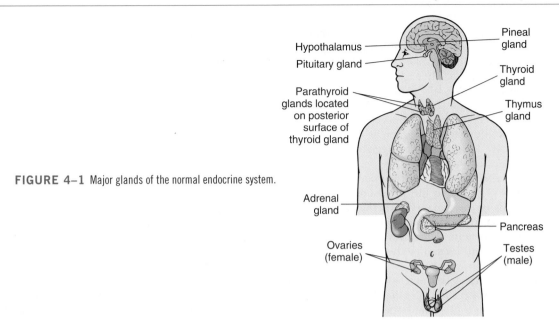

FIGURE 4–1 Major glands of the normal endocrine system.

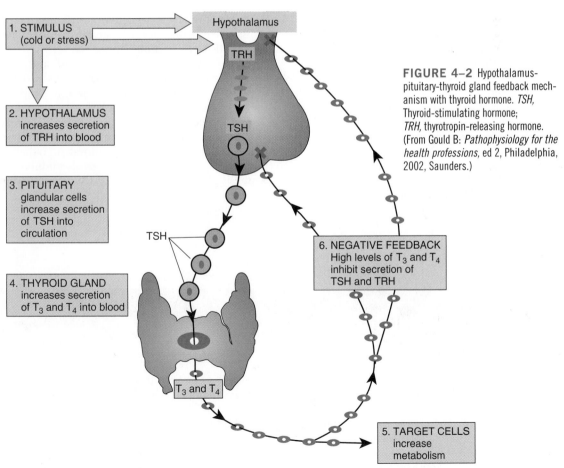

FIGURE 4–2 Hypothalamus-pituitary-thyroid gland feedback mechanism with thyroid hormone. *TSH,* Thyroid-stimulating hormone; *TRH,* thyrotropin-releasing hormone. (From Gould B: *Pathophysiology for the health professions,* ed 2, Philadelphia, 2002, Saunders.)

1. STIMULUS (cold or stress)

2. HYPOTHALAMUS increases secretion of TRH into blood

3. PITUITARY glandular cells increase secretion of TSH into circulation

4. THYROID GLAND increases secretion of T_3 and T_4 into blood

5. TARGET CELLS increase metabolism

6. NEGATIVE FEEDBACK High levels of T_3 and T_4 inhibit secretion of TSH and TRH

Hormones that stimulate secretion of other hormones are called *tropic* hormones. For example, the **gonadotropins** stimulate ovarian hormones. In diagnostic analysis, when excessive hormones are produced by an ectopic source (e.g., a malignant tumor), the tropic hormones are low. Other secreting cells that perform endocrine functions may be scattered in the tissue, such as in the digestive tract, where local hormones regulate the motility and secretions of the tract.

Endocrine diseases result from an abnormal increase or decrease in the secretion of hormones. Symptoms of disease vary with the degree of increase or decrease in hormonal secretion and the age of the patient. This divergence from normal hormone quantities may be the result of *hyperplasia, hypertrophy,* or *atrophy* of an endocrine gland. Changes in gland size that affect the gland's production and secretion of a hormone often result from an insult to the gland, such as infection, radiation, trauma, surgical intervention, and inflammation. Dysfunction of an endocrine gland is associated with many physical and mental symptoms. Some common symptoms are:

- Growth abnormalities
- Emotional disturbances or psychiatric problems
- Skin, hair, and nail changes
- Edema
- Hypertension or hypotension
- *Arrhythmia*
- Changes in urine output
- Muscle weakness and atrophy
- Menstrual irregularity or amenorrhea
- Impotence or changes in libido
- Sterility
- Sharp changes in energy level

To appreciate the effect of endocrine gland function on health and disease, review the main glands and their primary hormones (Table 4–1). The pituitary gland, intimately related to the hypothalamus, plays a central role in regulating most of the endocrine glands; it has a cascading effect on the glands it stimulates. The **hypothalamus,** a part of the brain that also has endocrine functions, controls many activities of the pituitary gland via neural and chemical stimuli. Pituitary dysfunction can affect some or all of the glands that are targets of pituitary hormones, thereby indirectly affecting body structure and function (Fig. 4–3).

Diagnosing endocrine disorders requires correctly matching the patient's symptoms with a specific hormone dysfunction and obtaining laboratory confirmation of overproduction or underproduction of a particular hormone or hormones. Hormone levels usually are detected by blood tests, **radioimmunoassay** (RIA), and 24-hour urine tests. Scans, ultrasound, and magnetic resonance imaging (MRI) can help determine the type and location of a lesion. Biopsy is used to determine whether a lesion is malignant.

After an endocrine problem is identified, treatment is initiated to replace the hormone deficit or reduce a lesion by surgical removal or radiation therapy. Newer medical therapies also inhibit the synthesis of hormones. However, therapeutic drugs may have substantial side effects.

TABLE 4–1
Major Endocrine Gland Secretions and Functions

ENDOCRINE GLAND	HORMONE	TARGET ACTION
Anterior pituitary	Growth hormone (GH)	Promotes bone and tissue growth
	Thyrotropin (thyroid-stimulating hormone [TSH])	Stimulates thyroid gland and production of thyroxine
	Corticotropin (adrenocorticotropic hormone [ACTH])	Stimulates adrenal cortex to produce glucocorticoids

TABLE 4-1
Major Endocrine Gland Secretions and Functions—cont'd

ENDOCRINE GLAND	HORMONE	TARGET ACTION
Anterior pituitary—(cont'd)	Gonadotropins	
	Follicle-stimulating hormone (FSH)	Initiates growth of eggs in ovaries; stimulates spermatogenesis in testes
	Luteinizing hormone (LH)	Causes ovulation; stimulates ovaries to produce estrogen and progesterone; stimulates testosterone production
	Prolactin	Stimulates breast development and formation of milk during pregnancy and after delivery
	Melanocyte-stimulating hormone (MSH)	Regulates skin pigmentation
Posterior pituitary	Vasopressin (antidiuretic hormone [ADH])	Stimulates water resorption by renal tubules; has antidiuretic effect
	Oxytocin	Stimulates uterine contractions, stimulates ejection of milk in mammary glands; causes ejection of secretions in male prostate gland
Thyroid	Thyroxine (T_4) and triiodothyronine (T_3)—thyroid hormone (TH)	Regulates rate of cellular metabolism (catabolic phase)
	Calcitonin	Promotes retention of calcium and phosphorus in bone; opposes effect of parathyroid hormone
Parathyroid	Parathyroid hormone (parathormone, PTH)	Regulates metabolism of calcium; elevates serum calcium levels by drawing calcium from bones
Adrenal cortex	Mineralocorticoids (MC), primarily aldosterone	Promote retention of sodium by kidneys; regulate electrolyte and fluid homeostasis
	Glucocorticoids (GC): cortisol, corticosterone, cortisone	Regulate metabolism of carbohydrates, proteins, and fats in cells
	Gonadocorticoids: androgens, estrogens, progestins	Govern secondary sex characteristics and masculinization
Adrenal medulla	Catecholamines: epinephrine and norepinephrine	Produce quick-acting "fight or flight" response during stress; increase blood pressure, heart rate, and blood glucose level; dilate bronchioles
Pancreas	Insulin	Regulates metabolism of glucose in body cells; maintains proper blood glucose level
	Glucagon	Increases concentration of glucose in blood by causing conversion of glycogen to glucose
Ovaries	Estrogens	Cause development of female secondary sex characteristics
	Progesterone	Prepares and maintains endometrium for implantation and pregnancy
Testes	Testosterone	Stimulates and promotes growth of male secondary sex characteristics and is essential for erections
Thymus	Thymosin	Promotes development of immune cells (gland atrophies during adulthood)
Pineal gland	Melatonin	Regulates daily patterns of sleep and wakefulness Inhibits hormones that affect ovaries; other functions unknown

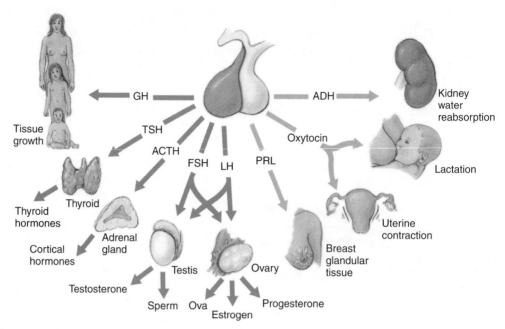

FIGURE 4–3 The effect of pituitary hormones on target tissues. *GH,* Growth hormone; *TSH,* thyroid-stimulating hormone; *ACTH,* adrenocorticotropic hormone; *FSH,* follicle-stimulating hormone; *LH,* luteinizing hormone; *PRL,* prolactin; *ADH,* antidiuretic hormone. (From Applegate EJ: *The anatomy and physiology learning system,* ed 2, Philadelphia, 2000, Saunders.)

Pituitary Gland Diseases

– Hyperpituitarism

Hyperpituitarism, a chronic and progressive disease, is caused by excessive production and secretion of pituitary hormones, particularly human growth hormone (hGH). The excessive hGH produces one of two distinct conditions, gigantism or acromegaly, depending on the time of life at which the dysfunction begins.

Gigantism
DESCRIPTION
Gigantism describes an abnormal pattern of growth and stature.

■ ICD-9-CM Code **253.0**

SYMPTOMS AND SIGNS
When the hypersecretion of hGH (growth hormone, **somatotropin**) occurs before puberty, the result is gigantism, a proportional overgrowth of all body tissue (Fig. 4–4). The child experiences abnormal and accelerated growth, especially of the long bones, because **epiphyseal** closure has not begun. The very young child may have an arched palate and slanting eyes. Sexual and mental development often are retarded.

PATIENT SCREENING
Symptoms usually appear over time; signs of the condition may be discovered during a routine examination. Follow office policy for referral to an endocrinologist.

ETIOLOGY
An anterior pituitary *adenoma* is often the cause of oversecretion of hGH that results in gigantism.

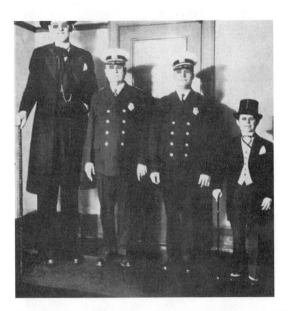

FIGURE 4-4 Effects of growth hormone. Comparison of (left to right) gigantism, normal, and dwarfism. (From Thibodeau GA: *Anatomy and physiology,* ed 5, St. Louis, 2003, Mosby. Courtesy of Dr. Edmund Beard, Cleveland, Ohio.)

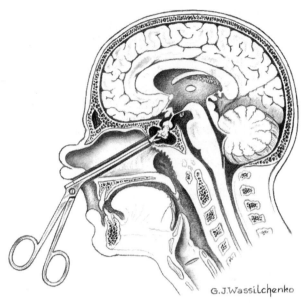

FIGURE 4-5 Transsphenoidal approach to removing a pituitary tumor. (From Rudy E: *Advanced neurological and neurosurgical nursing,* St. Louis, 1984, Mosby.)

Although a genetic link has not been identified, gigantism sometimes affects multiple members of a family. Hypogonadism may lead to gigantism by delaying puberty and closure of the *epiphyses.*

DIAGNOSIS

The clinical picture of abnormal growth in a prepubescent child leads the physician to perform diagnostic investigations. Levels of hGH are elevated on RIA. Various means of imaging the skull, such as radiography, computed tomography (CT), and arteriography, suggest the presence of a pituitary lesion. Bone radiographic films show thickening of the cranium and long bones.

TREATMENT

The object of treatment is to reduce the amount of hGH that is secreted. This is performed by either radiation of the pituitary gland or surgical intervention to reduce its size (Fig. 4-5). Appropriate gonadal hormones may be needed in children or adolescents exhibiting hypogonadism. Yearly follow-up examinations are recommended.

PROGNOSIS

Correction of the disorder prevents further physical disfigurement.

PREVENTION

No prevention is known.

PATIENT TEACHING

Explain the diagnostic tests and surgical interventions as appropriate. Give the child and parents visual aids depicting the pituitary gland and its functions. Emphasize the importance of getting follow-up care and adhering to a precise dosage schedule for medication.

Acromegaly
DESCRIPTION

Acromegaly is a chronic metabolic condition of adults caused by hypersecretion of growth hormone (hGH).

 ICD-9-CM Code 253.0

SYMPTOMS AND SIGNS

When the hypersecretion of hGH occurs after puberty and epiphyseal closure, acromegaly (an overgrowth of the bones of the face, hands, and feet) occurs, along with an excessive overgrowth of soft tissue (Fig. 4–6). It is often seen in people 30 to 40 years old after they experience years of excess growth hormone. The patient notices that he or she must wear larger gloves, shoes, or both. The jaw grows, causing larger spaces between the teeth. He or she may experience joint pain resulting from osteoarthritis and a host of other clinical features in the body systems.

PATIENT SCREENING

Symptoms usually appear over time; signs of the condition may be discovered during a routine examination. Follow office policy for referral to an endocrinologist.

ETIOLOGY

As with gigantism, a pituitary tumor or adenoma often is the cause of acromegaly. It affects women and men with equal frequency.

DIAGNOSIS

The clinical picture of abnormal thickening of the bones of the face, hands, and feet leads the physician to perform diagnostic tests. Levels of hGH are elevated on RIA. Various methods of imaging the skull, such as radiography, MRI, and arteriography, suggest the presence of a pituitary lesion along with a thickening of the bones.

TREATMENT

The object of treatment is to reverse or prevent tumor mass effects and reduce the amount of hGH secreted. Correcting the disorder prevents further disfigurement and reduces the mortality that results from production of excess growth hormone. This is performed by either radiation of the pituitary gland (less recommended) or surgical intervention to reduce its size (see Fig. 4–5). The success of medical therapies depends on the response of tumor cells to the intervention.

PROGNOSIS

Reducing levels of GH is associated with an improvement in symptoms and signs.

PREVENTION

No prevention is known.

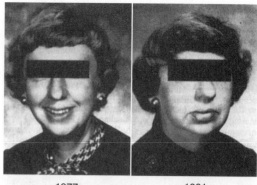
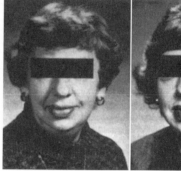
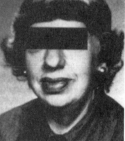

1977   1981

1983   1988

FIGURE 4–6 Clinical features of acromegaly. (From Bennett JC, Plum F: *Cecil textbook of medicine,* ed 20, vol 2, Philadelphia, 1996, Saunders.)

PATIENT TEACHING

Give visual aids that explain the anatomy and function of the pituitary gland and its hormones. Explain the purpose of the required diagnostic tests. Describe the surgical procedures if appropriate. Explain the medication dosage schedule and the possible adverse effects to report. Encourage the patient to express concerns and questions about changes in body image.

Hypopituitarism

DESCRIPTION

Hypopituitarism is a condition caused by a deficiency or absence of any of the pituitary hormones, especially those produced by the anterior pituitary lobe.

 ICD-9-CM Code 253.2

SYMPTOMS AND SIGNS

Because the anterior pituitary secretes several major hormones, the syndrome can be complex and marked by metabolic dysfunction, sexual immaturity, or growth retardation. Physical findings vary with the specific hormone deficiency. A deficiency of pituitary hormones that stimulate other endocrine glands can result in the atrophy of those glands. When **thyrotropin** (thyroid-stimulating hormone [TSH]) secretion is reduced, the functioning of the thyroid gland is affected and the patient experiences symptoms of hypothyroidism. When the secretion of corticotropin (adrenocorticotropic hormone [ACTH]) dwindles, salt balance and nutrient metabolism are affected. Gonadotropin deficiency impairs sexual functions, including sexual development, menstruation, and libido.

Hypopituitarism produces growth retardation in children. Headache and blindness are signs of tumor infringement on the optic nerve.

PATIENT SCREENING

Symptoms of the complex syndromes associated with this disorder usually have an insidious onset. Schedule a complete medical evaluation and follow office policy for referral to an endocrinologist.

ETIOLOGY

The cause of hypopituitarism may be a pituitary tumor or a tumor of the hypothalamus. Some causes are congenital deficiencies. In some instances, hypopituitarism results from damage to the pituitary gland caused by radiation or surgical removal or from *ischemia* of the gland caused by *infarct,* tumor, or basilar skull fracture. If the ischemia is severe and not reversed, permanent destruction of glandular tissue begins. Destruction of the entire anterior lobe is termed **panhypopituitarism,** and none of the important anterior pituitary hormones are secreted. The condition is most common in women, and sometimes the cause is unknown.

DIAGNOSIS

When the patient presents with the clinical symptoms of hyposecretion of any of the anterior pituitary hormones, a complete medical evaluation is necessary to pinpoint the diagnosis. A history of head trauma, previous radiation, or a surgical procedure to the gland or nearby tissue contributes to the diagnosis. Plasma levels of all or some of the pituitary hormones are low. Radiographic films of the skull, cranial CT, and MRI scans are used to identify tumors. The clinical investigation must rule out disease of the target glands themselves.

TREATMENT

The age of the patient, the severity and type of deficiency, and the underlying cause of hypopituitarism determine the course of treatment. When *neoplasia* is the cause, removal of the tumor eases the symptoms. Replacement therapy with hormonal supplements, including **thyroxine,** cortisone, sex hormones, or somatrem or somatropin (hGH), is usually effective. Hormone levels must be continually monitored during hormone replacement therapy.

PROGNOSIS

The prognosis varies because of the many possible causes of hypopituitarism and the complex functions of the pituitary gland itself.

PREVENTION

No prevention is known.

PATIENT TEACHING

Give the patient visual aids depicting the pituitary gland, and describe the features of the major pituitary hormones. Explain the diagnostic procedures and any planned surgical intervention. Emphasize the importance of following any instructions given by the endocrinologist regarding hormone replacement therapy, and list warning signs of overreplacement. Emphasize the importance of follow-up visits to monitor the results of therapy and adjust the dosage.

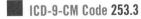
Dwarfism

DESCRIPTION

Dwarfism is the abnormal underdevelopment of the body, or hypopituitarism, occurring in children.

■ **ICD-9-CM Code 253.3**

SYMPTOMS AND SIGNS

Hyposecretion of the pituitary gland hormones, especially hGH, results in growth retardation. As a result, the child is extremely short, with a body that is small in proportion (see Fig.4–4). The prepubescent child does not develop secondary sex characteristics.

The condition may be linked to other defects and a varying degree of mental retardation.

PATIENT SCREENING

Children deficient in growth hormone require regular follow-up appointments during therapy. Follow office policy for referral to an endocrinologist.

ETIOLOGY

Dwarfism can be congenital or the result of a cranial hemorrhage after the birth process. Occasionally, there is no identifiable cause. A deficiency of the growth-hormone–releasing hormone (GH-RH) produced by the hypothalamus is termed secondary hypopituitarism and results from head trauma, tumor, or infection.

DIAGNOSIS

Physical examination shows that the child fails to grow at a normal rate and is short in stature. The child's general health appears to be good. However, secondary tooth eruption is delayed, and fat deposits may be noted in the lower trunk area. Persistently low serum hGH levels are found. A CT scan may confirm the presence of a cranial tumor.

TREATMENT

Somatotropin (hGH) is administered until the child reaches a height of 5 feet. These children also may need replacement of thyroid and adrenal hormones. As they approach puberty, sex hormones are administered if necessary.

PREVENTION

Known causes are not preventable, except that common precautions may be taken against head trauma and infection.

PROGNOSIS

Clinical manifestations of GH deficiencies depend on the time of onset and the degree of hormone deficiency. Growth hormone replacement is effective in children with well-documented GH deficiency. Treatment is essential to help reach final adult height.

PATIENT TEACHING

Give the patient and family visual aids to familiarize them with the pituitary gland and the hormones that affect growth and maturation. Explain the regimen of GH treatment, which may include frequent injections, and emphasize the importance of patient compliance to achieve the desired therapeutic goal.

Diabetes Insipidus

DESCRIPTION

Diabetes insipidus is a disturbance of water metabolism resulting in extreme thirst and excessive secretion of dilute urine.

 ICD-9-CM Code 253.5

SYMPTOMS AND SIGNS

Diabetes insipidus is a deficiency in the release of **vasopressin** (antidiuretic hormone [ADH]) by the posterior pituitary gland, resulting in the excretion of copious amounts of colorless and dilute urine **(polyuria).** The patient experiences excessive thirst **(polydipsia)**, fatigue, and symptoms of dehydration, including dry mucous membranes, hypotension, dizziness, constipation, and poor skin turgor. The onset of symptoms may be abrupt.

PATIENT SCREENING

An abrupt onset of excessive thirst and excessive urination together with the symptoms of dehydration merits prompt medical attention.

ETIOLOGY

In diabetes insipidus, the posterior pituitary gland releases reduced amounts of vasopressin. The condition may be hereditary, or it may be the result of an insult to the hypothalamus or to the pituitary gland resulting from head trauma, cerebral edema, or an intracranial lesion. Nephrogenic diabetes insipidus results from renal tubular resistance to the action of vasopressin. More common in men than women, this disease may occur in childhood or early adulthood. In many cases, the cause is unknown. When the amount of vasopressin is insufficient, the distal tubules of the nephron do not reabsorb water from the filtrate back into the blood stream; consequently, the volume of urine is excessive.

DIAGNOSIS

The presence of polyuria and polydipsia leads the clinician to investigate the composition of the urine through laboratory tests. Urinalysis that reveals almost colorless urine that has a low specific gravity (<1.005) suggests diabetes insipidus as a diagnosis. To confirm the diagnosis of diabetes insipidus, the patient is given a water-restriction test, during which the kidneys exhibit the inability to concentrate urine when the patient is deprived of fluid intake for several hours. After the patient has lost 3% of his or her body weight or hypotension becomes severe, vasopressin (antidiuretic hormone [ADH]) is administered. Urine volume is compared with specific gravity. Reduced output and increased specific gravity of urine after the administration of vasopressin indicate diabetes insipidus.

TREATMENT
Treatment consists of vasopressin injections or nasal spray therapy with lypressin (Diapid) or desmopressin acetate (DDAVP). Thiazide diuretics block the ability of the kidneys to excrete free water by inhibiting reabsorption of sodium and chloride and increasing the excretion of sodium, chloride, and water. Any underlying cause should be identified and treated. When the excessive diuresis is the result of trauma to the pituitary gland, the symptoms begin to subside as the insult resolves and inflammation decreases.

PROGNOSIS
Individuals with uncomplicated diabetes insipidus respond to treatment and return to normal lives.

PREVENTION
The causes and contributing factors cannot be prevented.

PATIENT TEACHING
Give the patient guidelines for monitoring fluid intake and output to ensure adequate water replacement. Instruct the patient to notify the physician of any increase in symptoms, including weight loss or gain. Demonstrate the procedure of checking the specific gravity of urine. Discuss the side effects or toxic effects of prescribed medications. Encourage the patient to wear a Medic Alert bracelet (Fig. 4–7).

Thyroid Gland Diseases

Thyroid diseases present as functional disturbances that produce excessive or reduced secretions of thyroid hormones thyroxine (T_4) and

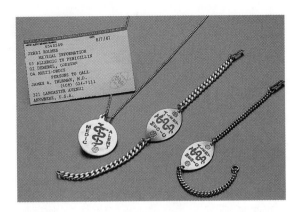

FIGURE 4–7 Medic Alert. (From Judd RL, Ponsell PP: *Mosby's first responder,* ed 2, St. Louis, 1988, Mosby.)

triiodothyronine (T_3) and mass lesions of the thyroid. Table 4–2 lists thyroid diseases with their signs and symptoms. Fortunately, diseases of the thyroid gland may be resolved through medical and surgical intervention.

The thyroid gland is the endocrine organ that most often produces pathology. Under the control of thyroid-stimulating hormone (TSH) from the pituitary gland, the thyroid gland produces two types of hormones: thyroxine (T_4) and triiodothyronine (T_3). Released into systemic circulation, thyroid hormones affect the metabolism of all body tissues, the function of the pituitary's essential growth hormone, and many body systems. The size and superficial location of the thyroid gland in the neck make it uniquely available for inspection and palpation. A goiter is often the first sign of thyroid disease.

Simple Goiter

DESCRIPTION
The term goiter refers to any enlargement of the thyroid gland.

> **ICD-9-CM Code   240.0** *Goiter (specified as simple)*
> **240.9** *Goiter (unspecified)*
> *Disorders of the thyroid gland are coded according to the underlying pathology. Refer to the physician's diagnosis and then to the current edition of the ICD-9-CM coding manual to ensure the greatest specificity of pathology and any appropriate modifiers.*

TABLE 4–2
Comparison of Hypothyroid and Hyperthyroid Disorders

	HYPOFUNCTION OF THYROID	HYPERFUNCTION OF THYROID
Names or Types	Congenital, untreated can become cretinism or thyroid dwarfism	Hyperthyroidism
	Thyroiditis–Myxedema	Thyrotoxicosis
	Hashimoto disease	Graves' disease–autoimmune with or without exophthalmos
	Iodine deficiency–simple goiter	Toxic nodular hyperplasia
	Idiopathic hypothyroidism	Toxic adenoma, thyroid tumors
Symptoms and Signs	Decreased activity, sleepiness, lethargy	Restlessness, irritability, easy fatigability, nervousness
	Reduced mental alertness, easy fatigability	Tremors
	Dry skin and hair, decreased sweating	Moist skin, increased sweating
	Cold intolerance	Heat intolerance
	Bradycardia	Tachycardia and palpitations
	Constipation	Diarrhea
	Weight gain	Weight loss, increased appetite
	Edema, bloated face, puffy eyelids	Polydipsia
	Poor circulation, extremity edema	Loss or thinning of hair
	TSH levels increased	TSH levels decreased
	T_3, T_4 levels decreased	T_3, T_4 levels increased
	I^{131} uptake decreased	I^{131} uptake increased

I^{131}, Radioactive iodine; T_3, triiodothyronine; T_4, thyroxine; *TSH*, thyroid-stimulating hormone.

SYMPTOMS AND SIGNS
Simple goiter, a hyperplasia of the thyroid gland, may be *asymptomatic* in the early stages. The patient, who is usually female, may be unaware of the condition until the anterior aspect of the neck enlarges with a conspicuous swollen mass called a goiter (Fig. 4–8). As the hyperplasia increases, it presses on the trachea, producing *dyspnea,* and on the esophagus, producing difficulty in swallowing. A large goiter can cause dizziness or **syncope.**

PATIENT SCREENING
The patient who complains of an enlargement in the area of the thyroid gland, with or without accompanying discomfort in the area, should be scheduled for a thorough patient history and physical examination.

ETIOLOGY
Simple, or nontoxic, goiter results from a shortage of iodine in the diet. Iodine is necessary for the synthesis of both triiodothyronine (T_3) and thyroxine (T_4). These are known together as thyroid hormone and are produced by the thyroid gland. The inadequate blood level of thyroid hormone causes the anterior pituitary gland to increase its secretion of thyrotropin. Thyrotropin keeps attempting to stimulate the thyroid gland to produce thyroid hormone. This continued stimulation in turn causes the thyroid gland to increase in size.

In the past, geographic regions in which the soil had low levels of iodine and where seafood was not readily available had high rates of simple goiter. The advent of rapid refrigerated transport of seafood and fresh vegetables from areas in which soil and water iodine levels are high has reduced the *endemic* aspects of this condition. Simple goiter can appear sporadically as a result of ingestion of large amounts of *goitrogenic* foods such as turnips and cabbage or drugs such as lithium.

DIAGNOSIS
Diagnosis is made by examination of the neck, noting the enlargement of the thyroid gland (goiter).

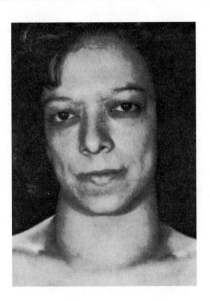

FIGURE 4–8 Endemic goiter. (From Wilson JD, Foster DW: *Williams textbook of endocrinology,* ed 8, Philadelphia, 1992, Saunders.)

Blood studies indicate elevated thyrotropin levels and reduced levels of T_3 and T_4.

TREATMENT

Treatment in the early stages is simple: the administration of one drop per week of saturated solution of potassium iodide. Prevention calls for the addition of iodine to the diet, including the use of iodized salt. Sporadic goiter requires avoidance of goitrogenic drugs or food.

PROGNOSIS

The prognosis is good when treatment to reduce the goiter is successful. When a large goiter is unresponsive to treatment, a subtotal *thyroidectomy* may be required.

PREVENTION

Adequate dietary intake of iodized salt (or 150 to 300 mcg of iodine) prevents this deficiency. Some individuals should be advised to avoid goitrogenic drugs or foods.

PATIENT TEACHING

Instruct the patient to take prescribed thyroid hormone medication at the same time each day to maintain a constant level of the medication in the

blood. Make sure the patient and the family know the symptoms of adverse effects of a thyroid preparation that should be reported to the physician: palpitations, increased pulse rate, anxiety, insomnia, sweating, and tremors.

Hashimoto Disease

DESCRIPTION

Hashimoto disease (chronic thyroiditis) is a chronic disease of the immune system that attacks the thyroid gland.

ICD-9-CM Code 245.2

In some coding books this disease may be spelled Hashimoto's Disease.

SYMPTOMS AND SIGNS

The condition occurs in women eight times as often as in men, is most common between 45 and 65 years of age, and is the leading cause of nonsimple goiter and hypothyroidism. The outstanding clinical feature is the gradual and painless enlargement of the thyroid gland, which causes a feeling of pressure in the neck and difficulty with swallowing. Symptoms of hypothyroidism, such as sensitivity to cold, weight gain, and mental apathy, appear as the disease progresses.

PATIENT SCREENING

Schedule a physical examination for a patient presenting with a "lump in the throat" or swelling in the neck. Follow office policy for referral to an endocrinologist.

ETIOLOGY

The cause of Hashimoto disease is unknown, but a genetic factor is suspected. Autoimmune factors play a prominent role because antibodies appear to destroy thyroid tissue instead of stimulating it. The gland enlarges as a result of an inflammatory process, with massive infiltration by lymphocytes and plasma cells. As a result, gland tissue is replaced by fibrous tissue.

DIAGNOSIS

Thyroid function is measured by a radioactive iodine uptake (RAIU) test. Serum thyroid-stimulating hormones are elevated. Autoantibodies against thyroid tissue are found in the blood. In Hashimoto disease, characteristic changes can be seen in the thyroid gland through needle biopsy and examination of the gland tissue.

TREATMENT

The treatment is lifelong replacement of thyroid hormone. This also prevents further growth of the goiter.

PROGNOSIS

Mild hypothyroidism is common and usually responds well to thyroid-replacement therapy.

PREVENTION

No prevention is known.

PATIENT TEACHING

Explain each diagnostic test and procedure. Review the purpose and dosage schedule of prescribed medication and the adverse effects to report. Emphasize the importance of follow-up visits to monitor thyroid-replacement therapy. Encourage the patient to expect improvement in symptoms with treatment.

Hyperthyroidism
Graves' Disease burn 6,000 calories

DESCRIPTION

Graves' disease, a condition of primary hyperthyroidism, occurs when the entire thyroid gland hypertrophies, resulting in a diffuse goiter.

■ **ICD-9-CM Code 242.0**
Refer to the physician's diagnosis and then to the current edition of the ICD-9-CM coding manual to ensure the greatest specificity of pathology and any appropriate modifiers.

SYMPTOMS AND SIGNS

Overproduction of thyroid hormone causes increased metabolism and multisystem changes. The patient has rapid heartbeat and palpitations, nervousness, excitability, and insomnia. Despite excessive appetite and food consumption, the patient loses weight. Profuse perspiration and warm, moist skin cause the person to be intolerant of hot weather. Other symptoms include excessive thirst, nausea and vomiting, muscular weakness, and dermopathy. General hyperactive behavior, tremor, and loss of hair are noted. As the condition advances, the eyes develop exophthalmos, an outward protrusion, which gives the patient a staring expression (Fig. 4–9). A sudden exacerbation of symptoms may signal **thyrotoxicosis,** or thyroid storm, which can be life threatening.

PATIENT SCREENING

A patient with mild or vague symptoms should be scheduled for a medical history and physical. An acute manifestation of severe symptoms (e.g., marked tachycardia, manic behavior, vomiting, confusion, coma) can indicate a life-threatening condition. Prompt consultation with the physician is appropriate.

ETIOLOGY

The cause of Graves' disease is uncertain; however, it is believed to be an autoimmune response. Antibodies to thyroid antigens stimulate the hyperactivity of the thyroid gland. There is a familial predisposition that strongly suggests genetic causation.

DIAGNOSIS

Taking the clinical picture and a thorough history are the first steps in the diagnosis. Serum T_3 and T_4 levels are elevated, and a thyroid scan indicates increased uptake of radioiodine. Blood tests may reveal elevated levels of certain antithyroid immunoglobulins.

TREATMENT

The goal of treatment is to reduce the formation and secretion of thyroid hormone. Treatment

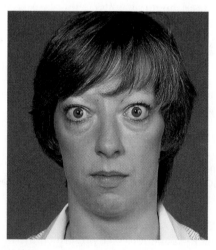

FIGURE 4–9 Graves' disease. (From Stevens A, Lowe J: *Pathology—illustrated review in color,* ed 2, St. Louis, 2000, Mosby.)

begins with the administration of antithyroid drugs such as propylthiouracil and methimazole (Tapazole) to block the synthesis of thyroid hormone. Beta-blockers such as propranolol hydrochloride (Inderal) and atenolol (Tenormin) are given to treat *tachycardia* and hypertension. In nonresponsive or severe cases, radioactive iodine therapy or surgery (thyroidectomy) is used to reduce the activity of the thyroid gland. Patients require ongoing medical supervision to monitor thyroid hormone levels. Some patients need help in coping with the anxiety and physical discomforts associated with Graves' disease.

PROGNOSIS

Therapeutic intervention often restores the balance of thyroid in the body and relieves symptoms. Some cases are more difficult to treat, and complications may arise. On the other hand, some cases experience spontaneous remission. Relapses do occur; thus lifelong follow-up is recommended.

PREVENTION

Precise causes are not understood, so prevention is unidentified.

PATIENT TEACHING

Give the patient visual aids that explain the location and function of the thyroid gland. Explain the effects of hyperthyroidism on the body and on emotional stability. Discuss diagnostic procedures and their purpose. Explain the dosage schedule of medications and the adverse effects to report. Give preoperative and postoperative instructions as appropriate. Emphasize the importance of follow-up appointments to monitor treatment. Special instructions are required for skin care and eye care.

Hypothyroidism

Hypothyroidism can strike either sex and at any age. Much of the world's population lives at high risk in iodine-deficient areas, resulting in congenital hypothyroidism, a major cause of mental deficiency.

Cretinism
DESCRIPTION

Cretinism is a hypothyroidism developing in infancy or early childhood.

■ **ICD-9-CM Code 243**

SYMPTOMS AND SIGNS

Cretinism is a congenital hypothyroid condition in which the thyroid gland is absent or thyroid hormone is not synthesized by the thyroid gland; this causes mental and growth retardation in the infant or young child. The child develops as a dwarf, stocky in stature with a protruding abdomen. Other physical characteristics include a short forehead, a broad nose, small wide-set eyes with puffy eyelids, a wide-open mouth with a thick, protruding tongue, an expressionless face, and dry skin. The sex organs fail to develop. Growth and physical and mental capabilities are retarded. A lack of muscle tone contributes to an inability to stand or walk.

PATIENT SCREENING

Follow office policy for referral of newborns or children with endocrine conditions or with suspected developmental disorders.

ETIOLOGY

An error in fetal development may cause the thyroid gland to fail to develop or to fail to function. The patient may have a congenital absence of one of the enzymes necessary for T_3 and T_4 synthesis. Maternal thyroid deficiency or antithyroid drugs taken during pregnancy may be an etiologic factor.

DIAGNOSIS

A blood test that indicates an absence or abnormally low amount of T_4 in the presence of an elevated level of thyrotropin indicates cretinism. A thyroid scan shows reduced levels of iodine uptake and confirms the absence of thyroid tissue. If cretinism is not detected during the neonatal period, the infant will be slow to smile and eventually will be developmentally retarded.

TREATMENT

Early treatment with thyroid hormone promotes normal physical growth but may not prevent mental retardation. This replacement therapy must continue throughout the life of the patient.

PROGNOSIS

The prognosis is good when cretinism is discovered early in life and thyroxine replacement is begun. Even skeletal abnormalities are reversible with treatment. The condition may be associated with other endocrine abnormalities.

PREVENTION

The use of iodized salt greatly reduces the incidence of cretinism in a population. Public education about the importance of good prenatal care that manages any maternal endocrine disease is important.

PATIENT TEACHING

Explain the importance of regular monitoring of the therapeutic response to hormone replacement. The response to the hormone replacement takes time; give the parent reasonable expectations for the child taking the medication. Give the parents or caregivers educational materials and referrals to support appropriate to their individual needs.

Myxedema

DESCRIPTION

Myxedema is severe hypothyroidism developing in the older child or adult.

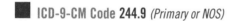 ICD-9-CM Code **244.9** *(Primary or NOS)*

SYMPTOMS AND SIGNS

Myxedema, severe hypothyroidism with reduced levels of T_4, has its onset in the older child or in adult life. Clinical manifestations vary with the age of onset. As levels of T_4 decrease, metabolism is slowed and there is the insidious onset of systemic conditions. The patient, who is usually female, experiences *menorrhagia*. The skin becomes dry and scaly, with little or no perspiration. The face becomes bloated, the tongue thick, and the eyelids puffy (Fig. 4–10). Muscular weakness, excessive tiredness, and fatigue are common symptoms. Weight gain, loss of hair, constipation, and intolerance to cold are experienced. Speech becomes slow and slurred, with mental apathy, and there are diminished physical capabilities. In severe cases, myxedema coma, a rare but life-threatening emergency, can occur; this is best treated with intensive care.

PATIENT SCREENING

Complaints will vary with the age of onset. A parent reporting slowing of physical and mental activity in a child, or an adult reporting the same, needs an appointment for a complete physical. Keep in mind symptoms may mimic depression.

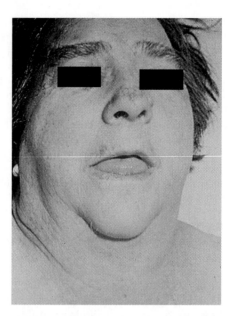

FIGURE 4–10 Myxedema facies. (From Seidel HM et al: *Mosby's guide to physical examination,* ed 5, St. Louis, 2003, Mosby. Courtesy Paul W. Ladenson, MD, The Johns Hopkins University and Hospital, Baltimore.)

ETIOLOGY

The thyroid gland's ability to synthesize T_4 is impaired. This can be the result of reduced amounts of thyrotropin, radiation destruction of the thyroid gland, surgical removal of the gland without T_4 replacement therapy, tumor, or failure of the thyroid gland to function. The disorder also may be secondary to failure of the pituitary to produce thyrotropin. A common cause for hypothyroidism in children and teens is Hashimoto disease.

DIAGNOSIS

The clinical features of myxedema in the adult or the retardation of physical and mental development in the child lead the physician to perform diagnostic tests. Blood studies indicate abnormally low levels of T_4, thyrotropin, or both. Radioactive iodine uptake tests may indicate the absence of response to thyrotropin.

TREATMENT

Levothyroxine sodium (T_4), a therapeutic agent, is administered. The goal of medical management is to achieve normal thyroid function with the lowest possible dose. The patient should be told that replacement therapy likely will be required for the rest of his or her life.

PROGNOSIS

The response to hormone replacement therapy is usually good, and the symptoms improve. Left untreated, severe hypothyroidism affects almost every body system.

PREVENTION

Endocrinologists and other health-care providers recommend screening (testing for TSH levels) in identified high-risk groups and at age 35 and every 5 years thereafter as part of a periodic health examination.

PATIENT TEACHING

Patients on medications should be taught the importance of taking the medication at the same time each day on an empty stomach and the signs of overmedication. Inform the patient that a clinical response to the medication may take several weeks to appear and that blood tests will be required to monitor for therapeutic blood levels of the medication. Demonstrate and encourage periodic self-examination of the thyroid gland.

Thyroid Cancer

DESCRIPTION

Thyroid cancer occurs in the thyroid gland, a bilobed structure below and anterior to the larynx.

> ### ICD-9-CM Code 193
> *Refer to the physician's diagnosis and then to the current edition of the ICD-9-CM coding manual to ensure the greatest specificity of pathology and any appropriate modifiers.*

SYMPTOMS AND SIGNS

Thyroid malignancies often do not cause symptoms until the disease is advanced. Palpation of a hard, painless lump or nodule on the thyroid gland, vocal cord paralysis, obstructive symptoms, and cervical-lymph adenopathy all indicate cancer. Hormone secretion by the tumor can lead to systemic symptoms such as diarrhea, facial flushing, and Cushing syndrome. Some patients exhibit dysphagia or hoarseness resulting from compression of the upper aerodigestive tract.

PATIENT SCREENING

Schedule patients complaining of persistent hoarseness or difficulty swallowing, or who notice a painless lump in the neck, for an appointment with the physician as soon as possible.

ETIOLOGY

Thyroid cancer accounts for only about 6% of all thyroid nodules. Other causes include multinodular goiter, Hashimoto thyroiditis, cysts, and follicular adenomas. Women are nearly three times more likely to develop thyroid cancer than are men. Relatives of thyroid cancer patients have a 10-fold higher incidence of thyroid cancer, which indicates a genetic basis for tumor susceptibility. Previous head and neck radiation exposure, especially in early childhood, is the only other established risk factor, but hormonal and reproductive factors in women may play a role as well.

The four main types of thyroid cancer are papillary, follicular, medullary, and anaplastic. Papillary and follicular carcinomas are the most common and are classified as differentiated neoplasms. They grow slowly, especially in people younger than 45, and are associated with high survival rates even when cancer has spread to nearby lymph nodes. A diet deficient in iodine may contribute to follicular cancer. Although 80% of cases of medullary carcinoma are sporadic, some are due to inherited genetic mutations that lead to multiple endocrine neoplasia (MEN) type 2 (a rare, heritable disorder characterized by various types of endocrine tumors). Inherited medullary cancer usually presents in the third decade of life. *Anaplastic* tumors are undifferentiated and rare and occur mainly in patients over the age of 60. They often arise from nodular goiters or from differentiated carcinomas. They typically do not respond to treatment. Other cancers found in the thyroid include metastases from breast, colon, kidney, or skin cancers.

DIAGNOSIS

Thyroid nodules are usually discovered by the patient or found incidentally on physical examination or radiologic procedure. Nodules can be evaluated through high-resolution thyroid ultrasonography or through radionuclide scanning. Ultimately, fine-needle aspiration and histological examination of the nodule tissue are needed to confirm the diagnosis of cancer and to type and stage the tumor. Medullary thyroid carcinomas are tumors of the parafollicular cells, so they often secrete calcitonin and occasionally secrete carcinoembryonic antigen (CEA), both of which can serve as tumor markers. Although many staging systems have been developed for the differentiated thyroid cancers, no system is universally accepted. Most use some combination of tumor size, number of metastases, and patient age to stage the patient. Tests used for staging include a CT scan of the neck and a chest x-ray. With medullary carcinoma, the TNM (Tumor, Node, Metastasis) system is used for staging. All anaplastic tumors are considered to be stage IV (see Chapter 1 for discussion of staging cancer).

TREATMENT

The primary therapy mode for papillary, follicular, and medullary thyroid cancers is surgery. Most patients undergo total thyroidectomy with removal of any involved lymph nodes, followed by the administration of radioiodine to destroy any remaining thyroid tissue and tumor and to image any recurrent disease. Aggressive initial therapy yields lower rates of local and regional recurrence and lower overall mortality. Thyroid surgery is associated with the risk of vocal cord paralysis resulting from damage to the recurrent laryngeal nerve and the risk of hypoparathyroidism. After surgery, patients are started on thyroxine therapy to suppress the serum thyrotropin (TSH) concentration, to prevent potential TSH stimulation of tumor growth, and to prevent hypothyroidism. However, thyroxine therapy carries risks of accelerated bone loss, atrial fibrillation, and cardiac dysfunction, so the amount of thyroxine administered is carefully regulated and linked to the tumor stage at the time of diagnosis.

For anaplastic tumors, nonsurgical treatment such as radiotherapy and/or chemotherapy may prolong survival. Total thyroidectomy is indicated to reduce symptoms caused by the tumor mass if the disease is confined to the local area.

Most recurrences of any type of thyroid neoplasm appear within 5 years of initial treatment, although they can occur decades afterward. All patients should undergo a physical examination and thyroid testing periodically after treatment.

PROGNOSIS

Most patients with differentiated thyroid carcinomas do not die of their disease. The most important prognostic factors are age at diagnosis, size of the primary tumor, and the presence of tissue inva-

sion or metastases. The overall 5-year survival rate is 95%. Many patients with medullary carcinoma have metastatic disease at the time of diagnosis. Despite this metastasis, some patients survive for years, depending largely on the age of the patient. The 5-year survival rate is 95% for patients under age 40 and 65% for those over 40. For anaplastic tumors, 5-year survival is very poor. Death often results from local cancer in the neck within months of diagnosis.

PREVENTION

Patients who have been exposed to radiation should receive follow-up screening for thyroid cancer development depending on their estimated risk level. Those at low risk should undergo thyroid palpation every year or every other year. Those at high risk should undergo annual palpation and thyroid ultrasonography every 3 to 5 years. Those at high risk usually have been exposed to high-dose radiation of the thyroid at a young age, are female, and have had another radiation-related tumor or a sibling with a radiation-related tumor.

PATIENT TEACHING

Give the patient preoperative instructions and encourage the patient to ask questions about the risks the surgeon identifies. Tell the patient what to expect after surgery, including temporary loss of the voice. Explain postoperative instructions, including hormone therapy, chemotherapy, and/or radiotherapy as prescribed by the physician. Refer the patient to the attending physician for questions about the prognosis after treatment. Emphasize the need for follow-up appointments, and review the schedule for these appointments.

Parathyroid Gland Diseases

Hyperparathyroidism

DESCRIPTION

Hyperparathyroidism is a condition caused by overactivity of one or more of the four parathyroid glands and results in the overproduction of parathyroid hormone (parathormone [PTH]).

ICD-9-CM Code 252.0

SYMPTOMS AND SIGNS

Hyperparathyroidism increases the breakdown of bone (demineralization) through the subsequent release of excessive calcium into the blood (hypercalcemia) and extracellular fluid. Hypercalcemia produces the symptoms of hyperparathyroidism. Hypercalcemia reduces the irritability of nerve and muscle tissue, and this causes the patient to experience muscle weakness and atrophy, gastrointestinal pain, and nausea and vomiting. High serum calcium levels can produce conduction defects in the heart. An increased deposit of calcium in soft tissue causes low-back pain and *renal calculi*. Bone tenderness, arthritis-type pain, and easy fracturing of the bones are the result of demineralization of the bone.

PATIENT SCREENING

Some patients may present with vague symptoms such as fatigue, weakness, or mental disturbance. Schedule a complete physical examination. A patient experiencing symptoms of hypercalcemia is very ill and requires prompt medical intervention.

ETIOLOGY

The cause of primary hyperparathyroidism is increased activity of the parathyroid gland, usually as a result of a parathyroid tumor (adenoma) or an *idiopathic* hyperplasia of the gland. The incidence rises sharply after age 40 and is twice as common in women. Secondary hyperparathyroidism may be caused by an increased secretion of PTH induced by a low level of serum calcium caused by renal disease or other disorders.

DIAGNOSIS

A high concentration of serum PTH is noted on RIA. Blood calcium, chloride, and alkaline phosphatase levels are elevated, and serum phosphorus levels are reduced. The calcium level in urine is increased. Diffuse demineralization of bones and bone cysts are evident on radiographic films; cortical bone absorption also is noted along with erosion of the middle phalanx.

TREATMENT

The treatment plan for hyperparathyroidism varies with the cause and is highly individualized. If the hypersecretion of PTH is caused by an adenoma, the tumor is removed. If hypertrophy is the cause of the hypersecretion, part or all of a gland is removed. Limiting the dietary intake of calcium is helpful, as is *diuresis* by forced fluid intake and administration of loop diuretics (furosemide [Lasix] or ethacrynic acid [Edecrin]), with resulting excretion of calcium and sodium. When the condition is secondary, the underlying cause must be treated and the blood serum calcium levels reduced. Drugs that increase the excretion of calcium by the kidneys or inhibit the reabsorption of calcium from bone may be used. Lifelong vitamin D supplementation may be indicated after surgery.

PROGNOSIS

After successful surgery, **hypocalcemia** is usually mild and allows skeletal remineralization in patients with bone disease.

PREVENTION

No prevention is known.

PATIENT TEACHING

Give the patient a visual aid explaining the location and function of the parathyroid glands. Explain hyperparathyroid disease and the treatment plan. Give preoperative and postoperative instructions as indicated. Explain the dosage schedule for prescription medication and the adverse side effects to report. Caution against using over-the-counter medications containing calcium. Refer the patient to a dietitian as required.

Hypoparathyroidism

DESCRIPTION

Hypoparathyroidism is the condition in which the secretion of parathormone (PTH) by the parathyroid glands is greatly reduced.

 ICD-9-CM Code 252.1

SYMPTOMS AND SIGNS

PTH increases the blood calcium level by stimulating bone demineralization and increasing absorption of calcium in the digestive tract and kidneys. When the level of this hormone is insufficient, circulating levels of calcium are reduced, resulting in hypocalcemia, with excessive deposit of calcium into bone tissue. A consequence of the hypocalcemia is a hyperexcitable nervous system, resulting in an overstimulation of the skeletal muscles. Initial symptoms include numbness and tingling of fingertips, toes, ears, or nose, followed by muscular spasms or twitching of

Adrenal Gland Diseases

the hands and feet. *Tetany,* or severe, sustained muscular contractions, may develop. The patient may experience emotional changes, confusion, and irritability. Sustained hypocalcemia leads to laryngospasm, arrhythmias, respiratory paralysis, and death.

PATIENT SCREENING

Acute, symptomatic hypocalcemia requires emergency treatment.

ETIOLOGY

The cause may rest in the parathyroid gland itself or may stem from raised blood calcium levels, which, by negative feedback, cause decreased PTH output. Acquired hypoparathyroidism can result from injury to one or more of the parathyroid glands, ischemia from an infarct, accidental radiation, *neoplasia,* or various disease processes. Accidental surgical removal of the parathyroid gland during thyroidectomy can induce hypocalcemia. The condition may result from an *autoimmune* genetic disorder or from a congenital absence of the glands.

DIAGNOSIS

The clinical picture of neuromuscular hyperexcitability along with a history of possible insult to the parathyroid glands leads the physician to further investigation. The presence of *Trousseau's phenomenon* is a sure indication of hypocalcemia. Blood studies indicate reduced serum calcium levels and increased serum phosphate levels. Increased bone density is evident on radiographic films. An *electrocardiogram* shows increased QT and ST intervals. PTH levels are reduced on RIA.

TREATMENT

Calcium replacement therapy with vitamin D reduces hypocalcemia. This replacement therapy is usually lifelong unless the condition is reversible. In the case of a life-threatening deficiency (tetany), calcium gluconate is administered intravenously. The patient is encouraged to follow a high-calcium, low-phosphorus diet.

PROGNOSIS

Reversible forms of the condition respond to appropriate treatment. Some cases are transient.

PREVENTION

No known prevention is known.

PATIENT TEACHING

Answer questions about the location and function of the parathyroid gland. Explain hypocalcemia and the way it affects the nervous system. Refer the patient to a dietitian as indicated. Emphasize the importance of follow-up care to monitor renal function and serum and urine levels of calcium.

Adrenal Gland Diseases

Cushing Syndrome

DESCRIPTION

Cushing syndrome is a condition of chronic hypersecretion of the adrenal cortex, which results in excessive circulating cortisol levels.

 ICD-9-CM Code 255.0
In some coding books this syndrome may be spelled Cushing's syndrome.

SYMPTOMS AND SIGNS

The patient with Cushing syndrome experiences fatigue, muscular weakness, and changes in body appearance. Fat deposits form in the scapular area (buffalo humps) and in the trunk, causing a protruding abdomen (Fig. 4–11). Salt and water retention results not only in hypertension and edema, but also in the characteristic moon face noted in the patient with Cushing syndrome. The patient may show clinical evidence of *hyperlipidemia,* osteoporosis, and atherosclerosis. Psychiatric problems are common. The skin becomes thin, has a tendency to bruise easily, and develops red or purple striae (stretch marks). The individual is predisposed to infection resulting from suppression of the immune response. Other symptoms include excessive hair growth, amenorrhea, and impotence. The affected individual also may have diabetes mellitus.

PATIENT SCREENING

Early manifestations include weight gain, hypertension, and emotional instability. These symptoms warrant a medical evaluation. Follow office policy for referral to an endocrinologist.

ETIOLOGY

Excessive levels of circulating cortisol can be caused by hyperplasia of the adrenal gland, exces-

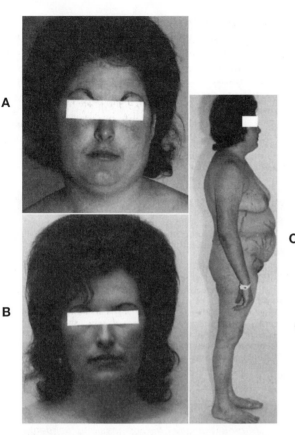

FIGURE 4-11 The appearance of a patient with Cushing syndrome. **A,** Before; **B,** 1 year after removal of an adrenal adenoma; **C,** profile before transplant. (From Wyngaarden J, Smith L, Bennett J: *Cecil textbook of medicine,* ed 19, Philadelphia, 1992, Saunders.)

TREATMENT

Treatment of Cushing syndrome depends on the cause of the oversecretion of cortisol. When a tumor is the cause, surgical removal or radiation of the tumor is indicated. Drug therapy to suppress ACTH secretions can be used separately or as an adjunct to radiation.

PROGNOSIS

The prognosis depends on the underlying cause. Without treatment, or when the condition is due to ectopic carcinoma, the prognosis is poor.

PREVENTION

Generally there is no prevention; however, the patient on large doses of glucocorticoids is monitored closely.

PATIENT TEACHING

If surgery is indicated, give the patient information about the procedures and what to expect after surgery. Give careful instructions about medication if hormone replacement is planned; the medication must be taken exactly as directed and never discontinued abruptly. Refer the patient to a dietitian as indicated. Teach the patient the symptoms of adrenal hypofunction: apathy, fatigue, weakness, and syncope.

Addison Disease

DESCRIPTION

Addison disease is partial or complete failure of adrenocortical function.

■ **ICD-9-CM Code 255.4**
In some coding books this disease may be spelled Addison's disease.

sive secretion of **corticotropin** (ACTH) from the pituitary gland, a tumor of the adrenal cortex, or production of corticotropin in another organ (because of extrapituitary tumors). Iatrogenic conditions such as prolonged administration or large doses of glucocorticoids used to treat other diseases can induce Cushing syndrome.

DIAGNOSIS

The typical picture of the moon face, buffalo hump, and gross obesity of the trunk, particularly the abdomen, leads the physician to further investigation. Continuous elevation of serum cortisol levels is found in Cushing syndrome. Free cortisol levels are elevated in 24-hour urine collections. CT or MRI may detect adrenal tumors.

SYMPTOMS AND SIGNS

Addison disease, adrenal insufficiency or hypoadrenalism, is manifested as symptoms of fatigue, weakness, anorexia, weight loss, and gastrointestinal disturbances. A typical bronze skin color is exhibited. The patient can experience cardiovascular difficulties, including irregular pulse, reduced cardiac output, and orthostatic (postural) hypotension. Depression, anxiety, and emotional distress are often experienced. Reduced levels of aldosterone cause an inability to retain salt and water. When dehydration, **hyperkalemia,** and electrolyte imbalance occur, the condition is life threatening.

PATIENT SCREENING

The onset is usually gradual over weeks or months. However, when complications such as fever, profound weakness, or confused behavior prompt the call, life-threatening conditions may follow, requiring emergency care.

ETIOLOGY

The onset of Addison disease is usually gradual, with progressive destruction of the adrenal gland and reduction in its many important hormones. The destruction can result from an autoimmune process, tuberculosis, hemorrhage, fungal infections, *neoplasms,* or surgical removal. There are familial tendencies. The disease also can be secondary to hypopituitarism, in which there is a reduced output of corticotropin.

DIAGNOSIS

Blood and urine cortisol levels are low, as are serum sodium and fasting glucose levels. Serum potassium, blood urea nitrogen, lymphocyte, and eosinophil levels and *hematocrit* are elevated. Adrenal calcification is identified by radiographic film, as is a smaller-than-normal heart.

TREATMENT

Treatment includes replacement of the natural hormones with glucocorticoid and mineralocorticoid drugs, increased fluid intake, control of salt and potassium intake, and a diet high in carbohydrate and protein. Hormone replacement therapy with close medical supervision must continue for life. The patient must be educated about the symptoms of overdosage and underdosage and the role of stress and infection in Addison disease. Insufficiency or a sudden decrease in adrenocortical hormone levels, such as from a sudden withdrawal of glucocorticoid therapy, can result in a life-threatening emergency, called an *addisonian crisis.*

PROGNOSIS

Early diagnosis and strict adherence to the treatment regimen can result in a good prognosis.

PREVENTION

There is no prevention for the onset of the disease. After diagnosis, the individual with adrenal hypofunction requires lifelong steroid replacement.

PATIENT TEACHING

The goal of patient teaching is good compliance to prevent adrenal crisis and to promote general well-being. Refer the patient to a dietitian to ensure adequate nutrient and fluid intake. Give the patient instructions on detecting signs of electrolyte imbalance or adrenal crisis. Give careful instructions on taking medication, and warn the patient not to discontinue medication abruptly. Emphasize the importance of getting follow-up care from the healthcare provider.

Endocrine Dysfunction of Pancreas

—Diabetes Mellitus

DESCRIPTION

Diabetes mellitus is a chronic disorder of carbohydrate, fat, and protein metabolism caused by inadequate production of insulin by the pancreas or faulty utilization of insulin by the cells.

ICD-9-CM Code 250.90

Diabetes mellitus is coded in the fourth digit according to clinical manifestations and with a fifth-digit modifier for non–insulin-dependent or insulin-dependent state. Refer to the physician's diagnosis and then to the current edition of the ICD-9-CM coding manual to ensure the greatest specificity of pathology and any appropriate modifiers.

SYMPTOMS AND SIGNS

The functional pancreas secrets insulin and maintains glucose levels in a precise range. Insulin normally reduces blood glucose levels by transporting glucose into the cells for use as energy and storage as glycogen. A reduction in insulin results in **hyperglycemia** and deprives cells of fuel. Cells begin to metabolize fats and proteins; this process allows wastes called ketone bodies to accumulate in the blood (ketosis). Ketonuria develops as excess ketone bodies are excreted in the urine. This leads to **acidosis.** Hyperglycemia and ketosis then are at the root of the principal symptoms: polyuria, **polyphagia,** polydipsia, weight loss, and fatigue. The patient may have **pruritus,** especially in the genital area, and a fruity odor to the breath may be noted.

Diagnostic tests of the blood and urine point to the common signs of diabetes mellitus.

There are two primary forms of diabetes mellitus:

1. Type 1 (formerly known as "juvenile onset" diabetes or "insulin-dependent diabetes mellitus" [IDDM]) has an early, abrupt onset, usually before 30 years of age, with little or no insulin being secreted by the patient, and can be difficult to control.

2. Type 2 (formerly known as "adult onset" diabetes or "non–insulin-dependent diabetes mellitus" [NIDDM]), the more common form, has a gradual onset in adults older than 30, and more often in people over the age of 55. In this form, some pancreatic function remains, permitting control of symptoms by dietary management; in addition, an oral hypoglycemic medication is necessary in some cases.

Untreated or poorly managed diabetes has many systemic complications. Even with good compliance with treatment, diabetics are prone to retinopathy, which leads to blindness. Other complications include neuropathy, atherosclerosis, renal failure, myocardial infarction, and cerebrovascular accidents. Hyperglycemia delays healing and impairs resistance to infection. Diabetics require careful attention to foot care to prevent the damage that can result from circulatory disorders and infections (Fig. 4–12).

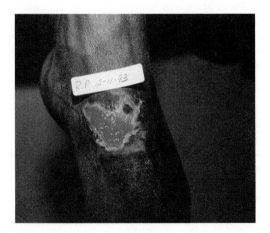

FIGURE 4–12 Diabetic ulcer, dorsal aspect of the foot. (From Hill MJ: *Skin disorders—Mosby's clinical nursing series*, St. Louis, 1994, Mosby.)

PATIENT SCREENING

Individuals known to be at high risk require frequent screening for the signs of diabetes as part of regular medical check-ups. Known diabetics presenting with warning signs of diabetic coma or insulin reaction need instructions for immediate medical intervention (Table 4–3). Anyone complaining of weight loss, excessive thirst, excessive hunger, and frequent urination needs a prompt appointment for diagnostic evaluation.

TABLE 4–3
Warning Signs and Interventions for Diabetic Coma and Insulin Reaction

DIABETIC COMA	INSULIN REACTION
CAUSES	
Undiagnosed diabetes	Excessive insulin
Skipped insulin dose	Delayed meal
Excessive food	Insufficient food
Infection or stress	Excessive exercise
SYMPTOMS AND SIGNS	
Slow onset	Rapid onset
Thirst	Hunger
Increased urination	Trembling and paleness
Nausea and vomiting	Feeling of faintness
Abdominal pain	Cold sweat
Drowsiness	Headache
Lethargy	Anxiety
Flushed appearance	Rapid heartbeat
Dry skin	Irritability
Fruity breath odor	Impaired vision
Dehydration	Hypoglycemia
Heavy respirations	Confusion
Dilated, fixed pupils	Seizures
Hyperglycemia	Loss of consciousness
Ketoacidosis	
Loss of consciousness	
Coma	
INTERVENTION	
Give insulin, fluids, and salt	If awake, give simple sugar, candy, orange juice, or soda
If severe, give intravenous fluids, insulin, and sodium bicarbonate	If unconscious, give intravenous dextrose or glucagon

ETIOLOGY

The disease is often familial but may be acquired. Metabolic abnormalities can induce the diabetic disease process, causing insulin resistance, abnormal insulin secretion by the pancreas, or inappropriate glucose production by the liver. Although diabetes mellitus is an ancient disease, in most cases the cause is unknown. Both forms seem to be linked genetically. In type 1, an infection early in life may trigger an autoimmune process that produces antibodies that destroy the beta cells of the pancreas. Type 2 tends to occur in older, overweight adults. Destruction of the pancreas by tumor, trauma to the pituitary gland, or other endocrine disorders can induce diabetes mellitus. Some drugs also may suppress insulin production. Some genetic disorders render the body's insulin receptors insensitive to insulin.

DIAGNOSIS

The diagnosis of diabetes mellitus is straightforward, beginning with a patient history. The patient is assessed carefully for the cardinal symptoms. At least two positive tests of fasting blood plasma glucose and the presence of glucose and acetone in the urine confirm the diagnosis. Other tests include blood insulin level determination and an ophthalmic examination for diabetic retinopathy.

TREATMENT

The goal of treatment is to normalize blood glucose levels and thus prevent complications. Management of diabetes is multifactorial, including a well-balanced diet closely integrated with insulin administration (if needed), exercise, blood and urine testing, and hygienic measures. Patient compliance and education are vital to the control of symptoms and complications.

Type 1 diabetics may require insulin replacement therapy that correlates closely with calculated caloric intake on a regular schedule and consistent, moderate exercise. Methods of insulin delivery include injection, open-loop infusion pumps, injection ports, and insulin infuser pens. Insulin preparations can be short-acting, intermediate-acting, long-acting, or premixed insulins. Researchers are investigating other insulin delivery methods, including rapid-acting pulmonary insulins and a liquid oral insulin.

Type 2 diabetics usually do not require insulin injections to control blood glucose levels. Their therapeutic regimen includes restricted caloric intake and exercise, although some require oral hypoglycemic medications.

Various forms of oral drug therapy currently are used to treat type 2 diabetes. The sulfonylureas (oral hypoglycemic drugs), such as glipizide (Glucotrol) and glyburide (DiaBeta or Micronase) stimulate the pancreas to produce insulin. These medications are usually taken once a day, and blood glucose levels must be monitored on a strict schedule. Because sulfonylureas stimulate the pancreas to increase insulin production, the increased insulin levels tend to lower blood glucose levels, often resulting in symptoms and complications of hypoglycemia.

Metformin hydrochloride (Glucophage) approaches with a trilateral concept. It prevents the liver from producing hepatic glucose, reduces intestinal absorption of glucose, and increases the utilization of available insulin. Under normal circumstances, metformin hydrochloride does not elevate blood insulin levels and therefore does not produce hypoglycemia.

Acarbose (Precose), an alpha-glucosidase inhibitor, works in the gastrointestinal tract to delay the digestion of carbohydrates and lengthens the time needed to convert carbohydrates to glucose, mainly affecting blood sugar levels after eating. An annoying side effect is the formation of intestinal gas and resulting flatus.

Pioglitazone (Actos) and rosiglitazone maleate (Avandia) of the thiazolidinediones approach the treatment of type 2 diabetes mellitus by increasing the body's sensitivity to insulin. They reduce the cell's resistance to insulin, thereby increasing the cell's usage of available insulin. Avandia also slows the liver's production of glucose (gluconeogenesis). (See the Alert box for special information and warnings about hypoglycemic agents.)

PROGNOSIS

Today people with diabetes mellitus are living longer than they were. When people with diabetes mellitus practice appropriate self-care, the symptoms are eased, blood glucose levels are controlled, and they experience fewer complications and have fewer hospitalizations. Without treatment and when blood sugar levels remain high over a long period, the eyes, blood vessels, kidneys, and nerves sustain serious damage.

PREVENTION

The precise causal mechanism of diabetes mellitus remains unknown; however, screening for diabetes

ALERT
GLUCOPHAGE: INFORMATION AND WARNINGS

Glucophage, an antidiabetic agent, should not be taken by patients with a history of kidney disease, congestive heart failure, liver disease, or alcoholism. Patients should be instructed to stop taking Glucophage before undergoing any imaging procedures with injectable contrast agents. In addition, patients must notify the surgeon of Glucophage use before any surgery so that the surgeon may decide whether to discontinue the medication until after the surgical procedure.

A rare but serious side effect of Glucophage is lactic acidosis. Therefore patients for whom Glucophage is prescribed must be cautioned about symptoms and signs of lactic acidosis and must be warned of certain side effects.

The symptoms and signs of lactic acidosis are weakness, fatigue, unusual muscle pain, dyspnea, unusual stomach discomfort, dizziness or lightheadedness, and bradycardia or cardiac arrhythmias. With any of these symptoms, *stop* the Glucophage immediately and contact the physician.

---

mellitus is recommended for those with risk factors such as genetic susceptibility, obesity, a history of gestational diabetes, and an age of 45 or older.

PATIENT TEACHING
Diabetic control is monitored daily mainly by measuring blood glucose levels through the use of a device for that purpose, and by testing of urine glucose and acetone levels. These monitoring techniques are taught to patients so that they can use them at home. With experience, the patient can interpret the results and make simple modifications in insulin dosage and caloric intake to maintain precise blood glucose control. All diabetic patients are encouraged to reach and maintain appropriate body weight. In addition, patients must be taught that the balance between insulin and glucose requirements is upset easily by trauma and infection. Regular medical supervision is encouraged, especially for insulin-dependent patients. Patient and caregiver are taught the proper techniques of insulin administration. The patient and family members must be educated to recognize the symptoms of diabetic coma (high blood glucose levels) and insulin shock (excessive insulin) and to take immediate action to correct these serious complications (see Table 4–3).

The patient must understand the importance of preventing infection and avoiding injury. Give the patient written material that explains the importance of skin care, foot care, and dental care. Instruct the patient to carry some form of fast-acting sugar, such as hard candy or sugar packets, to combat the onset of hypoglycemia. Advise the patient to obtain a Medic Alert bracelet (see Fig. 4–7). Refer the patient to counseling and support to help him or her adapt to the challenges of long-term disease.

NOTE: A more accurate assessment of overall blood glucose control may be obtained with the glycosylated hemoglobin test (designated Hgb A *1c*). A home test kit is available to diabetic patients. The test is performed every 5 to 6 weeks, and there are no dietary or medication restrictions.

Gestational Diabetes

DESCRIPTION
Gestational diabetes mellitus (GDM), or type 3 diabetes, is a condition of damaged ability to process carbohydrate that has its onset during pregnancy.

 ICD-9-CM Code 648.80 *(Mother)*

SYMPTOMS AND SIGNS
Gestational diabetes is detected between 24 and 28 weeks of gestation. The pregnant patient may be asymptomatic or she may exhibit the usual signs of diabetes mellitus: polyuria, polydipsia, and polyphagia. Routine urine screening, performed during each prenatal visit, indicates the presence of glucose.

ETIOLOGY
Signs indicate that destruction of insulin by the placenta plays a role in causing GDM. Increased maternal insulin production results in increased placental production of human placental lactogen (hPL). This is followed by the reduced effective-

ness of maternal insulin. The fetus takes its glucose from the mother, stressing the balance of glucose production and glucose utilization. Elevated levels of estrogen and progesterone block the action of insulin. Risk factors include a family history of diabetes, obesity, and age over 25 years.

DIAGNOSIS
The first indication of GDM is a routine prenatal urine glucose test demonstrating the presence of glucose in the urine. A fasting blood glucose determination indicates elevated levels of glucose. Other serum tests are glucose tolerance tests, 2-hour *postprandial* (oral glucose tolerance) tests, and glycated hemoglobin tests. Elevations above normal levels yield a positive diagnosis.

TREATMENT
The medical management of GDM is similar to the treatment of any diabetes, with close surveillance of mother and fetus because of the increased risk of complications, control of the diet, and limits on the intake of simple sugars. Consistent moderate exercise, such as walking, is encouraged. Oral hypoglycemic agents may be prescribed, or insulin may be indicated. The patient is instructed to monitor blood glucose levels frequently with finger sticks and glucometer testing. If delivery of the infant and placenta does not terminate the condition, a therapeutic diabetic regimen must continue.

PROGNOSIS
The risk of cesarean delivery and neonatal complications, including large body size and hypoglycemia, is increased. The condition usually disappears within 6 weeks after delivery. Thirty to forty percent of women who have had GDM develop type 2 diabetes within 5 to 10 years of GDM.

PREVENTION
GDM is a common enough complication of pregnancy to warrant regular monitoring of glucose levels in the urine and blood during gestation.

PATIENT TEACHING
Emphasize the importance of regular prenatal check-ups to monitor weight, proper nutrition, and blood and urine glucose levels. This is even more important for women who have a family history of diabetes. Teach self-monitoring of blood glucose and insulin administration as required. Dietary

management depends on the severity of the disease and the amount of insulin therapy required. Make sure the patient has instructional material on the specific prescribed diet, or refer her to a dietitian.

Hypoglycemia

DESCRIPTION
Hypoglycemia is an abnormally low glucose level in the blood.

 ICD-9-CM Code 251.2 *(Unspecified)*

SYMPTOMS AND SIGNS
Hypoglycemia, a deficiency of glucose (sugar) in the blood, can be a serious condition. It occurs when excessive insulin enters the bloodstream or when the glucose release rate falls below tissue demands. This condition may occur despite adequate food intake. The symptoms include sweating, nervousness, weakness, hunger, dizziness, trembling, headache, and palpitations. Because glucose is the primary fuel of the brain, the consequences of hypoglycemia can be severe. Extremely low blood glucose levels can cause central nervous system manifestations, including confusion, visual disturbances, behavior that may be mistaken for drunkenness, stupor, coma, and seizures. Hypoglycemic syndromes are classified as drug induced (the most common) or non–drug induced.

PATIENT SCREENING
An individual with severe symptoms of acute reactive hypoglycemia requires emergency medical attention. The individual experiencing milder episodes of hypoglycemia should be scheduled as early as possible for a diagnostic evaluation of the cause. Follow office policy for referral of an infant or child to a pediatrician.

ETIOLOGY
The major cause of drug-induced hypoglycemia (or reactive hypoglycemia) is insulin overdosage in a diabetic subject. Failure to eat a meal or excessive exercise also can trigger hypoglycemia in the insulin-dependent diabetic. A person with a significantly elevated blood alcohol level can experience alcoholic hypoglycemia. *Sulfonylureas* can induce hypoglycemia. Non–drug-induced hypoglycemia can result from fasting, delayed or excessive secretion of insulin by the pancreas,

adenoma or carcinoma of the pancreas, gastrointestinal disorders, or various hereditary or endocrine disorders.

DIAGNOSIS

The diagnosis requires evidence that the symptoms correlate with a low blood glucose level and are remedied by raising the blood glucose level. The glucometer, or a blood reagent strip, can be used as a quick screening test for abnormally low blood glucose levels in patients with symptoms of hypoglycemia. The blood glucose level is further evaluated through a glucose tolerance test. An abnormally low plasma glucose level usually is defined as less than 40 mg/dl in men and less than 45 mg/dl in women after a period of fasting. The diagnosis is uncomplicated when the initial assessment suggests a probable cause, such as a history of insulin use, excessive ingestion of alcohol, and the use of sulfonylureas in treatment.

TREATMENT

In acute hypoglycemia, the priority is to restore a normal blood glucose level through intravenous infusion of glucose. The hormone glucagon also may be given to counteract the effects of insulin. As the patient's condition is stabilized, a complex-carbohydrate and protein snack is given to keep the blood glucose level within normal limits. Hypoglycemia associated with tumors may require surgery. The diet is modified to correct hereditary fructose intolerance or gastrointestinal conditions that provoke symptoms.

PROGNOSIS

The underlying cause of hypoglycemia dictates the long-term management of the disorder. In most cases the signs and symptoms of hypoglycemia resolve with the ingestion of food or glucose to increase the glucose level in the blood.

PREVENTION

The most common cause of episodic hypoglycemia is prevented by the proper adjustment of diet, insulin, and exercise in the diabetic individual.

PATIENT TEACHING

Teach the patient to watch for the signs of hypoglycemia. Instruct the insulin-dependent diabetic always to be prepared to counter an attack of hypoglycemia by carrying glucose tablets to take at the first sign of hypoglycemia. Address the effects

of alcohol intoxication and adverse reactions to medication on hypoglycemia, as appropriate. Refer the patient to a dietitian as indicated.

Precocious Puberty

Precocious Puberty in Boys

DESCRIPTION

Precocious puberty in boys is defined as the onset of puberty before the age of nine.

 ICD-9-CM Code 259.1 *(Precocious sexual development and puberty not elsewhere classified)*

SYMPTOMS AND SIGNS

Precocious, or earlier than expected, sexual maturity in the male is manifested by early development of secondary sex characteristics, gonadal development, and spermatogenesis. The patient's history may include altered growth pattern or emotional disturbances. Pubic hair and the beard begin to grow, the gonads and the penis increase in size, and sebaceous gland activity increases. Male puberty normally begins between 13 and 15 years; an onset before 9 years of age is considered precocious.

PATIENT SCREENING

Schedule a physical examination with the health-care provider. Then follow office policy regarding referral to an endocrinologist.

ETIOLOGY

Idiopathic precocity may be transmitted genetically. The hypothalamus normally initiates puberty by stimulating the pituitary gland. Because the pituitary gland secretes vital gonadotropic hormones that stimulate the testes to produce sex hormones, many problems involving sexual development can be traced to pituitary dysfunction. Intracranial pituitary or hypothalamic neoplasia can cause excessive or premature secretion of gonadotropin. Testicular tumors and other endocrine disorders can induce precocious development. The history may reveal inadvertent ingestion of sex steroids through therapeutic medications or deliberate ingestion of sex steroids.

DIAGNOSIS

Obvious physical and emotional signs of precocity are noted. Diagnostic tests include MRI, blood tests for elevated hormone levels, brain scans, electroencephalographic (EEG) studies, skull and bone radiographic studies, chromosomal *karyotype* studies, and testing of a 24-hour urine specimen for steroid excretion levels.

TREATMENT

The therapy depends on the cause of precocious puberty. When the boy's condition is idiopathic, no specific treatment may be needed. Taking hormones known as progestogens may suppress sexual maturation until the appropriate time for the onset of puberty. When the cause is testicular tumor or brain tumor, the treatment is more invasive, and the prognosis is guarded. Other endocrine disorders may require lifelong hormone therapy.

PROGNOSIS

Early diagnosis and treatment of true precocious puberty offers a positive outcome. More complicated cases have a guarded prognosis.

PREVENTION

In almost all cases no prevention is known.

PATIENT TEACHING

Emphasize the importance of following the exact medication regimen and keeping follow-up appointments. Refer the patient to genetic counseling and psychological support as indicated by the treatment plan.

Precocious Puberty in Girls

DESCRIPTION

Precocious puberty in girls is defined as the onset of puberty before the age of eight.

■ ICD-9-CM Code **259.1** *(Precocious sexual development and puberty not elsewhere classified)*

SYMPTOMS AND SIGNS

Precocious, or earlier than expected, sexual maturity in the female is marked by increased growth rate, breast enlargement, and the appearance of pubic hair and underarm hair before 8 years of age; the onset of menstruation (menarche) may oc-

cur before 10 years of age. Ovarian function makes pregnancy a possibility. Emotional problems may occur.

PATIENT SCREENING

Schedule a physical examination with the healthcare provider. Then follow office policy about a referral to an endocrinologist.

ETIOLOGY

In most cases, precocious puberty in girls is idiopathic, without associated abnormalities. Uncommon causes include intracranial tumors, encephalopathy, *meningitis,* and endocrine disorders. The ingestion of oral contraceptives, other estrogen-containing drugs, or meat with high estrogen content is a rare cause. Hormone-secreting ovarian or adrenal neoplasms infrequently are causes.

DIAGNOSIS

Blood serum levels of follicle-stimulating hormone (FSH), luteinizing hormone (LH), and sex steroids are in the normal adult range. Urinalysis of hormone levels and excretion of 17-ketosteroids shows elevated levels. RIA for both FSH and LH demonstrates elevated concentrations of the hormones in blood plasma. Other diagnostic studies to determine the cause include ultrasonography, electroencephalography, CT, and MRI.

TREATMENT

As in male precocity, the treatment of precocious female puberty depends on the cause. Tumors, if treatable, may require surgery or radiation. Hormone therapy may be used to suppress the secretion of gonadotropins and to prevent menstruation in true precocious female puberty. The girl and her family may benefit from mental health counseling to develop coping skills for handling emotional problems. Parents must understand that physical maturity may occur with psychological immaturity, and that precocious puberty does not necessarily trigger sexual behavior.

PROGNOSIS

The outcome depends on the early diagnosis and treatment of true precocious puberty; certain causes prompt a more guarded prognosis.

PREVENTION

In almost all cases, no prevention is known.

PATIENT TEACHING

Emphasize the importance of following the exact medication regimen and keeping follow-up appointments. Refer the patient to genetic counseling and psychological support as indicated by the treatment plan.

REVIEW CHALLENGE

Answer the following questions:

1. Name the major glands of the endocrine system.
2. What are some ways in which the endocrine system affects health and disease?
3. Describe two conditions that are the result of increased production and secretion of pituitary human growth hormone (hGH).
4. What pathologic changes may result from hypopituitarism? Why is the age of the individual significant?
5. What causes diabetes insipidus?
6. What causes the thyroid gland to enlarge in the patient with a simple goiter?
7. Which hypothyroid condition (or chronic thyroiditis) is thought to be caused by autoimmune factors?
8. Describe the signs and symptoms of Graves' disease.
9. Explain the relationship of hypoparathyroidism to hypocalcemia.
10. What disease may be induced by prolonged administration or large doses of corticosteroids?
11. What are the possible causes of Addison disease?
12. Compare the cause and treatment of type 1 and type 2 diabetes mellitus.
13. Distinguish between diabetic coma and insulin shock.
14. How are hypoglycemic syndromes classified?
15. Name the important prognostic factors for thyroid malignancy.
16. What are the possible causes of precocious puberty in boys and girls?

REAL-LIFE CHALLENGE

Hypothyroidism

A 40-year-old female reports tiredness, loss of hair, and weight gain. She has not had a menstrual period for 3 months. Her skin appears dry and scaly. On questioning, the patient reports episodes of constipation and tells of being unable to tolerate cold. Her speech is somewhat slow and slurred. A blood test for thyroid functioning shows low thyrotropin levels. Thyroid scan shows no uptake of thyrotropin. The diagnosis of this patient is hypothyroidism.

QUESTIONS

1. Hypothyroidism with onset at maturity is often called *myxedema*. What is the term describing hypothyroidism with onset in infancy or early childhood?
2. What causes the insidious onset of the various complaints and conditions of the patient with hypothyroidism?
3. What can be the cause of the reduced production of T_4 by the thyroid gland?
4. Hormone replacement is the usual drug therapy of choice. Research levothyroxine sodium (Synthroid) and explain its side effects.
5. For patient teaching, how long will the patient be instructed to take the medication?

REAL-LIFE CHALLENGE

Diabetes Mellitus

A 50-year-old man became lethargic and drowsy with flushed dry skin after eating a large meal. His family became concerned when he was difficult to rouse, and he had a fruity odor to his breath. He was transported to an emergency facility, where he gave a history of extreme thirst, hunger, and frequent urination. He recently had an upper-respiratory infection that was slow to clear. Adult-onset diabetes mellitus is suspected.

QUESTIONS

1. Which blood test would be ordered?
2. What are normal blood glucose levels?
3. What are some of the possible causes of adult-onset type 2 diabetes mellitus?
4. In addition to the symptoms previously described, what else might be observed?
5. What determines the course of the treatment prescribed?
6. Why is glucose-level monitoring important?
7. What patient teaching should be considered?
8. Why is diet important?
9. Explain how insulin works.
10. What is the therapeutic action of the sulfonylureas?
11. How does metformin hydrochloride (Glucophage) reduce blood glucose levels?

INTERNET ASSIGNMENTS

1. Choose a related topic (an endocrine disorder) from the National Institute of Diabetes and research the latest health information on that topic. Review the easy-to-read and/or Spanish language options.

2. Visit the American Thyroid Association website and report on a recent public health statement related to the treatment of thyroid disease.

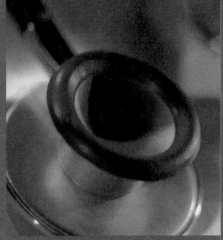

Diseases and Disorders of the Eye and Ear

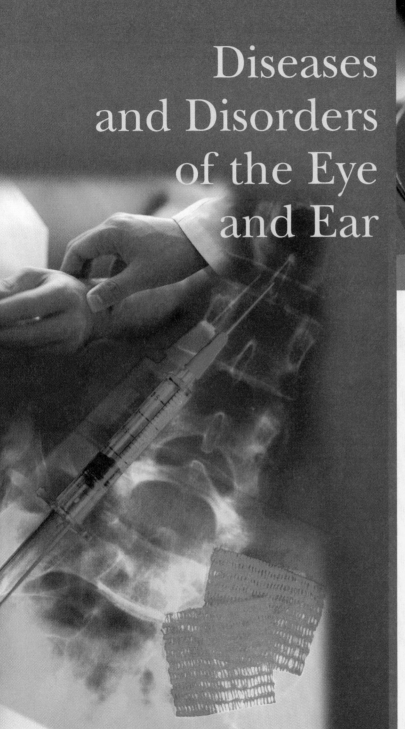

DISORDERS OF THE EYE, *179*
FUNCTIONING ORGANS
  OF VISION, *179*
REFRACTIVE ERRORS, *182*
  Hyperopia (Farsightedness), *182*
  Myopia (Nearsightedness), *182*
  Astigmatism, *183*
  Presbyopia, *183*
NYSTAGMUS, *185*
STRABISMUS, *185*
DISORDERS OF THE EYELID, *187*
  Hordeolum (Stye), *187*
  Chalazion, *187*
  Keratitis, *188*
  Blepharitis, *189*
  Entropion, *190*
  Ectropion, *190*
  Blepharoptosis, *191*
  Conjunctivitis, *192*
DISORDERS OF THE GLOBE
  OF THE EYE, *193*
  Corneal Abrasion or Ulcer, *193*
  Scleritis, *194*
  Cataract, *194*
  Glaucoma, *195*
  Macular Degeneration, *197*
  Diabetic Retinopathy, *198*
  Retinal Detachment, *199*
  Uveitis, *200*
  Exophthalmos, *201*

Continued

Chapter Outline—Cont'd

Learning Objectives

After studying Chapter 5, you should be able to:

1. Describe the processes of vision and hearing.
2. Recall and define the four main refractive errors of vision.
3. Compare the pathology and etiology of nystagmus with that of strabismus.
4. Explain the importance of early treatment of glaucoma.
5. Name the possible causes of conjunctivitis.
6. List the causes of cataracts.
7. Explain the susceptibility of diabetics to diabetic retinopathy.
8. Characterize the visual disturbance caused by macular degeneration.
9. Explain why early diagnosis and treatment is important in retinal detachment.
10. Compare conductive hearing loss with sensorineural hearing loss.
11. List the symptoms of otitis externa.
12. Describe the treatment of otitis media.
13. Explain the signs and symptoms of Ménière disease.
14. Discuss the importance of preventing sensorineural hearing loss.

Key Terms

amblyopia (**am**–blee–**OH**–pee–ah)
blepharitis (**blef**–ar–**RIE**–tis)
cryotherapy (kry–o–**THER**–ah–pee)
diplopia (dih–**PLO**–pee–ah)
iridotomy (ir–ih–**DOT**–oh–me)
labyrinth (**LAB**–ih–rinth)
macula (**MACK**–you–la)
meibomian (my–**BO**–mee–an)
myringotomy (mir–in–**GOT**–oh–me)

otoscopy (oh–**TOSS**–ko–pee)
retinopathy (ret–ih–**NOP**–ah–thee)
seborrhea (seb–oh–**RHEE**–ah)
sensorineural (**sen**–so–ree–**NEU**–rol)
tinnitus (tih–**NIE**–tus)
tonometry (tohn–**AHM**–eh–tree)
tympanoplasty (**tim**–pan–oh–**PLAS**–tee)
vertigo (**VER**–tih–go)

DISORDERS OF THE EYE

FUNCTIONING ORGANS OF VISION

MAJOR ORGANS OF SPECIAL senses include the eye and the ear. The functional process of vision takes place in the presence of light in the following manner: (1) an image is formed on the retina; (2) the rods and cones are stimulated; and (3) nerve impulses are conducted to the brain. The area of the brain that involves the sense of sight is much larger than the areas involved with the other senses. Before discussing the pathophysiology of ocular disease, a review of the complex structure of the eye is in order (Fig. 5–1).

The eyeball, similar in shape to a sphere, is composed of a wall of primary structures in three concentric layers—the sclera, the choroid, and the retina—and is connected to the brain by way of the optic nerve.

The sclera, the outermost layer, consists of tough fibrous connective tissue that is visible as the white of the eye. Attached to the sclera are the extrinsic muscles that move the eye (Table 5–1). The cornea, the colorless transparent structure on the front of the eye, is continuous with the sclera on the anterior aspect of the globe. This transparent structure, the window of the eye, helps focus the light rays as they enter the eye.

Next to the sclera is the middle layer of tissue called the *choroid*. The choroid has dark pigment cells that function to absorb excess light rays that interfere with vision. This layer is continuous with the ciliary body and the iris. These vascular structures supply the tissues of the eye with oxygen and nutrients. Anteriorly, the choroid joins the ciliary body, which contains ciliary muscles used to focus the lens of the eye. The ciliary processes in the ciliary body secrete aqueous humor, the fluid found in the anterior portion of the eye. The ciliary body is connected by suspensory ligaments to the biconvex, transparent lens of the eye. Contraction of the ciliary muscles causes the suspensory ligaments to relax. The lens then bulges, allowing the focusing that is necessary for close vision.

Also attached to the ciliary body is the iris, or colored portion of the eye, which helps regulate the amount of light entering the eye. In a brightly lit environment, the iris contracts, causing the opening in the center of the iris, the pupil, to become smaller. In limited light conditions, the iris relaxes and the pupil enlarges, permitting more light to enter the eye.

The innermost layer, covering the posterior three quarters of the eye, is called the *retina*. The retina is a light-sensitive layer made up of sensor-receptive cells called *rods and cones*. The rods function best in dim light, thereby enabling night vision, whereas the cones function in bright light and also detect color and fine detail. Within the rods and cones, the image initiates a chemical reaction and sends a message through the nerve fiber layer of the retina to the optic nerve. The optic nerve penetrates the fibrous layers at the optic disk and continues on to the brain. The optic disk contains no receptor cells and often is called the "blind spot" of the eye. The optic nerve transmits the image to the portion of the brain that is used for vision. The brain interprets the impulses from each eye and produces a single three-dimensional image. The **macula** lutea, a yellow spot, lies lateral to the optic disk. In the center of the macula lutea is the fovea centralis, the area that produces the sharpest image.

Covering the anterior externally visible portion of the sclera is a thin transparent membrane called the *conjunctiva*. It begins at the edge of the cornea, extends over the exposed sclera, and folds anteriorly to line the inside portion of the lids. This creates both a superior cul-de-sac and an inferior cul-de-sac where the conjunctiva reflects from the sclerae to the lids. The space between the iris, the colored portion of the eye, and the anterior clear cornea is called the *anterior chamber*. The fluid occupying both the anterior and posterior chambers is a watery substance called the *aqueous humor*, which is produced by the ciliary body and the fluid exits the anterior chamber through a drainage system located at the junction of the base of the iris and the cornea. Appropriate pressure within the eye is maintained by the aqueous humor, which ultimately enters the general circulation of the body. The large cavity behind the lens is the vitreous body; it contains a jelly-like fluid called the *vitreous humor*, which helps maintain the globular shape of the eyeball and facilitates the refraction of images.

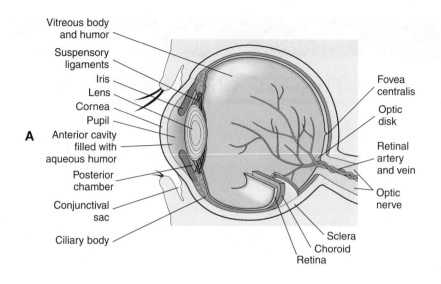

A

- Vitreous body and humor
- Suspensory ligaments
- Iris
- Lens
- Cornea
- Pupil
- Anterior cavity filled with aqueous humor
- Posterior chamber
- Conjunctival sac
- Ciliary body
- Fovea centralis
- Optic disk
- Retinal artery and vein
- Optic nerve
- Sclera
- Choroid
- Retina

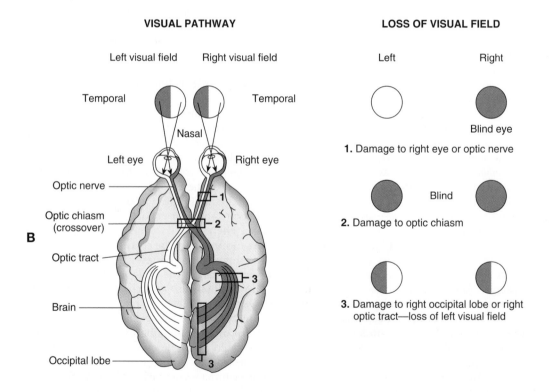

VISUAL PATHWAY

Left visual field   Right visual field

Temporal   Temporal

Nasal

Left eye   Right eye

- Optic nerve — 1
- Optic chiasm (crossover) — 2
- Optic tract

B

- Brain
- Occipital lobe — 3

LOSS OF VISUAL FIELD

Left   Right

Blind eye

1. Damage to right eye or optic nerve

Blind

2. Damage to optic chiasm

3. Damage to right occipital lobe or right optic tract—loss of left visual field

FIGURE 5–1 **A,** Normal eye. **B,** The visual pathway. (**B** from Gould B: *Pathophysiology for the health professions,* ed 2, Philadelphia, 2002, Saunders.)

TABLE 5–1
The Extrinsic Muscles of the Eye

MUSCLE	FUNCTION	CRANIAL INNERVATION
Inferior rectus	Rotates eyeball downward and medially; adducts	Oculomotor nerve (III)
Lateral rectus	Rotates eye laterally; abducts eyeball	Abducens nerve (VI)
Medial rectus	Rotates eye medially; adducts eyeball	Oculomotor nerve (III)
Superior rectus	Causes eye to look up	Oculomotor nerve (III)
Inferior oblique	Rotates eyeball upward and outward; abducts	Oculomotor nerve (III)
Superior oblique	Rotates eyeball downward and outward; abducts	Trochlear nerve (IV)

The internal lens of the eye is elastic and therefore can focus images whether viewed close by or at a distance. The focusing is accomplished by contraction and relaxation of the muscles of the ciliary body. This action makes it possible for the lens to assume either a more rounded spherical shape or a flatter elongated shape, depending on the focus required. The lens is attached to the ciliary body by small strands of tissue called *zonules*. These are attached at points all the way around the lens. When the ciliary body relaxes, the zonules are pulled, causing a flattening of the lens, the configuration needed for focusing on a distant image.

Light rays are the key to sight. The light rays enter the eye and pass through the cornea, aqueous humor, lens, and finally the vitreous humor. These rays can travel in a straight line or be bent at an angle. The process of bending lights rays is known as *refraction*. The cornea, aqueous humor, lens, and vitreous humor are all capable of bending or refracting the light rays so that they can be focused on the retina. The image that forms on the retina is backward and upside down. The image is turned right side up and forward in the brain as the brain interprets the visual concept. Another step in the process of vision involves accommodation. Adjustments must be made in the eye to facilitate focusing or "sharpening" of the image in relation to the viewer's distance from the object. The process of accommodation involves changing the shape of the lens, making it either flat or bulb shaped. The ciliary muscle and the suspensory ligaments contract and relax in opposition to accomplish this task.

Each eye has six extrinsic muscles that control the movements of the eye; these muscles pull on the eyeballs, making the two move together to converge on one visual field (see Table 5–1). Normally, the eyes work together in unison, so an assessment of the functioning of these muscles often is included in a neurologic assessment. Table 5–2 summarizes the functions of the major parts of the eye.

Some eye disorders are signs of systemic diseases, such as hypertension, diabetes mellitus, or certain autoimmune arthritic diseases. Common symptoms of eye diseases and conditions that should be called to the attention of the physician include the following:

- Redness of the eye
- Pain, itching, or burning in or around the eye
- Swollen red eyelids
- Drainage from the eyes
- Lesions/sores in or around the eyes
- Visual disturbances
- Unequal pupils, sudden loss of vision, persistent pain or other symptoms associated with eye injury
- Repetitive, involuntary movements of the eye
  Diagnostic tests for eye diseases and conditions include the following:
- Eye charts, such as the Snellen chart, to measure visual acuity
- Visual field tests to check central and peripheral vision
- **Tonometry** to indirectly measure intraocular pressure
- Eye cultures to identify viral or bacterial infectious agents
- Electronystagmography (ENG) to measure the direction and degree of nystagmus
- Electroretinography to measure electric activity of the retina in response to flashing of light

TABLE 5–2
Functions of the Major Parts of the Eye

STRUCTURE	FUNCTION
Sclera	External protection
Cornea	Light refraction
Choroid	Blood supply
Iris	Light absorption and regulation of pupillary width
Ciliary body	Secretion of vitreous fluid; in addition, its smooth muscles change the shape of the lens
Lens	Light refraction
Retinal layer	Light receptor that transforms optic signals into nerve impulses
Rods	Means of distinguishing light from dark, and perceiving shape and movement
Cones	Color vision
Central fovea	Area of sharpest vision
Macula lutea	Blind spot
External ocular muscles	Movement of the globe
Optic nerve (cranial nerve II)	Transmission of visual information to the brain
Lacrimal glands	Secretion of tears
Eyelid	Eye protection

From Damjanov I: *Pathology for the health-related professions,* ed 2, Philadelphia, 2000, Saunders.

Refractive Errors

Refractive errors that result in the eye being unable to focus light effectively on the retina are identified as hyperopia, myopia, astigmatism, and presbyopia.

Hyperopia (Farsightedness)

DESCRIPTION
Hyperopia (farsightedness) occurs when light that enters the eye is focused behind the retina rather than on the retina, which requires refocusing by the internal lens or the use of an external corrective lens to reposition the viewed object on the retina to sharpen the image. With this condition, near vision is impaired whereas distance vision is usually clear. Hyperopia occurs when the eyeball is abnormally short as measured from front to back (Fig. 5–2).

■ ICD-9-CM Code **367.0**

Myopia (Nearsightedness)

DESCRIPTION
Myopia (nearsightedness) is the result of light rays entering the eye being focused in front of the retina, causing vision to be blurred. Near objects can be seen clearly, but distant objects are blurry, and the image being viewed cannot be sharpened by the internal lens of the eye. Myopia occurs when the eyeball is abnormally long as measured from front to back (Fig. 5–3).

■ ICD-9-CM Code **367.1**

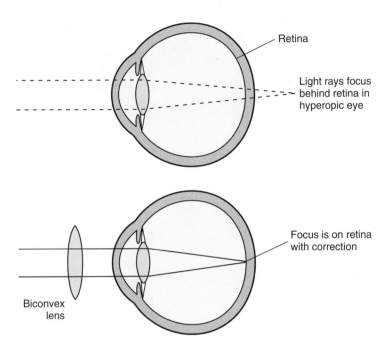

Retina

Light rays focus
behind retina in
hyperopic eye

Focus is on retina
with correction

Biconvex
lens

FIGURE 5–2 Hyperopia and correction.

Astigmatism

DESCRIPTION

Astigmatism is an irregular focusing of the light rays entering the eye. It usually is caused by the cornea not being spherical. The front of the cornea may be more egg shaped than spherical, thereby causing light rays to be unevenly or diffusely focused across the retina. This causes some images to appear clearly defined, whereas others appear blurred.

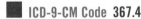 **ICD-9-CM Code 367.20** *(Unspecified)*
Refer to the physician's diagnosis and then to the current edition of the ICD-9-CM coding manual to ensure the greatest specificity of pathology and any appropriate modifiers.

Presbyopia

DESCRIPTION

Presbyopia is the inability of the internal lens of the eye to focus and then refocus quickly to accommo-
date variations in distance because of a gradual loss of muscle elasticity, which generally is the result of aging. This condition usually occurs in people in their mid-40s.

■ **ICD-9-CM Code 367.4**

SYMPTOMS AND SIGNS

The primary symptoms of a refractive error are blurred vision and eye fatigue, which can lead to squinting, frequent rubbing of the eyes, and headaches.

PATIENT SCREENING

Schedule a comprehensive optometric examination for a patient complaining of changes in visual acuity or clearness or sharpness of visual perception.

ETIOLOGY

Some refractive errors seem to be familial, which suggests a genetic link.

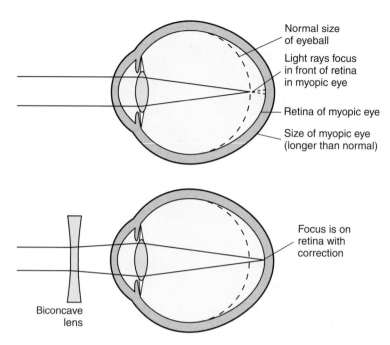

Normal size
of eyeball

Light rays focus
in front of retina
in myopic eye

Retina of myopic eye

Size of myopic eye
(longer than normal)

Focus is on
retina with
correction

Biconcave
lens

FIGURE 5–3 Myopia and correction.

DIAGNOSIS

Eye health history, tests for visual acuity, *ophthalmoscopic* examination, and evaluation of visual deficit are used to diagnoses refractive errors. Usually the pupils are dilated with eyedrops and the eyes are then evaluated for refractive error with a retinoscope. The optimal lens adjustment needed to correct the deficit is determined by having the patient look through a series of corrective lenses of different powers.

TREATMENT

Correcting refractive errors involves fitting the patient with artificial lenses in the form of eyeglasses or contact lenses or performing corrective surgery. Radial keratotomy, a surgical procedure used to reshape the eye, has been replaced by laser surgery, which results in more precise visual correction and has fewer complications. The following refractive surgical procedures can be done to correct myopia, hyperopia, and astigmatism: LASIK (a laser surgical procedure), PRK (photo refractive keratotomy), and intraocular contact lenses (lens permanently placed in the eye). Laser surgery can not improve presbyopia.

PROGNOSIS

Excellent results can be expected with correctly prescribed eyeglasses or contact lenses. Elective refractive surgical procedures can benefit those individuals who are medically eligible. The risks for complications are generally low.

PREVENTION

Refractive errors cannot be prevented.

PATIENT TEACHING

When a patient is to have refractive surgery, describe the procedure and advise the patient as to when to expect visual recovery, how to use preoperative and postoperative medications, and when return to a regular work schedule is likely. Explain the importance of follow-up visits to monitor progress.

Nystagmus

DESCRIPTION

Nystagmus (also called *nystaxis*) is involuntary, repetitive, rhythmic movements of one or both eyes.

ICD-9-CM Code 379.50 *(Unspecified)*
Refer to the physician's diagnosis and then to the current edition of the ICD-9-CM coding manual to ensure the greatest specificity of pathology and any appropriate modifiers.

SYMPTOMS AND SIGNS

Any repetitive or involuntary movement of one or both eyes is a sign of nystagmus. The eye movements can be horizontal, vertical, or circular, or a combination of these. Blurred or decreased vision also can be associated with nystagmus.

PATIENT SCREENING

Schedule a comprehensive optometric examination for a patient complaining of changes in visual acuity or of any involuntary or "jerky" movements of the eye. *Acquired nystagmus always necessitates a complete neurologic evaluation.*

ETIOLOGY

Brain tumors and cerebrovascular lesions can cause nystagmus. Acquired nystagmus results when a disease process produces lesions in the brain or inner ear. Alcohol use and abuse of certain drugs also may cause this condition. Congenital nystagmus is manifested before 6 months to 1 year of age and is the most common type. Nystagmus is not necessarily associated with brain lesions and may instead be the result of abnormal development of the retina.

DIAGNOSIS

Nystagmus usually can be diagnosed clinically by external examination of the eyes and observa-

tion of any involuntary movements. Other, more specific, complex tests are available as well when needed for definitive diagnosis.

TREATMENT

Acquired nystagmus is managed by treating the underlying cause of the condition. Congenital nystagmus often can be lessened by using the Kestenbaum procedure in which the eyes are surgically rotated towards the null point of the eye.

PROGNOSIS

The outcome of acquired nystagmus depends on the treatment of the underlying cause. Surgical intervention for congenital nystagmus attempts to minimize nystagmus when the eyes are looking straight ahead.

PREVENTION

No specific method of prevention is known.

PATIENT TEACHING

In acquired nystagmus the patient benefits from understanding the underlying cause and treatment of the nystagmus. Parents of the child with congenital nystagmus are given support and clear explanations about the condition and the surgical treatment, if indicated.

Strabismus

DESCRIPTION

Strabismus is failure of the eyes to look in the same direction at the same time, which primarily occurs because of weakness in the nerves stimulating the muscles controlling the position of the eyes (Fig. 5–4).

ICD-9-CM Code 378.9
Refer to the physician's diagnosis and then to the current edition of the ICD-9-CM coding manual to ensure the greatest specificity of pathology and any appropriate modifiers.

SYMPTOMS AND SIGNS

In esotropia (convergent strabismus, or cross-eye), both eyes turns inward; in exotropia (divergent strabismus, or wall-eye), both eyes turn outward.

Strabismus

With either form, the main symptom is **diplopia** if strabismus is acquired as an adult. Diplopia is usually not present when the strabismus is congenital.

PATIENT SCREENING

Schedule a comprehensive optometric examination for a patient complaining of changes in visual acuity, clearness or sharpness of visual perception, or double vision. Parents may report the noted appearance of "crossed eyes" in an infant or young child.

ETIOLOGY

Esotropia usually develops in infancy or early childhood and may be associated with **amblyopia.** Amblyopia is reversible until the retina is fully developed at about 8 years of age. In almost all cases, esotropia that develops in adults is caused by a condition or disease elsewhere in the body. Either the nerves between the brain and the eye muscles or the muscles themselves are affected. These diseases and conditions include diabetes mellitus, temporal arteritis, muscular dystrophy, high blood pressure, trauma, aneurysm, or an intracranial lesion.

DIAGNOSIS

To discover the underlying cause, the physician performs a complete ophthalmic examination and orders various appropriate radiographic studies and blood and urine tests.

TREATMENT

Strabismus should be treated as soon as possible. Early intervention is the key. Corrective glasses, amblyopia treatment, or surgery to restore the eye muscle balance may be used in the course of the treatment.

PROGNOSIS

In most cases children respond well to early treatment. Adults with acquired strabismus have a guarded prognosis depending on the underlying cause.

PREVENTION

No specific method of prevention is known.

PATIENT TEACHING

Give parents of children with strabismus an explanation of the condition and the cause if known. Reinforce the importance of early treatment to help prevent visual loss. The adult with acquired strabismus can benefit from an explanation of the relationship of the eye condition to the identified underlying cause.

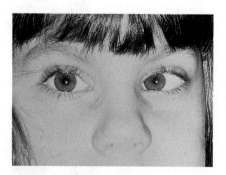

FIGURE 5–4 Strabismus. (From Zitelli BJ, Davis HW: *Atlas of pediatric physical diagnosis,* ed 4, St. Louis, 2002, Mosby.)

Disorders of the Eyelid

Hordeolum (Stye)

DESCRIPTION
Hordeolum (styes) are inflammatory infections of the hair follicles or sebaceous glands of the eyelids (Fig. 5–5).

■ **ICD-9-CM Code** **373.11** *(Hordeolum externum)*
373.12 *(Hordeolum internum)*
373.13 *(Abscess of the eyelid)*

SYMPTOMS AND SIGNS
Styes occur most often at the outside edge of the lid. Pain, swelling, redness, and the formation of pus at the site are the main symptoms of a stye. Patients may report a feeling of having "something in the eye."

PATIENT SCREENING
Patients complaining of a lesion of the eyelid, with or without purulent drainage, require an appointment with their health care provider for a visual examination of the affected area. Follow office policy for referral to an ophthalmologist.

ETIOLOGY
Often styes are the result of a staphylococcal infection and can be associated with and secondary to **blepharitis** (see Blepharitis).

DIAGNOSIS
Visual examination alone is usually sufficient for making the diagnosis. A culture may be taken to confirm that the infection is caused by staphylococci; however, this is usually not necessary.

TREATMENT
To hasten relief of pain, hot compresses may be applied to the eye as soon as the inflammation is evident. If recurrence becomes a problem, topical or systemic antibiotics may be needed.

PROGNOSIS
The prognosis is good but recurrence is common.

PREVENTION
No specific method of prevention is known.

PATIENT TEACHING
Instruct the patient regarding the correct technique of applying an eye compress as prescribed. Inform the patient concerning the correct application and usage of topical or systemic antibiotic therapies.

Chalazion

DESCRIPTION
A chalazion is a small, painless, localized swelling on the margin or body of the eyelid; it occurs with occlusion of the **meibomian** glands (Fig. 5–6).

■ **ICD-9-CM Code** **373.2**

SYMPTOMS AND SIGNS
A chalazion can vary in size from being barely visible to being the size of a pea. Chalazions can become infected, producing redness, swelling, and pain.

PATIENT SCREENING
A brief visual examination is scheduled for diagnosis of a lesion of the eyelid. Follow office policy for referral to an ophthalmologist.

ETIOLOGY
Chalazions are caused by a blockage of fluid originating from one of the meibomian glands, which lubricate the eyelid margin.

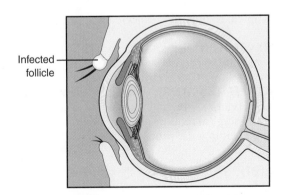

Infected follicle

FIGURE 5–5 Hordeolum (stye).

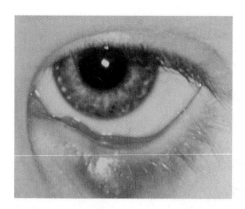

FIGURE 5–6 Chalazion. (From Zitelli BJ, Davis HW: *Atlas of pediatric physical diagnosis,* ed 4, St. Louis, 2002, Mosby.)

DIAGNOSIS
Visual examination and patient history are all that is necessary to make the diagnosis.

TREATMENT
Small chalazions usually disappear spontaneously over a month or two. Resolution may be facilitated by antibiotic treatment. Larger pea-sized chalazions do not spontaneously disappear and need to be removed surgically. This is a minor procedure that often can be done in the ophthalmologist's office or in an outpatient setting.

PROGNOSIS
Complete resolution is expected.

PREVENTION
No method of prevention is known.

PATIENT TEACHING
The patient may be told a chalazion is not malignant. If surgical removal is recommended, reassure the patient that the procedure is minor.

Keratitis

DESCRIPTION
Keratitis is any inflammation that causes superficial ulceration of the cornea.

ICD-9-CM Code 370
Keratitis has many forms and therefore many ICD-9-CM codes. Refer to the physician's diagnosis and then to the current edition of the ICD-9-CM coding manual to ensure the greatest specificity of pathology and any appropriate modifiers.

SYMPTOMS AND SIGNS
Symptoms are decreased visual acuity, irritation, tearing, *photophobia,* and mild redness of the conjunctiva. Pain or numbness of the cornea may soon follow and is a significant sign.

PATIENT SCREENING
The patient experiencing the symptoms listed above is scheduled for a prompt ophthalmic examination. Follow office policy for referral to an ophthalmologist.

ETIOLOGY
Keratitis often is caused by an infection resulting from the herpes simplex virus. This is especially likely when the keratitis is preceded by an upper respiratory infection (URI) with facial cold sores (see Herpes Simplex [Cold Sores] in Chapter 8). Certain bacteria and fungi also can be responsible for keratitis. Other forms of keratitis can be caused by corneal trauma, contact lens wear, or exposure of the cornea to dry air or intense light, as occurs during welding. Cultures may be taken to identify the causative organism.

DIAGNOSIS
Examination of the cornea using a slit lamp confirms the diagnosis. Medical history may indicate a recent URI, and visual acuity may be decreased.

TREATMENT
Ophthalmic ointments and eyedrops may be prescribed, and the administration of a broad-spectrum antibiotic can effectively eradicate the infection. An eye patch may be needed to relieve discomfort caused by photophobia. However, this is contraindicated in cases of fungal infection or contact lens wear.

PROGNOSIS
Prompt treatment of the condition decreases the risk of ulceration that can erode the cornea and cause formation of scar tissue that may interfere with vision.

PREVENTION

Following the recommended instructions for contact lens wear and care, such as proper handling and cleaning of the lenses, can reduce the risk of infection. Avoiding hand to eye contact can lessen transfer of infection to the eye from contaminated medication, makeup, or contact lenses.

PATIENT TEACHING

Explain how a herpes simplex virus infection from the mouth can be transferred to the eyes by the fingers. Encourage the contact lens wearer to follow all directions for use. Teach the patient the proper technique for instillation of ophthalmic ointment and eyedrops as prescribed; emphasize the importance of hand washing before doing the procedure.

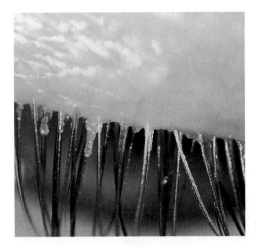

FIGURE 5–7 Blepharitis. (From Zitelli BJ, Davis HW: *Atlas of pediatric physical diagnosis*, ed 4, St. Louis, 2002, Mosby.)

Blepharitis

DESCRIPTION

Blepharitis is inflammation of the margins of the eyelids involving hair follicles and glands. It can be either ulcerative or nonulcerative.

■ **ICD-9-CM Code 373.00** *(Unspecified)*
373.01 *(Ulcerative blepharitis)*
373.02 *(Squamous blepharitis)*
Refer to the physician's diagnosis and then to the current edition of the ICD-9-CM coding manual to ensure the greatest specificity of pathology and any appropriate modifiers.

SYMPTOMS AND SIGNS

Blepharitis causes an unattractive, persistent redness and crusting on and around the eyelids (Fig. 5–7). Symptoms may include itching, a burning sensation, or a feeling of a foreign body being present in the eye. In severe cases, *ulcers* can develop on the eyelid margins, eyelashes can fall out, and the scales can flake from the eyelids and get into the eye, causing conjunctivitis (see Conjunctivitis).

PATIENT SCREENING

The patient experiencing irritation of the eyelids with crusts, itching, and burning needs a prompt clinical evaluation.

ETIOLOGY

The ulcerative form of blepharitis is usually the result of a staphylococcal infection. Nonulcerative blepharitis can be caused by allergies or exposure to smoke, dust, or chemicals. This condition also can be secondary to **seborrhea** of the eyelid's sebaceous glands, and often the patient has a history of repeated hordeolum (see Hordeolum [Stye]) and chalazions (see Chalazion).

DIAGNOSIS

Visual examination of the eyelids and the presence of collarettes (dried secretions) can determine the presence of staphylococci.

TREATMENT

If the condition does not improve within 2 weeks after the patient has cleaned the eyes twice a day with warm compresses, a physician should be consulted. Antibiotic or sulfonamide ophthalmic ointments may be needed.

PROGNOSIS

The condition can sometimes be resistant to treatment and may become chronic if not properly treated.

PREVENTION

It is prudent to protect the eyes from infection by adhering to proper hygiene.

PATIENT TEACHING

Warn the patient not to rub the eyes because that action can spread infection from the mouth or throat to the eyes. Teach the patient the proper technique for instilling ophthalmic ointment and eyedrops as prescribed; emphasize the importance of hand washing before the procedure. Some patients benefit from the use of seborrheic dermatitis medicated shampoos.

Entropion

DESCRIPTION

In the case of entropion, the eyelid margins (more often the margin of just the lower lid) turn inward, causing the lashes to rub the conjunctiva (Fig. 5–8).

> ■ **ICD-9-CM Code 374.00** *(Entropion, unspecified)*
> *Refer to the physician's diagnosis and then to the current edition of the ICD-9-CM coding manual to ensure the greatest specificity of pathology and any appropriate modifiers.*

SYMPTOMS AND SIGNS

The patient has the sensation of a foreign body in the eye, tearing, itching, and redness. Chronic epithelial defects may cause conjunctivitis (see Conjunctivitis) or corneal ulcers (see Corneal Abrasion or Ulcer). Entropion damages the cornea and causes vision problems if not corrected.

PATIENT SCREENING

Schedule a same-day appointment for the patient reporting the discomforting symptoms mentioned above.

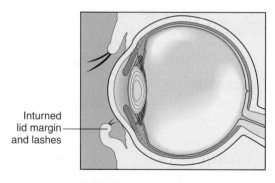

Inturned
lid margin
and lashes

FIGURE 5–8 Entropion.

ETIOLOGY

Entropion most often affects older people. With aging, the fibrous tissue on the lower eyelids becomes loose, resulting in excessive contraction of the eyelid muscle. This excessive contraction causes the eyelids to turn inward, thereby allowing the lashes to irritate the conjunctiva.

DIAGNOSIS

Visual examination reveals the inversion of the eyelid. The lashes are visible on the conjunctiva, as is the redness that results from the irritation.

TREATMENT

If the condition does not clear up on its own, the patient should be seen by a physician. A minor surgical procedure on the eyelid usually corrects the problem.

PROGNOSIS

Treatment brings complete relief.

PREVENTION

No specific method of prevention is known.

PATIENT TEACHING

Advise the patient not to rub the eyes to avoid infection. If surgery is required to correct the condition, explain the minor procedure.

Ectropion

DESCRIPTION

Ectropion is a condition in which the lower eyelid everts from the eyeball, and the exposed surface of the eyeball and the lining of the eyelid become dry and irritated (Fig. 5–9).

> ■ **ICD-9-CM Code 374.10** *(Ectropion, unspecified)*
> *Refer to the physician's diagnosis and then to the current edition of the ICD-9-CM coding manual to ensure the greatest specificity of pathology and any appropriate modifiers.*

SYMPTOMS AND SIGNS

Eversion of the eyelid exposes the conjunctival membrane lining the eyelid. Tears are diverted away from the tear duct and run down the cheeks instead. The patient reports dryness in the eye and tearing.

PATIENT SCREENING

Schedule the first available appointment for a medical evaluation for a patient experiencing the symptoms listed above.

ETIOLOGY

This condition usually occurs in the elderly as a result of muscles in the lower eyelid. Ectropion also can be caused by a scar on the eyelid or cheek that contracts and pulls the eyelid downward.

DIAGNOSIS

The problem can be detected easily by visual examination, and a history of symptoms confirms the diagnosis.

TREATMENT

Ectropion rarely disappears without treatment; therefore, a physician should be consulted. A minor surgical procedure is all that is needed to correct the condition.

PROGNOSIS

If it is not treated, ectropion can cause the development of corneal ulcers and permanent damage to the cornea.

PREVENTION

No method of prevention is known.

PATIENT TEACHING

Assure the patient, who often times is elderly, that a minor surgical procedure can correct the problem. Teach the patient the proper technique for instilling ophthalmic ointment and eyedrops as pre-

scribed; emphasize the importance of hand washing before performing the procedure.

Blepharoptosis

DESCRIPTION

Blepharoptosis, also called *ptosis,* is a permanent drooping of the upper eyelid, such that it partially or completely covers the eye (Fig. 5–10).

> ■ **ICD-9-CM Code 374.30** *(Ptosis of the eyelid, unspecified)*
> *Refer to the physician's diagnosis and then to the current edition of the ICD-9-CM coding manual to ensure the greatest specificity of pathology and any appropriate modifiers.*

SYMPTOMS AND SIGNS

Blepharoptosis usually affects one eye, but both can be involved. The condition can vary in severity throughout the day. Blepharoptosis can occur at any age, is often familial, and if severe, obstructs the vision of the affected eye.

PATIENT SCREENING

When vision is affected, or a previously normal upper eyelid has begun to droop, a physician should be consulted. Schedule the first available appointment.

ETIOLOGY

This condition is caused either by weakness of the third cranial nerve or weakness of the muscle that raises the eyelid. Blepharoptosis also can occur

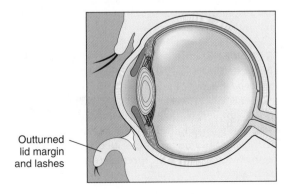

Outturned
lid margin
and lashes

FIGURE 5–9 Ectropion.

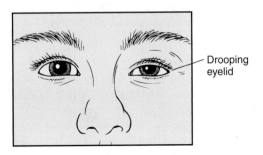

Drooping
eyelid

FIGURE 5–10 Blepharoptosis.

when the muscle of the eyelid or the nerve that controls the muscle is damaged. Several diseases, such as diabetes mellitus, muscular dystrophy, myasthenia gravis, and brain tumor, can cause ptosis.

DIAGNOSIS

In addition to an ophthalmic examination, blood tests and imaging may be ordered to rule out underlying disease.

TREATMENT

An operation can be performed to strengthen the muscle of the eyelid, or a support to keep the eyelid raised can be incorporated into eyeglasses.

PROGNOSIS

Successful treatment of any underlying disease should help correct the blepharoptosis.

PREVENTION

No specific method of prevention is known.

PATIENT TEACHING

Explain the relationship between the ptosis and the underlying disease, if known. If surgery is scheduled, describe the procedure to the patient and provide written postoperative instructions, if appropriate.

Conjunctivitis

DESCRIPTION

Inflammation of the conjunctiva, the mucous membrane that covers the anterior portion of the eyeball and also lines the eyelids, is called *conjunctivitis*.

■ **ICD-9-CM Code 372.30** *(Conjunctivitis, unspecified)*
Refer to the physician's diagnosis and then to the current edition of the ICD-9-CM coding manual to ensure the greatest specificity of pathology and any appropriate modifiers.

SYMPTOMS AND SIGNS

Conjunctivitis can be either unilateral or bilateral and is common. Symptoms include redness, swelling, and itching of the sclera and conjunctiva. The eyes may tear excessively and be extra sensitive to light. In cases of infectious conjunctivitis, pus is

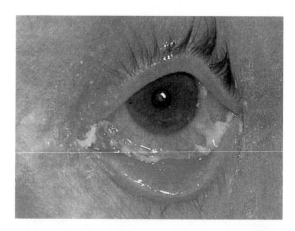

FIGURE 5–11 Acute conjunctivitis. (From Newell FW: *Ophthalmology: principles and concepts,* ed 8, St. Louis, 1996, Mosby.)

discharged from the eye, and this condition (pinkeye) is highly contagious (Fig. 5–11).

PATIENT SCREENING

Schedule a prompt ophthalmic examination for the patient presenting with swollen, red, itching eyes; a discharge from the eyes also may be present.

ETIOLOGY

Conjunctivitis can be caused by infection, either viral or bacterial, and also by irritation resulting from allergies or chemicals. Infections often are transmitted when contaminated fingers, washcloths, or towels touch the eyes.

DIAGNOSIS

Ophthalmic examination reveals inflammation of the conjunctiva. To identify bacterial or viral organisms, samples of the discharge are taken for culture and sensitivity tests.

TREATMENT

The treatment varies depending on the causative agents. The eyes should be kept free from discharge. This can be accomplished with cool compresses applied to the eyes 3 or 4 times a day for about 10 to 15 minutes at a time. For bacterial infections, antibiotics are prescribed. They can be in the form of ophthalmic preparations or systemic medications.

PROGNOSIS

Except in rare instances, conjunctivitis is usually not a serious condition, although recurrences are common. Superficial infections have a good prognosis. Usually, 1 to 2 weeks of treatment clears up this type of infection. Viral infections usually are self-limiting.

PREVENTION

If the determined cause is irritants or allergens, implementing measures of environmental control can be a means of prevention. Some causes of infectious conjunctivitis can be controlled by having the patient avoid contaminated washcloths or by refraining from touching the eyes with contaminated fingers.

PATIENT TEACHING

Give the patient written instructions on how to apply cool compresses and on the dosage schedule to be followed for medications. Teach the patient the proper technique for instilling ophthalmic ointment and eyedrops as prescribed; emphasize the importance of hand washing before performing the procedure.

Disorders of the Globe of the Eye

Corneal Abrasion or Ulcer

DESCRIPTION

A corneal abrasion and/or ulceration is the painful loss of surface epithelium, or outer layers of the cornea.

■ ICD-9-CM Code **918.1**
371.82 *(Corneal injury due to contact lens)*

SYMPTOMS AND SIGNS

The transparent outer covering of the eye is called the *cornea*. Because of its location, it is susceptible to injury and infection. Symptoms of abrasion and ulcer include pain, redness, and tearing. The patient may describe a sensation of having something foreign in the eye constantly and may report vision impairment as well. The patient may have a history of having had a foreign body in the eye or of recent ocular trauma.

PATIENT SCREENING

The patient with corneal abrasion may be experiencing significant pain in the eye that lasts more than 30 minutes. Prompt medical care within 2 hours is indicated. The physician should be consulted for instructions immediately after documenting a thorough history of what chemicals the eye has been exposed to. Follow office policy for referral to an ophthalmologist.

ETIOLOGY

Abrasions may be caused by foreign bodies being trapped between the cornea and the eyelid, by direct trauma to the cornea, such as being poked by a fingernail, or by the wearing of contact lenses that are scratched or poorly cleaned. Poorly fitting contact lenses also can cause corneal abrasions. If abrasions are not treated promptly, an ulcer can develop. A corneal ulcer is always a serious problem, and the patient should be referred to an ophthalmologist immediately in such a case.

DIAGNOSIS

The diagnosis is confirmed by the presence of characteristic symptoms as well as by a visual examination of the patient. Corneal abrasions and ulcerations stain with fluorescein, which makes them readily detectable.

TREATMENT

If a foreign body is present, it must be removed promptly to prevent further ulceration and infection. An ophthalmic antibiotic ointment often is prescribed to prevent a secondary infection in cases of corneal abrasion. Application of an eye dressing may be needed to promote healing if an abrasion is present. The dressing reduces movement of the cornea against the eyelid. Corneal ulcers need to be treated with intensive broad-spectrum antibiotic therapy immediately.

PROGNOSIS

Early treatment of superficial corneal abrasions results in healing and regeneration of tissue. Complications can include secondary infection and scaring of tissue that may necessitate a corneal transplant.

PREVENTION
Abrasions can be prevented by wearing protective eyewear while working in hazardous situations or when engaging in sports that might put a person at risk for ocular injuries.

PATIENT TEACHING
Teach the patient the proper care of an eye dressing and the technique for instilling ophthalmic ointment and eyedrops as prescribed; emphasize the importance of hand washing before performing the procedure. Stress the importance of keeping follow-up appointments to monitor the treatment.

Scleritis

DESCRIPTION
Inflammation of the sclera, the white outermost covering of the eyeball, is called *scleritis*.

> ■ **ICD-9-CM Code 379.00** *(Unspecified)*
> *Refer to the physician's diagnosis and then to the current edition of the ICD-9-CM coding manual to ensure the greatest specificity of pathology and any appropriate modifiers.*

SYMPTOMS AND SIGNS
Scleritis can affect either one or both eyes; symptoms include dull pain and intense redness in one or more areas of the sclera. Inflammation can occur in the posterior portion of the eye, which may cause some loss of vision. If scleritis is left untreated, perforation of the globe and loss of the eye are possible outcomes.

PATIENT SCREENING
Eye pain and redness indicate the need for an ophthalmic examination as soon as possible.

ETIOLOGY
The inflammation of scleritis often is associated with rheumatoid arthritis (see Rheumatoid Arthritis in Chapter 3) and certain digestive disorders, such as Crohn disease (see Crohn Disease [Regional Enteritis] in Chapter 8).

DIAGNOSIS
The patient should see an ophthalmologist as soon as possible if symptoms develop because of the possibility of perforation. A thorough ophthalmic examination is needed, and blood tests may be necessary to determine any underlying causes.

TREATMENT
Mild cases of scleritis usually respond well to instillation of topical eyedrops. For severe cases, *immunosuppressive* drugs may be prescribed. Perforation of the sclera necessitates a surgical repair called a *scleroplasty*.

PROGNOSIS
The prognosis is good for mild cases.

PREVENTION
No method of prevention is known.

PATIENT TEACHING
Teach the patient the proper technique for instilling ophthalmic ointment and eyedrops as prescribed; emphasize the importance of hand washing before performing the procedure. If surgery is required, use visual aids (if possible) to describe the anatomy of the eye to the patient and explain the procedure of surgical repair. Describe the postoperative regimen, and stress the importance of follow-up care.

Cataract

DESCRIPTION
A cataract is a cloudy or opaque area in an otherwise normal lens of the eye.

> ■ **ICD-9-CM Code 366**
> *Additional digits are required. Refer to the physician's diagnosis and then to the current edition of the ICD-9-CM coding manual to ensure the greatest specificity of pathology and any appropriate modifiers.*

SYMPTOMS AND SIGNS
Cataracts usually develop slowly and progressively reduce visual acuity. The primary symptom is the deterioration of vision in the affected eye. Blurring of vision and photosensitivity are also common. In advanced cases, the cataract may become readily visible, giving the pupil a white, opaque appearance and blocking light, thereby impairing vision (Fig. 5–12).

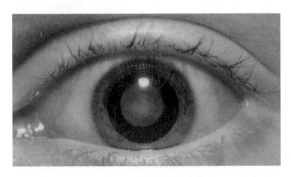

FIGURE 5–12 Cataract. (From Black JM, Hawks JH, and Keene AM: *Medical-surgical nursing: clinical management for positive outcomes,* ed 6, Philadelphia, 2001, Saunders. Courtesy Ophthalmic Photography, University of Michigan WK Kellogg Eye Center, Ann Arbor.)

PATIENT SCREENING

Cataracts often are noted during a routine ophthalmic examination. Patients reporting changes in visual acuity and/or photosensitivity should be given the first available appointment for an ophthalmic examination. Follow office policy for referral to an ophthalmologist.

ETIOLOGY

The most common cause of cataracts is deterioration of the lens caused by the aging process. They also may be congenital or may result from ocular trauma, lightning injury, drug toxicity (prolonged high-dose corticosteroid administration), or from systemic disease such as diabetes mellitus, or as a complication of other ocular diseases. Cataracts often have a familial occurrence; however, they also are a common condition in the general population.

DIAGNOSIS

Examination by an ophthalmologist should be considered if vision becomes distorted or seems to be deteriorating. Ophthalmoscopy with dilation of the eye and a simple penlight or slit-lamp examination confirms the presence of a cataract.

TREATMENT

The treatment depends on the amount of visual impairment and the age, health, and occupation of the patient. Surgery is advised when the cataracts begin to interfere with the lifestyle of the patient. The most common method of removing a cataract is phacoemulsification. Contrary to general belief, at present, cataracts are not removed routinely with the laser. In extracapsular surgery, the nucleus, or center, of the cataract is removed in one piece. This necessitates a larger incision and more sutures. With phacoemulsification, an ultrasonic probe vibrates to break up the cataract, which subsequently is aspirated through the small incision. With this method, often no sutures are required for wound closure.

In both extracapsular cataract extraction and phacoemulsification, the posterior capsule of the lens is left in place. This membrane helps to support an artificial lens, which is placed into the eye after removal of the cataract. Often, the posterior membrane becomes cloudy 1 to 3 years after surgery, which again reduces the visual acuity. If this does occur, a laser can be used to make an opening in the center of the cloudy membrane, thus immediately restoring good vision. This outpatient procedure usually entails local anesthesia.

PROGNOSIS

After cataract surgery, the patient will need a change in eyeglass prescription. Cataract surgery currently is quite successful; however, as with all surgery, significant complications are possible.

PREVENTION

Being primarily associated with the aging process, no method of prevention is known. It is prudent for patients and physicians to consider the risk of cataracts associated with drug toxicity from certain medications.

PATIENT TEACHING

Explain the preoperative tests and medications as prescribed. Discuss the postoperative need for a protective eye shield at night and the purpose of postoperative medications administered to prevent increasing ocular pressure. Give the patient written instructions regarding the technique for instilling eyedrops and all other medications, how to apply the eye shield carefully, and any limitation of activities during recovery. Stress the importance of regular follow-up visits.

Glaucoma

DESCRIPTION

Glaucoma is damage to the optic nerve, often caused by elevated intraocular pressure.

■ **ICD-9-CM Code 365**

Additional digits are required. Refer to the physician's diagnosis and then to the current edition of the ICD-9-CM coding manual to ensure the greatest specificity of pathology and any appropriate modifiers.

Glaucoma is one of the most common and severe ocular diseases and is a major cause of blindness. It is more common in patients older than 60 years of age; however, it can occur at any age. The ciliary body in the eye continually produces fluid called the *aqueous humor.* Normally this fluid circulates freely between the posterior and anterior chambers of the eye and passes through the trabecular meshwork and drains into the general circulation. Several different pathologic causes and abnormalities in fluid drainage lead to glaucoma. Risk factors include age older than 60 years, nearsightedness, blood relatives with glaucoma, and African-American descent.

The many types of glaucoma include chronic open-angle and acute angle-closure glaucoma (Fig. 5–13).

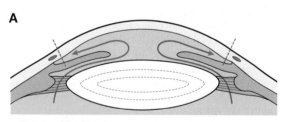

A

Open-angle glaucoma

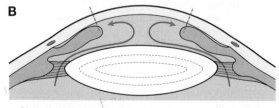

B

Closed-angle glaucoma

FIGURE 5–13 Glaucoma. **A,** In open-angle glaucoma, the obstruction occurs in the trabecular meshwork. **B,** In closed-angle glaucoma, the trabecular meshwork is covered by the root of the iris or adhesions between the iris and the cornea. (From Damjanov I: *Pathology for the health-related professions,* ed 2, Philadelphia, 2000, Saunders.)

PATIENT SCREENING

Encourage patients, especially those with the risk factors listed above, to have a regular ophthalmic examination and appropriate testing. Patients reporting the onset of headaches, changes in visual acuity, photophobia, nausea and vomiting, and/or eye pain need to see their ophthalmologist immediately; their condition should be treated as an emergency.

Chronic Open-Angle Glaucoma

■ **ICD-9-CM Code 365.10** *(Open-angle glaucoma, unspecified)*

Refer to the physician's diagnosis and then to the current edition of the ICD-9-CM coding manual to ensure the greatest specificity of pathology and any appropriate modifiers.

SYMPTOMS AND SIGNS

Chronic open-angle glaucoma, a silent disease, is the most common form of glaucoma and is the most treatable cause of blindness. Patients can have open-angle glaucoma for a significant period of time before symptoms appear. By the time symptoms do appear, considerable damage usually has occurred. The best way to detect glaucoma is by having periodic routine ophthalmic examinations, which include intraocular pressure readings as well as optic nerve evaluations. If the intraocular pressure is somewhat elevated or the optic nerve shows signs of becoming atrophic, glaucoma needs to be considered as a possibility. If chronic open-angle glaucoma goes untreated, the patient gradually loses peripheral (side) vision. The central vision may remain clear for a considerable period of time. However, if the condition progresses, the central vision is also lost, causing complete blindness.

ETIOLOGY

In chronic open-angle glaucoma, a block at the level of the trabecular meshwork impairs aqueous humor reabsorption. Chronic open-angle glaucoma can occur secondary to trauma, even years later. Overuse of topical steroids also can cause the condition.

DIAGNOSIS

The diagnosis of open-angle glaucoma is determined by patient history, ophthalmic examination with tonometry, examination of the optic nerves, and visual field analysis.

TREATMENT

Early treatment of glaucoma is essential; if not treated promptly, the disease can lead to blindness because any vision lost as a result of the disease generally cannot be regained. This condition usually is treated with medication to decrease the production of aqueous humor (carbonic anhydrase inhibitors, beta blockers, and alpha-adrenergic agents) or increase uveoscleral outflow (prostaglandin analogs). Laser treatment also can be beneficial in opening the drainage system; occasionally, surgery is necessary to bypass the chronically defective draining system. Fortunately, most of the time chronic open-angle glaucoma can be controlled with eyedrops.

Acute Angle-Closure Glaucoma

ICD-9-CM Code 365.2 *(Primary angle-closure glaucoma)*
Refer to the physician's diagnosis and then to the current edition of the ICD-9-CM coding manual to ensure the greatest specificity of pathology and any appropriate modifiers.

SYMPTOMS AND SIGNS

Acute angle-closure glaucoma usually is associated with blurred vision, severe pain, headaches, and redness of the eye. The patient becomes photophobic and sees "halos" around light. With the full attack of acute glaucoma, the symptoms persist and become worse. Often severe pain develops that is associated with nausea and vomiting. The cornea of the eye becomes hazy because of the elevated pressure. The elevation of pressure in acute angle-closure glaucoma is usually significantly higher than that associated with chronic open-angle (simple) glaucoma. If acute angle-closure glaucoma is left untreated, the patient can lose his or her vision.

ETIOLOGY

In acute angle-closure glaucoma, the mouth or opening of the drainage system is narrow and can close completely, causing a marked increase in the intraocular pressure (IOP) during a short time.

DIAGNOSIS

The diagnosis is made based on the patient's history and a marked increase in the IOP. With a special lens called a *goniolens,* the ophthalmologist can view directly the opening of the drainage system to determine whether it is open or closed. The eye is usually red, and the cornea can be hazy.

TREATMENT

Treatment of acute angle-closure glaucoma is done primarily by laser **iridotomy,** which creates a small opening between the anterior and posterior chambers, allowing the filtering angle to open. Often the IOP is lowered with medication before the laser treatment. However, the definitive treatment of angle-closure glaucoma is virtually always a laser iridotomy.

PROGNOSIS

The prognosis depends on the type of glaucoma, how early the condition is recognized and treatment is begun, and patient compliance with therapeutic regimens. Untreated glaucoma is a major cause of blindness.

PREVENTION

Regular ophthalmic examinations with testing appropriate to age and risk factors are recommended.

PATIENT TEACHING

Explain the type of glaucoma and the treatment regimen. Teach the patient the proper technique for instilling ophthalmic ointment and eyedrops as prescribed; emphasize the importance of hand washing before performing the procedure. Review the symptoms and signs that should be reported to the physician: severe eye pain, headache, blurred vision, halos, nausea and vomiting. Stress the importance of good compliance with medication regimen and follow-up care. Provide referrals for support services.

Macular Degeneration

DESCRIPTION

Macular degeneration is a progressive deterioration of the macula of the retina.

 ICD-9-CM Code 362.50 *(Senile, unspecified)*
Refer to the physician's diagnosis and then to the current edition of the ICD-9-CM coding manual to ensure the greatest specificity of pathology and any appropriate modifiers.

SYMPTOMS AND SIGNS

The area of the retina near the optic nerve in the center of the field of vision that defines fine details is known as the *macula lutea*. An early symptom of macular degeneration may be a mild distortion of central vision. The condition is usually painless, develops slowly, and does not affect the peripheral vision. In most cases, both eyes are affected, either at the same time or one right after the other. As the condition worsens, reading and activities that require sharp vision become impossible. Eventually, the central vision may disappear altogether.

PATIENT SCREENING

Macular degeneration is often considered to be age related; therefore the mature adult is encouraged to have regular ophthalmic examinations. Patients reporting changes in visual acuity, or loss of sharpness in central vision, are scheduled for a prompt ophthalmic examination. Follow office policy for referral to an ophthalmologist.

ETIOLOGY

Although this condition usually is age related, it may be secondary to several diseases. Genetic factors and environmental exposure to ultraviolet rays and drugs are considered etiologic components. When age-related, macular degeneration usually is caused by degenerative changes in the pigment epithelium of the retina. Associated atherosclerotic changes in the vessels may occur as well. Hemorrhage also may occur in some cases. As a result, the macula does not receive sufficient blood, causing it to degenerate and central vision to become blurred.

DIAGNOSIS

The diagnosis of macular degeneration is made after a thorough examination by an ophthalmologist, using ophthalmoscopy and *fluorescein angiography,* and the patient history are reviewed.

TREATMENT

No definitive medical cure is known; however, a recent study shows that vitamin supplements, especially vitamins A, C, E, and zinc, can help slow deterioration of moderate dry macular degeneration. The wet form of this disease may be lessened somewhat with a procedure called *laser photocoagulation.* Visual aids, such as strong magnifying lenses in eyeglasses, also may be beneficial.

PROGNOSIS

No cure is known and the success of treatment has been limited.

PREVENTION

Vitamin therapy and protecting the eyes from ultraviolet rays are considered prudent measures.

PATIENT TEACHING

Patients benefit from an explanation of why their vision and depth perception have changed and how they can use visual aids to improve vision. Instruct the patient to contact the physician if a sudden worsening of vision is noted. Provide emotional support.

Diabetic Retinopathy

DESCRIPTION

Diabetic retinopathy is a disorder of the retinal blood vessels.

ICD-9-CM Code	362.0
	250.5 *(Code first diabetes)*

Refer to the physician's diagnosis and then to the current edition of the ICD-9-CM coding manual to ensure the greatest specificity of pathology and any appropriate modifiers.

SYMPTOMS AND SIGNS

Diabetic **retinopathy** is characterized by microaneurysms, hemorrhages, dilation of retinal veins, and the formation of abnormal new vessels (neovascularization). This condition usually occurs in both eyes, affecting the sharpness and clarity of vision. Diabetic retinopathy is a major cause of blindness.

PATIENT SCREENING

The diabetic patient is encouraged to have frequent ophthalmic examinations. Any sudden change in visual acuity is regarded as an emergency and is to be reported to the attending physician immediately.

ETIOLOGY

Diabetic retinopathy usually occurs about 8 to 10 years after the onset of diabetes mellitus. It occurs most often in those with diabetes who do not control their blood glucose levels, but all persons with diabetes are susceptible. Diabetes causes some of the tiny blood vessels in the retina to become constricted and die. The remaining vessels may leak blood into the retina and cause a permanent reduction in the sharpness of vision. Sometimes, fragile new blood vessels (neovascularization) can grow on the retina and, in turn, leak blood into the vitreous humor. This may markedly reduce vision. In either case, the blood usually is reabsorbed by the choroid; however, scar tissue forms on the retina and may cause partial or permanent loss of vision (Fig. 5–14).

DIAGNOSIS

Complete ophthalmoscopic examination detects the retinal effects of diabetes. As with other ocular disorders, a thorough ophthalmic examination should be done regularly, especially when diabetes is a factor.

TREATMENT

Treatment with laser photocoagulation is usually effective in controlling retinopathy. The condition has a tendency to recur, but with treatment, vision often may be maintained. In cases of vitreous hemorrhage or proliferative disease, a vitrectomy may be necessary.

PROGNOSIS

Diabetic retinopathy can be controlled with treatment; however, the prognosis is guarded.

PREVENTION

Maintaining good control of the diabetic condition can retard the progression of diabetic retinopathy.

PATIENT TEACHING

Stress the importance of good diabetic care to help prevent the complication of diabetic retinopathy and possible loss of vision.

Retinal Detachment

DESCRIPTION

A retinal detachment is an elevation (separation) of the retina from the choroid (Fig. 5–15).

ICD-9-CM Code 361.9 *(Retinal detachment unspecified)*
Refer to the physician's diagnosis and then to the current edition of the ICD-9-CM coding manual to ensure the greatest specificity of pathology and any appropriate modifiers.

SYMPTOMS AND SIGNS

Retinal detachment may be partial or complete and usually is associated with a retinal tear, or a hole in the retina. Early symptoms of detachment consist of the patient seeing many new floaters and light flashes. This persists and worsens and is followed by seeing a dark shadow that extends from the periphery inward. This may begin in either the lower or upper field of vision or in one of the side fields of vision. If the detachment extends to the central retina, the central vision also is blocked. The detachment often happens suddenly and without pain.

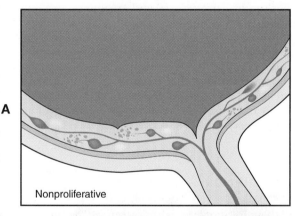

A

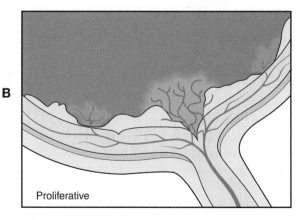

B

FIGURE 5–14 Diabetic retinopathy. **A,** Nonproliferative retinopathy shows edema, microaneurysm, and exudates. **B,** Proliferative retinopathy shows new blood vessel formation. (From Damjanov I: *Pathology for the health-related professions,* ed 2, Philadelphia, 2000, Saunders.)

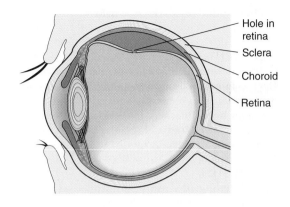

- Hole in retina
- Sclera
- Choroid
- Retina

FIGURE 5–15 Retinal detachment.

PATIENT SCREENING

The patient reporting light flashes, painless changes in vision, and visualization of new floating spots is brought to the physician's attention immediately.

ETIOLOGY

People who are extremely nearsighted are more susceptible to retinal detachments than the general population. Ocular trauma also can predispose a person to retinal detachments. A retinal detachment usually begins with a tear in the retina. Fluid then leaks under the retina and separates it from the choroid. After the retina is separated from the choroid, that portion of the retina no longer functions visually. As the retina continues to elevate, more and more vision is lost.

DIAGNOSIS

An ophthalmoscopic examination readily reveals the retinal detachment.

TREATMENT

Early treatment is advised; intervention is imperative. Treatment of a retinal detachment consists of either photocoagulation or surgery. This should be done without delay to prevent additional portions of the retina from detaching. When the detached retina is repositioned, it regains most of its function. If the detachment has extended to the macula, the central retina, some permanent reduction in central acuity often occurs. Photo-coagulation or **cryotherapy** can be used to treat retinal tears if no associated detachment occurs. Photocoagulation is a relatively simple procedure, which can be used to seal retinal tears before the development of retinal detachment. Early diagnosis is important in such cases.

PROGNOSIS

Irreversible blindness can result from untreated retinal detachment.

PREVENTION

No specific method of prevention is known.

PATIENT TEACHING

Use visual aids to explain the condition and the treatment to the patient. Prepare the patient for postsurgical procedures and treatments, including instruction on wearing a protective patch over the eye, applying cool compresses, taking pain medications, and executing measures to avoid raising intraocular pressure. Teach the patient the proper technique for instilling ophthalmic ointment and eyedrops as prescribed; emphasize the importance of hand washing before performing the procedure.

Uveitis

DESCRIPTION

Uveitis denotes inflammation of the uveal tract, including the iris, ciliary body, and choroid.

> ■ **ICD-9-CM Code 364.3** *(Unspecified)*
> *Refer to the physician's diagnosis and then to the current edition of the ICD-9-CM coding manual to ensure the greatest specificity of pathology and any appropriate modifiers.*

SYMPTOMS AND SIGNS

Uveitis is usually unilateral but may be bilateral. Pain, photophobia, blurred vision, redness, and pupillary constriction can occur. The photophobia is often intense.

PATIENT SCREENING

Having a complete ophthalmic examination performed, as soon as possible, is necessary for a patient experiencing the symptoms mentioned above. Follow office policy for referral to an ophthalmologist.

ETIOLOGY

Uveitis can be associated with autoimmune disorders; juvenile rheumatoid arthritis (see Chapter 3) and ankylosing spondylitis (see Chapter 3) are especially likely to be associated with uveitis. Infections such as syphilis, tuberculosis, toxoplasmosis, and histoplasmosis also may be causative. Often an exact cause for uveitis cannot be determined.

DIAGNOSIS

A complete examination with the slit lamp is necessary for the diagnosis to be made. To detect some forms of disease, skin tests for tuberculosis, *toxoplasmosis,* and *histoplasmosis* may be needed. Certain blood tests also may aid in confirming the diagnosis.

TREATMENT

Treatment is specific for the particular type of uveitis and consists largely of topical or, in severe cases, systemic immunosuppression. Any underlying cause should be treated. Cycloplegic agents and steroids are often beneficial in treating inflammation.

PROGNOSIS

The prognosis is variable depending on the clinical type and the underlying cause.

PREVENTION

No method of prevention is known.

PATIENT TEACHING

Use visual aids to demonstrate what structure(s) of the eyes are involved in the inflammation. Explain the medical treatment. Teach the patient the proper technique for instilling ophthalmic ointment and eyedrops as prescribed; emphasize the importance of hand washing before performing the procedure.

Exophthalmos

DESCRIPTION

Exophthalmos is an abnormal protrusion of the eyeballs.

 ICD-9-CM Code 376.2 *(First code underlying thyroid disorder)*
Refer to the physician's diagnosis and then to the current edition of the ICD-9-CM coding manual to ensure the greatest specificity of pathology and any appropriate modifiers.

SYMPTOMS AND SIGNS

Exophthalmos exposes an abnormally large amount of the anterior eye. Patients report dryness and a gritty feeling in the affected eye or eyes. They also may note double vision and eye movement restriction. In severe cases, vision becomes seriously blurred.

PATIENT SCREENING

Schedule a prompt appointment for a complete medical evaluation and ophthalmic examination. Follow office policy for referral to an ophthalmologist.

ETIOLOGY

Exophthalmos is caused by multiple factors including enlarged extraocular muscles, retrobulbar mass or edema of the soft tissue that lines the bony orbit of the eye. This condition may be associated with hyperthyroid, hypothyroid, or euthyroid (normal thyroid) stare (see Hyperthyroidism in Chapter 4). Sudden unilateral onset is usually a sign of hemorrhage or inflammation.

DIAGNOSIS

A complete ophthalmic examination, along with blood tests, radiographic studies, computed tomography (CT), and echography, is done to determine the underlying cause.

TREATMENT

The diagnosis determines the therapy. If the condition is caused by hyperthyroidism, the underlying disorder needs to be corrected. Severe cases may require surgical decompression of the orbit, and systemic steroids are beneficial in controlling edema.

PROGNOSIS

The prognosis depends on the successful treatment of the underlying cause.

PREVENTION

No method of prevention is known.

PATIENT TEACHING

Explain how exophthalmos relates to the underlying cause as diagnosed. Explain the purpose and dosage schedule of prescribed medication. Give emotional support, as the patient is likely to be distressed by the cosmetic effect of "bulging eyeballs."

Cancer of the Eye

DESCRIPTION

Cancer of the eye may involve the eyeball (ocular tumors), the orbit (the bone surrounding the orbital cavity and the soft tissues and muscles that lie between the globe and the bone), the optic nerve, or the eyelids. Neoplasms may be benign, malignant, or metastatic from another location (secondary tumors).

> ■ **ICD-9-CM Code 239.8** *(Unspecified)*
> *Neoplasms of the eye must be specified for location and type. Therefore it is not possible to list all applicable ICD-9-CM codes for neoplasms of the eye. Refer to the physician's diagnosis and then to the current edition of the ICD-9-CM coding manual to ensure the greatest specificity of pathology and any appropriate modifiers.*

SYMPTOMS AND SIGNS

Tumors of the eyelid generally present as visible lesions. (See Chapter 6 for a discussion of basal cell carcinoma, squamous cell carcinoma, and malignant melanoma lesions.) Squamous papilloma presents as a skin tag (skin projection) on the eyelid. Sebaceous cell carcinoma often looks like a recurring chalazion (see Chalazion in this chapter). Primary ocular, orbital, and optic nerve tumors may have symptoms, depending on the tumor type and location, of exophthalmos, strabismus, nystagmus, and impaired vision. In addition to decreased visual acuity, secondary eye tumors are usually associated with pain, thereby distinguishing them from primary ocular melanoma.

PATIENT SCREENING

Patients reporting visible lesions around or "in" the eye, or those experiencing any usual appearance or movement of the eye(s), with or without pain, need a timely appointment for a medical evaluation and an ophthalmic examination.

ETIOLOGY

Ocular tumors include retinoblastoma, the most common primary malignancy of the eye in children (Fig. 5–16), and ocular (or uveal tract) melanoma in adults. Retinoblastoma is a neoplasm of the retina that affects 1 in 18,000 to 30,000 live births. It is most often due to a heritable mutation on chromosome 13, although only 8% of affected children have a positive family history of retinoblastoma. Almost all cases of ocular melanoma are found in Caucasians. Orbital tumors are more rare and include rhabdomyosarcoma (malignant) and capillary hemangioma (benign) in children. Eyelid tumors include cutaneous neoplasms (usually caused by sun exposure to the eyelid), as well as benign squamous papillomas and the rare sebaceous cell carcinomas. Basal cell carcinoma is the most common malignant eyelid tumor (85% to 90% of eyelid lesions). Melanoma, on the other hand, accounts for only 1% of eyelid tumors, but over 65% of all deaths caused by neoplasms of the eyelid. Squamous papilloma is the most common benign eyelid tumor and is caused by human papillomavirus (HPV) infection. Optic pathway glioma is a low-grade tumor of the optic nerve or chiasm that usually occurs in children under the age of 20 years. Approximately 1200 new cases of primary eye cancer occur each year, and 200 deaths result from this type of cancer. The most common tumor of the eye is cancer that has metastasized to the eye. Approximately 30,000 cases of secondary eye cancer occur per year. The most common sites of origin are the lung in men and the breast in women, but many other types of cancer also are known to metastasize to the eye.

DIAGNOSIS

The lesions of ocular melanoma may be first identified on routine eye examination, before symptoms arise. Eyelid tumors are diagnosed after biopsy of the lesion. Other types of eye tumors may be seen on fundoscopic examination, but magnetic resonance imaging (MRI), with or without a biopsy (depending on the tumor location), is used for definitive diagnosis and evaluation of the extent of disease.

TREATMENT

Treatment may involve excision of the tumor, eyeball removal, or radiation therapy. The treatment of optic pathway glioma usually involves a period of observation to see whether any changes in tumor size or visual function occur over time because spontaneous regression is possible. If treatment is

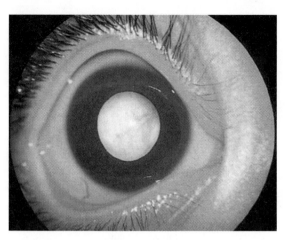

FIGURE 5–16 Retinoblastoma. (From Michelson JB, Friedlaender MH: *The eye in clinical medicine,* London, 1996, Times Mirror International Publishers.)

PROGNOSIS

Overall 5-year survival rate for patients with primary eye neoplasms is generally good but largely depends on tumor size and stage at diagnosis. Although many children survive retinoblastoma with appropriate treatment, they are at risk for developing secondary malignancies, especially osteosarcoma, later in life.

PREVENTION

No methods of prevention are known for orbital and ocular eye tumors. The skin neoplasms of the eyelid may be prevented by wearing sunglasses and wide-brimmed hats to reduce sun exposure to that area.

PATIENT TEACHING

Information given to the patient is determined by the type of neoplasm, the treatment, and the prognosis. Patients, or the parents of children, benefit from clear explanations of all ongoing diagnostic and therapeutic procedures. In all cases, but especially with children, emotional support is imperative.

necessary, it usually involves amputation of the optic nerve or radiation therapy. Treatment of secondary eye cancer rarely improves patient survival, but chemotherapy or radiation therapy may be given for palliation of symptoms.

DISORDERS OF THE EAR

FUNCTIONING ORGANS OF HEARING

THE EAR IS THE ORGAN OF BALANCE as well as the organ of hearing. The ear is composed of three sections: the outer, the middle, and the inner ear (Fig. 5–17).

The outer section is made up of the external ear, also called the *pinna* or *auricle*, and the external auditory canal. The latter's function is to collect sound waves, or vibrations, from the air or environment and channel them to the *tympanic membrane* (eardrum), which then begins to vibrate.

The middle section contains the tympanic membrane and three ossicles (tiny bones) called the *malleus* (hammer), the *incus* (anvil), and the

stapes (stirrup). Also in the middle ear is a canal, called the *eustachian tube,* which leads to a cavity (the pharynx) at the back of the nose. At the innermost region of the middle ear is the oval window, the opening to the inner ear. The middle ear receives the sound waves from the vibrating eardrum and relays them along the three bones to the oval window.

The inner ear contains two membrane-lined chambers, each filled with fluid, called the *cochlea* and the **labyrinth.** The cochlea contains tiny hairs that change the sound waves in the fluid into nerve impulses, which then are transmitted to the

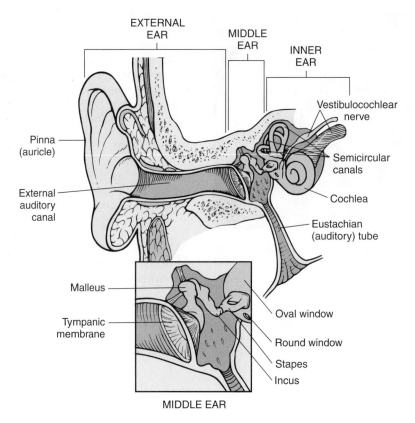

EXTERNAL EAR

MIDDLE EAR

INNER EAR

Vestibulocochlear nerve

Pinna (auricle)

Semicircular canals

External auditory canal

Cochlea

Eustachian (auditory) tube

Malleus

Tympanic membrane

Oval window

Round window

Stapes

Incus

MIDDLE EAR

FIGURE 5–17 Normal ear.

brain via the auditory nerve. The labyrinth is responsible for maintaining balance. It consists of three connected tubes bent into half circles, called the *semicircular canals*. Their function is to detect movement of the head and relay this information to the brain.

Common symptoms of ear diseases and conditions that should receive attention from healthcare professionals include the following:

- Hearing loss
- Ear pain or pressure
- **Tinnitus** (ringing or buzzing noise)
- **Vertigo** (dizziness)
- Nausea and vomiting

Hearing loss or deafness is denoted as two basic types: conductive loss and **sensorineural** loss. Conductive deafness is caused by an impairment of the eardrum or bones in the middle ear, which conduct sound waves to the cochlea in the inner ear. Sensorineural, or nerve, deafness results from impairment of the cochlea or the auditory nerve (see the Enrichment box on Cochlear Implants).

Central deafness results when the central nervous system (CNS) cannot interpret impulses because of a cerebrovascular accident (CVA) or brain tumor (see the Alert box on Ototoxicity for chemical causes of temporary or permanent hearing loss).

ALERT
OTOTOXICITY

Ototoxicity occurs when a drug or chemical causes damage to the eighth cranial (acoustic) nerve or to the inner ear, resulting in temporary or permanent hearing loss or disturbances in balance. Symptoms and signs of ototoxicity usually have an insidious onset and include tinnitus, a feeling of fullness or pressure in the ears, hearing loss, vertigo, and occasionally nausea.

Drugs that can cause ototoxicity include salicylates (aspirin and aspirin-containing products), nonsteroidal antiinflammatory drugs (NSAIDs), certain antibiotics (aminoglycosides, erythromycin, vancomycin), loop diuretics (furosemide [Lasix], bumetanide [Bumex], ethacrynic acid [Edecrin]), chemotherapeutic agents (cisplatin, vincristine, vinblastine), and quinines (quinidine and quinine). The physician should be notified of any of the aforementioned symptoms when the individual is taking or going to receive any of the previously mentioned medications.

Discontinuing aspirin, aspirin-containing products, and NSAIDs often reverses the ototoxic effects of these drugs. Any of the other drugs should not be discontinued unless so ordered by the physician. Quinine ototoxicity, like aspirin-induced ototoxicity, usually can be reversed when the medication is stopped. Large dosages of antibiotics that may be ototoxic usually are administered in life-threatening situations.

Chemotherapeutic agents are monitored for any ototoxic side effects. In normal dosages, the loop diuretics usually have very few ototoxic side effects; it is when they are given in massive doses for treatment of acute kidney failure or acute hypertension that ototoxicity may occur.

Environmental chemicals include, but are not limited to, butyl nitrite, carbon disulfide, hexane, styrene, toluene, trichloroethylene, and xylene.

Once damage has occurred, it cannot be reversed. Hearing loss may be helped somewhat by hearing aids or cochlear implants. When the patient experiences loss of balance, physical therapy may be needed to help the patient regain the ability to balance.

ENRICHMENT
COCHLEAR IMPLANTS

INDIVIDUALS WHO EXPERIENCE severe sensorineural hearing loss that is not helped by hearing aids may have partial hearing restored by means of cochlear implants. Cochlear implants are electronic devices that use minute electrical currents to stimulate the auditory nerve and help the currents travel to the auditory cortex to be perceived as sound.

Cochlear implant systems are complex and include an electrode array, a receiver, a speech processor, a transmitting coil, and a microphone. The electrode array is placed surgically in the cochlea, and the receiver is implanted and fixed to the skull behind the mastoid bone. The surgical incision is allowed to heal for 4 to 6 weeks, after which the external components (the microphone, transmitting coil, and speech processor) are fitted to the patient. Fitting includes calibration of the transmitting coil and programming of the speech processor. Auditory and speech training are provided to the implant recipient.

Cochlear implants do not restore normal hearing; however, they can improve a deaf person's functioning in a hearing world. Candidates for the implants are selected carefully and should have a severe to profound bilateral sensorineural hearing loss and be older than 2 years of age. Many still employ lip reading and American Sign Language (ASL) as adjunct therapies in order to communicate.

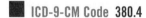

Disorders of Conduction

Impacted Cerumen

DESCRIPTION
Impacted cerumen is an atypical accumulation of cerumen in the canal of the outer ear. The "ear wax" that has accumulated hardens and has a tendency to prevent sound waves from reaching the tympanic membrane (eardrum), resulting in decreased hearing (Fig. 5–18).

■ **ICD-9-CM Code 380.4**

SYMPTOMS AND SIGNS
The normal, soft, yellowish brown, waxlike secretion produced by the glands of the external ear canal is called cerumen, or "ear wax." If this secretion accumulates excessively, a gradual loss of hearing may occur, and the patient may have a feeling that the ear is plugged and may experience tinnitus or sometimes an earache (otalgia). Impacted cerumen is a common cause of conductive hearing loss.

PATIENT SCREENING
Individuals complaining of ear pain should be seen as soon as possible. Many times the only complaint will be one of reduced hearing level. Schedule an appointment as soon as possible. Referral to an audiologist may be indicated. Awareness of the incidence of impacted cerumen may come about during a routine examination or during the course of an office visit for some other reason.

ETIOLOGY
Abnormal accumulation of cerumen can be caused by dryness and scaling of the skin or by excessive hair in the ear canal. Some people have abnormally narrow ear canals, which may predispose them to this condition.

DIAGNOSIS
The physician or specialist does an otologic examination, and the patient history of symptoms confirms the diagnosis.

TREATMENT
If impacted cerumen is found, it must be removed. If the cerumen adheres to the wall of the ear canal, it may have to be softened first with oily drops or hydrogen peroxide and then irrigated with water to accomplish removal (Fig. 5–19). Any hearing loss caused by the impaction is alleviated after removal of cerumen.

PROGNOSIS
The prognosis for removal is positive. Hearing usually improves once the ear canal is clear of the im-

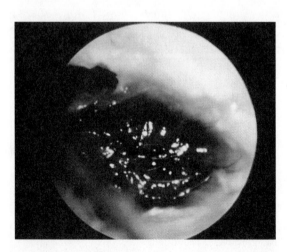

FIGURE 5–18 Impacted cerumen. (From Sigler B: *Ear, nose, and throat disorders—Mosby's clinical nursing series*, St. Louis, 1994, Mosby.)

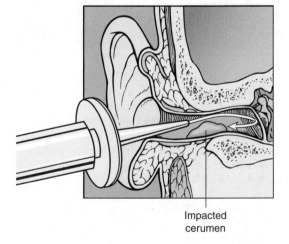

Impacted cerumen

FIGURE 5–19 Irrigation of the ear for impacted cerumen. Irrigation of the ear also is used to remove foreign bodies.

pacted ear wax. Recurrence is likely so periodic examinations may be necessary.

PREVENTION

Prevention includes routine cleansing of the ear canal by the primary care physician or an ear care specialist. Other prevention includes avoiding placing any object in the ear canal that may push the ear wax down into the ear canal. Use of cotton-tipped applicators in the ear is often times the cause of cerumen being packed into the ear canal.

PATIENT TEACHING

Patient teaching involves reinforcement of not putting anything into the ear that would have the ability to push or pack the earwax down into the outer ear canal. Providing written information concerning proper ear care to the patient and family is helpful.

Infective Otitis Externa

DESCRIPTION

Inflammation of the external ear canal is called *otitis externa*. This condition is usually accompanied by an infectious process.

■ **ICD-9-CM Code** **380.1** *(Infective otitis externa)*
380.10 *(Infective otitis externa, unspecified)*
380.1 or 380.10 are the usual codes used for otitis externa. Designation by the physician of any special circumstances will determine the applicable code. Refer to the physician's diagnosis and then to the current edition of the ICD-9-CM coding manual to ensure the greatest specificity of pathology and any appropriate modifiers.

SYMPTOMS AND SIGNS

Severe pain; a red, swollen ear canal; hearing loss; fever; and *pruritus* are common symptoms of otitis externa. Drainage from the ear may be either watery or *purulent*.

PATIENT SCREENING

Individuals reporting pain in the ear accompanied by drainage require prompt attention.

ETIOLOGY

Accumulation of cerumen in the ear canal, when mixed with water, acts as a culture medium for bacteria or fungi. Otitis externa also may be caused by dermatologic conditions such as seborrhea and psoriasis. Trauma to the ear canal, caused by attempts to clean or scratch inside the ear with a foreign object, or frequent use of earphones and earplugs or hearing aids can predispose a person to the development of otitis externa.

DIAGNOSIS

An otologic examination and a history of symptoms confirms the diagnosis (Fig. 5–20). If a bacterial infection is suspected, a culture of the material found in the canal may be needed to determine how to properly treat the infection.

TREATMENT

The ear canal must be kept clean and free from water. Antibiotic or steroid eardrops and systemic antibiotics may be prescribed, depending on the severity. Otitis externa tends to recur and can become chronic.

PROGNOSIS

The prognosis is positive with treatment. Chronic otitis externa may develop with repeated irritation by earphones, earplugs, or hearing aids.

PREVENTION

Preventive measures include keeping the ear clean and dry. It is important to also keep earphones, earplugs, and hearing aids clean. Additionally, the use of another's earphones or earplugs is discouraged.

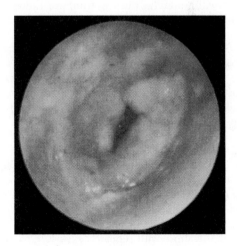

FIGURE 5–20 External otitis.

If this is a usual practice, any shared object placed in the ears should be disinfected before use.

PATIENT TEACHING
Provide the patient or family with pictures of the anatomy of the ear. Demonstrate how moisture trapped in the ear by earphones, earplugs, or hearing aids can contribute to infective otitis externa. Explain why sharing of objects that are placed in the ear may cause infective otitis externa.

Swimmer's Ear
DESCRIPTION
Inflammation and resulting infection of the outer ear canal after water has been entrapped during swimming is termed *swimmer's ear*.

 ICD-9-CM Code 380.12 *(Acute swimmer's ear)*

SYMPTOMS AND SIGNS
Similar to infectious otitis externa, severe pain; a red, swollen ear canal; hearing loss; fever; and pruritus are common symptoms of swimmer's ear. Any drainage from the ear may be either watery or purulent. Typically, the onset of the condition occurs after the patient has been swimming.

PATIENT SCREENING
Individuals reporting pain in the ear accompanied by drainage require prompt attention.

ETIOLOGY
Accumulation of cerumen in the ear canal, when mixed with water (as during swimming), acts as a culture medium for bacteria or fungi.

DIAGNOSIS
An otologic examination and a history of symptoms confirms the diagnosis. If a bacterial infection is suspected, a culture of the material found in the canal may be needed to determine how to properly treat the infection.

TREATMENT
It is important for the ear canal to be kept clean and to be dried after swimming. Antibiotic or steroid eardrops and systemic antibiotics may be prescribed, depending on the severity of the condition. Swimmer's ear tends to recur and can become chronic for those with repeated exposure to water as in swimming.

PROGNOSIS
Prognosis is positive with treatment. Swimmer's ear has a tendency to recur with subsequent exposure to water during swimming or other water-related activities.

PREVENTION
Preventive measures include keeping the ear clean and dry. Ear plugs may be used during water activities and swimming. Thorough drying of the ear canal after exposure to water is important.

PATIENT TEACHING
Provide the patient or family with pictures of the anatomy of the ear. Demonstrate how moisture in the ear can contribute to swimmer's ear. Encourage compliance of any drug therapy prescribed.

Otitis Media
DESCRIPTION
Otitis media is inflammation of the normally air-filled middle ear with the accumulation of fluid behind the tympanic membrane (eardrum), occurring either unilaterally or bilaterally.

ICD-9-CM Code 381.4 *(Nonsuppurative otitis media, not specified as either acute or chronic)*
382 *(Suppurative and unspecified otitis media)*
Refer to the physician's diagnosis and then to the current edition of the ICD-9-CM coding manual to ensure the greatest specificity of pathology and any appropriate modifiers.

SYMPTOMS AND SIGNS
Otitis media is the most common reason for visits to physicians by children and also can be experienced by adults.

Otitis media is classified as either serous or suppurative, according to the composition of the accumulating fluid. In serous (nonsuppurative) otitis media, the fluid is relatively clear and sterile. With suppurative otitis, the fluid is purulent. Symptoms vary according to the type. With serous otitis media, the only symptoms may be a feeling of fullness or pressure and some degree of impaired hearing. Suppurative otitis media, however, is painful. General symptoms of infection, fever, chills, nausea, and vomiting usually accompany this type. Children often rub or pull at the affected ear and lean the head sideways toward the affected side. Dizziness can be a symptom in either type. Muffled hearing may be present, or a significant loss of hearing may occur.

PATIENT SCREENING

The febrile individual or child experiencing ear pain and possible diminished hearing requires prompt assessment and pain relief. If it is not possible to see the patient the same day as the initial phone contact, refer the patient to another medical care facility where prompt assessment can be provided.

ETIOLOGY

Serous otitis media may be either acute or chronic. With acute serous otitis media (Fig. 5–21), the cause is usually a virus from a URI that has spread through the eustachian tube into the middle ear. It can occur spontaneously or may result from an allergic reaction. Chronic otitis media (Fig. 5–22) can develop from an acute attack, hypertrophy of the adenoids, or chronic sinus infections. Suppurative otitis media (Fig. 5–23) is caused by bacteria, which also can enter the middle ear through the eustachian tube from the nose or

throat or from a ruptured tympanic membrane. This condition often follows a bout of influenza or mumps. Variations in the normal structure of the eustachian tube can predispose a person to this disease. Often times an allergic response is responsible for swelling of the eustachian tube and the resulting otitis media.

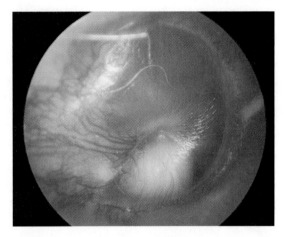

FIGURE 5–22 Chronic otitis media. (From Damjanov I, Linder J: *Pathology: a color atlas,* St. Louis, 1999, Mosby.)

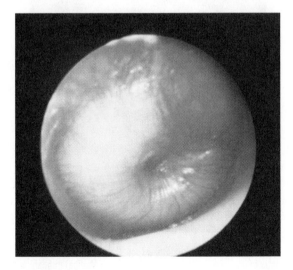

FIGURE 5–21 Acute otitis media. (From Sigler B: *Ear, nose, and throat disorders—Mosby's clinical nursing series,* St. Louis, 1994, Mosby.)

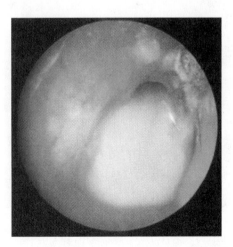

FIGURE 5–23 Suppurative otitis media. (From Sigler B: *Ear, nose, and throat disorders—Mosby's clinical nursing series,* St. Louis, 1994, Mosby.)

DIAGNOSIS

Otoscopy reveals the presence of a fluid-filled middle ear. The normally pearl-gray eardrum (Fig. 5–24) is inflamed and may be bulging. Fluid bubbles may be visible through the membrane. If a culture of the fluid taken from the ear shows bacteria and the *white blood cell (WBC) count* is elevated, suppurative otitis media is present. Audiometry may reveal mild to severe hearing loss. Measurement of the pressure in the middle ear by a tympanogram provides the physician with an estimation of how well the eustachian tube is functioning.

TREATMENT

Analgesics and decongestants may be ordered to provide pain relief and to promote drainage in both types of otitis media. Antibiotics are ordered for cases of suppurative otitis media. In severe cases, or in patients who fail to respond to medical treatment, surgical evacuation of the fluid **(myringotomy)** is necessary to prevent permanent hearing loss and the possible development of mastoiditis (see Mastoiditis) or a cholesteatoma (see Cholesteatoma). To keep the

middle ear air filled and to prevent fluid from accumulating, myringotomy tubes (Fig. 5–25) may need to be inserted after the myringotomy (Fig. 5–26). Diagnosis and treatment of any allergic response involved is necessary. Removal of hypertrophic adenoids is a therapeutic measure.

PROGNOSIS

Prognosis is positive with drug therapy. Otitis media often recurs; thus any indication of returning symptoms requires prompt attention. Surgical intervention with placement of myringotomy tubes usually helps promote a positive outcome. Identification of allergic mediated responses and removal of enlarged adenoids is also helpful for a positive outcome.

PREVENTION

Prompt treatment of upper respiratory infection helps prevent the occurrence of otitis media. When the otitis is a result of an upper respiratory allergic reaction, diagnosis and control of allergic response is helpful, as is the surgical removal of hypertrophied adenoids.

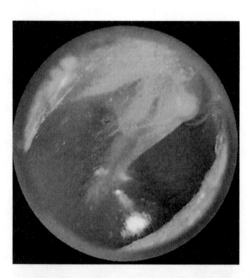

FIGURE 5–24 Normal tympanic membrane. (From Seidel HM et al: *Mosby's guide to physical examination,* ed 5, St. Louis, 2003, Mosby. Courtesy Richard A. Buckingham, Clinical Professor, Otolaryngology, Abraham Lincoln School of Medicine, U of IL, Chicago.)

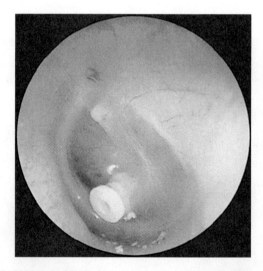

FIGURE 5–25 Myringotomy tube. (From Fireman P, Slavin RG: *Atlas of allergies,* ed 2, London, 1996, Gower Medical Publishing.)

PATIENT TEACHING

If surgery is scheduled, provide patients and family with information regarding the care of the ear with myringotomy tubes in place. Stress the importance of drug therapy compliance and completion of prescribed antibiotic regimen.

Otosclerosis

DESCRIPTION

Otosclerosis primarily affects the stapes or third bone or ossicle of the middle ear as the individual ages. Movement of the ossicles is impaired, which causes diminished conduction of sound waves and resulting hearing loss.

■ **ICD-9-CM Code 387.9** *(Unspecified)*
Designation by the physician of any special circumstances will determine the applicable code. Refer to the physician's diagnosis and then to the current edition of the ICD-9-CM coding manual to ensure the greatest specificity of pathology and any appropriate modifiers.

SYMPTOMS AND SIGNS

With this condition, an abnormal growth of spongy bone forms around the oval window, causing *ankylosis* of the stapes, the third ossicle (small bone) in the middle ear. Ankylosis produces conductive deafness because the ossicles cannot conduct the sound vibrations as they enter the ear. Symptoms of otosclerosis are a gradual hearing loss of low or soft sounds, which may be unilateral at first, but usually affects both ears at some point, and tinnitus. Patients usually report not being able to hear as well with the affected ear when talking on the telephone. Relatives may notice that patients turn their heads to hear better. Otosclerosis is a young person's disease, with

FIGURE 5–26 Myringotomy and insertion of a tympanoplasty tube as a treatment for otitis media.

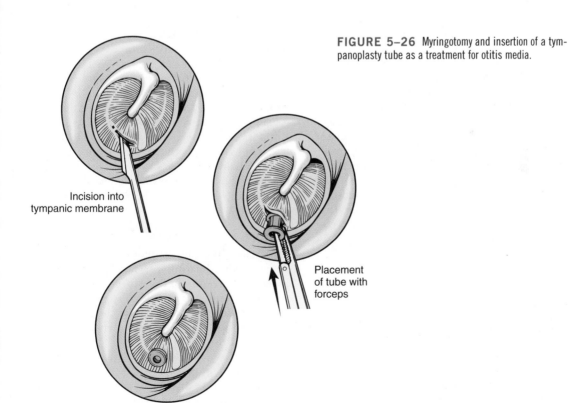

Incision into tympanic membrane

Placement of tube with forceps

Tube in place

onset usually beginning after puberty and before 35 years of age.

PATIENT SCREENING

Individuals requesting an appointment for evaluation of decreased hearing are scheduled for the next available appointment that is convenient for them. It is important to realize that patients experiencing hearing loss may be anxious.

ETIOLOGY

Otosclerosis is *idiopathic,* but there is evidence of familial tendency, suggesting genetic factors. The condition seems to be more prevalent in women and can be aggravated by pregnancy.

DIAGNOSIS

A diagnosis of otosclerosis is made by the physician using an *audiogram,* the patient history, and otoscopy. The audiogram will show a moderate to severe hearing loss, especially for loss in the low range.

TREATMENT

The only treatment that cures otosclerosis is a surgical procedure called a *stapedectomy.* A stapedectomy involves the removal of the diseased stapes and replacement with a prosthesis. The composition of the prosthesis may be metal or a ceramic or plastic material. Use of a ceramic or plastic is likely because these materials facilitate visualization by MRI for the purpose of diagnosing and because of the inability to perform an accurate test of the patient's hearing if the prosthesis is made of metal. If the condition is bilateral, only one ear is operated on at a time so the success of the procedure can be evaluated. Generally, hearing improves soon after the surgery. If surgery is not an option for the patient, a hearing aid can be tried.

PROGNOSIS

Surgical intervention usually has a positive outcome.

PREVENTION

Because this is an idiopathic condition, no method of prevention is known.

PATIENT TEACHING

Provide patients and families with information concerning postsurgical care for surgical interven-

tion. Assist patients and families in locating and contacting community support groups for those with diminished hearing.

Ménière Disease

DESCRIPTION

Ménière disease is a chronic disease of the inner ear that affects the labyrinth.

> **ICD-9-CM Code 386.00** *(Ménière disease, unspecified)*
> *There are specific codes for various states and sites of Ménière disease. Once the physician has established the pathologic evolvement of Ménière disease, refer to the physician's diagnosis and then to the current edition of the ICD-9-CM coding manual to ensure the greatest specificity of pathology and any appropriate modifiers.*

SYMPTOMS AND SIGNS

Ménière disease is marked by a recurring syndrome of vertigo, tinnitus, progressive hearing loss, and a sensation of fullness or pressure in the affected ear. Symptoms have a sudden onset. Nausea, vomiting, sweating, and loss of balance can follow an acute attack of vertigo. These attacks can last from a few hours to several days and may become increasingly serious with each recurrence. Ménière disease usually affects just one ear, but eventually both ears may become involved. The disease usually manifests in individuals between 40 and 50 years of age.

PATIENT SCREENING

Individuals reporting symptoms of vertigo, tinnitus, progressive hearing loss, and the sensation of fullness and pressure in the ear require prompt assessment and intervention. If an appointment time is not immediately available, refer the patient to an emergency facility for evaluation. Suggest that the patient not drive.

ETIOLOGY

The cause of this disease is unknown; however, the disease process seems to involve destruction of the tiny hair cells inside the cochlea. Predisposing factors for Ménière disease are middle ear infections, head trauma, dysfunction in the autonomic nervous system, noise pollution, and premenstrual edema.

DIAGNOSIS

When the four main symptoms are present (recurring vertigo, tinnitus, progressive hearing loss, and a sensation of fullness in the ear), the diagnosis is easy. If symptoms are less obvious or pronounced, additional testing with audiometry, balance studies, radiographic studies including MRI, and ENG (electronystagmography) may be necessary. Electro-cochleograph (EcoG) studies, a recent addition to the available diagnostic techniques, are used to measure inner ear fluid pressure.

TREATMENT

For acute attacks of Ménière disease, the physician usually prescribes medication to control the nausea and vomiting. Long-term treatment could include following a salt-free diet, restricting fluid intake, and using diuretics, antihistamines, anticholinergics and mild sedatives. If the disease does not respond to dietary restrictions and medications, surgical intervention may be needed. Surgical destruction of the affected labyrinth, using ultrasound, relieves the symptoms but also causes permanent hearing loss unless the cochlea is preserved.

PROGNOSIS

No cure for Ménière disease is known. The goal of treatment is to improve or control symptoms. This condition has a tendency to recur.

PREVENTION

At the present time, no etiology has been established, and therefore, no preventive measures have been identified. Prompt treatment of otitis media is a prudent action and hopefully can ameliorate the condition.

PATIENT TEACHING

Provide patients and family with information regarding the condition and its possible outcomes. Assist patients and families with locating and contacting appropriate community resource agencies for those with decreased hearing.

Labyrinthitis

DESCRIPTION

Labyrinthitis is an inflammation or infection of the labyrinth of the inner ear.

 ICD-9-CM Code 386.3
     386.30 *(Labyrinthitis, unspecified)*
Additional digits will be required. Once the physician has designated the pathology and type of labyrinthitis, refer to the physician's diagnosis and then to the current edition of the ICD-9-CM coding manual to ensure the greatest specificity of pathology and any appropriate modifiers.

SYMPTOMS AND SIGNS

The labyrinth is a group of three fluid-filled chambers (the semicircular canals) in the inner ear that control balance (Fig. 5–27). Inflammation or infection of these chambers is called *labyrinthitis*. The onset of infection is often acute and is associated with fever, with temperatures of 100° to 101° F. The main symptom of this disease is extreme vertigo. Balance is affected, and nausea and vomiting may occur in some cases.

PATIENT SCREENING

Individuals reporting sudden onset of fever, vertigo, balance problems, and nausea and vomiting require prompt assessment. Refer the patient to an emergency facility for assessment to rule out a severe neurologic infection.

ETIOLOGY

Labyrinthitis is usually the result of a virus but can be caused by a bacterial infection that has spread from the middle ear. It also may be a result of meningitis.

DIAGNOSIS

The diagnosis of labyrinthitis is based on the results of several tests, including audiometry and blood, neurologic, caloric, and, possibly, imaging studies.

TREATMENT

Bed rest for several days may be necessary. Prescriptions for a tranquilizer, an antiemetic agent, and an antibiotic may be necessary if a

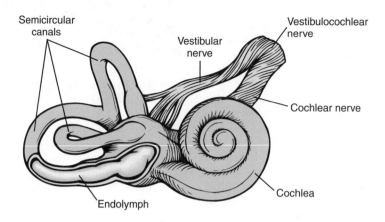

FIGURE 5–27 Labyrinth or inner ear. Labyrinthitis is caused by a disturbance in the fluid in the semicircular canals.

bacterial infection is present. When properly treated, labyrinthitis is not a dangerous condition; however, it can be debilitating, and the labyrinth is a delicate and easily damaged organ.

PROGNOSIS
In most cases, labyrinthitis completely clears up within 1 to 3 weeks; however, a result of bacterial labyrinthitis may be permanent hearing deficiency or loss and/or balance problems.

PREVENTION
Prevention involves prompt medical treatment for otitis media or any other ear infection.

PATIENT TEACHING
Stress the importance to patients and families to seek medical treatment for any type of ear infection. Provide written information about the condition.

Ruptured Tympanic Membrane (Ruptured Eardrum)

DESCRIPTION
Any type of tear or injury to the eardrum causes a breach in the integrity of the membrane. This may be the result of pressure, force, or insult from the exterior aspect, or it may be caused by increased pressure within the middle ear.

ICD-9-CM Code 384.2
                384.20 *(Perforation of tympanic membrane, unspecified)*
Refer to the physician's diagnosis and then to the current edition of the ICD-9-CM coding manual to ensure the greatest specificity of pathology and any appropriate modifiers.

SYMPTOMS AND SIGNS
Symptoms of a ruptured tympanic membrane (eardrum) are usually slight pain and partial loss of hearing and may include a slight discharge or bleeding from the ear. When an infectious process is involved, the drainage usually is purulent in nature. These symptoms may last only a few hours. The major risk is that an infection may develop in the middle ear.

PATIENT SCREENING
Individuals calling with complaints of diminished hearing, pain in the ear, ear infections, history of abrupt force or pressure being incurred, and drainage from the ear require prompt assessment.

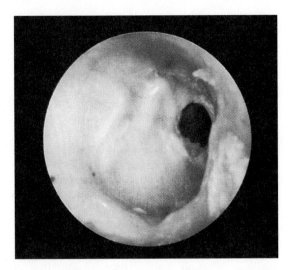

FIGURE 5–28 Ruptured tympanic membrane. (From Sigler B: *Ear, nose, and throat disorders—Mosby's clinical nursing series*, St. Louis, 1994, Mosby.)

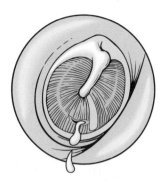

FIGURE 5–29 Ruptured tympanic membrane with purulent discharge.

ETIOLOGY

The four most common causes of a ruptured eardrum are insertion of sharp objects into the ear canal, a nearby explosion (including lightning strikes), a severe middle ear infection, and a blow to the ear. A ruptured eardrum also can occur as a result of a fractured skull. The eardrum occasionally ruptures spontaneously.

DIAGNOSIS

A visual examination of the ear with an otoscope confirms the diagnosis of a ruptured eardrum (Fig. 5–28). Purulent drainage is usually present during an episode of suppurative otitis media complicated by rupture of the tympanic membrane (Fig. 5–29). Audiometry also may be used.

TREATMENT

An antibiotic may be prescribed to prevent infection, and a patch may be applied to the eardrum to aid healing and to improve hearing. This procedure is similar to a **tympanoplasty** (tympanoplasty involves actual grafting of tissue for eardrum repair).

PROGNOSIS

Prognosis is good after treatment of the underlying cause. The eardrum heals naturally in about 1 to 2 weeks. After the eardrum has healed, hearing loss is minimal.

PREVENTION

Prompt intervention in otitis media may help prevent a buildup of pressure in the middle ear. It is not possible to prevent many environmental causes of otitis media.

PATIENT TEACHING

Provide an explanation and demonstration of the mechanism of ruptured tympanic membrane. Encourage patients and families to seek early treatment for otitis media.

Cholesteatoma

DESCRIPTION

A cholesteatoma is a pocket of skin cells, normally shed by the eardrum, that collect into a cyst-like mass or ball and become infected. As the infected material accumulates, the bone lining the middle ear cavity erodes, and the ossicles become damaged.

ICD-9-CM Code 385.3 *(Cholesteatoma of the middle ear and mastoid)*
Cholesteatomas are located at various sites in the ear and therefore have specific ICD-9-CM codes for various sites. Refer to the physician's diagnosis

and then to the current edition of the ICD-9-CM coding manual to ensure the greatest specificity of pathology and any appropriate modifiers.

SYMPTOMS AND SIGNS

The most common symptom of cholesteatoma is a mild to moderate hearing loss. A purulent substance may drain from the affected ear, and earache, headache, vertigo, and some weakness of the facial muscles also may be present.

PATIENT SCREENING

Individuals with cholesteatomas usually have a history of otitis infections and are scheduled for routine reassessments. Often the condition will be recognized during a routine follow-up examination. As with other ear conditions, drainage from the ear and diminished hearing requires prompt assessment. The patient should be scheduled for the next available appointment on the day the patient calls.

ETIOLOGY

This condition begins to develop in infancy. The eustachian tube from the middle ear to the pharynx either fails to open properly or becomes blocked with material from recurring middle ear infections (see Otitis Media). As a result, this normally air-filled chamber develops a weak vacuum, causing the eardrum to become retracted. This forms the pocket in the eardrum that allows the cholesteatoma to develop.

DIAGNOSIS

Patient history, otoscopy, and audiometry enable the physician to make the diagnosis. Radiographic studies also may be useful, and a culture of the purulent drainage may be necessary to determine the most effective antibiotic for treatment.

TREATMENT

If the cholesteatoma is discovered early, before eroding begins, it can be removed fairly simply by a thorough cleaning of the middle ear cavity. Inflation of the eustachian tube may produce some improvement, and treatment with steroids and antibiotics helps to prevent recurrence. If the cholesteatoma is discovered in an advanced stage, its removal becomes much more complicated. Damage to the middle ear structures may be extensive, necessitating surgical reconstruction of these structures. Badly damaged hearing may be improved with the use of a hearing aid. Untreated, a cholesteatoma erodes the roof of the middle ear cavity, making the development of an epidural *abscess* or *meningitis* possible.

PROGNOSIS

Surgical intervention usually leads to a positive outcome.

PREVENTION

Early development of the condition begins in infancy. Prompt attention to otitis infections and problems of eustachian tube drainage helps to delay the onset of this condition. Total prevention is not considered possible.

PATIENT TEACHING

Encourage parents of children with chronic otitis media to schedule routine examinations that include audiology testing. Explain the origin and progression of the condition so families have an understanding of how early intervention can help relieve this condition.

Mastoiditis

DESCRIPTION

Mastoiditis, whether acute or chronic, is inflammation of the mastoid bone, or mastoid process.

ICD-9-CM Code **383.9** *(Unspecified)*
383.0 *(Acute mastoiditis)*
383.1 *(Chronic mastoiditis)*
Refer to the physician's diagnosis and then to the current edition of the ICD-9-CM coding manual to ensure the greatest specificity of pathology and any appropriate modifiers.

SYMPTOMS AND SIGNS

The mastoid is a round process of the temporal bone that can be felt immediately behind each ear and is porous or honeycombed in appearance. Pain and occasionally edema are present over and around the mastoid. Fever and chills may be present. A profuse discharge from the external canal is likely because of the middle ear involvement.

PATIENT SCREENING

Individuals reporting discharge from the ears accompanied by fever, chills, and pain in the mastoid region require prompt assessment. Schedule an appointment that same day or if none is available, refer the patient to a facility where prompt assessment is possible.

ETIOLOGY

Acute mastoiditis is the result of neglected acute otitis media. *Streptococcus* is the usual causative organism, but certain pneumococci and *Staphylococcus aureus* also may be involved. Chronic mastoiditis, necessitating radical or modified radical mastoidectomy, is associated with cholesteatoma.

DIAGNOSIS

The diagnosis is made from patient history, otoscopy, audiometry, radiographic studies of the mastoid, and the results of blood and culture studies.

TREATMENT

The treatment is based on the results of the sensitivity studies. Antibiotic or sulfonamide therapy is prescribed. Mastoiditis not responding to this treatment necessitates a surgical procedure, called *simple mastoidectomy,* to prevent further complications and to preserve hearing. A radical mastoidectomy may be needed for chronic mastoiditis.

PROGNOSIS

Prognosis is variable and depends on the degree of infection, extent of tissue involvement, and response to antibiotic and drug therapy. Surgical intervention usually corrects chronic involvement.

PREVENTION

Because acute mastoiditis is the result of neglected acute otitis media, prompt medical intervention for otitis media is essential in preventing complications.

PATIENT TEACHING

Stress the importance of prompt medical treatment of otitis media as well as completion of prescribed antibiotic regimen.

Sensorineural Hearing Loss

DESCRIPTION

In sensorineural hearing loss (deafness), also often referred to as *occupational hearing loss,* sound waves reach the inner ear but are not perceived because the nerve impulses are not transmitted to the brain.

 ICD-9-CM Code 389.1 *(Sensorineural hearing loss)*
Refer to the physician's diagnosis and then to the current edition of the ICD-9-CM coding manual to ensure the greatest specificity of pathology and any appropriate modifiers.

SYMPTOMS AND SIGNS

Symptoms include tinnitus and partial to severe hearing loss.

PATIENT SCREENING

Sensorineural hearing loss usually has an insidious onset. Many times the hearing loss is detected during a routine medical examination or pre-employment screening. An abrupt onset of hearing loss is possible after sudden exposure to a loud explosive type noise or nearby lightning strike. Consider the anxiety level of these individuals when making an appointment for prompt assessment.

ETIOLOGY

The cause of sensorineural hearing loss is nerve failure or damage to the cochlea or the auditory nerve. This can be the result of the aging process; however, loud music, machinery noise, or sometimes the side effects of medications can cause such damage at any age (Fig. 5–30, *A* and *B* and Table 5–3).

DIAGNOSIS

The patient history and audiometry findings are usually all that is needed to make the diagnosis. Physicians are concerned that sensorineural hearing loss, tinnitus, and vertigo may be symptoms of a space-occupying mass such as a tumor or an aneurysm; therefore, these symptoms are investigated further to rule out such masses.

TREATMENT

Regardless of the amount of damage to the cochlea, steps *must* be taken to prevent further damage. Reducing noise levels by implementing measures such as turning down the volume on loud music and wearing ear protectors at rock concerts or in work areas with high noise levels can prevent further or future damage to the ears.

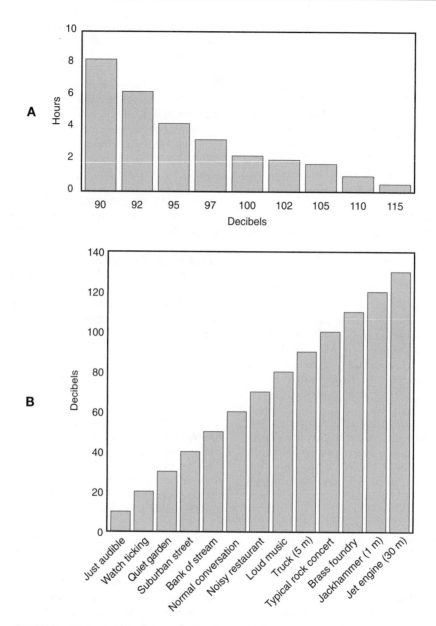

FIGURE 5–30 A, Maximum occupational noise exposure (in hours per day) allowed by U.S. Occupational Safety and Health Administration (OSHA) regulations. **B,** Examples of decibel levels in everyday situations.

PROGNOSIS

Sensorineural hearing loss that is caused by damage to the cochlea is *irreversible*. Prevention is essential.

PREVENTION

No method of preventing hearing loss that results from the aging process is known. Prevention of exposure to constant and extensive loud noise is essential in the prevention of sensorineural hearing loss. Use of ear protection at rock concerts and in work areas with high noise levels is helpful.

PATIENT TEACHING

Provide patients with information about noise pollution and preventive measures that can be taken,

TABLE 5-3
Changes in Hearing Caused by Aging*

CHANGES IN STRUCTURE	CHANGES IN FUNCTION
Cochlear hair cell degeneration	Inability to hear high-frequency sounds (presbycusis, sensorineural loss); interferes with understanding speech; hearing may be lost in both ears at different times
Loss of auditory neurons in spiral ganglia of organ of Corti	Inability to hear high-frequency sounds (presbycusis, sensorineural loss); interferes with understanding speech; hearing may be lost in both ears at different times
Degeneration of basilar (cochlear) conductive membrane of cochlea	Inability to hear at all frequencies but more pronounced at higher frequencies (cochlear conductive loss)
Decreased vascularity of cochlea	Equal loss of hearing at all frequencies (strial loss); inability to disseminate localization of sound
Loss of cortical auditory neurons	Equal loss of hearing at all frequencies (strial loss); inability to disseminate localization of sound

From McCance KL, Huether SE: *Pathophysiology: the biological basis for disease in adults and children,* ed 4, St. Louis, 2002, Mosby.
*Hearing loss affects about one third of older people.

including wearing ear protection when exposure to loud noise is possible. Stress the importance of avoiding high volume on the radio or other audio equipment. Discuss sources of every day noise pollution.

Cancer of the Ear

DESCRIPTION

Tumors of the ear can occur in any part of the ear and may be benign or malignant. They include the cutaneous tumors of the external ear, cerumenal gland neoplasms, acoustic and facial neuromas, and glomus tumors. Many cancers from other locations in the body may metastasize to the ear, resulting in secondary ear cancer.

ICD-9-CM Code **239.2** *(Neoplasms of the ear, unspecified)*
171.0 *(Cartilage of ear, primary malignancy)*
198.89 *(Other specific sites, secondary malignant neoplasm)*

Neoplasms of the ear must be specified for location and type. Therefore it is not possible to list all applicable ICD-9-CM codes for neoplasms of the ear. Refer to the physician's diagnosis and then to the current edition of the ICD-9-CM coding manual to ensure the greatest specificity of pathology and any appropriate modifiers.

SYMPTOMS AND SIGNS

Symptoms of these neoplasms commonly include progressive hearing loss, chronic otic discharge, a visible mass or lesion on ear examination, loss of equilibrium, and tinnitus. Some cancers, such as squamous cell carcinoma of the middle ear, are quite painful. Glomus tumors cause a pulsatile tinnitus, that is, hearing a pulsing sound in the ear that has the tumor as a result of the tumor pressing on the bones of hearing.

PATIENT SCREENING

Symptoms may have an insidious onset with recognition of diminished hearing being thought of as troublesome rather than an acute symptom. Drainage from the ear, loss of equilibrium, and tinnitus require prompt assessment. Schedule patients with these symptoms for the next available appointment on the day of call. It is also important to consider the anxiety experienced by these patients and their families with the onset of this type of symptomology.

ETIOLOGY

Benign tumors of the ear include acoustic neuromas, facial neuromas, and glomus tumors. Acoustic neuroma arises from the eighth cranial nerve, whereas facial neuroma is a tumor of the facial nerve. These tumors put pressure on the nerve fibers as they expand, causing hearing loss or facial paralysis, respectively, among other symptoms. Glomus tumors are the most common tumors of the middle ear and arise from the glomus bodies (tiny structures that serve as baroreceptors).

The most common malignant tumors of the external ear are the skin cancers, basal cell carcinoma (BCC) and squamous cell carcinoma (SCC). BCCs are more common and usually begin as a circular raised area of skin with a central, crater-like ulceration. They are slow growing and often are caused by years of sun exposure. SCC lesions may look like BCC in the early stages, but SCC grows faster and is more aggressive (see Chapter 6 for further discussion of these skin cancers). Another type of tumor found in the external auditory canal is the cerumenal gland neoplasm—a tumor arising from the glands producing cerumen—which can be either malignant or benign. Malignant tumors of the middle ear are very uncommon. Squamous cell carcinoma may arise in this location because of chronic inflammation of the middle ear or mastoid.

DIAGNOSIS

Tumors of the ear are often first identified because of the symptoms they cause. Examination of the ear may reveal a BCC or SCC lesion, a mass in the external ear canal, or evidence of one of the other neoplasms. Biopsy is often performed to confirm the nature of the lesion, and CT scan and MRI are used to evaluate the extent of disease.

TREATMENT

Treatment for all of these tumors is surgical excision. Radiation therapy is used if the tumor is known to be aggressive. A nerve graft may be performed after surgical excision of a neuroma.

PROGNOSIS

Prognosis for many of these tumors is good after the patient receives appropriate treatment. However, SCC of the middle ear has a very poor prognosis because it is often at an advanced stage at the time of diagnosis.

PREVENTION

No methods for prevention of most ear neoplasms are known. The skin cancers of the external ear may be prevented by reducing sun exposure to that area.

PATIENT TEACHING

Encourage patients to be compliant with prescribed therapy. Provide information for postoperative care of any surgical excision site.

REVIEW CHALLENGE

Answer the following questions:

1. How does the process of normal vision take place?
2. What are the four main errors of refraction?
3. What is the difference between nystagmus and strabismus?
4. Name a common etiologic factor in hordeolum and blepharitis.
5. What are the pressing symptoms and signs of conjunctivitis? Is the condition contagious?
6. Name some possible causes of corneal abrasions.
7. How do cataracts interfere with vision?
8. Differentiate between the two primary types of glaucoma.
9. How is diabetic retinopathy detected and treated?
10. Explain the pathology involved in retinal detachment. How is this condition treated?
11. What are the possible causes of exophthalmos?
12. What is the primary symptom of refractive errors?
13. Name the etiologic factors of macular degeneration.
14. What is the best way to help control diabetic retinopathy?
15. Describe some ways cancer can affect the eye and adjacent structures.
16. Describe the three separate parts of the ear.
17. How does impacted cerumen cause deafness?
18. Precisely define otitis media. How is it classified? How is it diagnosed?
19. What is myringotomy?
20. What symptoms may an individual with Ménière disease experience?
21. Name the major symptom of labyrinthitis.
22. List common causes of a ruptured eardrum.
23. What causes occupational deafness?

REAL-LIFE CHALLENGE

Acute Angle-Closure Glaucoma

A 61-year-old man presents with sudden onset of blurred vision, head and eye pain, and nausea and vomiting. Upon questioning, he admits to seeing "halos" around lights and being especially sensitive to light. The physician examination confirms blurred vision and photosensitivity. Intraocular pressure (IOP) measures greater than 20 mm Hg on the tonometer.

The patient is diagnosed with acute angle-closure glaucoma and referred to an ophthalmologist for immediate treatment.

QUESTIONS

1. Compare the symptoms of chronic open-angle glaucoma and acute angle-closure glaucoma.
2. Compare the reason for a buildup of IOP in chronic open-angle glaucoma and acute angle-closure glaucoma.
3. What history would suggest this patient is at risk for glaucoma?
4. Which type of treatment would you expect the ophthalmologist to institute?
5. If this were chronic open-angle glaucoma, which types of medications would you expect to be prescribed?
6. How would these medications help to treat the disorder?
7. What is the danger of untreated glaucoma?

REAL-LIFE CHALLENGE

Otitis Media

A 18-month-old male child has been brought to the physician's office by his parents, who say that he has been fussy and crying for the last 10 hours. The mother says she is having difficulty getting him to eat and she has noticed he sits with his head held to the right side. He has a history of a cold in the past few days with a runny nose and watering eyes.

Examination reveals a temperature of 103° F, pulse of 116, and respirations of 32. The otoscopic examination was used to evaluate the condition of the tympanic membranes. The physician examined the left ear first, a method employed to see what the asymptomatic ear looked like. It revealed a normal translucent pearl-gray tympanic membrane. Examination of the right or symptomatic ear disclosed a red, bulging eardrum. The mucous membrane of the nasal passages appeared inflamed, as did the back of the throat.

An antibiotic (amoxicillin trihydrate [Amoxil] 125 mg qid × 10 days) was prescribed. The parents were instructed to give acetaminophen or ibuprofen (Motrin) for a temperature greater than 101° F and to call if the fever and pain persisted beyond 24 hours. The child was scheduled for a follow-up visit in 1 week.

QUESTIONS

1. Why is it important to note that the child sits with his head held to the side?
2. What effect does the elevated temperature have on the other vital signs?
3. Why did the physician examine the left eardrum first?
4. What patient teaching would you offer the parents about the medication suggested for the elevated temperature?
5. What patient teaching would you offer the parents about the antibiotics?
6. Why are treatment and follow-up important?
7. Which surgical procedure may be indicated?
8. What long-term effects may the child experience if the otitis does not respond to treatment?

INTERNET ASSIGNMENTS

1. Research facts about aging and vision by exploring the website of the American Foundation for the Blind (AFB). Choose a subject that considers older individuals and vision loss.
2. Visit the National Institute on Deafness and Other Communication Disorders website, choose the *News and Events* option, and research a current subject such as new state guidelines for screening infant hearing.
3. Research a current topic, such as the danger of using illegal contact lenses, by visiting the American Academy of Ophthalmology website.

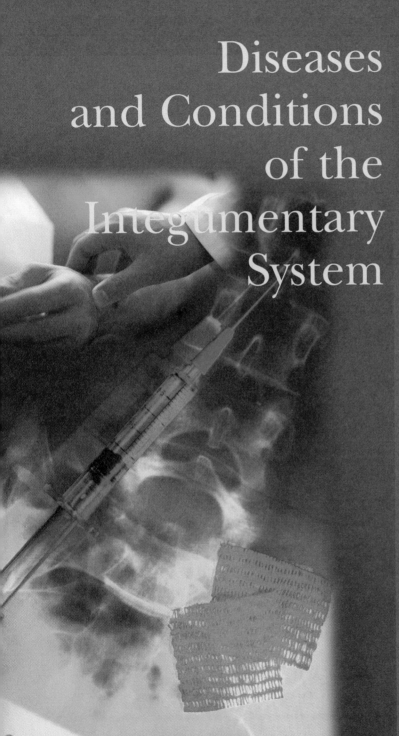

CHAPTER 6

Diseases and Conditions of the Integumentary System

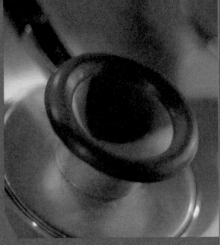

Chapter Outline

Continued

Orderly Functioning of the Integumentary System

Chapter Outline—Cont'd

Learning Objectives

After studying Chapter 6, you should be able to:

1. Explain the functions of the skin.
2. Recognize common skin lesions.
3. Describe how seborrheic dermatitis affects the skin.
4. Discuss the possible causes of contact dermatitis, atopic dermatitis, and psoriasis.
5. Describe the treatment of acne vulgaris.
6. Explain the pathologic course of herpes zoster.
7. Name the etiology of impetigo.
8. Explain why the treatment of cellulitis is important.
9. Cite examples of the classifications of fungal infections of the skin.
10. List preventive measures for decubitus ulcers.
11. Name the two most common parasitic insects to infest man. Describe how infestation can occur.
12. Name two common premalignant tumors.
13. Differentiate the three types of skin cancer.
14. Describe the guidelines for avoiding excessive sun exposure.
15. List some conditions that are caused by the abnormal development or distribution of melanocytes.
16. Name some possible causes of alopecia.
17. State the cause of warts.
18. List some of the likely causes of deformed or discolored nails.

Key Terms

bulla (**BUL**–la)
cellulitis (sell–you–**LIE**–tis)
comedo (**KOM**–ee–doe)
debride (dah–**BREED**)
dermatome (**DER**–mah–tome)
electrodesiccation (ee–leck–tro–**des**–ih–**KA**–shun)
erythema (**eh**–rih–**THEE**–ma)
exudate (**EKS**–you–date)
exudative (**EKS**–you–**day**–tive)
fissure (**FIS**–ur)

keratolytic (ker–ah–toe–**LIT**–ik)
keratosis (ker–ah–**TOE**–sis)
nevus (**NEE**–vus)
papule (**PAP**–youl)
plaques (plaks)
sebaceous (seh–**BAY**–shus)
vesicle (**VES**–ih–kl)
vesicular (veh–**SIK**–you–lar)
wheal (**WHEEL**)

ORDERLY FUNCTIONING
OF THE INTEGUMENTARY SYSTEM

THE SYSTEM COMPRISING the skin and its accessory organs (hair, nails, and glands) is called the integumentary system. The skin, one of the largest organs, protects the body from trauma, infections, and toxic chemicals. When exposed to sunlight, the skin synthesizes vitamin D. Within the skin are millions of tiny nerve endings called receptors. These receptors sense touch, pressure, pain, and temperature. In addition to the skin's roles in protection, sensation, and synthesis of vitamin D, it assists in the regulation of body temperature and in excretion.

The skin has three main structural layers (Fig. 6–1). The epidermis (outer layer) is a thin, cellular, multilayered membrane that is responsible for the production of *keratin* and *melanin*. The dermis, or corium (middle layer), is a dense, fibrous layer of connective tissue that gives skin its strength and elasticity. Within the dermis are blood and lymph vessels, nerve fibers, hair follicles, and sweat and **sebaceous** glands. Third is the subcutaneous layer, a thick, fat-containing section that insulates the body against heat loss.

Skin diseases frequently are manifested by cutaneous lesions, or alterations of the skin surface (Table 6–1). The diagnosis of a cutaneous disease often is based on the appearance of a specific type of lesion or group of lesions (Fig. 6–2).

Common presenting symptoms that need attention from health-care professionals include:
- Cutaneous lesions or eruptions
- Pruritus (itching)
- Pain
- Edema (swelling)
- **Erythema** (redness)
- Inflammation

Many skin conditions are known to be aggravated by stress. Cosmetically, the skin is important to appearance. Much time and money is spent pursuing "beauty" and disguising the aging of the skin. Patients with skin conditions may feel anxious about their appearance. The treatment of many skin diseases is tedious, requiring strict compliance. Patient education and psychological support reduce the patient's anxiety and encourage good adherence to the treatment plan.

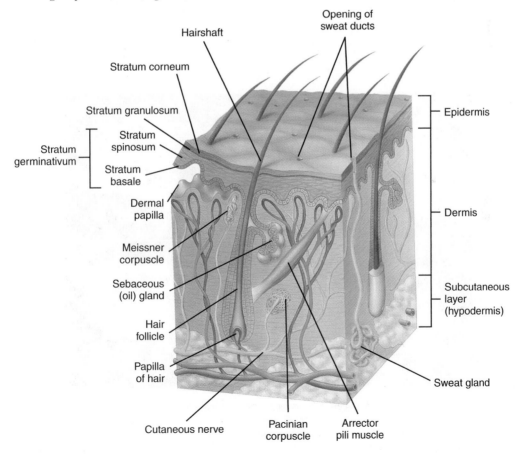

FIGURE 6–1 Normal skin. (From Patton KT, Thibodeau GA: *Mosby's handbook of anatomy and physiology*, St. Louis, 2000, Mosby.)

TABLE 6–1
Description of Some Skin Lesions

Macule	Small, flat circumscribed lesion of a different color than the normal skin
Papule	Small, firm, elevated lesion
Nodule	Palpable elevated lesion; varies in size
Pustule	Elevated, erythematous lesion, usually containing purulent exudate
Vesicle	Elevated, thin-walled lesion containing clear fluid (blister)
Plaque	Large, slightly elevated lesion with flat surface, often topped by scale
Crust	Dry, rough surface or dried exudate or blood
Lichenification	Thick, dry, rough surface (leather-like)
Keloid	Raised, irregular, and increasing mass of collagen resulting from excessive scar tissue formation
Fissure	Small, deep, linear crack or tear in skin
Ulcer	Cavity with loss of tissue from the epidermis and dermis, often weeping or bleeding
Erosion	Shallow, moist cavity in epidermis
Comedone	Mass of sebum, keratin, and debris blocking the opening of a hair follicle

From Gould, B: *Pathophysiology for the health professions,* ed 2, Philadelphia, 2002, Saunders.

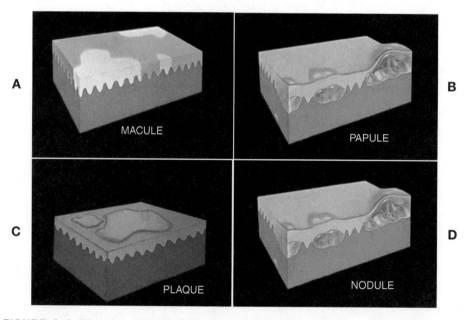

A, MACULE
B, PAPULE
C, PLAQUE
D, NODULE

FIGURE 6–2 Skin lesions. **A,** Macule. A flat, colored lesion that may be white (hypopigmented), brown (hyperpigmented), or red (erythematous and purpuric). **B,** Papule. A small elevated lesion less than 0.5 cm in diameter. **C,** Plaque. A plateau-like elevated lesion greater than 0.5 cm in diameter. **D,** Nodule. A marble-like lesion greater than 0.5 cm in depth and diameter.

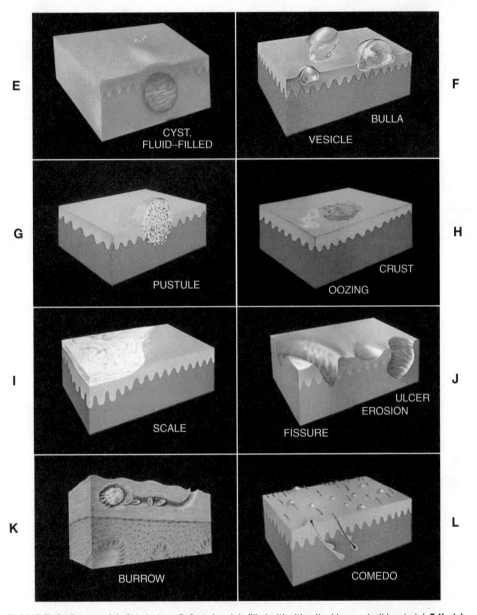

FIGURE 6-2, cont'd Skin lesions. **E,** Cyst. A nodule filled with either liquid or semisolid material. **F, Vesicle** and **bulla.** Blisters containing clear fluid. Vesicles are less than 0.5 cm in diameter, and bullae are greater than 0.5 cm in diameter. **G,** Pustule. A vesicle containing purulent or cloudy fluid. **H,** Crust. Liquid debris dried on the skin's surface, resulting from ruptured vesicles, pustules, or bullae. **I,** Scale. A thickened outer layer of skin that is dry and whitish colored. **J,** Fissure, erosion, and ulcer. A **fissure** is a thin tear. An erosion is a wide but shallow fissure. An ulcer involves the epidermis and dermis. **K,** Burrow. A tunnel or streak caused by a burrowing organism. **L,** Comedo. A lesion of acne. (From Lookingbill D, Marks J: *Principles of dermatology,* ed 3, Philadelphia, 2000, Saunders.)

Dermatitis

Dermatitis

Inflammation of the skin, or dermatitis, occurs in many types or forms. They all are manifested by pruritus, erythema, and the appearance of various cutaneous lesions. The more common forms are seborrheic dermatitis, contact dermatitis, and atopic dermatitis (eczema). All forms of dermatitis can be acute, subacute, or chronic.

Seborrheic Dermatitis

DESCRIPTION

Seborrheic dermatitis, one of the most common skin disorders, is an inflammatory condition of the sebaceous, or oil, glands.

■ **ICD-9-CM Code** **690.10** *(Seborrheic dermatitis, unspecified)*
690.11 *(Seborrhea capitis) (cradle cap)*
690.12 *(Seborrheic infantile dermatitis)*
690.18 *(Other seborrheic dermatitis)*

SYMPTOMS AND SIGNS

Seborrheic dermatitis is marked by a gradual increase in the amount of, and a change in the quality of, the *sebum* produced by the sebaceous glands. The inflammation occurs in areas with the greatest number of sebaceous glands. These include the scalp, eyebrows, eyelids, sides of the nose, the area behind the ears, and the middle of the chest. Affected skin is reddened and covered by yellowish, greasy-appearing scales (Fig. 6–3). Itching may occur but is usually mild.

Seborrheic dermatitis can occur at any age but is most common during infancy, when it is called cradle cap. Cradle cap usually clears without treatment by 8 to 12 months of age. Seborrheic dermatitis occurs at a higher rate in adults with disorders of the central nervous system, such as Parkinson disease. Patients who are recovering from stressful medical conditions, such as a myocardial infarction (heart attack); patients who have been confined to hospitals or nursing homes for long stays; and those who have immune system disorders such as acquired immunodeficiency syndrome (AIDS) appear to be more prone to this dis-

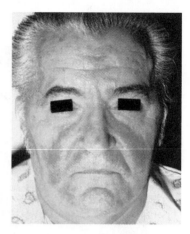

FIGURE 6–3 Seborrheic dermatitis. (From Lookingbill D, Marks J: *Principles of dermatology*, ed 3, Philadelphia, 2000, Saunders.)

order. More intense forms of seborrheic dermatitis can be seen in patients with psoriasis (see Psoriasis). Mild forms are mainly cosmetic problems that can be easily treated or may disappear spontaneously.

PATIENT SCREENING

This condition has a gradual onset. The irritation becomes troublesome, and the patient or parent calls to request an appointment. Schedule the patient to be seen at the earliest convenient time or next available appointment.

ETIOLOGY

This condition is *idiopathic;* however, heredity may predispose an individual to the condition, and emotional stress may be a precipitating factor. Evidence suggests that this skin disorder may be perpetuated or intensified by the yeast-like organism, *Pityrosporum,* which is normally found on the skin in small numbers. Whether diet or food allergies play a role in the development of seborrheic dermatitis in infants is still unknown.

DIAGNOSIS

In most patients, blood, urine, or allergy tests are not necessary. In the rare case of chronic seborrheic dermatitis that does not respond to treatment, a skin *biopsy* or more extensive testing may be performed to rule out the possibility of another disease.

TREATMENT

One of the more effective methods of treatment is the use of a low-strength cortisone or hydro-cortisone cream, applied topically to the affected area. *Caution:* Prolonged use of these medications should be avoided because of the possible side effects of using steroids. When the scalp is involved, causing dandruff, the frequent use of nonprescription shampoos containing tar, zinc pyrithione, selenium sulfide, sulfur, and salicylic acid also is recommended. Patients not responding to these treatments should consult a dermatologist who can prescribe stronger medications.

PROGNOSIS

Most episodes will resolve with treatment. Those who do not respond positively should be referred to a dermatologist for additional drug therapy. Whether treated or not, this condition tends to recur.

PREVENTION

No known prevention is known.

PATIENT TEACHING

Teach the patient to properly apply the prescribed medication. For infants with cradle cap, instruct parents to shampoo the scalp daily and possibly apply gentle massage to the area with a toothbrush.

Contact Dermatitis

DESCRIPTION

Contact dermatitis is an acute inflammation of the skin.

ICD-9-CM Code 692

Contact dermatitis has more than one form and therefore more than one ICD-9-CM code. The general code is 692. Refer to the physician's diagnosis and then to the current edition of the ICD-9-CM coding manual to ensure the greatest specificity of pathology and any appropriate modifiers. A list of some of the specific codes follows.

> *Contact dermatitis:*
> **692.0** *(Due to detergents)*
> **692.1** *(Due to oils and greases)*
> **692.2** *(Due to solvents)*
> **692.3** *(Due to drugs and medicines in contact with skin)*
> **692.4** *(Due to chemical products)*

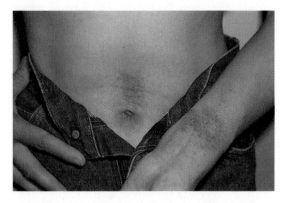

FIGURE 6–4 Contact dermatitis. (From Lookingbill D, Marks J: *Principles of dermatology,* ed 3, Philadelphia, 2000, Saunders.)

> **692.5** *(Due to food in contact with skin)*
> **692.6** *(Due to plants, except food)*
> **692.72** *(Due to solar radiation)*
> **692.8** *(Due to other specified agents)*
> **692.9** *(Unspecified cause)*

SYMPTOMS AND SIGNS

Contact dermatitis is caused either by the action of irritants on the skin's surface or by contact with a substance that causes an allergic reaction. Symptoms include erythema, edema, and small vesicles that ooze, itch, burn, or sting (Fig. 6–4).

PATIENT SCREENING

The patient reporting symptoms of contact dermatitis will feel the characteristic itching, burning, and stinging. These patients should be scheduled at the earliest possible time the same day they call. If this is not possible, the prudent step for patient comfort is to refer the patient to another facility.

ETIOLOGY

Many substances can induce contact dermatitis, including plants such as poison ivy, oak, or sumac. Poison ivy may be spread as an airborne irritant by burning plants. Other irritants are dyes used in soaps and facial and toilet tissue, other dyes, latex, furs, preservatives, drugs, detergents, cleaning compounds, cosmetics, chemicals, acids, and certain metals (e.g., nickel) used to make jewelry. Solar radiation and other forms of radiation, including exposure through a tanning bed, may cause the dermatitis. If an irritant remains in constant contact with the skin, the dermatitis spreads.

Contact dermatitis develops in three ways.

First, it can develop through irritation, either chemical or mechanical, such as by latex gloves and wool fibers. If the irritant is strong, a single exposure may cause a severe inflammatory reaction.

Second, contact dermatitis may develop by sensitization. This means that the first contact with a substance causes no immediate inflammation. However, after the skin becomes sensitized, future contact or exposure results in inflammation.

Third, another interesting but uncommon mechanism for the development of this form of dermatitis is photoallergy. Some chemicals found in perfumes, soaps, suntan lotions containing *para*-aminobenzoic acid, or medications (e.g., tetracycline) can sensitize the skin to sunlight. The next time the individual uses the products and is exposed to sunlight, a rash develops.

DIAGNOSIS

Diagnosis of a contact dermatitis is based on the appearance of the affected area, a medical history, including prior outbreaks and their locations; and identification of the specific irritant or allergen with a *patch test*.

TREATMENT

If a patient has come in contact with a known irritant, thoroughly cleaning the skin surface should be the first step. This should be followed by the topical application of a steroid cream. An oral steroid such as methylprednisolone (Medrol) may be prescribed for 6 days, with a decreasing dosage. Some physicians believe that 6 days is typically not a long enough treatment for many contact dermatitis conditions. Poison plant dermatitis nearly always needs at least 12 days of medication. Sometimes dermatitis rebounds after short-course steroids.

PROGNOSIS

The prognosis varies depending on the amount of skin area involved as well as the likelihood that the causative agent can be removed. The response to drug therapy is usually positive when combined with removal of the offending substance.

PREVENTION

Identification of the offending or causative substance is primary in preventing recurrences. After the substance is identified, contact must be avoided. Should accidental contact occur, immediate intervention by removing the source and seeking drug therapy may reduce the intensity of the condition.

PATIENT TEACHING

Encourage patients to avoid substances or situations that trigger contact dermatitis. Give information about proper methods of cleansing the skin after contact with offending substances. Instruct patients to refrain from scratching affected skin to prevent additional damage or infection from developing in the skin tissue.

Atopic Dermatitis (Eczema)

DESCRIPTION

Atopic dermatitis (eczema) is an inflammation of the skin that tends to occur in patients with a family history of allergic conditions.

 ICD-9-CM Code 691.8

SYMPTOMS AND SIGNS

A rash, with **vesicular** and **exudative** eruptions in children and dry, leathery vesicles in adults, develops (Figs. 6–5 and 6–6). The rash occurs in a characteristic pattern on the face, neck, elbows, knees, and upper trunk of the body and is accompanied by pruritus.

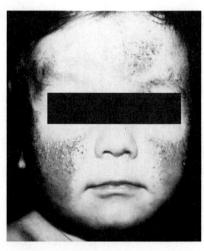

FIGURE 6–5 Infantile atopic dermatitis. (From Zitelli BJ, Davis HW: *Atlas of pediatric physical diagnosis*, ed 4, St. Louis, 2002, Mosby.)

PATIENT SCREENING

When the individual calls for an appointment, consider the discomfort he or she is experiencing and schedule the patient to be seen at the earliest possible time. If a prompt appointment is not possible, referral is indicated.

ETIOLOGY

Eczema is an idiopathic disease. The tendency of this condition to develop is inherited, and an allergic connection is assumed. Eczema in some infants is believed to be traceable to sensitivity to milk, orange juice, or some other foods.

A flare-up of eczema can be triggered by stress, anxiety, or conflict. Stress actually can make the condition worse. Climate, especially sudden or extreme changes in temperature, can affect or aggravate the condition. High humidity also may aggravate eczema.

Eczema in infants usually subsides by the age of 2 years. The rash may resolve during adolescence or persist into adulthood. Eczema generally tends to improve with time.

DIAGNOSIS

A medical history, including family history, along with examination of the skin, confirms the diagnosis. Skin testing for specific allergies occasionally is indicated to identify underlying causes.

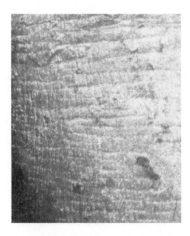

FIGURE 6–6 Atopic dermatitis. (From Lookingbill D, Marks J: *Principles of dermatology,* ed 3, Philadelphia, 2000, Saunders.)

TREATMENT

The main objective in treating atopic dermatitis is reducing the frequency and severity of eruptions and relieving the pruritus. Unfortunately, no medications can eliminate eczema. Topical ointments and creams containing a cortisone derivative are the primary treatment for eczema. In addition, two new agents, Protopic (tacrolimus) and Elidel (pimecrolimus), are prescribed specifically to treat eczema. Local and systemic medications, such as antihistamines, tranquilizers, and other sedatives, may be prescribed to prevent or control the pruritus. Secondary bacterial or viral infections can result from scratching of the rash or lesions. A secondary bacterial infection is the most common complication. The physician usually prescribes an antibiotic to control the infection. A more serious complication of eczema can be caused by infection with certain viruses, especially herpes simplex virus.

PROGNOSIS

Reducing the frequency and severity of eruptions and relieving pruritus is a positive outcome. There is no cure, and eczema cannot be eliminated by medication. Medications are prescribed to control the itch-scratch cycle that aggravates the condition. Many occurrences resolve spontaneously but recur later.

PREVENTION

As an idiopathic disease with a tendency to be inherited and possibly with an allergic connection, eczema has no known prevention. One should attempt to prevent the secondary bacterial or viral infections that result from scratching of the rash or lesions.

PATIENT TEACHING

Teach the patient the importance of not scratching the involved area. In young adults and older people, explain how scratching irritates the condition.

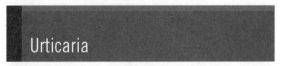

Urticaria

DESCRIPTION

Urticaria, or hives, is associated with severe itching followed by the appearance of redness and an area of swelling **(wheal)** in a localized area of skin (Fig. 6–7).

ICD-9-CM Code 708

Urticaria has more than one form and therefore more than one ICD-9-CM code. The general code for urticaria is 708. Refer to the physician's diagnosis and then to the current edition of the ICD-9-CM coding manual to ensure the greatest specificity of pathology and any appropriate modifiers. Some of the specific codes follow.

708.0 *(Allergic urticaria)*
708.1 *(Idiopathic urticaria)*
708.2 *(Urticaria due to cold and heat)*
708.3 *(Dermatographic urticaria)*
708.4 *(Vibratory urticaria)*
708.5 *(Cholinergic urticaria)*
708.8 *(Other specified urticaria)*
708.9 *(Urticaria, unspecified)*

SYMPTOMS AND SIGNS

Hives of various sizes can erupt as a few lesions anywhere on the skin and often are scattered over the body or mucous membrane. In gastrointestinal involvement, the patient complains of abdominal colic. When hives develop in the pharyngeal mucosa, the airway can become obstructed, causing asphyxiation. When the swelling involves deeper tissues, the condition is called *angioedema* and is more serious. Urticaria is common, often acute, and self-limiting, lasting a few hours. In other cases, hives continue over months or years, becoming a chronic condition.

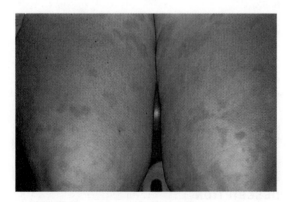

FIGURE 6–7 Urticaria. (From Murphy GF, Herzberg AJ: *Atlas of dermatopathology,* Philadelphia, 1996, Saunders.)

PATIENT SCREENING

Hives can develop into a life-threatening condition if they involve the respiratory system. Anyone experiencing respiratory difficulties should be brought into the emergency medical system for immediate assessment and intervention. Cutaneous symptoms make the individual very uncomfortable, and the patient should be seen immediately or referred to another facility for prompt assessment.

ETIOLOGY

Urticaria affects the dermis and results from an acute hypersensitivity and the release of histamine. This causes local inflammation and vasodilation of capillaries with marked edema. Allergic reactions to foods (such as shellfish, strawberries, or peanuts), drugs (such as penicillin), or insect stings (frequently from a bee) are some common causes. Infection can cause an attack of hives, as can some inhalants, sunlight, and temperature extremes. Sometimes the cause is not identified.

DIAGNOSIS

Visual inspection of the urticaria is diagnostic. A prior episode in conjunction with a particular exposure to a known allergen is significant in the patient's history. If the medical history is void of clues to the cause, sensitivity testing and blood tests for antibodies may help distinguish the causative agent.

TREATMENT

If known, the antigenic factor is removed and then avoided if possible. Antihistamines bring quick relief of symptoms. An injection of epinephrine is used in more severe cases. In persistent cases, a course of prednisone is therapeutic.

PROGNOSIS

Immediate drug therapy usually resolves the allergic response, and the hives disappear. Another exposure to the same allergen will probably elicit the same response, so the triggering allergen must be avoided.

PREVENTION

Prevention depends on identifying the offending allergen and avoiding it.

PATIENT TEACHING

Teach patients the importance of avoiding the causative allergen and seeking proper and prompt medical intervention in the recurrence of the condition.

Psoriasis

DESCRIPTION

Psoriasis is a chronic skin condition marked by thick, flaky, red patches of various sizes, covered with characteristic white, silvery scales (Fig. 6–8).

ICD-9-CM Code **696.1** *(Psoriasis NOS)*
696.0 *(Psoriasis arthropathy)*
696.2 *(Parapsoriasis)*
Psoriasis has more than one form and therefore more than one ICD-9-CM code. The general code for psoriasis is 696. Refer to the physician's diagnosis and then to the current edition of the ICD-9-CM coding manual to ensure the greatest specificity of pathology and any appropriate modifiers.

SYMPTOMS AND SIGNS

Psoriasis is an inflammatory chronic and recurrent skin condition with silvery scales. These scales develop into dry **plaques** (see Fig. 6–2, *C*), sometimes progressing to *pustules* (see Fig. 6–2, *G*). They usually do not cause discomfort but might be slightly itchy or sore. Affected skin typically appears dry, cracked, and encrusted. The most common areas in which psoriasis develops are the scalp; the outer sides of the arms and legs, especially the elbows and knees; and the trunk of the body. In addition, the palms of the hands and soles of the feet may be affected. In some patients, psoriasis spreads to the nail beds, causing the nails to thicken and crumble. Psoriasis can occur at any age but is more common between 10 and 30 years of age. It is noninfectious and does not affect general health.

PATIENT SCREENING

Symptoms of psoriasis are troublesome. The patient calling for an appointment for these symptoms should be scheduled for the next convenient appointment.

ETIOLOGY

The cause of psoriasis is unknown, but it seems to be genetically determined. Psoriasis may be an *autoimmune* disorder and is more common among the white race. Precipitating factors for the development of psoriasis include hormonal changes such as those occurring with pregnancy, climate changes, emotional stress, and a period of generally poor health.

DIAGNOSIS

The white, silvery scales of psoriasis are recognizable, making the condition easy to diagnose. A careful patient history, observation of the skin, or a skin biopsy may help when the scales are not evident, as with patients who bathe and scrub frequently. Scratching the lesions reveals the telltale scales.

TREATMENT

The goal of treatment is to reduce inflammation and to slow the rapid growth of skin cells that cause the condition. Keeping the involved skin moist and lubricated is beneficial. Treatment options include exposure to ultraviolet light to help to retard cell reproduction, the use of steroid creams (methoxsalen) in combination with ultraviolet light, the application of coal tar preparations, the administration of low-dosage antihistamines, and oatmeal baths. Severe cases of psoriasis may require chemotherapy with methotrexate or the use of etretinate, which is related to vitamin A. *Caution:* Pregnant women and nursing mothers should never take etretinate. Antibiotics also may be prescribed.

PROGNOSIS

No cure for psoriasis is known, but it is controllable. Remissions and *exacerbations* occur often, and the condition may require treatment for a lifetime.

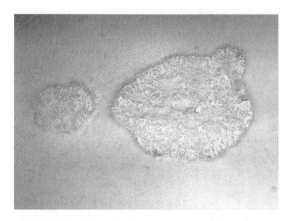

FIGURE 6–8 Psoriasis. (From Lookingbill D, Marks J: *Principles of dermatology,* ed 3, Philadelphia, 2000, Saunders.)

Advise patients to consider counseling for stress reduction because stress may cause recurrence of the disorder.

PREVENTION

With no identifiable etiology, no prevention is known. Keeping the skin moist and lubricated, avoiding cold, dry climates, avoiding stress and anxiety, limiting alcohol intake, and not scratching and picking the skin help to prevent recurrence of the condition.

PATIENT TEACHING

Explain the concept of exposure to ultraviolet light and methods of timing the exposure. Demonstrate application of steroid creams, coal tar preparations, and other skin creams.

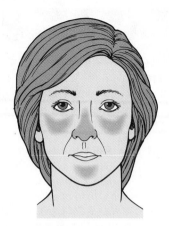

FIGURE 6–9 Rosacea.

Rosacea

DESCRIPTION

Rosacea, a disorder of the facial skin, causes redness, primarily in the areas where individuals blush or flush.

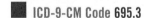 ICD-9-CM Code **695.3**

SYMPTOMS AND SIGNS

The onset of rosacea is insidious and often is mistaken for a complexion change, a sunburn, or even acne. The redness becomes more noticeable and does not go away. The skin then may begin exhibiting dryness and pimples that may become inflamed or pus filled. In addition, small blood vessels of the cheeks and face enlarge and show through the skin as red lines even after the redness diminishes (Fig. 6–9). Small knobby bumps occasionally appear on the nose, causing it to look swollen, mostly in the male with rosacea.

ETIOLOGY

The etiology of rosacea, a chronic and often cyclic condition, is unknown. A possible correlation with the frequency of the individual's blushing or facial flushing has been suggested. Those with lighter complexions appear to have a greater incidence of the disorder, and rosacea possibly may be inherited. Rosacea is not considered to be infectious or contagious and is not spread by skin contact.

DIAGNOSIS

Rosacea is diagnosed from the history of facial blushing and flushing. Although rosacea often has many of the same symptoms as acne, the individual experiencing episodes of rosacea does not have the blackheads or whiteheads (**comedones**) typical of acne. A dermatologist should be consulted for a definite diagnosis.

TREATMENT

Rosacea has no cure, but symptoms can be controlled through medical treatment with Finacea 15% (azelaic acid) and change of lifestyle. The patient is urged to identify situations that cause him or her to blush or experience facial flushing and attempt to avoid these triggers. These events may be different for various rosacea sufferers, so the patient would be wise to avoid sunlight, hard exercise, extreme heat or cold, stress, spicy foods, hot drinks, and alcohol. Sun exposure, hot weather, cold weather, and wind all have been identified as triggers, as have abrupt changes of season and weather extremes. The physician may prescribe medications to control the redness. Antibiotics sometimes are prescribed. Mild cleansers should be used, and moisturizers that do not contain alcohol or drying agents should be applied routinely. Sunscreens help. Consistent treatment is necessary to avoid flare-ups.

PROGNOSIS

As previously mentioned, rosacea has no cure, but the patient may be able to control symptoms with medical treatment and modification of lifestyle.

Rosacea

PREVENTION

The etiology is unknown, so prevention is not possible. Identifying situations with the potential to cause blushing or facial flushing and attempting to avoid these triggers are helpful. Avoiding sunlight, hard exercise, extreme heat or cold, stress, spicy foods, hot drinks, and alcohol also helps. The patient also is urged to avoid triggers such as sun exposure, hot weather, cold weather, and wind as well as abrupt changes of the seasons and weather extremes.

PATIENT TEACHING

Work with patients to identify causative factors and discuss ways to avoid these factors. Assist them in locating and contacting support groups for this disorder.

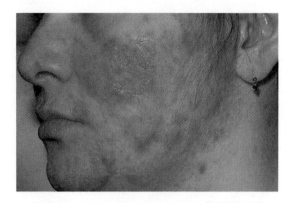

FIGURE 6–10 Acne. Inflammatory acne is characterized by erythematous papules and pustules, with the possibility of eventual scarring. (Cotran R et al: *Robbins pathological basis of disease,* ed 6, Philadelphia, 1999, Saunders.)

Acne Vulgaris

DESCRIPTION

Acne vulgaris is an inflammatory disease of the sebaceous glands and hair follicles. **Papules,** pustules, and comedones are usually present (Fig. 6–10).

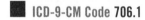 ICD-9-CM Code **706.1**

SYMPTOMS AND SIGNS

Acne vulgaris is marked by the appearance of papules, pustules, and comedones (see Fig. 6–2, *B, G,* and *L*). Deeper, boil-like lesions called nodules sometimes can occur. Scars may develop if the chronic irritation and inflammation continue for a long period. Acne is found most often on the face but also can occur on the neck, shoulders, chest, and back (Fig. 6–11). Acne can appear at any age but is more common in adolescents. In girls, it is usually at its worst between the ages of 14 and 17 years. In boys, it reaches its peak in the late teens.

PATIENT SCREENING

Many calls requesting appointments for treatment of acne-type conditions will be for teenagers. Acne is not a medical emergency, but an individual experiencing its symptoms may be feeling emotional stress. Therefore the physician should schedule these patients for the next available appointment.

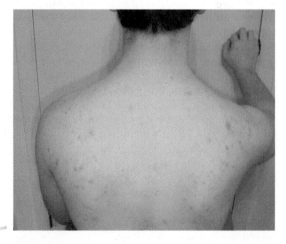

FIGURE 6–11 Photo of teenage acne. (Courtesy David Frazier, 2003.)

ETIOLOGY

The cause of acne vulgaris is unknown. Research on the cause, however, links it to hormonal changes of adolescence that affect the activity of the sebaceous glands. Hereditary tendencies also are known to be predisposing factors. Precipitating factors may include food allergies, endocrine disorders, psychological factors, fatigue, and the use of steroid drugs.

Sebum, an oily substance produced by the sebaceous glands, reaches the skin surface through the hair follicle. Overproduction of the oil seems to stimulate the follicle walls, causing a faster shedding of skin cells. This causes the cells and sebum to stick together and to form a plug, which promotes the growth of bacteria in the follicles. This is the process by which pimples and nodules form.

DIAGNOSIS

Examination of the characteristic lesions and patient history confirm the diagnosis.

TREATMENT

Therapy may include the use of topical or systemic antibiotics or both. Topically applied **keratolytic** agents may prove appropriate for many cases of acne. Topical application of medications chemically related to vitamin A (e.g., tretinoin [Retin-A]) reduces the skin's natural oils and promotes drying and peeling of the acne lesions. Antibiotics are prescribed to kill bacteria residing on the skin or in the lesions. Long-term antibiotic use for acne treatment, however, may have side effects. Isotretinoin (Accutane) helps to reduce the amount of sebum the body manufactures. Low-dose estrogen is prescribed to balance hormone levels. Optimal results usually are obtained by incorporating medications. Caution must be taken in the use of isotretinoin because it may produce serious psychological side effects, including depression, psychosis, and even suicide.

PROGNOSIS

The prognosis varies depending on the extent of the acne and the individual's compliance with the medication regimen, including all topical and ingested medications prescribed.

PREVENTION

The etiology is unknown, so no prevention is known.

PATIENT TEACHING

Give patients information about acne and its care. Teach patients the methods of applying dermal medications. Encourage patients to report any side effects resulting from oral medications. Emphasize the importance of not squeezing any pimples or pustules. In addition, emphasize the importance of good hand washing after touching involved skin areas.

Herpes Zoster (Shingles)

DESCRIPTION

Herpes zoster, or shingles, is an acute inflammatory dermatomal eruption of extremely painful vesicles.

ICD-9-CM Code 053.9

Herpes zoster has more than one form and location and therefore more than one ICD-9-CM code. The code for herpes zoster without mention of complication is 053.9. Refer to the physician's diagnosis and then to the current edition of the ICD-9-CM coding manual to ensure the greatest specificity of pathology and any appropriate modifiers.

SYMPTOMS AND SIGNS

Shingles occurs in a band-like unilateral pattern along the course of the peripheral nerves or **dermatomes** that are affected and does not cross the midline of the body (Fig. 6–12). Pain begins about 2 or 3 days before the appearance of the lesions and sometimes is accompanied by a fever. The eruptions begin as a rash that rapidly develops into vesicles. The skin that overlies the affected dermatome or dermatomes becomes reddened and blistered. These vesicles often are grouped on a reddened area of the skin. After several days, the vesicles appear pustular, develop a crust, and then develop a scab.

The incubation period is from 7 to 21 days. The duration of the disease, from onset to recovery, is usually 10 days to 5 weeks. If all the vesicles appear within 24 hours, the total duration is usually shorter. Although the commonly affected site is the skin overlying thoracic dermatomes (see Fig. 6–12), any area of the body may be affected. Shingles occasionally occurs on the face, neck, and scalp. When nerves supplying the eye are involved, the disease may cause serious damage to the eye structure.

PATIENT SCREENING

Patients experiencing the onset of herpes zoster often experience excruciating pain in the affected area. Prompt assessment and intervention are required. An appointment should be scheduled as soon as possible for the day of the call. When no appointment is available, refer to a facility where the patient can be seen promptly. Drug therapy be-

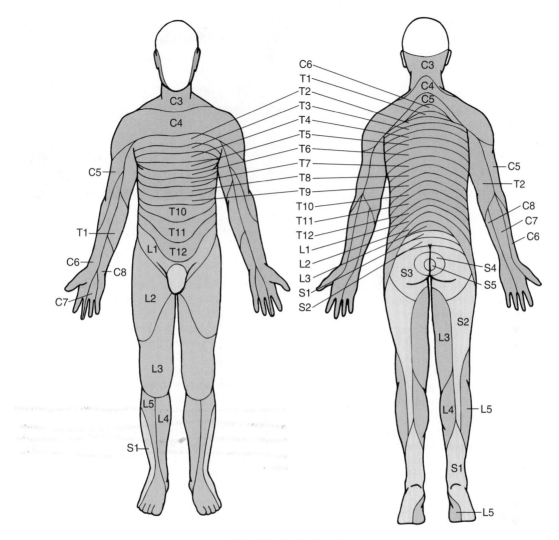

FIGURE 6–12 Dermatomes.

ginning immediately helps to reduce the severity of symptoms.

ETIOLOGY
The cause is the herpes varicella-zoster virus (VZV), the same virus that causes chickenpox. For unknown reasons, after lying dormant in the dorsal root ganglia, it becomes reactivated in later years. Stress appears to be a precipitating factor.

DIAGNOSIS
Shingles is diagnosed by its characteristic pattern and painful vesicles. One can confirm the diagno-

sis by culturing the virus from vesicle scrapings. A blood sample containing the varicella-zoster antibodies also aids in the diagnosis. Although shingles can affect any age group, those older than 55 are more frequently affected.

TREATMENT
Treatment of shingles is directed toward making the patient comfortable. Analgesics, mild tranquilizers or sedatives, antipruritics, steroids (e.g., methylprednisolone, prednisone, and betamethasone [Celestone Soluspan]), and a drying agent to be applied directly to the vesicles may be prescribed. Acyclovir

(Zovirax) used orally, parenterally, or topically also is prescribed and is quite effective. Other antiviral agents that may be prescribed include famciclovir (Famvir), valacyclovir (Valtrex), or foscarnet sodium (Foscavir). Antibiotic therapy may be necessary to prevent a secondary infection. If the eye is affected, early treatment with idoxuridine is necessary. An ophthalmologist should supervise the latter therapy.

When the pain is intolerable, injections of lidocaine and nerve-block agents may be attempted. If these steps do not provide relief, permanent nerve blocks via alcohol or nerve resection may be used as a last resort. Shingles occasionally recurs at later dates.

PROGNOSIS

Most cases resolve within a month. A common complication for some patients is postherpetic neuralgia. This chronic pain may persist from a month to years after the skin lesions have healed. Patients with chronic postherpetic neuralgia are often referred to pain clinics for treatment.

PREVENTION

No prevention currently is known. Research is being conducted to determine the effectiveness of the chickenpox vaccine in preventing subsequent incidence of shingles. Shingles is not contagious, but exposure to fluid in the blisters by an individual who has never had chickenpox may cause that individual to develop chickenpox. Immunocompromised patients should avoid contact with individuals diagnosed with shingles.

PATIENT TEACHING

Give patients information about the disorder. Encourage patients to take medications, including pain medications, as prescribed.

Impetigo

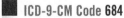

DESCRIPTION

Impetigo is a common, contagious, superficial skin infection. It manifests with early vesicular or pustular lesions that rupture and form thick yellow crusts (Fig. 6–13).

■ **ICD-9-CM Code 684**

Impetigo has more than one form or location and therefore more than one ICD-9-CM code.

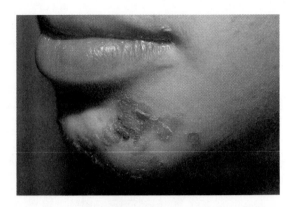

FIGURE 6–13 Impetigo. (From Lookingbill D, Marks J: *Principles of dermatology,* ed 2, Philadelphia, 1993, Saunders.)

> *The general code for impetigo is 684. Refer to the physician's diagnosis and then to the current edition of the ICD-9-CM coding manual to ensure the greatest specificity of pathology and any appropriate modifiers.*

SYMPTOMS AND SIGNS

Impetigo lesions usually develop on the legs and are found less often on the face, trunk, and arms. Small vesicles are surrounded by a circle of reddened skin and usually are accompanied by pruritus. Adjacent lesions may develop as a result of autoinoculation resulting from scratching, but systemic symptoms are uncommon. Ulcerations with erythema and scarring also may result from scratching or abrading of the skin.

PATIENT SCREENING

Discovering the impetigo infection can be distressing to the individual or parent of the child. Urgent attention also is needed because impetigo can spread among children or contacts. Because of this contagious nature of impetigo, the child's school may require immediate attention to the situation. Schedule the patient for the next available appointment, and if none is available that day or the next, refer the patient to an open facility (emergency department or clinic) for prompt assessment and treatment.

ETIOLOGY

Impetigo is caused by either *Streptococcus* or *Staphylococcus aureus*. The infection is thought to originate from insect bites, scabies infestation, poor hygiene, anemia, and malnutrition. It is also highly contagious so may be spread from child to child in the school or childcare environment. Cases of impetigo are common in temperate climates and occur more often in warm weather.

DIAGNOSIS

The diagnosis is based on the appearance of the characteristic lesions. To differentiate impetigo from other skin diseases, a *Tzanck test* and a *Gram stain* may be useful.

TREATMENT

Systemic use of antibiotics and proper cleaning of lesions two or three times a day are effective treatments for impetigo. Bactoban ointment or cream along with erythromycin or dicloxacillin are used in treatment. Avoiding infected individuals is essential.

PROGNOSIS

With treatment, prognosis is good. Most children recover without difficulty.

PREVENTION

Good hygiene is essential in preventing impetigo. Frequent and thorough hand washing is the first line of defense, as in many contagious conditions. Instruct children not to share towels, bedding, clothing, or other personal items.

PATIENT TEACHING

Give parents or caregivers information about impetigo and the ways it spreads. Encourage them to teach children good hygiene.

Furuncles and Carbuncles

DESCRIPTION

A furuncle, or boil, is an abscess that involves the entire hair follicle and adjacent subcutaneous tissue. A carbuncle is either an unusually large furuncle or multiple furuncles that develop in adjoining follicles, connected by many drainage canals.

ICD-9-CM Code 680.9 *(Unspecified site)*
Furuncles and carbuncles are coded by the site or location. The code above is for unspecified site. Refer to the physician's diagnosis and then to the current edition of the

ICD-9-CM coding manual to ensure the greatest specificity of pathology and any appropriate modifiers.

680.0 *(Face)*
680.1 *(Neck)*
680.2 *(Trunk)*
680.3 *(Upper arm and forearm)*
680.4 *(Hand)*
680.5 *(Buttock)*
680.6 *(Leg, except foot)*
680.7 *(Foot)*
680.8 *(Other specified sites)*

SYMPTOMS AND SIGNS

Furuncles begin as the inflamed hair follicle becomes infected and the infection extends beyond the follicle. The affected area is red, swollen, and painful (Fig. 6–14, *A* and *B*). Eventually, over several days, the abscess either bursts through the skin or, less often, discharges internally. In either case, the pain is relieved and the boil heals. Erythema and edema may persist at the site for several more days or weeks.

Boils are extremely common. They can affect almost everyone at some time. Carbuncles are much more rare. Both tend to recur.

PATIENT SCREENING

The individual reporting the symptoms of a furuncle or carbuncle will convey the degree of urgency to be seen. Give the patient some possible appointment times and schedule to his or her convenience. When the patient reports pain and swelling, suggest the next available appointment.

ETIOLOGY

The most common cause of furuncles and carbuncles is bacterial infection with *Staphylococcus*, usually *S. aureus*. Both are localized infections and usually heal uneventfully. Predisposing factors include diabetes mellitus, nephritis, and other underlying diseases (e.g., digestive or gastrointestinal conditions). In some cases, furuncles and carbuncles result from poor resistance to infection or poor hygiene.

DIAGNOSIS

One makes the diagnosis by observing the characteristic lesion. An abscess may be cultured to isolate the causative organism. If recurring boils are a problem, the physician may order blood and urine analyses to rule out any underlying disease.

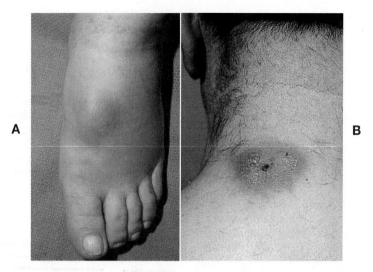

FIGURE 6–14 **A,** Furuncle. **B,** Carbuncle. (**A** from Lookingbill D, Marks J: *Principles of dermatology,* ed 2, Philadelphia, 1993, Saunders; **B** from Lawrence CM, Cox NH: *Physical signs in dermatology: color atlas and text,* London, 1993, Mosby Europe.)

TREATMENT

Applying hot compresses every few hours helps to relieve the discomfort and to hasten the draining. Surgical incision and drainage (I and D) may be necessary. Antibiotic treatment also may be needed for several weeks.

PROGNOSIS

Most furuncles and carbuncles resolve with drainage and antibiotic therapy.

PREVENTION

Prevention requires thorough cleansing of the skin and good hand-washing techniques. Patients should be urged not to squeeze the lesions.

PATIENT TEACHING

Give patients information on skin infections and their spread. Demonstrate good hand-washing techniques.

Cellulitis

DESCRIPTION

Cellulitis is an acute, diffuse, bacterial infection of the skin and subcutaneous tissue.

ICD-9-CM Code 682.9 *(Diffuse)*
Cellulitis appears in many forms and locations and thus has more than one ICD-9-CM code. The code for diffuse cellulitis is 682.9. Refer to the physician's diagnosis and then to the current edition of the ICD-9-CM coding manual to ensure the greatest specificity of pathology and any appropriate modifiers.

SYMPTOMS AND SIGNS

Cellulitis occurs most often in the lower extremities, but any part of the body can be affected. Clinically, erythema and pitting edema develop, and the skin becomes tender and hot to the touch (Fig. 6–15). The infection develops and spreads gradually over a couple of days. Red lines or streaks may appear proximal to the infection and run along lymph vessels to nearby lymph glands. If the lymph glands become edematous, systemic symptoms of fever and malaise may be present.

PATIENT SCREENING

An individual reporting symptoms of skin that is edematous, reddened, and hot along with streaks of red radiating from the site requires prompt assessment. If the individual cannot be seen in the office within a few hours, refer him or her to a med-

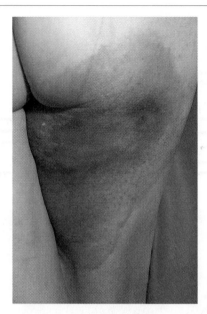

FIGURE 6-15 Cellulitis. (From Lookingbill D, Marks J: *Principles of dermatology,* ed 3, Philadelphia, 2000, Saunders.)

ical facility where prompt and immediate evaluation and treatment may be obtained.

ETIOLOGY

The cause of cellulitis is either *Streptococcus* or *Staphylococcus* that enters the skin's surface via a small cut or lesion. The bacteria produce enzymes that break down the skin cells. As a result of the release of enzymes, the infection spreads locally. These enzymes prevent body responses that normally would reduce local spread of infection by closing off the site.

DIAGNOSIS

An examination of the affected body part, a check for pitting edema and other symptoms, and a blood culture aid the physician in making the diagnosis.

TREATMENT

The affected limb should be immobilized and elevated. Cool magnesium sulfate (Epsom salt) solution compresses may be used for discomfort. Warm compresses should be applied to increase circulation to the affected part. Systemic antibiotics, with penicillin being the drug of choice, are prescribed for the infection. Aspirin or acetaminophen alone

or in combination with codeine is given for pain. Hospitalization is indicated when cellulitis is severe.

PROGNOSIS

The prognosis is good with prompt intervention and drug therapy. Hospitalization with IV drug therapy often will be required to produce the positive outcome.

PREVENTION

Good hand washing is essential for prevention. Attention to small nicks and cuts helps prevent this infection.

PATIENT TEACHING

Give patients information about skin infections and the importance of seeking medical attention promptly for an infected cut or scrape.

Dermatophytoses

DESCRIPTION

Dermatophytosis (tinea) is a chronic superficial fungal infection of the skin.

 ICD-9-CM Code 110.9 *(Of unspecified site)*
There are many ICD-9-CM codes for dermatophytosis, depending on site. Refer to the physician's diagnosis and then to the current edition of the ICD-9-CM coding manual to ensure the greatest specificity of pathology and any appropriate modifiers. The code for site unspecified is 110.9.

SYMPTOMS AND SIGNS

Dermatophyte infections are classified by the body region they inhabit. All dermatophytosis lesions are characterized by an active border and are marked by scaling with central clearing. Dermatophytosis occurring on the scalp is called tinea capitis; the body, tinea corporis (cradle cap); the nails, tinea unguium; the feet, tinea pedis (athlete's foot); and the groin region, tinea cruris.

PATIENT SCREENING

Dermatophytosis is troublesome, worrisome, and annoying. The individual calling for an appointment for these symptoms should be scheduled to be seen at the next convenient appointment.

Tinea Capitis

■ **ICD-9-CM Code 110.0**

Tinea capitis is characterized by round, gray, scaly lesions on the scalp (Fig. 6–16). It is contagious and often epidemic among children. The infected child may have a slight pruritus of the scalp or may be *asymptomatic*.

Tinea Corporis (Ringworm)

■ **ICD-9-CM Code 110.9** *(Ringworm unspecified)*

Tinea corporis is characterized by lesions that are round, ringed, and scaled with vesicles (Fig. 6–17). This infection can occur in anyone who has skin contact with infected domestic animals, especially cats. It is more common in rural settings and in hot and humid climates.

Tinea Unguium

■ **ICD-9-CM Code 110.1**

Tinea unguium frequently begins at the tip of toenails, affecting one or more nails at a time. It also can affect fingernails, but this is less common. The affected nail or nails appear hypertrophic or thickened, brittle, and lusterless.

Tinea Pedis (Athlete's Foot)

■ **ICD-9-CM Code 110.4**

Tinea pedis is characterized by intense, burning, stinging pruritus between the toes and on the soles of the feet (Fig. 6–18). The skin can become inflamed, dry, and peeling, and fissures (see Fig. 6–2, *J*) may develop. This condition is rare in children.

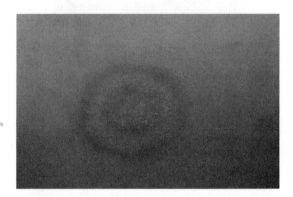

FIGURE 6–17 Tinea corporis (ringworm). (From Callen J, Greer K, Hood A, et al: *Color atlas of dermatology,* Philadelphia, 1993, Saunders.)

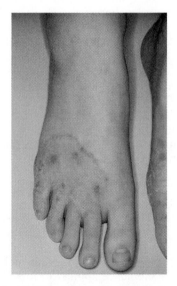

FIGURE 6–18 Tinea pedis (athlete's foot). (From Callen J, Greer K, Hood A, et al: *Color atlas of dermatology,* Philadelphia, 1993, Saunders.)

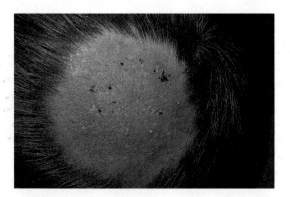

FIGURE 6–16 Tinea capitis. (From Callen J, Greer K, Hood A, et al: *Color atlas of dermatology,* Philadelphia, 1993, Saunders.)

Tinea Cruris (Jock Itch)

■ ICD-9-CM Code 110.3

Tinea cruris is characterized by raised, red, pruritic vesicular patches, with well-defined borders, located in the groin area (Fig. 6–19). It can be associated with athlete's foot and occurs more often in adult men. Flare-ups are frequent in summer months and are aggravated by physical activity, perspiration, and tight-fitting clothes.

ETIOLOGY

Dermatophytosis is caused by several species of fungi that can invade the skin or nails, especially if the integrity of the skin is compromised. The infection is transmitted by direct contact with the fungus or its spores.

DIAGNOSIS

The diagnosis is based on the appearance and location of the lesions. To isolate the causative fungus, a culture of the lesions is necessary.

TREATMENT

Antifungal medications are prescribed either for topical application (ointment) or for oral use, depending on the severity of the infection. The agents usually prescribed for treatment are as follows: tinea capitis, Nizoral shampoo (ketoconazole 2%); tinea pedis, tinea corporis, and tinea cruris, Lamisil (terbinafine hydrochloride), Lotrimin Ultra (butenafine), and griseofulvin. The affected skin must be kept as clean and dry as possible, clothing should be loose-fitting and clean, and exercise should be limited to prevent excessive perspiration. Because all forms of dermatophytosis tend to be persistent and chronic, meticulous management is needed to correct this condition.

PROGNOSIS

The prognosis is good with treatment that includes drug therapy and good skin care, but because the condition tends to be chronic, recurrence is likely.

PREVENTION

The wearing of loose-fitting cotton clothing helps prevent the condition. The patient must dry the skin after bathing or swimming, with special attention to drying the skin between the toes and in folds of the skin.

PATIENT TEACHING

Give the patient information about the disorder. Encourage the patient to dry the skin after exposure to moisture, especially in the areas between the toes and in the folds of the skin. Explain the importance of wearing cotton clothing that absorbs moisture from the body. Advise diabetics or patients with compromised peripheral circulation to seek medical attention for athlete's foot.

Decubitus Ulcers

DESCRIPTION

A decubitus ulcer, commonly called a pressure ulcer or bed sore, is a localized area of dead skin that can affect the epidermis, dermis, and subcutaneous layers (Fig. 6–20).

■ ICD-9-CM Code 707.0

Skin ulcers can occur in many locations. The code for decubitus ulcers is 707.0. Refer to the physician's diagnosis and then to the current edition of the ICD-9-CM coding manual to ensure the greatest specificity of pathology and any appropriate modifiers.

SYMPTOMS AND SIGNS

An early sign of a decubitus ulcer is shiny, reddened skin appearing over a bony prominence in

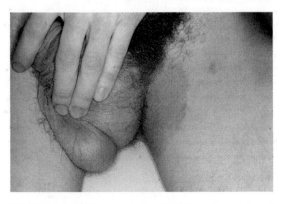

FIGURE 6–19 Tinea cruris (jock itch). (From Callen J, Greer K, Hood A, et al: *Color atlas of dermatology*, Philadelphia, 1993, Saunders.)

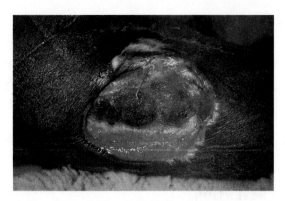

FIGURE 6–20 Decubitus ulcer. (From Callen J, Greer K, Hood A, et al: *Color atlas of dermatology*, Philadelphia, 1993, Saunders.)

individuals with prolonged immobilization. Other signs that eventually occur include blisters, erosions, necrosis, and ulceration. If the decubitus ulcer becomes infected, a foul-smelling, purulent discharge is present. Pain may or may not accompany a decubitus ulcer.

PATIENT SCREENING
Most patients experiencing decubitus ulcers are confined to a bed or are generally immobile. These patients may not be capable of going to the office for a visit and therefore will be seen in the hospital, nursing care facility, or home. Make arrangements for those who are immobile to be visited by a physician in their environment. Schedule the mobile patient to be seen at the earliest available time.

ETIOLOGY
Decubitus ulcers are caused by impairment or lack of blood supply to the affected area of skin. This is the result of constant pressure against the surface of the skin, as seen in people who are debilitated, paralyzed, or unconscious.

DIAGNOSIS
Visual examination of the ulcer is sufficient for a diagnosis. If infection is suspected, culture and sensitivity testing may be needed to isolate the causative organism.

TREATMENT
If not treated vigorously, the ulcer progresses from a simple erosion of the skin to complete involvement of all layers of skin. Eventually, the ulcer extends to the underlying muscle and bone tissue, and osteomyelitis and/or gangrene may result.

Topical agents that have proved effective in the treatment of decubitus ulcers include absorbable gelatin sponges, granulated sugar, karaya gum patches, antiseptic irrigations, **debriding** agents, and antibiotics (when infection is present).

PROGNOSIS
The prognosis is fair. Resolution and healing of the lesion depends on the patient's general health and potential for mobility and removal of pressure on the lesion site.

PREVENTION
Preventive measures include frequent inspection of the skin for signs of breakdown, alleviation of pressure points over bony prominences, good skin care, early ambulation when possible, position changes every 2 hours, passive range-of-motion exercises, and the use of special pads and mattresses.

PATIENT TEACHING
Most teaching will be directed to the care provider. Encourage preventive measures and prompt reporting of any signs of impending skin breakdown.

Scabies and Pediculosis

DESCRIPTION
Itch mites (scabies) and lice (pediculosis) are the two most common parasitic insects to infest humans. Human scabies infestations are caused by the human itch mite, *Sarcoptes scabiei* (Fig. 6–21, *A*). The three species of human lice are the head louse, *Pediculus humanus capitis* (Fig. 6–22, *A*); the body louse, *P. humanus corporis;* and the pubic, or crab, louse, *Phthirus pubis* (Fig. 6–23, *A*). Lice resemble insects, but they are wingless parasites with sucking mouths to feed on human blood. They prefer to lay their eggs on body hair but also lay them in folds of clothing.

■ **ICD-9-CM Code 132.9** *(Infestation)*
133.0 *(Human itch mite, Sarcoptes scabiei)*
132.0 *(Head louse, Pediculus humanus capitis)*

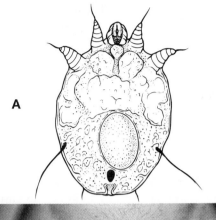

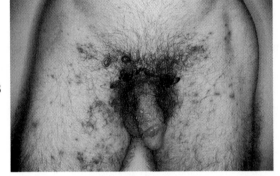

A

B

FIGURE 6–21 **A,** Itch (scabies) mite. **B,** Scabies rash.
(**B** from Callen J, Greer K, Hood A, et al: *Color atlas of dermatology,*
Philadelphia, 1993, Saunders.)

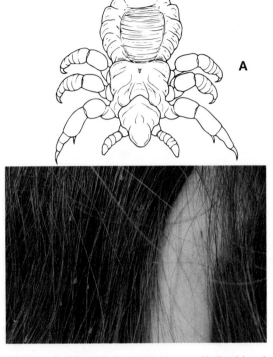

A

B

FIGURE 6–22 **A,** *Pediculus humanus capitis* (head louse).
B, Lice in hair. (**B** from Callen J, Greer K, Hood A, et al: *Color atlas
of dermatology,* Philadelphia, 1993, Saunders.)

132.1 *(Body louse,
P. humanus corporis)*
132.2 *(Pubic, or crab,
louse, Phthirus pubis)*
*Five codes are listed. Scabies and lice ICD-9-
CM codes should be confirmed for accuracy
with a coding manual. Refer to the physician's
diagnosis and then to the current edition of the
ICD-9-CM coding manual to ensure the greatest
specificity of pathology and any appropriate
modifiers.*

SYMPTOMS AND SIGNS

Both scabies and pediculosis are *highly* contagious.
They produce intense pruritus and a sensation of
something crawling on the skin. With scabies, the
most common symptom is a rash (Fig. 6–21, *B*) accompanied by intense itching that worsens at
night. Scabies can occur anywhere on the body but

usually is found on hands, breasts, armpits, waist-
line, and the genital area. Lice also can produce a
rash or wheals, but the most common sign or symptom is the presence of nits (eggs) on hair shafts,
skin, or clothing (see Figs. 6–22, *B,* and 6–23, *B*).

PATIENT SCREENING

Patients reporting symptoms of scabies or lice
should be seen as soon as possible. The infestation
in children may have been detected at a child-care
facility or school. These children must be assessed
and treatment must be prescribed and started as
soon as possible. Although not a life-threatening
condition, scabies or lice can be spread to others
through close contact, and the offending mites and
lice should be brought under control quickly.

ETIOLOGY

Itch mites and lice can infest anyone at any
age. Both are spread easily from one person to

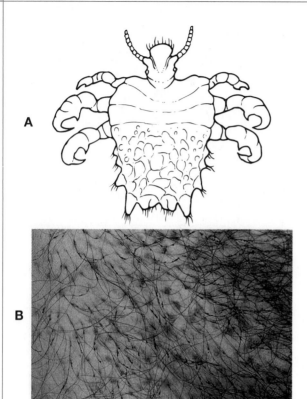

FIGURE 6–23 A, *Phthirus pubis* (pubic, or crab, louse). **B,** Pubic lice rash. (**B** from Callen J, Greer K, Hood A, et al: *Color atlas of dermatology,* Philadelphia, 1993, Saunders.)

another by close physical contact. Transmission occurs most often between children playing together, family members, and sexual partners. In addition to physical contact, transmission may occur indirectly via infected clothing, bed sheets, towels, and hair combs or brushes. Although the scabies mite can infest other mammals, it is not transmitted from pets to humans. Pubic lice, however, have been known to infest dogs and then migrate to humans. Both scabies and pediculosis are common in overcrowded areas that have inadequate facilities and where poor personal hygiene is practiced.

DIAGNOSIS

Visual examination can identify lice and nits on the hair, body, and clothing. Other skin disorders such as atopic dermatitis (see Atopic Dermatitis), con-tact dermatitis (see Contact Dermatitis), and psoriasis (see Psoriasis) must be ruled out when scabies is suspected. A similar rash occurring about the same time in several family members should suggest scabies.

TREATMENT

The goals of treatment of scabies and pediculosis are to remove the mites, lice, and nits; to eliminate the pruritus; to provide emotional support to the patient, family, and contacts; and to treat the environment to prevent reinfestation.

To kill head lice, a special shampoo must be used and then repeated in 7 to 10 days to ensure that all the nits are dead. The patient must follow this with meticulous combing with a special fine-toothed comb to dislodge the nits. Body lice are removed with soap and water or the same shampoo used for head lice. Pubic lice may be treated with shampoo, creams, or lotions. Directions must be followed when using the shampoos because they may have residual toxic effects.

Scabies treatment includes the use of special shampoos, creams, sulfur preparations, and topical steroids. Because of the intense pruritus and the scratching associated with scabies and lice infestations, a secondary infection may occur, necessitating treatment with oral antibiotics.

With both scabies and pediculosis, family members and others who have had direct contact with the infected person must be treated as well. All clothing and bedding belonging to the infected person must be washed in hot water or dry-cleaned. Any furniture that the person has been using also should be cleaned either with a surface cleaner or by vacuuming.

PROGNOSIS

The prognosis is good with treatment and appropriate disinfection or decontamination of clothing, bedding, and furniture. Those who have had contact with the patient must be made aware of the infestation and be treated in a similar manner to prevent reinfestation.

PREVENTION

Prevention is difficult with the close contact among people in our society. Recommend that family members, including children, not share hats and hair-grooming equipment. Pubic lice are considered an STD, and suggested precautions are discussed in Chapter 12.

PATIENT TEACHING

Give patients written information about recognizing scabies and lice. Pictures of the offending organisms help in recognition. Explain the importance of laundering clothing and bedding appropriately. Emphasize the importance of notifying all persons in contact with the patient about the infestation so they can seek treatment. Teach the correct methods of using shampoo or scabicide.

Benign and Premalignant Tumors

DESCRIPTION

Noncancerous growths or tumors of the skin fall into two categories: benign and premalignant. Benign tumors are usually a cosmetic problem only. Premalignant tumors must be identified and treated as early as possible to prevent them from developing into malignancies. Common benign tumors include seborrheic keratoses, dermatofibromas, keratoacanthomas, keloids and hypertrophic scars, epidermal (sebaceous) cysts, acrochordons (skin tags), actinic keratoses, and nevi.

SYMPTOMS AND SIGNS

Symptoms and signs vary according to the conditions experienced. Moles are the most common premalignant tumors. Following is a discussion of the conditions.

PATIENT SCREENING

Although benign tumors are usually only a cosmetic problem, they still present a source of anxiety to the patient. Premalignant tumors require early identification and treatment to prevent their development into malignancies. Recognize the patient's anxiety level and schedule an appointment at the earliest convenient time.

Seborrheic Keratosis

■ **ICD-9-CM Code 702.11** *(Inflamed seborrheic keratosis)*
702.19 *(Other seborrheic kerotosis) (NOS)*

Seborrheic **keratoses** are benign growths originating in the epidermis, clinically appearing as tan-brown, greasy papules or plaques (see Fig. 6–2, *B*

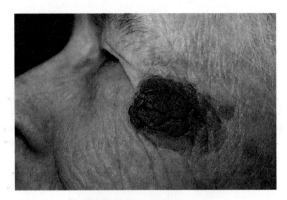

FIGURE 6–24 Seborrheic keratosis. (From Callen J, Greer K, Hood A, et al: *Color atlas of dermatology*, Philadelphia, 1993, Saunders.)

and *C*) and having the appearance of being pasted onto the skin (Fig. 6–24). They are, for the most part, asymptomatic but may cause pruritus, especially in elderly people. The cause of seborrheic keratoses is unknown, and although they have no potential for developing into malignancy, they should be differentiated from other potentially malignant tumors. The appearance of a sudden increase in the number or size of these growths on uninflamed skin could indicate the presence of an internal malignancy, most commonly of the stomach.

Dermatofibroma

■ **ICD-9-CM Code 216.9** *(Skin, site unspecified)*
Dermatofibromas can have more than one site and therefore more than one ICD-9-CM code. The code for skin, site unspecified, is 216.9. Refer to the physician's diagnosis and then to the current edition of the ICD-9-CM coding manual to ensure the greatest specificity of pathology and any appropriate modifiers.

Dermatofibromas are benign and asymptomatic and can be found on any part of the body, particularly on the front of the lower leg. They are more common in women and are thought to be caused by fibrous reactions to viral infections. These growths also can be caused by a reaction to insect bites and trauma. Dermatofibromas are scaly, hard growths that are slightly raised and pinkish brown (Fig. 6–25).

Keratoacanthoma

■ ICD-9-CM Code 238.2

Keratoacanthoma is a benign epithelial growth that may be caused by a virus and generally is seen in people in their 60s. The growth is a smooth, red, dome-shaped papule with a central crust that usually appears singly but may occur in multiple (Fig. 6–26). Keratoacanthoma can disappear spontaneously, but scarring is common. It must be differentiated from squamous cell carcinoma.

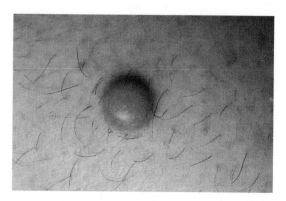

FIGURE 6–25 Dermatofibroma. (From Callen J, Greer K, Hood A, et al: *Color atlas of dermatology,* Philadelphia, 1993, Saunders.)

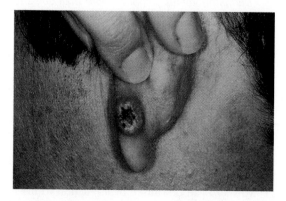

FIGURE 6–26 Keratoacanthoma. (From Callen J, Greer K, Hood A, et al: *Color atlas of dermatology,* Philadelphia, 1993, Saunders.)

Keloids and Hypertrophic Scars

■ ICD-9-CM Code 701.4

Keloids and hypertrophic scars occur secondary to trauma or surgery. A keloid first appears normal, but after several months, it becomes noticeably larger and thicker (Fig. 6–27). Keloids are harmless, but they can cause pruritus and sometimes deformities. They are more common in black-skinned people. Keloids extend beyond the wound site and do not regress spontaneously. Hypertrophic scars, however, do not extend but stay confined to the site and generally regress over time. Keloids can be addressed surgically.

Epidermal (Sebaceous) Cyst

■ ICD-9-CM Code 706.2

Sebaceous cysts develop when a sebaceous gland slowly fills with a thick fluid. This process can take many years but is usually painless and harmless. Some cysts, usually small ones, have a blackhead in

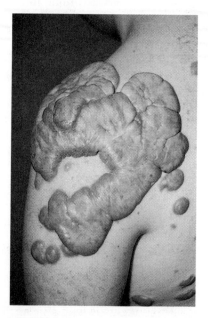

FIGURE 6–27 Keloid. (From Callen J, Greer K, Hood A, et al: *Color atlas of dermatology,* Philadelphia, 1993, Saunders.)

the pore connecting the cyst to the skin's surface. Larger cysts most often are closed on the surface. The cysts are palpable and moveable and range in size from millimeters to several centimeters (Fig. 6–28). Sebaceous cysts commonly are found on the scalp, on the face, at the base of the ears, and on the chest. They also can develop in any area of the body that contains sebaceous glands. If bacteria enter the pore, the cyst becomes infected and enlarges, and inflammation and tenderness occur. The cyst eventually may burst, releasing a foul-smelling pus. Inflammation recedes, but the cyst remains and can become reinfected at another time.

Acrochordon (Skin Tag)

■ ICD-9-CM Code **701.9** *(Unspecified)*

Acrochordons are common benign skin growths or tags. They are found mainly in the axilla, on the neck, and on inguinal areas of the body. They can be brown or skin colored, and are attached to the body by a short stalk (Fig. 6–29).

Actinic Keratosis

■ ICD-9-CM Code **702.0**

Actinic keratoses are common premalignant lesions and are seen on sun-exposed areas of the body. They are caused by long-term exposure to sunlight, and their numbers increase with age. Light-skinned

people have a higher risk. Actinic keratosis initially appears as an area of rough, vascular skin, which later forms a yellow, adherent crust (Fig. 6–30).

ETIOLOGY
The causes of these lesions vary with the particular lesion.

DIAGNOSIS
The diagnosis of these lesions is made by visual examination; a biopsy of the tissue may be necessary to confirm the findings.

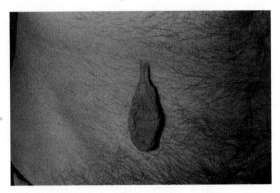

FIGURE 6–29 Acrochordon (skin tag). (From Callen J, Greer K, Hood A, et al: *Color atlas of dermatology*, Philadelphia, 1993, Saunders.)

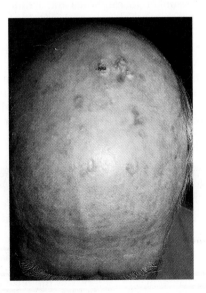

FIGURE 6–30 Actinic keratoses. (From Callen J, Greer K, Hood A, et al: *Color atlas of dermatology*, ed 2, Philadelphia, 2000, Saunders.)

FIGURE 6–28 Epidermal (sebaceous) cyst. (From Lookingbill D, Marks J: *Principles of dermatology*, ed 3, Philadelphia, 2000, Saunders.)

TREATMENT

Treatment of these lesions varies depending on the specific type of lesion. Seborrheic keratoses are treated with cryosurgery and curettage. Keratoacanthoma is treated by surgical excision, adrenocorticosteroids applied topically, and, for multiple lesions, oral isotretinoin and etretinate administration. Keloids and hypertrophic scars are treated with corticosteroids injected into the lesion once every 4 weeks or surgery with scar compression. Epidermal, or sebaceous, cysts are excised surgically and treated with antibiotics if infected. Acrochordons (skin tags) also are treated by excisional surgery. Actinic keratosis is treated with topical agents—tretinoin (Retin-A) alone or in combination with fluorouracil—and by curettage and desiccation. Chloasma can be treated with Retin-A in an attempt to lighten the affected skin.

PROGNOSIS

The prognosis varies depending on the condition, the age of the condition, the amount of skin involved, and the physical condition of the patient. Biopsy reports will indicate a possible outcome.

PREVENTION

Most of these lesions cannot be prevented. Avoiding direct exposure of the skin to sunlight helps prevent keratoacanthoma and actinic keratosis. The use of sunscreen is encouraged.

PATIENT TEACHING

Give patients information about various benign and premalignant tumors. Encourage consistent use of sunscreen as well as regular evaluation of suspicious skin lesions by a physician. Explain that many patients will be referred to a dermatologist for follow-up care.

Skin Carcinomas

Collectively, the skin cancers, basal cell carcinoma (BCC), squamous cell carcinoma (SCC), and malignant melanoma, represent the most common type of malignancy. In fact, BCC is the most prevalent form of cancer worldwide. Because BCC and SCC usually do not metastasize, however, they often are not included on most cancer registries. Left un-treated, however, these non-melanoma skin cancers can be extremely locally destructive and can invade and destroy nerves, lymphatics, blood vessels, cartilage, and bone.

Non-Melanoma Skin Cancers

DESCRIPTION

Basal cell carcinoma (BCC) and squamous cell carcinoma (SCC) affect more than one million Americans each year. BCC arises in the basal (deepest) layer of the epidermis, and SCC arises in the epithelial (outer) layer.

> ■ **ICD-9-CM Code** *(Refer to the Neoplasm Table in the current edition of the ICD-9-CM coding manual)*
> *Skin cancers are coded by body site and type. Refer to the physician's diagnosis and then to the current edition of the ICD-9-CM coding manual to ensure the greatest specificity of pathology and any appropriate modifiers. A morphology code is also required and is listed in the current edition of the ICD-9-CM coding manual.*

SYMPTOMS AND SIGNS

BCC and SCC lesions can appear anywhere on the body. The most common sites are the sun-exposed areas: face, scalp, ears, back, chest, arms, and back of the hands. About 70% of BCC lesions occur on the face (25% to 30% on the nose) (Fig. 6–31). Five warning signs suggest the presence of basal cell cancer:

- A shiny bump or nodule that is pearly white, pink, red, or translucent. Blood vessels may appear on the surface.
- A sore that bleeds, heals, and recurs. It may be associated with ulceration and crusting.
- A reddish, irritated area, usually on the back, shoulders, extremities, or chest that may or may not be painful or cause pruritus.
- A smooth growth with an indented center and elevated, rolled edge, or border.
- A scar-like area, often with poorly defined edges, that is white, yellow, or waxy in appearance.

SCC lesions often present as a crusted or scaly area with a red, inflamed base; as a growing tumor; as a non-healing ulcer; or as a raised, firm papule (Fig. 6–32). The ulcerated lesions may be painful.

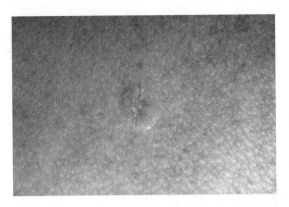

FIGURE 6–31 Basal cell carcinoma. (From Lookingbill D, Marks J: *Principles of dermatology,* ed 3, Philadelphia, 2000, Saunders.)

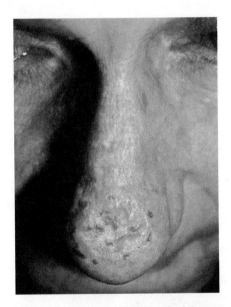

FIGURE 6–32 Squamous cell carcinoma of the nose. (From Friedman RJ et al: *Cancer of the skin,* Philadelphia, 1991, Saunders.)

PATIENT SCREENING

Patients reporting any of the following should be scheduled to be seen at the next available appointment: skin lesions such as a sore that bleeds, heals, and recurs; a reddish, irritated area, usually on the back, shoulders, extremities, or chest, that may or may not be painful or cause pruritus; or a smooth growth with an indented center and elevated, rolled edge or border or a scar-like area, often with poorly defined edges, that is white, yellow, or waxy in appearance. Although most of these conditions at an early stage are not life-threatening, the patient's anxiety probably is quite high. Giving the patient the earliest possible appointment for assessment and treatment of the condition is a prudent aspect of total patient care.

ETIOLOGY

These forms of skin cancer can develop in anyone, especially those with a history of chronic sun exposure. People at highest risk have fair skin and light-colored hair and eyes. Chronic exposure to the ultraviolet (UV) radiation in sunlight has two main effects that can lead to tumor formation. First, it causes mutations in DNA. Second, it suppresses the skin's immune system, weakening the immune system's ability to fight any tumors that do form. Additional risk factors include therapeutic radiation treatment, immunosuppression, and chronic exposure to arsenic. SCC often arises from actinic keratosis, and occasionally from scar tissue. Although non-melanoma skin cancers are not likely to metastasize, some forms of SCC are more aggressive and will spread to distant locations in the body. Both types will cause local destruction if left untreated.

DIAGNOSIS

Unusual skin lesions are often identified by the patient or by the physician on examination of the skin. A biopsy (usually a punch biopsy) of the lesion is required for definitive diagnosis.

TREATMENT

Treatment consists of surgical excision (90% of cases), cryosurgery (tissue destruction by freezing), **electrodesiccation** (tissue destruction by heat), or radiotherapy. Having non-melanoma skin cancer increases one's risk of getting another BCC or SCC and of developing malignant melanoma. Patients should be followed periodically for 5 years after treatment to check for recurrence, metastasis, or a new skin cancer.

PROGNOSIS

The overall 5-year survival rate for non-melanoma skin cancer is 95%. SCC carries a worse prognosis if it occurs on the lip, ear, or scalp or is larger than 2.5 cm in diameter.

PREVENTION

Minimizing sun exposure is the key to prevention, especially during childhood, because people generally receive most of their lifetime UV exposure before adulthood. Any suspicious skin lesions should be evaluated by a physician.

PATIENT TEACHING

Give the patient written information about skin cancer. Help them find additional resources for more information. After excision of any lesion, give the patient information about care of the site. Encourage the consistent use of sunscreen on exposed skin, and recommend that the patient limit the duration of exposure. Emphasize the importance of regular follow-up examinations.

Malignant Melanoma

DESCRIPTION

Malignant melanoma is the most serious of the three types of skin cancer, but it is not as common. It arises in epidermal melanocytes, cells that make the brown pigment, melanin.

ICD-9-CM Code

Refer to the physician's diagnosis and then to the current edition of the ICD-9-CM coding manual for "Melanoma, Malignant by body site" to ensure the greatest specificity of pathology and any appropriate modifiers.

SYMPTOMS AND SIGNS

Most melanomas occur as solitary lesions. They can be found anywhere on the skin, but are most common on the backs of men and the legs of women. The most common symptom is change, either a newly pigmented area of the skin or a change in a mole that may have been present since birth or childhood (Fig. 6–33, *A–B*). Changes that may indicate the presence of malignant melanoma are:

- Change in size, especially sudden or continuous enlargement
- Change in color, especially multiple shades of tan, brown, and black; mixing of red, white, and blue; or spreading of color from the border into adjacent skin
- Change in shape, especially the development of an irregular, notched border of an area with a previously regular border
- Change in the elevation of a previously flat pigmented area
- Change in the surface: scaliness, erosion, oozing, crusting, or bleeding
- Change in the surrounding skin: redness, swelling, or the development of colored areas adjacent to but not part of the pigmented area
- Change in sensation: tenderness, pain, or pruritus
- Change in consistency: softening or hardening

These changes are incorporated into a list known as the ABCDs of melanoma (see the Enrichment box).

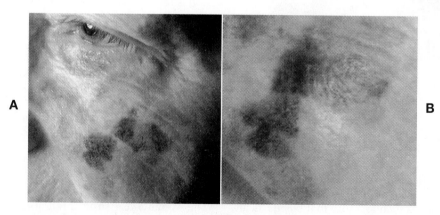

FIGURE 6–33 A, A fully developed malignant melanoma of the left cheek in an elderly man. **B,** Close-up of the lesion. (From Friedman RJ et al: *Cancer of the skin,* Philadelphia, 1991, Saunders.)

PATIENT SCREENING

Patients who report the previous warning signs or symptoms should be scheduled to be seen at the next available appointment. Consider that the patient's anxiety level is probably quite high. Giving the patient the earliest possible appointment for assessment and treatment of the condition is a prudent aspect of total patient care.

ETIOLOGY

About 95% of all skin carcinomas result from chronic overexposure to the sun. Geographic location also is a factor. The frequency of melanoma also is higher in people who live closer to the equator. It affects all adult age groups but is rare in children. The median age for diagnosis is 53. Risk factors include a sun-sensitive skin type (fair skin, light-colored hair and eyes, skin that burns easily), history of severe sunburn (especially during childhood), and use of tanning beds. Intermittent, intense exposures to UV light increase one's risk more than a continuous exposure. Apart from sun/UV-radiation exposure, other factors also make certain people more prone to malignant melanoma:

- A family history of malignant melanoma
- A previous case of malignant melanoma or non-melanoma skin cancer
- More than 50 common moles or more than 10 atypical (irregular shape or color) moles
- Xeroderma pigmentosum—a genetic disorder associated with defects in DNA repair, leading to multiple skin cancers at a young age

DIAGNOSIS

If a patient observes any of the ABCDE warning signs or notices an unusual growth, he or she should see a physician immediately. More than 50% of melanomas are first identified by the patient. A biopsy, usually an excisional or punch biopsy, is needed for histological diagnosis and for staging. The staging system for melanoma was recently developed by the American Joint Committee on Cancer. It relies on tumor thickness rather than level of invasion, uses ulceration as a prognostic indicator, emphasizes the number of positive nodes rather than nodal size, and uses serum LDH level to stratify level-IV disease (normal LDH level correlates with better survival in stage-IV disease). Staging is performed through a full physical exam, chest x-ray, liver function tests, and serum LDH measurement. If distant metastases are expected, CT scans may be ordered. Serum levels of S-100 B protein may be measured, because they are often elevated in melanoma.

TREATMENT

The treatment of choice is complete excision of the cancerous lesion, often with wide margins. Lymph node is dissected if nodal involvement is suspected. For metastatic cancer, chemotherapy or radiation therapy may improve survival. High-dose interferon alpha-2b may benefit these patients as well. Because surgical excision includes removal of skin tissue, scarring is inevitable. Cosmetically acceptable results are achieved if the tumors are small. Reconstructive surgery in the form of skin grafts or flap rotations may be required after excision of larger tumors.

ENRICHMENT
ABCDs OF MALIGNANT MELANOMA

- A = Asymmetry (lack of equality in the diameter)
- B = Border (notched, scalloped, or indistinct)
- C = Color (uneven, variegated—ranging from tan, brown, or black to red and white)
- D = Diameter (usually larger than 6 mm)

Adapted from *The ABCDs of moles and melanoma*, New York, The Skin Cancer Foundation, Copyright 1985.

PROGNOSIS

Overall 5-year survival for all stages of melanoma is 89%, although the presence of distant metastasis reduces this rate to only 12%. Poorer prognosis is associated with the presence of an ulcerated lesion, axial location of the melanoma, higher number of positive lymph nodes, age greater than 60, and male sex. In addition, the prognosis can be accurately correlated to tumor thickness (called the Breslow thickness). The correlation ranges from a thickness of less than 0.76 mm carrying a 97% 5-year survival, to a thickness of greater than 8.0 mm carrying a 32% 5-year survival.

PREVENTION

Increased awareness of skin cancer and education about the dangers of sun exposure greatly improve the prevention and early detection of skin carcinomas and save lives. Adults should perform regular skin self-examinations. People at very high risk (those with familial melanoma syndromes, multiple atypical or common moles, or excessive sun exposure) should see their physicians for a biannual whole-body examination to look for early melanoma lesions.

PATIENT TEACHING

As with basal cell and squamous cell carcinoma, give the patient written information about skin cancer. Help the patient find additional sources of information. After excision of any lesion, give the patient information about care of the site. Encourage the consistent use of sunscreen on exposed skin and recommend limiting the time of exposure. Emphasize the importance of regular follow-up examinations. Encourage patients to ask questions about the effects of chemotherapy and radiation therapy.

See Chapter 15 for a discussion of sunburn.

Abnormal Skin Pigmentation

DESCRIPTION

The skin normally contains special cells called melanocytes that produce melanin, a black pigment that gives color to the skin. Several conditions cause the melanocytes to develop abnormally or to be distributed abnormally. Melanocytes sometimes are fewer in number or less active than normal. This results in a pale area of skin that does not tan when exposed to sunlight. When melanocytes are more numerous or more active than normal, a darker area of skin that tans easily results. These abnormal conditions include albinism, vitiligo, melasma (chloasma), nevi (moles), seborrheic warts, pityriasis, and abnormal suntan.

PATIENT SCREENING

Abnormal skin pigmentation presents a cosmetic problem. The individual calling for an appointment for these symptoms should be scheduled for the next convenient appointment.

Albinism

■ **ICD-9-CM Code 270.2**

Albinism is a rare inherited condition in which the melanocytes are unable to produce melanin. The

---

ENRICHMENT

GUIDELINES FOR PROTECTING THE SKIN AGAINST EXCESSIVE SUN EXPOSURE

- Avoid sunlight between 10 AM and 3 PM, when ultraviolet rays are the strongest.
- Plan outdoor activities for early morning or late afternoon.

- Wear protective clothing, especially a hat.
- Use a sunscreen with a sun protection factor (SPF) of at least 15, applied 15 to 30 minutes before exposure and again after getting wet, especially after swimming.

Abnormal Skin Pigmentation

patient is pale skinned, with white hair and generally pink or pale blue eyes (Fig. 6–34). A rare disorder occurring in all races, albinism often is accompanied by eye problems. Eye problems may include myopia, hyperopia, astigmatism, nystagmus, strabismus, and photophobia. Patients with albinism must avoid the sun to prevent their eyes and skin from burning. This genetic disorder has no cure, but many of the eye problems can be treated. Counseling may help the child or young adult deal with social problems created by the lack of understanding in society about the disorder.

Vitiligo

■ ICD-9-CM Code **709.01**

Possibly an immune condition, vitiligo produces pale irregular patches of skin, often evenly located on one side of the body (Fig. 6–35). The patches may enlarge, shrink, or stay the same size. Vitiligo can occur on any area of the body and affects all races. Vitiligo often follows a stressful incident. Vitiligo has no cure, but cosmetics may be used to cover the affected skin areas. Patients with vitiligo should be encouraged to use sunscreen.

Melasma (Chloasma)

■ ICD-9-CM Code **709.09**

Melasma occurs in some women during hormonal changes, such as during pregnancy or with oral contraceptive use. Patches of darker skin develop on the face, especially over the cheeks (Fig. 6–36). This condition disappears after childbirth or when the oral contraceptive use is discontinued.

Hemangiomas

■ ICD-9-CM Code **228.00**
Hemangiomas are coded by sites and types. The general code for hemangioma is 228.00. Refer

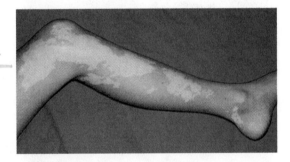

FIGURE 6–35 Vitiligo. (From Callen J, Greer K, Hood A, et al: *Color atlas of dermatology*, Philadelphia, 1993, Saunders.)

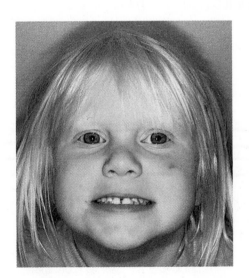

FIGURE 6–34 Albinism. (From Callen J, Greer K, Hood A, et al: *Color atlas of dermatology*, Philadelphia, 1993, Saunders.)

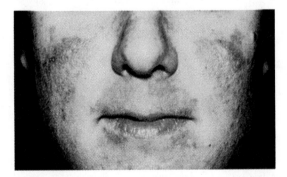

FIGURE 6–36 Melasma (chloasma). (From Callen J, Greer K, Hood A, et al: *Color atlas of dermatology*, Philadelphia, 1993, Saunders.)

to the physician's diagnosis and then to the current edition of the ICD-9-CM coding manual to ensure the greatest specificity of pathology and any appropriate modifiers.

Hemangiomas are benign lesions of proliferating blood vessels in the dermis that produce a red, blue, or purple color. Examples of hemangiomas are the **nevus** flammeus (port-wine stain), which is dark red to purple and usually is located on the face (Fig. 6–37, *A*); the strawberry hemangioma, which is bright red and has a protruding, rough surface (Fig. 6–37, *B*); and the cherry hemangioma, which is red to purple and is a smooth, dome-shaped, small papule 2 to 5 mm in diameter (Fig. 6–37, *C*).

Nevi (Moles)

■ **ICD-9-CM Code** *(Refer to Neoplasm, Skin, Benign in the current edition of the ICD-9-CM coding manual)*
There are many codes for nevus. Refer to the physician's diagnosis and then to the current edition of the ICD-9-CM coding manual to ensure the greatest specificity of pathology and any appropriate modifiers.

Moles are small dark areas of skin composed of dense collections of melanocytes; some may contain hair. A mole occasionally may become malignant (see Malignant Melanoma).

Seborrheic Warts

■ **ICD-9-CM Code 078.10**
There are several ICD-9-CM codes for wart. The code for warts (common) is 078.10. Refer to the physician's diagnosis and then to the current edition of the ICD-9-CM coding manual to ensure the greatest specificity of pathology and any appropriate modifiers.

Seborrheic warts are not true warts but are round or oval patches of darkly pigmented skin 1 to 3 cm across. They often develop after middle age and have a crusty, greasy-looking surface.

Pityriasis

■ **ICD-9-CM Code 696.5**
Pityriasis may be coded according to location or form. The 696.5 is a general code. Refer to the physician's diagnosis and then to the current edition of the ICD-9-CM coding manual to ensure the greatest specificity of pathology and any appropriate modifiers.

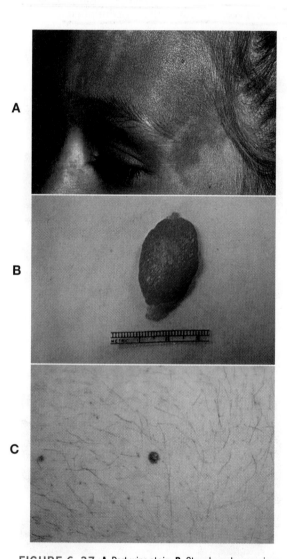

A

B

C

FIGURE 6–37 A, Port wine stain. **B,** Strawberry hemangioma. **C,** Cherry hemangioma. (**A** from Callen J, Greer K, Hood A, et al: *Color atlas of dermatology,* Philadelphia, 1993, Saunders. **B** and **C** from Lookingbill D, Marks J: *Principles of dermatology,* ed 3, Philadelphia, 2000, Saunders.)

Pityriasis is a fungal infection that causes patches of flaky, light, or dark skin to develop on the trunk of the body. This is an uncommon condition.

Abnormal Suntan

■ ICD-9-CM Code 995.2

Abnormal suntan is an unspecified adverse effect resulting from a proper drug, medicinal, or biological substance properly administered. Some drugs and certain diseases such as Addison disease can produce a suntan without exposure to sunlight.

ETIOLOGY

The causes of abnormal skin pigmentation vary according to the abnormality.

DIAGNOSIS

Most of these conditions are harmless, and visual examination by a physician confirms the diagnosis. Moles may cause concern, especially if size or shape has changed. The physician may recommend a biopsy to rule out a malignancy.

TREATMENT

When any of these conditions produce skin color variations, nonprescription depigmenting creams may be used to lighten the affected skin. Vitiligo may be improved by ultraviolet lamp treatments combined with drug therapy. Pityriasis can be cured by the application of antifungal ointments. Moles can be removed surgically, and other skin blemishes can be covered with special cosmetics. Laser surgery may be used to treat hemangiomas.

PROGNOSIS

The prognosis varies and depends on the condition and its extent. When drug therapy and surgical intervention are not appropriate or successful, cosmetics may be used to conceal the pigmentation problem.

PREVENTION

The etiology varies, and so prevention varies. Hereditary conditions cannot be prevented. Most of these conditions occur without warning.

PATIENT TEACHING

Help patients locate and use the available resources for their condition. Support groups often are available for certain cases. Encourage patients to recognize their self-worth.

Alopecia (Baldness)

DESCRIPTION

Alopecia is the loss or absence of hair, especially on the scalp.

■ ICD-9-CM Code 704.00 *(Unspecified)*
Alopecia has four ICD-9-CM codes. Refer to the physician's diagnosis and then to the current edition of the ICD-9-CM coding manual to ensure the greatest specificity of pathology and any appropriate modifiers.

> **704.01** *(Alopecia areata)*
> **704.02** *(Telogen effluvium)*
> **704.09** *(Other)*

SYMPTOMS AND SIGNS

Alopecia can be either temporary or permanent. It can appear gradually, as with aging, or suddenly, occurring all at once or in patchy areas, as with alopecia areata (Fig. 6–38, *A*).

PATIENT SCREENING

Alopecia is a troublesome and worrisome condition. It also may be the sign of an underlying health problem. Schedule this patient to be seen when convenient for all involved.

ETIOLOGY

In most cases, baldness is a result of the aging process or heredity. It can, however, be a consequence of certain systemic illnesses, such as thyroid diseases and iron deficiency anemia. Certain forms of dermatitis (see Dermatitis) also can cause alopecia. Chemotherapy, radiation therapy used to treat cancer, and some other types of medications may lead to thinning and loss of hair. The hair often grows back after treatment has been completed. More often, however, hair loss is not attributed to any specific disease process.

In men, alopecia tends to be part of the aging process and have a familial occurrence on the mother's side. The typical pattern is for the front hairline to recede and for the hair on the top of the head to thin. In some men, these areas eventually

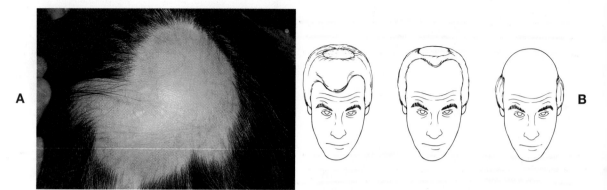

FIGURE 6–38 A, Alopecia areata. **B,** Androgenetic alopecia (male pattern baldness). (**A** from Callen J, Greer K, Hood A, et al: *Color atlas of dermatology,* Philadelphia, 1993, Saunders.)

meet, leaving hair on only the sides of the head. This pattern of hair loss is called androgenetic alopecia (male pattern baldness) (Fig. 6–38, *B*). Most women experience a gradual but slight loss of hair throughout life. Some women experience thinning of their hair about 3 months postpartum. This is a fairly common occurrence and corrects itself within a few months.

Finally, a more severe but rare form of alopecia causes permanent hair loss over the entire body, including the eyebrows and eyelashes.

DIAGNOSIS
Visual examination may be all that is needed for the diagnosis, but the cause also should be investigated. Blood and thyroid studies are needed to rule out thyroid disease and anemia.

TREATMENT
Treatment of alopecia varies according to the cause. Effective treatment of any underlying disease usually restores hair growth to normal. To treat male pattern baldness, minoxidil (Rogaine) preparations used topically in cream and spray forms have shown promise. Finasteride (Propecia) is an additional drug therapy. Other options include wearing a toupee or wig or having a hair transplant. Transplantation is effective for certain types of hair loss, especially male pattern baldness, but transplantation and the use of minoxidil are expensive and can have side effects. The minoxidil must be continued indefinitely, or hair will begin to fall out again.

PROGNOSIS
The prognosis varies depending on the cause. Alopecia resulting from the aging process or heredity will not improve. As previously stated, treatment of an underlying medical cause may result in improvement.

PREVENTION
No prevention is known for alopecia.

PATIENT TEACHING
Those who have baldness resulting from the aging process or heredity should be encouraged to accept the condition. Offer information about alopecia and permanent or temporary hair replacement.

Folliculitis

DESCRIPTION
Folliculitis is an inflammatory reaction of the hair follicles that produces erythemic, pustular lesions (Fig. 6–39).

◼ **ICD-9-CM Code 704.8**

SYMPTOMS AND SIGNS
The pustules of folliculitis are individual and do not combine. They usually are found on the thighs and buttocks but also can occur in the beard area and on the scalp. Some patients may

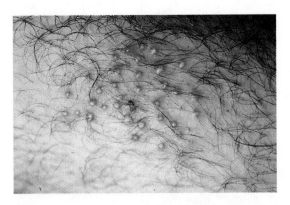

FIGURE 6–39 Folliculitis. (From Callen J, Greer K, Hood A, et al: *Color atlas of dermatology,* Philadelphia, 1993, Saunders.)

report mild discomfort, mainly pruritus, associated with the pustules, but folliculitis is usually asymptomatic.

This is a relatively common condition that affects primarily young adults. It can be chronic or recurrent.

PATIENT SCREENING

As with many other skin disorders, folliculitis is a troublesome and worrisome condition. Schedule the patient to be seen at the next available appointment.

ETIOLOGY

Folliculitis is a bacterial infection caused by *Staphylococcus aureus.* The bacteria enter the skin through the opening of the hair follicle and cause a low-grade infection within the epidermal layer. Shaving with a straight razor is a common precipitating factor.

DIAGNOSIS

The diagnosis of folliculitis is based on the presence of hairs within the pustular lesions. It is confirmed when a culture of the purulent material shows the presence of *S. aureus.*

TREATMENT

For most mild cases of folliculitis, a topical antiseptic cleanser, such as povidone-iodine (Betadine), used daily or every other day for several weeks, manages the problem. More extensive involvement requires a systemic antibiotic, such as eryth-

romycin, taken 4 times a day for 10 days, in addition to the topical cleansers.

Folliculitis occasionally results in the development of a furuncle that requires incision and drainage (see Furuncles and Carbuncles).

PROGNOSIS

With treatment, the prognosis is good.

PREVENTION

Avoid the use of a straight razor. Good hygiene always helps combat any infectious condition.

PATIENT TEACHING

Give patients information about the disorder. Encourage them not to squeeze any resulting pustules.

Corns and Calluses

DESCRIPTION

Corns and calluses are extremely common, localized hyperplastic areas of the stratum corneum layer of the epidermis.

 ICD-9-CM Code 700

SYMPTOMS AND SIGNS

Corns have a glassy core, are small (less than ⅕ inch), are more painful than calluses, and develop on the toes. Calluses are larger (up to 1 inch) and commonly develop on the ball of the foot and the palms of the hands. Tenderness and pain over the affected area are the common symptoms.

PATIENT SCREENING

Patients with corns and calluses usually report painful feet when requesting an appointment. Schedule the next available appointment that is convenient for all involved.

ETIOLOGY

Both conditions may be due to pressure or friction caused by ill-fitting shoes, orthopedic deformities, or faulty weight-bearing. People who play stringed instruments and manual laborers are prone to calluses caused by repeated trauma. In addition, people with impaired circulation in their feet resulting from peripheral neuropathy (sometimes caused by diabetes mellitus) are more prone to the development of corns and calluses.

DIAGNOSIS

It is unusual for corns and calluses to become so painful that the patient consults a physician. When the patient does consult a physician, a physical examination of the affected area and brief history are sufficient for diagnosis.

TREATMENT

Relieving pressure and friction points as soon as possible is the goal of treatment. Many self-help measures are available, such as pads and sponge rings, chemical agents to soften and loosen corns, and pumice stone to rub off dead skin resulting from calluses. If these treatments are ineffective, a physician can trim the corn or callus surgically or with strong chemicals. *Warning:* Patients with diabetes mellitus should not use self-help measures but should seek the help of a podiatrist to treat corns and calluses.

PROGNOSIS

Most corns and calluses will resolve with treatment and removal of the offending pressure source.

PREVENTION

Properly fitting shoes help prevent corns and calluses. Some calluses caused by repeated trauma cannot be prevented.

PATIENT TEACHING

Give patients information about the etiology of corns and calluses. Recommend the wearing of proper footwear. Encourage diabetics and those with impaired circulation to seek professional foot care on a regular basis.

Verrucae (Warts)

DESCRIPTION

Verrucae are elevated growths of the epidermis that result from hyperplasia (Fig. 6–40).

■ **ICD-9-CM Code 078.10** *(Viral warts, unspecified)*
Warts have several ICD-9-CM codes. The code for viral warts, unspecified, is 078.10. Refer to the physician's diagnosis and then to the cur-

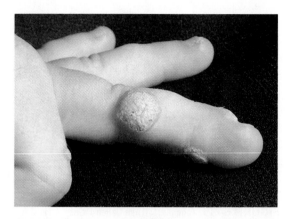

FIGURE 6–40 Verruca (common wart). (From Lookingbill D, Marks J: *Principles of dermatology,* ed 3, Philadelphia, 2000, Saunders.)

rent edition of the ICD-9-CM coding manual to ensure the greatest specificity of pathology and any appropriate modifiers.

SYMPTOMS AND SIGNS

Of the several types of warts, the most common is the plantar wart. This wart is a small, hard, white or pink lump with a cauliflower-like surface. Inside the wart are small, clotted blood vessels that resemble black splinters.

A verruca can develop anywhere on the body but is most likely to appear on the hands or the soles of the feet. For the most part, the wart is painless, but a wart on the sole of a foot (plantar wart) can feel as if one has a stone in the shoe. Pruritus also can accompany a wart. Verrucae are common among teenagers and children, but no serious health risks are associated with these warts.

ETIOLOGY

Warts are caused by viruses and are spread by touch or contact with the skin shed from a wart. Each of the five viruses known to cause warts tends to infect a different part of the body.

DIAGNOSIS

Diagnosis is made by visual examination. There are two cases of warts in which a physician should be consulted. One is penile or vulvar warts, and the other is a wart that develops after the age of 45 years. What looks like a wart actually could be a serious skin condition such as skin cancer.

TREATMENT

Most warts disappear naturally over time. Many self-help remedies are available in the form of paints, creams, or plasters. These medications contain chemicals that destroy the abnormal skin cells, but they also damage the surrounding healthy cells. Care must be taken to minimize soreness. Warts located on the face or genitals should not be treated with these chemicals. A physician can remove persistent warts by surgical excision, cryosurgery, or electrodesiccation. Treatment is often painful and tedious.

PROGNOSIS

With medical intervention, the prognosis for most warts is good. Some warts tend to recur.

PREVENTION

Warts are contagious, and a wart may shed cells along with the virus when it is touched. Prevention of venereal warts is discussed in Chapter 12.

PATIENT TEACHING

Give patients information about warts and how they are spread. Advise them to wear shower shoes when using a public bathing facility.

Deformed or Discolored Nails

DESCRIPTION

Nails with any unusual thickening, shape, or color that deviates from normal are classified as deformed or discolored nails.

 ICD-9-CM Code 703.9

SYMPTOMS AND SIGNS

Any unusual thickening, color variation, and change in the shape of either the fingernails or the toenails can be symptoms of an underlying disease or disorder.

PATIENT SCREENING

Patients reporting deformities, odd shapes, or discoloration of nails are usually scheduled for an appointment that fits their convenience. The physician must remember that any sudden deviation from normal may be the result of underlying disease process.

ETIOLOGY

Injury to the nail bed caused by continuous pressure from ill-fitting shoes or poor circulation caused by arteriosclerosis can lead to thickening of the whole nail. Many disorders can produce nail deformities. Psoriasis, lichen planus, and chronic paronychia can cause the end of the nail to separate from the underlying skin. Bacteria can enter this space and make the nail turn a blackish green. Iron deficiency anemia can cause spooning of the nails. Congenital heart disorders and lung cancer can cause clubbing, or knobby ends of the fingers or toes, and then cause the nails to grow around these ends.

Nail discoloration is caused by many illnesses. With anemia, the nail bed appears pale. A person with chronic hepatic disease has white nail beds. Small, black, splinter-like areas appear under the nails with infections of the cardiac valves, systemic lupus erythematosus, and dermatomyositis.

Vitamin or mineral deficiencies and injury to a nail may cause one or more white patches to develop in the nail. The nail of the big toe sometimes can curve under at the sides and dig into the skin, causing pain as it grows. This is known as an ingrown toenail.

DIAGNOSIS

Examination of the affected nail or nails and a medical history may be all that is needed for a diagnosis. A blood chemistry profile detects any underlying condition or illness.

TREATMENT

Deformities and discolorations caused by underlying illnesses resolve when the illness is corrected. Nails damaged by injury usually grow back in or grow out again in about 9 months. The patient can practice several self-help measures with an ingrown toenail, such as wearing loose-fitting shoes, keeping the area clean and dry to prevent infection, and cutting the nail straight across the top. If these measures do not help, the patient should see a physician. The physician can remove the ingrowing edge of the nail and the toe's nail fold and apply a chemical to the edge to relieve the discomfort and prevent the edge from ingrowing again.

PROGNOSIS

As previously mentioned, deformities and discolorations caused by underlying illnesses usually resolve when the illness is corrected. Nails damaged by injury usually grow back in or grow out again in about 9 months. Treatment for ingrown toenails usually has a positive outcome.

PREVENTION

Trimming toenails straight across helps prevent ingrown toenails. Malformations of the nails often are the result of injury to the nails or nail beds or the sequela to certain disease processes and cannot be prevented.

PATIENT TEACHING

Give patients information about proper care and trimming of nails. Encourage those with ingrown toenails to select shoes with sufficient toe space.

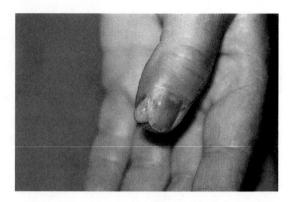

FIGURE 6–41 Paronychia. (From Callen J, Greer K, Hood A, et al: *Color atlas of dermatology,* Philadelphia, 1993, Saunders.)

Paronychia

DESCRIPTION

A paronychia is an infection of the skin around a nail.

ICD-9-CM Code 681.02

The ICD-9-CM code 681.02 applies to paronychia of the finger. There are several ICD-9-CM codes listed for paronychia, so refer to the physician's diagnosis and then to the current edition of the ICD-9-CM coding manual to ensure the greatest specificity of pathology and any appropriate modifiers. Additional codes are required to identify the causative organism.

SYMPTOMS AND SIGNS

With an acute paronychia, the cuticle or nail fold becomes edematous, red, and painful. If the cuticle lifts away from the base of the nail, purulent material may be expressed from beneath. When the nail fold is affected, a blister of pus called a whitlow develops beside the nail (Fig. 6–41). Chronic infections produce similar symptoms, and often several nails are affected. With the cuticle lifted, the nail roots no longer are protected and become damaged. This produces deformed or discolored nails.

PATIENT SCREENING

The patient experiencing a paronychia may also feel pain in the hand. If an appointment cannot be promptly scheduled, refer the patient to a medical facility that can provide prompt assessment and treatment.

ETIOLOGY

The infection may be caused by bacteria or fungi. Bacteria usually cause acute infections, whereas fungi usually cause chronic infections. The chronic infections develop slowly and are less painful but are also more persistent. Paronychia occurs particularly in people who have their hands in water for long periods.

DIAGNOSIS

A physician can diagnose a paronychia on examination of the affected areas and with a history of the symptoms. A culture of the **exudate** is needed to identify a bacterial or fungal origin.

TREATMENT

Antibiotics correct a bacterial infection, and if the infection is chronic, an antifungal cream or paint (ciclopirox [Penlac]) is prescribed.

PROGNOSIS

Drug therapy usually helps the infection to resolve. Several months of treatment may be required for the swelling to subside and the raised cuticle to return to normal.

PREVENTION

Encourage good hand-washing technique along with thorough drying of the hands after washing or being in water for extended periods of time.

PATIENT TEACHING

Demonstrate proper hand-washing technique. Emphasize the importance of drying the hands after exposure to water.

REVIEW CHALLENGE

Answer the following questions:

1. What are the functions of the integumentary system?
2. What is the difference between a macule and a cyst? A plaque and a fissure? A comedo and a pustule?
3. How is cradle cap related to seborrheic dermatitis?
4. What factors might induce the inflammation of contact dermatitis?
5. How is the skin likely to appear in a person diagnosed with atopic dermatitis?
6. Where on the body are the lesions of psoriasis most likely to appear?
7. What treatment might the physician prescribe for acne vulgaris?
8. What is the clinical course of herpes zoster?
9. Is impetigo contagious?
10. Are there any conditions considered predisposing to furuncles and carbuncles? If so, what are they?
11. Is cellulitis always a local infection?
12. How are dermatophytoses classified?
13. What are the early signs of a decubitus ulcer?
14. What is the comprehensive treatment plan for a human scabies infestation, or for lice?
15. What are two of the most common premalignant skin tumors?
16. What is the most serious type of skin cancer? What are the characteristics of such a lesion?
17. Besides the aging process, what are other possible causes of alopecia?
18. What are the ABCDs of malignant melanoma?

REAL-LIFE CHALLENGE

Shingles

A 57-year-old woman presents with severe pain in the left occipital region, in the left side of her neck, and in the left scapular region. The onset was approximately 36 hours ago. She describes the pain as intermittent, sharp, shooting, and severe. She has been taking ibuprofen for the pain, with little relief. She noticed small blisters forming along the painful areas in the last few hours. She is afebrile and appears quite uncomfortable.

On examination, small blister-like eruptions are noted along the left side of the neck, left anterior shoulder, and clavicular area. Some eruptions also appear at the base of the skull just in the hairline. These eruptions do not cross the midline on either the front or back of the body.

The patient is diagnosed with shingles, along the C-2, C-3, C-4 peripheral nerve or dermatome area. On questioning, the patient confirms having chickenpox in childhood at about 8 years of age.

Medications prescribed include famciclovir (Famvir) 500 mg tid for 7 days. Acyclovir (Zovirax) cream also was prescribed for topical application to the affected areas and hydrocodone bitartrate with acetaminophen (Vicodin) for pain.

QUESTIONS

1. What is the significance of the previous occurrence of chickenpox?
2. What is the causative agent of chickenpox? Of shingles?
3. Why is the fact that the eruptions do not cross the midline important?
4. Identify other medications that may be prescribed for shingles.
5. What might the patient expect as an outcome of this condition?
6. What is meant by postherpetic neuralgia?

REAL-LIFE CHALLENGE

Malignant Melanoma

A 35-year-old fair-skinned woman has noticed the enlargement of a mole on her right lower arm. The mole has been present as long as she can remember. In the past month, it appears to have doubled in size and has become darker.

The patient admits to having been exposed to direct sunlight for the past several years. She lives in southern Texas and spends several hours a day in the sun while doing garden work. She has not consistently applied sunscreen to her lower arms and hands.

Visual examination shows a slightly elevated, 7-mm, irregularly shaped, dark multicolored lesion on the dorsal aspect of the right lower arm, about 3 inches above the wrist. Closer examination shows the lesion to be asymmetrical, with a notched border.

Family history reveals that the patient's mother had three lesions removed from her arms and face that were diagnosed as malignant melanoma. In addition, two maternal aunts have had malignant melanomas. One aunt recently died from metastatic cancer. The patient remembers having incurred several sunburns with blistering as a child.

Surgical excision of the lesion is performed, and the biopsy confirms the diagnosis of malignant melanoma. The patient is referred to an oncologist for possible chemotherapy.

QUESTIONS

1. What characteristics does the patient have that suggest she may have malignant melanoma?
2. What symptoms distinguish malignant melanoma from basal cell or squamous cell carcinomas?
3. What is the prognosis for a patient with malignant melanoma, such as this patient?
4. What patient teaching would you offer to patients about extensive exposure to sunlight?
5. What is the importance of a good family history?
6. Why was the patient referred to an oncologist?
7. Would this patient be a candidate for further surgical procedures? If so, what procedures and why?
8. List the warning signs of malignant melanoma.

INTERNET ASSIGNMENTS

1. Research actinic keratosis at the American Academy of Dermatology and write a report on its connection with squamous cell carcinoma.

2. Research the incidence of malignant melanoma and its treatment at The Melanoma Research Foundation. Investigate the mortality and morbidity rates of this condition

Diseases and Conditions of the Musculoskeletal System

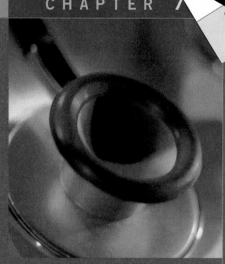

Continued

Chapter Outline—Cont'd

Learning Objectives

After studying Chapter 7, you should be able to:

1. List the functions of the normal skeletal system.
2. Distinguish among the pathologic features of lordosis, kyphosis, and scoliosis.
3. Describe the signs and symptoms of the most common form of arthritis.
4. Explain the importance of early diagnosis and treatment of Lyme disease.
5. Describe the treatment of bone tumors, both benign and malignant.
6. Discuss the specifics of a physical examination when fibromyalgia is suspected.
7. Explain why joint disability results from gout.
8. Describe the clinical picture of osteomyelitis and explain how it is treated.
9. Describe the disability that results from advanced osteoporosis.
10. Explain why osteomalacia is termed a metabolic bone disease.
11. Distinguish between hallux valgus and hallux rigidus.
12. Differentiate between a strain and a sprain.
13. Explain the importance of proper treatment of dislocations.
14. Describe the cause of shin splints.
15. List some factors that contribute to the development of plantar fasciitis.
16. Explain how torn meniscus is treated.
17. Describe the signs and symptoms of rotator cuff tears.

Key Terms

avulsion (ah–**VUL**–shun)
bursae (**BURR**–see)
calcitonin (**kal**–sih–**TOE**–nin)
crepitation (krep–ih–**TAY**–shun)
fascia (**FASH**–ee–ah)
hematopoiesis (**heem**–ah–toe–poy–**EE**–sis)

meniscus (meh–**NIS**–kuss)
metatarsophalangea (**met**–ah–**tar**–so–fah–**LAN**–jee–al)
ossification (**oss**–ih–fih–**KAY**–shun)
osteogenesis (**oss**–tee–oh–**JEN**–eh–sis)
synovial (sin–**OH**–vee–al)
tenorrhaphy (teh–**NOR**–ah–fee)

THE MUSCULOSKELETAL SYSTEM

USCLES, BONES, LIGAMENTS, tendons, cartilage, and the joints they form, provide the body with a supportive framework that allows flexibility of movement and protects the internal organs. The tissues of the musculoskeletal system also give shape to the body; act partially as a storage and supply area for minerals; and serve as sites for the formation of blood cells.

When the tissues are unable to perform their usual functions because of trauma or rheumatic, inflammatory, or degenerative conditions, a person's physical support, protection, mobility, and ability to perform in normal activities are affected. Trauma is a major cause of musculoskeletal disorders; automobile accidents and injuries (strains, sprains, dislocations, and fractures) are the leading causes of disabilities and death.

All muscles are composed of a basic cellular unit called the *muscle fiber,* which is made of protein. Muscles of the skeleton are collections or masses of tissue that cover bones, providing bulk to the body while also helping to hold body parts together and to move various joints (Fig. 7–1).

All movement, including the movement of the body itself and of the internal organs, is performed by muscle tissue. For example, movement of the extremities is accomplished through the contraction and relaxation of certain skeletal muscles, which

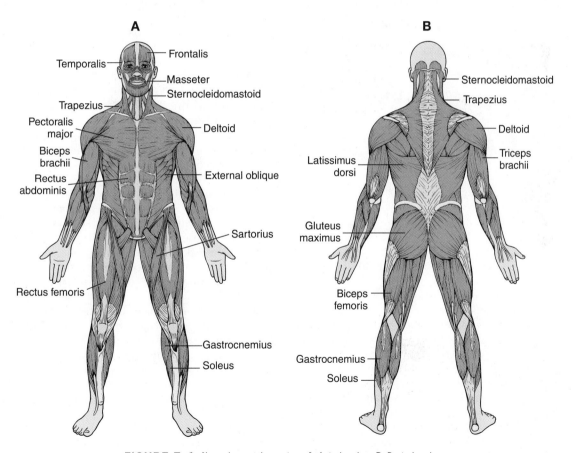

FIGURE 7–1 Normal muscular system. **A,** Anterior view. **B,** Posterior view.

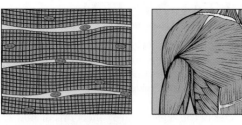

Striated (skeletal) muscle

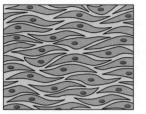
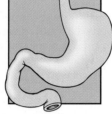

Nonstriated (smooth) muscle

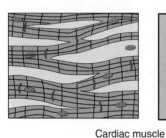
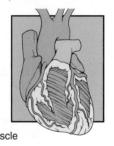

Cardiac muscle

FIGURE 7–2 Types of muscles.

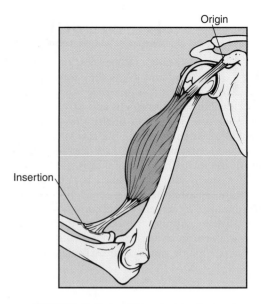

FIGURE 7–3 Insertion and origin of a muscle.

have been stimulated by nerves at the request of the brain.

The three types of muscle are striated (skeletal), nonstriated (smooth), and cardiac (Fig. 7–2); they are classified as either voluntary or involuntary. Skeletal muscle is voluntary and is under the control of the conscious mind; this includes the muscles used to move the limbs, arms, and legs. Smooth muscle and heart muscle are involuntary and function without conscious control or awareness. Examples are the muscles that move the bowels and create the heartbeat of the heart. The point of attachment of a muscle to a stationary bone is referred to as the *origin* of the muscle, and the point of attachment to a bone that is moved by the muscle is referred to as its *insertion* (Fig. 7–3).

The skeletal system is composed of 206 bones that provide an important support system for the many parts of the body and enable a person to stand erect (Fig. 7–4).

Some bones encase and protect specific organs (e.g., the skull protects the brain, and the rib cage and the backbone protect the heart and lungs). In coordination with muscles and joints, bones assist body movement. The blood cells are formed in the bone marrow in a process called **hematopoiesis.** Bones are not lifeless structures, but instead are structures infused with living cells arranged in a hard framework of minerals (calcium and phosphorus). These cells are continuously forming new bone; bone formation is counter-balanced by bone reabsorption. Normally, the balance of these two processes prevents bones from becoming excessively thick, as with Paget disease of bone, or too thin, as with osteoporosis.

Bones are complete organs; they are composed mainly of connective tissue with a rich supply of blood vessels and nerves. They develop through a process called **osteogenesis,** and the complete skeleton is formed by the end of the third month of gestation. The fetal skeleton is composed of cartilage tissue, which is replaced gradually by bone cells in a process called **ossification.** Ossification depends on an adequate supply of calcium and phosphorus getting to the bone tissue.

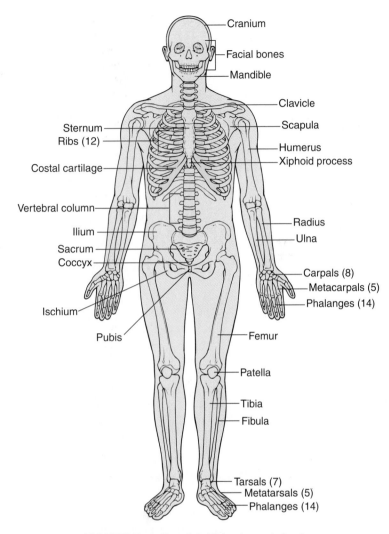

Cranium
Facial bones
Mandible
Clavicle
Scapula
Sternum
Ribs (12)
Humerus
Xiphoid process
Costal cartilage
Vertebral column
Radius
Ilium
Ulna
Sacrum
Coccyx
Carpals (8)
Metacarpals (5)
Phalanges (14)
Ischium
Pubis
Femur
Patella
Tibia
Fibula
Tarsals (7)
Metatarsals (5)
Phalanges (14)

FIGURE 7–4 Normal skeletal system, anterior view.

Several different types of bone make up the skeleton. Long bones are strong and have broad ends and large surface areas for muscle attachment. They are found in the humerus (upper arm), the ulna and radius (lower arm, or forearm), the femur (thigh), and the tibia and fibula (lower leg). Short bones have small, irregular shapes and include the carpal (wrist) and the tarsal (ankle) bones. Flat bones cover soft body parts; they include the scapula (shoulder), ribs, and pelvic bones. Sesamoid bones are small and rounded and are found near joints. The patella (kneecap) is an example.

Joints, or articulations, are body structures in which bones are joined or the surfaces of two bones come together for the purpose of creating motion. With the help of ligaments, joints hold bones firmly together yet allow movement between them. Joints are classified by the type of material found between the bones: fibrous, cartilaginous, and **synovial.** Joints also are classified according to the degree of movement (Fig. 7–5) they can make. Immovable (synarthrodial) joints (e.g., suture joints between the bones of the skull) are connected by fibrous tissue; slightly movable (amphiarthrodial) joints (e.g., the intervertebral joints

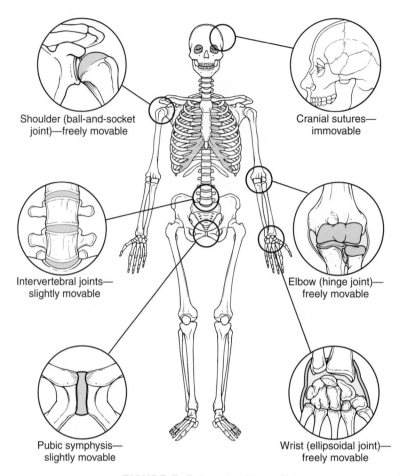

Shoulder (ball-and-socket joint)—freely movable

Cranial sutures—immovable

Intervertebral joints—slightly movable

Elbow (hinge joint)—freely movable

Pubic symphysis—slightly movable

Wrist (ellipsoidal joint)—freely movable

FIGURE 7–5 Examples of types of joints.

and the pubic symphysis) are connected by cartilage; and freely movable (diarthrodial) joints (e.g., the knee and the elbow) are called *synovial joints* because they are lined with the fluid-producing synovial membrane. Within synovial joints also are bones, cartilage that covers the ends of the bones, ligaments that hold bones together, synovial fluid, blood and lymph vessels, and nerves.

Most joints are the freely movable type. The amount or degree of movement that a joint has is referred to as its range of motion (ROM). Only the freely movable joints can execute a wide range of movements.

Ligaments are tough, dense, fibrous bands of connective tissue that hold bones together, either around a joint capsule (e.g., the hip joint) or across a joint (e.g., the knee [Fig. 7–6]). They allow movement in some directions while restricting it in other directions, thereby providing some stability. Injury to ligaments can occur in several ways; they can be overstretched and sustain partial or complete tears (sprains) or be torn completely loose from their attachment to a bone, an injury called an **avulsion.**

Tendons are strong, tough strands, or cords, of dense connective tissue. They serve to attach muscles to bones and other parts (see Fig. 7–6). Tendons are nonelastic and are capable of withstanding great forces from contracting muscles without sustaining damage to themselves. Injury to a tendon is called a *strain.*

Fascia is a specialized flat band of tissue located just below the skin that covers and separates underlying tissues, commonly muscle layers. Inflamed or injured fascia is referred to as *fasciitis.*

Cartilage is a semi-smooth, dense, supporting connective tissue that is found at the ends of bones. It forms a cap over the ends of bones and provides support and protection when they are engaged in weight-bearing activities. Cartilage absorbs the energy force of weight pressed or thrust against joints to prevent injury to joints, bones, and the cartilage itself; in effect, it functions as a "shock absorber." To remain healthy, cartilage at the joints must receive nutrients from the joint fluid and maintain normal joint movement and weight-bearing activities.

Also necessary to the functioning of the musculoskeletal system are the **bursae,** closed sacs or cavities of synovial fluid lined with a synovial membrane. Positioned between tissues such as tendons, bones, and ligaments, bursae make it possible for these tissues to glide over each other without creating friction. Bursae are located in the shoulder (see Fig. 7–15), elbow, and knee joints.

Another substance found throughout the musculoskeletal system is a fibrous protein called *collagen.* Collagen is the major supporting element, or glue, in the connective tissues that holds the cells together. In adults, collagen makes up one third to one half of the total body protein (see Chapter 3).

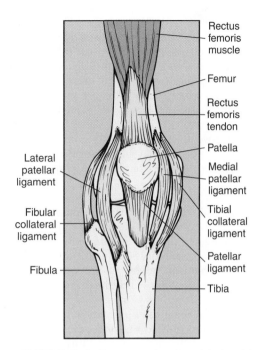

FIGURE 7–6 Ligaments and tendons of the knee joint.

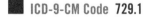

Fibromyalgia

DESCRIPTION
Fibromyalgia is a chronic pain condition associated with stiffness and tenderness that affects muscles, tendons, and joints throughout the body. Fibromyalgia is also characterized by restless sleep, depression, fatigue, anxiety, and bowel dysfunction.

■ ICD-9-CM Code **729.1**

SYMPTOMS AND SIGNS
Fibromyalgia, one of the most common diseases affecting the muscles, causes chronic pain in muscles and soft tissues surrounding joints. Fatigue is extremely common in patients with this condition. Patients also may report diffuse aching or burning in the muscles, stiffness, disturbed sleep patterns, poor concentration, irritability, and depression. They may note extreme tenderness of various areas of the body. Other nonspecific symptoms include headaches, jaw pain, and sensitivity to odors, bright lights, and loud noises. Some patients experience symptoms of irritable bowel syndrome or "spastic colon," including nausea, diarrhea, constipation, or abdominal pain with gas and distention. Urinary symptoms, when present, include urinary urgency or frequency brought on by bladder spasms and irritability. Often patients experiencing fibromyalgia wake up feeling tired, even if they have slept all through the night. Others sleep lightly and wake up during the night.

PATIENT SCREENING
Schedule the patient complaining of persistent fatigue and unexplained muscle pain and tenderness for an appointment within 2 days or at earliest convenience.

ETIOLOGY
The cause of fibromyalgia is unknown. Patients experience pain in response to stimuli that are normally not perceived as painful. Researchers have found elevated levels of a nerve growth factor and a chemical signal, called *substance P,* in the spinal

fluid of patients with fibromyalgia. The amount of serotonin, a chemical produced in the brain that affects nerves, is relatively low in these patients. Furthermore, those with fibromyalgia experience impaired non–rapid eye movement (non-REM) sleep, which likely explains the common feature of waking up feeling fatigued and unrefreshed. The onset of fibromyalgia has been associated with psychologic distress, trauma, and infection. The condition may be aggravated by poor posture, inappropriate exercise, and smoking.

DIAGNOSIS

Many medical conditions can cause pain in multiple areas of the body, thus mimicking fibromyalgia. Blood testing and physical examination are important to *exclude* conditions such as hypothyroidism, hypoparathyroidism, other muscle diseases, bone diseases, virus infections, and cancer.

No specific laboratory or imaging studies that can be used to diagnose fibromyalgia are known. Testing is done only to exclude other causes of muscle pain. The diagnosis of fibromyalgia is made purely on clinical grounds based on the thorough history and physical examination to reveal widespread tenderness and pain or aching in at least 11 of 18 specific tender points (Fig. 7–7). Usually found on both sides of the body in all four quadrants, the widespread pain should exist for a minimum of 3 months before being diagnosed as fibromyalgia. The 18 sites of tender points cluster in the regions of the neck, shoulders, chest, hips, knees, and elbows. Additionally, the occurrence of sleep disorders helps to confirm the diagnosis.

TREATMENT

Although no cure for fibromyalgia is known, treatment can help alleviate symptoms and restore function. Treatment involves patient education, stress reduction, physical activity, and medications. Attempts are made to reduce pain and improve the quality of sleep. Medications that can improve sleep patterns may be prescribed, such as low doses of the antidepressant amitriptyline (Elavil). For muscle and joint soreness, nonsteroidal antiinflammatory drugs (NSAIDs) and/or muscle relaxants can be helpful. Stress reduction, relaxation techniques, massage therapy, acupressure, and exercise also have been found to be beneficial. Exercises that are helpful in reducing pain include walking, biking, swimming, or water aerobics.

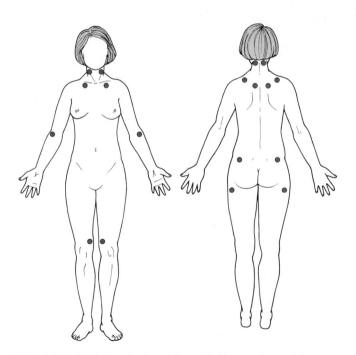

FIGURE 7–7 Eighteen tender points used to diagnose fibromyalgia.

PROGNOSIS

With a good understanding of the concepts of the symptoms and methods of treatment available, patients generally can control their condition and return to normal function. Despite potentially disabling body pain, patients with fibromyalgia do not develop musculoskeletal damage or deformity. Fibromyalgia also does not cause damage to internal body organs.

PREVENTION

To prevent initiating or worsening symptoms, patients should work toward minimizing stressful situations, perform aerobic exercise regularly, and under the guidance of their health-care practitioners, consider taking medications that can lessen symptoms.

PATIENT TEACHING

Optimal management of fibromyalgia involves maximizing the patient's understanding of all known concepts of the illness. The patient and the caregiver then develop the ideal treatment strategy, which is customized for each unique patient.

Spinal Disorders

Lordosis

DESCRIPTION

Lordosis is an exaggerated inward curvature of the spine. Lordosis is sometimes referred to as a swayback or saddleback deformity.

■ **ICD-9-CM Code 737.20**

SYMPTOMS AND SIGNS

The lumbar spine normally curves inward. This normal anterior curve of the lumbar spine can become exaggerated by a variety of conditions. Excessive inward curvature, or lordosis, occurs as the person compensates for added abdominal girth caused by pregnancy, obesity, or large abdominal tumors. Lordosis also can occur developmentally for unknown reasons. Lordosis may cause no symptoms, or the patient may experience low back pain because of strains on the muscles and ligaments. As compared with normal spine posture (Fig. 7–8), lordosis results in a protruding abdomen and buttocks and an arched lower back (Fig. 7–9).

PATIENT SCREENING

Schedule the patient complaining of persistent low back pain, and no history of injury or symptoms of infection, for the first convenient appointment.

ETIOLOGY

Excessive abdominal weight gain and mass cause an individual to compensate by unconsciously tightening muscles in the low back to maintain balance when standing. Lordosis often is noted in prepubescent girls. One possible cause is rapid skeletal growth that occurs without the necessary natural stretching of the posterior soft tissues. Osteoporosis, with resulting loss of bone mass, may cause lordosis in the older population.

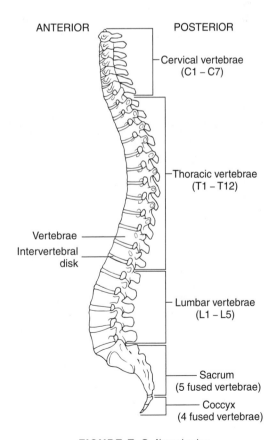

ANTERIOR   POSTERIOR

Cervical vertebrae (C1 – C7)

Thoracic vertebrae (T1 – T12)

Vertebrae
Intervertebral disk

Lumbar vertebrae (L1 – L5)

Sacrum (5 fused vertebrae)

Coccyx (4 fused vertebrae)

FIGURE 7–8 Normal spine.

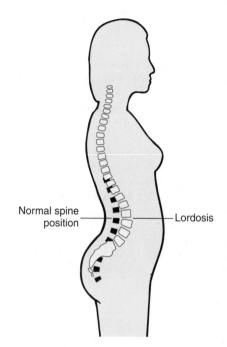

FIGURE 7–9 Lordosis.

DIAGNOSIS

Patients who present with persistent low back pain should be evaluated for degenerative and congenital diseases of the spine, as well as inflammation of the spine (spondylitis) and conditions involving adjacent internal organs, such as the kidneys, prostate gland, aorta, and pancreas.

Observation of the spine in various postural positions and an examination of the lower spine are the primary steps in diagnosis. When the condition is a result of pregnancy, no additional information usually is required to make the diagnosis. Further investigation can include radiographic studies to determine the extent of lordosis, along with a thorough history and physical examination to discover the underlying cause of the condition.

TREATMENT

When lordosis is caused by pregnancy, delivery of the infant usually resolves the condition. When obesity is the cause, weight loss and exercises to strengthen abdominal muscles are beneficial. Performing pelvic tilt exercises and maintaining good posture help to correct the condition. Progressive untreated lordosis can lead to degenerative lumbar disk disease or ruptured lumbar disks. Additional treatment of the condition can include the use of a brace. For severe lordosis, spinal fusion and displacement osteotomy are considered. This latter procedure requires the surgical division of a vertebra with shifting of the bone segments to change the alignment of, or alter weight-bearing stress on, the spine.

PROGNOSIS

Lordosis may never cause symptoms, but patients who do have symptoms usually respond to conservative management techniques.

PREVENTION

Optimal prevention measures center around developing ideal posture habits, exercises, and support devices such as braces and lumbar support when seated.

PATIENT TEACHING

Patients can benefit from a brief review of the normal anatomy of the affected areas as well as specific exercise instructions. Recommendations on proper posturing and adjustments to their specific sitting environments can be extremely valuable.

Kyphosis

DESCRIPTION

Kyphosis is an abnormal outward curvature of the spine (convexity backward).

ICD-9-CM Code 737.10

SYMPTOMS AND SIGNS

Kyphosis, an excessive posterior curve of the thoracic spine, often has an *insidious* onset and is *asymptomatic* until the hump becomes obvious. As the curve progresses, the patient begins to experience mild pain, fatigue, tenderness along the spine, and decreasing mobility of the spine. The shoulders appear rounded, and the head protrudes forward (Fig. 7–10, *A*).

PATIENT SCREENING

Schedule the individual complaining of persistent upper back pain, without history of injury or symptoms of infection, for an appointment at his or her convenience.

Normal spine position — Lordosis

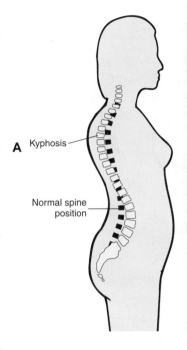

A

Kyphosis

Normal spine position

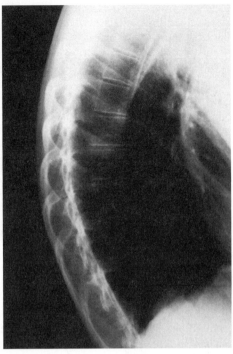

B

FIGURE 7–10 **A**, Kyphosis. **B**, Kyphosis associated with Scheuermann disease. (**B** from Mourad LA: *Orthopedic disorders—Mosby's clinical nursing series,* St. Louis, 1991, Mosby.)

ETIOLOGY

Kyphosis that occurs in very young children has no specific cause and is felt to be developmental. Adolescent kyphosis usually is related to Scheuermann disease, a degenerative deformity of the thoracic vertebrae (Fig. 7–10, *B*). Additional disease processes that contribute to the occurrence of kyphosis include tumors or tuberculosis of the vertebral bodies and ankylosing spondylitis. Osteoporosis is often responsible for the hunchback that develops in the older person, particularly the postmenopausal woman. Wearing away of the anterior portion of the vertebrae in a wedge-type manner (anterior wedging) or deterioration of the vertebrae, from whatever cause, results in the excessive curvature of kyphosis.

DIAGNOSIS

Visual inspection of the spine discloses the excessive curve in the thoracic region. Radiographic films and bone scan document the concave curvature of the thoracic spine along with the wedging of the anterior aspect of the vertebral bodies (see Fig. 7–10, *B*). Older patients with osteoporosis have a loss of bone density.

TREATMENT

Exercises to strengthen the muscles and ligaments are prescribed. Back braces also are used to stabilize the condition. The underlying cause must be determined and treated. When other measures fail to produce results and when the respiratory and cardiac systems are compromised, spinal fusion with instrumentation and temporary immobilization is performed. Kyphosis that is caused by a sudden collapse of a vertebra because of osteoporosis is sometimes treated with a new procedure called *vertebroplasty,* in which a balloon is inflated within the vertebra and methylmethacrylate is inserted to provide a "cement" foundation to maintain reestablished vertebral height.

PROGNOSIS

The outlook for patients with kyphosis depends on the cause. Optimal outcome results from accurate diagnosis and early treatment.

PREVENTION

Optimal prevention measures center around developing ideal posture habits, exercises, and support devices such as braces and back support when seated. Medications may be needed for osteoporosis or inflammation of the spine.

PATIENT TEACHING

Patients with kyphosis who are found to have significant osteoporosis should be instructed regarding exercise programs, calcium supplementation, and medications.

Scoliosis

DESCRIPTION

Scoliosis is a lateral (sideways) curvature of the spine. Scoliosis typically is congenital, but some diseases also can cause it.

▪ **ICD-9-CM Code**   **737.30** *(Acquired; postural)*
                     754.2 *(Congenital)*

SYMPTOMS AND SIGNS

Scoliosis, a lateral curvature of the spine, often has an insidious presentation, possibly going unnoticed for years before detection. In women, for example, the first indication is often unequal bra strap lengths. The patient, usually an adolescent female, reports back pain, fatigue, and sometimes shortness of breath with exertion. Observation of the back reveals a lateral curve of the spine, one shoulder higher than the other, one scapula more prominent than the other, one hip higher than the other, and when the patient bends over, an enlarged muscle mass on one side of the back (Fig. 7–11).

PATIENT SCREENING

Referrals may come from school scoliosis screening programs that have detected possible scoliosis.

ETIOLOGY

Idiopathic scoliosis is the most common form; however, the cause is postulated to be genetic in some cases. Other suggested causes of scoliosis are deformities of the vertebrae, uneven leg lengths, and muscle degeneration or paralysis from diseases such as poliomyelitis, cerebral palsy, and muscular dystrophy.

DIAGNOSIS

Patients with scoliosis are evaluated for muscle disease and weakness, congenital conditions, neurologic disorders, and degeneration of the bones and disks of the spine. Diagnosis is made from visual ex-

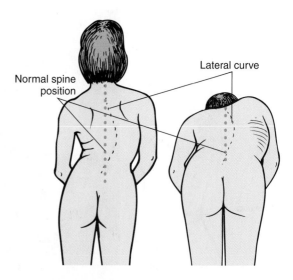

FIGURE 7–11 Scoliosis.

amination of the back, which reveals uneven shoulder and hip heights, a prominent scapula on one side, an enlarged muscle mass on one side, and a definite torsional curve of the vertebral column. It is important to examine the lengths of the lower limbs, because discrepancy of the leg lengths can lead to spinal curvature. Radiographic films not only confirm the diagnosis but also provide the physician with a means of measuring the degree of curvature.

TREATMENT

Treatment depends on the extent and cause of the curve. Mild scoliosis is treated with exercise to strengthen the weak muscles. Bracing of the back with a Milwaukee brace or a molded plastic clamshell jacket, along with an exercise program, is the suggested course of treatment for the growing girl or boy. This bracing may take from 2 to 5 years to prevent further curvature. Curves that do not respond to the bracing or that are severe (greater than 40 degrees) need surgical intervention to decrease the curve and to realign and stabilize the spine. These procedures include fusion of the vertebrae and internal fixation with instrumentation by means of rods, wires, or plates and pedicle screws. Some patients are placed in body casts or plastic jackets to maintain the integrity of the fixation until the fusion heals. The respiratory and cardiac systems may be compromised if the curvature is left untreated.

PROGNOSIS

The outlook for patients with scoliosis depends primarily on the severity of the curvature. Optimal outcome results from accurate diagnosis and early treatment.

PREVENTION

Prevention measures center around developing ideal posture habits, performing beneficial exercises, and wearing support devices such as the braces described above. Timely surgical intervention is key for severely affected children.

PATIENT TEACHING

Posture training, regular use of proper bracing, and instructions for avoiding stresses to the affected spine are keys to ideal management. Children with significant scoliosis should avoid aggressive contact sports, such as football and rugby.

Osteoarthritis

DESCRIPTION

Osteoarthritis is a type of arthritis that results from the breakdown and eventual loss of the cartilage of one or more joints.

 ICD-9-CM Code 715.90
Osteoarthritis is coded according to site. Refer to the physician's diagnosis and then to the current edition of the ICD-9-CM coding manual for most accurate specificity.

SYMPTOMS AND SIGNS

Osteoarthritis, also known as *degenerative joint disease* or *degenerative arthritis,* is by far the most common form of arthritis. It develops as a result of normal wear and tear on the joints and is most common in the elderly, being almost universal in those older than 75 years. Osteoarthritis occurs mainly in the large weight-bearing joints, especially the knees and hips (Figs. 7–12 and 7–13). The tendency is for the smallest joints at the ends of the fingers to be affected by spur formation that leads to the classic bony enlargement referred to as a Heberden node. To a lesser degree, involvement of the joints of the fingers at the proximal interphalangeal joints (Bouchard nodes)—wrists, elbows, and ankles—can occur. Degenerative changes in the spinal vertebrae and the joints of the pelvis can lead to abnormal curvature and local pain.

The onset of osteoarthritis is usually insidious, and the symptoms vary with the severity of the disease. Joint soreness, aching, and stiffness, especially in the morning and with changes in the weather; edema; dull pain; and deformity are some of the common symptoms. Stiffness is noted, particularly after the patient has been immobile for a period of time. Clicking or crackling sounds **(crepitation)** often are heard with joint movement. Decreased ranges of motion, joint instability, and an increase in pain with use of the joints are also common.

PATIENT SCREENING

When a patient develops a persistent joint problem, a thorough history and physical examination is essential. Schedule the first available appointment. Subsequently follow office policy for referral to a rheumatologist.

ETIOLOGY

The exact cause of most osteoarthritis is unknown, but it appears to be generally associated with aging. The tendency toward developing osteoarthritis is sometimes inherited. In some persons, osteoarthritis may follow injury to the joint, or be associated with hormonal disorders or underlying diseases, such as diabetes and obesity.

DIAGNOSIS

Patients must be evaluated to exclude the over 100 other forms of arthritis, and any underlying diseases or conditions must be detected as well. The diagnostic investigation begins with physical examination and patient history. Radiographic films, *computed tomography (CT)* scans, and *magnetic resonance imaging (MRI)* scans confirm the presence of and document the severity of osteoarthritis. Plain radiographic testing can be very helpful for excluding other causes of pain in a particular joint. Radiographic tests also can assist in deciding when surgical intervention should be considered.

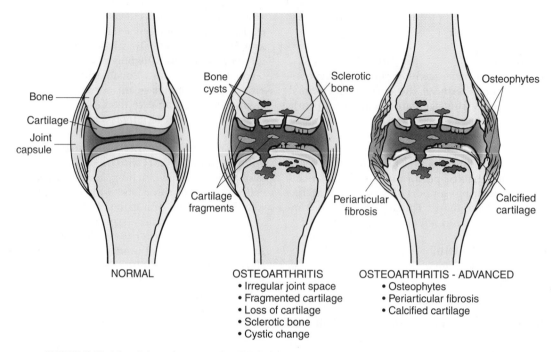

Bone

Cartilage

Joint capsule

Bone cysts

Sclerotic bone

Cartilage fragments

Osteophytes

Periarticular fibrosis

Calcified cartilage

NORMAL

OSTEOARTHRITIS
• Irregular joint space
• Fragmented cartilage
• Loss of cartilage
• Sclerotic bone
• Cystic change

OSTEOARTHRITIS - ADVANCED
• Osteophytes
• Periarticular fibrosis
• Calcified cartilage

FIGURE 7–12   Schematic presentation of the pathologic changes in osteoarthritis. Fragmentation and loss of cartilage denude the subchondral bone, which undergoes sclerosis and cystic change. Osteophytes form on the lateral sides and protrude into the adjacent soft tissues, causing irritation, inflammation, and fibrosis. (From Damjanov I: *Pathology for the health-related professions,* ed 2, Philadelphia, 2000, Saunders.)

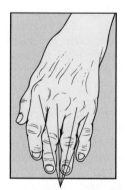

Bouchard's nodes

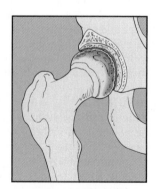

Degenerative process— worn cartilage and roughened bone

FIGURE 7–13 Osteoarthritis.

TREATMENT

Because osteoarthritis cannot be cured, the goal of treatment is to reduce inflammation, to minimize pain, and to maintain functioning joints. Treatment of osteoarthritis involves physical and drug therapy, nutritional management, and supportive care. Surgery also may be needed in severe cases. Physical therapy includes range-of-motion exercises, alternation of moist heat and cold applications, massage therapy, and the use of elastic bandages and splints for limb support. Drug therapy can include the use of analgesics, muscle relaxants, and NSAIDs. Intraarticular steroid injections may be used for specific or individual joints. Fish oils have been suggested to have some antiinflammatory properties. Food supplementation with glucosamine and chondroitin can reduce pain and stiffness in some patients. For supportive care, it may be necessary to use a cane, walker, or crutches to lessen the strain on some joints. Restricting physical activity or resting affected joints also may be necessary. Surgery for osteoarthritis may involve total joint replacement. Joints commonly replaced are the hip and the knee. Ankle, wrist, elbow, and shoulder joints also can be replaced. Joint fusion may be done to increase stability for the cervical and lumbar vertebrae.

PROGNOSIS

The outlook for patients with osteoarthritis depends primarily on the severity and location of the involved joints. Optimal outcome results from accurate diagnosis and early management.

PREVENTION

Avoiding injury and reinjury to joints is important in preventing future osteoarthritis. Persons with flaccid (overstretched) ligaments may require support devices to engage in some activities. Early contact with health-care practitioners can optimize long-term health.

PATIENT TEACHING

Providing specific guidance on food supplementation, medications, and proper exercise can significantly improve the quality of life for these patients.

Lyme Disease

DESCRIPTION

Lyme disease is an infectious disease caused by the bacterium *Borrelia burgdorferi,* a bacterium of the spirochete family. Ticks that bite the skin spread Lyme disease, by injecting the bacterium from their gut into the human body. Lyme disease can affect the skin, joints, heart, and nervous system.

■ ICD-9-CM Code **088.81**

SYMPTOMS AND SIGNS

Lyme disease, also known as *Lyme arthritis,* was first detected in 1975 in Lyme, Connecticut. Lyme disease is more prevalent in the northeast part of the Unites States, especially New York, New Jersey, and Connecticut, where large areas of forests and fields provide habitat for ticks. The disease has been found, however, in all 50 states and on five continents.

Lyme disease can occur in any age group, and no one is immune to the infection. Approximately half of all patients with Lyme disease have a characteristic red, itchy rash with a red circle center resembling the bull's eye on a target (target lesion) (Fig. 7–14, A). Lyme disease can masquerade as arthritis and cause influenza-like symptoms such as headache, fever, fatigue, joint pain, and general *malaise.* If the person does not seek medical attention for the symptoms, complications of muscle weakness, paralysis, and neurologic conditions (e.g., learning difficulties, excessive fatigue, and muscle coordination problems) can develop as the bacterium spreads internally unchecked. Encephalitis, gastritis, or carditis may develop in some patients.

PATIENT SCREENING

Early detection of Lyme disease is imperative. In areas where the deer tick is prevalent and/or the patient reports a "target lesion," a visual inspection and diagnostic laboratory tests are necessary. Likewise, if a patient reports flu-like symptoms 2 to 4 weeks after receiving a tick bite, an appointment for prompt diagnostic evaluation is indicated.

ETIOLOGY

Lyme disease is caused by the spirochete *Borrelia burgdorferi,* which is transmitted to humans by a bite from a small tick (Fig. 7–14, B) that is carried by mice or deer. The disease is usually transmitted to humans while they are camping or hiking in woods, fields, or other areas that ticks inhabit. After infiltrating the skin, the bacterium can infect internal organs of the body, causing a variety of symptoms, which often leads to delay in making the correct diagnosis.

DIAGNOSIS

The evaluation of patients with the nonspecific symptoms of early Lyme disease such as headache,

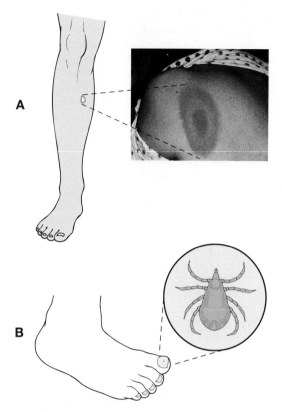

FIGURE 7–14 **A,** Target lesion of Lyme disease. **B,** Tick that causes Lyme disease. (Photo from Stone DR, Gorbach SL: *Atlas of infectious diseases,* Philadelphia, 2000, Saunders.)

TREATMENT

Treatment of Lyme disease begins with removal of the tick, if it is found on skin or clothing. Early treatment is imperative because treatment in the early stages of disease leads to complete cure with simple oral antibiotics. Lyme disease in the later stages requires intravenous antibiotics for cure. Antipyretics are given for headache and fever. Bed rest is necessary if neurologic symptoms are present, and physical therapy is prescribed for impaired musculoskeletal mobility. Joint symptoms are often treated with antiinflammatory medications.

PROGNOSIS

Lyme disease is curable with antibiotics. The outlook for patients with Lyme disease is a function of how early it is detected. Early stage Lyme disease involves a minor skin rash with muscle aching that easily resolves with antibiotics. Later stage Lyme disease can cause residual damage to the joints, heart, or nervous system. Optimal outcome results from accurate diagnosis and early treatment.

PREVENTION

Avoiding tick bites is the best prevention of Lyme disease. When inhabiting locations known to harbor ticks, wear long clothing to protect the skin. Carefully examine all clothing first and then the entire body, including the scalp, to detect the presence of ticks after being in high-risk areas. Close inspection of children and pets is especially important. Ticks can be removed gently with tweezers and saved in a jar in case identification of the vector is needed later. Bathing the skin and scalp, and washing clothing after possible exposure to ticks may prevent the bite and subsequent transmission of the disease. Vaccines were once available, but these have been removed from the market. Further studies of vaccines are needed.

PATIENT TEACHING

Community awareness of tick-avoidance measures is essential for prevention. Patients who develop Lyme disease should be instructed to closely follow the specific instructions provided by their qualified health-care practitioners regarding therapeutic medications.

fever, fatigue, joint pain, and general malaise can be exhaustive. A complete history and physical examination as well as laboratory tests are important for excluding other infectious diseases, forms of arthritis, immune diseases, muscle diseases, and even cancer.

The diagnosis of Lyme disease can be based on physical examination (the discovery of a tick on the skin), the presence of the classic target lesion, and the patient history. Confirmation is attained by positive test results for the Lyme *antibodies* or directly identifying the bacterium in the infected skin via biopsy.

Bursitis

DESCRIPTION

Bursitis is inflammation of a bursa. A bursa is a tiny fluid-filled sac that functions as a gliding surface to reduce friction between tissues of the body. Bursae are found between muscles and tendons and cover bony prominences to facilitate movement. They can become inflamed, infected, or traumatized. The major bursae are located adjacent to the tendons of the large joints, such as the shoulders, elbows, hips, and knees.

■ **ICD-9-CM Code** **727.3**
727.2 *(Specific bursitis often of occupational origin)*

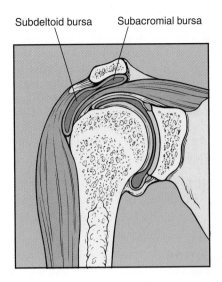

Subdeltoid bursa   Subacromial bursa

FIGURE 7–15 Bursae of the shoulder.

SYMPTOMS AND SIGNS

The classic symptoms of bursitis are tenderness, pain when moving the affected part, flexion and extension limitation, and edema at the site of inflammation. The most frequently affected bursae are those of the shoulder (Fig. 7–15), elbow, knee, and hip, and those between the tendons and muscles of the tibia. Point tenderness may be present, in which case the patient actually can point to the spot of greatest tenderness. If bursae are continually or chronically irritated and inflamed, calcifications can develop. In addition, adhesions can occur around an affected bursa, which limits the movement of the tendons.

PATIENT SCREENING

Pain, swelling, or limitation of motion in any joint, with or without previous injury, requires an appointment for diagnostic evaluation. Early treatment and relief from pain are important measures.

ETIOLOGY

Bursitis can result from continual or excessive friction between the bursae and the surrounding musculoskeletal tissues. Systemic diseases (e.g., gout and rheumatoid arthritis) and infection can lead to the development of bursitis. In addition, repeated trauma, from overuse of a joint, can cause bursitis (see Cumulative Trauma in Chapter 15).

DIAGNOSIS

Bursitis is generally a straightforward diagnosis that can be made after evaluating information gained from the history and physical examination. However, in patients with bursitis that is not associated with injury, possible underlying gout or arthritis should be considered. In patients with abrasion of the overlying skin, infection also must be considered. Range of motion may be impaired, and the pain is acute. MRI indicates an enlarged bursa, and radiographic films may show calcified deposits at the affected site when the bursitis is chronic. Aspiration of fluid from an inflamed bursa can assist in diagnosing infectious bursitis (septic bursitis).

TREATMENT

The treatment for traumatic bursitis may include avoidance of activities until acute pain subsides, the application of moist heat, immobilization of the affected part, the use of aspirin or acetaminophen for pain, the administration of nonsteroidal antiinflammatory agents (e.g., ibuprofen and indomethacin), and local injection of corticosteroid. If infection is present, drainage of the inflamed bursa and the use of antibiotics specific to the infectious microbe are critical. Active range-of-motion exercises to prevent adhesions and to maintain or regain motion are needed after the acute pain subsides. Surgical excision of the bursa and any accompanying calcified deposits can be required for either chronic noninfectious and infectious bursitis.

PROGNOSIS

Bursitis is curable. With treatment and proper attention to any underlying cause, the outlook is excellent.

PREVENTION

Actions that initiate or promote tissue inflammation, such as repetition of a throwing motion in the case of shoulder bursitis, prolonged leaning on the elbow in the case of elbow bursitis, or prolonged kneeling in the case of knee bursitis should be avoided.

PATIENT TEACHING

Patients can benefit from being given specific information regarding the cause of the inflamed bursa and from instructions regarding aggravating factors to avoid. For any recurrent inflammation, patients should be instructed to immediately apply ice packs to the area so that inflammation can be minimized.

Osteomyelitis

DESCRIPTION

Osteomyelitis is a serious infection of bone that requires aggressive antibiotic treatment.

■ **ICD-9-CM Code 730.20** *(Unspecified, site unspecified)*
Refer to the physician's diagnosis and then the current edition of the ICD-9-CM coding manual for greatest specificity of site and stage (acute or chronic) of bone infection.

SYMPTOMS AND SIGNS

Inflammation, swelling, localized heat, redness, pain, and local tenderness over and around the affected bone are characteristic signs of osteomyelitis. Other symptoms of osteomyelitis include chills, fever, sweating, and malaise. As the infection progresses, a *purulent* material called a subperiosteal *abscess* may develop, causing pressure and eventual fracturing of small pieces of the bone. These fractured, dead pieces of bone may in turn become surrounded by the purulent material and form a *sequestrum* (Fig. 7–16).

The most commonly involved bones in osteomyelitic infections are the upper ends of the humerus and tibia, the lower end of the femur, and occasionally, the vertebrae.

Osteomyelitis most often begins as an acute infection; however, it can remain undetected for months or years and evolve into a chronic condition. Both the acute and chronic forms can present the same clinical picture.

PATIENT SCREENING

Patients with localized bone inflammation and pain must be evaluated for possible fractures and bone tumors before the diagnosis of osteomyelitis can be ascertained.

ETIOLOGY

Staphylococcus aureus is the bacterial organism responsible for 90% of osteomyelitic infections. Streptococcal bacteria account for the next largest number of infections. Viruses and fungi also have been known to cause osteomyelitis. Osteomyelitis can develop when blood-borne pathogens are deposited in the metaphyseal area of a bone after physical trauma or surgery.

Diabetes mellitus or peripheral vascular disease may predispose individuals to the development of osteomyelitis, as can the presence of prosthetic hardware (e.g., rods, screws, and plates within the bone) and total joint replacement. Osteomyelitis in infants and children develops as a secondary infection from streptococcal pharyngitis (strep throat). Persons with sickle cell disease, *immunodeficiency,* or malignancies are also at increased risk for the development of osteomyelitis.

The possible development of osteomyelitis must be the concern of any person who has an open wound, sore (strep) throat, or a systemic infection that could be transmitted to the bones.

DIAGNOSIS

Aspiration and culture of material taken from the site of the infection are essential to isolating the causative organisms. A blood culture, a *white blood cell (WBC) count*, and an *erythrocyte sedimentation rate (ESR)* are also helpful for determining diagnosis and monitoring treatment. MRI, CT, or bone scans aid in determining the site and extent of acute or chronic infection.

TREATMENT

Osteomyelitis usually requires extensive, long-term antibiotic treatment with follow-up care to prevent recurrent infections. Parenteral or locally administered antibiotics (e.g., aqueous penicillin, cephalosporin, erythromycin [for penicillin-allergic individuals], tetracycline, and ampicillin), at a dosage specific to the patient's age and the pathogenic organism involved, are needed. Additional measures include increased intake of proteins and vitamins A, B, and C to promote cell regeneration, bed rest as needed to conserve energy, control of chronic conditions (e.g., diabetes), immobilization of the affected part to prevent fracture of weakened bones, and analgesics. Surgical drainage to remove purulent material and sequestrum also may be necessary, along with bone grafting. Hyperbaric oxygen treatments may prove beneficial as well.

PROGNOSIS

Osteomyelitis is curable. The long-term outcome depends on the amount of bone and/or joint damage as a result of the infection. Damaged bone can lead to deformity and impaired function, especially if growth plates are affected in children.

PREVENTION

For most patients, osteomyelitis cannot be prevented because it occurs randomly. However, patients with diabetes mellitus and sickle cell disease, as well as those with impaired immune systems, should be particularly diligent about reporting to their doctors any signs of infections.

PATIENT TEACHING

Patients must be instructed on the specific details and importance of their antibiotic management.

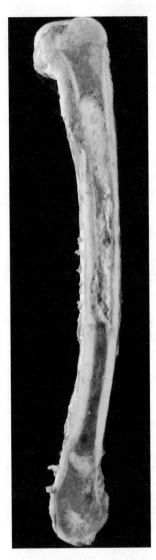

FIGURE 7–16 Osteomyelitis. (From Cooke RA, Stewart B: *Colour atlas of anatomical pathology,* ed 2, London, 1995, Churchill Livingstone. Copyright North Brisbane Hospitals Board, Brisbane, Australia.)

Long-term antibiotic treatments administered intravenously can require special catheters, such as a peripherally inserted central catheter ("PICC line"), which must be cared for according to specific guidelines.

Gout

Gout

DESCRIPTION

Gout is a chronic disorder of uric acid metabolism that manifests as an acute, episodic form of arthritis; chronic deposits of uric acid form hard nodules in tissues.

ICD-9-CM Code 274.9 *(Unspecified)*
Gout is coded according to site and type of pathologic involvement. Refer to the physician's diagnosis and then to the current edition of the ICD-9-CM manual for greatest specificity.

SYMPTOMS AND SIGNS

Gout involves an overproduction or decreased excretion of uric acid and urate salts. This leads to high levels of uric acid in the blood and also in the synovial fluid of joints. Deposits of other urate compounds can be found in and around the joints of extremities, often leading to joint deformity and disability (Fig. 7–17, *A* and *B*).

Typically, gout affects the first metatarsal joint of the great toe, causing severe to excruciating pain when an attack occurs. The joints of the feet, ankles, and knees also can be affected. Pain usually peaks after several hours, and then subsides gradually. A slight fever, chills, headache, or nausea may accompany an acute attack. Between attacks, the person is characteristically free from any symptoms. Gout also is characterized by renal dysfunction, *hyperuricemia*, and renal calculi (kidney stones).

The disease is uncommon in children; gout generally appears in people older than 30 years. Men are affected more often than women. In women, gout often appears after menopause. Gout also can develop secondary to cell breakdown resulting from drug therapy, especially with chemotherapy for malignant diseases (e.g., leukemia).

PATIENT SCREENING

The patient with gout may complain of severe, acute joint pain and possibly mild systemic symptoms. Schedule a timely appointment so treatment can begin and medication that will relieve the pain can be prescribed.

ETIOLOGY

The cause of this disorder is most often an inherited abnormality of metabolism. It may result from a lack of an enzyme needed to completely metabolize purines in foods for excretion from the kidneys. This incomplete metabolism leads to the buildup of uric acid, which is a breakdown product of purines. Renal gout is caused by some forms of kidney dysfunction. The body may produce levels of uric acid that are normal, but kidney function is insufficient to remove the product from the blood. Excessive weight gain, leukemias and lymphomas, and certain drugs including diuretics and tuberculosis medications also can precipitate gout.

DIAGNOSIS

Patients with new-onset joint inflammation are evaluated for many types of arthritis, such as rheumatoid arthritis, spondylitis, reactive arthritis, and joint infection. Microscopic examination of aspirated synovial joint fluid shows the presence of urate crystals (see Fig. 7–17, *B*). Urinalysis and a serum uric acid test almost always indicate hyperuricemia. Radiographic films may be used to assess the amount of damage to affected joints.

TREATMENT

General treatment of an acute attack of gout could involve bed rest to lessen pressure on affected joints, immobilization of the affected limb, and the application of ice to the inflamed joints, if the patient is able to tolerate the pressure of an ice bag. An antiinflammatory agent (NSAIDs) and corticosteroids taken orally or injected into the gouty area are options that can be implemented to reduce inflammation. Dietary modifications include a low-purine diet and frequent fluid intake. For chronic gout, after the acute attack has subsided, the patient may be given antihyperuricemic medications (e.g., probenecid and allopurinol). Gradual weight reduction can be helpful in those patients who are overweight.

PROGNOSIS

With proper management, potential damage to the bones and joints can be avoided. Chronic gouty deposits of uric acid (tophi) can be difficult to treat, and, if they do not shrink with medication, can be surgically resected.

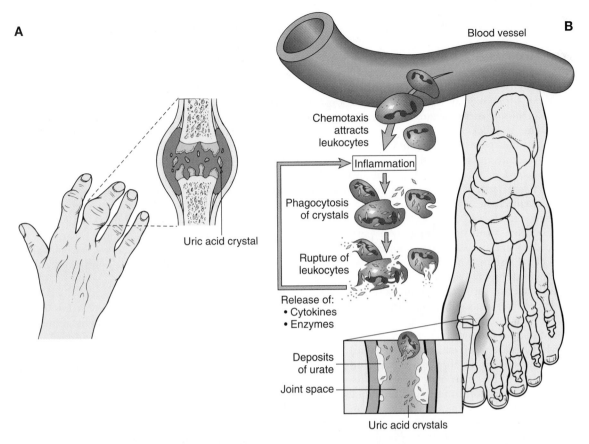

FIGURE 7–17 A, Gout. **B,** Gouty arthritis. Deposits of uric acid crystals in the connective tissue have a chemotactic effect and cause exudation of leukocytes into the joint. The inflammation most often affects the **metatarsophalangeal** joint. (**B** from Damjanov I: *Pathology for the health-related professions,* ed 2, Philadelphia, 2000, Saunders.)

PREVENTION
Limiting alcohol intake, avoiding dehydration, and eating a proper diet are keys to prevention of gout attacks.

PATIENT TEACHING
Patients should understand that early measures to treat inflammation, such as ice packs and antiinflammatory medication, may help them avoid prolonged pain and dysfunction. Specific dietary instructions should be given to any patient with gout.

Paget Disease (Osteitis Deformans)

DESCRIPTION
Paget disease is a chronic bone disorder that typically results in enlarged, deformed bones resulting from irregular breakdown and formation of bone tissue. Paget disease can cause bones to weaken and may result in bone pain, arthritis, bone deformities, and fractures. Paget disease is also known as *osteitis deformans.*

■ **ICD-9-CM Code 731.0**

SYMPTOMS AND SIGNS

In patients with Paget disease, affected areas of bone produce new bone tissue faster than the old bone can be broken down. Paget disease occurs characteristically in two stages. The initial stage is called the *vascular stage.* Bone tissue is broken down, but the spaces left are filled with blood vessels and fibrous tissue instead of new strong bone. In the second, or *sclerotic,* stage, the highly vascular fibrous tissue hardens and becomes similar to bone but is fragile instead of strong. This can lead to pathologic fractures.

This disease can occur in only a part of one bone, all of one bone, or many bones throughout the skeletal system. The most common sites of the disease are the pelvis and the tibia. Other sites often affected are the femur, spine, skull, and clavicle. Paget disease usually affects individuals older than 40 years of age and becomes increasingly more common with advancing age.

Paget disease often causes no symptoms. When symptoms do occur, they usually include local bone pain. The pain can become disabling. Aching is almost continuous and is often worse at night. Some patients may have edema or deformity in one of the bones or may notice that they need a larger hat size because the bones of the skull have enlarged. If the ossicles of the ear are involved, hearing loss or deafness may occur. Other complications of Paget disease can include frequent fractures, spinal cord injuries, hypercalcemia, renal calculi, and infrequently a serious form of cancer, bone sarcoma.

PATIENT SCREENING

A patient presenting with bone pain must be evaluated for fracture and infection of bone.

ETIOLOGY

The cause of Paget disease is not known.

DIAGNOSIS

A physical examination and a history of the patient's symptoms are needed. The physician then orders several tests and blood work. Radiographic imaging, bone scanning, and possibly a bone marrow biopsy assist in the diagnosis. Blood analysis will indicate an elevated serum concentration of alkaline phosphatase, and urinalysis reveals an elevated hydroxyproline concentration. Both of these findings are produced by the high rate of bone production.

TREATMENT

Patients with Paget disease who have no symptoms require no treatment. With symptoms, treatment options include analgesics, antiinflammatory drugs, cytotoxic agents, or injections of a hormone called **calcitonin**. Calcitonin is produced naturally by the thyroid gland and works with parathyroid hormone (parathormone) and vitamin D to regulate the level of calcium in the blood. Increased amounts of calcitonin can reduce pain for some patients and prevent bone loss. Eating a high-protein, high-calcium diet, with vitamin D supplementation, may be advised as well. Newer treatments include bisphosphonate medications, such as alendronate, risidronate, tiludronate, andpamidronate.

PROGNOSIS

For most patients with Paget disease, few if any symptoms are noted. If needed, medications can relieve persistent bone pain. Complications including hypercalcemia, fractures, heart failure, gout, and bone cancer (sarcoma) can lead to increased morbidity.

PREVENTION

Patients with Paget disease should receive 1000 to 1500 mg of calcium, adequate exposure to sunshine, and at least 400 units of vitamin D daily. This is especially important for patients being treated with bisphosphonates. Patients with a history of kidney stones should discuss calcium and vitamin D intake with their physician.

PATIENT TEACHING

Exercise is an important part of maintaining skeletal health, as is avoiding weight gain, and maintaining joint mobility. Because undue stress on affected bones should be avoided, patients should discuss any planned exercise program with their physician before beginning.

Marfan Syndrome

DESCRIPTION

Marfan syndrome is a group of inherited conditions featuring abnormal connective tissue with weakness of blood vessels and excessive length of the extremities (Fig. 7–18).

■ ICD-9-CM Code 759.82

SYMPTOMS AND SIGNS

Marfan syndrome is characterized by abnormally long extremities and digits. Additional deformities include *subluxation* of the lens of the eyes and heart and vascular anomalies. This condition may go undetected until harmful complications are precipitated. The person with Marfan syndrome is tall and slender with long, narrow digits. An asymmetry of the skull may be noted. Visual difficulties are encountered when lens involvement includes dissociation. Scoliosis is another manifestation. Joints can be hyperextensible in those with Marfan syndrome. Mitral valve prolapse and thickening of the heart valves and aortic aneurysm may be present but go undetected (see Valvular Heart Disease in Chapter 10). Often, the first indication of the syndrome occurs during exercise that precipitates rupture of an aortic aneurysm with catastrophic results.

PATIENT SCREENING

A patient diagnosed with Marfan syndrome may develop serious complications of the eyes or cardiovascular system requiring immediate medical attention. Defer to the health-care provider for direction.

ETIOLOGY

This syndrome results from an *autosomal* dominant genetic disorder. The affected gene is on the long arm of chromosome 15. The defective gene can be inherited as follows: The child of a person who has Marfan syndrome has a 50% chance of inheriting the gene. The defective gene is determines the structure of fibrillin, a protein that is an important component of connective tissue. Although everyone with Marfan syndrome has the same defective gene, not everyone experiences the same symptoms. This is referred to as "variable expression" of the gene.

DIAGNOSIS

Patients with Marfan syndrome may sometimes be confused with those who have homocystinuria (an amino acid disorder) because connective tissue abnormalities and abnormal movement of the lens of the eye are present in both conditions. A person with Marfan syndrome is born with the disorder,

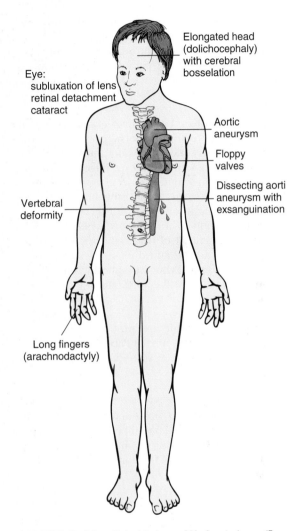

FIGURE 7–18 Typical features of Marfan syndrome. (From Damjanov I: *Pathology for the health-related professions,* ed 2, Philadelphia, 2000, Saunders.)

although it may not be diagnosed until later in life. The diagnosis is made based on the family history, the physical examination findings of abnormal length of the limbs and lens abnormality in the eye, and tests of the heart and blood vessels. Diagnosis of the syndrome in early childhood is possible when the lens dissociation and mitral valve prolapse anomalies are detected. The clinical picture

Musculoskeletal Tumors

of a rapid growth spurt and scoliosis, coupled with the visual disturbance and mitral valve prolapse, leads to further investigation. *Echocardiographic* measurements of the aortic diameter aid in detecting potential aortic dissection. Patients at risk for impending aortic dissection may be asymptomatic or may experience chest pain that is tearing in nature and radiates to the neck, back, and arms.

TREATMENT

Treatment involves controlling excessive height with hormones before puberty, preventing glaucoma, controlling blood pressure, and preventing aortic dissection. Ophthalmic examinations should be conducted on a routine basis to detect any problem at an early stage. Monitoring blood pressure and maintaining it at a normal level are essential. Close observation of aortic status is necessary, and surgical replacement of diseased portions may be indicated. Aortic and mitral valves may need to be replaced surgically. Echocardiography is used on a regular basis to assess the aortic status.

PROGNOSIS

The major risks to life are rupture of blood vessels, particularly the aorta. Patients can be disabled because of severe spine abnormalities and joint dislocations.

PREVENTION

The key measures to prevent complications include avoiding elevated blood pressure and trauma that could cause bleeding or bone and joint injury. Monitoring the status of the aorta with echocardiograms is essential.

PATIENT TEACHING

Patients should be educated about the anomalies in their own anatomy and physiology so they will understand the need to minimize high-risk activities and to report any signs of problems to their caregivers.

Musculoskeletal Tumors

DESCRIPTION

Musculoskeletal tumors are abnormal growths, whether benign or malignant, within the muscles

or bones. Benign neoplasms are much more common than malignant tumors.

Bone Tumors

DESCRIPTION

The term *bone tumor* describes any abnormal growth, whether benign or malignant, in the bone. The definition includes chondrogenic (from cartilage), osteogenic (from bone), and fibrogenic (from fibrous tissue) tumors.

 ICD-9-CM Code *(Refer to the Neoplasm table in the current edition of the ICD-9-CM coding manual)*
Neoplasms of the bone are coded according to anatomic site, classified as benign or malignant or designated as unspecified. Refer to the physician's diagnosis and then to the current edition of the ICD-9-CM coding manual for greatest specificity.

SYMPTOMS AND SIGNS

Often bone tumors produce no symptoms and are detected incidentally when radiographic imaging is performed for some other reason. Radiographic studies can reveal osteonecrosis or increased ossification and calcification. The bone tumor weakens the bone and makes it susceptible to fracture when subjected to the slightest strain. This is called a *pathologic fracture* (see Fig. 7–25). A pathologic fracture is often one of the first indications of the presence of metastatic disease, and it commonly occurs in the acetabulum or the proximal femur. Other possible symptoms are a palpable mass, pain that may be dull or severe and is localized to the affected area, and limitation of movement. A parent may notice a child begin to limp or curtail physical activity.

For benign bone tumors (e.g., osteochondroma, osteoid osteoma, and giant cell tumor), pain is the most common presenting complaint. The pain may be the result of tumor invasion of soft tissue or a resulting pathologic fracture. Local swelling may be evident as the neoplasm enlarges. Muscle atrophy or muscle spasm may be present. Different varieties of malignant tumors have characteristic signs and symptoms. Osteosarcoma presents with pain and swelling of short duration and a "sunburst" appearance on radiograph. Patients with Ewing sarcoma, in addition to pain and swelling, have systemic symptoms such as fever, fatigue and pallor caused by anemia, and leukocytosis. The Ewing sarcoma lesion has an "onion skin" appearance on radiograph. Chondrosarcomas present with a slow-growing mass; dull, intermittent pain; and a lobular pattern on radiograph.

PATIENT SCREENING

Bone pain, with or without local swelling and muscle spasm, requires a timely medical evaluation. Systemic symptoms also may be present and indicate the need for the earliest possible appointment.

ETIOLOGY

Benign bone tumors are usually slow growing. Many types have an onset in childhood, but may not be discovered until adulthood. Malignant tumors may be primary or secondary in origin. Primary tumors account for over 85% of bone tumors in children but are rarely seen after the age of 30. Males are affected more often than women. Metastatic, or secondary, tumors in bones occur more often than do primary tumors and are more common in older age groups. Cancers that commonly metastasize to the bones include breast, lung, prostate, thyroid, and kidney cancer. The bones affected most often are the pelvis, vertebrae, ribs, hip, femur, and humerus.

Osteosarcoma is the most common type of primary bone neoplasm (Fig. 7–19). Peak incidence is between the ages of 10 and 15 years. Osteosarcoma develops most often in the distal femur, followed by the proximal tibia and the humerus. Metastasis to the lung within 2 years of treatment is common and often results in death. Additional risk factors include Paget disease of the bone and radiation therapy received for other forms of cancer. Ewing sarcoma most often involves the pelvis and lower extremity. The peak incidence occurs between the ages of 4 and 25 years. The tumor is not encapsulated and often extends into soft tissue. Metastasis to the lungs and other bones happens early in the disease. Chondrosarcoma often arises in the pelvis and proximal femur. It primarily affects individuals between the ages of 30 and 60 years. It grows more slowly than other malignant tumors of the bone and is locally invasive.

DIAGNOSIS

Patients with local bone pain are evaluated for injury, fracture, hematoma, and local bone infection. Paget disease of bone can mimic or be associated with bone cancer. The diagnosis is made based on the complete patient history, physical examination, laboratory studies, and diagnostic procedures. Many diagnostic procedures, including radiographic studies, CT scan, and MRI scan greatly aid in determining the diagnosis and in evaluating the extent of soft tissue involvement by the tumor. Other markers may be useful in identification of tumor type. Malignant bone tumors of osteoid origin generally have an elevated serum alkaline phosphatase level. Some patients with secondary bone cancer have an elevated serum calcium level. A biopsy is necessary for definitive diagnosis and to determine the tumor type. Bone cancers are usually staged using the TNM (Tumor, Node, Metastasis) system or a system that relies on tumor grade, tumor site, and presence of metastases. The biopsy findings aid in staging, as do CT scans of the chest and regional lymph nodes to evaluate for metastatic spread. For Ewing sarcoma, bone marrow aspiration is performed to check for metastasis to the bone marrow.

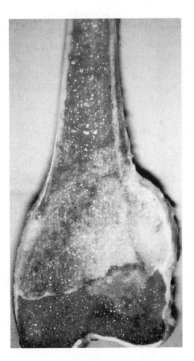

FIGURE 7–19 Osteosarcoma. (From Kumar V, Cotran RS et al: *Robbins basic pathology,* ed 7, Philadelphia, 2003, Saunders.)

TREATMENT

Bone tumors, whether benign or malignant, are treated by surgical excision. The surrounding muscle, bone, and other tissue often are removed also, and bone grafting may be needed. Depending on the tumor site and extent, limb amputation may be required. Isolated metastases to the lungs may be amenable to surgical resection as well. Surgery alone is enough to treat benign tumors, whereas treatment of malignant neoplasms usually includes administration of chemotherapy and/or radiation therapy. Treatment choice depends on tumor type. For example, Ewing sarcoma is usually chemosensitive, whereas chondrosarcomas are generally chemoresistant.

PROGNOSIS

The overall 5-year survival rate for patients with primary bone cancer is about 70%. Poor prognostic indicators are a high-grade tumor, large tumor size, and presence of metastasis. The anatomic location of the affected bone also affects prognosis, depending on the tumor type.

PREVENTION

Prevention is difficult because few risk factors have been identified. Bone pain and masses should be evaluated promptly to reduce the risk of complications such as fractures, deformity, and need for amputation. No type of routine screening is recommended, even for those with risk factors for bone tumor development.

PATIENT TEACHING

Patients require specific instructions as to use and rehabilitation of involved extremities. Managing the timing and intensity of weight bearing with leg involvement, for example, is crucial for avoiding injury.

Muscle Tumors

DESCRIPTION

Neoplasms of muscle include benign tumors or malignant sarcomas that may arise at any site in the body. The most commonly affected areas are the extremities, head and neck, trunk, and retroperitoneum.

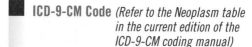

ICD-9-CM Code *(Refer to the Neoplasm table in the current edition of the ICD-9-CM coding manual)*
Neoplasms of the muscle are coded according to anatomic site, classified as benign or malignant or designated as unspecified. Refer to the physician's diagnosis and then to the current edition of the ICD-9-CM coding manual for greatest specificity.

SYMPTOMS AND SIGNS

Muscle tumors often present as a painless lump of a few weeks' or months' duration. In some instances, pain and tenderness may be present secondary to pressure effects on a nerve from the mass.

PATIENT SCREENING

A child or adult presenting with a lump or painless swelling in a muscle should be scheduled for a visual inspection and medical evaluation.

ETIOLOGY

Muscle neoplasms are exceedingly rare. When they do occur, they are almost always benign and not life threatening (e.g., leiomyomas [tumors of smooth muscle] and rhabdomyomas [tumors of striated muscle]). A malignant growth is a serious, life-threatening matter because the tumor grows and metastasizes rapidly and is difficult to treat (e.g., leiomyosarcomas and rhabdomyosarcomas). The relative incidence of benign to malignant tumors is roughly 100:1. Malignant muscle tumors grow by local extension and infiltration along tissue planes. They only rarely traverse fascial planes or bone. The presence of metastasis at diagnosis is uncommon but often develops within 24 months of initial diagnosis. The most common site of metastasis is the lungs. In contrast to primary bone tumors, muscle sarcomas occur most often in patients over the age of 50 years. The exception is the small peak of incidence in early childhood, mainly accounted for by rhabdomyosarcoma. Risk factors may include radiation treatment for previous cancer and exposure to chemicals such as vinyl chloride gas and arsenic.

DIAGNOSIS

An MRI is the most effective imaging technique for muscle tumors. Radiographs are taken to evaluate the status of the adjacent bone. A radiograph and CT scan of the chest are often performed to look for metastasis to the lungs. The biopsy method can affect subsequent treatment and should be carefully planned using the information gained from imaging studies. The histologic grade of the tumor is determined from the biopsy specimen. Tumor grade is very important in determining stage and prognosis. Although several staging systems are in existence, the one used most often is a variation of the TNM (Tumor, Node, Metastasis) system that also incorporates grade into the stage grouping.

TREATMENT

Surgical resection of the tumor is performed for all tumors, benign or malignant. For benign tumors, complete surgical resection is usually all that is required for treatment. For sarcomas, surgery is often combined with radiation therapy. Amputation of the affected limb may be necessary. Chemotherapy is used as an adjunct to surgery in children with rhabdomyosarcoma. Resection of pulmonary metastases may offer survival benefit and possible cure. Because lung metastasis can be clinically silent, frequent follow-up imaging studies are indicated for all patients after initial treatment.

PROGNOSIS

Prognosis worsens significantly with increasing tumor grade. Other poor prognostic indicators include deep anatomic tumor location, large tumor size, and presence of metastases. The 5-year survival rate ranges from 30% to 95% based on subtype and grade.

PREVENTION

No methods of prevention are known.

PATIENT TEACHING

Explain the scheduled diagnostic procedures to the patient and describe what is normally experienced during the tests. Tell the patient when to expect the results. If surgery is necessary, explain preoperative and postoperative procedures. Address patient concerns if the tumor is malignant, within the guidelines suggested by the physician. Give a full explanation of the radiation and/or chemotherapy regimen and what side effects may occur. Offer sensitive support to parents when the patient is a child and make appropriate referrals for additional support.

Osteoporosis

DESCRIPTION

Osteoporosis is a condition that features loss of the normal bone density. Osteoporosis leads literally to porous bone that can be described as being "compressible" like a sponge rather than being dense like a brick (Fig. 7–20, *A* and *B*).

 ICD-9-CM Code 733.00 *(Unspecified)*
Osteoporosis may be coded according to cause or onset. Refer to the current edition of the ICD-9-CM coding manual for greatest specificity.

SYMPTOMS AND SIGNS

Osteoporosis is a condition in which there is wasting or deterioration of bone in mass and density. It occurs more often in women than men, especially in postmenopausal women. Women who are small boned; who come from northern European or Asian backgrounds; and those who have a family history of the disease are at the greatest risk for osteoporosis.

Unless it occurs in the vertebrae or weight-bearing bones, osteoporosis usually does not produce symptoms. Osteoporosis is a silent disease until a bone break causes pain. Spontaneous fractures, especially in vertebrae of the mid to lower thoracic spine, and loss of height are the most common signs (Fig. 7–21).

PATIENT SCREENING

Unrecognized osteoporosis may first be discovered when the patient sustains a fracture. Emergency care is required for difficulty breathing, severe pain, bone protruding through the skin, or numbness in a limb.

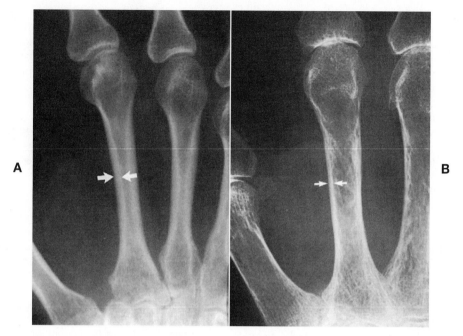

FIGURE 7-20 A, Normal metacarpal bone. **B,** Osteoporotic metacarpal bone. (From Helms CA: *Fundamentals of skeletal radiology,* ed 2, Philadelphia, 1995, Saunders.)

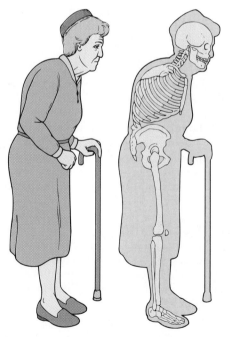

FIGURE 7-21 Typical posture in osteoporosis.

ETIOLOGY

Osteoporosis is the most common metabolic bone disease. It is caused by the imbalance between the breakdown of old bone tissue and the manufacture of new bone. Metabolic bone diseases primarily originate from hormonal or dietary factors or disuse, but trauma also may cause the development of this condition. Osteoporosis also can be caused by radiation treatments, malabsorption, smoking, immobility, and chronic disease such as rheumatoid arthritis. *Senile* and postmenopausal osteoporosis, usually resulting from a lack of estrogen, are the most common forms. Osteoporosis also can result from use of medications, such as heparin, phenytoin, and the cortisone medications prednisone and prednisolone.

DIAGNOSIS

Patients with spontaneous bone fracture are screened for cancer in the involved bone thorough radiographic testing. When osteoporosis is detected, patients are further evaluated for hormone imbalances, kidney disease, diet inadequacy, and medication use, including cortisone medications such as prednisone and prednisolone.

The diagnosis of osteoporosis is based on the results of blood serum studies, radiographic films, urinalysis, CT scan, and bone scan. The best test for osteoporosis is a dual energy x-ray absorptometry (DEXA) scan. If more specific diagnostic data are needed, a bone biopsy may be ordered.

TREATMENT

Osteoporosis can cause permanent disability if not arrested, and treatment varies depending on the cause. Increased dietary intake of calcium, calcium carbonate, calcium carbonate with sodium fluoride, phosphate supplements, and vitamins, especially vitamin D, may be prescribed. Estrogen replacement therapy may be attempted for postmenopausal osteoporosis. For women not wishing to use estrogen replacement therapy, bisphosphonate medications, such as alendronate sodium (Fosamax) and risedronate (Actonel) may be prescribed. Calcitonin (Miacalcin) nasal spray and parathyroid hormone (Forteo) are other options. Exercise can help to minimize osteoporosis by slowing the loss of calcium. Moderate exercise in the form of walking, swimming, or riding a stationary bicycle is best. Physical therapy exercises for persons who are immobilized or paralyzed are necessary. If, however, the bones have become brittle, exercise of any type may be limited. To alleviate pain and muscle spasms, analgesics and muscle relaxants may be prescribed.

PROGNOSIS

The outlook for patients with osteoporosis depends on many factors including their age and mobility, the severity of bone loss, underlying causes, and complications related to fractures.

PREVENTION

Prevention is absolutely the key to osteoporosis management. Bone density testing should be performed in all women over the age of 65 years, in all postmenopausal women with risk factors for osteoporosis, and postmenopausal women who sustain fractures. Women should consult their caregivers regarding adequate calcium intake and regular exercise programs.

PATIENT TEACHING

Patients must be instructed regarding diets that promote bone health, smoking cessation, calcium and vitamin D intake, and exercise programs.

Osteomalacia and Rickets

DESCRIPTION

Osteomalacia is a disease characterized by a defective mineralization of the bones.

 ICD-9-CM Code 268.2 *(Unspecified)*
Additional codes may be required to identify the nature or cause of osteomalacia. Refer to the physician's diagnosis and then to the current edition of the ICD-9-CM coding manual for greatest specificity.

SYMPTOMS AND SIGNS

Osteomalacia causes the bones to become increasingly soft, flexible, and deformed. When the disorder occurs in children, it impacts the growing skeleton and is called *rickets*. In adults, it usually is referred to as osteomalacia.

Early symptoms may include general fatigue; progressive stiffness; tender, painful bones; backaches; muscle twitches and cramps; and difficulty in standing up. As the disease progresses, the patient may experience fractures, bowing of the legs, chest deformity, and shortening of the spine that leads to an overall reduction in height.

PATIENT SCREENING

The early symptoms mentioned above require an appointment for a medical assessment.

ETIOLOGY

Osteomalacia is a metabolic bone disease resulting from a deficiency or ineffective use of vitamin D, which is essential to the process of bone formation. Without vitamin D, the body cannot absorb the bone-building minerals (calcium and phosphorus).

Other causes of this disorder may include an inadequate exposure to sunlight, which prevents the body from synthesizing its own vitamin D; intestinal malabsorption of vitamin D; and chronic renal diseases.

DIAGNOSIS

Children presenting with skeletal abnormalities suggestive of rickets are evaluated for genetic disorders and disease of the kidneys and bowels.

Adults with osteomalacia are screened for metabolism disorders, as well as kidney and bowel disease.

The diagnosis of osteomalacia can involve a series of blood tests (e.g., serum calcium, serum alkaline phosphatase, and vitamin D levels) and erythrocyte sedimentation rate (ESR), radiographic studies, bone scan, and possibly a bone biopsy.

TREATMENT

Treatment involves taking vitamin D supplements and adding vitamin D, calcium, and calcitonin to the diet. Exposure to sunlight increases vitamin D metabolism and absorption, especially for elderly persons. Any underlying disorder, such as kidney or bowel disease, causing the deficiency must be treated as well.

PROGNOSIS

The outlook for patients with osteomalacia depends to a great extent on how early the condition is detected. The severity of the disorder, underlying causes, and complications, such as fracture of bone, are each important factors affecting the long-term outlook.

PREVENTION

Prevention focuses on early diagnosis and avoiding bone injury.

PATIENT TEACHING

Patients are instructed regarding vitamin D and calcium metabolism, dietary requirements, and the role of ultraviolet radiation in sunlight in producing natural vitamin D within the body.

Hallux Valgus (Bunion)

DESCRIPTION

A bunion is a localized area of enlargement of the inner portion of the metatarsophalangeal joint at the base of the big toe (Fig. 7–22).

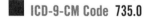 **ICD-9-CM Code 735.0**

SYMPTOMS AND SIGNS

Bunions progressively enlarge over time. If an inflamed bursa develops, secondary to pressure and inflammation at the joint, it can become painful. At times, the great toe may override or undercut the second toe. This causes crowding of the other toes and the possible development of hammer, claw, or mallet toe. Bunion development is more common among women and adolescent girls.

PATIENT SCREENING

Schedule an appointment for a visual examination for a patient complaining of a painful large toe.

ETIOLOGY

Bunion is usually the result of a foot disorder known as *hallux* valgus, in which the great toe is positioned toward the midline of the body. The condition also has been associated with rheumatoid arthritis. A flatfoot also contributes to hallux valgus and the development of a bunion because of the fallen, or dropped, longitudinal arch of the foot. The wearing of improperly fitting or high-heeled shoes aggravates hallux valgus. There is also a familial tendency for developing this condition. Bunions are common in ballet dancers.

DIAGNOSIS

Patients with bunions are evaluated for underlying forms of arthritis, particularly osteoarthritis and gout. Footwear should be closely scrutinized. A physical examination of the foot, along with history of the symptoms, may be sufficient for the diagnosis. Radiographic studies confirm the lateral displacement of the great toe and any degenerative arthritic joint changes.

TREATMENT

Management of a bunion can include wearing shoes with a roomy "toe box" to avoid crowding the toes together; wearing shoes with lower heels; using padding between the toes or around the bunion to relieve pressure; applying ice to the bunion to reduce the inflammation and lessen the pain; and resting the affected joints.

Analgesic–*antipyretic* medications (e.g., aspirin and acetaminophen) are given for pain. Intraarticular (joint) injections of corticosteroid may be helpful as well.

There are many different surgical procedures for the treatment or correction of hallux valgus. Bunionectomy, osteotomy, and arthroplasty are the more common procedures.

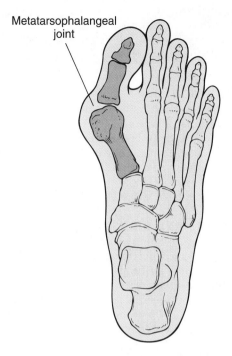

Metatarsophalangeal joint

FIGURE 7–22 Bunion—hallux valgus.

PROGNOSIS

With proper footwear, bunions often can be tolerated without surgical intervention. For those with persistent pain, surgical treatments can be curative.

PREVENTION

Proper footwear to minimize trauma to the toe and metatarsophalangeal joint is essential for the best outcome.

PATIENT TEACHING

Patients can benefit by learning about the anatomy of the foot and the affected joint. They should be alerted to the potential for secondary infection if the bunion is abraded by footwear; if such is the case, antibiotics are instituted if needed.

Hallux Rigidus

DESCRIPTION

Hallux rigidus is a stiff big toe that develops as a result of degeneration of the cartilage of the first metatarsophalangeal (MTP) joint.

■ **ICD-9-CM Code 735.2**

SYMPTOMS AND SIGNS

Hallux rigidus causes pain and loss of motion in the joint. The MTP joint becomes painful, stiff, and swollen. The onset may be insidious, with the limitation of movement being gradual.

PATIENT SCREENING

An appointment for visual inspection and probable radiographic studies is indicated for a patient complaining of pain in the large toe.

ETIOLOGY

Degeneration of the MTP joint can occur as a result of injury or underlying arthritis, such as osteoarthritis. Over a period of time, constant wear and tear on the joint or repetitive minor trauma to the joint causes the articular cartilage of the joint to degenerate, resulting in raw bone surface rubbing against raw bone surface. This degenerative arthritic type of process allows for the formation of bone spurs or osteophytes in the joint space that restricts joint motion.

DIAGNOSIS

Diagnosis is made from the history of pain, either continuous or when walking, and restriction of motion of the MTP joint of the great toe. Physical examination usually reveals a straight hallux with an enlarged and tender joint with limited dorsiflexion (Fig. 7–23). Radiographic studies confirm the degenerative process, and the joint space is diminished. Advanced conditions may show chips of the cartilage in the joint space, which may eventually calcify.

TREATMENT

Conservative treatment includes drug therapy with antiinflammatory agents and wearing of shoes with thick hard soles and low heels. When

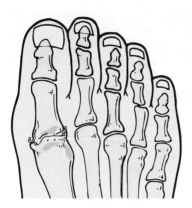

FIGURE 7–23 Hallux rigidus.

surgical intervention is indicated, a *cheilectomy* to remove bone spurs and degenerative changes of the joint is considered. During cheilectomy, a portion of the dorsal aspect of the metatarsal head also is removed. This is followed by rehabilitation with ROM exercises. When the progression of the condition is extensive, *arthrodesis,* or fusion of the joint, may be the only method of pain relief. Some surgeons may perform an *arthroplasty* and replace the destroyed joint with a plastic prosthesis or an artificial joint. The problem with this procedure is that the lifetime of the joint usually is limited, making it possible that future procedures will be needed.

PROGNOSIS

With proper footwear and medication to relieve intermittent pain, hallux rigidus often can be tolerated without surgical intervention. For those with persistent pain, surgical treatments can be curative.

PREVENTION

Proper footwear to minimize trauma to the toe and metatarsophalangeal joint is essential for the best outcome.

PATIENT EDUCATION

Patients can benefit by learning about the anatomy of the foot and the affected joint. Repeated impact loading of the affected joint can lead to progressive worsening.

Hammer Toe

DESCRIPTION

A hammer toe is a condition of the toe in which the toe bends upward like a claw because of an abnormal flexion of the proximal interphalangeal (PIP) joint; it can occur in any one of the four lesser toes (Fig. 7–24, *A*).

 ICD-9-CM Code 735.4 *(Acquired)*

SYMPTOMS AND SIGNS

Hammer toe usually occurs in the second toe, manifested by a hyperextension of the MTP joint. This deformity can be painful and often causes abrasion and inflammation where the flexed toe rubs against footwear. It can lead to the formation of a corn on the top of the affected toe and callus formation on the sole of the foot.

PATIENT SCREENING

Patients with hammer toes are evaluated for underlying forms of arthritis, such as rheumatoid arthritis and psoriatic arthritis.

ETIOLOGY

Many factors may contribute to the occurrence of hammer toe. Although a congenital tendency of a long second metatarsal bone may exist, often shoes that are too short and have pointed toes or high heels may be the contributing factor. Nerves supplying the muscles of the toe are subjected to repeated insult, resulting in muscle imbalance in the foot and the development of the hammer toe. Underlying arthritis from diseases such as rheumatoid arthritis and psoriatic arthritis can lead to the formation of hammer toes.

DIAGNOSIS

History of pain in the affected toe along with visual inspection is usually sufficient for determining diagnosis (Fig. 7–24, *B*). Imaging studies confirm the diagnosis and rule out forms of arthritis.

TREATMENT

If the patient presents early in the onset of symptoms, often switching to shoes that fit properly and allow enough space for the second toe can reverse

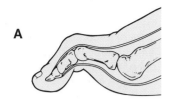

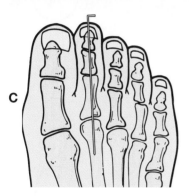

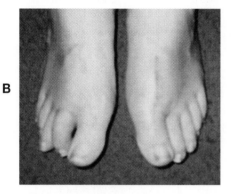

FIGURE 7–24 **A,** Hammer toe. **B,** Hammer toe of second lesser toe, right foot. **C,** Pin in place after surgical arthroplasty and fusion of proximal interphalangeal (PIP) joint.

the process, and the toe will eventually straighten. Splinting of the affected toe and performing therapeutic exercises can be helpful. The more advanced conditions in which a contracture exists require surgical arthroplasty and possible fusion of the PIP joint (Fig. 7–24, *C*).

PROGNOSIS

Proper footwear and monitoring for secondary infection improve outcome. For those with persis-

tent pain and irritation, surgical treatments can be curative.

PREVENTION

Proper footwear to minimize trauma to the toe is essential for the best outcome. Box-toed shoes can be very helpful.

PATIENT TEACHING

Patients can benefit by learning about the anatomy of the foot and the affected toe. They should be instructed regarding the care of the foot and toenails as well as how to monitor for signs of secondary infection.

Traumatic and Sports Injuries

Fractures

DESCRIPTION

Fractures, or broken bones, are caused by stress on the bone resulting from a traumatic insult to the musculoskeletal system, severe muscle spasm, or bone disease. They can occur in any bone in the body and are classified by the nature of the fracture, which is the result of the mechanism of injury (Fig. 7–25, *A-O*).

ICD-9-CM Code 800-829

Fractures are classified and coded according to site, type, multiple fractures of sites, and cause of injury, and subclassified by factors such as the occurrence of complications and late effects. Refer to the physician's diagnosis and then the current edition of the ICD-9-CM coding manual for greatest specificity.

Fractures are described by specific names or by location:
- Colles fracture is fracture of the distal head of the radius, with possible involvement of the ulnar styloid. Colles fractures usually result from a fall in which the person attempts to break the fall with an extended arm and open hand. Pain and swelling are experienced. Treatment includes closed reduction of the fracture and immobilization of the arm, including the elbow, with a cast.

- Fracture of the humerus involves an obvious displacement of the bone of the upper arm along with shortening of the extremity and an abnormal mobility of the upper arm. Closed reduction of the fracture is followed by immobilization in a hanging arm cast and sling and swathe.
- Fracture of the pelvis is usually the result of a motor vehicle accident or a fall, in the case of an elderly person. Complications of this fracture include lacerated colon, paralytic ileus, bladder and urethral injury, and intrapelvic hemorrhage. Treatment includes bed rest, possible immobilization with a pelvic sling or skeletal traction, and open reduction and repair.
- A fractured hip is usually the result of a fall. This fracture occurs most often because of osteoporosis in women older than 60 years. An outward rotation along with a shortening of the affected extremity is noted. Repair is accom-

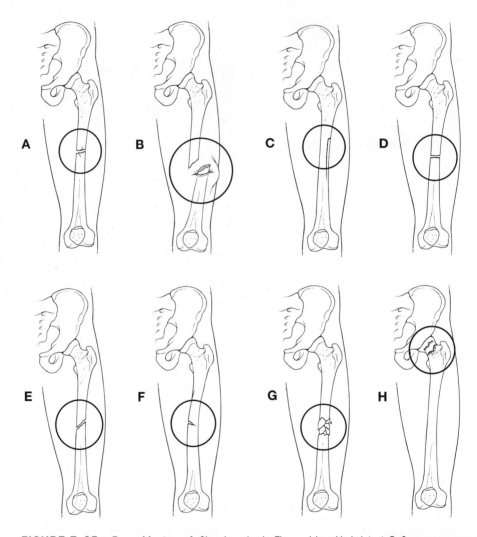

FIGURE 7–25 Types of fractures. **A,** Closed, or simple. The overlying skin is intact. **B,** Open, or compound. The skin overlying the bone ends is not intact. **C,** Longitudinal. The fracture extends along the length of the bone. **D,** Transverse. The fracture is at right angles to the axis of the bone. **E,** Oblique. The fracture extends in an oblique direction. **F,** Greenstick. The fracture is on one side of the bone; the other side is bent. **G,** Comminuted. The bone is splintered or crushed. **H,** Impacted. The fractured ends of the bone are driven into each other.

plished by surgery that involves the insertion of a prosthesis or pins, or both.

- Fracture of the femoral shaft is more common in young adults and usually is the result of a severe direct impact related to motor vehicle accidents or severe trauma. A marked angulation deformity and shortening of the affected leg is present. The patient is unable to move the knee or hip. The fracture is stabilized by skeletal traction or internal fixation with a rod or a plate and screws.
- Fracture of the tibia results from a strong force exerted on the lower leg that causes soft tissue damage in addition to the fracture. Open or closed reduction is employed, followed by immobilization with a cast.
- Vertebral fracture, usually occurring in the cervical region, is the result of acceleration-deceleration trauma. Immediate immobilization is imperative to prevent spinal cord damage and resulting paralysis. Thoracic and lumbar vertebrae also can be fractured. Immobilization may be followed by surgical repair and possible insertion of surgical hardware (rods, plates) for stabilization.
- Basilar skull fracture is fracture of the floor of the cranial vault (see Fig. 13–11 in Chapter 13).

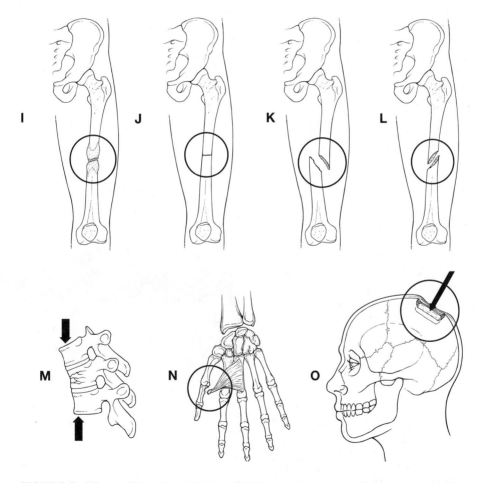

FIGURE 7–25, cont'd Types of fractures. **I,** Pathologic. The fracture results from weakening of the bone by disease. **J,** Nondisplaced. The bone ends remain in alignment. **K,** Displaced. The bone ends are out of alignment. **L,** Spiral. The fracture results from a twisting mechanism, causing the break to wind around the bone in a spiral. **M,** Compression. Excessive pressure causes the bone to collapse. **N,** Avulsion. Tearing away of a muscle or a ligament is accompanied by tearing away of a bone fragment. **O,** Depression. Bone fragments of the skull are driven inward.

It is usually the result of massive trauma to the head from a motor vehicle accident.

- Le Fort fracture, bilateral horizontal fracture of the maxilla, often results when the face is forced against the steering wheel in a motor vehicle accident.
- In Pott fracture, the lower part of the fibula is fractured. The lower tibial articulation sustains serious injury.
- Clavicular fracture is fracture of the clavicle (collar bone). It is a common sports injury, usually involving bicycling accidents, and occurs often in children of all ages.

SYMPTOMS AND SIGNS

Pain accompanies most fractures. Edema, tenderness, discoloration, and inability to move the affected part follow. In some instances, a deformity of the affected part is noted. The location of the fracture and the type of the fracture are determining factors in the symptoms and signs.

PATIENT SCREENING

Severe pain, deformity, inability to move an extremity, bone protruding through the skin, numbness or tingling in a joint, or difficulty breathing are indications for emergency care. NOTE: In some diseases fractures are not associated with injury, but are "spontaneous fractures."

ETIOLOGY

Any force, external or internal, that disrupts the continuity of the bone causes a fracture. Diseases such as neoplasms, tuberculosis of the bone, and osteoporosis cause pathologic fractures, which occur without significant external trauma.

DIAGNOSIS

The major issues in assessing patients' injuries include defining the extent of the fracture and any complications resulting from the fracture and also detecting any underlying disease of the bone. A complete history and physical examination are followed by radiographic studies of the affected structure. Bone scans and MRI aid in determining diagnosis. Underlying pathologic change is investigated and diagnosed; sometimes this requires a bone biopsy.

TREATMENT

Treatment depends on the location, severity, type, and cause of the fracture as described above. Simple fractures of long bones are reduced and immobilized. Compound fractures are cleaned, *debrided,* reduced, and immobilized. Immobilization is accomplished by splinting (including the use of posterior splints), casting, taping, and external or internal fixation. Internal fixation (open reduction) includes the use of surgically implanted pins, wires, rods, plates, screws, or other devices. Some fractures are placed in traction, to hold the ends of the bones in proper alignment until healing takes place.

Complications of fractures include compartment syndrome, in which the circulation to the area is compromised because of edema; nonunion and malunion of bones; infection; *necrosis;* fat emboli; and pulmonary emboli.

PROGNOSIS

The outlook for a patient with a fracture depends on the location, severity, complications, and presence of underlying disease. Fractures that damage the epiphyseal plate ("growth" plate) in the child may have long-term residual effects such as stunted growth or osteoarthritis.

PREVENTION

Wearing protective gear when playing contact sports and engaging in conditioning exercises can decrease the risk for fractures.

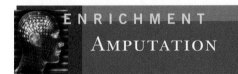

ENRICHMENT

AMPUTATION

MOST LIMB AMPUTATIONS INVOLVE the legs and are necessary because of peripheral vascular disease from atherosclerosis and consequent gangrene. Trauma, malignancy, and congenital defects are additional reasons for amputation. Many upper extremity amputations are the sequelae of trauma including crushing injuries, open fractures, and thermal or electrical burns. Infection and malignancy also may necessitate the amputation. The extent of the amputation can range from removal of a portion of a digit to a complete disarticulation at the hip or shoulder.

Rehabilitation is important and is attempted as soon as possible to afford the patient independence. Many customized prostheses are available for both upper and lower extremities.

PATIENT TEACHING

Patient education should be focused on appropriate conditioning programs to avoid future fractures. After a patient has experienced a fracture, instructions on cast or brace care, activity limitations, and gradual rehabilitation exercises are essential.

To ensure optimal rehabilitation of the involved body areas, explain the exact condition and long-term goals to the patient.

Strains and Sprains

DESCRIPTION

A strain is an injured tendon, muscle, or other tissue resulting from overuse, overstretching, or excessive forcible stretching of the tissue beyond its functional capacity.

A sprain is an acute partial tear of a ligament (Fig. 7–26). They are classified as first-, second-, or third-degree, or grade.

ICD-9-CM Code 840-848

Strains and sprains are classified and coded according to such factors as site, occurrence of injury and involvement of adjacent structures. Refer to the physician's diagnosis and then the current edition of the ICD-9-CM coding manual for greatest specificity.

SYMPTOMS AND SIGNS

Strains and sprains can be an acute injuries or can be the result of chronic overuse (cumulative trauma). Symptoms may include localized pain, weakness, numbness, and possibly edema around the site of the injury. With both strain and sprain injuries, using, moving, or bearing weight on the affected limb or part is difficult or sometimes nearly impossible for the patient. Sprains may include damage to blood vessels and nerves, and edema, ecchymosis, and sharp, transient pain may develop. When sprains and strains are caused by chronic overuse, they typically cause stiffness, tenderness, and soreness.

PATIENT SCREENING

Ankle injury accompanied by obvious deformity, bone protruding through the skin, or bleeding requires emergency care. Schedule a same-day appointment for an individual with a painful ankle injury that involves inability to bear weight or walk.

ETIOLOGY

Strains and sprains can be caused by acute trauma (e.g., automobile accidents) or cumulative trauma (e.g., overuse, such as with sports-related injuries).

DIAGNOSIS

A physical examination and medical history of a recent injury resulting from physical activity, an accident, or repetitive overuse may suggest the diagnosis. Patients with obvious significant physical trauma should be evaluated for possible associated

ENRICHMENT

PHANTOM LIMB AND PHANTOM LIMB PAIN

PHANTOM LIMB SENSATION is an unpleasant complication that sometimes follows an amputation, especially of a leg, and is difficult to treat. It is the feeling that the limb still is attached. Phantom limb pain of the leg can present as a burning sensation of the foot or as a feeling of having the toes stepped on when no limb exists.

Both conditions usually disappear with time and with the realization that the limb is gone. Phantom limb pain may necessitate injection or removal of troublesome nerve endings that are located in the stump.

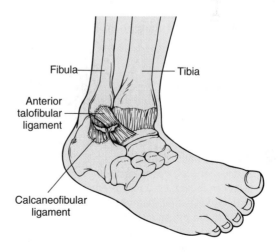

FIGURE 7–26 Ankle sprain.

fractures. Radiographic studies are ordered to rule out the possibility of a fracture.

TREATMENT

The treatment of both strains and sprains is similar and depends on the degree, or grade, of the injury. The sprain, being the more serious injury, requires more intense treatment. Treatment of sprains and strains entails elevation and rest of the affected limb and the application of ice to control edema. Immobilization of the limb with an elastic bandage, soft cast, or splint may be necessary. Analgesics and possibly antiinflammatory agents are used to control pain and inflammation. Surgery may be indicated if the injury involves a large tear or if it heals improperly.

PROGNOSIS

Healing of a strain or sprain usually requires 2 to 4 weeks, longer with the more serious degrees of strain or sprain. The outlook is best when the patient participates in a progressive rehabilitation program.

PREVENTION

Recognizing personal physical limitations, following safety precautions, and taking time to warm up the muscles by slow, easy stretching before engaging in exercise or physical activity all help to prevent sprains and strains. Sometimes support bracing is necessary when engaging in strenuous activities after incurring one of these injuries.

PATIENT TEACHING

Encourage compliance with the treatment plan and rehabilitation program. Discuss the prevention measures mentioned above to avoid reinjury.

Dislocations

DESCRIPTION

A dislocation is the forcible displacement of a bone from its joint, thereby causing loss of joint function (Fig. 7–27).

ICD-9-CM Code 830-839

Dislocations are coded according to site, type (open or closed, etc.), occurrence of injury, and nature (congenital, pathologic, recurrent, etc.). Refer to the physician's diagnosis and then the current edition of the ICD-9-CM coding manual for greatest specificity.

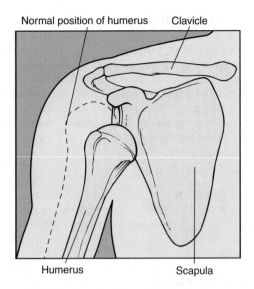

Normal position of humerus   Clavicle

Humerus   Scapula

FIGURE 7–27 Dislocation of the shoulder.

SYMPTOMS AND SIGNS

A joint that is dislocated appears misshapen, is extremely painful, and rapidly becomes edematous, ecchymotic, and immovable. Injury to the ligaments and capsule of the joint is present. Other symptoms are a function of the extent of damage to the surrounding tissues, nerves, and blood vessels.

Dislocation of spinal vertebrae can result in damage to the entire spinal cord and cause paralysis below the injured area. A dislocation of a shoulder or hip can damage the nerve supply and cause paralysis of the limb. Some joints that have been dislocated tend to be susceptible to developing osteoarthritis in later years.

PATIENT SCREENING

Traumatic dislocations require *immediate* emergency medical care.

ETIOLOGY

The cause of a dislocation is usually a severe injury (e.g., a fall, automobile accident, or sports-related trauma) that exerts force great enough to tear the joint ligaments. Occasionally, the injury that causes the dislocation also causes a fracture.

Dislocations not caused by injury may be congenital or may result from a complication of arthritis. They can happen repeatedly, without apparent cause, to a joint already weakened by an earlier injury. The jaw and shoulder joints are especially susceptible to recurring dislocation.

A rare cause of recurrent dislocations is the inherited connective tissue disorder Ehlers-Danlos syndrome, which is characterized by joint and skin laxity.

DIAGNOSIS
The obvious abnormal appearance of the affected joint, the history of the injury, and the physical examination may be all that is necessary to determine the diagnosis. A radiographic study can confirm whether a dislocation has occurred and whether any fractures are present. Patients also must be evaluated for nerve and blood vessel injury.

TREATMENT
An untrained individual never should attempt to reduce a dislocation; to do so may cause extensive damage. A physician should be seen within 15 to 30 minutes for proper repositioning of the joint. After that time, a dislocated joint may be so edematous and painful that reduction may have to be performed with the patient under general anesthesia. If dislocation is a recurring problem, patients may be taught how to reposition the joint themselves.

Surgery is sometimes necessary to achieve satisfactory reduction. If a joint has become weakened from repeated dislocation, surgery to tighten the ligaments that hold the adjoining bones may be recommended.

PROGNOSIS
The outlook for a dislocated joint depends on the amount of damage to the tissues of the joint and the overall strength of the adjacent muscles. Surgical procedures can stabilize the joint, but sometimes limit range of motion.

PREVENTION
Persons who have suffered a dislocation to a joint may require use of stabilization splints when engaging in activities. Repeated dislocation is potentially damaging to the joint.

PATIENT TEACHING
Teaching the proper use of splinting devices and proper timing of resumption of activities is essential for optimal outcome.

Adhesive Capsulitis (Frozen Shoulder)

DESCRIPTION
Adhesive capsulitis is a condition in which a shoulder is significantly limited in its range of motion as a result of inflammation, scarring, thickening, and shrinkage of the capsule that surrounds the normal shoulder joint. Adhesive capsulitis is commonly called "*frozen shoulder.*"

 ICD-9-CM Code 726.0

SYMPTOMS AND SIGNS
A frozen shoulder presents as a shoulder that has become stiff and painful, making normal movement impossible. The pain can be either localized in the shoulder itself or spread out encompassing the upper arm or neck. It is often severe enough to disrupt sleep. Symptoms become gradually worse during the first few months after injury, then remain at a constant degree of discomfort for a couple more months, and then finally begin a period of gradual improvement. With time the pain subsides, but the mobility of the shoulder often remains permanently impaired, or frozen.

PATIENT SCREENING
Regular follow-up appointments are important for patients undergoing treatment for frozen shoulder.

ETIOLOGY
Frozen shoulder is caused by inflammation of the capsule of the joint with secondary scarring. It usually begins after a slight injury or minor problem, such as bursitis and *tendinitis,* which prevents normal use of the joint. Disuse of the shoulder leads to more and more stiffness, pain, and increased disuse.

DIAGNOSIS
The symptoms alone are usually enough to identify this condition. However, a review of the patient history may indicate a recent injury that precipitated bursitis or tendonitis. Patients with frozen shoulder are evaluated for underlying arthritis, injury, and diabetes.

Radiographic tests can be helpful for detecting underlying problems in the shoulder and can demonstrate calcification that would indicate past chronic inflammation.

TREATMENT

A stiff shoulder must be kept in motion, as much as possible, to prevent permanent immobility. A physical or occupational therapist may be needed to teach and assist the patient with ROM exercises. Analgesics, antiinflammatory agents, and often an injection of a steroid medication into the joint are needed. If the condition is severe and persistent, the physician may suggest shoulder manipulation, under general anesthesia, to increase mobility.

PROGNOSIS

The outlook for a patient with a frozen shoulder depends on the severity, the duration of the condition, and the presence of underlying joint disorders. Longstanding frozen shoulders tend to be less responsive to treatments.

PREVENTION

Persons who have had chest surgery, including heart and breast procedures, should perform upper body exercises to minimize the risk of developing a frozen shoulder.

PATIENT TEACHING

Patients are instructed on the details and importance of ROM exercises to restore joint function. Avoiding reinjury is key for optimal outcome.

Severed Tendon

DESCRIPTION

Tendons are long, fibrous cords that connect muscles to bones (e.g., the Achilles tendon connects the gastrocnemius muscle to the calcaneus bone at the back of the heel). A severed tendon is torn completely in tow and thus prevents the muscle from performing its function of moving a body part.

 ICD-9-CM Code 848.9

SYMPTOMS AND SIGNS

A severed tendon produces immediate, severe pain, inflammation, and immobility of the affected parts (Fig. 7–28).

PATIENT SCREENING

Injury followed by pain and immobility of the affected area requires prompt medical care.

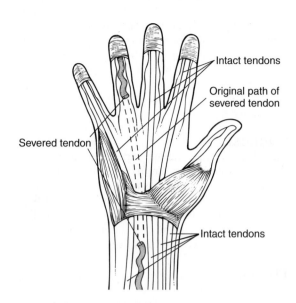

FIGURE 7–28 Severed tendon of the hand.

ETIOLOGY

The cause of a severed tendon is an injury or laceration. It involves the forearm, hand, calf of the leg, or foot. The injury may extend partially or completely through one or more tendons.

DIAGNOSIS

Physical examination of the injured site and the patient's inability to move the affected parts are usually sufficient for determining the diagnosis. A radiographic study rules out a fracture as the cause of the immobility. A person with a severed tendon must be closely evaluated for possible infection and foreign objects or materials in the wound site.

TREATMENT

Tendons are under tension, so if they become severed, the two ends snap away from each other and are difficult to retrieve. A surgeon may attempt to suture the two ends of the tendon together (**tenorrhaphy**) immediately or may wait for the injury to heal, depending on the extent of the injury. A large incision may be necessary to locate the ends of the tendon, before the tenorrhaphy can be attempted. To repair the damaged tendon, it may be necessary to insert a piece of tendon from elsewhere in the body.

The outcome of a tenoplasty is usually satisfactory. However, in some cases, the affected parts may be stiff and have less mobility after the surgery than before the injury. Physical therapy ensures as much mobility as possible.

PROGNOSIS

The prognosis depends on the tendon involved and the results of surgery. Infection will potentially complicate the outcome. Permanent muscle atrophy can result from tendon damage.

PREVENTION

Persons with lacerated tendons should receive tetanus vaccination.

PATIENT TEACHING

Patients are instructed on the details of rehabilitation and progressive exercise, beginning with gentle ROM exercises.

Shin Splints

DESCRIPTION

Shin splints are a painful condition involving inflammation of the periosteum, the extensor muscles in the lower leg, and the surrounding tissues.

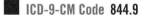 **ICD-9-CM Code 844.9**

SYMPTOMS AND SIGNS

Inflammation, edema, pain, and tenderness along the inner aspect of the tibia are common symptoms of shin splints. The pain worsens with exercise and then disappears with rest. Shin splints occur most commonly during the first weeks of a new exercise program or after a sudden increase in the amount of exercise in an on-going program.

This disorder is especially common in sports and fitness enthusiasts who jog, run, or engage in high-impact aerobics and is most often bilateral.

PATIENT SCREENING

A physical examination is required to evaluate the cause of pain and identify tenderness along the tibia.

ETIOLOGY

Overuse and overpronation are the most common factors that predispose an individual to shin splints. Pronation of the foot is an inward rotation of the ankle that causes the inner arch of the foot to sag

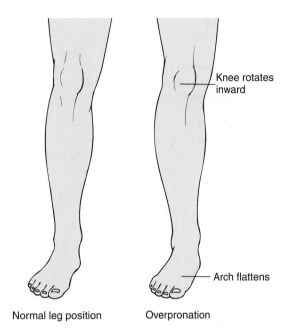

FIGURE 7–29 Excessive pronation of the foot.

and the ankle joint to tip upward (Fig. 7–29). All people pronate when they walk to some degree; however, excessive pronation places abnormal stress on the calf muscles. This leads to the development of shin splints and tendon and ligament strain around the ankles and knees.

Improper conditioning and running on hard surfaces also can contribute to the development of shin splints.

DIAGNOSIS

The diagnosis is based on physical examination and history of pain that worsens with exercise and disappears after rest. A patient with symptoms of shin splints also can have stress fracture of the tibia bone. This can be detected with bone scanning and is considered when pain and tenderness are severe.

TREATMENT

The key to successful treatment of shin splints is rest. Applications of ice or heat, or both alternately, are essential in the treatment. Aspirin or stronger NSAIDs may be ordered to relieve the pain and to reduce inflammation. Specially designed shoes to correct overpronation or the use of an orthotic device in existing shoes may be recommended.

PROGNOSIS

The prognosis is generally very good for complete recovery, although this can sometimes be prolonged for serious athletes. Shin splints are painful but not dangerous, unless they are ignored and consequently result in stress fractures.

PREVENTION

Proper conditioning and gradual stretching of the legs before exercise, jogging or running on grass or other soft surfaces, performing aerobic exercises on mats, and ensuring that exercise shoes are well padded for support can help prevent this condition.

PATIENT TEACHING

Patient education is focused on proper footwear and conditioning and gradual return to exercise while incorporating a stretching and strengthening program.

Plantar Fasciitis (Calcaneal Spur)

DESCRIPTION

Plantar fasciitis, also known as *calcaneal,* or *heel, spur syndrome,* is an inflammatory response at the bottom of the heel bone (calcaneus). There the flat tissue (fascia) that acts like a bowstring for the arch of the foot attaches to the bottom of the heel.

■ **ICD-9-CM Code 728.71**

SYMPTOMS AND SIGNS

Plantar fasciitis is a common problem among people who are active in sports, especially runners. The problem begins as a dull, intermittent pain on the bottom of the foot, which can progress to a sharp persistent pain. Characteristically, the pain is worse on getting out of bed and taking the first few steps in the morning, after sitting for a time, after standing or walking, and when beginning a sporting activity. Plantar fascia injury also can occur at mid sole or near the toes.

The plantar fascia is a thick fibrous material on the bottom of the foot. It is attached to the calcaneus, fans forward toward the toes, and acts like a bowstring to maintain the arch of the foot.

PATIENT SCREENING

Patients with plantar fasciitis are evaluated for possible reactive arthritis, inflammatory bowel disease, ankylosing spondylitis, and diffuse idiopathic skeletal hyperostosis.

ETIOLOGY

The problem usually occurs when part of the inflexible fascia is repeatedly placed under tension (e.g., when running). This constant tension causes an inflammatory response, usually at the point where the fascia is attached to the calcaneus. The result is pain and the development of the spur.

Factors contributing to the development of plantar fasciitis include:
- Flat (pronated) feet
- High-arched, rigid feet
- Toe running or hill running
- Running on soft terrain (e.g., sand)
- Poor shoe support
- Sudden increase in activity level
- Sudden weight increase
- Increasing age
- Familial tendency

Underlying diseases including reactive arthritis, inflammatory bowel disease, ankylosing spondylitis, and diffuse idiopathic skeletal hyperostosis.

The inflammatory response at the calcaneus can produce spike-like projections of new bone called *calcaneal* (heel) *spurs* (Fig. 7–30, *A*). They do not cause the initial pain, nor do they cause the initial problem; they are a result of the problem.

DIAGNOSIS

Physical examination and the patient history of symptoms usually provide sufficient information for making the diagnosis. The bottom of the foot is typically very tender, particularly at the heel. Radiographic films sometimes show the spur (Fig. 7–30, *B*).

TREATMENT

The initial treatment of heel spurs consists of resting, applying ice to the sore area, taking antiinflammatory or analgesic medication, using heel pads (doughnut-shaped pads that equalize and absorb the shock on the heel and ease pressure on the plantar fascia), and wearing a shoe with good support. Sometimes local cortisone injection can reduce inflamed tissues. In addition, the physician may tape the foot to maintain the arch and help take some of the tension off the plantar fascia. Shoe inserts called *orthotics* also may be prescribed.

After the inflammation has subsided, physical therapy to strengthen the small muscles of the foot can begin. If done regularly, this helps prevent reinjury. Surgery rarely is required for the correc-

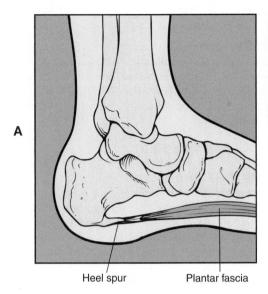

A

Heel spur   Plantar fascia

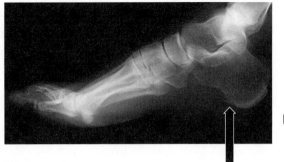

B

FIGURE 7–30 A, Calcaneal (heel) spur. **B,** Radiographic appearance.

tion of heel spurs. It is considered only if all forms of more conservative treatment fail and the pain still is incapacitating after several months of treatment. When performed, surgery involves removing the bone spur and releasing the plantar fascia.

PROGNOSIS

The prognosis is generally very good in response to conservative management. Surgical procedures are usually unnecessary.

PREVENTION

The key to prevention is the use of proper footwear. Any underlying associated medical condition should be optimally managed.

PATIENT TEACHING

Understanding the anatomy of the foot and what causes the condition can benefit affected patients as they undertake measures to promote healing.

Ganglion

DESCRIPTION

A ganglion is a benign sac-like swelling or cyst that is filled with a colorless, jelly-like fluid. A ganglion is formed from the tissue that lines a joint or tendon.

■ **ICD-9-CM Code 727.43** *(Unspecified)*

SYMPTOMS AND SIGNS

A ganglion most commonly develops on the back of the wrist as a single, smooth lump, just under the surface of the skin (Fig. 7–31). It can, however, develop near other joints, such as around the ankle joint, behind the knee, and on the fingers. Also, ganglia may appear as multiples or in clusters. Most are about the size of a pea, but others may grow as large as an inch or more in diameter. Ganglia may be soft to the touch or firm, and they are usually either painless or only somewhat bothersome. Pain may occur on occasion when moving the wrist, especially if the growth is large or inflamed.

PATIENT SCREENING

A visual examination by the health-care giver is indicated for a cystic swelling on a joint.

ETIOLOGY

Although some physicians believe that ganglia are caused by repetitive minor injuries, the underlying cause usually is unknown. A ganglion is sometimes a sign of arthritis of the adjacent joint. Whatever triggers the ganglion's development, it usually arises either in the joint capsule or in a tendon sheath.

DIAGNOSIS

The primary concern in evaluating a patient with a ganglion is whether or not underlying arthritis is

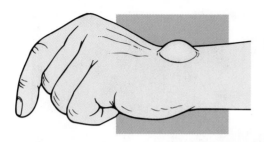

FIGURE 7–31 Ganglion.

present. A ganglion usually can be diagnosed by palpation and by observation of the appearance of the lump and the characteristic site. If in doubt, the physician can perform a needle aspiration to withdraw some of the fluid for laboratory analysis.

TREATMENT

If the ganglion does not cause pain and is not large enough to cause disfigurement or to interfere with wrist function, treatment is unnecessary. However, if the ganglion is causing pain, disfigurement, or impairment of the ROM, several options are available. The physician may try to rupture the ganglion by applying firm pressure. Needle aspiration may be used to remove as much fluid as possible, followed by instillation of a steroid, such as cortisone, or a *sclerosing* solution that helps to prevent recurrences. The physician may recommend a surgical procedure called a *ganglionectomy* to remove the ganglion.

Ganglia that originate in the wrist joint may be difficult to remove completely and therefore tend to recur. Even after surgical excision, approximately 10% recur. Over a period of months, ganglia often disappear on their own.

PROGNOSIS

Ganglia are usually harmless and do not impair function.

PREVENTION

The key to prevention is the identification of underlying arthritis.

PATIENT TEACHING

Simple reassurance that the condition can be resolved along with an explanation of the nature of the ganglion is generally helpful to patients.

Torn Meniscus

DESCRIPTION

A **meniscus** is a semilunar cartilage found in the knee joint. There are two menisci within the joint, a medial and a lateral (Fig. 7–32). A tear of the meniscus is a crack or fissure that is usually a result of wear or injury.

 ICD-9-CM Code 836.2

SYMPTOMS AND SIGNS

The medial meniscus is larger and more restricted in movement than the lateral meniscus and therefore is injured more often, or torn. Anterior and posterior cruciate ligament tears may accompany meniscal tears because the menisci are attached to the ligaments.

A person with a torn meniscus has acute pain when putting full weight on the affected leg and knee. The person may report that the knee "locks" or "gives way." Snapping or clicking sounds (crepitus) may be heard on flexion or extension. Full flexion of the affected knee may be difficult, and pain increases with full extension.

PATIENT SCREENING

Patients experiencing acute knee pain should be seen by the health-care provider as soon as possible.

ETIOLOGY

Most torn menisci are related to sports injuries. Participants in football, baseball, and soccer are especially susceptible to this type of injury. Tears in the meniscus usually result from sudden twisting or external rotation of the leg while the knee is flexed.

DIAGNOSIS

Patients with symptoms suggestive of a meniscal tear are evaluated for ligament injury and arthritis of the affected joint. Physical examination of the knee indicates the limitation of movement. Radiographic studies and MRI, which is the preferred procedure, are ordered; MRI may show the exact injury to the meniscus and, if any, to the ligaments.

TREATMENT

The injured knee should be immobilized immediately and elevated, with ice applied to slow bleeding and edema. No weight-bearing should be al-

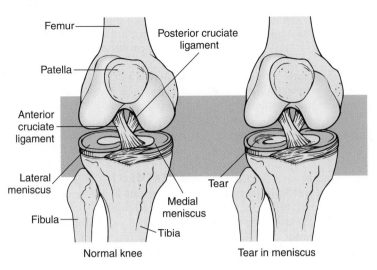

Normal knee   Tear in meniscus

FIGURE 7-32 Torn meniscus.

E N R I C H M E N T

ARTHROSCOPY

ARTHROSCOPY IS A SURGICAL PROCEDURE used to examine the structures within a joint using a tube-like viewing instrument called an arthroscope. The arthroscope is a small tube that contains optical fibers and lenses. It is passed through tiny incisions in the skin into the joint to be examined. The arthroscope is connected to a video camera that allows the interior of the joint to be seen on a television monitor. The size of the arthroscope used varies with the size of the joint being examined.

Arthroscopy can be used for diagnosis and/or treatment. When procedures are performed in addition to examining the joint with the arthroscope, this is referred to as arthroscopic surgery. A number of procedures are done in this fashion. When a procedure can be done arthroscopically instead of by traditional open surgical methods, it usually causes less tissue trauma and therefore results in less pain. This tends to promote a quicker recovery.

Arthroscopy is performed by orthopedic surgeons, generally in an outpatient setting. After the procedure, patients usually can return home and begin a rehabilitation program.

---

lowed, and the physician should be seen as soon as possible. The physician orders antiinflammatory or analgesic medications as needed.

The treatment of a torn meniscus usually can be done arthroscopically with the patient under anesthesia, unless injury to the cruciate ligaments also has occurred. Ligament tears require more extensive surgery to expose and repair them.

Total excision or partial excision of the torn meniscus is called a *meniscectomy*. A total meniscectomy usually is not done because it predisposes the knee to degenerative changes and instability.

PROGNOSIS
Meniscal tears respond very well to surgical treatments.

PREVENTION

The key to prevention is the early care of underlying arthritis.

PATIENT TEACHING

A customized, extensive, progressive exercise program begins after the initial postoperative period and continues during the subsequent months.

Rotator Cuff Tears

DESCRIPTION

The four tendons of the rotator cuff, formed by the muscles of the shoulder, partially surround the head of the humerus and stabilize it in the glenoid cavity or socket. The infraspinatus muscle rotates the humerus externally, and the subscapularis muscle rotates the humerus internally. Other muscles involved in the rotator cuff are the supraspinatus and the teres minor. Tears in any of the rotator cuff tendons limit the function of the shoulder.

 ICD-9-CM Code 840.4

SYMPTOMS AND SIGNS

Tears in the tendons of the rotator cuff muscles produce an immediate snapping sound and acute pain and leave the person unable to *abduct* the arm. Range of motion becomes limited to varying degrees depending on the severity of the particular tear.

PATIENT SCREENING

Patients presenting with *acute* shoulder pain and limited mobility of the shoulder require medical attention as soon as possible

ETIOLOGY

Tears can result from acute trauma (most common) or from degenerative changes with age. Calcium deposits may develop in the insertion sites because of the degenerative changes and may predispose the tendons to tears or rupture. Also, steroid injections into the tendon areas can predispose them to tears or rupture.

DIAGNOSIS

Diagnosis is based on physical examination and the patient history. The shoulder may have limited and painful ROM. Confirmation is made by the results of an arthrogram or MRI scan. Patients are screened for bursitis and arthritis of the shoulder.

TREATMENT

Acute pain is managed with narcotic medication (e.g., codeine). Acetaminophen is given for moderate pain, and antiinflammatory medication is given for the inflammation. With rest and conservative therapy, including gradual physical therapy, minor tears can heal with restoration of function.

Significant acute tendon tears are surgically repaired immediately to preserve strength of the muscles and to restore motion of the shoulder. After surgery, the affected arm is placed in a shoulder immobilizer or abduction splint for approximately 3 weeks. Extensive, active exercises are begun when the cast is removed.

PROGNOSIS

Minor tears can heal in response to conservative measures. Major tears require surgical repair.

PREVENTION

Conditioning and stretching exercises are the best prevention for rotator cuff tears.

PATIENT TEACHING

Rubber band shoulder exercises and stretching are keys to long-term rehabilitation of the rotator cuff. A customized, extensive, progressive exercise program begins after the initial postoperative period and continues during the subsequent few months.

REVIEW CHALLENGE

Answer the following questions:

1. What are the functions of the normal skeletal system?
2. What procedures are employed in diagnosing scoliosis?
3. What pathology is characteristic of osteoarthritis?
4. The symptoms of Lyme disease mimic which disease?
5. Are any preventive measures recommended for Lyme disease?
6. What is the clinical picture of a patient with osteomyelitis?
7. What causes joint deformity in gout?
8. Which disease is characterized by a high rate of bone production?
9. What would the treatment plan for a patient with osteoporosis include?
10. How is vitamin D deficiency related to osteomalacia?
11. What specific findings from a physical examination are typical of fibromyalgia?
12. What causative factors contribute to hallux valgus (bunion)? Hallux rigidus? Hammer toe?
13. How are fractures classified?
14. How would you describe Colles fracture?
15. What is meant by phantom limb?
16. What methods are used to immobilize fractures?
17. Why is a sprain considered more serious than a strain?
18. What joints are more susceptible to dislocation?
19. What conditions result in a "frozen shoulder"?
20. What is the relationship of overpronation to shin splints?
21. Under what conditions might plantar fasciitis (spur syndrome) develop?
22. What acute symptoms is a person with torn meniscus likely to describe? A person with rotator cuff tear?

REAL-LIFE CHALLENGE

Osteoporosis

A 72-year-old woman recently experienced midthoracic back pain following a minor fall. Imaging studies confirm fractures of T-7 and T-8. Measurement of this small-boned woman revealed a loss of 1 inch in height, with a current measurement of 5 feet 1 inch compared with 5 feet 2 inches at the last physical exam 14 months ago. Serum calcium is elevated. The CT scan indicates osteoporosis.

According to history, the patient does not include many dairy products in her diet and takes no dietary supplements. In addition, she has never taken any form of estrogen replacement and does not exercise regularly.

QUESTIONS

1. In what type of individual would you expect to find the greatest incidence of osteoporosis?
2. What bones other than vertebrae are prone to fracture in osteoporosis?
3. Why would serum calcium be elevated in osteoporosis?
4. What is meant by the description of osteoporosis as a metabolic bone disease?
5. What should be included in a diet to prevent or slow the onset of osteoporosis?
6. Why is daily exercise important in preventing osteoporosis?
7. What type of drug therapy may be prescribed for the patient?

REAL-LIFE CHALLENGE

Lyme Disease

A 27-year-old man has been experiencing flu-like symptoms for 4 days. He reports headache, fatigue, joint pain, and "just not feeling well." Vital signs are temperature of 102.2° F, pulse of 96, respirations of 20, and blood pressure of 132/86. Physical examination reveals two areas on the left lower leg that have a fading red rash in a circle-type pattern. The center of each circle is pale, and there is a possible spot in the center of each.

Questioning discloses that the patient was deer hunting 5 days ago, walking through tall grass. He remembers experiencing itching on the lower left leg. Lyme disease is suspected. A blood test to detect antibodies to the spirochete *Borrelia burgdorferi* is ordered. Antibiotics are prescribed, as is acetaminophen for the fever, pain, and aches. The patient is encouraged to rest and return for recheck in a few days.

QUESTIONS

1. In what region of the country would you expect this patient to live?
2. What precautions should be taken by people who will be out walking in tall grass?
3. What should individuals who think they have been bitten by a tick do as soon as they discover the bite?
4. If Lyme disease is not diagnosed in its early stages, what complications may develop?
5. What is the causative agent of Lyme disease?
6. Discuss the prevention of Lyme disease, including vaccines.

INTERNET ASSIGNMENTS

1. Visit the American Lyme Disease Foundation website to research the latest statistics on Lyme disease; also gather information on other tick-borne diseases.

2. Research the "News and Events" page at the National Osteoporosis Foundation website and report on recent findings.

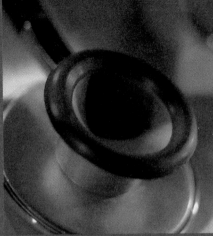

CHAPTER 8

Diseases and Conditions of the Digestive System

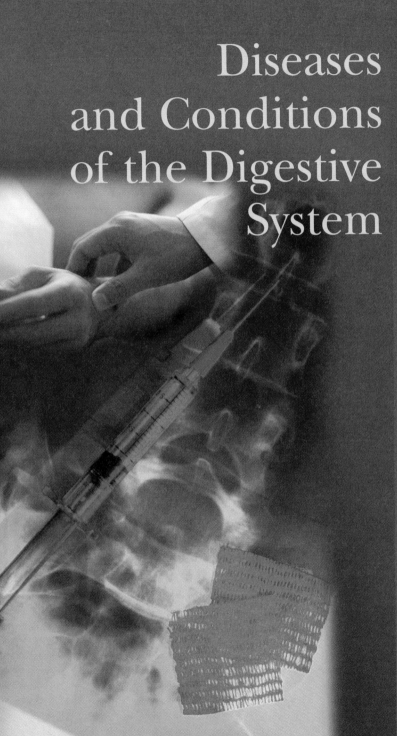

Chapter Outline—Cont'd

Learning Objectives

After studying Chapter 8, you should be able to:

1. Trace the process of normal digestion and absorption.
2. Discuss the importance of normal teeth and a normal bite.
3. Describe the presenting symptoms of temporomandibular joint syndrome.
4. Compare the etiology of herpes simplex to the etiology of thrush.
5. Name a serious complication of esophageal varices.
6. Explain the clinical significance of Barrett's esophagus.
7. Describe the pathology of peptic ulcers and identify the etiology.
8. Explain the diagnosis of gastric cancer.
9. Describe a hiatal hernia.
10. Distinguish the types of abdominal hernias.
11. Explain the differences between the pathology of Crohn disease and that of ulcerative colitis.
12. Describe the etiology of gastroenteritis.
13. Explain the difference between a functional and a mechanical obstruction of the bowel.
14. Discuss the pathologic conditions that may result in intestinal obstruction.
15. Distinguish between diverticulosis and diverticulitis.
16. Discuss the screening program for and treatment of colorectal cancer.
17. Explain the relationship between broad-spectrum antibiotics and pseudomembranous enterocolitis.
18. List the causes of inflammation of the peritoneum.
19. Explain the pathologic symptoms and signs of cirrhosis of the liver.
20. Name the most important etiologic factor for hepatocellular carcinoma and other additional risk factors.
21. Contrast the causes and preventive measures of hepatitis A and hepatitis C. Explain how health-care providers are at special risk for hepatitis B.
22. Name the most common bloodborne infection in the United States.
23. Describe the clinical picture of an individual with (a) biliary colic and (b) acute pancreatitis.
24. State the prognosis of pancreatic cancer.
25. Describe the clinical manifestations of malnutrition and malabsorption.
26. Explain the diagnostic criteria for celiac disease.
27. List some ways one can lower the risk of food poisoning.
28. Distinguish between the clinical picture of the patient with anorexia and that of the patient with bulimia.
29. State the components of a successful weight-loss program.

Key Terms

adenocarcinoma (**ad**–ih–no–**kar**–sin–**OH**–ma)
anastomosis (ah–**nas**–toh–**MOH**–sis)
antiemetic (**an**–tih–ee–**MET**–ik)
aphthous (**AF**–thus)
ascites (ah–**SIGH**–teez)
cholinergic (**ko**–lin–**ER**–jik)
endoscopy (en–**DOS**–ko–pee)
fistula (**FIS**–tew–lah)
fulminant (**FUL**–mih–nant)
gastroscopy (gas–**TROS**–koh–pee)
gingivitis (jin–jih–**VIE**–tis)
hematemesis (hem–ah–**TEM**–eh–sis)

hepatomegaly (**hep**–ah–toh–**MEG**–ah–lee)
hypokalemia (**high**–poh–ka–**LEE**–me–ah)
inguinal (**ING**–gwih–nal)
intussusception (in–tah–sus–**SEP**–shun)
periodontitis (**per**–ee–oh–don–**TIE**–tis)
peritonitis (**per**–ih–toh–**NIE**–tis)
proctoscopy (prock–**TAHS**–ko–pee)
pseudomembranous (**soo**–doe–**MEM**–brah–nus)
sigmoidoscopy (**sig**–moy–**DOS**–ko–pee)
temporomandibular (**tem**–poh–roh–man–**DIHB**–you–lar)
varices (**VAR**–ih–seez)

ORDERLY FUNCTION OF THE DIGESTIVE SYSTEM

THE DIGESTIVE SYSTEM COMPRISES the alimentary canal and the accessory organs of digestion (Fig. 8–1). Each unit of the system must be normal in structure and function to regulate the ingestion, digestion, and absorption of nutrients. The alimentary canal processes and transports the products of digestion. The accessory organs, located outside the gastrointestinal (GI) tract, manufacture and secrete endocrine and exocrine enzymes, secretions that are essential to the digestion and absorption of nutrients.

Diseases of the GI tract affect health and threaten life because they interfere with the critical functions of ingestion and digestion of food, absorption of nutrients for metabolism, and elimination of wastes. General categories of diseases and conditions of the digestive system include erosion of tissue, inflammation, infection, benign and malignant tumors, obstruction, interference with blood or nerve supply, malnutrition, and malabsorption syndromes.

Diseases and Conditions of the Oral Cavity and Jaws

The function of the teeth is mastication (chewing) to break down food into pieces that can be swallowed and digested easily (Fig. 8–2, *A* and *B*).

Hindrance of the chewing function caused by decay, infection of the teeth or gums, *malocclusion*, or missing teeth can interfere with this phase of the digestive process.

Most disorders affecting the mouth or the tongue are not serious, and treatment is simple and effective. Because malignant tumors are possible, a dentist or a physician should see any lump or change in the mouth or on the tongue that persists for longer than 10 days.

Missing Teeth

DESCRIPTION
Permanent teeth are missing.

ICD-9-CM Code 525-10 (*Acquired absence of teeth, unspecified*)
Loss of teeth is coded by causative factors. Refer to the physician's diagnosis and then to the current edition of the ICD-9-CM coding manual to ensure the greatest specificity of pathology and any appropriate modifiers.

SYMPTOMS AND SIGNS
The loss of permanent teeth, after the loss of primary teeth, can cause serious dental problems later in life (Fig. 8–3). Missing teeth can alter the bite, that is, how the teeth come together

ACCESSORY ORGANS

MAIN ORGANS

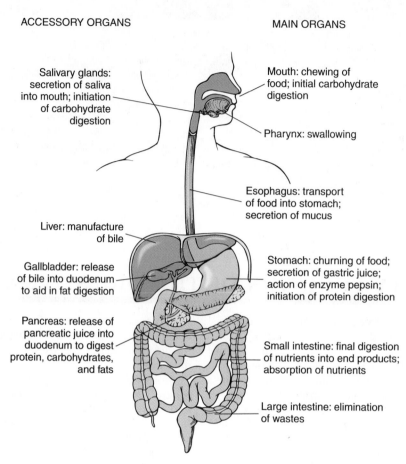

Salivary glands: secretion of saliva into mouth; initiation of carbohydrate digestion

Mouth: chewing of food; initial carbohydrate digestion

Pharynx: swallowing

Esophagus: transport of food into stomach; secretion of mucus

Liver: manufacture of bile

Gallbladder: release of bile into duodenum to aid in fat digestion

Stomach: churning of food; secretion of gastric juice; action of enzyme pepsin; initiation of protein digestion

Pancreas: release of pancreatic juice into duodenum to digest protein, carbohydrates, and fats

Small intestine: final digestion of nutrients into end products; absorption of nutrients

Large intestine: elimination of wastes

FIGURE 8–1 Main and accessory organs of the normal digestive system. (Redrawn from Miller M: *Pathophysiology: principles of disease,* Philadelphia, 1983, Saunders.)

(occlusion). Malocclusion eventually leads to jaw pain, called **temporomandibular** joint disease (see Temporomandibular Joint Syndrome), if not corrected.

PATIENT SCREENING

Schedule the patient for an initial evaluation by the dentist.

ETIOLOGY

There are three causes of missing permanent teeth. The most common is loss from decay or accident. Teeth also may be congenitally missing, or they may be impacted and prevented from erupting by the root of an adjacent tooth.

DIAGNOSIS

Diagnosing missing teeth may be as simple as performing an oral examination and obtaining radiographic films to determine whether the tooth is absent or impacted.

TREATMENT

Treatment is aimed at restoring the occlusion. This is accomplished by placement of a permanent or removable prosthesis (false tooth), by *orthodontics,* or by use of a surgical implant.

PROGNOSIS

The prognosis is good when a prosthesis or surgical implant provides replacement.

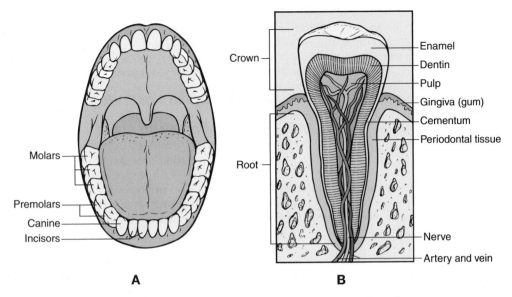

FIGURE 8–2 **A,** Thirty-two permanent teeth. **B,** Structure of a tooth.

PREVENTION
General good dental hygiene to prevent tooth decay and loss of teeth is the only method of prevention.

PATIENT TEACHING
Emphasize the importance of complying with the individualized treatment plan. Teach proper cleaning techniques to prevent decay when the patient has a dental appliance in place. Make sure the patient knows what to expect after any surgical procedure.

Impacted Third Molars

DESCRIPTION
An impacted third molar is malpositioned, thereby preventing normal eruption.

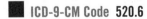 **ICD-9-CM Code 520.6**

SYMPTOMS AND SIGNS
Third molars, also known as wisdom teeth, are the last teeth in the back of the mouth. They begin developing between the ages of 8 and 10 years and erupt between the ages of 17 and 21 years. In some people, one or more of these teeth never erupt. There are usually no symptoms until these teeth begin to emerge. Even when wisdom teeth develop

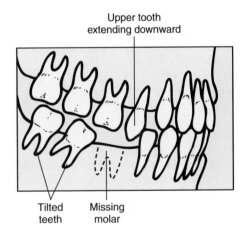

FIGURE 8–3 Missing molar.

normally, they are difficult to clean because of their position at the back of the mouth. Because of this, they decay much more often than other teeth, and pain results.

PATIENT SCREENING
Schedule the initial consultation with a dentist for a diagnostic evaluation.

ETIOLOGY

These molars become impacted when they do not have enough room to erupt because of bone structure or because adjacent teeth block eruption (Fig. 8–4). Sometimes they erupt at an angle, creating a space in which food can become trapped. This can lead to *pericoronitis* around the tooth, which in turn causes pain when biting and a foul taste in the mouth. The gum around the tooth becomes red and swollen.

DIAGNOSIS

Radiographic studies are needed to determine the position of the tooth if it is not completely erupted. An examination also is performed to search for the presence of infection.

TREATMENT

The dentist is likely to prescribe an antibiotic (penicillin, Amoxicillin) to clear up any infection that is present and an analgesic (Darvocet N-100, Vicodin) to relieve pain temporarily. After the infection clears up and pain has lessened, the impacted tooth must be extracted to prevent recurrence.

PROGNOSIS

Treatment of the infection and extraction of the impacted tooth solve the problem.

PREVENTION

No prevention is known.

PATIENT TEACHING

Emphasize the importance of taking the entire course of antibiotics as prescribed. Explain the procedure of tooth extraction and what to expect after surgery.

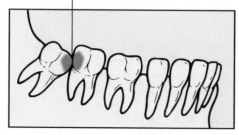

Site of impaction

FIGURE 8–4 Impacted wisdom tooth.

Dental Caries

DESCRIPTION

Dental caries is considered an infection resulting in erosion of tooth surface.

 ICD-9-CM Code 521.00 *(Unspecified)*

SYMPTOMS AND SIGNS

The main symptom in the early stage of dental caries, also known as tooth decay, is a mild toothache, with hypersensitivity to sweets and temperature extremes in food or beverages. If caries is left untreated, an unpleasant taste in the mouth results from the accumulation of food and bacteria in the cavity. Eventually, the pulp becomes inflamed, and the pain may become persistent or feel like a stabbing pain in the jaw. As the tooth continues to die, an **abscess** may form (see Tooth Abscesses).

PATIENT SCREENING

Schedule the patient for a dental examination.

ETIOLOGY

Dental caries occurs when bacteria in *plaque* break down the sugar found in food. This process forms acid, and this acid erodes the calcium in the tooth's enamel, causing the formation of a cavity (Fig. 8–5). In addition, episodes of purging in the patient with bulimia can contribute to the breakdown of tooth enamel and erosion of the teeth and gums.

DIAGNOSIS

The dentist examines the teeth for signs of cavity formation and may obtain radiographic films to determine the extent of the decay.

TREATMENT

In early treatment, one removes the diseased portion of the tooth enamel and pulp and fills the cavity to prevent further decay. If the decay has advanced into the pulp, the dentist may perform a root canal procedure. In this procedure, the infected pulp tissue is removed and then the canals in the roots of the tooth are filled and sealed. Tooth extraction may be necessary if root canal therapy fails or if the tooth is beyond saving.

PROGNOSIS

The prognosis is good with treatment.

PREVENTION

Caries may be prevented with good oral hygiene and regular professional cleaning of the teeth. The limiting of sweets is suggested.

PATIENT TEACHING

Demonstrate good brushing and flossing techniques. Explain what causes dental caries. Professional cleaning of the teeth and regular dental examinations are recommended.

Discolored Teeth

DESCRIPTION

In this condition, teeth are discolored.

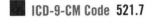 **ICD-9-CM Code 521.7**

SYMPTOMS AND SIGNS

Symptoms of discolored teeth are obvious, and colors may range from a slight yellow to brown and gray. Some teeth may have brown spots, patches, and dark lines in or on them.

PATIENT SCREENING

Schedule the patient for a dental consultation.

ETIOLOGY

Discoloration of teeth can have many causes. Age alone causes a slight yellowing of the teeth. Smoking turns teeth surfaces brown, and a dead tooth often turns gray. Certain drugs (e.g., tetracyclines) taken in large quantities during childhood can cause the formation of defective, discolored enamel (Fig. 8–6). Severe attacks of pertussis (whooping cough) and measles in children can cause discolored patches to form on the teeth. Naturally occurring fluoride can, in excessive amounts, produce white or brown spots in the teeth.

DIAGNOSIS

The dentist performs an oral examination. A pertinent history includes recent illness, medications, and trauma to the teeth. Hereditary factors also are considered.

TREATMENT

The extent of treatment varies and depends on whether the discoloration is superficial or deep within the enamel. Superficial discoloration can be removed or reduced by polishing with a rotary polisher. Deeper discolorations can be treated by capping or crowning and by bonding a synthetic veneer to the tooth.

PROGNOSIS

Resolution of the discoloration is possible within a range of treatments.

PREVENTION

Dental hygienists suggest avoiding smoking and drinking of coffee, tea, or red wine to prevent staining

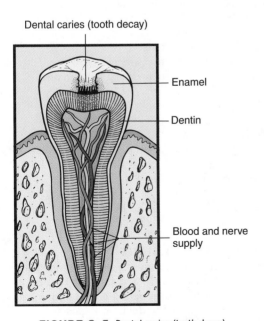

Dental caries (tooth decay)

— Enamel

— Dentin

Blood and nerve supply

FIGURE 8–5 Dental caries (tooth decay).

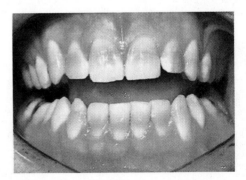

FIGURE 8–6 Discolored teeth. (From Christensen GJ: *A consumer's guide to dentistry,* St. Louis, 1994, Mosby.)

of the teeth. Many products on the market claim to whiten teeth and use various forms of peroxide as a bleaching agent. Intrinsic causes may or may not be preventable.

PATIENT TEACHING
In addition to the preventive measures mentioned previously, the dentist may suggest treatment for deeper discoloration. Explain the planned dental procedures to help reduce anxiety.

Gingivitis

DESCRIPTION
Gingivitis is inflammation and swelling of the gums (Fig. 8–7).

■ **ICD-9-CM Code** **523.0** *(Acute gingivitis)*
523.1 *(Chronic gingivitis)*

SYMPTOMS AND SIGNS
Gums that are normally pale pink and firm become red, soft, and shiny. They bleed easily, even with gentle toothbrushing. If gingivitis is not treated, it leads to destruction of the gums and bone disease called **periodontitis** (see Periodontitis).

PATIENT SCREENING
Schedule the patient for a dental examination and consultation.

ETIOLOGY
The most common cause of gingivitis is plaque. Plaque is a sticky deposit of mucus, food particles, and bacteria that builds up around the base of the teeth as a result of inadequate brushing and flossing. As the gums become inflamed and swollen, the plaque causes a pocket to form between the gum

and the teeth, and that space becomes a food trap. Other causes of gingivitis include vitamin deficiencies, glandular disorders, blood diseases, viral infections, and the use of certain medications. Pregnant women and diabetics are particularly susceptible to gingivitis.

DIAGNOSIS
If symptoms develop, a dentist should be seen as soon as possible to confirm gingivitis and to begin treatment to prevent complications.

TREATMENT
Treatment includes removal of the plaque and **calculus** via professional cleaning, a process called scaling, and then teaching by the dentist or dental hygienist about the proper care of the teeth. In advanced cases of gingivitis, the dentist may prescribe an antibacterial mouthwash like chlorhexidine (Periogard), to help to clear up the infection.

PROGNOSIS
Identifying and treating underlying causes offers the best outcome.

PREVENTION
Prophylaxis includes good oral hygiene and removal of plaque at the gum line. Toothbrush trauma and excessive brushing should be avoided. Excessive use of abrasives is contraindicated.

PATIENT TEACHING
See the preventive measures listed above. Urge the patient to have regular dental examinations.

Periodontitis

DESCRIPTION
Periodontitis, also called periodontal disease, is destructive gum and bone disease around one or more of the teeth (Fig. 8–8).

■ **ICD-9-CM Code** **523.3** *(Acute)*
523.4 *(Chronic)*

SYMPTOMS AND SIGNS
Periodontitis is the end result of gingivitis (see Gingivitis) that was treated too late or not at all. The pockets that form between the teeth and gums in gingivitis gradually deepen, exposing the root. Plaque develops there, causing unpleasant tastes in the mouth and offensive breath (halitosis). As

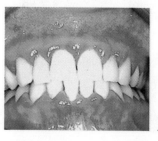
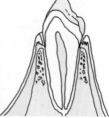

FIGURE 8–7 Gingivitis. (From Murray PR et al: *Medical microbiology,* ed 2, St. Louis, 1994, Mosby.)

more root is exposed, the tooth or teeth become extremely sensitive to temperature extremes in food and painful during chewing. Abscesses can form (see Tooth Abscesses), and eventually a tooth or several teeth become loose and possibly fall out.

PATIENT SCREENING
Schedule a complete dental examination and consultation without delay.

ETIOLOGY
The cause of periodontitis is unchecked gingivitis. Over a period of years, the bacteria in plaque destroy the bone surrounding and supporting the teeth. Contributing factors include smoking, chemotherapy, diabetes, and HIV infection.

DIAGNOSIS
To determine the stage of the periodontal disease, the dentist measures the depth of the pockets and obtains radiographic films. Radiographic films reveal the condition of the underlying bone, and this knowledge aids the dentist in deciding how to treat the disease.

TREATMENT
Conservative treatment includes thorough cleanings of root surfaces of teeth and also multiple daily sessions of brushing and flossing of teeth. Periodontal surgery may be required if the pockets have become deep. The procedure, called a gingivectomy, requires the dentist to trim the gums to reduce the depth of the pockets and to remove any damaged bone.

PROGNOSIS
The prognosis varies with the extent of the disease process, the presence of complications, and the effectiveness of treatment.

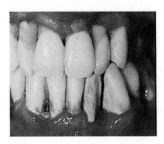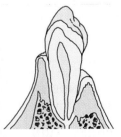

FIGURE 8–8 Advanced periodontitis. (From Murray PR et al: *Medical microbiology*, ed 2, St. Louis, 1994, Mosby.)

PREVENTION
Frequent professional cleaning and examination of the teeth is of primary importance. Smoking and other contributing factors that result in gingivitis are avoided if possible. In some cases medication and periodontal surgery prevent loss of teeth.

PATIENT TEACHING
Reinforce the advice of the dentist about following an ongoing dental-care plan. Emphasize the long-term advantages of early detection and treatment to save teeth.

Oral Tumors

DESCRIPTION
Oral tumors are neoplasms that are benign or malignant, localized or invasive.

 ICD-9-CM Code 210 *(Benign neoplasm of lip, oral cavity, and pharynx)*
Benign oral tumors have code modifiers according to location. Refer to the physician's diagnosis and then to the current edition of the ICD-9-CM coding manual to ensure the greatest specificity of pathology and any appropriate modifiers. See oral cancer for coding of malignant oral tumors.

SYMPTOMS AND SIGNS
Tumors can develop anywhere in or on the surface of the mouth, gums, cheeks, or palate, but not on the teeth. They begin as single, small, pale lumps, in or on the mouth, that bleed easily. There are two types of tumors: benign, or noncancerous, and malignant, or cancerous. Benign tumors grow slowly over several years, do not *metastasize,* and are not life-threatening. Malignant tumors are generally not painful until they reach advanced stages. (See Oral Cancer.)

PATIENT SCREENING
The lesion should be evaluated without delay. Biopsy of the lesion may be required.

ETIOLOGY
The cause of benign and malignant oral tumors is unknown, although certain factors, such as tobacco use, seem to affect a tumor's development into a malignancy.

DIAGNOSIS
An oral surgeon or a physician should be consulted if the patient has a lump, an ulcer, or a color

change in or on the surface of the mouth that does not clear up within 10 days. If a tumor is discovered, a biopsy is needed to determine whether it is benign or malignant.

TREATMENT

If the tumor has been determined to be benign, it should be observed periodically to ensure that it has not become malignant. Benign tumors must be excised if they interfere with the fit of a denture. (See Oral Cancer for discussion on malignant oral tumors.)

PROGNOSIS

Benign tumors are usually curable with excision.

PREVENTION

Avoid chronic irritation to the lips and mouth. Any mouth lesion that does not heal should be evaluated and treated.

PATIENT TEACHING

Lesions that result from chronic irritation require the patient's understanding of the cause and the course of action to take to promote healing.

Malocclusion

DESCRIPTION

Malocclusion describes specific angles of malposition and contact of the maxillary and mandibular teeth.

 ICD-9-CM Code 524.4 *(Unspecified)*

SYMPTOMS AND SIGNS

The relationship of the upper and lower teeth when the mouth is closed is called occlusion, or bite; a faulty bite is called malocclusion (Fig. 8–9). Signs of malocclusion include a protrusion or a recession of the jaw, and teeth that are turned or twisted out of position because of crowding. The patient usually experiences some degree of difficulty with mastication.

PATIENT SCREENING

Schedule a dental examination and consultation. Inform the patient that radiographic studies may be indicated.

DIAGNOSIS

A visual examination and radiographic studies clearly identify the malocclusion.

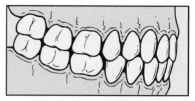
Normal teeth

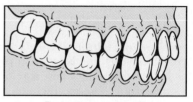
Protruding upper teeth

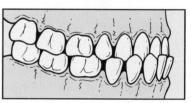
Receding upper teeth

FIGURE 8–9 Malocclusion.

ETIOLOGY

Malocclusion results from the characteristics inherited from the parents. Few people have perfectly aligned teeth. Heredity is not the only cause of malocclusion, however; crowding can result from the early loss of primary teeth. Other teeth may shift to fill the space left by this loss of teeth, causing the loss of space where the permanent tooth normally would erupt.

TREATMENT

Several treatments are used to correct this problem. These include the application of braces for a minor problem, extraction of one or more teeth, and surgical removal of portions of the jaw. The last approach is used for problems of protrusion and recession of the jaw. Another possible treatment is combining crowns or bridges to replace the missing teeth.

PROGNOSIS

The prognosis is favorable with treatment.

PREVENTION

Because of the hereditary component, no specific prevention is known.

PATIENT TEACHING

Special care is needed to avoid developing caries while wearing corrective dental appliances. The patient should practice thorough, regular cleaning of the teeth and avoid candy and gum.

Temporomandibular Joint (TMJ) Syndrome

DESCRIPTION

TMJ is a symptom complex related to inflammation, disease, or dysfunction of the temporomandibular joint.

 ICD-9-CM Code 524.60 *(Unspecified)*

SYMPTOMS AND SIGNS

The *synovial* joints between the condyles of the mandible and the temporal bones of the skull are known as the temporomandibular joints. When these joints are inflamed or diseased, jaw movement is markedly limited. The patient reports hearing clicking sounds during chewing or experiencing severe pain or aching that is made worse by chewing. This pain and limitation of movement is usually unilateral. *Tinnitus* and even deafness may be present. A reduced ability to open the jaw not only interferes with chewing but also prevents adequate cleaning of the teeth and treatment of cavities. It also may prevent the making of dentures because of the inability to take impressions of the teeth.

PATIENT SCREENING

Significant pain usually prompts a request for medical treatment.

ETIOLOGY

Temporomandibular disorders can be caused by a number of conditions, including malocclusion; poorly fitting dentures; rheumatoid, degenerative, or traumatic arthritis; and *neoplastic* diseases. Emotional stress, with accompanying clenching and grinding of the teeth, is also a contributing factor.

DIAGNOSIS

The diagnosis of temporomandibular joint syndrome is made by oral examination, the patient history, and radiographic studies. In the case of a neoplasm, a biopsy may be needed to rule out a malignancy.

TREATMENT

Treatment is aimed at the cause of the condition or disease. Symptoms of rheumatoid or traumatic arthritis often subside after 3 to 5 days of immobilization of the mandible. For cases in which inflammation causes TMJ, nonsteroidal antiinflammatory drugs often are used to treat the condition. Some patients wear special appliances to prevent them from grinding their teeth. If TMJ is caused by jaw misalignment, a plastic bite plate called a splint may be used to better align the jaw. The splint is worn over the teeth and establishes proper alignment, which can eliminate jaw locking, pain, and clicking sensations associated with TMJ. Intraarticular injections of hydrocortisone may be needed in more severe cases of rheumatoid or degenerative arthritis. When the teeth experience premature contact, the dentist adjusts the occlusion by grinding the surfaces of the teeth.

PROGNOSIS

Mild cases respond well to resting of the joint. More complicated chronic cases require extended treatment of the underlying cause.

PREVENTION

Regular dental checkups can identify underlying conditions. Treatment of these conditions can prevent the onset of TMJ.

PATIENT TEACHING

When the dentist prescribes an appliance, tell the patient what kind of initial discomfort he or she may expect. The patient is encouraged to use the appliance exactly as directed and is urged to report unusual discomfort during treatment.

Tooth Abscesses

DESCRIPTION

A tooth abscess is a pus-filled sac that develops in the tissue surrounding the base of the root.

 ICD-9-CM Code 522.5

SYMPTOMS AND SIGNS

An abscessed tooth aches or throbs persistently and can be extremely painful when biting and chewing food. Glands in the neck and face on the affected side may become swollen and tender. Fever also can develop, along with a feeling of general malaise.

PATIENT SCREENING

Tooth abscesses require prompt medical attention.

ETIOLOGY

An abscess forms when a tooth is decayed or dying or when the gums have severely receded, exposing the root. The dead pulp, along with invading bacteria, can infect the surrounding tissues, even after a root canal procedure, and form an abscess.

DIAGNOSIS

If any of the symptoms or signs are present, the patient should see the dentist as soon as possible. Swelling in the neck or face must be treated immediately to prevent the infection from spreading further.

TREATMENT

Antibiotic therapy is prescribed, and if this does not correct the problem, an apicectomy may be necessary. In this procedure, the dentist or oral surgeon makes an incision into the gum and removes the bone that covers the tip of the root and the infected tissue as well. If this fails to clear up the infection, the tooth must be extracted.

PROGNOSIS

Early intervention with a favorable response to antibiotic therapy offers the best prognosis.

PREVENTION

Prophylaxis includes good oral hygiene and regular dental checkups.

PATIENT TEACHING

Tell the patient that neglecting a tooth abscess can result in serious complications resulting from infection that spreads to the bone and may become systemic.

Mouth Ulcers

DESCRIPTION

An ulcer in the mouth is a lesion on the mucous membrane, exposing the underlying sensitive tissue.

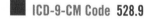 **ICD-9-CM Code 528.9**

SYMPTOMS AND SIGNS

Mouth ulcers (sometimes called canker sores) are common and look alike but vary considerably in their cause and seriousness. The two most common types of ulcers are **aphthous** ulcers (Fig. 8–10), which occur during stress or illness, and traumatic ulcers, which result from injury and are caused by a hot food burn, a rough denture, or even a toothbrush. Ulcers appear as pale yellow spots with red borders. Aphthous ulcers usually occur in clusters and last for 3 or 4 days. Traumatic ulcers are usually single and larger and last for a week or longer.

PATIENT SCREENING

Ulcers that do not heal require a physician's attention.

ETIOLOGY

A viral cause for aphthous ulcers has not been established. Acute ulcerations are usually the result of mechanical trauma, viral and bacterial infections, stress, or illness. In rare instances, an ulcer may be the first sign of a tumor in the mouth, anemia, or leukemia.

DIAGNOSIS

If an ulcer does not heal within 10 days or keeps returning, the patient should consult a dentist or physician. Blood tests and possibly a biopsy of the ulcer are needed to determine whether some underlying condition or disease is causing the ulcer. When the ulcer results from trauma, it does not heal until the cause is found and corrected.

TREATMENT

Self-treatment of ulcers includes using antiseptic mouthwashes, rinsing with warm salt water, and avoiding spicy or acidic foods and hot food or drinks. Topical analgesics such as benzocaine as

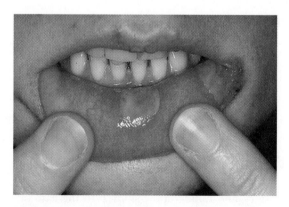

FIGURE 8–10 Mouth ulcers. (From Stevens A, Lowe J: *Pathology: illustrated review in color,* ed 2, London, 2000, Mosby.)

well as soothing agents like spirit of camphor can be used to reduce painful irritation. The dentist or physician may prescribe a steroid mouthwash or topical cream to speed the healing process.

PROGNOSIS

Most ulcers heal spontaneously in a week.

PREVENTION

No specific prevention is known, except when the ulcer is attributed to mechanical trauma that can be corrected.

PATIENT TEACHING

Advise the patient to use the self-help measures listed previously under Treatment.

Herpes Simplex (Cold Sores)

DESCRIPTION

Herpes simplex is a recurrent viral infection that affects the skin and mucous membranes. Herpes type 1 commonly produces cold sores and fever blisters (Fig. 8–11).

■ **ICD-9-CM Code 054.9**

SYMPTOMS AND SIGNS

Herpes simplex (cold sore) blisters can develop on the lips and inside the mouth, producing painful ulcers that last a few hours or days. These ulcers also can form on the gums, causing them to become red and swollen. Tingling and numbness around the mouth may precede or follow their appearance. Although most infections are subclinical, constitutional symptoms can occur.

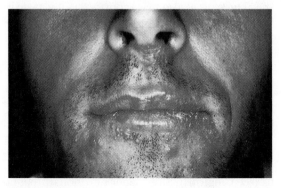

FIGURE 8–11 Herpes simplex 1. (From Damjanov I, Linder J: *Pathology: a color atlas,* St. Louis, 1999, Mosby.)

PATIENT SCREENING

A patient presenting with generalized symptoms like fever, anorexia, and lymphadenopathy should be seen by the physician at first opportunity. A pregnant woman is also given priority.

ETIOLOGY

The vesicles are caused by the herpes simplex virus type 1 (HSV-1) and are common. They tend to recur because the virus can lie dormant. Exposure to sunshine or wind or the presence of another infection, such as a common cold, can reactivate the virus.

DIAGNOSIS

An oral examination is usually sufficient for the diagnosis. Isolating the HSV-1 from local lesions can confirm the cause of the infection. The herpes simplex virus type 2 (HSV-2) causes a similar lesion in the oral cavity.

TREATMENT

Currently no cure is known. If the infection is mild, no treatment is necessary, but severe cases require medical attention. A herpes simplex infection usually does not cause serious risks to health, but rubbing the eyes after touching the ulcer could cause the formation of a herpetic corneal ulcer, and the infection can produce severe illness in an *immunocompromised* patient. The dentist or physician may advise resting, taking aspirin, and using an *anesthetic* mouthwash and a topical cream to relieve the pain and to heal the sores. Creams proven to shorten the duration of herpes sores and speed healing of cold sores are Abreva and Novitra. Both contain particles that bind to the virus and inhibit further spreading.

PROGNOSIS

Cold sores usually clear up uneventfully. Lesions tend to recur when reactivated by trauma or stress.

PREVENTION

Early treatment with an antiviral medication controls the outbreak and reduces the risk of transmission.

PATIENT TEACHING

Avoid close contact like kissing because the virus can remain in saliva after the vesicle has healed. When the patient has multiple lesions in the oral cavity, anesthetic mouthwashes reduce pain, enabling the patient to eat.

Thrush

DESCRIPTION
Thrush is candidiasis of the oral mucosa, involving the mouth, tongue, palate, and gums.

 ICD-9-CM Code 112.0

SYMPTOMS AND SIGNS
Thrush is a fungal infection of relatively short duration that produces sore, slightly raised, pale yellow patches in the mouth and sometimes the throat. These lesions cause a burning sensation in the mouth and become painful when rubbed by dentures, toothbrushes, or food when eating. Some patients suffering from severe cases of thrush have the smell of yeast in their breath. Thrush most often develops in young children, in immunodeficient people, and in the elderly, but it can occur at any age.

PATIENT SCREENING
If the patient also complains of fever or other systemic symptoms, he or she should see the physician promptly.

ETIOLOGY
The fungus *Candida albicans* causes most cases of thrush. Normally present in the mouth in small numbers, the fungus can multiply out of control. This may occur during lowered resistance or as a result of prolonged treatment with antibiotics, which upsets the normal number of protective microbes. Other predisposing factors are cancer chemotherapy, diabetes, or the taking of glucocorticoids. The infection rarely becomes systemic or infectious. This same fungus can cause vaginitis.

DIAGNOSIS
Diagnosis is made by the dentist or physician with an oral examination and laboratory analysis of a sample taken from a lesion. Blood tests also may be needed to rule out a serious underlying disease, such as iron deficiency anemia or early HIV.

TREATMENT
Thrush is treated successfully with an antifungal medication for 14 days. The antifungals used most often are nystatin, an antifungal suspension that is swished and then swallowed, and fluconazole (Diflucan), an oral tablet.

PROGNOSIS
The infection tends to recur in some patients. In all cases, treatment must begin as soon as possible because thrush can extend into the esophagus, causing esophagitis.

PREVENTION
Those who have had treatment with antibiotics should report any signs of thrush. Those using inhaled corticosteroids should rinse their mouths thoroughly after use to avoid the chance that thrush may form.

PATIENT TEACHING
Palliative care includes a soft diet and the use of a nonirritating mouthwash and a soft toothbrush for oral hygiene.

Necrotizing Periodontal Disease

(Formerly called acute necrotizing ulcerative gingivitis [trench mouth].)

DESCRIPTION
Necrotizing periodontal disease is a common infection affecting the gums and the anchoring structure of the teeth.

 ICD-9-CM Code 101

SYMPTOMS AND SIGNS
Necrotizing periodontal disease is a rare, painful ulceration and disease of the gums, particularly between the teeth, sometimes called Vincent's angina. The primary symptom is painful, red, swollen gums with ulcers that bleed. Gums also can appear grayish in areas of decomposing tissue. The patient also may report a metallic taste in the mouth and bad breath (Fig. 8–12). Mild systemic symptoms include fever and enlarged lymph nodes.

PATIENT SCREENING
Prompt medical treatment is advised.

ETIOLOGY
Anaerobic opportunistic bacteria cause necrotizing periodontal disease. It results from poor oral hygiene and bacterial infection secondary to gingivitis (see Gingivitis). Stress, poor nutrition, throat infections, smoking, and serious illness such as

leukemia are also contributing factors. Some cases have been linked to the use of oral contraceptives.

DIAGNOSIS

An oral examination by a dentist or physician is needed as soon as possible. Throat cultures and blood work may be necessary to rule out serious illness.

TREATMENT

The patient is given antibiotics, along with a hydrogen peroxide mouthwash to relieve pain and inflammation. After the disease has been halted, the teeth and gums must be professionally cleaned. A minor surgery on the gums, called a gingivectomy, also may be advised.

PROGNOSIS

With treatment, improvement can be expected within days.

PREVENTION

Prophylactic professional cleaning of the teeth, good oral hygiene, and avoidance of the contributing factors, such as smoking and poor diet, are recommended.

PATIENT TEACHING

Emphasize prevention as described above. Explain that particular medications and systemic diseases can aggravate periodontal disease.

Oral Leukoplakia

DESCRIPTION

Leukoplakia is hyperkeratosis or epidermal thickening of the buccal mucosa, palate, or lower lip.

■ **ICD-9-CM Code 528.6** *(Tongue, lip, mouth, buccal, gingiva)*

SYMPTOMS AND SIGNS

Leukoplakia or white plaque is a thickening and hardening of a part of the mucous membrane in the mouth (Fig. 8–13). It develops over several weeks and can vary in size. At first, the patient has no symptoms, but as it progresses, the mucous membrane becomes rough, hard, and whitish gray and is sensitive to hot or highly seasoned foods.

PATIENT SCREENING

Schedule the patient for an oral examination.

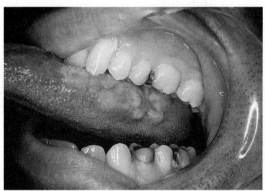
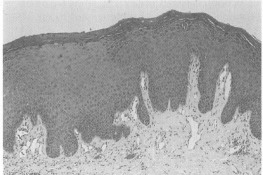

FIGURE 8–13 Leukoplakia. (From Kumar V, Cotran RS, Robbins SL: *Robbins basic pathology,* ed 7, Philadelphia, 2003, Saunders.)

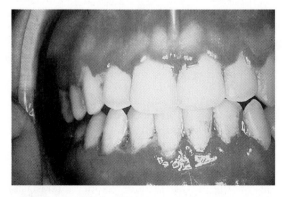

FIGURE 8–12 Necrotizing periodontal disease. (From Stevens A, Lowe J: *Pathology: illustrated review in color,* ed 2, London, 2000, Mosby.)

ETIOLOGY

Leukoplakia may develop at any age, but it is more common in the elderly. It usually results from chronic irritation such as the friction caused by a denture or a rough tooth that rubs an area raw. Leukoplakia also may be a reaction to the heat from tobacco smoke or local irritation from chewing tobacco.

DIAGNOSIS

An oral examination is needed. If the condition has not cleared up in 2 or 3 weeks, a biopsy is advised because about 3% of oral leukoplakia cases develop into oral cancers.

TREATMENT

The treatment of leukoplakia consists of finding and eliminating the source of the irritation. A rough tooth or denture may be smoothed, and giving up smoking may be advised. These measures are usually all that is needed to correct the condition. Until proven otherwise, the leukoplakia is considered precancerous.

PROGNOSIS

The lesions require monitoring because of the risk of malignant transformation.

PREVENTION

Although the cause is not always known, the patient is urged to eliminate tobacco and avoid exposure to persistent irritants.

PATIENT TEACHING

Avoid the common potentiating influences, including alcohol, tobacco (especially chewing tobacco), ill-fitting dentures, and frequent spicy foods.

Oral Cancer

DESCRIPTION

Oral cancer includes squamous cell carcinoma or **adenocarcinoma** of the lips, cheek mucosa, anterior tongue, floor of the mouth, hard palate, and upper and lower gingiva.

ICD-9-CM Code 145.9 *(Mouth, unspecified)*
Refer to the physician's diagnosis and then to the current edition of the ICD-9-CM coding manual for malignant neoplasm of other parts of the mouth to ensure the greatest specificity of pathology and any appropriate modifiers.

SYMPTOMS AND SIGNS

Oral cancer usually appears as a white, patchy lesion or an oral ulcer that fails to heal. If the cancer is on the lip or tongue, the ulcer is likely to be associated with pain. However, for most other locations of oral cancer, pain occurs very late in the disease process, which often leads to a delay in seeking medical treatment. Associated symptoms may include *dysphagia, odynophagia,* weight loss, bleeding, or referred pain in the ear or jaw. The patient also may have associated loosening of teeth or poor denture fit.

PATIENT SCREENING

Follow office policy for new referrals or oncology follow-up.

ETIOLOGY

More than 90% of oral cancers are squamous cell carcinomas, and most of the remaining 10% are adenocarcinomas. Oral cancers occur more often in men than women. The lip is the most common location of oral cancer. Use of alcohol and tobacco, especially cigarette smoking and snuff dipping, accounts for up to 80% of cases of oral cancer. Betel nut chewing, a practice common in Southeast Asia, produces an increased risk, as do poor oral hygiene, jagged teeth, and improperly fitting dentures. The lip has the additional risk factor of sun exposure.

Premalignant lesions of oral cancer include oral leukoplakia (see Fig. 8–13), a reactive process that presents as white patches of oral mucosa, and erythrodysplasia, a red patch of mucosa. The underlying abnormality of either lesion may be either benign or dysplastic. Microscopic analysis of a biopsy of the lesion is required to determine the type of abnormality. Some lesions with evident dysplasia will progress to invasive carcinoma.

DIAGNOSIS

Although the patient often notices the oral lesion, he or she often ignores it because the lesion is usually painless. Therefore the diagnosis of oral cancer is most often made in the dentist's office. The diagnosis is confirmed via *biopsy* of the persistent lesion. Oral tumors are classified and staged according to the TNM (Tumor, Node, Metastasis) classification system proposed by the American Joint Committee on Cancer. Staging of oral cancer is performed via contrast-enhanced CT scan to determine the extent of tumor infiltration. The CT scan also may detect bone and cartilage invasion. Neck dissection may be used to detect nodal metastases. Metastases to the lung, liver, and bone are the most common.

TREATMENT

The treatment for oral cancer depends on the stage. Early oral cancers are treated by radiotherapy and surgery, although the use of laser therapy in the excision of early-stage oral cancers has been increasing. Therapeutic irradiation is often employed for advanced tumors. Detecting recurrences after tumor removal is based on history, oral cavity examination, and CT imaging.

PROGNOSIS

Patients with large tumors or nodal metastases have a worse prognosis than do patients with small, localized tumors. Because oral cancer often is diagnosed late, the overall expected 5-year survival rate is about 51% and 10-year survival rate is 41%.

PREVENTION

Mouth examination to detect premalignant or early malignant lesions during routine visits to the dentist is recommended. Diets rich in vitamins A and C and carotenoids seem to protect against oral cancer. Avoiding the use of tobacco and alcohol is recommended.

PATIENT TEACHING

Review information about the treatment plan and encourage questions. Make certain the patient understands the plan for control of pain and side effects of any therapeutic intervention.

Diseases of the Gastrointestinal Tract

The alimentary canal, or GI tract, is a hollow continuous tube that extends from the mouth to the anus. It propels the products of digestion by peristalsis. It is also the site of the processes of mechanical and chemical breakdown of food. As the food passes through the tract, it is broken down into molecules that can be absorbed through the intestinal wall for distribution to body cells for metabolism.

Water and electrolytes are absorbed in the proximal colon; waste material is stored in the rectum, and indigestible wastes are voluntarily evacuated through the anus.

ENRICHMENT
DIGESTIVE DISTRESS SIGNALS

- Hiccup is an involuntary spasmodic contraction of the diaphragm in which the beginning of an inspiration is suddenly checked by closure of the glottis, resulting in the characteristic sound. It is usually transient.
- Indigestion is failure of digestion. The term frequently is used to denote vague abdominal discomfort after meals. Indigestion and eructation (belching) are common symptoms of upper GI tract disease.
- Heartburn is a sensation of retrosternal warmth or burning occurring in waves and tending to rise upward toward the neck; it may be accompanied by a reflux of fluid into the mouth (regurgitation).

- Nausea is an unpleasant sensation in the epigastrium. It often culminates in vomiting.
- Vomiting is the forcible expulsion of the contents of the stomach through the mouth.
- Colic is acute visceral pain caused by spasm, torsion, or obstruction of a hollow organ.
- Flatulence is the presence of extensive amounts of air or gases in the stomach or intestines, leading to distention of the organs.
- Diarrhea is abnormally frequent passage of loose stool.
- Constipation is a condition of infrequent bowel evacuation. It may be functional or organic.
- Fecal incontinence is an inability to control defecation.

Gastroesophageal Reflux Disease

DESCRIPTION

Gastroesophageal reflux disease (GERD) refers to clinical manifestations of regurgitation of stomach and duodenal contents into the esophagus, frequently occurring at night. Mild episodes may be described as heartburn by the patient.

 ICD-9-CM Code 530.81

SYMPTOMS AND SIGNS

The patient typically experiences belching that expresses vomitus into the mouth, with a burning sensation in the chest and mouth. A coughing spell and wheezing caused by irritation to the oropharynx or respiratory tree may follow. Chronic and frequent GERD may lead to dysphagia and erosive esophagitis with bleeding. Tooth enamel may become eroded, leading to caries. Other complications include esophageal stricture caused by scar tissue, ulceration of the mucosa, and pulmonary aspiration.

PATIENT SCREENING

The patient may present with symptoms that mimic angina pectoris or may report blood in the sputum. These are indications for prompt evaluation by the physician.

ETIOLOGY

Normal reflux can result from overeating, pregnancy, or weight gain. GERD that causes pathology frequently is associated with relaxation of the lower esophageal sphincter (LES) or an increase in intraabdominal pressure. Patients with hiatal hernia frequently experience GERD. Certain medications can contribute to GERD, including theophylline, calcium channel blockers, and meperidine. Some foods, coffee, and alcohol can irritate the condition. Even certain medications like birth control pills, antihistamines, antispasmodics, and some asthma drugs can reduce the strength of the esophageal sphincter, causing symptoms of GERD.

DIAGNOSIS

The history and clinical evidence of GERD are most important in establishing a diagnosis. Barium swallow detects gross changes, erosion, or other abnormalities of the esophagus. If results are abnormal, **endoscopy** with esophageal biopsy is next. Esophageal pH monitoring and scanning tests are other probative methods of diagnosis.

TREATMENT

When symptoms are mild and of short duration, simple measures to eliminate episodes of reflux are indicated. These include elevating the head of the bed about 6 inches, taking only a light evening meal 4 hours before bedtime (nothing eaten 3 hours before bedtime), and using antacids. Weight loss is indicated if the person is obese. Limiting or eliminating alcohol ingestion and stopping cigarette smoking are advised. When these measures fail, systemic medical management is initiated. The use of an *H$_2$-receptor antagonist* or a *proton pump inhibitor* inhibits acid secretion and allows for healing of the esophagus. Antireflux surgery is used conservatively. Symptomatic complications of chronic GERD are treated as required.

PROGNOSIS

When simple measures fail and the condition is chronic, symptoms typically improve with drug therapy.

PREVENTION

Preventive measures are directed at managing the causes that can be controlled.

PATIENT TEACHING

Explain how positional therapy uses gravity to reduce the onset of reflux. Instruct the patient not to recline until 4 hours after eating. List warning signs of complications, such as pulmonary symptoms, an increase in esophageal burning, or any bleeding.

Esophageal Varices

DESCRIPTION

Esophageal **varices** are varicose veins of the esophagus.

 ICD-9-CM Code   **456.1** *(Without mention of bleeding)*
                           456.0 *(With bleeding)*

SYMPTOMS AND SIGNS

The superficial veins lining the esophagus become swollen and twisted at the distal end of the esophagus (Fig. 8–14). Varices may produce no symptoms until they rupture, causing massive hemorrhage. With rupture, the patient experiences **hematemesis** and abdominal pain, and signs of **hypovolemic shock** may develop.

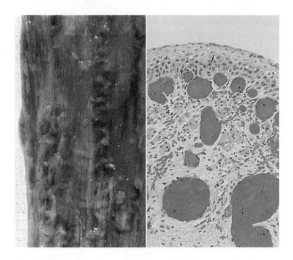

FIGURE 8–14 Esophageal varices. (From Damjanov I, Linder J: *Pathology: a color atlas,* St. Louis, 1999, Mosby.)

PATIENT SCREENING

Hemorrhage from ruptured esophageal varices is a medical emergency.

ETIOLOGY

Varices result from pressure within the veins. This pressure develops when the venous return to the liver is obstructed. Esophageal varices occur in about two-thirds of all patients with cirrhosis of the liver and are often associated with alcoholic cirrhosis. Esophageal varices are a common complication of cirrhosis of the liver because destruction of hepatic tissue interferes with emptying of the portal vein, resulting in portal hypertension.

DIAGNOSIS

Diagnosis is based on the clinical picture and history of hepatic disease, specifically cirrhosis. Radiographic examination is indicated to study obstruction of blood flow that causes back pressure in the esophageal vessels. Esophageal varices can be noted during endoscopic examination.

TREATMENT

The treatment of a patient with bleeding esophageal varices is the same as that for any patient with gross GI bleeding. Attempts are made to control or stop the bleeding by ice water *lavage* or epigastric *tamponade* with an epigastric balloon. Surgical interventions include endoscopic sclerotherapy and ligation of bleeding varices. Replacing the blood volume and maintaining the fluid and electrolyte balance restore *hemostasis.*

PROGNOSIS

The long-term prognosis is somewhat guarded because of the tendency to hemorrhage. Forty percent of patients die with the first episode of massive hemorrhage. Of those who survive, recurrent bleeding frequently occurs within 1 year, with a similar mortality rate for each episode.

PREVENTION

Esophageal varices are often associated with hepatic disease, which may or may not be preventable.

PATIENT TEACHING

Illustrate how obstruction of blood flow causes back pressure in the esophageal vessels. Teach the patient how to monitor for overt signs of upper-GI bleeding. When a procedure such as esophageal balloon tamponade is required to control bleeding, explain the procedure and its purpose.

Esophagitis

DESCRIPTION

Esophagitis is inflammation and tissue injury of the esophagus.

ICD-9-CM Code 530.1
Esophagitis is coded according to types and causes. Refer to the physician's diagnosis and then to the current edition of the ICD-9-CM coding manual to ensure the greatest specificity of pathology and any appropriate modifiers.

SYMPTOMS AND SIGNS

The main symptom that the patient experiences is burning chest pain (heartburn), which can make the patient believe that he or she is having a heart attack. The onset of pain typically follows eating or drinking. The patient even may have some vomiting of blood (hematemesis).

Corrosive esophagitis is severe inflammation of the esophagus resulting from ingestion of a caustic chemical (alkali or acid) that causes tissue damage (Fig. 8–15). In children, the ingestion is accidental; in adults the chemical ingestion often is a suicide attempt. The degree of damage to the esophageal tissue varies from pain and inability to swallow and speak, to perforation and even destruction of the esophagus.

PATIENT SCREENING

Acute cases caused by ingestion of a chemical require emergency care.

ETIOLOGY

The cause of esophagitis is *reflux* of the acid contents of the stomach resulting from a defect of the *cardiac sphincter*. The stomach acids irritate the esophageal lining, and this causes the inflammatory response. Erosive esophagitis can occur after one takes antibiotics such as tetracycline without drinking adequate amounts of water, and it can result from chemical injury. Esophagitis also can appear as a GI manifestation of human immunodeficiency virus (HIV) infection.

DIAGNOSIS

The diagnostic steps begin with a patient history, followed by a radiographic film of the upper GI tract to rule out an ulcer or hiatal hernia. An esophagoscopy helps the physician make the diagnosis and determine the extent of inflammation

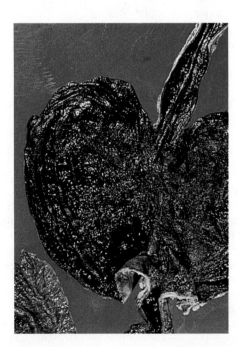

FIGURE 8–15 Corrosive esophagitis. (From Damjanov I, Linder J: *Pathology: a color atlas*, St. Louis, 1999, Mosby.)

and tissue damage. A history of chemical ingestion and the presence of redness and oropharyngeal burn point to caustic esophagitis.

TREATMENT

The treatment of esophagitis includes several weeks of a bland diet to calm the inflammation along with the use of strong antacids. Underlying causes of reflux, such as hiatal hernia, are addressed in the treatment plan. Sucralfate (Carafate) suspension sometimes is prescribed to relieve discomfort and to promote healing. Meals should be small and frequent, and alcohol must be avoided.

When there is an esophageal stricture, a dilation procedure may be indicated. Esophageal perforation requires emergency surgical repair.

PROGNOSIS

The prognosis for esophagitis is good if the patient follows the treatment the physician prescribes. Complications of chronic or caustic esophagitis are scarring and stricture of the esophagus.

PREVENTION

There is no known prevention for esophagitis, but avoiding alcohol, spicy foods, and caffeine helps to relieve the symptoms.

PATIENT TEACHING

Advise the patient that close monitoring of the condition is required during the treatment and healing process. Assess the need for psychological counseling, if contributing causes indicate this course of action.

Esophageal Cancer

DESCRIPTION

Esophageal cancer occurs in the esophagus, the muscular organ that carries food from the mouth to the stomach. It is lined for most of its length with squamous epithelium, which can give rise to squamous cell carcinoma (Fig. 8–16). The columnar epithelium near the esophagogastric junction may develop adenocarcinoma.

▮ **ICD-9-CM Code** **150.9** *(Unspecified)*
Esophageal cancer is coded according to the site of the lesion. Refer to the physician's diagnosis and then to the current edition of the ICD-9-CM coding manual to ensure the greatest specificity of pathology and any appropriate modifiers.

SYMPTOMS AND SIGNS

Symptoms may include dysphagia, weight loss, and a retrosternal discomfort or burning sensation. Iron-deficiency anemia may result from chronic esophageal blood loss. If the tumor involves the recurrent laryngeal nerve, hoarseness may result. A tracheoesophageal **fistula** may appear during the late stages of the disease, presenting with coughing or frequent pneumonias when saliva, liquids, or food spill into the lungs.

PATIENT SCREENING

Follow office policy for patient referrals and follow-up appointments.

ETIOLOGY

Squamous cell carcinoma (SCC) and adenocarcinoma occur at nearly equal rates. The incidence of SCC varies with geographic region, with the highest rates being found in Asia, Africa, and Iran. Risk factors for SCC include cigarette smoking, alcohol consumption, betel nut chewing (a practice common in some Asian countries), drinking of very hot beverages (greater than 65° C), eating of foods containing N-nitroso compounds (such as pickled vegetables), poor nutrition, and underlying esophageal disease such as achalasia or

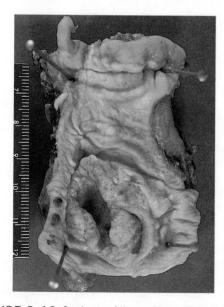

FIGURE 8–16 Carcinoma of the esophagus. (From Kumar V, Cotran RS, Robbins SL: *Robbins basic pathology*, ed 7, Philadelphia, 2003, Saunders.)

caustic strictures. Most SCCs are located in the midportion of the esophagus. The early lesions are subtle and easily missed on endoscopy.

Adenocarcinoma is largely a disease of Caucasians and males. The major risk factors are Barrett's esophagus and chronic gastroesophageal reflux disease (see the Enrichment box on Barrett's Esophagus). The risk of adenocarcinoma is greater in patients who smoke, are obese, and take drugs that reduce lower esophageal sphincter pressure, such as nitroglycerine, anticholinergics, beta-adrenergic agonists, aminophylline, and benzodiazepines.

Adenocarcinoma occurs near the gastro-esophageal junction. It may present as an ulcer, a nodule, or no abnormality on endoscopy. Because there is no serosal covering on the esophagus, unlike the rest of the gastrointestinal tract, both SCC and adenocarcinomas spread into adjacent mediastinal tissues early in the disease. Distant metastases to the liver, bone, and lung are seen in about 30% of patients.

DIAGNOSIS

Physicians detect most esophageal cancers incidentally on endoscopic exam or during screening of high-risk individuals by recognizing mucosal defects, nodules, ulcerations, or strictures on endoscopic exam. Among patients who have symptoms suggestive of esophageal cancer, a chest x-ray or double-contrast barium study may be used for the initial assessment. A biopsy is needed to confirm the diagnosis.

Initial patient evaluation after diagnosis includes assessment of operative risk as well as staging. (Staging systems for cancer are discussed in Chapter 1 and Table 1–4.) Esophageal tumors are staged according to the TNM (Tumor, Node, Metastasis) classification system proposed by the American Joint Committee on Cancer. Staging begins with a CT scan to evaluate for metastatic disease and to determine whether surgical resection of the tumor is a realistic option. If no metastases are seen, the patient undergoes endoscopic ultrasonography (EUS) for assessment of the cancer's progress through the esophageal wall and lymph node metastasis.

TREATMENT

Accurate staging is critical in selecting a treatment method. For patients with clinically localized cancer, the options are surgery and/or chemoradiotherapy. EUS is used to detect recurrence of the disease after successful tumor excision. For patients with advanced, unresectable disease, the therapeutic goal is to maintain the ability to swallow. Nonoperative measures may be used to palliate symptoms. Radiation, with or without chemotherapy, or endoscopic stent placement is used to treat dysphagia by shrinking the tumor or dilating the esophagus, respectively. These methods also reduce the risk of aspiration and weight loss, but rarely improve the survival of the patient.

PROGNOSIS

The prognosis is highly associated with the stage but is generally poor because esophageal cancer of both types has a high propensity for metastasis even in the earliest stages. The overall 5-year survival rate is about 14%.

PREVENTION

Screening endoscopies of the general population for SCC is not cost-effective in low-risk areas of the world such as the United States but has been effective in detecting early cancers in high-risk areas. It is, however, prudent to screen those with Barrett's esophagus for progression to adenocarcinoma. In addition, the patient should avoid practices associated with increased risk, such as the use of alcohol and tobacco.

PATIENT TEACHING

Assess the patient's knowledge of the diagnosis and treatment plan. Discuss possible side effects of radiation, chemotherapy, or surgery as appropriate. Encourage the patient to ask questions and discuss anxieties. Provide a list of local cancer support groups and other appropriate referrals.

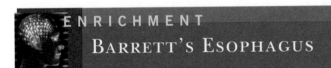

ENRICHMENT
BARRETT'S ESOPHAGUS

ONE OF THE MOST SEVERE CONSEQUENCES of chronic gastroesophageal reflux disease (GERD) is the replacement of the normal stratified squamous epithelium of the distal esophagus with abnormal columnar epithelium. This condition is known as Barrett's esophagus. In one sense, it is a protective *metaplastic* change produced because the columnar epithelium is more resistant to acid damage than the original stratified squamous epithelium, but at the same time, this adaptation predisposes to the development of adenocarcinoma of the esophagus and of the proximal stomach. About 10% of patients with chronic GERD develop Barrett's esophagus. Those with Barrett's have a risk 30 to 125 times that of the normal population of developing adenocarcinoma.

Barrett's esophagus is usually diagnosed during endoscopic examination of middle-aged and older adults. The mean age at the time of diagnosis is 55 years. It has a strong predilection for white or Hispanic males and is increasing in incidence in Western countries. The metaplasia itself causes no symptoms, and the condition is usually discovered as patients are being seen for symptoms of GERD, such as heartburn, regurgitation, and *dysphagia*.

The genetic changes leading from the development of Barrett's esophagus to adenocarcinoma are not completely understood. We do know that before the cells acquire enough DNA damage to become malignant, *dysplastic* morphologic changes appear. The use of acid-suppressive medications has been shown to slow the progression of the dysplasia.

Management of patients with Barrett's esophagus encompasses three main areas: treatment of the symptoms of GERD, endoscopic surveillance every 3 years to detect dysplasia, and treatment of the dysplasia. GERD is usually treated with acid-suppressive medications, antireflux surgery, or lifestyle changes. For patients found to have diffuse low-grade dysplasia on endoscopic exam, the endoscopy often is increased to every 6 months to 1 year. For patients with high-grade dysplasia, progress to adenocarcinoma is much more common but still varies. Therefore esophageal resection is a reasonable course of action to prevent cancer, but because of the risk of morbidity and mortality associated with the surgery, clinicians and their patients may choose to follow the path of watchful waiting (endoscopy every 3 months) before attempting such a procedure. Some techniques currently are being investigated for destroying Barrett's mucosa in the setting of high-grade dysplasia, but none are currently available in clinical practice.

Gastric and Duodenal Peptic Ulcers

DESCRIPTION

When the protective mucous membrane of the stomach or upper intestinal tract breaks down, the lining is prone to ulceration. These internal surface sores, or lesions, can be acute or chronic, clustered or singular, and shallow or deep. Deep sores involve the deep muscle layer of tissue (Fig. 8–17).

■ **ICD-9-CM Code** **531.90** *(Gastric)*
532.90 *(Duodenal)*
533.90 *(Peptic)*
Gastric, duodenal, and peptic ulcers are coded according to the pathology involved. Refer to the physician's diagnosis and then to the current edition of the ICD-9-CM coding manual to ensure the greatest specificity of pathology and any appropriate modifiers.

SYMPTOMS AND SIGNS

When the peptic ulcer occurs in the stomach (gastric ulcer), the patient reports heartburn, or indigestion, and *epigastric* pain. Some patients experience pain or a feeling of uncomfortable fullness after eating, which can cause them to avoid eating and thus lose weight.

The most common peptic ulcer is the duodenal ulcer (an ulcer of the first part of the small intestine), which causes symptoms that vary from subtle midepigastric pain and heartburn to intense pain in the upper abdomen with nausea and vomiting. The patient can be observed guarding the painful area by clutching the stomach, assuming a crouching position, or sitting with the knees drawn up to the chest. Some patients say that frequent eating helps to relieve discomfort; the attacks of most intense pain come about 2 hours after a meal.

If these ulcers bleed internally, occult (hidden) or frank (obvious) blood is found in the vomitus or stool. The situation is more serious if the lesion invades deeply and perforates, causing hemorrhage and leakage of the contents of the stomach or intestine into the abdominal cavity.

PATIENT SCREENING

Sudden onset of pain and vomiting with overt signs of bleeding presents an urgent need for medical care.

ETIOLOGY

Although the cause is not always clear, an area of breakdown of mucous membrane precipitates ulceration of the epithelial lining of the stomach or intestine. A crucial causal factor of peptic ulcers is *Helicobacter pylori* infection, thought to be the most common worldwide human bacterial infection (Fig. 8–18). When present, it produces inflammation in the mucous membrane of the GI tract. The second most common form of ulcer is related to use of nonsteroidal antiinflammatory drugs (NSAIDs). Ulcers related to stress are the next most common form. The less common gastric

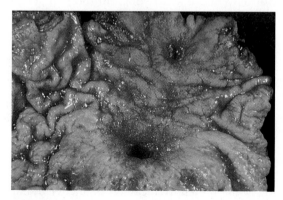

FIGURE 8–17 Peptic ulcer. (From Damjanov I, Linder J: *Pathology: a color atlas,* St. Louis, 1999, Mosby.)

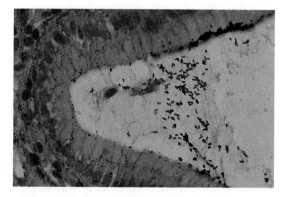

FIGURE 8–18 *Helicobacter pylori.* (From Cotran R et al: *Robbins pathologic basis of disease,* ed 6, Philadelphia, 1999, Saunders.)

ulcers follow chronic gastritis, in which the gastric mucosa becomes less able to defend itself against erosion. Some of the known contributing catalysts are the ingestion of gastric irritants; the use of ulcerogenic drugs, such as alcohol, aspirin, and other antiinflammatory agents; psychogenic stress; smoking; and the presence of a bacterial infection. Gastric ulcers are most common in middle-aged men.

Duodenal ulcers, which usually occur at 45 to 70 years of age, are associated with an increase of acid and gastric juice (pepsin). Predisposing factors include the presence of sustained anxiety and emotional stress, coupled with certain genetic factors.

DIAGNOSIS

The way a patient describes her or his illness can help to distinguish between a gastric and a duodenal ulcer. The diagnosis of peptic ulcer can be suspected based on the patient's history and physical examination. To confirm the diagnosis, the physician takes *barium* radiographic films of the upper GI tract to look for abnormal appearance and function. The ulcer may be visualized through upper-GI-tract endoscopy (Fig. 8–19). Diagnostic studies are available to identify *H. pylori*. Gastric contents are collected and analyzed for the level of acidity or the presence of blood in the secretions. The patient's stool also is checked for evidence of blood. When bleeding that causes anemia complicates the ulcer, blood tests show a reduced hemoglobin (Hb) concentration and reduced *hematocrit* (Hct). A biopsy, with microscopic study of the tissue, rules out or confirms the presence of cancer. Serum albumin and *transferrin* levels may be reduced if the patient has weight loss and malnutrition. Abdominal radiographic studies are performed to investigate the possibility of perforation or other abdominal conditions.

TREATMENT

The management of peptic ulcers requires rest, medication, changes in the diet, and adjustments in lifestyle. Surgery may be indicated in severe cases. If the cause is certain (e.g., the use of an ulcerogenic drug such as aspirin, nonsteroidal antiinflammatories, and alcohol), it must be eliminated. Reducing stress and physical activity promotes healing; sedatives and tranquilizers are prescribed if necessary. Drug therapy includes one or more of the following: histamine (H_2) receptor blocking agents to control gastric secretion

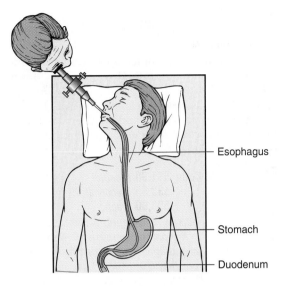

FIGURE 8–19 Upper gastrointestinal tract endoscopy. A flexible, lighted fiberoptic tube (endoscope) is inserted through the mouth to allow direct visualization of the upper gastrointestinal tract. A biopsy may be taken during the procedure when indicated.

(e.g., nizatidine [Axid], famotidine [Pepcid], cimetidine [Tagamet], and ranitidine [Zantac]); antacids (e.g., magnesium hydroxide–aluminum hydroxide [Maalox]) to reduce gastric acidity; coating agents (e.g., sucralfate) to protect the mucosa; and proton pump inhibitors (e.g., omeprazole [Prilosec] and lansoprazole [Prevacid]) to suppress secretion of gastric acid. When *H. pylori* is a causative factor, antibiotic therapy with clarithromycin (Biaxin) or azithromycin (Zithromax), combined with a proton pump inhibitor, may be prescribed. Small, frequent meals of soft, bland foods are better tolerated.

All these measures attempt to relieve symptoms and to encourage the healing process. Significant bleeding or perforation of the ulcer calls for more aggressive measures, such as surgical intervention, the administration of intravenous fluids, and blood replacement.

PROGNOSIS

Peptic ulcers can heal. Patients are instructed to follow the preventive measures even after healing because peptic ulcer disease tends to recur. Any nonhealing ulcer, especially a gastric ulcer, should be evaluated via endoscopy to rule out cancer.

PREVENTION

Limit ingestion of irritating, hot, spicy food. Drinking alcohol and smoking are not recommended. Follow directions when taking NSAIDs and aspirin, and report any GI side effects.

PATIENT TEACHING

Refer to a dietitian for nutritional counseling. Eliminate caffeine, alcohol, smoking, and any other known irritants. Reinforce the importance of strict adherence to a bland diet high in vitamin K. Instruct the patient to take prescribed analgesics or **antiemetics** 1 hour before meals to help control pain or nausea. Warn the patient to report signs of hematemesis and any occurrence of black or bloody stools.

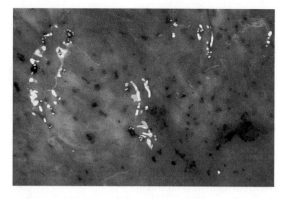

FIGURE 8–20 Chemical gastritis caused by aspirin. (From Damjanov I, Linder J: *Pathology: a color atlas,* St. Louis, 1999, Mosby.)

Gastritis

DESCRIPTION

Gastritis is an inflammation of the lining of the stomach; the acute form is a common disorder.

■ **ICD-9-CM Code 535.5** *(Unspecified)*
Gastritis is coded according to the pathology involved. Refer to the physician's diagnosis and then to the current edition of the ICD-9-CM coding manual to ensure the greatest specificity of pathology and any appropriate modifiers.

SYMPTOMS AND SIGNS

The mucous layer of the stomach normally acts as a physical barrier to resist injury, inflammation, and erosion. When the stomach lining becomes inflamed, the patient experiences epigastric pain, indigestion, and a feeling of fullness after meals. Other discomforts, such as nausea, belching, and fatty food intolerance, cause the patient to lose the appetite. When the gastric mucosa is inflamed and swollen, it can bleed, and the blood can be seen and detected in the patient's vomitus and stool. Chronic gastritis is more common in the elderly.

PATIENT SCREENING

Sudden onset of pain and hematemesis requires emergency medical care.

ETIOLOGY

As in peptic ulcers, the main cause of gastritis is inflammation associated with *H. pylori*. Many agents damage the gastric lining, including common medications such as aspirin and other antiinflammatory drugs, poisons, alcohol, smoking, infectious diseases, stress, and mechanical injury resulting from the swallowing of a foreign object (Fig. 8–20). The repeated ingestion of irritating foods or allergic reaction to foods irritates the gastric mucosa.

Chronic gastritis is associated with peptic ulcer disease and recurring exposure to irritating substances. It can also occur in patients with a history of chronic disease like pernicious anemia. A substantial number of patients have idiopathic gastritis. Paradoxically, gastritis also can result from the lack of production of gastric acids, which is sometimes associated with a vitamin B_{12} deficiency called pernicious anemia.

DIAGNOSIS

Gastroscopy allows visualization of the interior of the stomach, and radiographic films rule out other structural abnormalities. Samples of gastric juices and a biopsy specimen are obtained to determine the extent of disease. Blood counts and serum tests offer additional findings. Fecal occult blood tests may be positive as a result of gastric bleeding.

TREATMENT

Curing *H. pylori* infection with antibiotic therapy often rapidly resolves superficial gastritis. If any other source of irritation is known, it is eliminated or controlled. Gastric discomfort is relieved with the use of antacids and medications such as cimetidine and ranitidine hydrochloride to reduce the secretion of gastric acid. If the patient has bleeding, it is monitored and treated with medicine that constricts blood vessels. Antibiotics are given for infection, and antiemetics are given to help control nausea and vomiting. The patient is given a bland diet as tolerated, with vitamin and mineral supplements as needed. If the patient has a vitamin B_{12} deficiency, injections of vitamin B_{12} must be administered each month indefinitely.

PROGNOSIS

Acute mild cases of gastritis improve with conservative treatment and elimination of the known irritant. Chronic gastritis is monitored for complications.

PREVENTION

Preventive measures are the same as those for gastric and duodenal ulcer.

PATIENT TEACHING

When a patient has been under extreme stress because of a serious illness or emotional tension, counseling is part of the treatment plan. Teaching the patient about the relationship between his or her gastritis and contributing lifestyle factors can promote healing and prevent recurrences. (See Patient Teaching for gastric and duodenal peptic ulcer.)

Gastric Cancer

DESCRIPTION

Gastric cancer occurs in the stomach, an organ located in the upper abdomen that connects the esophagus and the small intestine (Fig. 8–21).

■ **ICD-9-CM Code 151.9**
Gastric cancer is coded according to the site of the lesion. Refer to the physician's diagnosis and then to the current edition of the ICD-9-CM coding manual to ensure the greatest specificity of pathology and any appropriate modifiers.

SYMPTOMS AND SIGNS

The patient with early carcinoma of the stomach is frequently *asymptomatic;* there are no specific symptoms, and pain is absent. As the disease progresses, the most common symptoms at initial presentation are weight loss and persistent abdominal pain, although nausea, *dysphagia, melena,* and *anorexia* are also seen. Anorexia occurs far more often with gas-

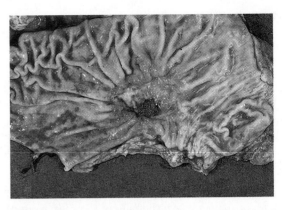

FIGURE 8–21 Ulcerative gastric carcinoma. (From Cotran R et al: *Robbins pathologic basis of disease,* ed 6, Philadelphia, 1999, Saunders.)

tric cancer than with ulcers. The most common physical finding is a palpable abdominal mass, which usually indicates advanced disease.

PATIENT SCREENING

The patient being treated for gastric cancer may experience a variety of complications resulting from surgery, chemotherapy, or radiation. Symptoms of GI obstruction or malnutrition also can occur. The patient is given priority in receiving the physician's advice or an appointment.

ETIOLOGY

Japan has the highest incidence of gastric cancer in the world. In general, cancer of the distal stomach is found more often in developing countries and favors those in urban areas and lower socioeconomic groups. It rarely occurs before age 40. Men are affected twice as often as women. *Helicobacter pylori* infection early in life is a definite cause of gastric cancer. Barrett's esophagus is the main risk factor for development of gastric cancer in the proximal stomach, which is more common in those of high socioeconomic status. Other risk factors are thought to include genetic predisposition (e.g., family history of gastric cancer, blood type A), dietary factors (i.e., diets rich in complex carbohydrates, which increase risk, as opposed to diets rich in fresh fruits and vegetables and in cereal fiber, which reduce risk), and acid hyposecretory conditions.

DIAGNOSIS

Cancer of the stomach usually begins as an ulcer in the lining of the stomach. Early lesions are rarely symptomatic and are rarely detected outside a screening program. When gastric cancer is suspected, a double-contrast barium meal and upper gastrointestinal endoscopy are used for diagnosis. A follow-up endoscopy in 8 to 12 weeks to verify healing of any ulcers detected on the initial test is recommended. Gastric cancer is staged using the TNM (Tumor, Node, Metastasis) classification system proposed by the American Joint Committee on Cancer. Staging is performed via physical examination; CT scan of the chest, abdomen, and pelvis to detect metastases; and an endoscopic ultrasound to assess the depth of tumor invasion and nodal involvement. Laparoscopy also may be used to directly visualize the surface of the liver, the peritoneum, and the local lymph nodes, the most likely sites of metastasis.

TREATMENT

The appropriate treatment regime is selected after accurate tumor staging. Gastric resection, usually followed by combined chemoradiotherapy with 5-fluorouracil and leucovorin, offers the best chance of long-term survival for patients with localized disease. Total gastrectomy is performed for lesions of the proximal stomach (upper third), and subtotal gastrectomy with resection of adjacent nodal tissue is usually sufficient for distal gastric cancer. Palliation is an important part of care for patients with gastric cancer because of the many who present with advanced disease and because of the high rate of recurrence after surgical resection. Palliative measures to relieve obstruction, pain, or bleeding may include resection, radiation therapy, endoscopic laser therapy, and endoscopic *stent* placement.

PROGNOSIS

The prognosis of gastric cancer has improved only slightly over the last few decades despite surgical advances and a decline in incidence. Most patients will develop metastases at some point during the course of their illness. Advanced, incurable cancer is present in about 50% of patients at initial presentation. Even those who undergo potentially curative surgery have high rates of local and distant recurrence. The overall combined 5-year survival rate is about 20%.

PREVENTION

The high mortality rate of gastric cancer is largely due to the prevalence of advanced disease at presentation. Therefore detection at the early stage is very important to survival. The cost-effectiveness of screening asymptomatic people, however, remains controversial. This practice has worked well in Japan, where the incidence of gastric cancer is high. In the United States, with a relatively low incidence of gastric cancer, screening is limited to those who are identified as "high-risk" because they have one of the following conditions: gastric adenomas, familial polyposis coli, or Barrett's esophagus. These patients should receive a screening endoscopy every 1 to 3 years, depending on their underlying condition.

PATIENT TEACHING

Assess the patient's knowledge of the disease process and the medical management prescribed by the physician. Address any related impairment to eating and nutrition. Encourage the patient to ask questions or express any feelings of anxiety. Discuss the side effects of chemotherapy or surgery. Make certain the patient understands all palliative measures and the warning signs to report to the physician or nurse. Provide referrals to cancer support groups.

Acute Appendicitis

DESCRIPTION

Appendicitis is an inflammation of the appendix, a narrow pouch about 3½ inches long that extends from the first part of the large intestine (cecum) (Fig. 8–22).

 ICD-9-CM Code 540
Appendicitis is coded according to the pathology involved. Refer to the physician's diagnosis and then to the current edition of the ICD-9-CM coding manual to ensure the greatest specificity of pathology and any appropriate modifiers.

SYMPTOMS AND SIGNS

The appendix has no known function in humans, and its only importance seems to be, unfortunately, that it can become inflamed. Classic symptoms include abdominal pain that usually starts as vague discomfort around the navel and, within a few hours, localizes in the right lower quadrant. As the

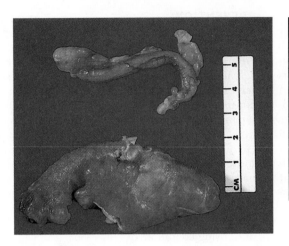
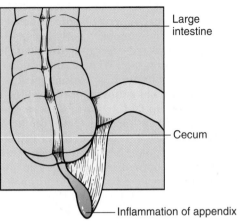

Large intestine

Cecum

Inflammation of appendix

FIGURE 8–22 Acute appendicitis. (From Cotran R et al: *Robbins pathologic basis of disease,* ed 6, Philadelphia, 1999, Saunders.)

condition worsens, the patient becomes nauseated and may vomit, runs a fever, and has diarrhea or constipation.

PATIENT SCREENING
Clinical signs vary but usually follow a sequence as described previously. A patient with low abdominal pain, fever, and nausea and vomiting requires immediate medical attention.

ETIOLOGY
The reason the appendix becomes swollen, inflamed, and abscessed is not completely understood. The condition may be initiated by obstruction with fecal material, neoplasm, a foreign body, or worms. Whatever the cause, the pathophysiology of the disease is the same. As bacteria multiply, they invade the wall of the appendix, and eventually the circulation to the appendix is compromised. Appendicitis is most common in the 20- to 40-year-old age bracket.

DIAGNOSIS
The physician makes a differential diagnosis of appendicitis to rule out other causes of right lower abdominal pain and acute abdomen. Appendicitis generally can be diagnosed based on the physical examination and the symptoms the patient describes; one significant diagnostic indicator is maximal tenderness of the abdomen at *McBurney's point.* Rebound tenderness on the opposite side

may be a sign of peritoneal irritation. A complete blood count (CBC) and urinalysis are performed and possibly repeated during hospital observation. Laboratory findings indicate an elevation of the *white blood cell (WBC)* count *(leukocytosis).* NOTE: the elderly may present with milder symptoms, delaying the diagnosis.

TREATMENT
Surgical removal of the appendix (appendectomy) is the best treatment and is performed as soon as appendicitis is confirmed. Broad-spectrum antibiotic therapy is initiated before surgery. If appendicitis is left untreated, necrosis and rupture of the appendix can result in **peritonitis,** a life-threatening complication.

PROGNOSIS
Complete recovery is expected with prompt medical and surgical intervention. Laparoscopic appendectomy allows quicker recovery.

PREVENTION
No prevention is known, but the appendix may be removed during unrelated abdominal surgery as a prophylactic measure.

PATIENT TEACHING
Local application of heat to the abdomen is contraindicated with the characteristic clinical symptoms of appendicitis. Postsurgical instructions in-

clude deep breathing and early ambulation to prevent complications. Review all postoperative instructions. Tell the patient to notify the physician if signs of infection appear at the incision site.

Hiatal Hernia

DESCRIPTION

A hiatal hernia is a defect in the diaphragm that permits a segment of the stomach to slide into the thoracic cavity.

 ICD-9-CM Code 553.3

SYMPTOMS AND SIGNS

Hiatal hernia is the condition in which the upper part of the stomach protrudes through the esophageal opening of the diaphragm and into the thoracic cavity (Fig. 8–23). The cardiac sphincter muscle at the top of the stomach malfunctions, allowing the contents of the stomach to regurgitate into the esophagus. This esophageal reflux (see Gastroesophageal Reflux Disease) can irritate the lining of the esophagus. The patient reports heartburn, which is usually worse when reclining. Symptoms of chest pain and difficulty in swallowing may suggest that a large portion of the stomach has slipped into the opening. Respiratory complications can develop as a result of aspiration.

Some hiatal hernias are asymptomatic.

PATIENT SCREENING

When patients report heartburn, excessive belching, or distention of the stomach, a routine appointment is scheduled. If the patient has substernal chest pain, dysphagia, or bleeding, he or she should be seen as soon as possible.

ETIOLOGY

Hiatal hernia, a common condition, can be caused by a congenital defect in the diaphragm or a weakness that develops in the diaphragm, allowing protrusion of part of the stomach into the thoracic cavity. The weakening of the muscle can result from obesity, old age, trauma, or intraabdominal pressure; sometimes the exact cause is uncertain.

DIAGNOSIS

Large hiatal hernias may show on a radiographic chest film. A diagnosis is based on barium radiographic studies of the esophagus and stomach. Endoscopy confirms the diagnosis and differenti-

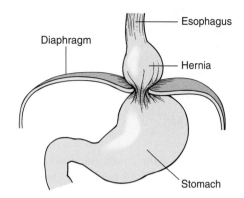

FIGURE 8–23 Hiatal hernia.

ates the condition from other diseases, such as peptic ulcer and malignant tumor. Additional diagnostic studies include measurement of reflux pH and examination of the reflux contents for the presence of blood.

TREATMENT

The first course is conservative treatment that relieves the symptoms and prevents complications. This includes dietary modification (smaller, more frequent meals of bland food). The patient is advised to minimize activities that increase intraabdominal pressure, such as straining and coughing. The obese patient is advised to lose weight.

Antacids and medications that control the acid secretions in the stomach are given. Drug therapy may include a **cholinergic** agent, which helps to control the episodes of reflux by strengthening the lower esophageal sphincter. Smoking is discouraged because it aggravates the heartburn. Because gravity plays a role in hiatal hernia, the patient is advised to avoid lying down for 4 hours after a meal; elevating the head of the bed on blocks also helps.

If these measures do not work or if the hernia becomes strangulated, surgical repair of the hiatus is the treatment of choice.

PROGNOSIS

Good compliance with conservative measures results in control of symptoms. If complications appear, antireflux surgical repair may be required.

PREVENTION

Prevention is not possible when the condition is due to congenital weakness or aging.

PATIENT TEACHING

Encourage the patient to follow the conservative measures listed above to control symptoms. Suggest ways to manage obesity and avoid any physical work that increases intraabdominal pressure.

Abdominal Hernia

DESCRIPTION

Abdominal hernia is the condition in which an organ protrudes through an abnormal opening in the abdominal wall.

 ICD-9-CM Code 553.9 *(Unspecified site)*

SYMPTOMS AND SIGNS

An abdominal hernia can occur when there is a weak spot in the muscles and membranes of the abdominal wall that allows an organ or part of an organ to break through the wall (herniate) or protrude. This can occur in a male or female and at any age. The signs and symptoms of abdominal hernias vary with the site and the size of the hernia.

The **inguinal** canal is a common site for hernias. A loop of bowel protrudes into the inguinal canal and, in a male, fills the scrotal sac (Fig. 8–24, *A*). The patient notices a lump or bulge in the inguinal area and may discover that pressing on the hernia to push it back into the abdomen can reduce it. A sharp pain in the groin is continuous or made worse when standing or straining.

If the patient has severe pain, the hernia may be trapped or strangulated (Fig. 8–24, *B*). This means that the blood flow to the herniated organ or bowel has been stopped, and *gangrene,* a serious condition, can set in. The umbilicus is another common site of herniation (Fig. 8–24, *C*).

PATIENT SCREENING

Unless the patient complains of severe pain, there is no urgency.

ETIOLOGY

An abdominal hernia begins when an abnormal opening develops in a weak area or when a congenital malformation exists in the containing structures of the abdominal cavity. Trauma or increased intraabdominal pressure resulting from heavy lifting or pregnancy also can cause a hernia. A hernia occasionally develops near the weakened site of a previous surgical scar.

DIAGNOSIS

A visible hernia can be palpated for size and inspected with the patient standing and then lying down. The physician listens for bowel sounds. An inguinal hernia can be detected in the male by asking him to perform *Valsalva's maneuver.* The medical assessment also might include radiographic studies of the abdomen and a white blood cell count.

TREATMENT

Therapeutic measures vary with the type of hernia as well as with the age and physical condition of the patient. If the hernia is uncomplicated and the hernial sac can be reduced back into the abdominal cavity, the patient can wear a device called a truss. If this measure keeps the patient comfortable and there are no signs of strangulation, surgical intervention may not be required. Surgical repair of the hernia (herniorrhaphy) is the treatment of choice in children and healthy adults.

PROGNOSIS

In uncomplicated cases, the prognosis is good. An incarcerated or strangulated hernia requires prompt surgical repair and a variable postsurgical recovery time.

PREVENTION

When the patient has known weakness in the abdominal wall, heavy lifting and trauma should be avoided. Smoking that causes coughing may contribute to hernias.

PATIENT TEACHING

Be sure the patient understands how to apply the device, a *truss,* recommended to reduce a hernia. Discuss any activity restrictions or allowance. When surgical repair (herniorrhaphy) is planned, review preoperative and postoperative procedures and discuss the warning signs of complications.

Crohn Disease (Regional Enteritis)

DESCRIPTION

Crohn disease is a chronic inflammatory disease of the alimentary tract. It is also called ileitis, regional enteritis, and ileocolitis.

 ICD-9-CM Code 555.9 *(NOS)*
In some coding books, this disease may be spelled "Crohn's Disease."

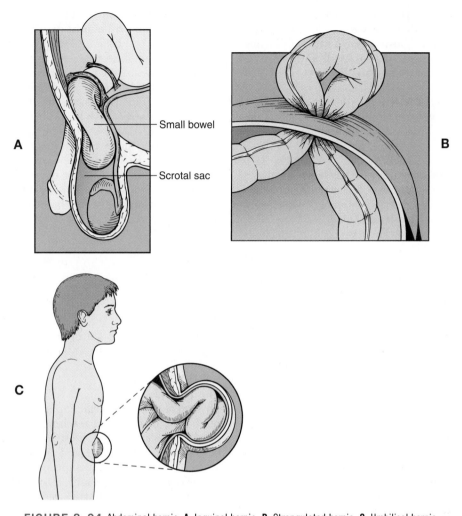

FIGURE 8–24 Abdominal hernia. **A,** Inguinal hernia. **B,** Strangulated hernia. **C,** Umbilical hernia.

SYMPTOMS AND SIGNS

Crohn disease is a fairly common chronic inflammatory disease of the alimentary canal in which all layers of the bowel wall are edematous and inflamed (Fig. 8–25). Any portion of the GI tract from mouth to anus can be affected. Patients with Crohn disease have chronic diarrhea along with cramping abdominal pain, often in the right lower quadrant of the abdomen. They also may experience weight loss, anorexia, fever, and abdominal fullness. If obstruction develops, patients have symptoms of an *acute abdomen.* The abdomen is tender and distended, and patients may vomit and experience blood in the stools. If the condition is

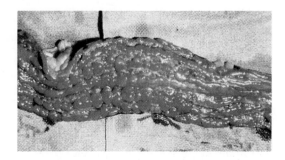

FIGURE 8–25 Crohn disease. (From Doughty DB, Jackson DB: *Gastrointestinal disorders—Mosby's clinical nursing series,* St. Louis, 1993, Mosby.)

chronic, signs and symptoms of malnutrition begin to materialize; perianal *fissures* and *fistulas* usually develop. Complications associated with the chronic inflammation include symptoms of bowel obstruction, adhesions, and abscesses.

PATIENT SCREENING

The acute symptoms of Crohn disease can mimic appendicitis, requiring prompt medical investigation.

ETIOLOGY

The etiology of Crohn disease has been greatly researched, but the cause is not known. Immunologic factors, infectious agents, psychosomatic illness, and dietary factors play a role; autoimmune factors, allergies, and genetic causes also have been investigated.

DIAGNOSIS

Diagnosis is based on symptoms, air-contrast barium enema radiographic studies, and flat-plate studies of the abdomen. The radiographic films reveal the diseased segments (strictures) separated by normal bowel in a characteristic distribution called "skip lesions." Anemia, leukocytosis, and *hypoalbuminemia* may be detected in blood tests. Electrolyte abnormalities reflect the severity of diarrhea. Colonoscopy (Fig. 8–26) and biopsy confirm the diagnosis.

TREATMENT

Crohn disease is considered a medically incurable condition. The general medical management includes nutritional support and control of symptoms. The patient may require dietary supplements of vita-

mins, minerals, protein, and calories. In cases of severe and prolonged bouts of diarrhea, intravenous nutrition may be necessary. Drug therapy with anticholinergics and narcotic agents relieves the cramping and diarrhea. If the disease includes bacterial involvement, the physician prescribes antibacterial agents, such as sulfasalazine. Sulfasalazine is a good treatment agent because it also has antiinflammatory properties. Corticosteroid therapy and *immunosuppressive* drugs also are used. If bowel obstruction, an abscess, or perforation develops, surgery to remove the affected portion of the intestine is indicated. Because this disease may be chronic, patients may benefit from counseling, participation in a support group, and physical rest.

PROGNOSIS

Crohn disease has a high rate of recurrence after treatment. The course of the disease varies. High stress levels cause exacerbations.

PREVENTION

Because the cause is uncertain, prevention is directed toward avoiding complications.

PATIENT TEACHING

The clinician is challenged to address the many physical and psychological implications of this type of chronic disease, and teaching may cover good nutrition, tolerable diet, lifestyle, the possibility of colectomy with ileostomy, and altered body image. Warn the patient that any signs of intestinal bleeding or a fever associated with increased abdominal tenderness must be reported to the physician.

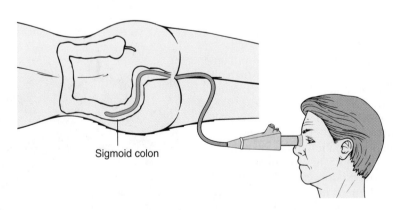

Sigmoid colon

FIGURE 8–26 Colonoscopy. A lighted fiberoptic endoscope is inserted through the anus to allow direct examination of the colon. This method is useful in differential diagnosis of bowel disease, to obtain biopsy, and in minor surgery such as polypectomy.

Ulcerative Colitis

DESCRIPTION

Ulcerative colitis is a chronic inflammatory bowel disease affecting the mucosa and submucosa of the rectum and colon (Fig. 8–27).

 ICD-9-CM Code 556.9 *(Unspecified)*

SYMPTOMS AND SIGNS

Ulcerative colitis, a common cause of serious bowel disease, can affect any age group. It is more common in young adults, especially women, and in the Jewish population. The symptoms result from a chronic, diffuse, continuous inflammation of the mucosa of the rectum and colon. The patient reports intermittent episodes of bloody diarrhea, abdominal cramping, urgency to defecate, and mucoid stools. As the disease progresses, the stools become looser and more frequent (10 to 20 per day), with cramping and rectal pressure; the patient also experiences weight loss, fever, and malaise. Some patients report diarrhea alternating with constipation. The watery stools contain blood, mucus, and pus resulting from mucosal ulceration of the bowel. If the disease is **fulminant,** major complications result from severe diarrhea, massive bleeding, and perforation.

PATIENT SCREENING

The hallmark sign that prompts an individual to contact a physician is frequent and bloody diarrhea. A prompt medical evaluation is appropriate.

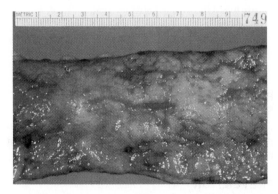

FIGURE 8–27 Ulcerative colitis. (From Doughty DB, Jackson DB: *Gastrointestinal disorders—Mosby's clinical nursing series,* St. Louis, 1993, Mosby.)

ETIOLOGY

The diseases has some familial tendency, but the cause is unknown. Current thinking suggests a relationship to an autoimmune response.

DIAGNOSIS

The diagnosis is based on the clinical picture, examination of the stool for blood, and laboratory values. The findings could include a reduced hemoglobin level and leukocytosis. Electrolyte abnormalities may be noted when diarrhea is severe. Plain films of the abdomen also are taken. Barium enema studies and colonoscopy are performed at the physician's discretion. Stool cultures are needed to rule out bacterial causes. Biopsy shows typical inflammatory changes in the mucosa.

TREATMENT

The patient is urged to consume a well-balanced diet devoid of foods that the patient finds irritating. The diet usually is low in fat and bulk and high in protein, vitamins, and calories. Anticholinergic drugs and occasionally antidiarrheal agents are prescribed. Sulfasalazine often is used for mild to moderate cases, and corticosteroid therapy is used in more severe cases. Surgical removal of the diseased colon is indicated for severe hemorrhage or perforation. The patient is examined annually because chronic ulcerative colitis is associated with an increased risk of colon cancer.

PROGNOSIS

The severity varies from mild to fulminant disease. The risk for colon cancer is higher with chronic ulcerative colitis.

PREVENTION

As in other types of irritable bowel syndrome (IBS), the cause of onset may be uncertain; thus the medical approach is to manage recurrent attacks and prevent complications.

PATIENT TEACHING

A team approach better addresses the multiple aspects of care in IBS. During an acute phase, encourage the patient to identify emotional or physical stressors. Discuss the results that the patient can expect from the prescribed regimen of diet, rest, and medication. Tell the patient to watch for signs of dehydration and GI bleeding. Severe episodes of bleeding require parenteral nutrition and perhaps surgical intervention. Referral to IBS support services is useful.

Gastroenteritis

DESCRIPTION

Gastroenteritis is a general term for acute inflammation of the lining of the stomach and intestines.

ICD-9-CM Code 558.9 *(Other and unspecified noninfectious gastroenteritis and colitis)*

SYMPTOMS AND SIGNS

The stomach and intestines usually are protected from infections and irritations by the presence of normal bacterial flora and acid secretions and by the healthy motility of the GI tract. When these mechanisms fail to rid the body of *toxins* or large numbers of disease-causing bacteria and viruses, the stomach and intestines become filled with the products of inflammation, and gastroenteritis results. The patient experiences increased intestinal motility, with the presence of mucus, pus, and blood in the stool. The body loses fluids too rapidly, causing dehydration with a disturbance in the body's electrolyte balance.

The common syndrome of gastroenteritis called traveler's diarrhea is characterized by varying degrees of anorexia, abdominal cramping, frequent loose stools, and nausea and profuse vomiting. If the infection is severe enough, fever and weakness follow. The same symptoms occur with intestinal influenza, food or chemical poisoning, allergic reactions to food, and some drug reactions.

PATIENT SCREENING

Weakness, dizziness, reduced urine output, and mental confusion are indications of dehydration. A patient who experiences acute vomiting and hematemesis or reports ingestion of a poisonous or corrosive agent should be treated as a medical emergency.

ETIOLOGY

Ingestion of disease-causing bacteria or parasites from contaminated food or water is the primary cause of traveler's diarrhea, whereas intestinal influenza is usually the result of a virus. Some bacteria produce toxins in food that cause food poisoning when ingested (see Food Poisoning). Ingestion of the poison in certain foods (e.g., poisonous mushrooms) or chemicals (e.g., arsenic) causes gastroenteritis. Other causes are chronic ingestion of spicy or irritating foods, alcohol, caffeine, aspirin, and other antiinflammatory agents. Gastroenteritis may be a complication of acute illness. In some people, gastroenteritis is stress induced.

DIAGNOSIS

The first important step in identifying the cause is to consider the medical history. Laboratory analysis and culture of the stool reveal the signs as well as the actual causes of infection or poisoning. The stool is inspected by electron microscopy for occult blood, leukocytes, erythrocytes, pus, abnormal bacteria, and viruses. The clinical evaluation includes blood studies for causative organisms, the presence of antibodies, abnormal blood cell counts, and serum electrolyte values. Endoscopy also may be performed but is contraindicated if a corrosive agent has been ingested.

TREATMENT

The treatment varies with the cause, the severity of the disease, and the age and general health of the patient. Gastroenteritis often is self-limiting, although it can become severe and life-threatening, with complications such as ulceration of the stomach or intestine. There is a danger of perforation and hemorrhage of these lesions. The very young, the elderly, and the chronically ill are most vulnerable to electrolyte imbalance resulting from dehydration, which can lead to death in a short time.

The goal of treatment is to control symptoms and to maintain a normal fluid and electrolyte balance. Direct management of the cause as diagnosed accomplishes this; the subsequent treatment includes the use of antiemetics, antibiotics, antacids, and either oral or intravenous rehydration solutions. The patient should rest and eat as tolerated. Antidiarrheal agents should not be used for treatment of traveler's diarrhea because they delay the body's elimination of organisms, which increases the duration of symptoms.

PROGNOSIS

Simple gastroenteritis is self-limiting; whereas chronic gastroenteritis carries a risk of serious complications such as perforation, abscess formation, and peritonitis.

PREVENTION

Education directed at eliminating the cause helps to prevent recurrences. Infection-control techniques, including frequent and thorough hand washing and avoidance of food that has not been well refrigerated and well cooked, are excellent preventive measures for the most common causes of gastroenteritis.

PATIENT TEACHING

Teach infection-control measures. Warn against ingesting aspirin, alcohol, and foods that cause gastric upset. Advise the patient to stop smoking. Explain the negative effects of extreme stress on the GI tract. Recommend relaxing before eating; taking smaller, more frequent meals; and eating slowly. Advise the patient that, when traveling, he or she should choose well-cooked foods over raw ones and drink purified bottled water.

Intestinal Obstruction

DESCRIPTION

Intestinal obstruction is mechanical or functional blockage of the intestines.

> **ICD-9-CM Code 560.9** *(Unspecified intestinal obstruction)*
> *Mechanical obstructions of the intestines are coded according to the nature of the obstruction. Refer to the physician's diagnosis and then to the current edition of the ICD-9-CM coding manual to ensure the greatest specificity of pathology and any appropriate modifiers.*

SYMPTOMS AND SIGNS

Intestinal obstruction occurs when the contents of the intestine cannot move forward because of a partial or complete blockage of the bowel. Although the cause and nature of the obstruction can vary, the patient's discomfort and the signs of blockage are characteristic and include severe pain, nausea and vomiting, and a bloated and painful abdomen without passage of stool or gas. Symptoms also include an electrolyte imbalance and an elevated WBC count. The bowel sounds can be hyperactive or missing, depending on the nature of the obstruction. This condition of the bowel can occur at any age but is more common in middle-aged and elderly people.

PATIENT SCREENING

The level of intestinal obstruction dictates the severity of the symptoms. A sudden increase in symptoms or an acute onset of symptoms requires urgent medical care.

ETIOLOGY

Mechanical blockage of the bowel narrows the normal lumen and prevents the flow of waste products. Mechanical causes of intestinal obstruction are many:
- Neoplasm (benign or malignant)
- Foreign bodies
- Fecal impaction
- Strictures
- Compression of the bowel
- Volvulus (a twisting of the bowel on itself) (Fig. 8–28)
- **Intussusception** (in which the bowel telescopes into itself) (see Fig. 8–28)
- Strangulated hernia (see Fig. 8–28)
- Adhesions that form tight bands of scar tissue on the bowel (see Fig. 8–28)

In some cases of mechanical obstruction, the blood supply to the affected area of intestine is blocked, which results in the death of tissue; this leads to the threat of perforation, with spillage of the intestinal contents into the abdominal cavity. This becomes a toxic condition that endangers the patient.

If the obstruction is nonmechanical (functional), it is called ileus. A paralytic condition of the small bowel, ileus can occur after abdominal surgery, when peristalsis and bowel sounds are absent. Normal peristalsis also can be inhibited by the use of certain medications (e.g., codeine, aluminum-containing antacids) or disease conditions such as peritonitis. The motility of the bowel often returns spontaneously. If it does not return within 48 hours, a syndrome of continuous pain, abdominal distention, vomiting of fecal material, and shock can be dangerous and life-threatening.

DIAGNOSIS

Barium swallow films of the abdomen show the point of obstruction of the bowel. A CBC shows an elevated WBC count; the patient also has electrolyte imbalances and acid–base disturbances.

TREATMENT

When the obstruction is mechanical, surgery is performed as soon as possible to remove the lesion or whatever is causing the blockage. If necessary, the diseased bowel is removed and the colon is reconstructed; an *ostomy* may be needed. A second surgical procedure is required to perform take-down of the ostomy and to rejoin the bowel.

In a nonmechanical or functional obstruction (ileus), the patient is not given anything by mouth and is fed intravenously until peristalsis has returned. A stomach tube is inserted to relieve distention and vomiting. Surgery is not usually indicated for functional obstruction. In cases of fecal impaction, a stool softener such as docusate sodium and a source of fiber are both used in treatment.

PROGNOSIS

The prognosis generally is good for mechanical obstructive bowel conditions treated with curative surgery. The outcome is guarded, however, with malignant tumors.

PREVENTION

Screening tests for colorectal cancer permit early detection and treatment of malignant tumors. Laxative therapy, especially for the elderly or bedridden person, helps prevent fecal impaction.

PATIENT TEACHING

Review the physician's explanations and discuss any anticipated surgical procedure. Give the patient a list of signs and symptoms that need to be reported to a doctor, such as any change in bowel habits or sign of GI bleeding. Refer a colostomy patient to an ostomy care nurse. Review any diet restrictions and urge adequate fluid intake. Obtain referrals for home health care as needed.

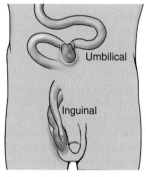

Herniation

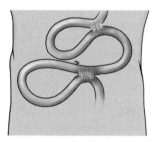

Adhesions

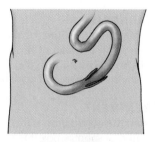

Intussusception

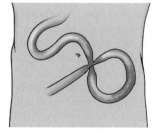

Volvulus

FIGURE 8–28 Schematic of intestinal obstructions. (From Cotran R et al: *Robbins pathologic basis of disease,* ed 6, Philadelphia, 1999, Saunders.)

Diverticulosis (Diverticular Disease)

DESCRIPTION

Diverticulosis is a progressive condition, common with age, characterized by defects in the muscular wall of the large bowel (Fig. 8–29).

■ **ICD-9-CM Code** **562.10** *(Without mention of hemorrhage)*
562.12 *(With hemorrhage)*

SYMPTOMS AND SIGNS

Diverticulosis is a condition in which out pouches (diverticula) of the mucosa penetrate weak points in the muscular layer of the large intestine. Diverticulosis occurs particularly in the distal part of the colon, the sigmoid colon (see Fig. 8–29). Diverticulosis usually causes no symptoms and brings no inflammation. Occasionally, the patient reports nonspecific abdominal distress, such as pain and flatulence, and difficulty in defecation. The patient may experience alternating constipation and diarrhea and even blood in the stool.

PATIENT SCREENING

Vague symptoms of intermittent abdominal pain and constipation are typical. Schedule a consultation with the physician.

ETIOLOGY

The causes are not clear. A diet that contains inadequate roughage and excessive amounts of highly refined foods is thought to contribute to diverticulosis. Lack of roughage produces small-caliber, drier stools, which fail to distend the bowel lumen. This luminal narrowing causes higher intraabdominal pressure during defecation, which in turn contributes to the small herniations or pouches through the mucosa of the muscular wall of the intestine. Diverticular disease can be progressive and is more common after the age of 35 years.

DIAGNOSIS

Diagnosis is based on the clinical picture and an air-contrast barium enema radiographic study.

TREATMENT

A diet that includes adequate fluids and roughage is indicated to produce a soft, formed stool daily; foods with kernels and seeds are omitted. Stress reduction is encouraged, and treatment should include rest and the administration of anticholinergic drugs.

PROGNOSIS

The prognosis is good unless the condition progresses to diverticulitis.

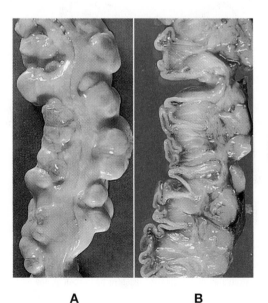
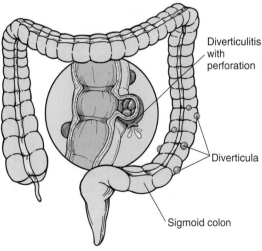

A **B** **C**

FIGURE 8–29 Diverticulosis. (**A** and **B** from Damjanov I, Linder J: *Pathology: a color atlas,* St. Louis, 1999, Mosby.)

PREVENTION

The onset cannot be prevented. Plenty of fluids, bran therapy, and a high-fiber diet rich in fruits and vegetables help prevent constipation and straining during defecation.

PATIENT TEACHING

Instruct the patient to follow the prevention measures mentioned above.

Diverticulitis

DESCRIPTION

Diverticulitis is an inflammation of one or more diverticula.

■ **ICD-9-CM Code** **562.11** *(Without mention of hemorrhage)*
562.13 *(With hemorrhage)*

SYMPTOMS AND SIGNS

When fecal matter becomes trapped in one or more diverticula, inflammation and infection can ensue, causing diverticulitis (see Fig. 8–29, *C*). The patient then has fever, nausea, and abdominal pain in the left lower quadrant, with distention. A palpable mass may be felt, and the patient reports changes in bowel function. The pain sometimes appears in the right lower quadrant or in the suprapubic area. Blood in the stools indicates small hemorrhages. Perforation into the abdominal cavity can produce symptoms of peritonitis, intestinal obstruction, and sepsis. Chronic diverticulitis can cause complications such as the formation of adhesions, abscesses, and fistulas.

PATIENT SCREENING

A patient previously diagnosed with diverticulitis can develop acute symptoms that require prompt medical attention. Warning signs may include persistent abdominal pain, rectal bleeding, fever, and weakness. Because diverticulitis carries the risk of bowel perforation and peritonitis, the condition may be a medical emergency.

ETIOLOGY

Diverticulitis, which is not nearly as common as diverticulosis, can develop when one or more diverticula become inflamed and perforate. Lack of dietary bulk, inadequate fluid intake, and constipation are thought to contribute. Fecal plugs in the diverticula can predispose patients to infection by colonic bacteria.

DIAGNOSIS

The patient is assessed for constipation, fiber and fluid intake, abdominal pain, and blood in the stools. **Sigmoidoscopy** or colonoscopy is performed to visualize the area and to rule out carcinoma. Barium enema study (contraindicated if there is perforation) and flat-plate radiographic examination of the abdomen may reveal the diverticular sacs and the narrowing of the colonic lumen. Blood tests may show leukocytosis, low hemoglobin level, and low hematocrit.

TREATMENT

Treatment is similar to that for diverticulosis and aims to prevent constipation and fight infection. Antibiotics are indicated until the inflammation has resolved, and medication can be used to control hemorrhage. Stool softeners are used, and a liquid diet is encouraged. If the symptoms are severe or if the bowel perforates, surgical intervention to remove the diseased portion of the colon is indicated.

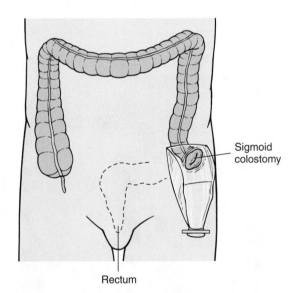

Sigmoid colostomy

Rectum

FIGURE 8–30 Colostomy. Colostomy is a surgical procedure that creates an opening for feces to pass through the abdominal wall. The opening in the colon is brought to the surface of the skin to divert feces into an external pouch worn by the patient. The colostomy may be temporary to promote healing or permanent if the distal bowel has been removed because of malignancy or other disease.

PROGNOSIS

Mild cases are self-limiting. Recovery is more complicated when surgery is required or there is infection, but the final outcome is usually favorable.

PREVENTION

Regular elimination of soft-formed stools is recommended, especially for a patient with diverticulosis.

PATIENT TEACHING

Explain the underlying contributing condition, diverticulosis. Surgical patients who have had a colon resection need to understand the progression to a normal diet and the schedule for antibiotic therapy. Those who have had a colon resection with a diverting colostomy can be referred to an enterostomy nurse for ostomy care and education (Fig. 8–30). Assess for signs of depression after surgery.

Colorectal Cancer

DESCRIPTION

Colorectal cancer is a cancer that arises in any part of the colon or the rectum (Fig. 8–31). It is the third-most-common site of cancer incidence and cause of cancer death in both men and women.

■ **ICD-9-CM Code** **154** *(Malignant neoplasm of rectum, rectosigmoid junction, and anus)*
Colorectal cancer is coded according to the site of the lesion. Refer to the physician's diagnosis and then to the current edition of the ICD-9-CM coding manual to ensure the greatest specificity of pathology and any appropriate modifiers.

SYMPTOMS AND SIGNS

Although symptoms in the early stages are often vague and nonspecific, most patients with colorectal cancer have one or more of the following symptoms at presentation: abdominal pain, change in bowel habits (diarrhea, constipation), bloody stools, rectal bleeding, and symptoms related to iron-deficiency anemia. Colon cancer should be considered in any older patient who develops iron-deficiency anemia. Later symptoms include indigestion, pain with tenderness in the lower abdomen, pallor, **ascites,** *cachexia, lymphadenopathy,* and **hepatomegaly.**

PATIENT SCREENING

Follow office policy for referrals and follow-up appointments.

ETIOLOGY

The risk of developing colon cancer increases with age. More than 90% of cases occur after the age of 50. The genetic disorders of familial adenomatous *polyposis* and hereditary nonpolyposis colorectal cancer predispose affected individuals to the early development of colorectal cancer. Risk factors also include a history of large adenomatous polyps, diabetes mellitus, ulcerative colitis, Crohn disease, or previous pelvic irradiation; a family history of colorectal cancer; cigarette smoking; physical inactivity; obesity; alcohol use; and consumption of red meat. The incidence of colon cancer varies widely from country to country. The highest incidences are in Western Europe and North America, possibly because of the higher average dietary fat intake in those countries.

Adenomas of the colon are thought to be the precursor lesion of colorectal cancer. Adenomas are composed of *dysplastic* epithelium that has proliferated to form a mass. Most colorectal carcinomas arise from adenomas over an average timeframe of 7 years. The vast majority of adenomas, however, do not develop into carcinoma.

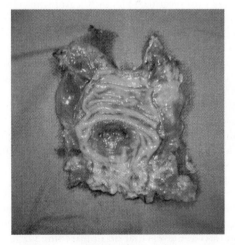

FIGURE 8–31 Adenocarcinoma of distal rectum. (From Doughty DB, Jackson DB: *Gastrointestinal disorders—Mosby's clinical nursing series,* St. Louis, 1993, Mosby.)

DIAGNOSIS

Many early-stage cases of colorectal cancer are detected within a screening program. The major screening tests currently available are the fecal occult blood test, double-contrast barium enema, sigmoidoscopy, and colonoscopy. Colonoscopy is the best test to use for symptomatic patients as well as for screening, as it allows the physician to visualize, sample, and remove lesions throughout the colon. The differential diagnosis of a colonic mass includes many benign and malignant disorders, so histological evaluation is necessary for a cancer and type diagnosis.

Although several staging systems have been proposed for colorectal cancer, physicians now prefer to use the TNM (Tumor, Node, Metastasis) classification system proposed by the American Joint Committee on Cancer. In the case of colorectal cancer, however, "T" reflects the depth of penetration by the tumor into or through the bowel wall rather than the size of the lesion. Clinical staging is determined by physical exam, CT scan of the abdomen and pelvis, and chest radiograph. For rectal cancers, endoscopic ultrasound also may be performed. The most common sites for distant metastases are the liver and lungs.

TREATMENT

Surgical resection of the affected part of the colon or rectum, as well as any affected lymph nodes, is the mainstay of treatment. A colostomy may be necessary if the surgeon cannot reconnect the parts of the colon (see Fig. 8–30). Adjuvant chemotherapy consisting of 5-fluorouracil and leucovorin is recommended for those with stage-III cancer. Metastatic colon cancer can be treated by surgery if the metastasis (usually to the liver) can be removed as well. Radiation therapy is useful in treating cancer confined to the rectum.

PROGNOSIS

The pathologic stage at diagnosis remains the best prognostic indicator. However, a serum tumor marker for colorectal cancer, carcinoembryonic antigen (CEA), also has been shown to have prognostic value. Patients with preoperative serum CEA of greater than 5 ng/ml have a worse prognosis, stage-for-stage, than those with lower levels. Elevated CEA levels that do not become normal after surgery indicate persistent disease. The overall 5-year survival rate is 61%.

PREVENTION

Relatively simple improvements in nutrition and physical activity and the use of available screening procedures could help prevent many cases of colorectal cancer and resulting deaths. A diet high in fruits and vegetables, regular exercise, and maintenance of a healthy weight reduce the risk of colorectal cancer, as do regular use of aspirin or NSAIDs, oral contraceptives, and estrogen-replacement therapy.

Screening for colorectal cancer has two functions. It enables the discovery and removal of adenomas to prevent incidence of cancer, and it detects cancer in the earlier, more curable stages. First, the patient's relative risk of developing colorectal cancer must be determined. A person is considered to be at high risk for colorectal cancer if he or she has hereditary nonpolyposis colon cancer, familial adenomatous polyposis, a previous history of colon cancer or polyps, a history of inflammatory bowel disease, or a family history positive for colorectal cancer. People at average risk for colorectal cancer are urged to start screening at age 50 with a fecal occult blood test every year and sigmoidoscopy every 5 years. Colonoscopy is urged for every 10 years. High-risk patients should start screening by age 40 rather than age 50. Patients with a history of colorectal cancer should receive surveillance colonoscopy at 1 year and then every 3 to 5 years to detect new cancer. Despite the availability and effectiveness of screening, however, fewer then half of adults age 50 or over participate in it.

PATIENT TEACHING

Assess the patient's knowledge of the disease process and the medical plan. Encourage the patient to ask questions and discuss the anxiety he or she feels. Answer questions about procedures. Discuss the side effects of surgery, chemotherapy, or intraoperative radiation therapy. Refer the patient to an ostomy nurse for stoma care. Give emotional support and refer the patient to cancer support groups. Encourage the patient to call the physician or nurse if complications occur.

Pseudomembranous Enterocolitis

DESCRIPTION

Pseudomembranous enterocolitis is acute inflammation with a plaque-like adhesion of necrotic debris and mucus adhered to the damaged superficial mucosa of the small and large intestines.

■ **ICD-9-CM Code 008.45** *(Clostridium difficile)*

SYMPTOMS AND SIGNS

Enterocolitis in which bowel mucosa has a membranous appearance is a disease marked by mild to severe diarrhea. The patient may have a fever, feel weak, and report abdominal cramping and tenderness. Some patients experience nausea and vomiting. If the diarrhea is severe enough, the patient has a dry mouth, is lightheaded and dizzy, and shows signs of dehydration and electrolyte imbalance. The urine is dark and concentrated, and the skin displays decreased *turgor.* Irritation develops around the anal area as a result of the frequent and watery stools; fecal incontinence can be a problem. Blood and mucus may be reported in the stools.

PATIENT SCREENING

A patient on an antibiotic regimen complaining of a sudden onset of copious watery diarrhea, abdominal pain, and fever should seek the advice of the physician prescribing the antibiotic.

ETIOLOGY

Pseudomembranous enterocolitis often is related to the use of broad-spectrum antibiotics; the patient either is taking the antibiotics or has been undergoing antibiotic therapy during the previous 6 weeks. Antibiotic therapy destroys the body's protective natural intestinal flora (along with the target pathogens) and allows a bacterial infection with *Clostridium difficile* to develop. This organism, a cytotoxic-producing strain of a normal gut organism, produces powerful toxins that cause the bowel wall to become inflamed, ulcerated, and necrotic (Fig. 8–32). The products of inflammation and dead tissue form a coating that is called a pseudomembrane.

This disease is more common in health-care facilities, where fecal contamination is more likely. Those who have had abdominal surgery are more susceptible.

DIAGNOSIS

Pseudomembranous enterocolitis is diagnosed when the causative bacteria are found in a stool culture or when *C. difficile* toxin is found in the stool; a rectal biopsy shows the pseudomembranous enterocolitis. The WBC count is elevated as a result of the immune response to the infection. In severe cases, the blood protein (serum albumin) levels are reduced and the serum electrolyte levels are abnormal. Abdominal radiographic films show a distended colon.

TREATMENT

One begins treatment by discontinuing the broad-spectrum antibiotic and substituting vancomycin to fight the infection. In milder cases, cholestyramine resin (Questran) is given to bind the toxins produced by the causative bacteria. Drugs that slow bowel activity are not recommended because they boost the retention of the toxins, thereby increasing damage to the bowel.

The general management of the patient includes monitoring of the fluid and electrolyte balance, with oral or intravenous supplement as needed. Surgery is rarely necessary. Careful hand washing and decontamination techniques are encouraged to prevent cross-infection.

PROGNOSIS

Some cases may require more than one course of antiinfection therapy. Severe cases, though rare, can be life-threatening.

PREVENTION

Prevention includes infection control in a healthcare facility and caution in prescribing broad-spectrum antibiotics to patients who have had abdominal surgery.

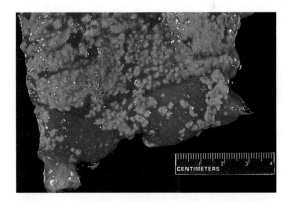

FIGURE 8–32 Pseudomembranous colitis. (From Kumar V, Cotran RS, Robbins SL: *Robbins basic pathology,* ed 7, Philadelphia, 2003, Saunders.)

PATIENT TEACHING

Warn the patient with pseudomembranous entero-colitis that medications that slow peristalsis are con-traindicated.

Short-Bowel Syndrome

DESCRIPTION

In short-bowel syndrome the small bowel fails to absorb nutrients because of inadequate absorptive surface.

 ICD-9-CM Code 579.3 *(Postsurgical, nonabsorption, unspecified, and other)*

SYMPTOMS AND SIGNS

Short-bowel syndrome is the result of an insufficient amount of functioning small bowel to absorb the nutrients, fluid, vitamins, and minerals that the body needs. Depending on the amount of missing or damaged bowel, significant signs of malnutrition are noted, including pathologic changes in other organs and body systems. Because there is insufficient small bowel to digest and absorb food adequately, diarrhea and abnormal stools occur. The patient loses weight and feels weak, tired, and dizzy. As the malnutrition continues, the hair and nails become brittle and rashes develop.

PATIENT SCREENING

The patient may require frequent follow-up appointments during recovery from bowel surgery and until nutritional status has stabilized.

ETIOLOGY

Short-bowel syndrome develops when the length of intact or functioning small bowel is altered significantly by disease or surgery. Crohn disease, intestinal infarction, and trauma are conditions that may cause extensive resection of the small intestine. This loss of functioning small bowel interferes with the digestion and absorption of needed nutrients.

DIAGNOSIS

The patient history initially may indicate the presence of bowel disease, with or without surgical intervention, that has reduced the length or function of part of the small bowel. In short-bowel syndrome, the results of blood tests reflect abnormal electrolyte levels, pH disturbance, and anemia. Stool studies show an increased amount of fat.

TREATMENT

The treatment plan depends on the cause of the syndrome and the particular manifestations of malnutrition. Medical management includes prescription of drugs for infection, diarrhea, vitamin and mineral deficiency, and pain as required. Food supplements are administered orally or intravenously as needed. Surgery may be performed to correct the underlying condition or to reconstruct the bowel. Postsurgical parenteral hyperalimentation is required for weeks or until the remaining gut adapts and becomes functional. Then oral feeding is gradually introduced.

PROGNOSIS

Many patients do quite well, even with extensive resection, as the remaining bowel adapts to increased nutrient absorption.

PREVENTION

After surgical resection of the small bowel, the patient is monitored closely for manifestations of malnutrition and weight loss.

PATIENT TEACHING

After surgery, the patient needs nutritional counseling as oral food is gradually reintroduced. Give instructions for controlling diarrhea with the prescribed agents.

Peritonitis

DESCRIPTION

Peritonitis, the inflammation of the peritoneum, can be acute or chronic and local or generalized.

 ICD-9-CM Code 567
Peritonitis is coded by etiology. Refer to the physician's diagnosis and then to the current edition of the ICD-9-CM coding manual to ensure the greatest specificity of pathology and any appropriate modifiers.

SYMPTOMS AND SIGNS

The large serous membrane that lines the abdominal cavity and folds over the visceral organs is normally transparent and sterile. When it is irritated or infected, the peritoneum becomes *hyperemic* and edematous, as fluid accumulates in the peritoneal space. The inflammatory process of peritonitis has the potential to cause abscesses and adhesions to form in the abdominal cavity (Fig. 8–33).

The patient reports abdominal pain, nausea and vomiting, weakness, and profuse sweating. Abdominal pain may be so severe that the patient may prefer not to move. The clinician who examines the patient finds fever, a tender and distended abdomen, and possibly paralytic ileus. In a fulminating case of peritonitis, the toxic exudate is absorbed by the body, leading to septicemia, shock, and death.

PATIENT SCREENING

A patient presenting with sudden, severe, and diffuse abdominal pain, fever, weakness, nausea, and vomiting requires emergency medical attention.

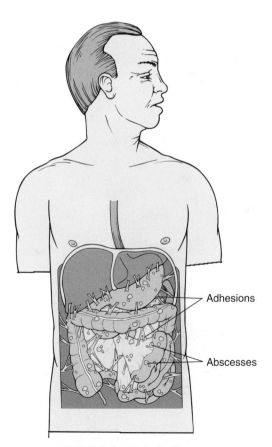

FIGURE 8–33 Peritonitis.

ETIOLOGY

Peritonitis can occur as a primary infection caused by blood-borne organisms or organisms originating in the genital tract. The infection is considered secondary if the source of infection is contamination by GI secretions resulting from a perforation of the GI tract or intraabdominal organs. For example, bacterial invasion could occur after surgery as a result of a breakdown of **anastomoses,** allowing contaminated intestinal secretions to spill into the abdominal cavity. A penetrating wound to the abdomen is another common cause. Systemic lupus erythematosus also can cause bouts of peritonitis as a result of continuous inflammation.

Noninfective secretions, such as bile from a ruptured, inflamed gallbladder, can cause an aseptic peritonitis resulting from chemical irritation of the membrane. Eventually, there is bacterial invasion. The organisms most often involved include *Escherichia coli,* anaerobic streptococci, and *Pseudomonas aeruginosa.*

DIAGNOSIS

Diagnostic findings include an elevated WBC, abnormal serum electrolyte levels (e.g., altered levels of sodium, potassium, and chloride), and gaseous distention of the bowel evident on radiographic examination of the abdomen. Radiographic studies also may reveal perforation of an abdominal organ and air in the abdominal cavity. Aspiration of peritoneal fluid shows cloudy peritoneal fluid and allows a culture and sensitivity study to identify the causative organism.

TREATMENT

The clinical manifestations of peritonitis must be assessed and the source of the irritation or infection identified. The patient is promptly and aggressively treated with broad-spectrum antibiotics, analgesics, and antiemetics. The patient is not given anything by mouth, and fluid and electrolyte losses are replaced parenterally. If there is a perforation, surgery is required to correct the source of infection and to drain the spilled contents. Continuous peritoneal lavage with a saline-antibiotic solution may be appropriate as part of the effort to eliminate the infection.

PROGNOSIS

Without prompt and aggressive medical intervention, peritonitis is life-threatening. The mortality rate was higher before antibiotics were introduced.

PREVENTION

Many of the underlying causes are not easily predicted.

PATIENT TEACHING

After the patient is stabilized by medical interventions, emphasize special instructions in writing about activity, medications, surgical wound care, and follow-up visits.

Hemorrhoids

DESCRIPTION

Hemorrhoids are varicose dilations of a vein in the anal canal or the anorectal area.

ICD-9-CM Code 455
The codes vary by the location and complications. Refer to the physician's diagnosis and then to the current edition of the ICD-9-CM coding manual to ensure the greatest specificity of pathology and any appropriate modifiers.

SYMPTOMS AND SIGNS

Hemorrhoids are tumor-like lesions in the anal area caused by dilated veins; hemorrhoids often are painless. If hemorrhoids are symptomatic, the patient experiences rectal pain, itching, protrusion, or bleeding, especially after defecation. The patient also may experience a mucous discharge from the rectum, a sensation of incomplete evacuation, and difficulty in cleaning the anal area.

PATIENT SCREENING

The patient reporting frequent, unrelieved urge to defecate, severe constipation, or bright red rectal bleeding needs a consultation with the physician.

ETIOLOGY

The veins in the rectal and anal area become varicose, swollen, and tender as a result of blockage. If they are within the rectal wall, these swollen and twisted varicosities are considered internal hemorrhoids; varicosities in the anal area are considered external hemorrhoids (Fig. 8–34). A large, firm subcutaneous lump indicates thrombosis of the external hemorrhoids. Constipation, straining, pregnancy, and any condition that increases pressure on the veins often exacerbate this condition.

DIAGNOSIS

The diagnosis is based on visual inspection of the anal area and **proctoscopy** to visualize internal hemorrhoids of the rectum. The patient's hemoglobin level and red blood cell (RBC) count may be below normal if the patient has experienced significant bleeding.

TREATMENT

Conservative treatment consists of measures to correct constipation and to prevent straining. Stool softeners and a diet high in fruits, vegetables, and whole-grain cereals are recommended. Warm sitz baths may be prescribed, along with a topical anesthetic ointment or witch hazel compresses. Products such as hydrocortisone acetate or pramoxine hydrochloride (ProctoCream-HC) may be applied locally to reduce inflammation. Shark liver oil is also used as a vasoconstrictor, which can reduce the size of hemorrhoids. If these measures do not help, *sclerotherapy* injections may be used to induce scar formation and to reduce prolapse. The hemorrhoids can be destroyed by ligation or by cryosurgery, a procedure that uses a probe to expose the hemorrhoids to extreme cold. Photocoagulation using an infrared device also is effective. Electrocoagulation and

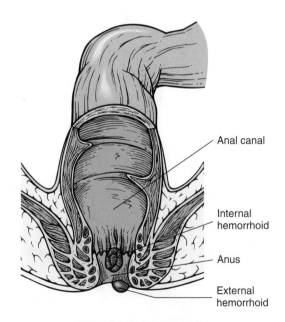

FIGURE 8–34 Hemorrhoids.

thermocoagulation are other alternatives. Lasers can be used, but this is more expensive and hazardous. When bleeding and other symptoms are severe, a hemorrhoidectomy is the best treatment.

PROGNOSIS
The procedures used to treat hemorrhoids produce good results. Complications are uncommon, and recurrences are unusual.

PREVENTION
To prevent exacerbation of the condition, the patient should avoid constipation, prolonged sitting at stool, straining during defecation, and heavy lifting. A high-bulk diet is recommended to promote regular bowel habits.

PATIENT TEACHING
Reinforce the preventive measures listed above. Also encourage adequate fluid intake. Urge good anal hygiene with gentle wiping after stools along with the other comfort measures listed under Treatment. Recommend weight loss for the obese patient. Give special consideration during pregnancy to minimize discomfort.

Diseases of the Liver, Biliary Tract, and Pancreas

The liver, gallbladder, and pancreas are accessory organs of digestion that introduce digestive hormones and enzymes into the alimentary canal, ensuring that the nutrients critical to life can be absorbed selectively by the small intestines into the bloodstream.

Cirrhosis of the Liver

DESCRIPTION
Cirrhosis of the liver is a chronic degenerative disease that is irreversible. It brings slow deterioration of the liver, resulting in the replacement of normal liver cells with hard, fibrous scar tissue, known as hobnail liver.

■ ICD-9-CM Code **571.2** *(Alcoholic cirrhosis of the liver)*

■ ICD-9-CM Code **571.5** *(Without mention of alcohol)*

SYMPTOMS AND SIGNS
Cirrhosis is twice as common in men as in women. As many as 40% of people with cirrhosis of the liver are asymptomatic.

In the early stages of the disease, the symptoms are vague and mild. As the liver is destroyed, the patient experiences loss of appetite and weight, nausea and vomiting, indigestion, abdominal distention (caused by ascites), and edema. The patient tends to bleed and bruise more easily, and frequent nosebleeds are common. The skin appears *jaundiced* and is dry with *pruritus.* Small, red, spidery marks (spider nevi) may appear on the face and body. Changes in the endocrine system cause testicular *atrophy, gynecomastia,* and loss of chest hair in the male (Fig. 8–35).

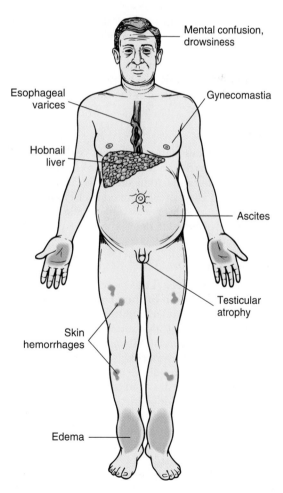

FIGURE 8–35 Cirrhosis of the liver (in the male).

As the cirrhosis advances, memory is impaired, and confusion and drowsiness occur and intensify. If cirrhosis is left untreated, hepatic failure and death eventually follow.

PATIENT SCREENING

The medical history determines the patient's degree of urgency to see the physician. The following changes in a patient diagnosed with cirrhosis should be reported to the physician immediately: changes in behavior or intellectual function, increased ascites, edema, shortness of breath, or GI bleeding.

ETIOLOGY

The causes of cirrhosis are many, but the most common cause is chronic alcoholism. Malnutrition, hepatitis (see Hepatitis A and Hepatitis C), parasites, toxic (poisonous) chemicals, and congestive heart failure are other possible causes of this disease. Inherited disorders such as Wilson disease and hemochromatosis can be predisposing conditions leading to cirrhosis of the liver. Cirrhosis also may be *idiopathic*.

DIAGNOSIS

On physical examination, the liver feels enlarged and firm to hard with a palpable blunt edge; abdominal radiographic films show this enlargement. Blood studies may reveal elevated liver enzyme and bilirubin levels. A liver scan and needle biopsy of the liver are essential to determine the type and extent of fibrosis.

TREATMENT

Treatment is directed at the cause of the disease in an attempt to prevent further damage to the liver. Regardless of the underlying cause, alcohol intake is prohibited. Malnutrition must be prevented, and adequate rest is essential. Vitamin and mineral supplements along with antacids are given. *Diuretics* reduce the excessive fluid (edema) that accumulates in the abdomen (ascites) and ankles. When the disease progresses to liver failure, liver transplantation is a viable option.

PROGNOSIS

Some early liver damage can be reversed. Chronic progressive hepatic disease is the eleventh-leading cause of death in the United States.

PREVENTION

Drinking alcohol only in moderation is the most effective prevention; about half of all cases are due to chronic alcoholism. Avoid chemical toxins such as arsenic and carbon tetrachloride. Shun exposure to infections known to damage the liver, such as those that cause hepatitis. Use caution when taking medications known to be hard on the liver.

PATIENT TEACHING

Because the cause and progression of symptoms vary, patient teaching is highly customized. Give the patient a written schedule explaining how to take prescribed medications. Advise the patient to inform any other physicians or the dentist he or she sees about the cirrhotic liver disease because of the resulting reduction in medication tolerance. Explain the importance of a low-sodium, highly nutritious diet, and give the patient a list of food and alcohol restrictions.

Viral Hepatitis

DESCRIPTION

Viral hepatitis is a systemic infection causing symptoms ranging from mild inflammation of the liver to severe involvement with destruction of hepatic cells. Viral hepatitis, a common cause of acute hepatitis, is endemic in much of the world. Most cases are caused by one of several viral agents described by letters of the alphabet. Some cases lead to chronic viral hepatitis, which is the tenth-leading cause of death among adults in the United States. The transmission of the disease varies with the type of virus: Hepatitis A moves through the fecal-oral route, hepatitis B is transmitted primarily through percutaneous and perimucosal routes, and hepatitis C is bloodborne. Similar symptoms occur with all forms of viral hepatitis. The differential diagnosis is based on laboratory tests. Treatment is symptomatic; some cases respond to antiviral agents.

PATIENT SCREENING

When the patient complains of an abrupt onset of fever, jaundice, malaise, dark urine, and/or yellowing of the sclera of the eyes, prompt medical evaluation is indicated.

NOTE: All universal precautions should be observed when the patient is seen. Hepatitis B vaccine is recommended for health-care workers who are likely to be exposed to bodily fluids.

SYMPTOMS AND SIGNS

Clinical manifestations of viral hepatitis can range from mild to chronic or severe. Many cases are self-limiting with complete recovery, but severe viral hepatitis can be life-threatening when liver function is destroyed and waste products accumulate in the blood. Because the liver has many functions, many abnormal findings are possible in blood and urine tests. The specific type of hepatitis can be established in laboratory tests that look for antibody and antigen markers.

Common symptoms in all forms of hepatitis include abrupt onset of headache, anorexia, malaise, fever, nausea, dark urine, and clay-colored stools. Jaundice and yellowing of the sclera of the eyes are noted. The patient may complain of abdominal discomfort and *myalgia.* Liver enlargement may be noted during physical examination. Some cases are asymptomatic, especially in children.

Hepatitis A

DESCRIPTION

Hepatitis A is highly contagious and causes mild liver infection. The incubation period varies from 15 to 50 days. The symptoms can be mild to severe. In most cases, the infection is self-limiting, liver function is fully recovered, and lifelong immunity to hepatitis A virus (HAV) is conferred.

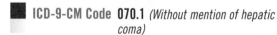 **ICD-9-CM Code 070.1** *(Without mention of hepatic coma)*

ETIOLOGY

The causative virus, HAV, is highly contagious and is transmitted by the fecal-oral route from contaminated food (including shellfish and contaminated strawberries), water, and stools. HAV is present in the stool before symptoms of the disease appear. This form of hepatitis is sometimes known as epidemic or infective hepatitis because it frequently occurs at schools, camps, or institutions.

DIAGNOSIS

A hepatitis profile is performed to identify the antibody and antigen markers and thereby establish the causative virus. Liver function studies are used to support the diagnosis. Blood tests show elevated serum levels of alanine transaminase (ALT) and aspartate transaminase (AST), usually found in the liver. The *prothrombin* time (PT) is prolonged, and the serum bilirubin level is elevated. Urine tests show *proteinuria* and *bilirubinuria.* The presence of antibody to hepatitis A in the serum confirms the diagnosis.

TREATMENT

General medical management includes rest and symptom control. Intramuscular administration of immune globulin is recommended within 2 weeks of exposure. The patient is isolated, and care is taken to prevent cross-infection. Medications to control nausea and pain are given as needed. Other measures taken while the liver heals are a low-fat, high-carbohydrate diet and restriction of physical activity. Alcohol should be avoided at all costs because of its potential to strain the liver.

PROGNOSIS

In adults the disease can be severe during the acute stage and lasts 4 to 8 weeks. Recovery is usually complete.

PREVENTION

A noninfectious vaccine called Havrix currently is recommended before travel into areas where hepatitis A is prevalent and where sanitation is poor. The vaccine should be received at least 2 weeks before potential exposure. One dose is sufficient for primary immunization, and a booster dose is given 6 to 12 months later. The duration of immunity has not been established.

Prevention includes education about proper sanitation, frequent and thorough hand washing, and proper cooking of food.

PATIENT TEACHING

Preventive measures and indications for inoculation with Havrix are recommended. The patient should habitually practice good hand washing, careful food preparation, and thorough cooking. The patient should dispose of fecal matter, including soiled diapers, properly. Person-to-person contamination is common in places like day-care centers.

Hepatitis B

 ICD-9-CM Code **070.30** *(Without mention of coma, also serum hepatitis)*

SYMPTOMS AND SIGNS

The symptoms and signs of hepatitis B, or serum hepatitis, are similar to those mentioned previously. Liver inflammation causes destruction of liver cells and necrosis. These changes can be detected in abnormal results of liver profile studies.

ETIOLOGY

Hepatitis B (HBV) is transmitted primarily through percutaneous and perimucousal routes. The mode of transmission includes contact with blood, semen, vaginal secretions, and saliva. Many infections result from sexual contact or blood exchange from the sharing of contaminated needles. Health-care providers are at risk of infection from accidental inoculation from a contaminated needle puncture or scratch, so all patients must be considered potential sources of the disease, and universal precautions must be practiced (see Chapter 3 or Chapter 12 for a list of universal precautions). An infected mother can transmit the virus during birth.

DIAGNOSIS

First, the patient's history may indicate how the disease was transmitted and the source of the infection. Laboratory tests as mentioned previously are ordered. The detection of hepatitis B surface antigen (HBsAG) and IgM antibody to hepatitis B core antigen (anti-HBc IgM) in the blood confirms the diagnosis. When HbsAg is detected in the blood for more than 6 months, chronic hepatitis is present. While the hepatitis B antigen is present in the blood, the disease is highly transmissible with exposure to blood and body fluids of the infected individual.

TREATMENT

Some cases are self-limiting; general medical management is the same as described previously for hepatitis A virus. Antiviral therapy may be employed in chronic cases when effective results are long lasting without relapses. Hepatitis B immune globulin (HBIG) is given to create passive immunity and is given to the exposed, nonimmune individual. Such exposure may occur through needle sticks or sex with an infected person. Interferon alfa, an antiviral agent, is used in treatment of persistent hepatitis B, but only a small percentage of those given this therapy show lasting benefits from it.

PROGNOSIS

Because HBV can be acute or chronic, the prognosis varies. Some people become chronic carriers because the virus remains in the blood. In most cases, however, the liver heals and regenerates, but this takes time, perhaps several months. Later in life, some patients with chronic hepatitis may be prone to cirrhosis and cancer of the liver.

PREVENTION

Hepatitis B is common enough to cause concern about unvaccinated health-care workers. Employers are required by OSHA to make hepatitis B vaccine available to workers in high-risk occupations. Among the general population, intravenous drug users, homosexual men, and inner-city heterosexuals are at greatest risk. Cases of hepatitis B must be reported to the state health department.

PATIENT TEACHING

Compliance with medical treatment and good follow-up care improve the possibility of a good outcome. Safe practices are taught for procedures that involve blood or body fluids to avoid transmission of HBV. High-risk behaviors and high-risk occupations should be discussed as indicated by the medical history or as needed. Not everyone who is infected with hepatitis is symptomatic, so it can be transmitted unknowingly. This makes awareness of safe practices very important.

Hepatitis C

ICD-9-CM Code **070.51** *(Acute or unspecified hepatitis C without mention of hepatic coma)*
070.54 *(Chronic hepatitis C without mention of hepatic coma)*

SYMPTOMS AND SIGNS

Hepatitis C (HCV), considered a widespread epidemic, is the most common bloodborne infection in the United States. About half of all people who become infected do not know how they were infected with HCV. Many people infected with HCV are asymptomatic and may infect others unknowingly. The incubation period varies from 2 weeks to 6 months. When present, symptoms resemble those of hepatitis A but are typically less severe and sometimes without jaundice. Chronic HCV results in gradual, insidious liver disease. Over a period of years the infection causes necrosis, fibrosis, and cirrhosis of the liver (Fig. 8–36).

Abnormal laboratory findings may include elevated serum levels of liver enzymes and bilirubin, although this evidence is inconclusive without a positive blood test for anti-HCV antibodies. Sometimes the liver is tender and enlarged on physical examination.

ETIOLOGY

Hepatitis C is caused by HCV, which is transmitted by blood and body fluids. Exposure may be traced to blood transfusions, especially those before 1990; kidney dialysis; an organ transplant before 1990; or behaviors involving contact with the blood of an infected person, including sexual contact. Other risk factors include working in the health-care environment, injecting illegal drugs, or sharing articles of personal hygiene with an infected person. When a person infected with HIV becomes infected with HCV, a more rapid progression to end-stage liver disease is likely and may lead to liver transplant. In many cases, the source of infection is not discovered.

DIAGNOSIS

A clinical history of possible exposure to HCV accompanied by symptoms of hepatitis may point to the diagnosis. An ultrasound of the liver may rule out other causes of liver disease. Laboratory findings include elevated serum levels of liver enzymes, elevated serum bilirubin, and bilirubinuria. HCV RNA serum tests detect circulating virus in the blood. A positive blood test result for the presence of anti-HCV antibodies indicates infection, past or present. Liver biopsy confirms the diagnosis.

TREATMENT

No cure for hepatitis C is known. Treatment aims at controlling symptoms and improving long-term liver function. Drug therapy may include gamma globulin, the antiviral agent interferon alfa, and glucocorticoids to reduce inflammation. Supportive measures include rest and a well-balanced diet. The increase in HCV infection (particularly when coinfection with HIV is present) has contributed to a high demand for liver transplants in the United States.

PROGNOSIS

Most patients recover completely. Some patients exhibit signs of chronic hepatitis and eventually, in about 20% of the cases, cirrhosis of the liver. As mentioned previously, coinfection with HIV presents a more complicated prognosis. Chronic hepatitis carries an increased incidence of liver cancer. Some patients die of liver failure.

PREVENTION

Standard universal precautions are strictly practiced. The risk factors of acute hepatitis C are employment in the health-care field, intravenous drug abuse, intranasal cocaine use, multiple sex partners, a history of sexually transmitted diseases, tattooing and body piercing with contaminated needles, and other factors mentioned previously. There is no vaccine for hepatitis C. HCV can exist in a carrier state, that is, without any active disease or in a low-grade infection. In the case of a known infection, every precaution must be taken to avoid transmission of the virus.

PATIENT TEACHING

The patient is taught the importance of diet and rest during the acute stage of infection with HCV. In the case of known infection, one should emphasize precautions to avoid transmission of the virus. Risk factors should be clearly identified. Patients addicted to alcohol or actively using IV drugs should delay treatment until these addictions are under control. When drug therapy is begun, the patient should be taught the possible side effects. Pregnancy is not contraindicated in HCV-infected women, and breast-feeding is considered safe. Medical follow-up and treatment may be recommended.

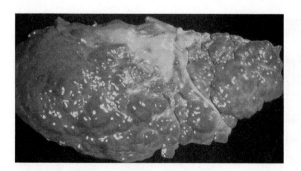

FIGURE 8–36 Cirrhosis of the liver resulting from hepatitis C. (From Cotran R et al: *Robbins pathologic basis of disease*, ed 6, Philadelphia, 1999, Saunders.)

Cancer of the Liver

DESCRIPTION

Hepatocellular carcinoma is a primary tumor of the liver that usually arises in the setting of chronic liver disease (Fig. 8–37).

 ICD-9-CM Code 155.0 *(Primary)*

SYMPTOMS AND SIGNS

Patients who develop hepatocellular carcinoma often have no symptoms other than those associated with their chronic liver disease. Symptoms may include upper abdominal pain, weight loss, early satiety, and a palpable abdominal mass. Physical findings may include ascites, splenomegaly, and jaundice.

PATIENT SCREENING

Schedule a patient with a history of cirrhosis for a prompt appointment on request.

ETIOLOGY

The most important etiologic factor in hepatocellular carcinoma worldwide is hepatitis B virus infection. Additional risk factors include cirrhosis resulting from any cause (e.g., hepatitis C and alcohol) and exposure to aflatoxins (toxins produced by molds that may contaminate food supplies such as corn, soybeans, and peanuts). The incidence of hepatocellular carcinoma varies widely with geographic location. Primary cancer of the liver is rare in more developed areas of the world and usually develops as a metastasis from another site in the body such as the colon, lung, breast, or prostate. However, hepatocellular carcinoma is the main cause of cancer death in Africa and Asia.

DIAGNOSIS

The diagnosis of hepatocellular carcinoma should be suspected in a patient with cirrhosis whose condition suddenly deteriorates. Neoplastic liver cells sometimes secrete alpha-fetoprotein (AFP) that can be detected in the serum. An increase in AFP level to greater than 500 g/L (normal value 10 to 20 g/L) in a high-risk patient is diagnostic of hepatocellular carcinoma. In any patient with an elevated AFP level, a CT scan or MRI of the liver is the next diagnostic procedure. Directed core biopsy can produce a definitive diagnosis, but it may be risky in patients with cirrhosis. Therefore it is attempted only in these patients when the result will affect disease management. Common sites of metastatic spread include bone, lungs, brain, peritoneum, and adrenal glands.

Although several staging systems for hepatocellular carcinoma are available, none has been universally accepted. A TNM (Tumor, Node, Metastasis) staging system has been developed, but it does not consider underlying liver disease, which is an important prognostic indicator. Two other systems, the Okuda system and the CLIP (Cancer of the Liver Italian Program), include measures for the severity of cirrhosis and are used more widely than TNM.

TREATMENT

Surgical resection (partial hepatectomy) of the liver is the treatment of choice for hepatocellular carcinoma, but many patients are not eligible because of tumor extent or underlying liver disease. For patients with a tumor size of less than 5 cm in diameter, no microvascular involvement, and no extrahepatic spread, liver transplantation is an op-

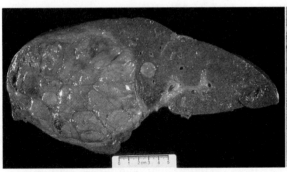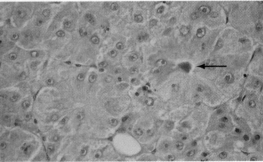

FIGURE 8–37 Hepatocellular carcinoma. (From Cotran R et al: *Robbins pathologic basis of disease,* ed 6, Philadelphia, 1999, Saunders.)

tion. Other nonsurgical options for nonmetastatic disease are *cryoablation* and percutaneous ethanol injection.

PROGNOSIS

The most important factors predicting survival are tumor size and severity of underlying liver disease. Because liver cancer often is detected late, the median survival after diagnosis is 6 to 20 months, and overall 5-year survival is only 5%. Patients living in high-incidence regions and those with higher AFP levels often have a worse prognosis.

PREVENTION

Vaccination against the hepatitis B virus could reduce the high rate of hepatocellular carcinoma worldwide. Despite a lack of evidence that screening programs are effective, there are programs that screen high-risk individuals with cirrhosis who would be candidates for surgical treatment if a cancer is detected. These programs measure the participant's AFP and perform ultrasonography every 6 months.

PATIENT TEACHING

The clinical effects of liver cancer present many indications for comprehensive support measures. Explain the need for special diet restrictions and total abstinence from alcohol. The treatment plan will be highly customized, depending on the therapies employed and the stage of the cancer.

Give written as well as oral directions. Preoperative and postoperative instructions may be indicated. Emotional support is of primary importance for the family as well as the patient.

Cholelithiasis (Gallstones)

DESCRIPTION

Cholelithiasis is a common condition in which there is an abnormal presence of calculi or gallstones that form in the bile.

■ **ICD-9-CM Code 574.20** *(Without cholecystitis and without mention of obstruction)*

SYMPTOMS AND SIGNS

The patient with cholelithiasis (gallstones) may be asymptomatic until the bile ducts become obstructed by the stones (Fig. 8–38, *A* and *B*). Colicky pain, or biliary colic, signals the obstruction of the cystic duct or the common bile duct by one or more stones. The pain is in the epigastric region or the right upper quadrant of the abdomen, often radiating to the right upper back in the area of the scapula. Nausea and vomiting accompany the pain. If the obstruction is prolonged, jaundice may appear.

PATIENT SCREENING

Biliary colic begins with sudden severe waves of pain in the upper right quadrant (URQ) of the

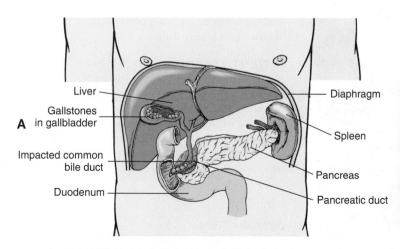

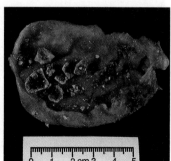

Liver —
Gallstones in gallbladder —
A
Impacted common bile duct —
Duodenum —
— Diaphragm
— Spleen
— Pancreas
— Pancreatic duct
B

FIGURE 8–38 A, Cholelithiasis. **B,** Cholesterol gallstones. (**B** from Kumar V, Cotran RS, Robbins SL: *Robbins basic pathology,* ed 7, Philadelphia, 2003, Saunders.)

abdomen that may radiate to the back. Initially, medication for pain is given as soon as possible. Ask about nausea and vomiting and note the presence of jaundice.

ETIOLOGY

Gallstones form in the gallbladder from insoluble cholesterol and bile salts; they vary in size and number. The reasons they form are not always clear, although they are more common with increasing age, with the high-calorie, high-cholesterol diet associated with obesity, and in the female population. Other risk factors are oral contraceptive use, pancreatitis, and ileal disease. People with alcoholic cirrhosis or biliary tract infection are also susceptible.

DIAGNOSIS

The clinical picture and ultrasonography of the gallbladder and biliary ducts are highly accurate in confirming the presence of cholelithiasis. Other diagnostic studies that reveal gallstones are radioisotope scan, oral *cholecystogram,* and intravenous *cholangiogram* (Fig. 8–39). One can estimate the size and type of stones with some accu-

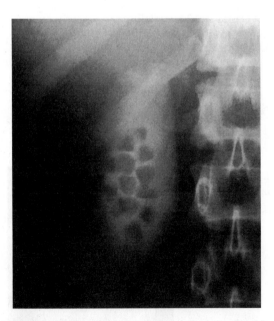

FIGURE 8–39 Oral cholecystogram. (From Doughty DB, Jackson DB: *Gastrointestinal disorders—Mosby's clinical nursing series,* St. Louis, 1993, Mosby.)

racy through test results. The serum bilirubin level is elevated with obstruction of the common bile duct.

TREATMENT

Asymptomatic gallstones are usually left alone. Fatty intake should be controlled through dietary changes. If the patient experiences recurring pain, surgical removal of the gallbladder (cholecystectomy) is indicated. A surgical procedure called laparoscopic cholecystectomy has shortened hospitalization and recovery time. The use of oral preparations called bile acids (chenodeoxycholic or ursodeoxycholic acid) to dissolve the gallstones may be attempted in some cases; it is most successful in patients with pure cholesterol gallstones that are less than one-half inch in diameter. It is usually not successful with calcified stones. Another nonsurgical treatment is called extracorporeal shock wave lithotripsy (ESWL). This method is considered safe and preserves the function of the gallbladder, but positive results have been limited.

PROGNOSIS

In mild cases diet modifications resolve symptoms. When there is infection, the recovery depends on a good response to antibiotics. Recovery varies with the method of treatment, as mentioned above. Nonsurgical interventions require more time to achieve results.

PREVENTION

A low-fat diet may help prevent attacks of biliary colic. Surgery may be required to prevent the complications of chronic obstructive disease of the gallbladder and biliary disease.

PATIENT TEACHING

Explain the risk factors, including a high-fat, high-calorie diet; hormone replacement therapy; obesity; diabetes; and liver disease. Emphasize the importance of the low-fat diet and the purpose of the prescribed medication. List the signs and symptoms that may indicate the onset of cholecystitis (see below).

Cholecystitis

DESCRIPTION

Cholecystitis is acute or chronic inflammation of the gallbladder, usually associated with obstruction of the cystic duct.

ICD-9-CM Code **575.12** *(Acute and chronic cholecystitis)*
Refer to the physician's diagnosis and then to the current edition of the ICD-9-CM coding manual to ensure the greatest specificity of pathology and any appropriate modifiers.

SYMPTOMS AND SIGNS

Cholecystitis, or inflammation of the gallbladder, usually is associated with cholelithiasis; infection often follows the inflammation (Fig. 8–40). The condition can become chronic.

The patient experiences acute colicky pain, which localizes in the right upper quadrant of the abdomen and becomes more severe while radiating around to the right lower scapular region. In addition, the patient experiences nausea and vomiting followed by guarding of the right upper quadrant muscles and shallow respirations. A fever may ensue. Other signs are jaundice, clay-colored stools, dark urine, and pruritis. In some cases, the acutely inflamed gallbladder ruptures, causing peritonitis. Otherwise, the cholecystitis may spontaneously subside, and the pain begins to abate in a few days.

PATIENT SCREENING

Acute onset of biliary colic with nausea, vomiting, chills, fever, and jaundice requires a swift medical evaluation.

ETIOLOGY

Most cholecystitis results from an obstruction of the biliary duct caused by gallstones. Trauma or other insult to the gallbladder, including infection, occasionally is the cause.

DIAGNOSIS

The diagnosis is based on the clinical picture and an ultrasonogram of the gallbladder and biliary ducts. Radiographic gallbladder studies that indicate a *nonvisualized* gallbladder indicate gallbladder disease. Other findings include an elevated WBC count and an increased serum bilirubin level.

TREATMENT

Treatment in uncomplicated cases consists of dietary modification with elimination of fatty foods. The acutely ill patient with persistent vomiting is given nothing by mouth, and a nasogastric tube is inserted. Intravenous feeding is given to replace fluids and electrolytes. When the patient is stabilized, surgical intervention to remove the gallbladder (cholecystectomy) is indicated. Medical management may include the administration of antibiotics, analgesics, and antiemetics.

PROGNOSIS

Mild and uncomplicated cases have a good prognosis. Chronic cholecystitis has been associated with fibrotic changes and may predispose the patient to adenocarcinoma of the gallbladder.

PREVENTION

Early medical attention and dietary modifications at the onset of symptoms related to inflammation of the gallbladder are the initial attempts to control the stages and complications of chronic gallbladder disease.

PATIENT TEACHING

Explain the relationship of a high-calorie, high-fat diet to the onset of gallstone disease that can in turn predispose to inflammation of the gallbladder. If a patient undergoes cholecystectomy, explain that the liver will continue to produce bile for fat digestion.

Acute and Chronic Pancreatitis

DESCRIPTION

Pancreatitis is acute or chronic inflammation of the pancreas with variable involvement of adjacent and remote organs.

ICD-9-CM Code **577.0** *(Acute pancreatitis)*
577.1 *(Chronic pancreatitis)*

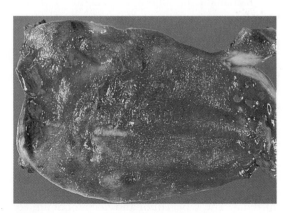

FIGURE 8–40 Cholecystitis. (From Damjanov I, Linder J: *Pathology: a color atlas*, St. Louis, 1999, Mosby.)

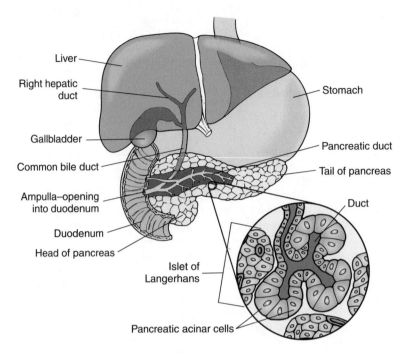

FIGURE 8–41 Location and structure of the pancreas.

SYMPTOMS AND SIGNS

Pancreatitis is inflammation of the pancreas (Fig. 8–41). It can range from a mild and self-limiting disease to a chronic and fatal destruction of pancreatic tissue. In pancreatitis, the pancreas, which functions as both an endocrine and an exocrine organ, becomes inflamed, edematous, hemorrhagic, and necrotic (Fig. 8–42). The patient with acute pancreatitis has a sudden onset of severe abdominal pain, which radiates to the back, along with nausea and vomiting. The patient is acutely ill, *diaphoretic*, and *tachycardic* and experiences shallow, rapid respirations. Blood pressure falls, and the temperature rises. The abdomen is tender, especially in the upper abdomen radiating to the lower abdomen. Bowel sounds are reduced. Many local and systemic complications (e.g., pancreatic abscess and pneumonia) are possible.

Chronic pancreatitis can present a more vague clinical picture. The patient may report constant pain in the back, with repeated mild episodes of the symptoms of acute pancreatitis. As pancreatic function deteriorates and the organ becomes fibrotic, signs of malabsorption and diabetes mellitus appear. Psychiatric disturbances have been reported.

PATIENT SCREENING

Acute pancreatitis is a life-threatening emergency. Systemic symptoms listed previously require emergency medical intervention.

ETIOLOGY

Several theories have been proposed for the mechanism that initiates acute pancreatitis and that triggers pancreatic autodigestion. Alcoholism, biliary tract disease, trauma, infection, structural anomalies, greatly elevated calcium levels in the blood, hemorrhage, *hyperlipidemia*, or drugs may cause pancreatitis. Gallstones often cause pancreatitis in the nonalcoholic individual. Less often, the cause is a metabolic or endocrine disorder. Some cases are idiopathic.

DIAGNOSIS

The diagnosis is based on the clinical picture, with dramatically elevated serum amylase and lipase levels on the first day of the attack. Serum amylase and lipase levels usually return to normal by the third day. The WBC count and hematocrit are elevated. Glucose levels may be high, indicating hyperglycemia. Radiographic films and ultrasono-

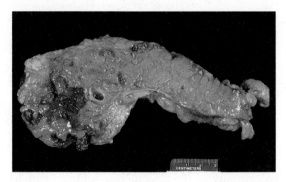

FIGURE 8–42 Acute pancreatitis. (From Cotran R et al: *Robbins pathologic basis of disease,* ed 6, Philadelphia, 1999, Saunders.)

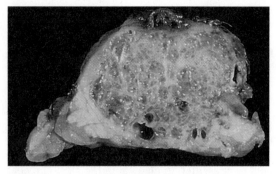

FIGURE 8–43 Pancreatic cancer. (From Cotran R et al: *Robbins pathologic basis of disease,* ed 6, Philadelphia, 1999, Saunders.)

gram may demonstrate stones in the biliary tract or dilation of the common bile duct, and the bilirubin level may be elevated. CT scan, with oral or intravenous contrast material, identifies pancreatic changes and complications.

TREATMENT

Most cases are mild without systemic and local complications, and treatment then consists of general supportive care. In other instances, acute pancreatitis may require emergency treatment consisting of intravenous fluid and electrolyte replacement. The patient is given nothing by mouth. The placement of a nasogastric suction tube with intermittent suction may be indicated for about 1 week. Pain medication, usually meperidine (Demerol) hydrochloride, is given generously. Antibiotics are administered to treat the bacterial infection, and anticholinergics are given to slow bowel motility and to reduce the pancreatic secretions. Laboratory blood values of electrolytes, serum amylase and lipase, hematocrit, glucose, and serum calcium are monitored.

In chronic pancreatitis, the patient also must be monitored closely for malabsorption, *steatorrhea,* and impaired glucose tolerance indicating diabetes mellitus. If the underlying cause of pancreatitis is an obstructed pancreatic duct, then surgery may be necessary to remove the obstruction.

PROGNOSIS

Eighty percent of mild cases resolve within a week. Severe cases with systemic complications or pancreatic necrosis face a variable outcome. The mortality rate varies from 15% to 100%.

PREVENTION

Preventive measures are based on the many clinical conditions, medications, and toxins associated with acute pancreatitis.

PATIENT TEACHING

Explain the measures needed to reduce recurrent episodes: forgoing alcohol, if the cause is alcohol related, and carefully managing gallstone disease. Teach the warning signs of endocrine and exocrine insufficiency: weight loss, digestive disturbance, and the signs and symptoms of hypoglycemia and hyperglycemia.

Pancreatic Cancer

DESCRIPTION

Cancer of the pancreas is a neoplasm, usually an adenocarcinoma, and occurs more often in the head of the pancreas (Fig. 8–43). Most neoplasms arise from the exocrine cells of the pancreas, while 1% to 2% involve the endocrine cells.

■ **ICD-9-CM Code 157.9** *(Part unspecified)*

SYMPTOMS AND SIGNS

Most patients with pancreatic cancer experience abdominal pain, weight loss, or jaundice. Nausea, vomiting, and steatorrhea are also common. On examination, the patient may have a palpable liver, abdominal tenderness, or a palpable gallbladder. As pancreatic tissue is infiltrated and destroyed, the patient can experience glucose intolerance increasing weakness, fatigue, and diarrhea.

Emotional disturbances and depression may appear in conjunction with a fear of fatal illness.

PATIENT SCREENING

The patient often reports feeling generally quite ill and experiencing the symptoms listed previously; a prompt appointment is indicated.

ETIOLOGY

Cancer of the pancreas is the fourth-leading cause of cancer-related death in the United States. It occurs twice as often in males as in females. The peak age of incidence is in the 40- to 60-year-old age group. Risk factors include cigarette smoking, a diet with a high intake of fat and/or meat, a history of chronic pancreatitis or diabetes, and a family history of pancreatic cancer.

DIAGNOSIS

Because of the retroperitoneal location of the pancreas, carcinoma is difficult to detect. The pancreas is inaccessible to palpation and insensitive to many diagnostic techniques. The diagnosis of pancreatic cancer is typically made radiographically and histologically. The initial study in a patient with suspected pancreatic cancer is either an abdominal ultrasound or a CT scan. Cancer is suggested by dilated bile ducts or a mass in the pancreas. If a mass lesion is present, the patient may be a candidate for surgery if the patient shows no evidence of distant metastases and no involvement of the major vessels. If the patient is unfit for surgical resection, a tissue diagnosis by endoscopic ultrasound-guided fine-needle aspiration biopsy is necessary to guide palliative treatment. Pancreatic tumors are classified and staged according to the TNM (Tumor, Node, Metastasis) classification system proposed by the American Joint Committee on Cancer. For this type of cancer, "T" reflects the presence and degree of tumor extension though the pancreatic capsule rather than the size of the lesion.

TREATMENT

Surgical resection is the only potentially curative treatment for pancreatic cancer. It is a viable option only for patients with disease confined to the pancreas and peripancreatic nodes. Because of late detection of the disease, however, only 15% to 20% of patients are candidates for surgery. For palliative treatment of advanced pancreatic cancer, chemotherapy with single-agent gemcitabine is the current standard of care. Stents can be placed to relieve bile-duct obstruction or gastric-outlet obstruction. Control of pain and treatment of depression are also important in the palliation of pancreatic cancer. Weight loss and malabsorption often are treated with pancreatic enzyme replacement.

PROGNOSIS

The prognosis is poor even after surgical resection; the 5-year survival rate is about 10% to 25%. The median survival is 8 to 12 months for those with locally advanced, unresectable disease and 3 to 6 months for those with metastatic disease. The overall 5-year survival rate is only 4%. The tumor can invade adjacent structures such as the duodenum, stomach, and liver, and death often results from these local effects.

PREVENTION

Cessation of cigarette smoking is recommended, as is ingestion of less meat and more vegetables. Although screening programs are available for people at high risk (those with family cancer syndromes or hereditary pancreatitis), no screening strategy has been shown to detect potentially curable, early pancreatic cancers in these patients.

PATIENT TEACHING

Give the patient and family both written and verbal instructions about surgery, pain management, and chemotherapy as indicated. Allow the time and opportunity for the patient and family to ask questions and express their feelings and anxiety. Make referrals for home care, hospice care, and social services, as needed.

Disorders of Nutrient Intake and Absorption

Proper nutrition is needed to enable the regulation and function of all body processes and to ensure that the body is healthy and has energy and nutrients to build and repair tissue. Nutritional deficiencies, excesses, or imbalances can affect the body's homeostasis. Any inability of the GI tract to digest or absorb nutrients can cause forms of malnutrition, even with adequate intake of food. Prolonged malnutrition or malabsorption results in anatomic lesions or disease entities.

ENRICHMENT

HYPERVITAMINOSIS

- Hypervitaminosis is a condition of toxicity resulting from an excess of any vitamin, but especially the fat-soluble vitamins A and D.
- The four fat (lipid)-soluble vitamins A, D, E, and K are stored in fat tissue.
- Symptoms of vitamin A toxicity include irritability, loss of hair, anorexia, enlargement of the liver and spleen, jaundice, skin changes, and psychiatric disorders. Vitamin A excess can be toxic to a developing fetus. Chronic toxicity in infants and children can cause increased pressure in the brain, tinnitus, pruritus, swelling of the optic nerve, and abnormal bone growth.
- Vitamin D is considered highly toxic, especially in infants and children. It can cause calcification of soft tissue, kidney damage, excessive thirst and urination, and mental changes.
- Very high doses of vitamin E may interfere with the blood-clotting action of vitamin K.
- Vitamin K toxicity is uncommon. Rapid infusion causes dyspnea, flushing, cardiovascular complications, red-blood-cell hemolysis, jaundice, and brain damage.
- Water-soluble vitamin C taken in excess causes nausea, diarrhea, and acidification of urine; niacin (B_3) may cause flushing, hyperglycemia, and liver damage; vitamin B_6 may cause photosensitivity and peripheral nerve damage.
- Overload of nutritional trace elements also produces toxicity.

Malnutrition

DESCRIPTION

Malnutrition is a disorder of nutrition caused by primary deprivation of protein energy (seen in poverty or self-imposed starvation) or secondary to deficiency diseases (such as cancer or diabetes).

 ICD-9-CM Code 263.9 *(NOS)*

SYMPTOMS AND SIGNS

Disturbances in nutrition can result from eating too much or too little food or from having an imbalanced diet. Even when diet is sufficient, however, if the body cannot absorb or use food properly, malnutrition results. Malnutrition disrupts the body's metabolic processes, disturbing normal physical structure and biologic function.

Malnourishment can cause many specific disease conditions, such as abnormal growth, with physical and intellectual impairment. The body deprived of adequate nutrition begins to manifest the loss of well-being externally and internally. The appetite may decrease or increase, resulting in emaciation or obesity. Signs and symptoms of malnutrition include loss of energy, diarrhea, drastic weight change, skin lesions, loss of hair, poor nails, and generalized edema; delayed healing and greasy stools may result from loss of fat. More advanced signs may include muscle wasting, enlarged glands, and hepatomegaly. Many abnormal findings of blood and urine tests are possible.

PATIENT TEACHING

A patient with a recent, unintended weight loss of 10 pounds should be scheduled for a complete physical examination.

ETIOLOGY

Various conditions and circumstances cause malnutrition, including famine, eating disorders, chronic illnesses, fad diets, poverty, biochemical disorders, certain medications, and various malabsorption syndromes. Without a special diet, a burn patient or a patient with severe trauma easily could experience inadequate nutrition.

When the body experiences prolonged deprivation of calories and nutrients, it begins to break down its own tissue to meet its caloric needs. Another syndrome results if caloric intake is adequate, but protein intake is low: The patient may not appear malnourished, but he or she loses important proteins.

DIAGNOSIS

Clinical evaluation of the patient includes a complete physical examination with special attention to weight and measurements of body fat and muscle mass. Laboratory diagnostic findings differ depending on the cause and type of malnutrition. Laboratory tests include blood protein levels, complete blood counts, and a 24-hour urine test for urea nitrogen. The tests may show evidence of mineral deficiency, anemia, abnormal protein metabolism, and other changes in metabolism related to malnourishment.

TREATMENT

The treatment of malnutrition is based on the underlying cause. After the patient's nutritional needs are assessed, nutritional supplements and replacement begin with appropriate oral and intravenous feedings. Certain pathologic condi-

tions may necessitate feedings through a nasogastric tube. Treatment may entail a combination of dietary modifications, including appropriate supplements of proteins, vitamins, and minerals. Diarrhea and infections are controlled with medications.

Surgery may be indicated when lesions of the GI tract cause the malnutrition. Patients with eating disorders require special counseling with medical treatment. The poor and elderly may require community services that make good nutrition available on a daily basis.

PROGNOSIS

The prognosis varies with the nature and severity of malnutrition. Severe cases have a high morbidity and mortality rate.

PREVENTION

Address the underlying cause to correct nutritional deficiencies, restore weight, and prevent complications.

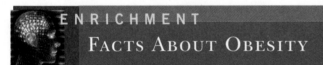

ENRICHMENT
FACTS ABOUT OBESITY

- About 34 million adult Americans are overweight despite the popularity of fad diets and sugar-free and fat-free products.
- More women are afflicted with obesity than men, especially as they age.
- Obesity is identified objectively by the use of height–weight tables and is defined as being 20% or more overweight.
- The causes of simple obesity are many and complex, but it often is associated with greater energy intake than output.
- Fatness and the regional distribution of fat have a strong genetic component.
- Factors that may contribute to obesity include overeating (sometimes linked to psychological stress or environment), a low rate of energy expenditure, inactivity, and more rarely, endocrine disorders.
- Obesity can lead to severe health problems, such as diabetes mellitus, hypertension, cardiovascular disease, sleep apnea, blood lipid abnormalities, and skin problems. Being overweight when younger than 45 years is more dangerous.

- Obesity can make a person feel self-conscious and can impair social relationships; overweight people sometimes experience prejudice and discrimination.
- Treatment goals are (1) to lose as much nonessential fat as possible while minimizing the loss of lean body mass and (2) to maintain a balance between energy intake and energy expenditure.
- Important elements in successful weight loss are active patient self-control, a supportive physician, a reduced-calorie, nutritionally adequate diet, and increased physical activity.
- Other controversial treatment modalities that have known risks, or lack proven long-term success, include extremely low-calorie diets, anorectic drugs, and surgical procedures.
- Many patients have great difficulty maintaining their reduced body weight. Exercise and control of food intake through behavior modification remain important.
- Consultation with a physician is recommended before a patient starts a substantial weight-loss program.

PATIENT TEACHING

After contributing factors have been identified, one can explain the treatment plan and the goals of therapy. Nutritional status is monitored, and the therapeutic diet is adjusted to allow for the patient's preferences. Address the psychological problems associated with eating disorders by making referrals for counseling and support.

Malabsorption Syndrome

DESCRIPTION

Malabsorption syndrome refers to a group of disorders in which intestinal absorption of dietary nutrients is impaired.

 ICD-9-CM Code 579.9 *(NOS)*

SYMPTOMS AND SIGNS

A person with malabsorption syndrome has impaired digestion and is unable to absorb fat or certain other components of diet. Symptoms include abdominal discomfort, bloating with gas, chronic diarrhea, and abnormal bowel movements. Stools may appear yellowish gray and may be greasy looking. The stools tend to float because of their high fat content. Over time, untreated malabsorption leads to weight loss, anemia, shortness of breath, and symptoms of vitamin and mineral deficiencies.

PATIENT SCREENING

The patient with malabsorption syndrome needs regular appointments for follow-up care until stable.

ETIOLOGY

The main cause of malabsorption syndrome is defective mucosal cells in the small intestine. Absorption also is hindered if the intestinal enzymes and chemicals are not properly assisting the digestive process. A diseased pancreas or a blocked pancreatic duct, which deprives the small intestine of *lipase,* may cause secondary malabsorption syndrome. Reduced secretion of bile, caused by hepatic disease or a bile-duct obstruction, also prevents lipid (fat) digestion. Metabolic or endocrine disorders such as *hyperparathyroidism* and diabetes mellitus are other possible causes of the syndrome. Severe parasitic and worm infestations, more common in underdeveloped countries, can cause malabsorption.

DIAGNOSIS

The physician usually orders several blood tests to determine the levels of proteins, fats, and minerals in the patient's bloodstream. A laboratory analysis of a stool sample also may be performed. Biopsy of the small bowel may reveal a primary condition responsible for malabsorption.

TREATMENT

The main task for the physician is to discover the underlying cause and to choose the course of treatment. Diet is controlled carefully. A high-protein, high-calorie diet with vitamin and mineral supplements, such as the fat-soluble vitamins A, D, E, and K, which are not being absorbed, aids the recovery.

PROGNOSIS

Improvement can be expected when the underlying causes are identified and successfully treated. When areas of the intestines are damaged or resected, the remaining bowel can adapt to absorb nutrients.

PREVENTION

Many specific and nonspecific therapies are available for malabsorption.

PATIENT TEACHING

Refer the patient to a dietitian for a nutrient-specific therapeutic diet. Give written instructions about prescribed vitamins and supplements. Instruct the patient to monitor his or her weight and return for follow-up testing for anemia.

Celiac Disease (Gluten Enteropathy)

DESCRIPTION

Celiac disease (celiac sprue) is a disease of the small intestine that is characterized by malabsorption, gluten intolerance, and damage to the lining of the intestine.

 ICD-9-CM Code 579.0

SYMPTOMS AND SIGNS

Symptoms include weight loss, anorexia, diarrhea, flatulence (gas), abdominal distention, intestinal bleeding, dermatitis, and the characteristically large, pale, greasy, foul-smelling stools. The end result of celiac disease is malabsorption and malnutrition.

PATIENT SCREENING

Assess the severity of symptoms to determine the patient's level of urgency to be seen by the physician.

ETIOLOGY

The cause of this disease may be either a toxic or an immunologic reaction to a component of gluten (a protein that is found in wheat and wheat products, barley, and oats). Celiac disease is linked to genetic factors because the occurrence is higher in siblings. Females are affected twice as often as males.

DIAGNOSIS

Celiac disease is often difficult to diagnose and differentiate from other intestinal diseases and disorders. For a positive diagnosis, two criteria are needed: (1) a biopsy of the small intestine showing changes or destruction in the mucosal lining and (2) improvement while on a gluten-free diet. Laboratory tests that may be ordered include blood tests for WBC count, platelet count, albumin level, and PT; and a glucose tolerance test. Upper-GI and small-bowel radiographic series demonstrate the characteristic abnormal patterns of barium passage.

TREATMENT

The patient must strictly adhere to a gluten-free diet. If the patient does not improve while on the diet, corticosteroid drugs may be used. Patients with this disease are more prone to develop abdominal lymphoma and cancer later in life, and they should be examined if GI symptoms develop.

PROGNOSIS

A gluten-free diet usually leads to gradual recovery.

PREVENTION

No known prevention for celiac disease is known.

PATIENT TEACHING

Refer the patient to a dietitian. For grains, the patient consumes corn and rice.

Food Poisoning

DESCRIPTION

Food poisoning is an illness resulting from the eating of foods that contain bacterial or toxic substances.

 ICD-9-CM Code 005.9 *(Unspecified)*

SYMPTOMS AND SIGNS

The symptoms of food poisoning are determined, in part, by the cause. The onset is sudden, with rumbling stomach sounds, nausea, vomiting, diarrhea with abdominal pain and cramps, malaise, and fever. The symptoms usually disappear within 24 to 48 hours. If an extreme case of food poisoning persists, the patient becomes disabled, and the situation becomes life-threatening.

PATIENT SCREENING

Screen the patient for severity of symptoms and signs of dehydration, mindful that the very young and the elderly are more prone to dehydration.

ETIOLOGY

True food poisoning includes poisoning from mushrooms, shellfish, foods contaminated with poisonous insecticides, and toxic substances such as lead and mercury. In addition, poisoning results from eating foods that have undergone putrefaction or decomposition and foods contaminated with bacteria or their toxins (Table 8–1).

DIAGNOSIS

The patient's history is important to diagnosis and can point to the cause. The physician may perform endoscopy. A stool or blood culture reveals the presence of any parasites or bacteria. The actual contaminated food also may be cultured.

TREATMENT

Most treatment is symptomatic. Bed rest is beneficial. To prevent or minimize fluid and electrolyte imbalances, nutritional support and fluid replacement are essential. These may have to be given intravenously if the patient becomes dehydrated. The physician may prescribe antidiarrheal and antiemetic agents.

PROGNOSIS

The prognosis for this condition varies with the cause. The prognosis generally is good if the cause has been determined and the treatment has begun. The earlier the diagnosis is made and treatment is begun, the better the chance is for a successful recovery. Many infections are mild and self-limiting.

PREVENTION

Food poisoning can be prevented by the fastidious practice of infection-control techniques as a first line of defense. Careful hand washing to avoid oral-

TABLE 8-1
Bacterial Causes of Food Poisoning

ORGANISM	MAJOR FOOD SOURCE(S)	PATHOPHYSIOLOGIC MECHANISM	
		TOXIN IN FOOD	INGESTION OF BACTERIA
Staphylococcus aureus	Cooked meat, cheese, pasta, cream buns, custard pies	Yes	No
Clostridium perfringens type A	Cooked meat, vegetable soup (prepared in bulk)	No	Yes (bacteria release enterotoxin in intestine)
Clostridium botulinum	Uneviscerated cured fish, preserved or fermented meat, home-preserved vegetables	Yes	No
Salmonella enteritidis/ Salmonella typhimurium	Raw eggs, mayonnaise, incompletely cooked meat and poultry	No	Yes
Salmonella dublin	Raw milk, unpasteurized cheese	No	Yes
Salmonella typhi/ Salmonella paratyphi	Food contamination by infected food handlers	No	Yes
Vibrio cholerae 01	Raw seafood	No	Yes
Vibrio cholerae non-01	Raw oysters	No	Yes
Vibrio parahaemolyticus	Raw seafood	No	Yes
Vibrio vulnificus	Raw seafood (especially oysters)	No	Yes
Listeria monocytogenes	Soft cheese	No	Yes
Shigella species	Food contamination during preparation	No	Yes
Escherichia coli 0157:H7	Ground beef	No	Yes
Campylobacter jejuni/ Campylobacter coli	Incompletely cooked poultry and other meats, raw milk	No	Yes
Bacillus cereus			
Heat-stable toxin	Fried rice	Yes	No
Enterotoxin	Meat products	Yes	No
Yersinia enterocolitica	Pork, raw milk	No	Yes

From Goldman L, Bennett JC: *Cecil textbook of medicine,* ed 21, vol. 1, Philadelphia, 2000, Saunders.

fecal transmission of disease-causing organisms is especially important in day-care centers and institutions. Avoid swimming in contaminated water and drinking untreated water. Careful handling of food and eating of well-cooked foods and those that are well refrigerated reduce the risk.

PATIENT TEACHING
Emphasize preventive measures listed above. Patients who are stabilized after a severe episode are given a diet as tolerated and are advised to rest.

Anorexia Nervosa

DESCRIPTION
Anorexia nervosa is linked to a psychological disturbance in which hunger is denied by self-imposed starvation, resulting from a distorted body image and a compulsion to be thin (Fig. 8–44).

 ICD-9-CM Code **307.1**
Refer to the current edition of the ICD-9-CM coding manual for exclusions.

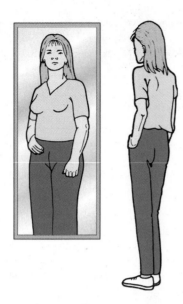

FIGURE 8–44 Anorexia nervosa. Persons with anorexia overestimate their body width, insisting that they are too fat despite profound weight loss.

SYMPTOMS AND SIGNS

The typical anorectic patient is a female adolescent who is meticulous, is a high achiever, and refuses food intake; she is preoccupied with obesity and obsessed with her weight. Although she experiences continued weight loss, she does not believe that anything is wrong. Concerned family members usually are the ones who bring the problem to the physician when the girl loses weight and body mass. She may have amenorrhea, constipation, bloating, or abdominal distress. This girl usually is hyperactive, exercises a great deal, is hypotensive, and experiences bradycardia and hypothermia. Bulimia sometimes occurs simultaneously.

PATIENT SCREENING

A parent or responsible party may be the first to report concern about a person's weight loss and anorexia; the patient frequently denies the condition until it is more advanced. Recommend a physical examination and consultation with the physician.

ETIOLOGY

Anorexia nervosa afflicts predominately younger, affluent females, although the prevalence among the male population is rising. The etiology is un-known, although it is believed that family and social factors may precipitate the condition. Current social and cultural factors promote thinness, which reinforces anorectic behavior. There may be a genetic predisposition. The patient often is intelligent, has a compulsive personality, and is driven to achieve.

DIAGNOSIS

The diagnosis is based on the clinical picture and history: The patient has lost significant weight and may appear emaciated, has intense fear of weight gain, and if female, has absent or irregular menstruation. The nutritional status and the electrolyte balance are evaluated through laboratory tests, including blood tests, urinalysis, and an *electrocardiogram*. Other disorders that cause physical wasting are ruled out.

TREATMENT

The goal of treatment is to promote normal weight and to restore nutrition. A team approach combining medical management, psychotherapy, behavior modification, family counseling, and nutritional counseling works best. The patient often is hospitalized to provide fluid and electrolyte replacement, to remove the patient from the home environment, and to place the patient in a controlled environment. Long-term emotional support is needed, and long-term psychiatric counseling often is indicated to correct any underlying dysfunction. Support groups for eating disorders help some patients.

PROGNOSIS

The outcome is more favorable when the patient seeks help willingly. Without medical intervention, life-threatening complications, such as cardiac arrest, are possible. Recovery is usually slow, and some patients become suicidal.

PREVENTION

Until the causes are known, there is no certain prevention.

PATIENT TEACHING

Establish a target weight. Give the patient as much control as possible over the foods and drinks preferred, while beginning an adequate diet. Encourage the patient to share her or his struggles in a "safe" setting such as an eating disorder support group.

Bulimia

DESCRIPTION

Bulimia is a behavioral disorder characterized by recurring episodes of binge eating followed by self-induced vomiting or purging, usually in secret.

 ICD-9-CM Code 307.51

SYMPTOMS AND SIGNS

The binge–purge eating pattern of bulimia is fueled by a morbid fear of becoming fat. The frequent presence of vomitus in the mouth causes erosion of the teeth. The patients also abuse laxatives and diuretics by using them excessively. Other signs are compulsive exercise, swollen salivary glands, and broken blood vessels in the eye. These patients, usually females, typically weigh more than anorectic patients and experience a wide fluctuation in weight. Some report feeling guilty about the binge–purge episodes.

PATIENT SCREENING

Be alert for the shame and denial associated with the disease. The patient may admit only to depression and resist medical intervention.

ETIOLOGY

Although the etiologic factors are similar to those of anorexia nervosa, the exact cause is uncertain. Psychosocial factors, depression, control issues, and conflict frequently are identified. The patient reports a typical disordered eating pattern with self-induced vomiting; the patient often denies this ritual and keeps it secret. Characteristic perfectionist personality traits are identified, as in anorexia nervosa. The condition is associated with depression and, in some cases, compulsion.

DIAGNOSIS

The diagnostic approach is similar to that for anorexia nervosa. Increased loss of electrolytes and metabolic acidosis are noted in laboratory testing. The patient exhibits a loss of muscle mass, cardiac irregularities, and dehydration. Anger and denial are part of the emotional state. Sudden death can result from hypokalemia and resulting cardiac arrhythmias.

TREATMENT

Treatment is similar to that of anorexia nervosa, with a multidimensional approach, including the administration of antidepressant drugs and partic-

ipation in a support group. After the patient has discontinued the bulimic behavior, she or he should be taught proper nutrition in the form of a balanced diet.

PROGNOSIS

Treatment may continue for years because recovery may be a slow process.

PREVENTION

No prevention is known.

PATIENT TEACHING

Encourage the patient's efforts to comply with medical management, psychotherapy, and self-help groups for eating disorders. Describe the risks of abusing laxatives and diuretics. Praise the patient for reaching goals in weight gain and behavior modification.

Motion Sickness

DESCRIPTION

Motion sickness is a loss of equilibrium experienced during motion.

 ICD-9-CM Code 994.6

SYMPTOMS AND SIGNS

During an episode of motion sickness, the patient experiences nausea and vomiting when riding in a motor vehicle, boat, airplane, or other means of transportation. Air hunger, excessive salivation, pallor, sweating, dizziness, or headache may precede the nausea and vomiting.

PATIENT SCREENING

A person susceptible to motion sickness needs a prescription before an airplane flight, car trip, or boating excursion.

ETIOLOGY

Motion sickness results from a disturbance in the sense of balance. The fluid in the semicircular canals of the ears becomes dislocated because of the motion. In addition, excessive stimulation of the vestibular apparatus in the inner ear is caused by repetitive acceleration and deceleration as well as by angular and linear motion.

DIAGNOSIS

The diagnosis is based on the clinical picture.

TREATMENT

The prevention of this condition is easier than the treatment. The patient is encouraged to sit in the vehicle in the position that has the least amount of motion and where he or she can see the horizon. The patient is urged to avoid foods and liquids before travel. If the patient must eat, only small amounts of food should be eaten. Prophylaxis with dermal patches of scopolamine (Transderm-Scop) often is employed. Dimenhydrinate (Dramamine) is another drug that helps to prevent, and also treats, motion sickness.

PROGNOSIS

The prognosis is good with prophylactic medication.

PREVENTION

Good results can be expected from taking an antiemetic in anticipation of a motion event.

PATIENT TEACHING

Refer to the comments listed previously under Treatment. Warn the patient about any possible adverse effects associated with the medication.

REVIEW CHALLENGE

Answer the following questions:

1. What are the accessory organs of digestion and their functions?
2. How does malocclusion lead to complications?
3. What problem may result from untreated gingivitis?
4. How would you describe the symptoms of temporomandibular joint (TMJ) disease?
5. What is the difference between an aphthous mouth ulcer and a "cold sore?"
6. What causes gastroesophageal reflux disease? How is it treated?
7. How does *Helicobacter pylori* relate to peptic ulcers and gastritis?
8. What is a serious possible complication of esophageal varices?
9. How are peptic ulcers treated?
10. What is the diagnostic value in (a) an endoscopy and (b) a colonoscopy?
11. Is pain usually the initial symptom of gastric cancer?
12. What is the diagnostic significance of McBurney's point?
13. What is a strangulated hernia?
14. What is the difference between ulcerative colitis and Crohn disease?
15. What is the goal in treatment of gastroenteritis?
16. What is the difference between a functional and a mechanical intestinal obstruction? Give an example of each.
17. How would you compare the pathology of diverticulosis to diverticulitis?
18. How is colorectal cancer detected?
19. What causes pseudomembranous enterocolitis?
20. If a person has peritonitis, what serious complications may occur?
21. What are the signs and symptoms of cirrhosis of the liver?
22. How do hepatitis A and hepatitis C compare in etiology? What are the preventive measures for each disease?
23. What are the presenting symptoms of a patient with (a) biliary colic and (b) acute pancreatitis?
24. What are the causes of pancreatitis?
25. What are some examples of disorders of nutrition caused by deficiencies and excesses?
26. In what ways do pathogens cause food poisoning?
27. What are two diagnostic criteria for celiac disease?
28. What are the similarities and differences between anorexia nervosa and bulimia?
29. What is the most common bloodborne infection in the United States?
30. What is the third-most-common site of cancer incidence and death in men and women?

REAL-LIFE CHALLENGE

Cholelithiasis

A 43-year-old woman is experiencing intermittent colicky-type pain in the right upper quadrant of the abdomen, radiating to the right scapular region. The onset was approximately 1 week ago. In the past few days, she has had nausea and vomiting, increasing in the past 24 hours. The pain is more severe today, and the emesis is bile colored. Vital signs are temperature, 99.6° F; pulse, 96; respirations, 26; and blood pressure, 144/92. Her skin is warm and dry, slightly jaundiced. The patient is somewhat obese and has been on oral contraceptives for 15 years.

Cholelithiasis is suspected. A CT scan of the gallbladder confirms the presence of stones in the gallbladder and also in the common bile duct. Serum bilirubin is elevated. The patient is scheduled for laparoscopic surgery.

QUESTIONS

1. When would a patient with gallstones be asymptomatic?
2. How do gallstones develop?
3. Which type of person would be most likely to develop gallstones?
4. Which diagnostic imaging studies would be ordered when gallstones are suspected?
5. Which blood studies would be ordered when gallstones are suspected?
6. What is the usual treatment for asymptomatic gallstones?
7. What is the treatment for symptomatic gallstones?
8. What is the difference between cholelithiasis and cholecystitis?

REAL-LIFE CHALLENGE

Ulcers

A 50-year-old man is experiencing midepigastric pain and heartburn along with nausea and vomiting, with the onset approximately 1 week ago. The patient says that the pain is better after eating and more severe 2 hours after eating. The patient is observed sitting slightly bent over with knees drawn up. Vital signs are temperature, 99.8° F; pulse, 104; respirations, 24; and blood pressure, 136/88. His skin is warm, dry, and pale. The physician suspects a duodenal ulcer. The abdomen is slightly distended and tender to palpation.

Diagnostic investigation includes Hb, Hct, gastric analysis, stool exam for occult blood, upper GI series, and a gastroscopy. Drug therapy includes antacid, histamine (H_2) blockers and an antibiotic. The patient is instructed to adhere to a bland diet including small and more frequent meals.

QUESTIONS

1. What population is most prone to develop ulcers?
2. Compare gastric, duodenal, and peptic ulcers.
3. Why would symptoms of gastric and duodenal ulcers vary?
4. Discuss theories of the cause of ulcers. Compare theories of stress versus ulcerogenic drugs versus bacterial origin.
5. What warnings should be given to patients taking NSAIDs?
6. Explain the complications of perforation.
7. Discuss the various forms of drug therapy available to treat ulcers.
8. What side effects might a patient on histamine (H_2) blockers experience?
9. What would a positive Guaiac test indicate?

INTERNET ASSIGNMENTS

1. Explore the American Dental Association website and report the latest news about the call for early detection of oral cancer. What do the relevant statistics suggest about oral cancer?
2. Visit the website of the National Eating Disorders Association and report on a relevant headline article. For example, what is being done to reach preteen children with a positive message about body image to avoid tragic deaths from eating disorders?
3. Research the latest approaches to the treatment of hepatitis C by searching the American Liver Foundation website and related links.

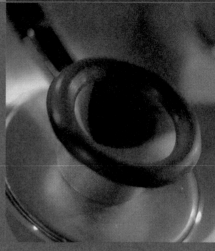

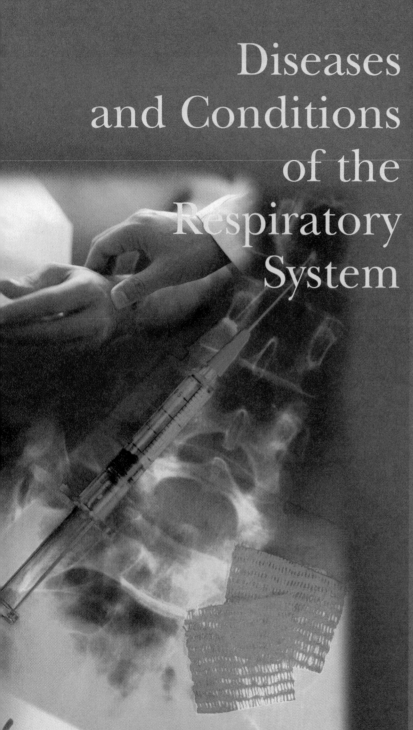

CHAPTER 9

Diseases and Conditions of the Respiratory System

Chapter Outline—Cont'd

Learning Objectives

After studying Chapter 9, you should be able to:

1. Explain the process of respiration.
2. Discuss the causes and medical treatment for (a) the common cold, (b) sinusitis, and (c) pharyngitis.
3. Name the treatment of choice for nasal polyps.
4. Discuss the prognosis of cancer of the larynx.
5. Define atelectasis and discuss some possible causes.
6. Name some systemic disorders that might cause epistaxis.
7. Compare the clinical pictures of (a) a patient with pulmonary embolism and (b) one with pneumonia.
8. List some possible causes of pulmonary abscess.
9. Compare legionellosis with Pontiac fever.
10. Explain who is at greatest risk for (a) respiratory syncytial virus pneumonia and (b) histoplasmosis.
11. List the groups recommended to receive prophylactic use of influenza vaccines.
12. Contrast the pathologic course of acute bronchitis with that of chronic bronchitis.
13. Compare the pathology involved in bronchiectasis with that of pulmonary emphysema.
14. Name and describe three causes of pneumoconiosis.
15. Explain the difference between pneumothorax and hemothorax.
16. Describe the presenting symptoms of pleurisy.
17. Discuss contributing factors to and concern about the rising prevalence of pulmonary tuberculosis.
18. Describe the clinical course of infectious mononucleosis.
19. Explain the pathologic changes of the lungs in adult respiratory distress syndrome (ARDS).
20. Name the leading cause of cancer deaths worldwide for both men and women.
21. Discuss the early findings concerning the threat of a SARS epidemic.
22. List some health hazards of common molds.

Key Terms

anosmia (an–**OZ**–me–ah)
anthracosis (an–thrah–**KOE**–sis)
aphonia (ah–**FOE**–nee–ah)
asbestosis (as–beh–**STOH**–sis)
aspiration (as–pih–**RAY**–shun)
circumoral cyanosis (sir–kum–**OH**–ral sigh–an–**OH**–sis)
dysphonia (dis–**FOE**–nee–ah)
epistaxis (**ep**–ih–**STAK**–sis)
exsanguination (eck–**sang**–win–**AY**–shun)
hemoptysis (he–**MOP**–tih–sis)

laryngectomy (lar–in–**JECK**–toh–me)
lymphadenitis (limf–**ad**–eh–**NIGH**–tis)
lymphadenopathy (limf–**ad**–eh–**NOP**–ah–thee)
pneumoconiosis (**nu**–moh–koh–nee–**OH**–sis)
rhonchi (**RONG**–ki)
silicosis (sill–ih–**KO**–sis)
sinusotomy (sigh–nus–**OT**–oh–me)
stridor (**STRY**–dor)
syncytial virus (sin–**SIGH**–shal virus)
tachypnea (**tach**–ip–**NEE**–ah)

ORDERLY FUNCTION
OF THE RESPIRATORY SYSTEM

THE PRIMARY FUNCTION of the lungs is respiration (Fig. 9–1). Respiration maintains life by supplying oxygen to cells and allowing for the removal of carbon dioxide (a waste product of metabolism). This process is made possible by ventilation (the bellows-like action of the chest) and healthy pulmonary tissue that is adequately perfused with blood. Breathing is controlled by the central nervous system; nerve stimulation of breathing begins in the medulla oblongata and pons. Pulmonary circulation is composed of pulmonary arteries that carry venous blood from the heart; pulmonary capillaries in which gas exchange occurs; and pulmonary veins, which return the freshly oxygenated blood to the heart for systemic circulation. Lung tissue itself is supplied with oxygen and nutrients by the blood supply that is carried to it by the bronchial arteries.

The lungs also have a major metabolic function: the maintenance of acid–base (pH) balance of the blood. Lack of oxygen with hypercapnia (increased carbon dioxide in the blood) causes respiratory acidosis; hyperventilation may produce hypocapnia (a decreased amount of carbon dioxide in the blood), causing respiratory alkalosis. In both conditions, arterial blood gases are abnormal.

In the lungs, oxygen inhaled from the air is exchanged with carbon dioxide from the blood; this process is called *external respiration. Internal respiration* refers to the exchange of gases between the blood and tissue cells. Carbon dioxide then is exhaled as a waste product. Inhaled and exhaled air passes through the respiratory tract, which includes the nose, pharynx, larynx, and trachea (Fig. 9–2).

In the chest, the trachea *bifurcates* into the bronchi. Each bronchus enters a lung, where it further divides into increasingly smaller air passages called *bronchioles*. At the end of each bronchiole is a sac-like cavity called an *alveolus*. There

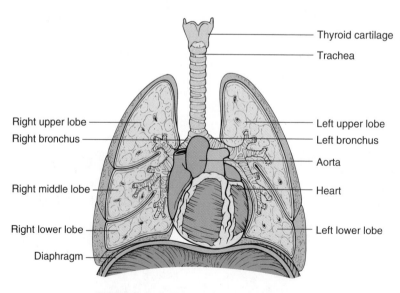

FIGURE 9–1 Normal lower respiratory system.

are approximately 300 million alveoli in each lung. The vital exchange of carbon dioxide for oxygen takes place through minute blood vessels in each alveolus.

A muscular, dome-shaped partition called the *diaphragm* attaches to the lower ribs and separates the thoracic cavity from the abdominal cavity. On inspiration, the diaphragm contracts, pulling downward and causing air to be sucked into the lungs. During expiration, the diaphragm relaxes, pushing upward and forcing air out of the lungs (Fig. 9–3).

The membrane called the *visceral pleura* encases the lungs, and the *parietal pleura* lines the inside of the pleural cavity. Approximately 5 to 6 ml of pleural fluid is contained in the space between the pleurae, preventing friction and allowing the pleurae to slide easily on each other. Between the lungs is the *mediastinum,* where the heart, great vessels, trachea, esophagus, and lymph nodes are located.

Respiratory failure can be caused by the inability to ventilate or impairment of alveolar–arterial gas exchange, as occurs in progressive lung disease. Diseases of the respiratory system result from infection, circulatory disorders, tumors, trauma, immune diseases, congenital defects, central nervous system damage or diseases, or environmental conditions.

Chief symptoms indicating respiratory tract disorders that should receive medical attention include:
- Chest pain
- Dyspnea (difficulty in breathing)
- Productive or nonproductive cough that is acute or chronic
- **Hemoptysis** (spitting up blood)
- **Dysphonia** (hoarseness)
- Chills
- Low- or high-grade fever
- Wheezing
- Fatigue

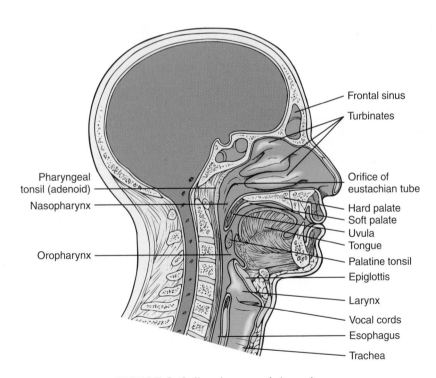

FIGURE 9–2 Normal upper respiratory system.

Frontal sinus
Turbinates
Orifice of eustachian tube
Hard palate
Soft palate
Uvula
Tongue
Palatine tonsil
Epiglottis
Larynx
Vocal cords
Esophagus
Trachea

Pharyngeal tonsil (adenoid)
Nasopharynx
Oropharynx

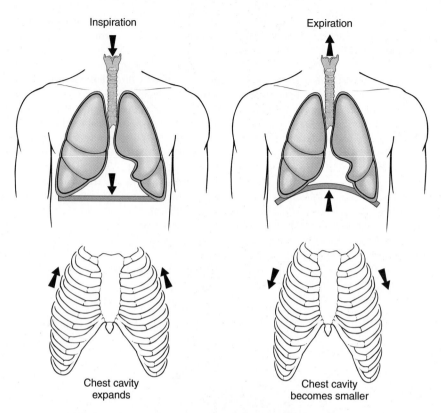

Inspiration

Expiration

Chest cavity
expands

Chest cavity
becomes smaller

FIGURE 9-3 Diaphragm and chest movement on inspiration and expiration.

Common Cold/ Upper Respiratory Tract Infection

DESCRIPTION

The common cold, also referred to as an *upper respiratory tract infection (URI)*, is an acute inflammatory process that affects the mucous membrane that lines the upper respiratory tract.

■ **ICD-9-CM Code** **460**

SYMPTOMS AND SIGNS

Although the common, or "head," cold is confined to the nose and pharynx, the same viruses can infect the larynx (see Laryngitis) and the lungs (see Acute and Chronic Bronchitis). The symptoms of a cold, to some extent, depend on which virus is responsible; they include nasal congestion and discharge, sneezing, watering eyes, sore throat, hoarseness of the voice, and coughing. When this highly contagious inflammatory process first begins, the nasal discharge is usually clear and thin. As the cold progresses, the discharge becomes greenish yellow and thick. *Cephalalgia,* a slight fever, and chills often accompany a cold. A high fever and *malaise,* however, are more likely to be symptoms of influenza (see Influenza).

PATIENT SCREENING

Symptoms of a cold that are prolonged or accompanied by fever, chest pain and congestion, earache, severe headache, stiff neck, decreased urine, or other complications, indicate the need for medical care within 24 hours.

ETIOLOGY

The common cold is a group of minor illnesses that can be caused by almost 200 different viruses. Rhinoviruses cause about one half of the colds in adults. (Some colds may result from *mycoplasma*, also transmitted by airborne respiratory droplets.) These viral infections sometimes are followed by bacterial infections of the pharynx, middle ear (see Otitis Media in Chapter 5), sinuses, larynx, or lungs. General poor health predisposes one to the common cold.

DIAGNOSIS

Diagnosis is made from the symptoms described by the patient. To rule out more serious disease, cultures of the nasal discharge and sputum, along with a complete blood count (CBC), may be needed.

TREATMENT

An ordinary cold should clear up in 4 or 5 days, and a bacterial infection should resolve in no longer than a week to 10 days. Nasal congestion may persist for an indefinite period. There is no cure for a cold. Resting, drinking plenty of fluids, using a vaporizer, and taking over-the-counter cold tablets, cough syrups, and mild analgesics can give temporary relief of symptoms. *NOTE: Aspirin is contraindicated for infants and children; acetaminophen is the drug of choice.*

The benefit to be gained from taking oral antihistamines to treat a cold is controversial. Antibiotics are of little value in treating viral infections; however, patients with recurring attacks of bronchitis (see Acute and Chronic Bronchitis) or frequent middle ear infections may receive some protection against these bacteria-caused complications by taking antibiotics.

PROGNOSIS

The common cold is usually benign and self-limiting. Patients who are immunocompromised may be more vulnerable to developing frequent colds and complications. Possible complications can include secondary bacterial infections as listed above under etiology.

PREVENTION

The mechanisms of transmission of cold viruses are not always clearly defined. Because, in many cases, the mode of transmission is airborne respiratory droplets and hand-to-hand contact, prevention is difficult.

PATIENT TEACHING

Colds are more common in children than adults and are a frequent cause of absenteeism. Once infected, children can easily transmit new strains to family members. Frequent, thorough hand washing, and isolation during the acute stage of illness are common sense measures that can help control transmission. Stress to the patient that antibiotics do not cure the common cold. Instruct the patient to avoid overuse of drugs such as nasal sprays and to take all medications only as instructed. List the warning signs of complications that should be reported to the health-care provider (i.e., shortness of breath, severe headache, chest pain, high fever, and symptoms of dehydration or stiff neck).

Sinusitis

DESCRIPTION

Sinusitis is acute or chronic inflammation of the mucous membranes of the paranasal sinuses.

ICD-9-CM Code 461.9 *(Acute, unspecified)*
473.9 *(Unspecified sinusitis, chronic)*
Sinusitis is classified by location, type, and extent of pathology. Refer to the physician's diagnosis and then to the current edition of the ICD-9-CM coding manual for greatest specificity.

SYMPTOMS AND SIGNS

The sinuses, cavities behind the facial bones that shape the nose, cheeks, and eye sockets, are normally air filled. In sinusitis, the frontal sinuses (located in the forehead above the eyes) and the maxillary sinuses (located under the maxillary bones in the face) are the most commonly involved sinuses (Fig. 9–4). When the frontal sinuses are affected, headache is common over one or both eyes, especially upon waking in the morning. Pain and tenderness, felt just above the eyes and usually intensifies

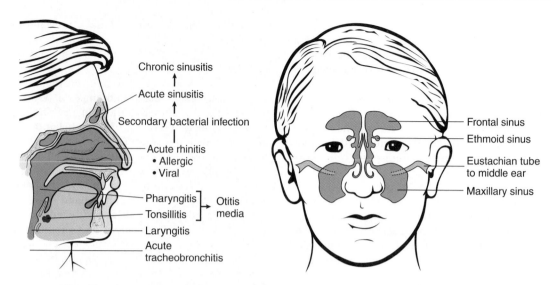

Chronic sinusitis
↑
Acute sinusitis
↑
Secondary bacterial infection

Acute rhinitis
• Allergic
• Viral

Pharyngitis
Tonsillitis } Otitis media

Laryngitis

Acute tracheobronchitis

Frontal sinus
Ethmoid sinus
Eustachian tube to middle ear
Maxillary sinus

FIGURE 9–4 Sinusitis. (From Damjanov I: *Pathology for the health-related professions,* ed 2, Philadelphia, 2000, Saunders.)

when bending over, are also common symptoms. Pain in the cheeks and upper teeth is a symptom of sinusitis in the maxillary sinuses. Drainage, if present, will be a thick and greenish yellow mucopurulent discharge. The course of acute sinusitis is 3 to 4 weeks.

PATIENT SCREENING

Individuals with symptoms of acute sinusitis (fever, sinus congestion, facial tenderness and pain, severe headache) are encouraged to seek medical attention as soon as possible.

ETIOLOGY

Sinusitis can be caused by either viral or, more commonly, bacterial infections that travel to the sinuses from the nose, often after the patient has been infected by a common cold. This occurs easily because the mucous membranes that line the nasal cavity extend into and also line the sinuses. One is predisposed to sinusitis by any condition that blocks sinus drainage and ventilation (e.g., a deviated nasal septum, or nasal polyps). Sinusitis also may result as a consequence of swimming or diving, tooth extractions, or tooth *abscess,* as well as allergies that affect the nasal passages. The cause of chronic sinusitis may never be determined; how-

ever, common variable immunodeficiency disease may be involved (see Chapter 3).

DIAGNOSIS

The diagnosis of sinusitis is made by evaluating the findings of a physical examination, the patient history, sinus radiographic studies, and endoscopic sinuscopy. Sinuses that are air filled appear as dark patches on a radiographic film, whereas fluid-filled sinuses appear as white areas. Bedside transillumination can suggest the presence of sinusitis. Additionally, a specimen of nasal secretions may be taken for culture to identify or rule out bacterial agents.

TREATMENT

Treatment consists of the use of a broad-spectrum antibiotic, decongestants, and antihistamines. Decongestants alleviate symptoms by shrinking the swollen mucous membranes and drying up the nasal discharge. This expands the airway and eases breathing. Treatment of allergic sinusitis includes allergy testing and appropriate desensitization with immunotherapy and corticosteroids. If the inflammation persists, a minor surgery called **sinusotomy** may be advised by the physician. With the patient under local anesthesia, the physician pierces the maxillary sinus, allowing drainage and relief of pressure. Often the physician instills sterile water into the sinus to flush out any residual material. Analgesics usually are given for pain relief.

PROGNOSIS

The prognosis for uncomplicated sinusitis is good. Chronic sinusitis can require more prolonged medical treatment with antibiotics.

PREVENTION

Management of conditions that predispose an individual to sinusitis may help prevent chronic sinusitis.

PATIENT TEACHING

Explain the importance of complying with the treatment plan. List the warning signs of complications, such as chills, fever, facial edema, severe headache, lethargy, or confusion. Prepare the patient for diagnostic testing or surgery by explaining each procedure and what to expect in terms of preparation and care afterwards.

Pharyngitis

DESCRIPTION

Pharyngitis is acute or chronic inflammation or infection of the pharynx.

■ **ICD-9-CM Code 462**

SYMPTOMS AND SIGNS

Pharyngitis may be acute or chronic and often involves inflammation of the tonsils, uvula, and palate. A sore throat with dryness, a burning sensation, or the sensation of a lump in the throat is common. Clinical manifestations vary with the type of pharyngitis. Generally chills, fever, *dysphonia, dysphagia,* and cervical **lymphadenopathy** are common. Upon examination of the throat, the mucosa of the pharynx is found to be red and swollen with or without tonsillar exudate, depending on the causative organism.

PATIENT SCREENING

An individual complaining of a persistent sore throat with systemic symptoms should be seen by a physi-

cian within 24 hours. Advise the patient not to initiate antibiotic therapy before the appointment because this can preclude accurate diagnostic testing.

ETIOLOGY

The most common cause of pharyngitis is a viral infection. In children, it is often an extension of a bacterial streptococcal infection from the tonsils, adenoids, nose, or sinuses. Persistent infection, or chronic pharyngitis, occurs when an infection (respiratory, sinus, or oral disease) spreads to the pharynx and remains. Acute pharyngitis may be secondary to systemic viral infections, such as chickenpox and measles, whereas chronic pharyngitis may accompany diseases such as syphilis and tuberculosis. Gonococcal pharyngitis may result from oral-genital sexual activity with an infected partner. Pharyngitis also can be caused by irritation and inflammation without infection. Occasionally, inhalation or swallowing of irritating substances, such as tobacco smoke and alcohol, is responsible for trauma to the mucous membranes of the pharynx; breathing in excessively heated air or chemical irritants and swallowing sharp objects (e.g., a large ice chip or hard candy) also can cause trauma. Seasonal allergies may induce pharyngitis.

DIAGNOSIS

Physical examination usually shows red, swollen mucous membranes. This, along with the patient history, is usually sufficient for determining the diagnosis of acute pharyngitis. For chronic pharyngitis, the physician needs to identify and locate the primary source of the infection or irritation. Further examination of the nasopharyngeal area, a complete blood count (CBC), and sinus radiographic films may be necessary.

TREATMENT

Home treatment using lozenges, mouthwashes, salt water gargles, an ice collar, and aspirin may be helpful for viral infections. *NOTE: Aspirin is not given to children because of the threat of Reye syndrome.* If symptoms persist for longer than a few days, a physician should be consulted. Acute bacterial infections necessitate systemic administration of antibiotics or sulfonamides. Documented streptococcal pharyngitis is treated with a 7- to 10-day course of antibiotics. Chronic tonsillitis, adenoiditis, and adenoid *hypertrophy* may be treated by surgical excision. Bed rest and copious amounts of fluids may be advised.

PROGNOSIS

Uncomplicated pharyngitis resolves within a few days. Bacterial causes are cured with appropriate antibiotics. Chronic cases may require eliminating the underlying cause, such as smoking or allergens, before improvement can be achieved.

PREVENTION

Prevention measures include maintaining general good health, avoiding infections, evading known irritants, and controlling allergies.

PATIENT TEACHING

Instruct the patient to take the entire course of antibiotic therapy and keep follow-up appointments to ensure a cure and help prevent complications. Provide a list of comfort measures such as safe use of analgesics, warm saline gargles, adequate fluid intake, and a soft diet. Advise patients with chronic pharyngitis to stop smoking; refer them to a support group.

Nasopharyngeal Carcinoma

DESCRIPTION

Nasopharyngeal tumors arise in the area of the pharynx that opens into the nasal cavity anteriorly and the oropharynx inferiorly. They are unique among head and neck cancers in that they are *not* strongly linked to tobacco use. Instead, they are linked to dietary intake and Epstein-Barr virus infection.

ICD-9-CM Code

Neoplasms are coded by such known factors as anatomic site, behavior, and nature (morphology). Greatest specificity is obtained by referring to the physician's diagnosis and then to the current edition of the ICD-9-CM coding manual.

SYMPTOMS AND SIGNS

Because of the anatomic location of the nasopharyngeal tumor, patients are often asymptomatic during the early stages of the disease. Neck mass is the most common symptom and occurs in over 90% of patients. The classic clinical triad of symptoms is neck mass, nasal obstruction with **epistaxis,** and serous otitis media. However, it is rare to find all three symptoms in a single patient. Other symptoms include hearing loss, tinnitus, pain, and impaired function of the cranial nerves.

PATIENT SCREENING

Provide the first available appointment to the individual reporting a neck mass or related symptoms.

ETIOLOGY

Although nasopharyngeal carcinoma is a rare disease in the United States and Western Europe, several populations do have a relatively high incidence. These include people from southern China, areas around the Mediterranean Sea, and southeastern Asia and North American Eskimos. It is two to three times more common in males than females, and has a peak incidence in persons between the ages of 50 and 60. Several known risk factors in the endemic areas include consumption of salted fish as a diet standard, foods with high levels of nitrates (such as processed meats), and Chinese herbs; infection with the Epstein-Barr virus (EBV); and having a first-degree relative with nasopharyngeal carcinoma.

DIAGNOSIS

Diagnosis is made following a full clinical examination of the head and neck and an endoscopic examination of the nasopharynx with biopsy of suspicious lesions. Fine needle **aspiration** biopsy of the neck mass also may be performed. Staging is determined according to the TNM (Tumor, Node, Metastasis) system, in which T reflects the extent of tumor invasion into adjacent structures and N incorporates lymph node location as well as size. An MRI of the head and neck, a bone scan, and a chest radiograph are used to aid in staging.

TREATMENT

Because of the anatomic constraints of the nasopharynx, surgery is usually not performed. Nasopharyngeal carcinoma commonly is quite radiosensitive, and most patients with early stage cancer are treated with radiation therapy. Those with recurrent or more advanced carcinomas are generally treated with chemoradiotherapy.

PROGNOSIS

Because early neoplasms rarely cause symptoms, most patients present with advanced carcinoma, and many already have distant metastases to the bone, lung, or liver. If the tumor has extended to involve one of the cranial nerves or metastasizes to the cervical lymph nodes, it indicates a worse prognosis.

PREVENTION

It is possible to detect EBV DNA in the nasopharynx by means of a brush biopsy. Still, screening for EBV is not currently performed, even in southern China where nasopharyngeal carcinoma is most prevalent.

PATIENT TEACHING

Prepare the patient for diagnostic testing by providing information about endoscopy of the nasopharynx and biopsy. Tell the patient when to expect results. After diagnosis, explain the treatment of choice and possible side effects. Encourage the patient to ask questions, and defer to the physician for prognosis. Provide information regarding cancer support groups.

Laryngitis

DESCRIPTION

Inflammation of the larynx, including the vocal cords, is called *laryngitis*.

ICD-9-CM Code 464
Laryngitis coding includes modifiers that specify causative agents and factors such as obstruction. Refer to the physician's diagnosis and then to the current edition of the ICD-9-CM coding manual for the appropriate modifiers.

SYMPTOMS AND SIGNS

Because the opening of the larynx is narrow, inflammation of the larynx sometimes interferes with breathing. Symptoms vary with the severity of the inflammation, but the main symptom of laryngitis is hoarseness, which causes **aphonia**. Fever, malaise, a painful throat, dysphagia, and other symptoms associated with influenza occur in more severe infections.

PATIENT SCREENING

Laryngitis associated with recent trauma requires immediate medical attention. A sensation of swelling in the throat, difficult breathing, and laryngitis is to be considered a medical emergency. An individual reporting persistent hoarseness and symptoms of infection should be seen in the medical office within 24 hours.

ETIOLOGY

The cause of laryngitis can be either viral or bacterial infection, and the condition can be either chronic or acute. URIs such as the common cold, tonsillitis, pharyngitis, and sinusitis are the most common causes of inflammation of the larynx. Laryngitis also occurs with bronchitis, pertussis, influenza, pneumonia, measles, mononucleosis, diphtheria, syphilis, and tuberculosis. Occasionally, laryngitis is caused by irritation without infection. Reflux laryngitis may result from repeated attacks of acid reflux. Inclement weather, tobacco smoke, drinking alcohol, inhalation of irritating materials, and excessive use of the voice are all predisposing factors, especially in the case of chronic laryngitis.

DIAGNOSIS

Laryngoscopic examination reveals mildly or highly inflamed mucosa, and vocal cord movement may be limited. If no inflammation is present, laryngitis is not the cause of dysphonia, and further diagnostic tests are needed to determine the underlying condition.

TREATMENT

Treatment of viral laryngitis includes the following palliative measures: absolute voice rest, bed rest in a well-humidified room, liberal fluid intake, no tobacco or alcohol consumption, and the use of lozenges and cough syrup. Improvement should be seen in 4 or 5 days. Antibiotic administration gives good results when laryngitis occurs in conjunction with another disease. When hoarseness persists for longer than 1 week, the condition may be chronic. Treatment of chronic laryngitis is based on elimination, as much as possible, of the causative factors.

PROGNOSIS

Recovery is generally complete within a week.

PREVENTION

Known irritants that cause laryngitis are avoided or treated if possible. Infections are difficult to prevent.

PATIENT TEACHING

Explain the importance of resting the voice and taking medications as prescribed, along with drinking plenty of fluids. When the cause of chronic laryngitis has been determined to be irritation from excessive alcohol intake or smoking, provide information on support groups that offer help to those with such addictions, if appropriate.

Deviated Septum

DESCRIPTION

A crooked nasal septum (the cartilage partition between the nostrils), is called a *deviated septum* (Fig. 9–5).

■ **ICD-9-CM Code 470** *(Acquired)*

SYMPTOMS AND SIGNS

Deviated septum causes narrowing and obstruction of the air passage, making breathing somewhat difficult. Other than mild breathing problems or a slightly increased tendency to develop sinusitis, no significant symptoms are associated with a deviated septum. The nose can appear normal on the exterior, with the deviation visible only on examination with a nasal speculum.

PATIENT SCREENING

Unless the deviated septum is severe, it may not be noted until inadvertently found as a consequence of a routine physical exam. The condition may be of no consequence until aggravated by trauma to the nose. In that case, schedule the first available appointment for evaluation.

ETIOLOGY

Congenital anomaly is usually the cause of minor deviation of the septum. Substantial septal deviation is uncommon and is usually the result of trauma to the nose.

DIAGNOSIS

A deviated septum may not be visible without the aid of a nasal speculum. The patient history and the amount of obstruction aid the physician in determining the diagnosis and treatment of this condition.

TREATMENT

Treatment is not usually necessary unless compromise of the air passage is noted. The septum can be straightened surgically to repair a significant obstruction or for cosmetic reasons. Straightening a deviated septum involves removing the cartilage (rhinoplasty or septoplasty). Once removed, the cartilage can be reshaped and repositioned in the nose, if needed, to maintain the nasal structure.

PROGNOSIS

This fairly common condition has a good prognosis.

PREVENTION

The only possible prevention is avoiding trauma to the nose.

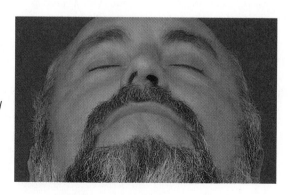

FIGURE 9–5 Deviated septum. (From Monahan FD, Neighbors M: *Medical-surgical nursing: foundations for clinical practice,* ed 2, Philadelphia, 1998, Saunders.)

PATIENT TEACHING

If surgical correction is scheduled, tell the patient what to expect after surgery, such as the use of nasal packing to control bleeding and analgesics for pain.

Nasal Polyps

DESCRIPTION

Nasal polyps are benign growths that form as a consequence of distended mucous membranes protruding into the nasal cavity (Fig. 9–6).

ICD-9-CM Code 471.9 *(Unspecified)*
Nasal polyps are coded by anatomic site and underlying pathology. Refer to the physician's diagnosis and then to the current edition of the ICD-9-CM coding manual for greatest specificity.

SYMPTOMS AND SIGNS

Nasal polyps are not harmful but can become large enough to obstruct the nasal airway, making breathing difficult. Polyps often affect or impair the sense of smell (see Anosmia). When polyps obstruct one of the sinuses, symptoms of sinusitis are present (see Sinusitis).

PATIENT SCREENING

Nasal polyps may be found in the patient exhibiting symptoms of allergic rhinitis and/or sinusitis. The degree of urgency for an appointment is based on severity of symptoms.

ETIOLOGY

Polyps are caused by the overproduction of fluid in the cells of the mucous membrane. This overproduction is often the result of a condition called *allergic rhinitis.* Some aspirin-sensitive persons have the triad of nasal polyps, asthma, and urticaria (hives).

DIAGNOSIS

The physician examines the inside of the nose using an instrument called a *nasal speculum.* Polyps appear as pearly gray lumps along the nasal passage.

TREATMENT

Surgical removal is the treatment of choice; however, considerable relief may be obtained through the injection of a steroid directly into the polyps. This procedure is repeated at 5- to 7-day intervals until relief is obtained. Removal of polyps is a minor procedure necessitating a local *anesthetic.* When the lining of the sinus also must be removed, a general anesthetic is used.

PROGNOSIS

The prognosis is good, although nasal polyps tend to recur.

PREVENTION

No specific preventive measures are known. Management of allergic rhinitis is beneficial.

PATIENT TEACHING

Instructions given to the patient are related to the treatment of choice. When appropriate, explain the relationship of allergic rhinitis to nasal polyps.

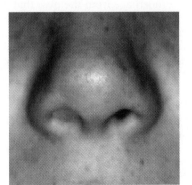

FIGURE 9–6 Nasal polyps. (From Lemmi FO, Lemmi CAE: *Physical assessment findings CD-ROM,* Philadelphia, 2000, Saunders.)

Anosmia

DESCRIPTION
Anosmia is the impairment or loss of the sense of smell.

 ICD-9-CM Code 781.1

SYMPTOMS AND SIGNS
The loss of smell that continues without an obvious cause is termed *anosmia*. The ability to taste liquids and food also is impaired or lost.

PATIENT SCREENING
The patient complaining of prolonged unexplained loss of the sense of smell is scheduled for a diagnostic evaluation.

ETIOLOGY
A chronic condition, such as nasal polyps and allergic rhinitis, is the most common cause of anosmia. Intranasal swelling accompanying an upper respiratory condition causes temporary anosmia. Sometimes a phobia concerning a particular odor accounts for a psychologic basis for anosmia. It may, however, be the result of damage to the olfactory nerves caused by head injury or, rarely, a symptom of a brain tumor.

DIAGNOSIS
If on examination the physician does not find any physical abnormality, or the patient history does not reveal recent head trauma or an allergic condition, a neurologist may be consulted to perform diagnostic tests.

TREATMENT
Treatment is aimed at the cause of the condition. When polyps are found, they are removed. Correction of nerve damage may not be possible. For allergic rhinitis, a series of injections containing increasingly stronger concentrations of the offending *allergen* is used to desensitize the patient.

PROGNOSIS
Anosmia is often related to an upper respiratory infection and is thus a temporary condition.

Other causes, as listed above, have a guarded prognosis.

PREVENTION
No means of prevention other than avoiding head injury is known.

PATIENT TEACHING
Patients may benefit from an explanation of how the olfactory nerve normally functions and how it is affected by the determined cause of anosmia.

Epistaxis (Nosebleed)

DESCRIPTION
Epistaxis is hemorrhage from the nose.

 ICD-9-CM Code 784.7

SYMPTOMS AND SIGNS
Hemorrhage from the nose, known as *epistaxis*, is a common, sudden emergency. Bleeding usually occurs from only one nostril, and often no apparent explanation for the bleeding is known. Most nosebleeds are seldom cause for concern. They are unlikely to be a symptom of any other disorders, unless injury has occurred or associated serious systemic conditions are present. With significant blood loss, systemic symptoms will occur, such as vertigo, increase in pulse, pallor, shortness of breath and drop in blood pressure. Epistaxis is more common in children than in adults.

PATIENT SCREENING
Hemorrhage from the nose that persists for 10 minutes or more after constant pressure is applied is considered severe and requires immediate emergency care. If the patient reports a severe headache at the onset of epistaxis, or is experiencing sequential nosebleeds, arrange for an immediate appointment.

ETIOLOGY
Common causes of epistaxis are colds and infections such as rhinitis, sinusitis, and nasopharyngitis, which can cause crusting that damages the

mucous membrane lining the nose or causes the rupture of tiny vessels in the anterior septum of the nose. Direct trauma to the nose, picking the nose, and the presence of a foreign body are the most common causes of epistaxis. Nasal hemorrhage also has been encountered in relation to many systemic disorders, such as measles, scarlet fever, pertussis, rheumatic fever, hypertension, congestive heart failure, and chronic renal disease. Epistaxis may be the foremost symptom of conditions such as hemophilia, *thrombocytopenia, agranulocytosis,* and leukemia. Risk factors include vitamin K deficiency, hypertension, aspirin ingestion, high altitude, and anticoagulant therapy. An infrequent cause of epistaxis is extensive hepatic disease.

DIAGNOSIS
The diagnosis of epistaxis is made on the basis of the patient history regarding the frequency of the nosebleeds, whether an injury has occurred, or whether the symptoms indicate that systemic disease may be present.

TREATMENT
Mild hemorrhage may be controlled by applying constant direct pressure on either side of the bridge of the nose for 5 to 10 minutes. Persistent bleeding is treated with local application of epinephrine followed by cauterization with silver nitrate or electric cauterization. If bleeding continues, a posterior nasal packing left in place for 1 to 3 days may be necessary. A mild sclerosing agent also may be injected into a bleeding vessel if it can be visualized by the physician. Additional measures such as surgical ligation of a bleeding artery may be necessary if other measures fail.

PROGNOSIS
The prognosis is generally good.

PREVENTION
Specific treatment of the underlying disease, if present, is of prime importance. Prevention includes instructing patients on how to avoid recurrences.

PATIENT TEACHING
Demonstrate first aid measures for controlling epistaxis—sitting with the head tilted forward while applying constant local pressure by compressing the side of the nose against the septum. Tell the patient to report repeated or severe nosebleed immediately to the health-care provider. Discuss measures for preventing recurrences.

Tumors of the Larynx

DESCRIPTION
Growths or tumors on the larynx may be either benign or malignant.

ICD-9-CM Code 140-239 *(Neoplasms)*
The above general code represents the broad category of neoplasms that are classified by such diagnostic criteria as malignant or benign, as primary or secondary, or according to site, function, and morphology. Refer to the physician's diagnosis and then to the current edition of the ICD-9-CM coding manual to ensure the greatest specificity of pathology and any appropriate modifiers.

SYMPTOMS AND SIGNS
Dysphonia is usually the only symptom of a tumor on the larynx. No influenza-like symptoms occur as with laryngitis (see Laryngitis), but when the tumor is malignant, dysphagia may be experienced. In children with tumors, a high-pitched crowing sound called **stridor** is present because of their small airways. Hoarseness caused by a benign tumor is usually intermittent, whereas that caused by cancer is continuous and gradually becomes worse. Neither type of laryngeal tumor is common, but malignant tumors are slightly more common in men than women.

PATIENT SCREENING
Unexplained, persistent hoarseness lasting longer than 2 weeks requires medical evaluation. Other symptoms related to the throat also may be present. The appointment can be made at the first available time or at the patient's first convenience.

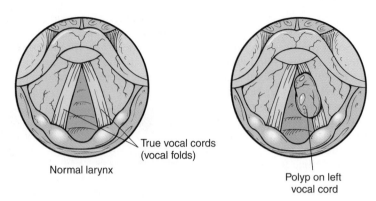

True vocal cords
(vocal folds)

Normal larynx

Polyp on left
vocal cord

FIGURE 9–7 Vocal cord polyp.

ETIOLOGY

There are two types of benign tumors: papillomas, which usually appear as multiples, and polyps, which usually appear singly (Fig. 9–7). These tumors are caused by misuse or overuse of the vocal cords. Malignant tumors occur more often in those who indulge in heavy tobacco use.

DIAGNOSIS

The physician or otolaryngologist thoroughly examines the larynx and vocal cords. When a tumor or tumors are found, a *biopsy* is done to determine whether a malignancy is present. Cancer of the larynx almost always can be cured if it is diagnosed early.

TREATMENT

Benign growths, whether papillomas or polyps, usually are excised with the patient under local anesthesia. Malignant tumors, if discovered early, often are treated and cured by radiation therapy. When the cancer has *metastasized*, a **laryngectomy** may be needed. After a laryngectomy, the patient needs extensive speech therapy to learn a substitute form of speech.

PROGNOSIS

The prognosis depends on the type of tumor and is therefore guarded.

PREVENTION

Avoidance of smoking or any chronic irritation of the larynx is recommended.

PATIENT TEACHING

Give the patient preoperative instructions and encourage the patient to express any concerns about treatment. When laryngectomy is necessary, provide every venue of psychologic support available to the family and patient.

Laryngeal Cancer

DESCRIPTION

Laryngeal cancer describes a neoplasm of the larynx, the part of the respiratory tract between the pharynx and the trachea that houses the vocal cords. Most laryngeal tumors are squamous cell carcinomas.

 ICD-9-CM Code 161.9 *(Larynx, unspecified)*
The above code is a nonspecific code and may be valid as a principal diagnosis, except for Medicare. Refer to the physician's diagnosis and then to the current edition of the ICD-9-CM coding manual to ensure the greatest specificity of pathology and any appropriate modifiers.

SYMPTOMS AND SIGNS

If the tumor involves the vocal cord area of the larynx, persistent hoarseness tends to occur early in the disease process and is the most common initial complaint. Hoarseness related to benign causes, such as a vocal cord polyp or nodule caused by chronic irritation or overuse, is usually intermittent, whereas that caused by a malignant neoplasm is continuous and gradually becomes worse over time. Other symptoms may include dysphagia, hemoptysis, chronic cough, referred pain to the ear, and stridor (a high-pitched crowing sound). Airway obstruction also may occur depending on the tumor location. No influenza-like symptoms as with laryngitis are present (see Laryngitis).

PATIENT SCREENING

Unexplained, persistent hoarseness lasting longer than 2 weeks requires medical evaluation. Other symptoms related to the throat also may be present. The appointment can be made at the first available time or at the patients' earliest convenience.

ETIOLOGY

Laryngeal cancer is most common in regions of the world where use of tobacco is extensive and consumption of alcohol is high, such as in central Asia, regions of France, central and Eastern Europe, and the United States. The combined effect of alcohol and tobacco in causing cancer is multiplicative, leading to heavy smokers and drinkers having a 200-fold greater risk of developing laryngeal cancer than nonsmokers and nondrinkers. Other risk factors include infection with HPV 16 or 18, occupational exposures to agents such as perchloroethylene (a dry cleaning agent) or asbestos, and having a first-degree relative with laryngeal cancer. Tumors of the larynx have a peak incidence in the sixth and seventh decades of life.

DIAGNOSIS

Laryngeal cancer is often diagnosed at an earlier stage than other head and neck cancers because hoarseness usually occurs early in the disease process. Flexible fiberoptic endoscopy allows visualization of the larynx and assessment of vocal cord mobility. Diagnosis of cancer requires a biopsy, which is usually done by fine needle aspiration. Staging is done using a TNM (Tumor, Node, Metastasis) system. A computed tomography (CT) scan or magnetic resonance imaging (MRI) scan is performed to evaluate depth and extent of tumor invasion and to look for nodal metastasis. A panendoscopy (laryngoscopy, esophagoscopy, and bronchoscopy) is generally done as well to look for other areas of tumor growth because tobacco and alcohol use often have widespread toxic effects on the aerodigestive tract.

TREATMENT

The larynx plays an important role in speech, swallowing, respiration, and protection of the lower airway. Therefore, quality of life issues are often incorporated into the treatment plan. For early stage cancer, often the physician will explain the risks and benefits of surgery and radiation therapy, both of which have a similar outcome, and let the patient decide on the therapy. Usually the patient will choose the option that preserves voice—radiation. Surgical options include partial laryngectomy, total laryngectomy, and endoscopic laser resection. The choice largely depends on tumor stage. Treatment of later stage (III and IV) cancers is more difficult. For patients with resectable tumors, treatment usually consists of surgery followed by radiation therapy or by radiation alone. Chemoradiotherapy may be tried in patients choosing an organ-sparing approach. For patients who do undergo a laryngectomy, follow-up care generally requires the services of a speech therapist for speech therapy and swallowing therapy.

PROGNOSIS

Because of the early manifestation of symptoms, laryngeal cancer is often diagnosed at a stage in which cure is possible. The most significant prognostic indicator is the status of the cervical lymph nodes. The overall 5-year survival rate is 65%, with early stage cancers having a 5-year survival rate of 83% and later stages having a 38% to 50% 5-year survival rate. Patients with laryngeal cancer are more likely to develop second primary cancers than patients with malignancies outside the head and neck because of the widespread carcinogenic effects of tobacco and alcohol in the head and neck area. The development of another primary tumor often indicates a worse prognosis.

PREVENTION

Cessation of smoking and reducing one's alcohol consumption are highly recommended. Periodic panendoscopy may be used to detect second primary cancers after treatment for laryngeal cancer.

PATIENT TEACHING

Encourage the patient to express any concerns about diagnostic procedures or the course of treatment chosen. Provide every venue of psychologic support available to the patient and the family. Give specifics about the postoperative care of laryngectomy, as appropriate. Help the patient plan alternate means of communication during speech rehabilitation.

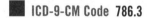

Hemoptysis

DESCRIPTION

Hemoptysis is the coughing or spitting up of blood from the respiratory tract.

■ ICD-9-CM Code 786.3

SYMPTOMS AND SIGNS

Blood-streaked sputum can be present with minor infections, or it can indicate a serious underlying condition. The patient coughs up bright or dark blood-streaked sputum from the pulmonary or bronchial circulation. Profuse bleeding is present in severe lung infections, a respiratory malignancy, or erosion of a pulmonary vessel.

PATIENT SCREENING

Blood of unknown origin in the sputum is a symptom that requires medical evaluation. If the bleeding is slight and associated with a known respiratory infection, schedule an appointment within 24 hours. Advise the patient experiencing profuse bleeding to seek emergency care, and inform the physician immediately.

ETIOLOGY

Trauma, erosion of a vessel, calcification, or tumors can cause bronchial bleeding, as can bronchitis or bronchiectasis. Venous hypertension and left-sided heart failure precipitate bleeding from pulmonary vessels. Additional origins of the bleeding can be fungal infections, pulmonary *infarcts,* tumors or *ulcerations* of the larynx or pharynx, and *coagulation* (clotting) defects.

DIAGNOSIS

Of primary importance is determination of the source of the bleeding. This is accomplished by visual examination of the mouth and nasopharynx; visualization of the larynx, trachea, and bronchi by **endoscopy;** and inspection of the lung fields by radiographic studies. Coagulation studies of the blood ascertain whether the problem is a clotting deficiency. A lung scan and a pulmonary angiogram may be indicated if previously mentioned investigations are inconclusive.

TREATMENT

After the location and the cause of the bleeding are determined, the source is treated. When the bleeding is severe, ligation or surgical removal or repair of the involved vessels is indicated. Measures are implemented to prevent asphyxiation by clotted blood in the air passages; to prevent obstruction of the bronchial tree by clots, with resulting lung collapse; and to prevent **exsanguination** of the patient. Patients are encouraged to cough to remove blood from the lungs. Postural drainage and inhalation of warm, moist air are beneficial. When bleeding results from an infection (e.g., tuberculosis), the infection is treated with antimicrobial agents.

PROGNOSIS

Figures may vary; however, in approximately 75% of cases, hemoptysis is not a sign of serious disease. The prognosis is good with treatment, but guarded if associated with a serious underlying illness.

PREVENTION

Hemoptysis is generally considered a symptom, so there is no directed prevention.

PATIENT TEACHING

Steps are taken to allay fear and anxiety that the patient might experience. Explain the diagnostic procedures and when to expect the results. Reassure the patient that hemoptysis may be expected following endoscopy. Reinforce the treatment regimen and encourage the patient to voice concerns.

Atelectasis

DESCRIPTION
Atelectasis is an airless or collapsed state of the pulmonary tissue.

ICD-9-CM Code 518.0

SYMPTOMS AND SIGNS
Atelectasis follows incomplete expansion of lobules or segments of the lung, with partial or complete collapse of the lung. The condition results in *hypoxia,* causing the patient to experience dyspnea. When only a small segment of the lung is involved, dyspnea may be the only clinical symptom. When a large area of the pulmonary tissue is involved, the area available for gas exchange is decreased, and the dyspnea becomes severe. *Substernal retraction* and *cyanosis* may be seen on physical examination, and diminished breath sounds over the affected area are noted upon auscultation. Radiographic chest films may indicate a mediastinal shift toward the side of collapse. Additionally, the patient experiences anxiety, *diaphoresis,* and *tachycardia.* Fever may be present because collapsed lung tissue is prone to infection. Atelectasis also can occur with incomplete expansion of the lungs at birth.

PATIENT SCREENING
The patient experiencing dyspnea requires prompt medical attention for evaluation. Severe dyspnea with or without a history of previous atelectasis is a medical emergency; instruct the patient to call an ambulance. The physician should be notified immediately.

ETIOLOGY
Atelectasis is caused by an obstruction in the bronchial tree; this can be a mucous plug, foreign body, or bronchogenic cancer. Compression atelectasis results when a tumor exerts pressure on the lung and does not allow air to enter that part. Inflammatory pulmonary disease can result in accumulation of fluid in the pleural cavity (pleural effusion) and induce atelectasis. Any condition that makes deep breathing difficult can lead to atelectasis (Fig. 9–8). Failure to breathe deeply postoperatively, or prolonged inactivity, also can induce the collapse of pulmonary tissue. In the newborn, causes include prematurity, *hyaline membrane* disease, decreased stimulus to breathe, narcotics that cross the placental barrier during labor, and obstruction of the bronchus by a mucous plug.

DIAGNOSIS
Radiographic chest films, a thorough history, and physical examination play important roles in the diagnosis. Lung scans may be necessary to detect subtle changes. Breath sounds are diminished over the affected area, and percussion is dull. *Bronchoscopy* may be indicated to evaluate obstruction by a foreign body or a neoplasm.

TREATMENT
Because postoperative patients are at high risk for atelectasis, they are encouraged to ambulate as soon as possible and to deep breathe and cough periodically. Other therapeutic measures include suctioning of the airway to remove any obstruction, spirometry, and the use of antibiotics to treat accompanying infection. Intermittent positive pressure breathing (IPPB) ensures adequate lung expansion. When atelectasis is chronic, surgical removal of the affected area may be necessary. Suctioning the trachea of the newborn is indicated to remove mucus and to facilitate a patent airway. Suctioning usually is followed by the administration of oxygen.

PROGNOSIS
The outcome depends on treatment of the primary cause. Mild cases may resolve spontaneously. More severe cases are prone to complications such as pneumonia and pneumothorax. Individuals with any chronic obstructive pulmonary disease are at higher risk.

PREVENTION
Early ambulation and good ventilation therapy, after surgery or for any condition that causes prolonged immobility, is important. Individuals with lung disease are strongly advised not to smoke.

PATIENT TEACHING
Discuss the diagnostic procedures and tell the patient when to expect results. Use visual aids depicting the respiratory system to explain atelectasis. Explain the importance of postoperative ambulation and ventilation therapy. Tell the patient to seek prompt medical care for respiratory infections.

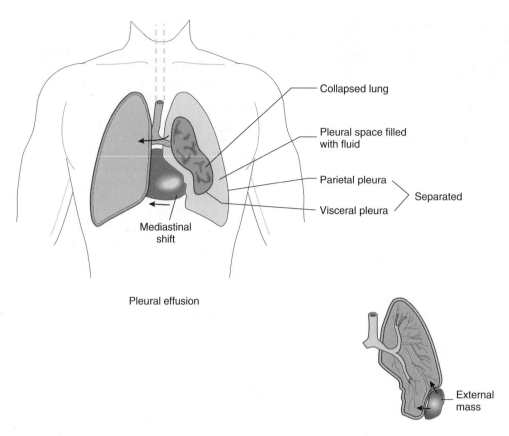

Collapsed lung

Pleural space filled with fluid

Parietal pleura

Visceral pleura

Separated

Mediastinal shift

Pleural effusion

External mass

Compression atelectasis

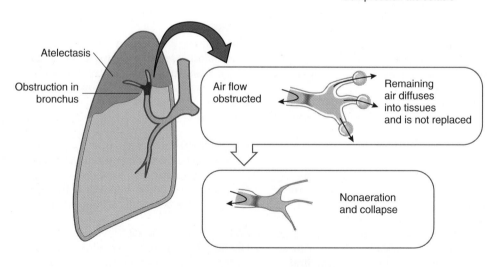

Atelectasis

Obstruction in bronchus

Air flow obstructed

Remaining air diffuses into tissues and is not replaced

Nonaeration and collapse

Obstructive atelectasis – Absorption atelectasis

FIGURE 9–8 Atelectasis. (From Gould B: *Pathophysiology for the health professions,* ed 2, Philadelphia, 2002, Saunders.)

Pulmonary Embolism

DESCRIPTION
A pulmonary embolism occurs when a clot of foreign material lodges in and occludes an artery in the pulmonary circulation (Fig. 9–9).

■ **ICD-9-CM Code** **415.19**

SYMPTOMS AND SIGNS
The size and location of the embolism, coupled with the general physical condition of the patient, determine the consequences of the interruption of blood supply to the area and the resulting symptoms and signs. The symptoms do not appear until the embolism has lodged in an artery and interrupts the blood flow. Apprehension is common. The patient with a small, uncomplicated embolism experiences a cough, chest pain, and a low-grade fever. The patient with a more extensive infarction experiences dyspnea, **tachypnea** (with a respiratory rate of at least 20 breaths per minute), chest pain, and occasionally hemop-tysis. Massive embolism leads to the sudden onset of cyanosis, shock, and death.

PATIENT SCREENING
Pulmonary embolism may present with symptoms that mimic a heart attack, with the onset of sudden chest pain and shortness of breath. He or she may be extremely apprehensive. Instruct the patient to call an ambulance and seek immediate emergency care. Notify the physician promptly. Individuals with milder symptoms of chest pain, fever, and dyspnea should be given prompt medical attention.

ETIOLOGY
Although most *emboli* are thrombi (blood clots) that have broken loose from a deep vein in the legs or pelvis, emboli also may be composed of air, fat globules, a small piece of tissue, or a cluster of bacteria. The mass moves through the venous circulation and is pumped by the right side of the heart to the pulmonary circulation, where it becomes lodged in a vessel, usually at a division of an artery where it narrows.

Stasis of blood flow from immobility, injury to a vessel, predisposition to clot formation, throm-

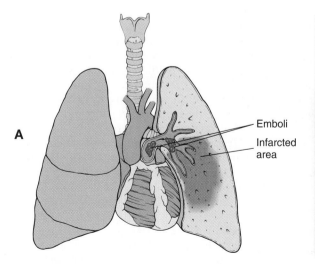

A

Emboli

Infarcted area

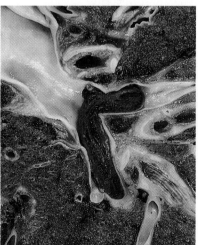

B

FIGURE 9–9 Pulmonary embolism. (**B** from Kumar V et al: *Robbins basic pathology,* ed 7, Philadelphia, 2003, Saunders.)

bophlebitis, cardiovascular disease, or pulmonary disease increases the risk of embolism formation. In pregnancy, multiple factors predispose individuals to venous thrombosis. Oral contraceptives high in estrogen, diabetes mellitus, and myocardial infarction are considered contributing factors.

DIAGNOSIS

The clinical picture, along with a history of physical immobility or other risk factors, leads to further investigation of respiratory status. Radiographic chest films, lung scans, and *magnetic resonance imaging (MRI)* scans are used to image the lung fields. Pulmonary angiography is the definitive method of making the diagnosis. *Auscultation* often reveals *rales* and pleural rub in the area of the embolism. Arterial blood gas determination shows reduced partial pressure of oxygen and carbon dioxide. Studies performed to find residual thrombi in the veins of the lower extremities are helpful in determining whether to use anticoagulants.

TREATMENT

Primary treatment is aimed at preventing a potentially fatal episode and maintaining cardiopulmonary integrity and adequate ventilation and *perfusion*. Oxygen therapy and *anticoagulant* administration are used to meet these goals. Heparin is the anticoagulant drug of choice in most cases. Additionally, thrombolytic drugs sometimes are administered to dissolve a clot.

Prevention is important; therefore, persons with cardiovascular disease and those who are immobile should be observed for early signs of any clot formation. Early ambulation and the use of thromboembolic disease (TED) stockings, or antiembolic stockings, are employed as preventive measures for patients who have had surgery.

PROGNOSIS

Mild cases can have a positive outcome with treatment. Mortality is high in cases of massive pulmonary embolism.

PREVENTION

Management of risk factors such as long-term immobility can prevent the formation of emboli that can potentially obstruct pulmonary circulation. Postoperative prophylactic measures are employed. Optimal management of systemic diseases such as

myocardial infarction, thrombophlebitis, and atrial fibrillation is beneficial.

PATIENT TEACHING

Explain anticoagulation therapy and the importance of regular blood monitoring to ensure that therapeutic levels of the anticoagulant are being maintained. Make the patient aware of side effects that should be reported to the health-care provider, such as nosebleeds, blood in the stool, or spontaneous bruising under the skin. Explain the postsurgical prevention measures prescribed to prevent venostasis, such as antiembolism stockings.

Pneumonia

DESCRIPTION

Pneumonia is an infective inflammation of the lungs.

■ **ICD-9-CM Code** **486** *(Organism unspecified)*

SYMPTOMS AND SIGNS

Pneumonia is not only a condition but also a general term applied to several types of inflammation of the lungs. The inflammation may be either unilateral or bilateral and involve all or only a portion of an infected lung (Fig. 9–10). The symptoms of pneumonia vary. The patient may have a cough, fever, shortness of breath even while at rest, chills, sweating, chest pains, cyanosis, and blood in the sputum. The infant or child exhibits "panting" or shallow rapid respirations. The larger the area of lung affected, the more severe the symptoms are. How quickly the symptoms develop and which symptoms are most evident vary with the cause.

Aspiration pneumonia results from aspiration of liquids, or other material, into the tracheobronchial tree. It tends to occur in patients who have serious problems with swallowing; among these are people afflicted with cancer or stroke.

PATIENT SCREENING

Cough, fever, and shortness of breath are symptoms that require a prompt, same-day appointment for medical evaluation. Parents of infants may report the child exhibits symptoms of a cold, with fever and fast respirations. The infant or child should be given top priority for a medical examination by a physician within 2 hours.

ETIOLOGY

Pneumonia usually is caused by viral or bacterial infections. Organisms commonly causing bacterial pneumonia are pneumococci, staphylococci, group A *hemolytic* streptococci, *Klebsiella pneumoniae* types 1 and 2, and other gram-negative organisms or *Legionella* (Legionnaires disease organism), *Haemophilus influenzae* type B, and *Francisella tularensis*. Viruses such as adenoviruses, influenza viruses, and respiratory **syncytial viruses** also can produce pneumonia. It also may be caused by damage to the lungs from inhalation of a poisonous gas such as chlorine or by aspiration of foreign matter. The pneumonia can range from a mild complication of URI to a life-threatening illness. Bacterial pneumonia can be community acquired (nosocomial).

DIAGNOSIS

The diagnostic evaluation begins with a physical examination, the patient history, and chest radiographic films to evaluate the pulmonary system. Further tests such as arterial blood gases, bronchoscopy, and sputum and blood cultures also are done.

TREATMENT

Treatment is based on the underlying cause of the pneumonia. Organism-specific antibiotics are prescribed for bacterial pneumonia. Penicillin is the drug of choice for a pneumococcal pneumonia. Tetracycline drugs, erythromycin, and sulfonamides may be administered. The use of *analgesics* such as aspirin helps to relieve chest pain, and oxygen therapy may be necessary for shortness of breath. Bed rest, increased fluid intake, a high-calorie diet, and postural drainage also prove beneficial.

PROGNOSIS

The prognosis is good for otherwise healthy individuals. Severely or chronically ill patients are more

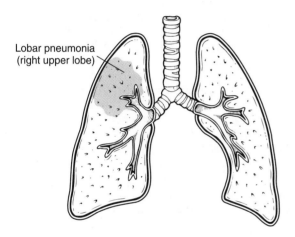

Lobar pneumonia
(right upper lobe)

FIGURE 9–10 Pneumonia.

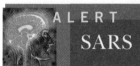

ALERT

SARS

At this writing, the Centers for Disease Control is investigating a mysterious respiratory illness called SARS (severe acute respiratory syndrome). A new mutation of a Corona virus, a genus of viruses that cause respiratory diseases, has been identified as the cause. The highly contagious disease has a sudden onset of fever, mild sore throat, muscle aches and a dry unproductive cough; chest radiographs may be normal at first. Lab tests may show lymphopenia, mild thrombocytopenia, and elevated liver enzymes. SARS symptoms vary from a simple febrile respiratory disease to severe pneumonia, with a significant mortality rate. At present no effective treatment for SARS is known, and relapses after recovery have been reported. The threat of an international epidemic resulted in the immediate isolation of suspected cases and travel warnings to China and Asia. Currently researchers at universities and government agencies are on a quest to find a reliable diagnostic test to seek out the newly discovered virus. All health care workers must protect themselves around known or suspected cases by using masks and standard precautions. Transmission is thought to be airborne and through environmental contamination.

Pneumonia

ALERT

HEALTH HAZARDS OF COMMON MOLDS

Recent concern about the health hazards of mold infestation in homes and other buildings has made its way into the public health media and medical arena. Toxic mold inside homes can cause allergic symptoms or unique or *rare* health conditions such as pulmonary hemorrhage or memory loss. Reported cases of illnesses from molds, in the indoor and outdoor environment, that contain mycotoxins (poisons produced by fungi) have prompted a plethora of questions from the public about how to determine mold infestation, what action to take, and when to seek medical attention. Listed below are some facts presented to the public by the Centers for Disease Control:

- Molds grow naturally in both the indoor and outdoor environments, especially where there is moisture. A constant supply of moisture is required for its growth.
- Large mold infestations usually can be seen or smelled.
- The hazards presented by molds that contain mycotoxins, such as *Stachybotrys chartarum,* should be considered the same as other common molds.
- Mold exposure does not always present a health problem.
- People with allergies may be more sensitive to molds. Possible allergic symptoms experienced are nasal stuffiness, eye irritation, and/or wheezing. Severe reactions may

occur among workers exposed to large amounts of molds in occupational settings.

- Those individuals who have decreased immunity, such as those with AIDS, or those with underlying lung disease or chronic diseases, are more susceptible to fungal infections.
- A common sense approach that includes routine measures of control should be used for any mold contamination existing inside homes and buildings. Decisions about treatment required for extensive mold infestations of homes or buildings are made individually; sometimes professional cleaning companies and reconstruction are employed.
- In most cases mold can be removed by a thorough cleaning with a weak (1:10) bleach and water solution. Moldy items are to be discarded.
- Recommendations for preventing mold infestation include ensuring adequate ventilation, using paint with mold inhibitors, cleaning bathrooms with mold-killing products, and promptly removing flooded carpets.
- A physician should be consulted for appropriate medical intervention when symptoms or illnesses are suspected to be the result of exposure to mold.

Modified from the CDC National Center for Environmental Health: *Questions and answers on* Stachybotrys chartarum *and other molds,* 2002, www.cdc.gov/nceh/airpollution/mold/stachy.htm.

predisposed to pneumonia. Pneumonia is the fifth leading cause of death in the United States.

PREVENTION

Antibiotic therapy for upper respiratory infections determined to be caused by bacteria such as streptococcus or staphylococcus can prevent pneumonia. Prophylactic measures against aspiration in stroke patients or those in an altered state of consciousness is prudent.

PATIENT TEACHING

Instruct the patient to take the full course of antibiotics and other medications as prescribed. Stress the importance of rest, plenty of fluid intake, and coughing to clear secretions. Counsel the patient to avoid smoking, limit alcohol intake, and not take over-the-counter medications. Tell the patient to seek prompt medical care for signs of respiratory infection in the

future, to stay away from persons with infections, and to take the influenza vaccine, if appropriate.

Pulmonary Abscess

DESCRIPTION

An area of contained infectious material in the lung is known as a *pulmonary abscess* (Fig. 9–11).

 ICD-9-CM Code 513.0

SYMPTOMS AND SIGNS

Abscesses are more common in the lower portions of the lungs and in the right lung because of its more vertical bronchus. The main symptoms are alternating chills and fever. Chest pain and a productive cough accompanied by *purulent,* bloody, or foul-smelling sputum and foul-smelling breath are also present.

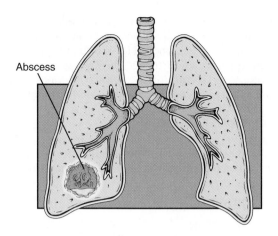

Abscess

FIGURE 9–11 Pulmonary abscess.

PATIENT SCREENING

Fever, bloody and/or foul smelling sputum, and chest discomfort indicate a serious respiratory infection that requires immediate medical care. The patient may report "a turn for the worse" while under treatment for pneumonia.

ETIOLOGY

Lung abscesses are often a complication of pneumonia caused by bacteria. Aspiration of food, a foreign object, bronchial *stenosis,* or *neoplasms* may cause pulmonary abscesses to form. A pulmonary abscess also may develop when a septic embolism is carried to the lung via the pulmonary circulation.

DIAGNOSIS

Decreased breath sounds are revealed on chest auscultation. The patient history may indicate recent aspiration. A radiographic chest film is necessary to locate the site of the affected portion of the lung. Blood and sputum cultures are used to detect the causative organism.

TREATMENT

The treatment of choice for an abscess is the use of antibiotics for a fairly long duration or until the abscess is gone. Surgical resection of the abscess and a portion of the affected lung may be required if the antibiotic therapy is not successful.

PROGNOSIS

The otherwise healthy individual who responds favorably to treatment has a good prognosis. Pro-

gnosis is guarded for the very young, the elderly, the immunocompromised, or the chronically ill.

PREVENTION

Some individuals (e.g., elderly patients) will benefit from taking the influenza vaccine.

PATIENT TEACHING

Explain to the patient the importance of taking medications exactly as prescribed, especially taking the entire course of antibiotics. Stress the importance of follow-up care until the condition is completely resolved.

Legionellosis (Legionnaires Disease and Pontiac Fever)

DESCRIPTION

Legionellosis is a pneumonia caused by the bacterium *Legionella pneumophila.*

 ICD-9-CM Code 482.84

SYMPTOMS AND SIGNS

This infection can evolve in two different forms, the more severe Legionnaires disease and the milder form, Pontiac fever. Legionnaires disease, an acute respiratory tract infection that produces severe pneumonia-like symptoms or possibly fatal pneumonia, was named after an epidemic outbreak at an American Legion convention in Philadelphia in July 1976. More than 200 people became ill, and 34 died of the disease.

Typical symptoms include general malaise, headache, and cough. These are followed rapidly by the onset of chills, fever, chest pain, dyspnea, *myalgia,* vomiting, diarrhea, and *anorexia.* The symptoms often mimic those of pneumonia. The incubation period for Legionnaires disease is 2 to 10 days, usually about 1 week. The symptoms of Pontiac fever are less severe and include a high fever and muscle aches, with a duration of 2 to 5 days. The incubation period of Pontiac fever is much shorter than Legionnaires disease, a few hours to 2 days.

PATIENT SCREENING

Initially the patient may experience multisymptom clinical features that progress to the more severe: headache, chills, high fever, dyspnea, restlessness, confusion, nausea, and vomiting. Schedule a prompt medical evaluation. Hospitalization may be required.

ETIOLOGY

Both disorders are caused by *L. pneumophila* and are not contagious. These bacteria thrive in warm aquatic environments and are inhaled from contaminated aerosolized water droplets. Air conditioning systems, cooling towers, whirlpool spas, showers, and the hot water plumbing of buildings in which the temperature of the water is between 95° and 115° F permit the reproduction of the bacterium. Predisposing factors include smoking, physical debilitation, especially among patients with chronic obstructive pulmonary disease (COPD), immunosuppression, and alcoholism. Pontiac fever usually occurs in otherwise healthy individuals.

DIAGNOSIS

A complete physical examination and patient history, along with radiographic chest studies and testing of blood samples, is done. Laboratory analysis of the blood indicates an elevation of the *white blood cell (WBC) count,* liver enzyme level, and *erythrocyte sedimentation rate (ESR).* A culture from the sputum to isolate the *Legionella* bacterium is necessary for confirmation of Legionnaires disease. The detection of the presence of bacteria in a urine sample indicates the disease. Evaluating convalescent serum samples to detect antibodies is the best diagnostic tool.

TREATMENT

Typically, antibiotic therapy is initiated before confirmation of the diagnosis is made because the response to treatment is usually slow. Erythromycin is the antibiotic most often used for treatment. Rifampin may be prescribed when the response to erythromycin is not as desired. Oxygen may be used for the dyspnea; *antipyretics, antiemetics,* and analgesics are also helpful.

Pontiac fever usually resolves itself in a few days, requiring no specific treatment. Legionellosis occurs worldwide. The National Center for Infectious Diseases monitors the incidence of legionellosis in the United States. Attempts are made to identify the sources of the disease transmission and recommendations for prevention and control measures are made.

PROGNOSIS

The prognosis is guarded in severe cases and in the immunocompromised.

PREVENTION

Prevention can be accomplished by the appropriate design of facilities to prevent stagnant water.

The temperature of the water in cooling towers and air conditioning units must be maintained either below 95° F or above 115° F, or it must have adequate chlorination to kill the *Legionella* bacillus. Monitoring of chlorine content of whirlpool baths and spas is a necessary obligation of the owners.

PATIENT TEACHING

Urge the patient to take the entire course of antibiotics as prescribed. Give the patient appropriate instructions regarding hospitalization when required.

Respiratory Syncytial Virus Pneumonia

DESCRIPTION

Respiratory syncytial virus (RSV) pneumonia, an inflammatory and infectious condition of the lungs, is most common in infants, young children, and the elderly.

 ICD-9-CM Code 480.1

SYMPTOMS AND SIGNS

RSV causes cold-like symptoms, including nasal congestion, *otitis media,* and coughing, in the mild upper respiratory tract form of infection. As the virus progresses downward to the lower respiratory tract, the patient experiences fever, malaise, lethargy, more frequent coughing, wheezing, and dyspnea.

PATIENT SCREENING

Infants with symptoms of a lower respiratory tract infection require prompt medical attention and close monitoring thereafter until well.

ETIOLOGY

Respiratory syncytial virus is the causative agent of RSV pneumonia. The greatest occurrence of these annual epidemic infections is during the winter months, December to March, and they most seriously affect children younger than 3 years of age and the elderly, especially patients whose respiratory systems already are compromised by underlying disease or predisposing factors. At greatest risk are infants who were premature or who have a congenital cardiac defect or a preexisting pulmonary disorder. Most people have experienced several RSV upper respiratory tract infections in their lifetimes, and most cases of mild RSV infection are self-limiting.

RSV is spread by contact with secretions of an infected person. Thorough hand washing and the use of disposable tissues for nasal secretions can prevent the spread of this disease.

DIAGNOSIS

Clinical findings, a thorough physical examination, and *lavage* of the nasal pharynx aid in determining the diagnosis of RSV pneumonia. The secretions obtained from the lavage are examined for the presence of RSV. When grown in tissue culture, RSV produces giant syncytial cells.

TREATMENT

Most cases of RSV infection involving the upper respiratory tract are self-limiting. Antipyretics are prescribed for fever, and antibiotics are given for otitis media. When the infection invades the lower respiratory tract of an infant or a young child, treatment may involve inhalation therapy. Hospitalization may be required for oxygen therapy and hydration.

PROGNOSIS

The prognosis is generally good. Infants are prone to the complication of otitis media.

PREVENTION

Adults with symptoms of respiratory infection should not handle infants. Strict hand washing is prudent, because the virus is transmitted by respiratory secretions.

PATIENT TEACHING

Infants are usually hospitalized so supportive therapy can be provided; thus parents need reassurance and support. Parents are encouraged to hold and interact with the infant. Inform the parents that the head of the crib or bed is elevated to prevent aspiration of secretions and aid respirations.

Histoplasmosis

DESCRIPTION

Histoplasmosis is a fungal disease originating in the lungs that is caused by inhalation of dust containing *Histoplasma capsulatum.*

 ICD-9-CM Code 115.90 *(Unspecified)*

SYMPTOMS AND SIGNS

Histoplasmosis may cause pneumonia or may become systemic. Many patients with histoplasmosis are *asymptomatic* at onset; it is not contagious. As the fungus disseminates throughout the pulmonary tissue, the patient reports dyspnea and loss of energy to the point of incapacitation. The patient becomes febrile. The spleen and lymph nodes become enlarged. In patients with acquired immunodeficiency syndrome (AIDS), histoplasmosis may occur as an opportunistic infection.

PATIENT SCREENING

The patient presenting with the above symptomatology should be seen for medical evaluation within 24 hours.

ETIOLOGY

Histoplasmosis is caused by the fungus *H. capsulatum,* which is carried by dust and is inhaled. The greatest occurrence of histoplasmosis is in the Midwestern United States. Often the fungus is found in soil contaminated by droppings from birds or bats specific to the area, which may be a source of the airborne fungus.

NOTE: Blastomycosis (also called Gilchrist disease) is a rare fungal infection caused by inhaling the fungus Blastomyces dermatitidis, which grows as a mold in moist soil and wood. It is found in specific endemic areas in North America and with greatest prevalence in the upper Midwest and southward along the Mississippi and Ohio riverbeds.

DIAGNOSIS

Diagnosis is made by evaluating the clinical findings, a positive skin test result, blood **serologic** findings specific for the fungus, or the identification of the fungus in pus, sputum, or tissue specimens. Radiographic chest films may be normal or may reveal patchy infiltrates and diffuse opacities.

TREATMENT

If the disease is self-limiting, no antifungal therapy is necessary. The antifungal drug amphotericin B is used to treat severe or progressive histoplasmosis.

PROGNOSIS

Spontaneous recovery is usual. Secondary infections are possible. Small calcifications remain in the lungs after infection. Progressive histoplasmosis can be fatal. Infection confers immunity.

PREVENTION

It is prudent to teach safety practices to workers in high-risk jobs that expose them to contaminated soil.

PATIENT TEACHING

Review appropriate prevention measures with individuals at risk because of poor health. Advise the patient to avoid contact with soil contaminated with bat or bird droppings.

Influenza

DESCRIPTION

Influenza is a generalized, highly contagious, acute viral disease that occurs in annual outbreaks.

ICD-9-CM Code 487

The above code is a nonspecific code and may be valid as a principal diagnosis, except for Medicare. Refer to the physician's diagnosis and then to the current edition of the ICD-9-CM coding manual to ensure the greatest specificity of pathology and any appropriate modifiers.

SYMPTOMS AND SIGNS

Influenza is characterized by inflammation of the upper and lower respiratory tract mucous membranes, a severe protracted cough, fever, headache, sore throat, and generalized malaise. The onset is usually sudden, marked by chills and a feverish feeling. In mild cases, the temperature may reach 101° to 102° F, and the fever may last for 2 or 3 days. In severe cases, a 103° to 104° F temperature is possible, lasting 4 or 5 days. Acute symptoms usually subside rapidly with decreasing fever. The weakness, sweating, and fatigue may continue for a few days to a few weeks; malaise may persist several days before full recovery.

Fever, cough, and other respiratory symptoms persisting for longer than 5 days may indicate a secondary bacterial pneumonia. Possible complications of influenza are bronchitis, sinusitis, otitis media, and cervical **lymphadenitis.**

ETIOLOGY

Known viruses that cause influenza are designated as orthomyxovirus types A, B, and C. However, many mutant strains also reproduce in both humans and animals. Acute uncomplicated influenza with recovery is the most frequently encountered type of this disease. Secondary bacterial pneumonia after influenza most often is caused by hemolytic streptococcus, staphylococcus, or pneumococcus.

Influenza outbreaks may be sporadic or epidemic. Epidemics occur every 1 to 4 years and spread rapidly because the incubation period is only 1 to 3 days. Transmission is by inhalation of the virus in airborne mucus discharge. Fatalities can occur in as short a time as 48 hours after the onset of symptoms.

PATIENT SCREENING

During a known epidemic, the health-care provider may give the telephone screener(s) guidelines to address callers with symptoms typical of influenza.

Individuals with severe symptoms or those who are at high risk for complications (i.e., the very young, the elderly, or those chronically ill) are given a prompt appointment for close medical monitoring.

DIAGNOSIS

Clinically, influenza may be indistinguishable from the common cold. When differentiating influenza from other respiratory tract infections, consideration should be given to the amount of time passed since onset, the presence of an epidemic in the community, and the severity of the patient's symptoms. Frequent recurrences of influenza-like syndromes may make the physician suspect tuberculosis (see Pulmonary Tuberculosis). A complicating pneumonia may be present if the patient has dyspnea, cyanosis, hemoptysis, or rales in the lungs. A WBC count may indicate *leukopenia* with relative *lymphocytosis.* Confirmation of the influenza diagnosis is made by isolation of the virus from a throat culture. A sputum culture isolates bacteria in secondary infections.

TREATMENT

Treatment is symptomatic; vaccines are useless after the disease is established. Bed rest, increased fluid intake, a light diet, and the use of antipyretic and analgesic drugs when needed are helpful. Amantadine, an antiviral agent, sometimes may be helpful in treating influenza. In less severe cases, treatment of respiratory tract symptoms may not be necessary; however, warm salt water gargles, steam inhalation, and the use of cough syrups may be comforting. Antibiotics are effective against bacterial pneumonia and other less serious complications such as sinusitis, otitis media, and lymphadenitis.

PROGNOSIS

Recovery is usually complete; however, complications such as pneumonia can occur. Those at highest risk are the young, the elderly, and the chronically ill. Epidemics can cause substantial morbidity, financial loss, and even death.

BOX 9-1
Target Groups for Influenza Immunization

GROUPS AT INCREASED RISK OF COMPLICATIONS

Persons aged 65 years and older

Residents of nursing homes and other chronic care facilities

Patients with chronic pulmonary (including asthma) or cardiac disorder

Patients with chronic metabolic disease (including diabetes), renal dysfunction, hemoglobinopathies, or immunosuppression

Children and teens receiving long-term aspirin

GROUPS IN CONTACT WITH HIGH-RISK PERSONS

Physicians, nurses, and other health care providers

Employees of nursing homes and chronic care facilities

Providers of home care to high-risk persons

Household members (including children) of high-risk persons

OTHER GROUPS

Providers of essential community services (e.g., police, fire)

International travelers

Students, dormitory residents

Anyone wishing to reduce risk of influenza

Modified from Advisory Committee on Immunization Practices, Centers for Disease Control and Prevention: MMWR 43(No RR-9):1, 1994. From Bennett JC, Plum F: *Cecil textbook of medicine,* ed 20, vol 1, Philadelphia, 1996, Saunders, p 1756.

PREVENTION

The *prophylactic* use of vaccines against influenza is effective in reducing the occurrence of the disease, especially for the elderly or infirm (Box 9–1). Because immunity from vaccination lasts only 1 year, annual booster doses are needed for optimal protection. After vaccination, about 2 to 4 weeks is required for immunity to develop.

PATIENT TEACHING

Reinforce the use of comfort measures, including antipyretics and analgesics as prescribed. *NOTE: Warn parents that aspirin is contraindicated for children because Reye syndrome can result.* Advise the patient to rest and take adequate fluids. Infection control including thorough and frequent hand washing is prudent to reduce the spread of the virus. Educate individuals at high risk about annual influenza immunizations.

Chronic Obstructive Pulmonary Disease

Chronic obstructive pulmonary disease (COPD), or chronic obstructive lung disease (COLD), encompasses several obstructive diseases of the lungs, including chronic bronchitis, bronchiectasis, asthma, emphysema, cystic fibrosis, and **pneumoconiosis**. Although the mechanism of the obstruction can vary, the consequence is the same; the patient with COPD is unable to ventilate the lungs freely, which results in an ineffective exchange of respiratory gases. This causes the patient's normal respiratory response to elevated carbon dioxide levels to become diminished.

Acute and Chronic Bronchitis

DESCRIPTION

Bronchitis is inflammation of the mucous membrane lining the bronchi.

 ICD-9-CM Code 491.21

SYMPTOMS AND SIGNS

A deep, persistent, productive cough is the main symptom. The patient has thick yellow to gray sputum. Other symptoms include shortness of breath, wheezing, a slightly elevated temperature, and pain in the upper chest, which is aggravated by the cough. Acute symptoms subside within a week, but the cough may continue for 2 to 3 weeks. Physical signs within the lungs are few or absent if the bronchitis is uncomplicated.

Scattered or occasional rales often are heard on auscultation.

Chronic bronchitis is similar to acute bronchitis, except that the inflammation persists and becomes worse. Mild forms may exist for many years, with the patient having only a slight cough in the mornings. Then the condition becomes aggravated when the patient contracts acute upper respiratory tract infections. As the condition progresses, obstructive and asthmatic symptoms appear, along with dyspnea. Chest expansion becomes diminished, and often, scattered rales and wheezing are heard. In the beginning stages of the disease, flare-ups of chronic bronchitis are likely to occur after the patient has experienced severe colds or influenza. In later stages, even a minor head cold can cause a severe attack. During the final stages, the coughing, shortness of breath and wheezing occur almost continuously. Prolonged, recurrent attacks cause gradual deterioration of the lungs.

For both acute and chronic bronchitis, the symptoms appear more troublesome during the winter months. Living or working in a cold, damp environment or in a polluted atmosphere can aggravate the condition.

PATIENT SCREENING

An individual complaining of a persistent, productive cough is advised to seek medical care if there has been no improvement. When the cough is described as chronic, with purulent sputum, and fever and/or wheezing are present, the patient should be examined by the health-care professional within 24 hours. Persons known to have chronic bronchitis should be seen promptly for suspected infections or sudden worsening of symptoms.

ETIOLOGY

Acute bronchitis is part of a general URI. It begins after a common cold or other viral infections of the nasopharynx and pharynx or occurs as a complication of bacterial infections. Recurring attacks in adults may indicate a focus of infection, such as chronic sinusitis (see Sinusitis), bronchiectasis (see Bronchiectasis), and pneumonia (see Pneumonia). In children, hypertrophied tonsils and adenoids may be the source of acute bronchitis. Allergens are also frequently predisposing factors.

No single or specific bacterium is responsible for chronic bronchitis; however, in many cases of recurrent infections, *Pneumococcus* or *H. influenzae* has been the main organism responsible. Chronic bronchitis often accompanies chronic asthma, pulmonary *fibrosis*, obstructive emphysema, pulmonary tuberculosis, or congestive heart failure. Chronic bronchitis often is associated with the cause of some forms of emphysema. Progressive and irreversible changes in the bronchi can result from constant irritation from smoking or exposure to industrial pollution.

DIAGNOSIS

Acute or chronic bronchitis can be suspected on the basis of the patient's symptoms and history. The presence of other diseases or their complications must be ruled out, especially if the symptoms are serious or prolonged. Diagnostic tests include radiographic chest studies, pulmonary function tests, arterial blood gases, and other blood and sputum analyses.

TREATMENT

Because acute bronchitis usually is caused by a viral infection, no specific treatment is prescribed, except for those measures that will relieve the symptoms. Aspirin may be used to control fever. Increased fluid intake, along with the use of a vaporizer and humidifier, helps to clear the nasal passages and bronchi. The physician may prescribe the use of a bronchodilator aerosol inhaler for wheezing and shortness of breath and a cough suppressant if the chest is sore from coughing. If a secondary bacterial infection is suspected, an antibiotic is prescribed.

The treatment of chronic bronchitis is based on the stage of the disease at the time the patient consults professional help. Prompt treatment of acute infections, when they occur, is of primary importance. Low-flow oxygen therapy may be administered as needed for hypoxemia. Postural drainage and percussion are techniques used to help loosen and expectorate thick mucus. Aerosolized corticosteroids may be ordered to control inflammation. The patient is advised to give up smoking, to avoid smoke-filled rooms, to stay away from people with colds, and to live in a warm, dry climate.

PROGNOSIS

Acute bronchitis resolves completely within a few days; however, a residual cough can remain for 2 to 3 weeks. Chronic bronchitis has a guarded prognosis because it may be progressive and involves airway obstruction and general debilitation.

PREVENTION
It is important for the patient to avoid the primary causative factors: smoking, chronic exposure to pollutants in the air, and recurrent respiratory infections.

PATIENT TEACHING
For acute bronchitis, the patient is advised to rest and take any palliative medications as prescribed. Patients with chronic bronchitis are advised not to smoke or expose themselves to known respiratory irritants. Demonstrate methods of chest physiotherapy. Explain the use of home equipment designed for oxygen therapy or inhalation therapy. Encourage smokers to take advantage of smoking cessation programs available in the community.

Bronchiectasis

DESCRIPTION
Bronchiectasis is the permanent, irreversible dilation or distortion of one or more of the bronchi, resulting from destruction of muscular and elastic portions of the bronchial walls (Fig. 9–12).

 ICD-9-CM Code 494.0

SYMPTOMS AND SIGNS
Bronchiectasis, a condition that takes many years to develop, is usually bilateral and involves the lower lobes of the lungs. A chronic cough producing large quantities of a purulent, foul-smelling sputum is the main symptom of bronchiectasis. Hemoptysis, dyspnea, wheezing, fever, and general malaise develop as the condition progresses. The patient also may experience chronic halitosis.

PATIENT SCREENING
Schedule the patient presenting with a chronic, highly productive cough for a clinical examination at his or her earliest convenience.

ETIOLOGY
Bronchiectasis may be caused by repeated damage to the bronchial wall caused by heavy smoking. It also can result from pneumonia, tuberculosis, bronchial obstruction, or inhalation of a corrosive gas. This condition is a common life-threatening complication of cystic fibrosis or other childhood

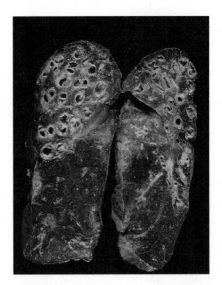

FIGURE 9–12 Bronchiectasis. (From Cotran R et al: *Robbins pathologic basis of disease,* ed 6, Philadelphia, 1999, Saunders.)

infections, such as measles and pertussis (whooping cough), and also may result from immune deficiency (e.g., hypogammaglobulinemia).

DIAGNOSIS
Initially, when symptoms are vague, determining the diagnosis of bronchiectasis may be difficult. Physical examination, history of symptoms, radiographic chest films, a high-resolution CT scan of the chest, bronchoscopy, sputum culture, and pulmonary function tests are of the most value in making the diagnosis.

TREATMENT
Antibiotics and bronchodilators are prescribed, and postural drainage is encouraged. Avoiding environmental irritants such as smoke, fumes, and large amounts of dust is important. If the patient has a great deal of hemoptysis, surgery to remove the affected part of the lung may be advised.

PROGNOSIS
The prognosis varies with the underlying cause. Serious respiratory and cardiac complications

such as pulmonary hypertension and cor pulmonale (see Chapter 10) develop with advanced bronchiectasis.

PREVENTION

Childhood immunizations and early treatment of respiratory infections are recommended for prevention, as is preclusion of smoking or exposure to any other respiratory irritants.

PATIENT TEACHING

The patient who smokes is strongly advised to cease smoking; offer a referral to a smoking cessation support group. Explain the medical management regimen, and demonstrate how to use home equipment for oxygen therapy and/or inhalation therapy. Teach the patient proper techniques for postural drainage and percussion and how to properly discard secretions.

Asthma

See Chapter 2 for a discussion of asthma. See Figure 9–13 for effects of smoking.

Pulmonary Emphysema

DESCRIPTION

Pulmonary emphysema is a chronic obstructive pulmonary disorder characterized by destructive changes in the alveolar walls and irreversible enlargement of alveolar air spaces.

> **ICD-9-CM Code　492.8** *(Other emphysema)*
> *The above code is a nonspecific code and may be valid as a principal diagnosis, except for Medicare. Refer to the physician's diagnosis and then to the current edition of the ICD-9-CM coding manual to ensure the greatest specificity of pathology and any appropriate modifiers.*

SYMPTOMS AND SIGNS

Pulmonary emphysema, a destructive disease of the alveolar septa, interferes with both the breathing process and gas exchange in the lungs. Alveoli become enlarged, which precipitates destruction of the alveolar walls and damage to the adjacent capillary walls. As a result of the decreased area for gas exchange and the trapped air, the patient experiences dyspnea. The onset of symptoms is insidious, with a gradual difficulty in breathing; dyspnea,

tachypnea, wheezing, and moist, persistent cough are the first indications of the disease. The inability to exhale carbon dioxide in a normal manner requires the patient with emphysema to use accessory muscles to force out air trapped in the alveoli and, subsequently, produces the characteristic barrel chest (Fig. 9–14). Shortness of breath and dyspnea increase, and the patient purses the lips to assist in exhaling. As the disease progresses, the patient develops **circumoral cyanosis,** symptoms of right ventricular heart failure (see Cor Pulmonale in Chapter 10), and digital clubbing.

PATIENT SCREENING

The patient who complains of an insidious onset of difficult breathing, wheezing, and/or persistent coughing should be given the first available appointment within 24 hours for clinical evaluation.

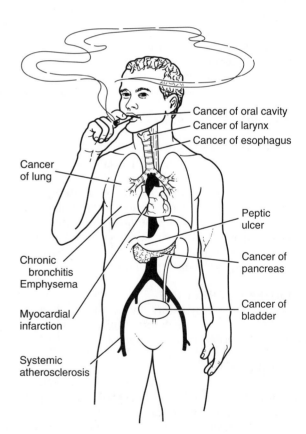

FIGURE 9–13 Effects of smoking. (From Kumar V et al: *Robbins basic pathology,* ed 7, Philadelphia, 2003, Saunders.)

ETIOLOGY

Although the etiology of pulmonary emphysema is not completely understood, long-term cigarette smoking appears to be a contributing factor. Repeated respiratory tract infections beginning in childhood and continuing throughout adulthood also may contribute to the increased occurrence of the disease. Additionally, irritants such as ozone, sulfur dioxide, and nitrogen oxides are thought to play a role in the etiology. The possibility of a familial tendency is supported by the increased frequency of the disease in families who experience an *antitrypsin* deficiency.

DIAGNOSIS

Diagnosis is based on a clinical examination and a thorough patient history, which usually shows a prolonged exposure to possible respiratory irritants, especially cigarette smoking. Pulmonary function studies indicate increased tidal volume and residual volume, along with decreased vital capacity and expiratory maneuver volumes. Radiographic chest studies show translucent-appearing lungs, a depressed or flattened diaphragm, and *cardiomegaly.* The patient exhibits tachypnea, tachycardia, hypertension, polycythemia, diminished breath sounds, and wheezing or **rhonchi.** Anteroposterior chest diameter is increased—producing a typical barrel chest appearance (see Fig. 9–8). Individuals with extensive progressive disease present with distended neck veins, *hepatomegaly,* peripheral edema, clubbed fingers, and cyanosis. *Blood gas* determinations in the advanced stages indicate decreased arterial oxygen tension and increased carbon dioxide.

TREATMENT

The patient is instructed and encouraged to avoid the inhalation of irritating substances, particularly cigarette smoke. Patients with pulmonary emphysema should take care to avoid exposure to possible respiratory tract infections and should receive influenza virus vaccination annually. A high-protein diet eaten in small portions and supplemental vitamins is recommended. Supplemental low concentrations of oxygen may help as well.

Drug therapy includes beta$_2$-adrenergic sympathomimetic drugs, such as albuterol (Ventolin and Proventil), terbutaline sulfate (Brethine), and metaproterenol sulfate (Alupent), for bronchodilation and antispasmodic activity; theophylline; expectorants; and antibiotics.

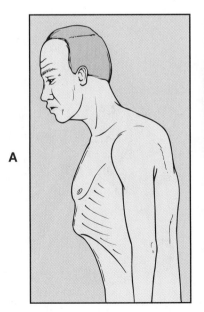
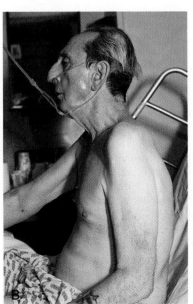

FIGURE 9–14 A, Note barrel chest of patient with emphysema and bluish discoloration around mouth. **B,** Note bolt upright position and pursed lip breathing. (**B** from Henry MC, Stapleton ER: *EMT prehospital care,* ed 3, Philadelphia, 2004, Saunders.)

PROGNOSIS

The prognosis for long-term disease is poor; in the United States, emphysema is the most common cause of death from respiratory disease.

PREVENTION

Education about the possible heath consequences of long-term smoking is imperative. It is helpful for patients to avoid exposure to respiratory irritants and to guard against repeated respiratory infections.

PATIENT TEACHING

The patient who smokes is strongly advised to cease smoking; offer a referral to a smoking cessation support group. Explain the medical management regimen, and demonstrate how to use home equipment for oxygen therapy and/or inhalation therapy. Demonstrate appropriate breathing techniques that maximize expiration and ventilation. Referral to a pulmonary rehabilitation program can be helpful as well.

Pneumoconiosis

DESCRIPTION

Pneumoconiosis is any disease of the lung caused by long-term dust inhalation.

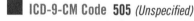 **ICD-9-CM Code 505** *(Unspecified)*

SYMPTOMS AND SIGNS

Pneumoconiosis means dust in the lungs. It refers to a number of occupational diseases that cause progressive, chronic inflammation and infection in the lungs. The onset of symptoms can be insidious, with dyspnea on exertion being the first symptom. In all types of dust-related disease, a dry cough, which later turns productive and becomes similar to the cough of chronic bronchitis, is typical. The patient may admit increasing effort is required for inspiration. Pulmonary hypertension, tachypnea, general malaise, and recurrent respiratory tract infections are common. Other symptoms may be associated with tuberculosis (see Pulmonary Tuberculosis) of the lungs. Family members are also at risk for pneumoconiosis if constantly exposed to dust particles in the worker's clothing.

PATIENT SCREENING

Persistent cough over a period of weeks or months and dyspnea are symptoms that require clinical evaluation; schedule the first available appointment. Inform the patient to call back for an immediate appointment if signs of infection occur or symptoms worsen.

ETIOLOGY

Pneumoconiosis is considered to be an occupational disease caused by inhaling inorganic dust particles over a prolonged period. It usually takes at least 10 years or longer of continual daily exposure for pneumoconiosis to develop; however, it may take as little as 2 years or as long as 30 years to develop.

Asbestosis is a form of dust disease caused by exposure to asbestos fibers. It is characterized by a slow and progressively diffuse fibrosis of the lungs. Asbestosis is the most commonly occurring type of pneumoconiosis.

Another form of pneumoconiosis is **anthracosis,** also known as black lung or coal miner's lung. Anthracosis is caused by the accumulation of carbon deposits in the lungs resulting from inhaling smoke or coal dust (Fig. 9–15).

Silicosis, another type of dust disease, affects workers who are stone masons or metal grinders or who work in quarries. Silicosis develops as a result of inhaling silica (quartz) dust and causes a dense

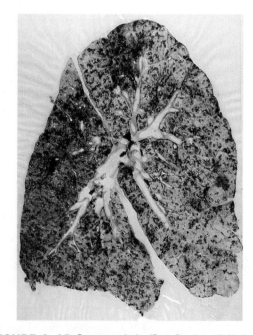

FIGURE 9–15 Pneumoconiosis. (From Damjanov I, Linder J: *Pathology: a color atlas,* St. Louis, 1999, Mosby.)

fibrosis of the lungs and emphysema with respiratory impairment.

Other workers who are also susceptible to dust diseases are those who work with aluminum, beryllium, iron, cotton, sugar cane, and a number of synthetic fibers.

DIAGNOSIS

A thorough patient history and a complete physical examination are essential for making the diagnosis. Radiographic chest studies, pulmonary function tests, and arterial blood gas determination confirm the diagnosis.

TREATMENT

The treatment of all pneumoconioses is directed toward relieving symptoms. Typically, this includes the administration of bronchodilators, oxygen therapy, chest physical therapy to help remove secretions and the use of corticosteroid drugs. A common complication, tuberculosis, must be treated aggressively.

PROGNOSIS

The damage to lung tissue is irreversible and infections are common.

PREVENTION

Pneumoconiosis is considered an environmental disease, thus dust reduction in the work place is essential. Smoking worsens the condition and embedded asbestos fibers increase the risk of lung cancer.

PATIENT TEACHING

Stress the importance of prompt treatment for infections. The patient is advised to end exposure to dust particles. Explain the medication dosage schedule and demonstrate the proper use of the inhaler and/or home oxygen therapy equipment. Offer a referral to a support group for cessation of smoking, if appropriate.

Pleurisy (Pleuritis)

DESCRIPTION

Pleurisy is an inflammation of the membranes surrounding the lungs and lining the pleural cavity (Fig. 9–16).

ICD-9-CM Code 511.0

SYMPTOMS AND SIGNS

The patient reports sharp, needle-like pain, which increases with inspiration and coughing. Additionally, this patient experiences a cough, fever, and chills. Inspirations are shallow and rapid.

PATIENT SCREENING

Usually, significant pain with inspiration is what prompts the call for medical intervention. Schedule the first available appointment within 24 hours.

ETIOLOGY

Pleurisy is usually secondary to other diseases or infections. The inflammation also may result from injury or the presence of a tumor.

Two types of pleurisy exist, wet and dry. When pleural fluid is present, the increased volume causes compression of the pulmonary tissue and dyspnea. Dry pleurisy occurs when the pleural fluid decreases in volume, resulting in a dryness between the pleura; the layers rub together and become congested and edematous.

DIAGNOSIS

Diagnosis is made from the symptoms, history, and physical examination. A pleural rub can be heard on auscultation of the lungs. Radiographic films

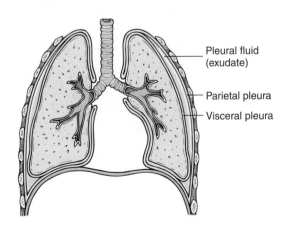

Pleural fluid (exudate)

Parietal pleura

Visceral pleura

FIGURE 9–16 Pleurisy.

may indicate the presence of pleural effusion and/or underlying pulmonary disease.

TREATMENT

Treatment is directed at the underlying cause. Antibiotic therapy and analgesics to control the pain may be given. Splinting of the chest and deep breathing exercises help promote good ventilation.

PROGNOSIS

Recovery is usually complete. In some cases, permanent adhesions may restrict lung expansion.

PREVENTION

No specific prevention is known.

PATIENT TEACHING

Explain to the patient the importance of deep breathing exercises for adequate lung expansion.

Pneumothorax

DESCRIPTION

Pneumothorax is a collection of air or gas in the pleural cavity that results in a collapsed or partially collapsed lung (Fig. 9–17).

ICD-9-CM Code 512.8

SYMPTOMS AND SIGNS

Collapse of a lung causes severe shortness of breath, sudden sharp chest pain, falling blood pressure, rapid weak pulse, and shallow and weak respirations. The patient may be cyanotic and appears anxious. Increased air pressure on the affected side causes a mediastinal shift to the unaffected side.

PATIENT SCREENING

The patient experiencing the crisis as described above requires urgent care and immediate transportation to the emergency room.

ETIOLOGY

Pneumothorax can be spontaneous or traumatic. Spontaneous pneumothorax occurs when an opening is present on the surface of a lung. Causative factors can be erosion of alveoli from tumor or disease, increased pressure from within the respiratory system (too great a force with artificial ventilation), or a spontaneous tear in the tissue. Traumatic pneumothorax occurs when the integrity of the pleural cavity is breached from without as the result of trauma, such as gunshot wound, stab wound, or crushing-type wound to the chest. The object (possibly the patient's own rib) penetrates the chest cavity, allowing air to enter from the atmosphere.

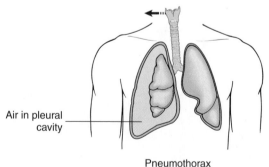

Air in pleural cavity

Pneumothorax

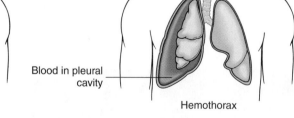

Blood in pleural cavity

Hemothorax

FIGURE 9–17 Pneumothorax and hemothorax.

DIAGNOSIS

Diagnosis is made after evaluating the history, the clinical findings, and radiographic studies. Radiographic films will show the air in the pleural cavity, the collapsed portion of the lung, and mediastinal shift. Breath sounds are diminished, and sucking air sounds are heard at the wound site. The patient is in acute distress.

TREATMENT

The patient is more comfortable in a *Fowler* or a semi-Fowler position and may require oxygen. An occlusive dressing is placed over any sucking wound to seal the portal of entry and to prevent additional air from entering the chest cavity. A *thoracentesis* is performed to withdraw air from the cavity. A closed drainage system is established if air continues to leak into the pleural space. This allows expansion and healing of the lung.

PROGNOSIS

Recovery depends on the degree of lung collapse, the cause, and prompt medical intervention.

PREVENTION

No specific measures of prevention are known.

PATIENT TEACHING

Throughout emergency care and after the patient is medically stable, offer support to the individual and family. Patients receiving conservative therapy are encouraged to rest during a period of close monitoring. More severe cases or those that result from trauma will require teaching about treatments used to expand the lungs.

Hemothorax

DESCRIPTION

Hemothorax is the accumulation of blood and fluid in the pleural cavity (see Fig. 9–17).

■ ICD-9-CM Code **511.8**

SYMPTOMS AND SIGNS

The patient experiences symptoms similar to those of pneumothorax. Signs of hemorrhage include pale and clammy skin, a weak and thready pulse, and falling blood pressure. The patient may experience chest pain and respirations are labored and shallow or gasping.

PATIENT SCREENING

Hemothorax is life threatening and requires emergency medical care.

ETIOLOGY

Blood enters the pleural space as the result of trauma or the erosion of a pulmonary vessel. This causes the lung to collapse.

DIAGNOSIS

Breath sounds are diminished or absent on the affected side, as is chest wall movement. Radiographic films show blood in the pleural space. Blood tests indicate hemorrhage; arterial blood gas analysis reflects respiratory failure. The patient is in acute distress.

TREATMENT

The treatment employed is similar to that for pneumothorax. The lung must be reexpanded, usually by thoracentesis with closed drainage to evacuate the blood. The underlying cause, once discovered, is treated, often necessitating surgical intervention to repair the wound. Vital signs are monitored, and blood loss is replaced.

PROGNOSIS

The prognosis for hemothorax is guarded, depending on the cause and the availability of effective treatment.

PREVENTION

No specific prevention measures are known.

PATIENT TEACHING

Every effort is made to reassure the patient while emergency and diagnostic measures are taking place. Once the patient is stabilized, explain the purpose of therapeutic procedures such as chest tube drainage and thoracentesis.

Flail Chest

DESCRIPTION

Flail chest is a condition of instability in the chest wall caused by multiple rib fractures; the sternum also may be fractured.

 ICD-9-CM Code 807.4

SYMPTOMS AND SIGNS

The patient with flail chest, a double fracture of three or more adjacent ribs, experiences severe pain and dyspnea and is cyanotic and extremely anxious. The segment of the chest involved moves inward during inspiration and outward during expiration; this is termed *paradoxical breathing*.

PATIENT SCREENING

Flail chest is a medical emergency and may be life-threatening.

ETIOLOGY

Direct trauma to the chest wall that fractures three or more adjacent ribs is the cause of flail chest. This trauma may be from direct compression by a heavy object, a motor vehicle accident (especially injury by the steering wheel), a hard fall onto a solid object, or an industrial accident. The paradoxical movement and instability of the chest wall occur when three or more adjacent ribs are broken in two places or break loose from the sternum while also being broken at another site (Fig. 9–18).

DIAGNOSIS

Diagnosis is made by noting history of chest trauma and observing the paradoxical movement of the chest wall. Radiographic chest films will confirm the diagnosis.

TREATMENT

First responder emergency care employs measures to stabilize the chest wall until surgical repair is possible. The treatment of flail chest involves allowing the rib fractures to heal while maintaining respiratory integrity. This may entail mechanical ventilation and sedation of the patient with an endotracheal tube in place. Pain medications such as morphine and meperidine hydrochloride (Demerol) are administered to keep the patient comfortable. Additionally, supplemental oxygen is administered.

PROGNOSIS

Emergency medical care and transport to the hospital as soon as possible helps to achieve a positive outcome. Delayed medical intervention and complications resulting from trauma can worsen the chance for recovery.

PREVENTION

Safety measures, such as wearing automobile seat belts, that protect the chest from trauma are prudent.

PATIENT TEACHING

Every effort is made to dispel the patient's anxiety during emergency measures to stabilize the chest wall. Continue to advise the patient of all procedures necessary to achieve respiratory integrity.

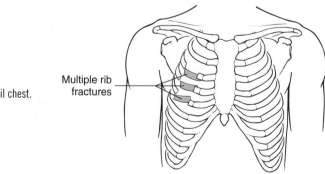

FIGURE 9–18 Flail chest.

Multiple rib fractures

Pulmonary Tuberculosis

DESCRIPTION

Pulmonary tuberculosis is a chronic, acute, or subacute infection of the lungs by *Mycobacterium tuberculosis*.

 ICD-9-CM Code 011.90

SYMPTOMS AND SIGNS

Pulmonary tuberculosis, an infectious and inflammatory disease of the lungs, is acquired by inhaling a dried droplet nucleus that contains the tubercle bacillus. These droplet nuclei may remain suspended in room air for many hours. The patient with a primary tuberculosis infection is often asymptomatic initially. When the infection is secondary, the patient experiences vague symptoms such as weight loss, reduced appetite, listlessness, vague chest pain, dry cough, loss of energy, and fever. As the disease progresses, the patient has productive cough with purulent sputum, the appearance of blood streaking or hemoptysis, fever, and night sweats.

PATIENT SCREENING

Schedule a prompt appointment for the patient complaining of a persistent cough with blood-tinged or purulent sputum. Constitutional symptoms such as fatigue, fever, and night sweats also may exist.

NOTE: All patients presenting with a cluster of symptoms that indicate a serious respiratory infection should be escorted upon arrival to the first available examination room. It is prudent to follow strict infection control.

ETIOLOGY

The tubercle bacillus *Mycobacterium tuberculosis* causes tuberculosis and is spread by droplet nuclei. The primary lesion usually is located in the lungs. The bacteria can survive in the dried form for months if not exposed to sunlight. Any tissue of the body can be affected; however, the lung is the typical site (Fig. 9–19).

The infection begins with a primary lesion in the lower area of the lung. As the body's defense mechanisms respond to the bacterial invasion, antigens are produced, which cause *necrosis* followed by fibrosis and calcification of the affected tissue. The infection then may be arrested and the disease becomes inactive, remaining so for years. If the infection is not arrested, the patient experiences progressive primary tuberculosis.

The patient's resistance to secondary tuberculosis depends on general health and environment. Malnutrition, poor health, an unsanitary and crowded living environment, and the presence of other illnesses tend to lower resistance to reinfection with the disease. The source of a secondary *exacerbation* of tuberculosis can be a reactivation of the previous primary infection or another infected person.

Human immunodeficiency virus (HIV) infection and the AIDS epidemic have contributed to an increase of tuberculosis in the United States.

DIAGNOSIS

The Mantoux test (purified protein derivative, or PPD test) is a standard intradermal test used to detect the presence of tuberculin antibodies. The test is interpreted in 48 to 72 hours; an induration of 8 to 10 mm indicates a sensitivity to the bacillus and is considered positive. The positive test result is followed by radiographic chest studies, examination of gastric washings, fiberoptic bronchoscopy and sputum cultures. The typical walled-off lesions (tubercles) can be seen in chest radiographic film. Apical pulmonary infiltrates with cavities are present in patients with tuberculosis. Final confirmation is positive culture of the sputum for the tubercle bacillus.

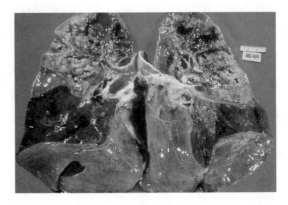

FIGURE 9–19 Tuberculosis. (From Kumar V et al: *Robbins basic pathology,* ed 7, Philadelphia, 2003, Saunders.)

TREATMENT

Persons with communicable tuberculosis must either be treated or quarantined; new cases must be reported to the local health department. Recently, concern has been raised over the increasing prevalence of drug-resistant tuberculosis and the resulting progression to complications.

Treatment of uncomplicated tuberculosis consists of drug therapy using multiple antituberculosis agents. Isoniazid (INH) is the drug of choice and is administered with rifampin, ethambutol, aminosalicylic acid, streptomycin, or cycloserine.

PROGNOSIS

Early and complete treatment affords an excellent prognosis. Drug therapy may continue for several months to a year. The prognosis is not as good for individuals infected with strains that are drug resistant. Risk factors exist for reactivation of infection.

PREVENTION

BCG vaccination has not been proven effective for preventing tuberculosis. All those who come in contact with infected patients are advised to have the tuberculin skin test, chest radiograph, and prophylactic isoniazid (INH).

PATIENT TEACHING

Tuberculosis is considered infectious and reportable to the local public health department; therefore, thorough, consistent hand-washing techniques and respiratory precautions must be practiced. Patient and family education about sources of contagion and transmission is indicated. A nutritious diet and sanitary living conditions are important for recovery. Provide information on adverse drug effects to report to the health-care provider. Stress the importance of regular follow-up care. Inform the care giver and/or family that the disease is no longer infectious when the sputum test is negative.

Infectious Mononucleosis: Epstein-Barr Virus Infection

DESCRIPTION

Infectious mononucleosis, also known as *glandular fever*, is an acute herpesvirus infection.

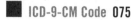 **ICD-9-CM Code 075**

SYMPTOMS AND SIGNS

The two main symptoms of this infection are lymphadenopathy and fever that typically peaks in the afternoon. Initially, symptoms are vague. They include general malaise, anorexia, and chills. As the infection progresses, symptoms include sore throat, fever, headache, fatigue, and cervical and generalized lymphadenopathy (Fig. 9–20). The syndrome causes a mild transient hepatitis and atypical lymphocytosis. The incubation period is from 5 to 15 days. This disease affects primarily adolescents and young adults. Infection is rare after the age of 35 years.

PATIENT SCREENING

Schedule a prompt appointment for a patient (likely to be a teenager or young adult) complaining of fever, sore throat, fatigue, and swollen glands.

ETIOLOGY

Mononucleosis is caused by the Epstein–Barr virus (EBV), a herpesvirus. The virus is carried in the saliva of previously infected individuals and may be transmitted through the oral pharyngeal route (e.g., during kissing) or through blood transfusions. After it is inside the body, the virus infects a type of white blood cell found in lymph, blood, and connective tissue.

DIAGNOSIS

A thorough patient history and physical examination are essential to rule out hepatitis and other

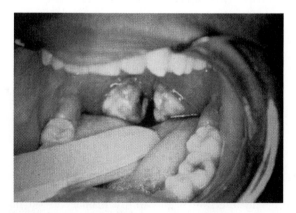

FIGURE 9–20 Tonsils coated with debris during infection of mononucleosis. (From Sigler B: *Ear, nose, and throat disorders—Mosby's clinical nursing series*, St. Louis, 1994, Mosby.)

lymphomatous disorders, such as leukemia, Hodgkin lymphoma, and lymphosarcoma. Two procedures of prime diagnostic importance are examination of a blood smear and immunologic study of the blood serum. Laboratory tests include infectious mononucleosis blood screening test, antinuclear antibody (ANA), total serum bilirubin, liver function tests, and Epstein-Barr (EBV) serology.

TREATMENT

The treatment is based almost entirely on the symptoms. During the acute phase of fever and malaise, bed rest should be enforced. Fluid intake should be forced orally, or if needed for high fever, intravenous fluids are indicated. Antipyretic medications such as acetaminophen are needed when the temperature becomes high (103° F in adults and 104° F in children). Secondary bacterial infections respond to treatment with sulfonamide or penicillin.

PREVENTION

Prevention is difficult because infectious mononucleosis can be transmitted by infected people before they have developed any symptoms. Carriers exist among the general population.

PROGNOSIS

Barring complications, recovery is complete within 3 to 4 months. Infection confers permanent immunity.

PATIENT TEACHING

Stress the importance of bed rest to prevent serious complications affecting the liver or spleen. Often, a soft bland diet is better tolerated. Advise the patient and care giver that although the disease is not highly infectious, strep throat also may be present; it is prudent to practice infection control during the recovery period.

Adult Respiratory Distress Syndrome

DESCRIPTION

Adult respiratory distress syndrome (ARDS) is severe pulmonary congestion characterized by acute respiratory distress and hypoxemia.

 ICD-9-CM Code 518.5

SYMPTOMS AND SIGNS

The sudden onset of severe hypoxemia, progressive *hypercapnia*, and *acidemia* in the patient who recently has experienced trauma, *septicemia*, shock, or insult to the lungs or the rest of the body is termed *adult respiratory distress syndrome (ARDS)*, or *shock lung*. The lungs are hemorrhagic, wet, boggy, congested, and unable to diffuse oxygen; atelectasis results. The onset of symptoms is usually 24 to 48 hours after medical or surgical insult to the body. Primary symptoms include sudden and severe dyspnea with rapid and shallow respirations. Inspiratory intercostal and suprasternal retractions are noted, along with cyanosis or mottled skin. During the Vietnam War, this condition was referred to as *Da Nang lung*. No improvement in the respiratory status is noted with the administration of supplemental oxygen. Rales, rhonchi, and wheezes may be present.

PATIENT SCREENING

The sudden onset of respiratory distress is a medical emergency. The patient is directed to call an ambulance for immediate transport to an emergency care facility. The physician is notified.

ETIOLOGY

Severe trauma or some agent of insult precipitates increased capillary permeability in the lungs, pulmonary edema, and resulting respiratory failure. Injury to the cells activates leukocytes and platelets in the capillaries to release products that cause additional injury. The alveoli fill with exudate 12 to 48 hours after the insult. The fluid-filled alveoli tend to collapse at the end of expiration, leaving less pulmonary tissue available for gas exchange. Consequently, low pulmonary compliance, pulmonary hypertension, decreased functional residual capacity, and hypoxemia result.

DIAGNOSIS

Patients with ARDS have an underlying cause, such as severe trauma, pneumonia, fulminating sepsis, aspiration of gastric contents, *hypovolemic shock,* a near-drowning episode, fat embolism, or cardiopulmonary bypass. Most patients appear to be doing well just before they experience dyspnea, and arterial blood gas determinations indicate reduced perfusion and increased pH. Radiographic chest films show diffuse bilateral alveolar infiltration with a normal cardiac silhouette.

TREATMENT

No cure for ARDS is known, therefore interventions are supportive only. Treatment of hypoxemia can be complicated because changes in the lung tissue leave less pulmonary tissue available for gas exchange, thereby causing inadequate perfusion. Efforts are made to correct the underlying cause of ARDS. Oxygenation may be accomplished by establishing an airway, administering humidified oxygen, and suctioning the air passages as necessary. When ventilation cannot be maintained, mechanical ventilation is attempted by *positive end-expiratory pressure (PEEP)*. Nutritional status and *cautious* hydration are maintained intravenously. The patient is observed for signs of renal failure and superinfection; intervention is undertaken if necessary. Arterial blood gases, blood pressure, and urine output are monitored.

PROGNOSIS

Prognosis is generally poor, depending on the cause. Some individuals do recover with no permanent lung damage.

PREVENTION

The onset of ARDS is generally unpredictable and therefore cannot be precluded.

PATIENT TEACHING

Patients are hospitalized where they will receive constant monitoring, reassurance, and meticulous care.

Lung Cancer

DESCRIPTION

Lung cancer is the most common cause of cancer death worldwide for both men and women, accounting for 28% of all cancer deaths. It is usually caused by repeated carcinogenic irritation to the bronchial epithelium, leading to increased rates of cell division (Fig. 9–21).

ICD-9-CM Code 162.9
The above code is a nonspecific code and may be valid as a principal diagnosis, except for Medicare. Refer to the physician's diagnosis and then to the current edition of the ICD-9-CM coding manual to ensure the greatest specificity of pathology and any appropriate modifiers.

SYMPTOMS AND SIGNS

The most common symptom is cough with or without sputum production. Because many patients diagnosed with lung cancer have coexisting chronic obstructive pulmonary disease (COPD) with a chronic cough, it is important to note any changes in the character of the cough. Other symptoms may include dyspnea, hemoptysis, chest pain (usually dull, intermittent pain on the side of the tumor), and weight loss. The brain is a common site for metastasis for some types of lung cancer. Symptoms of brain metastasis include headache, weakness, change in mental status, and seizures. Other common sites of metastasis are the liver, bone, and skin.

PATIENT SCREENING

A patient complaining of a chronic cough is scheduled for medical evaluation at the first available appointment.

ETIOLOGY

The four major histologic types of lung cancer include squamous cell carcinoma (30% of lung cancers), adenocarcinoma (40%), large cell carcinoma (10%), and small cell carcinoma (20%). The first three types are often collectively referred to as non–small cell lung cancer (NSCLC) because they behave and are treated similarly. Small cell lung cancer (SCLC) occurs almost exclusively in smokers, has a rapid growth rate, and metastasizes early in the disease process.

The primary risk factor for development of lung cancer is cigarette smoking. Smoking has been shown to be responsible for 87% of lung cancers, and smokers are between 10 and 30 times more likely to develop lung cancer than are nonsmokers. A smoker's risk for developing lung cancer is proportional to the total lifetime consumption of cigarettes. The risk does decrease after cessation of

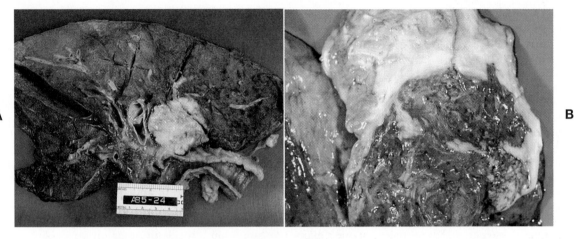

FIGURE 9-21 Examples of lung carcinomas. **A,** Centrally located tumor attached to bronchus. **B,** Mesothelioma on pleural surface. (From Damjanov I: *Pathology for the health-related professions,* ed 2, Philadelphia, 2000, Saunders.)

smoking, but it remains higher than in individuals who never smoked. Other factors that increase the risk of lung cancer include exposure to second-hand smoke, asbestos, radon, arsenic, air pollution, and radiation. Putative dietary and genetic factors are less well established.

DIAGNOSIS

Most patients are symptomatic at the time of diagnosis, although a minority of patients may be diagnosed incidentally following a chest radiograph. Advanced lesions of lung cancer can be seen on radiographic chest films. Sputum *cytologic* analysis that is positive for malignant cells is useful for diagnosis. A tissue biopsy specimen, taken during the bronchoscopy, is required for a definitive diagnosis. A mediastinoscopy looks for involvement of the lymph nodes in the mediastinum. CT scans of the chest, abdomen, and head and a bone scan are done to look for metastases. SCLC and NSCLC are staged differently. NSCLC is staged using the TNM (Tumor, Node, Metastasis) system. SCLC staging uses a two-stage system that involves distinguishing between disease that is confined to one side of the chest ("limited") versus disease that has spread to encompass the other lung or other parts of the body ("extensive").

TREATMENT

Treatment decisions are based on the type of tumor (small cell or non–small cell) and the stage of the tumor. For early stage NSCLC, surgical resection with or without radiation or chemotherapy is the preferred option and offers the best chance for survival. Surgery usually involves a lobectomy, removal of the portion of the lung affected by the tumor, or a pneumonectomy, removal of the entire affected lung. Later stage NSCLC is generally not treatable by surgical resection alone. A combined modality approach encompassing chemotherapy, radiotherapy, surgery, and/or palliative symptom control is used.

Because SCLC often metastasizes early in the disease process, it is usually treated using systemic chemotherapy (with cisplatin plus etoposide or irinotecan) or chemoradiotherapy rather than surgery even in the limited disease stage. Despite being initially responsive to both chemotherapy and radiotherapy, SCLC often relapses within 2 years. Recurrent SCLC may be responsive to a different chemotherapy regimen, but the prognosis is poor.

PROGNOSIS

The prognosis for patients with lung cancer is generally poor. The 5-year survival rate for all stages and types combined is just 15%. The 5-year survival rate for those with early stage lung cancer is 48%; with regionally advanced disease, 21%; and with metastatic disease, 3%. Some factors that have been shown to impact prognosis are the stage at the time of diagnosis, the histologic tumor type, the degree of differentiation of the tumor, the presence or absence of symptoms at diagnosis, and the presence and degree of weight loss.

PREVENTION

Early detection of lung cancer has not been proven to improve survival. Therefore, screening for lung cancer is not currently recommended by any major advisory organization. Cessation of smoking cannot be stressed enough, and reducing one's exposure to secondhand smoke is recommended. Also, it is important to emphasize the benefits of smoking cessation even to patients who already have

lung cancer, especially those with limited SCLC disease. If patients survive their lung cancer, relapse is much more likely in patients who continue to smoke.

PATIENT TEACHING

Explain diagnostic procedures, their purpose, and when to expect results. Encourage the patient to express concerns and offer to supply answers to any specific questions. After diagnosis, the patient benefits from explanation and clarification of the treatment regimen including verbal and written instructions. Offer referral to community support groups and information agencies such as the American Cancer Society and the American Lung Association. Provide information on smoking cessation programs when appropriate. Stress the importance of follow-up care.

REVIEW CHALLENGE

Answer the following questions:

1. What are the physical and chemical dynamics of normal respiration?
2. Why is the common cold so common?
3. How is sinusitis treated?
4. What are the possible causes of nasal polyps?
5. How is severe epistaxis treated?
6. What is the prognosis of malignant tumors of the larynx?
7. What are some causes of and risk factors for (a) atelectasis and (b) pulmonary embolism?
8. What determines the treatment of pneumonia?
9. Why does the patient with pulmonary abscess exhibit foul-smelling sputum?
10. Where does the causative organism of Legionnaires disease thrive?
11. What is the profile of individuals vulnerable to respiratory syncytial virus pneumonia?
12. How is histoplasmosis contracted?
13. Who would benefit from influenza immunization?
14. Why is influenza considered a serious infection?
15. To what does COPD refer?
16. How is chronic bronchitis associated with other pulmonary conditions?
17. Are emphysema and bronchiectasis reversible? What are some causes of both conditions?
18. Why is pneumoconiosis considered an occupational disease?
19. What is the treatment of hemothorax and pneumothorax?
20. Why is pulmonary tuberculosis more prevalent and difficult to treat today?
21. How would you describe the pathology in a patient with ARDS?
22. What steps are recommended to prevent lung cancer? How may the prognosis be improved?

REAL-LIFE CHALLENGE

Sinusitis

A 45-year-old man is experiencing headache over both eyes on awakening. The patient says he also experiences pain above the eyes when bending over. Tenderness above the eyes in the frontal area of the forehead and also in both cheeks is noted on palpation. A thick greenish-yellow mucous drainage is present. Sinus radiographs show cloudiness in the region of the maxillary and frontal sinuses.

Vital signs are temperature, 99.8° F; pulse, 90; respirations, 26; and blood pressure, 136/88. Mouth breathing is noted.

QUESTIONS

1. Compare symptoms and signs of sinusitis and of upper-respiratory-tract infection.
2. What are the causes of sinusitis?
3. Discuss the correlation between allergies and sinusitis.
4. What drug therapy might be prescribed for treatment of sinusitis.
5. What is the principle behind the use of decongestants for sinusitis?
6. How would radiographic films of air-filled sinuses appear?

REAL-LIFE CHALLENGE

Acute Bronchitis

A 39-year-old woman is experiencing a deep cough that produces a thick, yellow sputum. She is complaining of shortness of breath and pain in the upper chest. Audible wheezing is heard without a stethoscope. Vital signs are temperature, 100.2° F; pulse, 102; respirations, 32; and blood pressure, 134/88. Auscultation of the chest confirms the presence of bilateral wheezing and scattered rales.

The patient has a history of an upper-respiratory infection 2 weeks before the onset of coughing 3 days ago. Her husband is a cigarette smoker. Diagnostic studies ordered include chest radiographs, pulmonary studies, sputum analysis, CBC, and ESR. The patient is diagnosed with acute bacterial bronchitis.

QUESTIONS

1. Why would it be safe for the patient to take aspirin for control of the fever?
2. Why would increased fluid intake be recommended?
3. Which treatment would be recommended to relieve the wheezing?
4. Which treatment would be recommended to relieve the coughing?
5. Compare the symptoms and signs of chronic bronchitis with those of acute bronchitis.
6. Compare the etiology of chronic versus acute bronchitis.
7. How significant is the exposure to primary or secondary smoke to both acute and chronic bronchitis patients?
8. What would this patient's risk be for developing chronic bronchitis?

INTERNET ASSIGNMENTS

1. Research the American Lung Association for an update on SARS or another respiratory condition of your interest.
2. Visit the American Lung Association website. Go to the *Occupational Health* page and report on some of the work-related illnesses.
3. Explore the National Institute of Allergies and Infectious Diseases (NIAID) website and prepare a fact sheet on sinusitis for in-depth study on this common condition.

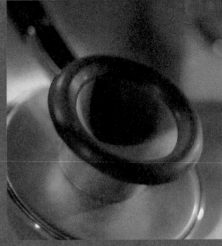

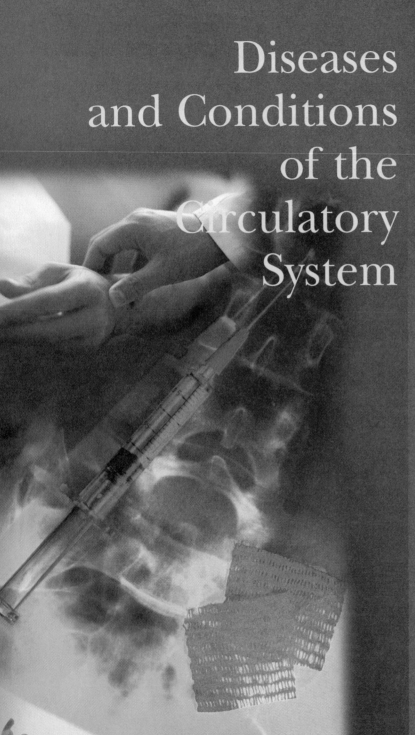

CHAPTER 10

Diseases and Conditions of the Circulatory System

Chapter Outline—Cont'd

Learning Objectives

After studying Chapter 10, you should be able to:

1. Name the common presenting symptoms in patients with cardiovascular disease.
2. Describe the pathology of coronary artery disease.
3. Name the contributing factors for coronary heart disease.
4. Explain what causes the pain of angina pectoris.
5. Explain the difference between myocardial infarction and angina pectoris.
6. Describe the treatment of myocardial infarction.
7. Name and describe the symptoms of the most prevalent cardiovascular disorder in the United States.
8. Explain what happens when the pumping action of the heart fails.
9. Compare right-sided heart failure with left-sided heart failure.
10. Name some causes of cardiomyopathy.
11. Distinguish among pericarditis, myocarditis, and endocarditis.
12. Explain why rheumatic fever is considered a systemic disease.
13. Recall the cardiac manifestations of rheumatic heart disease.
14. Explain the pathophysiology of valvular heart disease.
15. Name the causes of cardiac arrhythmias.
16. Describe the signs and symptoms of shock.
17. Explain the possible consequences of emboli.
18. Compare arteriosclerosis with atherosclerosis.
19. Describe an aneurysm and explain how it is diagnosed.
20. Explain the treatment for (a) thrombophlebitis and (b) varicose veins.
21. Describe the vascular pathology of Raynaud disease.
22. Define anemia and list the presenting symptoms.
23. Describe how anemias are classified and give some examples.
24. State the causes of agranulocytosis.
25. Describe the typical symptoms in all types of leukemias.
26. Distinguish between lymphedema and lymphangitis.
27. Explain the diagnostic significance of Reed-Sternberg cells in lymphoma.
28. Name the signs and symptoms of transfusion incompatibility reaction.
29. Explain the cause of classic hemophilia.

Key Terms

agglutination (ah–**glue**–tih–**NAY**–shun)
aggregation (**ag**–reh–**GAY**–shun)
angioplasty (**AN**–jee–oh–**plas**–tee)
arteriosclerosis (ar–**tee**–ree–oh–skleh–**ROW**–sis)
asystole (a–**SIS**–toh–lee)

atherosclerosis (**ath**–er–oh–skleh–**ROW**–sis)
bradycardia (brady–**KAR**–dee–ah)
bruit (**BREW**–ee)
cardiomegaly (**car**–dee–oh–**MEG**–ah–lee)
cardiomyopathy (**car**–dee–oh–my–**OP**–ah–thee)

Continued

Cardiovascular Diseases

Key Terms—Cont'd

cellulitis (sell–u–**LIE**–tis)

dyscrasia (dis–**CRAY**–zee–ah)

ecchymosis (ech–ih–**MO**–sis)

embolism (**EM**–boh–lizm)

hematopoiesis (**hem**–ah–toh–poy–**EE**–sis)

hemolytic (**hem**–oh–**LIT**–ik)

hypovolemia (**high**–poh–voh–**LEE**–mee–ah)

hypoxia (high–**POX**–see–ah)

ischemia (is–**KEY**–mee–ah)

orthopnea (**or**–**THOP**–nee–ah)

perfusion (per–**FYOU**–zhun)

petechiae (pee–**TEE**–kee–ee)

phlebotomy (phleh–**BOT**–oh–mee)

plaque (**PLACK**)

purpura (**PUR**–pu–rah)

syncope (**SIN**–ko–pee)

tachycardia (**tack**–ee–**CAR**–dee–ah)

tamponade (**tam**–pon–**ADE**)

thrombus (**THROM**–bus)

ORDERLY FUNCTION OF THE CIRCULATORY SYSTEM

CIRCULATION OF BLOOD is the primary function of the circulatory system. The heart is at the center of the circulatory system. Its steady beating pumps 5 quarts of blood through a complete vascular circuit of the body every minute in an adult; this is called the cardiac cycle. This circuit comprises a network of vessels: the arteries, veins, and capillaries (Figs. 10–1 and 10–2).

The heart consists of two side-by-side pumps, each divided into two chambers: two upper chambers called atria, and two lower chambers called ventricles. As blood returns to the heart from the body, it enters the right atrium, passes through the tricuspid valve, and with atrial contraction, enters the right ventricle. Heart valves prevent the blood from flowing backward. From the ventricle, blood is pumped through the pulmonary valve and, with ventricular contraction, into the pulmonary arteries and on to the lungs. In the lungs, carbon dioxide is removed and oxygen is added to the blood. Freshly oxygenated blood then returns to the heart via the pulmonary veins. It enters the left atrium, moves through the mitral (bicuspid) valve with atrial contraction, and enters the left ventricle. As the ventricle contracts again, the blood is forced out of the ventricle through the aortic valve, into the aorta, and on to the rest of the body (Figs. 10–3 and 10–4). This process is called the cardiac cycle (Fig. 10–5).

The heart is enclosed by the double-layered pericardium, which is composed of an inner serous layer (visceral pericardium or epicardium) and an outer fibrous layer (parietal pericardium). Between these layers in the pericardial cavity is a small amount of serous fluid that reduces friction during cardiac movements. Cardiac muscle tissue or myocardium is composed of striated muscle cells that can contract rhythmically on their own and characteristically are both voluntary and involuntary in response. Inside the cavities of the heart is a smooth serous lining called endocardium (Fig. 10–6). The entire conduction system of the heart coordinates the contraction and relaxation (cardiac cycle) of the heart by initiating impulses and distributing the impulses throughout the myocardium (see Fig. 10–32). Coronary arteries and a network of vessels continuously supply cardiac muscle tissue with oxygen (Fig. 10–7).

Cardiovascular Diseases

There are many and varied disorders of the heart and circulatory system. In some disorders, the rhythm of the heartbeats may become irregular, may enter **tachycardia** (become abnormally fast), or may enter **bradycardia** (become abnormally slow). Disorders of cardiac rhythm are called *arrhythmias* or *dysrhythmias*.

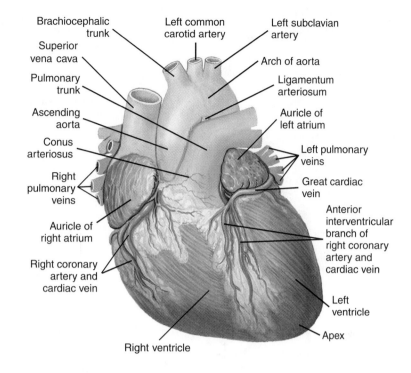

FIGURE 10–1 The heart and great vessels, anterior view. (From Patton KT, Thibodeau GA: *Mosby's handbook of anatomy and physiology,* St. Louis, 2000, Mosby.)

Brachiocephalic trunk

Left common carotid artery

Left subclavian artery

Superior vena cava

Arch of aorta

Pulmonary trunk

Ligamentum arteriosum

Ascending aorta

Auricle of left atrium

Conus arteriosus

Left pulmonary veins

Right pulmonary veins

Great cardiac vein

Auricle of right atrium

Anterior interventricular branch of right coronary artery and cardiac vein

Right coronary artery and cardiac vein

Left ventricle

Apex

Right ventricle

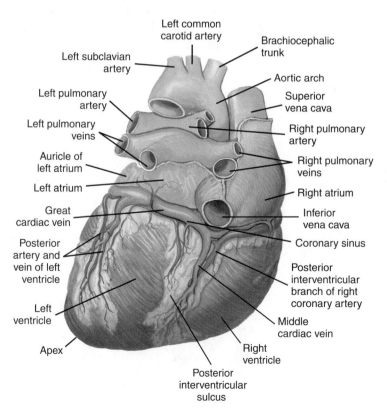

Left common carotid artery

Brachiocephalic trunk

Left subclavian artery

Aortic arch

Left pulmonary artery

Superior vena cava

Left pulmonary veins

Right pulmonary artery

Auricle of left atrium

Right pulmonary veins

Left atrium

Right atrium

Great cardiac vein

Inferior vena cava

Posterior artery and vein of left ventricle

Coronary sinus

Posterior interventricular branch of right coronary artery

Left ventricle

Apex

Middle cardiac vein

Right ventricle

Posterior interventricular sulcus

FIGURE 10–2 The heart and great vessels, posterior view. (From Patton KT, Thibodeau GA: *Mosby's handbook of anatomy and physiology,* St. Louis, 2000, Mosby.)

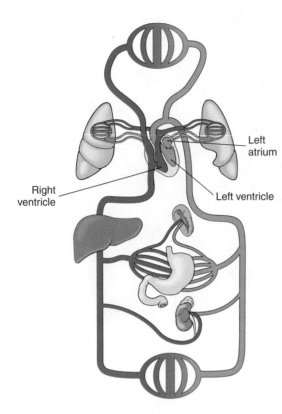

FIGURE 10–3 Circulation through the body.

Almost one-third of all deaths in Western countries are attributed to heart disease. Most of these deaths are caused by coronary artery disease and hypertension. Cardiovascular disorders such as *angina pectoris,* myocardial *infarction* (MI), congestive heart failure (CHF), cardiac arrest, shock, and cardiac **tamponade** also can result in death. Other diseases of the cardiovascular system include rheumatic fever, pericarditis, myocarditis, endocarditis, thromboangiitis obliterans (Buerger disease), Raynaud disease, and vascular (blood vessel) diseases.

Important presenting symptoms that tend to recur in patients with cardiovascular disease and need further investigation include:

- Chest pain
- *Dyspnea* (difficulty in breathing) on exertion
- *Tachypnea* (rapid breathing)
- Palpitations (rapid fluttering of the heart)
- *Cyanosis* (slight blue color)
- Edema
- Fatigue
- **Syncope** (fainting)

Lymphatic and Blood Disorders

See disorders under discussion of specific diseases.

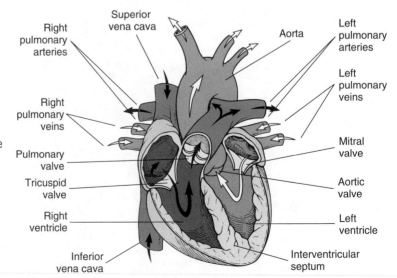

FIGURE 10–4 Circulation through the heart.

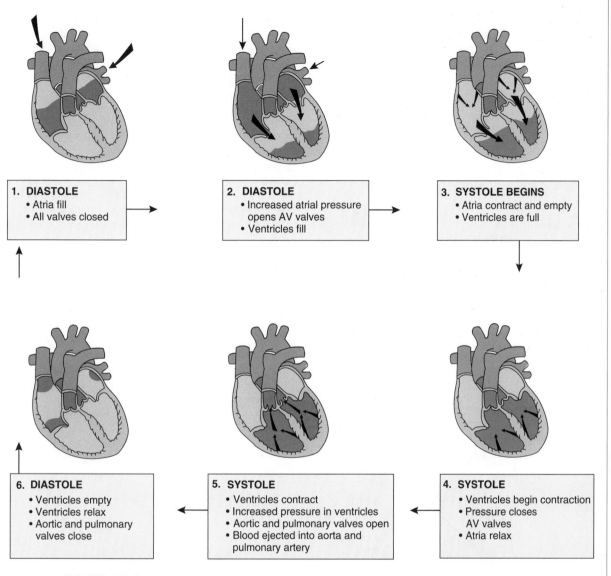

FIGURE 10–5 Cardiac cycle. (From Gould B: *Pathophysiology for the health professions,* ed 2, Philadelphia, 2002, Saunders.)

Coronary Artery Disease

DESCRIPTION

Coronary artery disease (CAD) is a condition involving the arteries supplying the myocardium (heart muscle) (see Fig. 10–7). The arteries become narrowed by atherosclerotic deposits over

time, causing temporary cardiac **ischemia** and eventually MI (heart attack).

ICD-9-CM Code 414.0
ICD-9-CM codes for coronary vascular disease are classified by location and type. The code for coronary heart disease or coronary atherosclerosis heart disease, atherosclerotic heart disease, coronary (artery) arteriosclerosis, arteritis or endoarteritis, atheroma, sclerosis, and stricture is 414.0. The

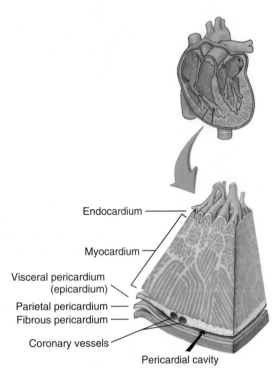

FIGURE 10–6 Layers of the heart wall. (From Applegate EJ: *The anatomy and physiology learning system,* ed 2, Philadelphia, 2000, Saunders.)

Endocardium

Myocardium

Visceral pericardium (epicardium)

Parietal pericardium

Fibrous pericardium

Coronary vessels

Pericardial cavity

code for chronic ischemic heart disease, unspecified, is 414.9. Refer to the physician's diagnosis and then to the current edition of the ICD-9-CM coding manual to ensure the greatest specificity of pathology and any appropriate modifiers.

SYMPTOMS AND SIGNS

Patients are *asymptomatic* initially, with the first symptom being the pain of angina pectoris (see Angina Pectoris). In advanced disease, the severe pain of MI is described as burning, squeezing, crushing, and radiating to the arm, neck, or jaw (see Myocardial Infarction). Nausea, vomiting, and weakness also can be experienced. Changes in the *electrocardiogram (ECG)* are recognized.

PATIENT SCREENING

Severe chest pain of sudden onset with or without previous diagnosis of angina is considered to be a cardiac event and has the potential for being catastrophic; therefore the patient should immediately be entered into the emergency medical system.

ETIOLOGY

Deposits of fat-containing substances called **plaque** in the lumen (opening) of the coronary arteries result in **atherosclerosis** and subsequent narrowing of the lumen of the arteries (Fig. 10–8). The myocardium

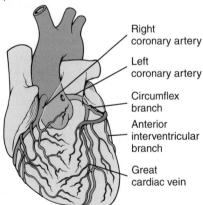

Right coronary artery

Left coronary artery

Circumflex branch

Anterior interventricular branch

Great cardiac vein

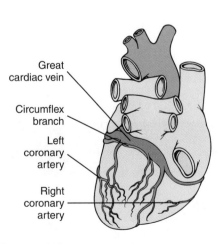

Great cardiac vein

Circumflex branch

Left coronary artery

Right coronary artery

FIGURE 10–7 Coronary arteries.

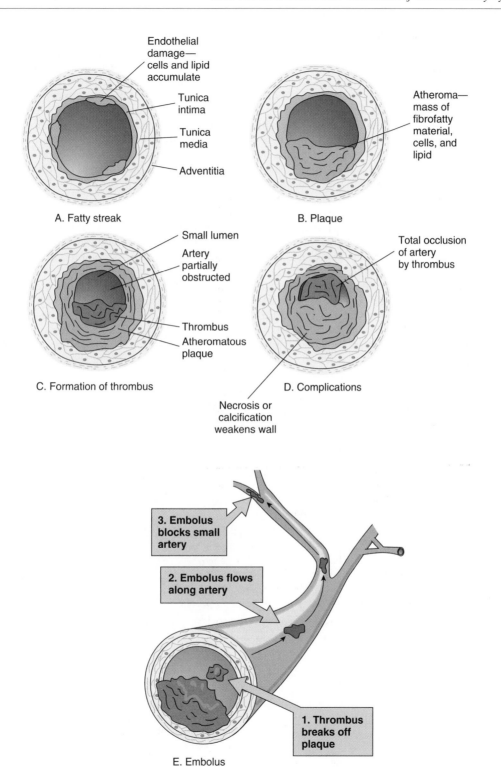

FIGURE 10–8 Development of an atheroma leading to arterial occlusion. (From Gould B: *Pathophysiology for the health professions,* ed 2, Philadelphia, 2002, Saunders.)

must have an adequate blood supply to function. The coronary arteries supply the cardiac muscle with blood but become constricted by atherosclerosis (Fig. 10–9).

Arteriosclerosis, commonly called "hardening of the arteries," is associated with the elderly and diabetics. The arteries eventually lose elasticity and become hard and narrow, resulting in cardiac ischemia. The cells in the myocardium gradually weaken and die. Replacement scar tissue forms, interfering with the heart's ability to pump, resulting in heart failure.

People at higher risk for CAD are those who have a genetic predisposition to the disease, those older than 40 years of age, men (slightly more than women), postmenopausal women, and Caucasians. Other factors contributing to increased risk of the disease include a history of smoking; residence in an urban society; the presence of hypertension, diabetes, or obesity; and a history of elevated serum cholesterol or reduced serum high-density lipoprotein (HDL) levels. Lack of exercise (a sedentary lifestyle) and stress are additional risk factors.

DIAGNOSIS

The patient usually does not experience chest pain from atherosclerosis until the coronary arteries are about 75% occluded. *Collateral* circulation often develops to supply the tissue with needed oxygen and nutrients (Fig. 10–10). An ECG shows ischemia (caused by a lack of blood supply) and possibly arrhythmias. Treadmill testing, *thallium scan,* cardiac catheterization, and angiograms are other tools of cardiac status evaluation used to detect insufficient oxygen supply and to confirm the diagnosis.

TREATMENT

Treatment consists of measures to restore adequate blood flow to the myocardium. Vasodilators are prescribed. **Angioplasty** is attempted in some instances to open the constricted arteries (Fig. 10–11). Claims of reduction of the plaque buildup with hypolipidemic drugs are being confirmed in some cases. Beta-blockers and anticoagulants are used to prevent blood clots from breaking off and lodging in cerebral arteries. When the blockage is severe or does not respond to drug therapy or angioplasty,

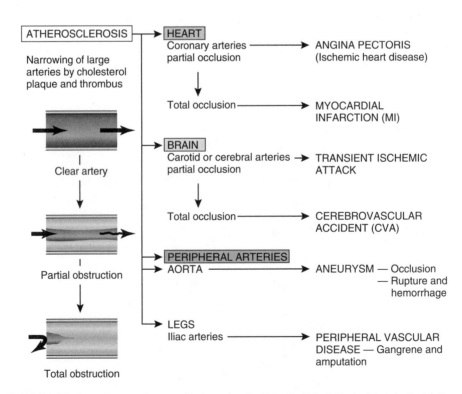

FIGURE 10–9 Possible consequences of atherosclerosis. (From Gould B: *Pathophysiology for the health professions,* ed 2, Philadelphia, 2002, Saunders.)

coronary artery bypass surgery may be indicated to restore circulation to the affected myocardium (Fig. 10–12). Stents must be placed in the arteries after angioplasty is performed if the patient is past the point of simple medications.

Experimental gene therapy uses injections of DNA directly into cardiac muscle to stimulate new growth of blood vessels.

PROGNOSIS

The prognosis varies and depends on the patient's response to the treatment, whether prescribed drug therapy, angioplasty, or coronary bypass surgery. An additional factor affecting the prognosis of smokers is the effect of smoking on the coronary arteries and whether they cease smoking.

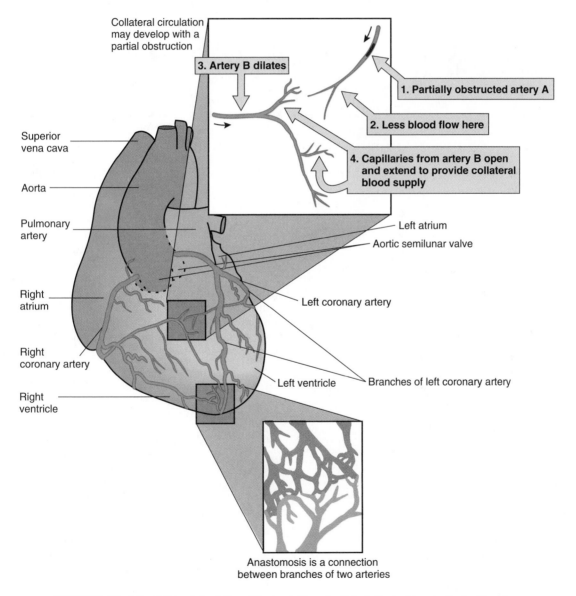

FIGURE 10–10 Collateral circulation of the heart. (From Gould B: *Pathophysiology for the health professions,* ed 2, Philadelphia, 2002, Saunders.)

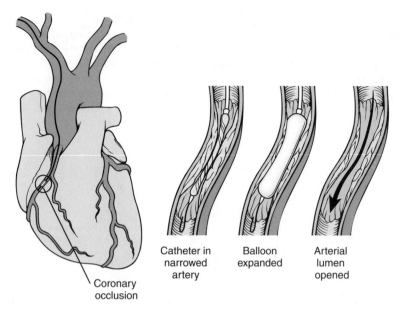

Coronary
occlusion

Catheter in
narrowed
artery

Balloon
expanded

Arterial
lumen
opened

FIGURE 10–11 Angioplasty.

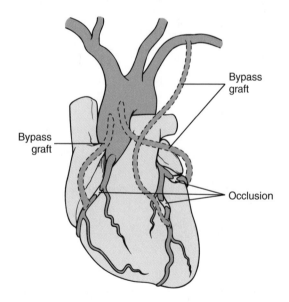

Bypass
graft

Bypass
graft

Occlusion

FIGURE 10–12 Coronary artery bypass.

PREVENTION

Measures to prevent CAD include a diet that is low in salt, fat, and cholesterol combined with exercise. Patients are encouraged to reduce stress and, if they smoke, to stop or reduce smoking.

PATIENT TEACHING

Give patients information about symptoms of impending myocardial infarction and encourage them to seek immediate emergency medical care at the first sign of any related symptoms. Offer printed information to all patients about the prevention or control of CAD and emphasize the importance of a low-fat diet, weight control, exercise, and cessation of smoking. Encourage follow-up cholesterol blood tests.

Angina Pectoris

DESCRIPTION

Angina pectoris, chest pain after exertion, is the result of reduced oxygen supply to the myocardium.

■ **ICD-9-CM Code 413.9** *(Other and unspecified angina pectoris)*
ICD-9-CM codes for angina pectoris are classified by type. The code for anginal decubitus (nocturnal angina) is 413.0, and the code for Prinzmetal angina (variant angina pectoris) is 413.3. The code for other and unspecified angina pectoris is 413.9. Refer to the physician's diagnosis and then to the current edition of the ICD-9-CM coding manual to ensure

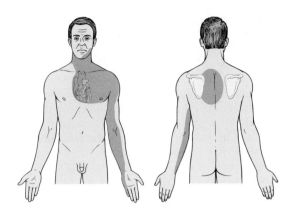

FIGURE 10–13 Common sites of pain in angina pectoris.

the greatest specificity of pathology and any appropriate modifiers.

SYMPTOMS AND SIGNS

The patient has a sudden onset of left-sided chest pain after exertion. The pain may radiate to the left arm or back (Fig. 10–13). The patient also may experience dyspnea. The pain usually is relieved by ceasing the strenuous activity and placing nitroglycerin tablets sublingually (under the tongue). The blood pressure may increase during the attack, and arrhythmias may occur.

PATIENT SCREENING

Patients experiencing symptoms of angina for the first time require immediate assessment. The sudden onset of chest pain could represent a life-threatening condition, and acute myocardial infarction must be ruled out. Those who have been diagnosed with angina pectoris, and in whom cessation of activity and use of vasodilating medications does not provide relief from the pain within 20 minutes, require immediate medical intervention through the emergency medical system.

ETIOLOGY

Atherosclerosis causes a narrowing of the coronary arteries, compromising the blood flow to the myocardium. Exertion requires increased blood flow to supply more oxygen, but the vessels cannot supply it. Spasms of the coronary arteries also may be a causative factor. Severe prolonged tachycardia, anemias, and respiratory disease also can cause cardiac ischemia.

DIAGNOSIS

The patient history reveals a previous exertional chest pain. An ECG taken during the anginal episode may show ischemia. Other diagnostic measures, such as those described for CAD, are performed.

TREATMENT

Treatment consists of cessation of the strenuous activity and the placing of nitroglycerin tablets under the tongue. Transdermal nitroglycerin helps in preventing angina. When angina persists after treatment or for more than 20 minutes, immediate medical attention is indicated.

PROGNOSIS

The prognosis varies and depends on the extent of the arterial involvement. When patients can stop the pain by ceasing strenuous activities and using vasodilating medications, the angina usually will diminish or disappear. The patient's ability to modify his or her lifestyle may improve the prognosis.

PREVENTION

Prevention is similar to that recommended for coronary artery disease. Recommendations focus on lifestyle modification, including appropriate exercise; a diet low in fat, cholesterol, and salt; control of hypertension; weight loss; and smoking cessation. Patients are encouraged to reduce stress.

PATIENT TEACHING

Patients and families should be given dietary information and suggestions for menu planning within the appropriate diet. Emphasize the importance of compliance with prescribed drug therapy. Help the patient and family locate and contact community services and support groups.

Myocardial Infarction

DESCRIPTION

Myocardial infarction is death of myocardial tissue caused by the development of ischemia.

■ **ICD-9-CM Code 410** *(Acute myocardial infarction)*
Acute myocardial infarction has many ICD-9-CM codes according to episode and location. The code can include a fifth-digit subclassification according to episode. ICD-9-CM codes for location have a fourth-digit code modifier and are as follows:

410.0 *(Of anterolateral wall)*
410.1 *(Of other anterior wall)*
410.2 *(Of inferolateral wall)*
410.3 *(Of inferoposterior wall)*
410.4 *(Of other inferior wall)*
410.5 *(Of other lateral wall)*
410.6 *(True posterior wall infarction)*
410.7 *(Subendocardial infarction)*
410.8 *(Of other specified sites)*
410.9 *(Unspecified site)*

NOTE: *The physician must designate the area of the infarction before a code is applied to the episode. Refer to the physician's diagnosis and then to the current edition of the ICD-9-CM coding manual to ensure the greatest specificity of pathology and any appropriate modifiers.*

SYMPTOMS AND SIGNS

An occlusion of a coronary artery resulting in ischemia and infarct (death) of the myocardium causes sudden, severe substernal or left-sided chest pain (Fig. 10–14). The pain is crushing, causing a feeling of massive constriction of the chest. This pain may radiate to the left arm, back, or jaw and is not relieved by rest or the administration of nitroglycerin. Irregular heartbeat, dyspnea, and *diaphoresis* often accompany the pain, and the patient usually exhibits denial and experiences severe anxiety (Fig. 10–15). MI occasionally is clinically silent.

PATIENT SCREENING

Early and immediate intervention improves the chance for survival and minimizes irreversible injury to the myocardium. Recent recommendations include calling 911 for entrance into the emergency medical system and chewing one 5 grain/325 mg aspirin tablet. Emergency intervention must be initiated immediately to control pain, stabilize heart rhythm, and minimize damage to the heart muscle. Most deaths caused by an MI result from primary ventricular fibrillation. Thus immediate ECG monitoring and possible defibrillation are of primary concern. The American Heart Association and the American Red Cross currently recommend defibrillation training for all certified first responders.

ETIOLOGY

Myocardial infarction (MI) results from insufficient oxygen supply, such as occurs when a coronary artery is occluded by atherosclerotic plaque, **thrombus,** or myocardial muscle spasm (Fig. 10–16). The pain is caused by ischemia, and if ischemia is not reversed within about 6 hours, the cardiac muscle dies. Coronary thrombosis is the most common cause of MI.

DIAGNOSIS

The diagnosis includes a thorough history, electrocardiogram (ECG), chest radiographic studies, and laboratory tests for cardiac enzyme levels. Changes in enzyme levels indicate the death of cardiac tissue and include (1) creatine phosphokinase (CPK), which is elevated in the first 6 to 24 hours after MI; (2) lactic dehydrogenase (LDH), which peaks at 48 hours after MI; and (3) aspartate aminotransferase (AST). When an elevation of these enzymes is detected, a study of cardiac isoenzymes is ordered to confirm the diagnosis. ECG changes in the PR and QRS complexes and in the ST segment correspond to the ischemic areas. Diagnostic confirmation is assisted by elevated cardiac enzyme levels and altered isoenzyme levels identified through blood tests.

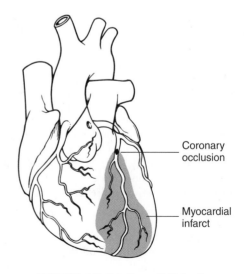

Coronary occlusion

Myocardial infarct

FIGURE 10–14 Myocardial infarction.

TREATMENT

Oxygen is administered, and morphine is given for pain. Aspirin is given as soon as possible to reduce the risk of additional damage to the heart and tissue by ischemia. Vasodilation is attempted by nitroglycerin drip. Lidocaine given by an intravenous drip, after a loading bolus, helps to control arrhythmias. Thrombolytic drugs, including tissue plasminogen activator (TPA), strepto-

kinase, or alteplase (Activase) may be administered as soon as possible after the diagnosis, unless there are contraindications. Within the 6-hour window before permanent damage, an attempt may be made to open the occlusion and to restore blood flow to the area by angioplasty (see Fig. 10–11), the administration of thrombolytic drugs, or coronary artery bypass surgery (Fig. 10–17).

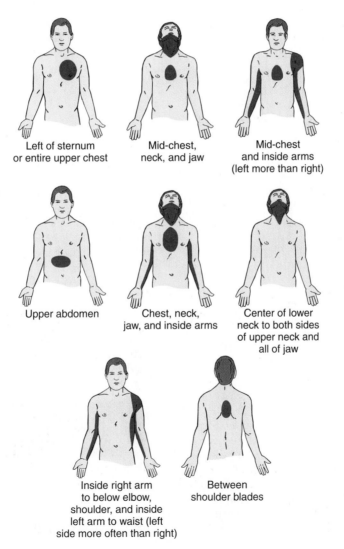

FIGURE 10–15 Locations of pain from myocardial infarction. (From *Mosby's medical, nursing, and allied health dictionary,* ed 6, St. Louis, 2002, Mosby.)

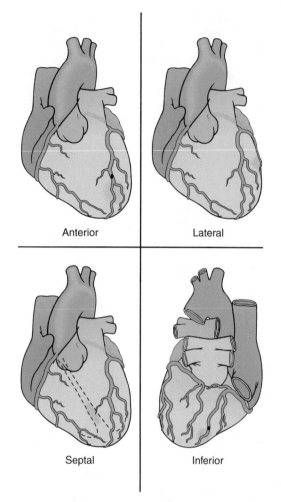

Anterior   Lateral

Septal   Inferior

FIGURE 10–16 Common locations of myocardial infarction. (From Lewis SM, Heitkemper MM, Dirksen SR: *Medical-surgical nursing: assessment and management of clinical problems,* ed 5, St. Louis, 2000, Mosby.)

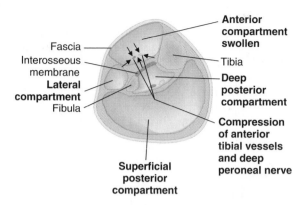

FIGURE 10–17 Anterior compartment syndrome. (From Black JM, Hawks JH, Keene AM: *Medical-surgical nursing: clinical management for positive outcomes,* ed 6, Philadelphia, 2001, Saunders.)

PROGNOSIS

About 65% of deaths caused by MI occur in the first hour. The prognosis is determined by immediate defibrillation for ventricular fibrillation. Late mortality depends on the extent of damage to the heart muscle and the occurrence of complications. Most late cardiac death is sudden, caused by the onset of a fatal arrhythmia.

PREVENTION

The prevention is similar to that recommended for coronary artery disease. Recommendations focus on lifestyle modification, including appropriate exercise; a diet low in fat, cholesterol, and salt; control of hypertension; weight loss; and smoking cessation. Patients are encouraged to reduce stress. Those surviving an MI are urged to take a daily aspirin dose as well as a beta-blocker or ACE inhibitor for life. Lipid-lowering medications are also recommended.

PATIENT TEACHING

Give patients and families dietary information and suggestions for menu planning within the appropriate diet. Emphasize the importance of compliance with prescribed drug therapy. Help the patient and family find and contact community services and support groups.

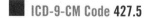

Cardiac Arrest

DESCRIPTION

Cardiac arrest is the sudden, unexpected cessation of cardiac activity.

■ **ICD-9-CM Code 427.5**

SYMPTOMS AND SIGNS

The patient is unresponsive, with no respiratory effort and no palpable pulse.

PATIENT SCREENING

Cardiac arrest is a true life-threatening emergency. Immediate intervention with instantaneous initiation of CPR and defibrillation may successfully restore contraction of the heart. The American Heart Association or American Red Cross protocol for caregivers in the field requires immediate contact of the emergency medical system by calling 911. Inpatient facilities use the "Code, Dr. Blue" message to alert personnel.

ETIOLOGY

Cardiac arrest results from anoxia (absence of oxygen to the tissue) or interruption of the electrical stimuli to the heart. It can be caused by respiratory arrest, arrhythmia, or MI. Electrocution, drowning, severe trauma, massive hemorrhage, or drug overdose also can cause cardiac arrest.

DIAGNOSIS

The diagnosis is based on the absence of respiratory effort and lack of palpable pulse. The ECG shows ventricular fibrillation or **asystole.**

TREATMENT

Cardiopulmonary resuscitation (CPR) must be instituted within 4 to 6 minutes of the cardiac arrest. Cardiac defibrillation is attempted by trained, advanced life-support personnel. Cardiac drugs, including epinephrine (Adrenalin) and isoproterenol (Isuprel) or dobutamine to stimulate the heart, are administered. Antiarrhythmic drugs, including lidocaine and bretylium, also may be administered.

PROGNOSIS

The prognosis varies depending on the length of time the individual has been in cardiac arrest. The earlier in the event that CPR and defibrillation are instituted, the greater possibility there is for survival. Within 1 to 2 minutes after cessation of cardiac activity, respiratory efforts will cease. At 4 to 6 minutes after the cessation of cardiac activity, brain cells will begin to die. At 10 minutes after the cardiac activity has ceased with no intervention, the brain will die and death is inevitable.

Successful resuscitation depends on immediate and complete intervention. Other factors that affect the final outcome of the event include the general health and age of the patient as well as the cause of the arrest. Successful interventions in cold water near-drowning and electrical shock have been recorded.

PREVENTION

Prevention of the catastrophic event of cardiac arrest is not likely. However, as in CAD and myocardial infarction, the same lifestyle modifications can reduce risk. One cannot predict near-drowning or electrical shock accidents, but the prudent individual will try to avoid situations that carry this risk.

PATIENT TEACHING

Encourage all possible candidates for CPR training to become certified. Help families of patients who do not survive cardiac arrest to find and contact support groups in the community. Emphasize safety guidelines to prevent drowning and electrical shock.

Encourage survivors of cardiac arrest to comply with the prescribed regimen of activities and drug therapy. Survivors also may need help in finding and contacting support groups for survivors of cardiac arrest.

Hypertensive Heart Disease

Hypertensive heart disease, the most prevalent cardiovascular disorder in the United States, is the result of chronically elevated pressure throughout the vascular system. Atherosclerosis, arteriosclerosis, renal disease, and any condition that creates increased vascular pressure cause the heart to work harder as it pumps against the increased resistance.

Essential Hypertension

DESCRIPTION

Essential, or primary, hypertension, a condition of abnormally high blood pressure in the arterial system, has an insidious onset, with the patient exhibiting few, if any, symptoms until permanent damage has occurred.

ICD-9-CM Code 401

Essential hypertension is listed in several ways under hypertensive heart disease. The code listed as essential hypertension is 401. Other mentions of hypertension are listed under hypertensive heart disease, hypertensive renal disease, hypertensive heart and renal disease, and secondary hypertension. Refer to the physician's diagnosis and then to the current edition of the ICD-9-CM coding manual to ensure the greatest specificity of pathology and any appropriate modifiers.

SYMPTOMS AND SIGNS

The patient may experience headaches, *epistaxis,* lightheadedness, or syncope. The hypertension generally is detected when blood pressure is taken during a physical examination or screening process. Hypertension is more common with increased age in all groups. If hypertension is accompanied by hyperlipidemia, it may lead to atherosclerosis.

PATIENT SCREENING

Many patients with essential hypertension have no indication of the condition. They may seek an appointment for a headache and should be scheduled for the next available appointment. Others may have recently had a blood pressure reading at a health screening or other event and have been advised to see their physician to report the elevated reading. These patients also should be scheduled for the next available appointment, preferably on the day of or the day after the call. Likewise, patients with a history of essential hypertension requesting an appointment for any hypertensive-related symptoms should be scheduled that day or the next day.

ETIOLOGY

The etiology is unknown, but many factors are thought to contribute to the condition. Stress is considered a major factor in hypertension. Age, heredity, smoking, obesity, and hyperactive personality or type A personality are possible causative factors in essential hypertension (Fig. 10–18).

DIAGNOSIS

Elevated blood pressure readings are the first indication of hypertension. A systolic reading of greater than 140 mm Hg and a diastolic reading of greater than 90 mm Hg indicate hypertension. Recent guidelines have established that systolic

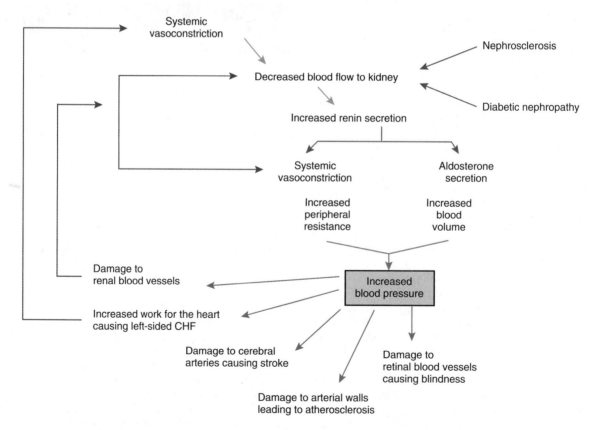

FIGURE 10–18 Development of hypertension. (From Gould B: *Pathophysiology for the health professions,* ed 2, Philadelphia, 2002, Saunders.)

readings of 120 to 140 mm Hg indicate borderline hypertension. The diagnosis is based on a series of blood pressure readings in which elevated values are obtained several times. A careful, complete medical history, physical examination, and laboratory evaluation should be performed before diagnosis is confirmed and therapy is initiated.

TREATMENT

Drug therapy used in the treatment of hypertension includes *diuretics* (to reduce circulating blood volume), beta-adrenergic blockers (to slow the heartbeat and to dilate vessels), vasodilators (to dilate vessels), calcium channel blockers (to slow the heartbeat, to reduce conduction irritability, and to dilate vessels), and *angiotensin-converting enzyme* (ACE) inhibitors (to produce vasodilation and to increase renal blood flow). These drugs may be prescribed singly or in combination. A program of drug therapy is designed to fit each patient's needs and response. Additional modes of therapy include limitation of sodium intake, dietary management, weight reduction, exercise, reduction of stressful situations, and cessation of smoking.

PROGNOSIS

The prognosis varies and depends on the patient's response to prescribed drug therapy and lifestyle modifications.

PREVENTION

With the etiology unknown, one cannot always prevent essential hypertension. The patient may be able to alter contributing factors by reducing stress levels, reducing sodium intake, controlling weight, and stopping smoking. Altering the individual's underlying personality, which plays a part in the condition, is difficult.

PATIENT TEACHING

Teaching the patient that this condition is not cured but only controlled by drug therapy is essential. Education reinforces the need to monitor the blood pressure on a regular basis and the need to continue drug therapy for life.

Malignant Hypertension

DESCRIPTION

Malignant hypertension, a life-threatening condition, is a severe form of hypertension.

ICD-9-CM Code **401.0**

Malignant hypertension is listed in several ways under hypertensive heart disease. The code listed as hypertension is 401.0. Other mentions of malignant hypertension are listed under hypertensive heart disease, hypertensive renal disease, hypertensive heart and renal disease, and secondary hypertension. Refer to the physician's diagnosis and then to the current edition of the ICD-9-CM coding manual to ensure the greatest specificity of pathology and any appropriate modifiers.

SYMPTOMS AND SIGNS

Severe headache, blurred vision, and dyspnea are symptoms that suggest the condition. The symptoms may have sudden onset.

PATIENT SCREENING

As with essential hypertension, many people with malignant hypertension are unaware of the condition. Some may report having been advised to contact their doctor for an elevated blood pressure reading. Others may complain of severe headache. Previously diagnosed essential hypertensive patients may complain of the sudden onset of a severe headache, blurred vision, and dyspnea. These patients are at risk for a cerebral vascular accident and require prompt assessment and intervention.

ETIOLOGY

The etiology of this severe form of essential hypertension is unknown, although extreme stress is thought to be a contributing factor.

DIAGNOSIS

Marked blood pressure elevation is considered malignant hypertension. In severe cases, the systolic pressure reading may be greater than 200 mm Hg and the diastolic pressure reading greater than 120 mm Hg.

TREATMENT

Aggressive intervention is indicated in severe malignant hypertension. Intravenous vasodilators such as diazoxide (Hyperstat) and sodium nitroprusside (Nipride) should be administered. After the condition is under control, blood pressure should be monitored on a regular basis and drug therapy continued for life.

PROGNOSIS

The prognosis varies and depends on the patient's response to drug therapy. These patients are at risk for a cerebrovascular accident (CVA), or stroke, and irreversible renal damage. When drug therapy is unsuccessful, the patient is likely to succumb to the condition after a cerebrovascular accident.

PREVENTION

With etiology being unknown, preventing this condition is difficult. Those who have been diagnosed as hypertensive, however, should comply with drug therapy and reduce their stress. The preventive measures suggested for essential hypertension also apply to malignant hypertension.

PATIENT TEACHING

Emphasize the importance of complying with drug therapy to patients and their families. Encourage patients to modify lifestyles to reduce stress in their lives. Give patients and families dietary information about low-fat, low-cholesterol, and low-sodium diets and management. Advise overweight patients about the importance of weight reduction and exercise.

Congestive Heart Failure

DESCRIPTION

Congestive heart failure (CHF) is an acute or chronic inability of the heart to pump enough blood throughout the body to meet the demands of homeostasis.

> ◼ **ICD-9-CM Code 428.0** *(Unspecified)*
> *The code for congestive heart failure, unspecified, and right-sided failure (secondary to left heart failure) is 428.0. Refer to the physician's diagnosis and then to the current edition of the ICD-9-CM coding manual to ensure the greatest specificity of pathology and any appropriate modifiers.*

SYMPTOMS AND SIGNS

CHF usually has an insidious onset with the patient experiencing gradually increasing dyspnea. Cardiac and respiratory rates increase, and the patient becomes anxious. As the condition progresses, the neck veins distend and edema is noted

in the ankles. When the right side of the heart fails, the liver and spleen enlarge and the peripheral edema is more prominent. Left-sided CHF causes increased pulmonary congestion and more pronounced respiratory difficulties (Fig. 10–19).

PATIENT SCREENING

Patients reporting unexplained chest discomfort, shortness of breath, or swelling of limbs require prompt medical assessment.

ETIOLOGY

Underlying conditions can compromise the pumping action of the heart, resulting in heart failure and inadequate **perfusion.** A common cause of acute congestive heart failure is myocardial infarction (Fig. 10–20). Some causes of chronic conges-

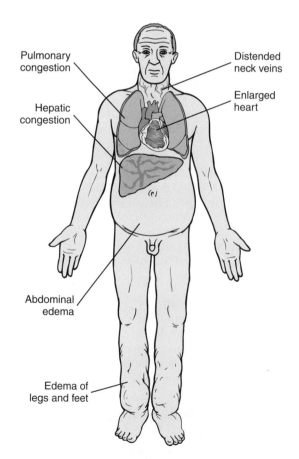

Pulmonary congestion

Distended neck veins

Enlarged heart

Hepatic congestion

Abdominal edema

Edema of legs and feet

FIGURE 10–19 Signs of congestive heart failure.

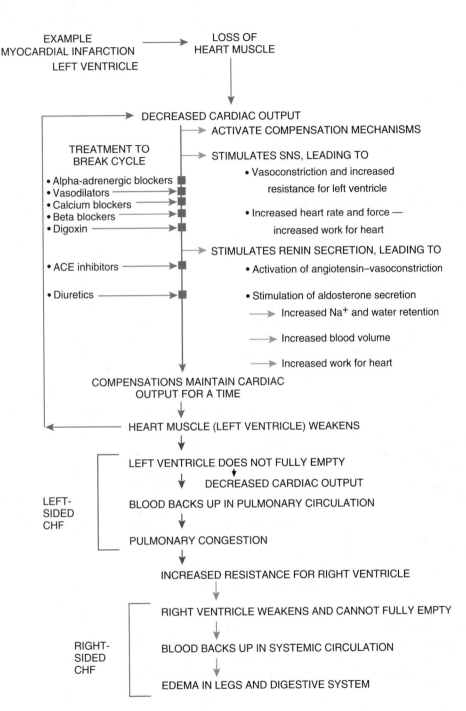

FIGURE 10–20 Course of congestive heart failure. (From Gould B: *Pathophysiology for the health professions,* ed 2, Philadelphia, 2002, Saunders.)

tive heart failure are hypertension, coronary artery disease (CAD), chronic obstructive pulmonary disease (COPD), cardiac valve damage, arrhythmias (dysrhythmias), and **cardiomyopathy.**

DIAGNOSIS

The diagnosis is made after a thorough history and physical examination. Breath sounds are diminished, and radiographic film indicates the presence of fluid in the lungs. An ECG is used to discover the underlying causes. An *echocardiogram* helps in evaluating cardiac chamber size, ventricular function, and disease of the myocardium, valves, cardiac structures (walls, septum, and papillary muscles), and pericardium (the covering of the heart) (Fig. 10–21). Catheterization can be used to monitor the pressures in the circulation.

TREATMENT

Treatment is directed at reducing the workload of the heart and increasing its efficiency. Digitalis preparations are administered to strengthen and slow the heartbeat. Beta-blockers and ACE inhibitors recently were approved for use in the treatment of CHF, mainly to increase blood flow. Diuretics help to reduce the volume of fluid in the body, and vasodilators help to reduce vascular pressure. Intake of fluid and sodium is restricted.

PROGNOSIS

The prognosis varies. Acute CHF usually responds well to medical interventions and therefore has a positive outcome. The patient with chronic CHF is vulnerable to major organ impairment and resulting complications.

PREVENTION

Public education about the contributors to heart health and control of blood pressure continue to produce positive statistical results, especially in the male population. Early medical intervention for CHF is important to prevent multiple organ complications.

PATIENT TEACHING

A primary goal is promoting good patient compliance with the medical treatment plan. Explain that many patients experience a quick improvement in symptoms when they take medications as prescribed, follow dietary instructions, and modify activities to allow required rest and to avoid fatigue. The use of diuretics requires patients to monitor their weight on a daily basis.

Cor Pulmonale

DESCRIPTION

Cor pulmonale, also known as right-sided heart disease, results in enlargement of the right ventricle as a sequela to primary lung disease.

 ICD-9-CM Code 416.9 *(Chronic, NOS)*

SYMPTOMS AND SIGNS

Cor pulmonale, or right-sided heart failure, causes the patient to experience dyspnea, distended neck veins, and edema of the extremities. The liver is enlarged and tender.

PATIENT SCREENING

Patients reporting unexplained chest discomfort, shortness of breath, or swelling of limbs require prompt medical assessment.

ETIOLOGY

Right-sided heart failure is an outcome of acute or chronic pulmonary disease and pulmonary hypertension. The diseased pulmonary blood vessels impair the flow of blood to pulmonary tissue. The increased pulmonary blood pressure increases the workload of the right side of the heart, causing the right ventricle to *hypertrophy* and thus to become less effective in pumping blood to the lungs. Chronic conditions causing cor pulmonale include emphysema and *fibrotic* pulmonary lesions, and the primary acute causative factor is pulmonary *emboli.* Chronic hypoxemia stimulates the bone marrow in an adaptive response to produce an increased number of red blood cells (RBCs) to carry additional oxygen. This condition of abnormally high levels of RBCs (polycythemia) increases the blood viscosity.

DIAGNOSIS

The diagnosis is based on a history of pulmonary disease and **hypoxia.** The patient's respiratory and cardiac status is assessed for neck vein distention and peripheral edema. Radiographic chest studies and echocardiography reveal pulmonary congestion and right-sided heart enlargement, and the ECG frequently shows arrhythmias. If polycythemia is present, the RBC count is elevated.

TREATMENT

Treatment entails relieving the causative factors in the pulmonary system and reducing hypoxemia.

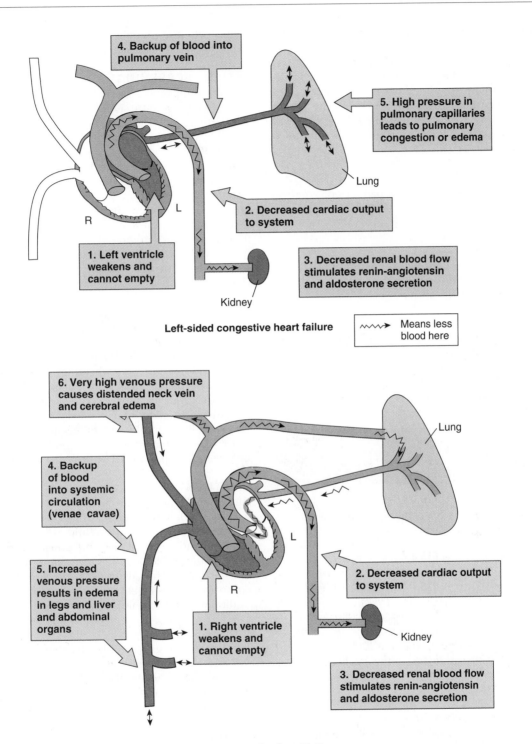

FIGURE 10–21 Effects of CHF. (From Gould B: *Pathophysiology for the health professions,* ed 2, Philadelphia, 2002, Saunders.)

Bronchodilators are administered. Supplemental oxygen provides additional comfort to the patient. Bed rest is encouraged, and digitalis preparations are administered to strengthen and slow the heartbeat. Diuretics are prescribed when edema is present. Anticoagulants are given to avoid the risk of thromboembolisms. **Phlebotomy** may be used when polycythemia is a problem. A low-salt diet is encouraged.

PROGNOSIS

The outcome depends on the patient's response to treatment of the many possible disorders that predispose to cor pulmonale.

PREVENTION

No direct prevention of this condition is known. Many of the predisposing factors have no preventive measures to be taken.

PATIENT TEACHING

Emphasize the instructions given by the physician. Explain the dosage schedule, and encourage compliance with drug therapy. Give patients information on possible side effects. Advise patients to report adverse effects from medications.

Pulmonary Edema

DESCRIPTION

Pulmonary edema is a condition of fluid shift into the extravascular spaces of the lungs.

ICD-9-CM Code **518.4** *(Acute pulmonary edema NOS)*
428.1 *(Acute with mention of heart disease or failure)*
514 *(Chronic or unspecified)*
Refer to the physician's diagnosis and then to the current edition of the ICD-9-CM coding manual to ensure the greatest specificity of pathology and any appropriate modifiers.

SYMPTOMS AND SIGNS

Pulmonary edema causes patients to experience dyspnea and coughing, **orthopnea,** increased cardiac and respiratory rates, and often bloody, frothy sputum. Blood pressure may fall, and the skin becomes cold and clammy. The symptoms often occur at night after the patient has lain down.

PATIENT SCREENING

Patients complaining of shortness of breath, typically when lying down, should be told to seek emergency care.

ETIOLOGY

Pulmonary edema is caused by left-sided heart failure, mitral valve disease, pulmonary embolus, systemic hypertension, arrhythmias, and renal failure. Head trauma, drug overdose, and exposure to high altitudes are other causes. Excessive fluid accumulates in the pulmonary tissue and air spaces of the lungs. The pulmonary circulation is overloaded with an excessive volume of blood (Fig. 10–22).

DIAGNOSIS

The clinical picture of dyspnea, orthopnea, and bloody, frothy sputum leads to further investigation. Breath sounds are diminished, with the presence of *rales, rhonchi,* and wheezing. Arterial *blood gas* measurement shows reduced oxygen saturation, increased carbon dioxide retention, increased bicarbonate levels, and decreased pH of the blood. Radiographic chest films show increased *opacity* of the pulmonary tissue, an enlarged heart, and prominent pulmonary vessels.

TREATMENT

The patient is placed in *Fowler's position* (sitting), and oxygen therapy is administered. Drug therapy includes diuretics to improve fluid excretion, digitalis preparations to increase the efficiency of the heart, morphine sulfate to induce venous dilation, and beta$_2$-adrenergic drugs to dilate bronchioles and to control bronchial spasms. Severe cases may require mechanical ventilation.

PROGNOSIS

Pulmonary edema is a life-threatening condition and is considered a medical emergency. The prognosis varies depending on the severity of the pulmonary edema and the patient's response to intervention.

PREVENTION

Certain causes are controlled by prevention of heart disease and avoidance of risk factors such as drug overdose.

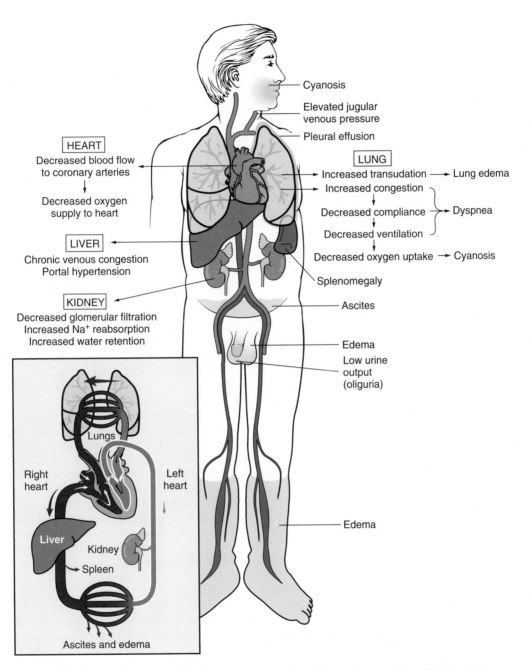

FIGURE 10–22 Chronic passive congestion. Left heart failure leads to pulmonary edema. Right ventricular failure causes peripheral edema that is most prominent in the lower extremities. (From Damjanov I: *Pathology for the health related professions,* ed 2, Philadelphia, 2000, Saunders.)

PATIENT TEACHING

Encourage compliance with drug therapy and follow-up care. Patients taking diuretics are instructed about the importance of monitoring weight on a daily basis.

Cardiomyopathy

DESCRIPTION

Cardiomyopathy is a noninflammatory disease of the cardiac muscle resulting in enlargement of the myocardium and ventricular dysfunction.

ICD-9-CM Code 425

Cardiomyopathy is coded according to type. Refer to the physician's diagnosis and then to the current edition of the ICD-9-CM coding manual to ensure the greatest specificity of pathology and any appropriate modifiers.

SYMPTOMS AND SIGNS

Cardiomyopathy causes the patient to experience symptoms of CHF, including dyspnea, fatigue, tachycardia, palpitations, and occasionally chest pain. Peripheral edema and hepatic congestion also may be present. Syncope and cardiac murmurs may occur. The symptoms and signs vary with the type and cause of this condition.

PATIENT SCREENING

Patients reporting dyspnea, fatigue, tachycardia, palpitations, and occasional chest pain require prompt assessment by a physician.

ETIOLOGY

Primary causes are mostly unknown. Cardiomyopathies are divided into three groups: dilated, hypertrophic, and restrictive. Dilated cardiomyopathy can be the result of chronic alcoholism, an autoimmune process, or viral infections. Regardless of the cause, dilated cardiomyopathies result in a diffuse degeneration of the myocardial fibers. This is followed by a decrease in contractile effort.

Hypertrophic cardiomyopathies are thought to be genetic and are considered *idiopathic.* The left ventricular wall hypertrophies, as does the interventricular septum, resulting in a small and elongated left ventricle and possible obstruction of the aortic valve.

Restrictive cardiomyopathies occur when any infiltrative process of the heart causes fibrosis and thickening of the myocardium.

DIAGNOSIS

The diagnosis includes a thorough patient history and a complete physical examination. **Cardiomegaly** at various stages is present, along with assorted cardiac murmurs. The radiographic chest film confirms the presence of cardiomegaly, and the ECG reveals rate and rhythm abnormalities. Echocardiograms and cardiac catheterization may help to identify the type of cardiomyopathy and the extent of the condition. *Biopsy* may be required.

TREATMENT

Treatment is determined by the type of cardiomyopathy. Therapy for dilated cardiomyopathies is aimed at appropriate control of the CHF, with the measures previously mentioned for treatment of CHF. Antiarrhythmic agents, digitalis, and *anticoagulant* drugs are prescribed. Activities are limited, with some patients restricted to bed rest. Treatment of hypertrophic cardiomyopathies also is aimed at reducing the workload of the heart. Beta-adrenergic blockers such as propranolol hydrochloride (Inderal) reduce the myocardial contractility, the heart rate, and the conductivity, thus preventing arrhythmias. Calcium channel blockers are prescribed to help reduce the blood pressure and relax the heart muscle. ACE inhibitors are used to help relax blood vessels and reduce the heart's workload. Treatment of restrictive cardiomyopathies also includes reducing the workload of the heart. The changes in the cardiac muscle caused by the infiltrates are irreversible, making the prognosis for these patients poor.

PROGNOSIS

Medication improves the survival rate of these patients. Some conditions can be fatal, with the only hope for survival being heart transplantation.

PREVENTION

In many cases, these conditions are idiopathic. Prevention is non-specific depending on the original underlying causative factor.

PATIENT TEACHING

Patient teaching focuses on improving the patient's compliance with the medical treatment plan. Patients are encouraged to avoid alcohol and to limit salt intake. Some patients benefit from support groups for people living with chronic disease.

Pericarditis

DESCRIPTION
Pericarditis is an acute or chronic inflammation of the pericardium (serosa), the sac enclosing and protecting the heart (Fig. 10–23).

ICD-9-CM Code 423.9 *(Unspecified)*
Pericarditis is coded by type. Refer to the physician's diagnosis and then to the current edition of the ICD-9-CM coding manual to ensure the greatest specificity of pathology and any appropriate modifiers.

SYMPTOMS AND SIGNS
The space between the outer parietal layer of pericardium and the inner visceral layer of epicardium (heart wall) normally is filled with a small amount of

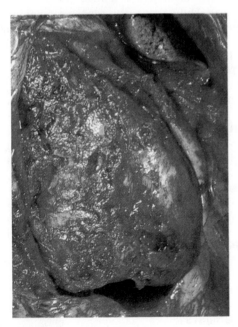

FIGURE 10–23 Pericarditis. (From Damjanov I: *Pathology for the health related professions,* ed 2, Philadelphia, 2000, Saunders.)

thin, lubricating serous fluid (see Fig. 10–6). When blood or inflammatory exudate is released into the pericardial sac, or pericardial space, friction and irritation between the layers result in pericarditis. Associated manifestations include fever, *malaise,* chest pain that fluctuates with inspiration or heartbeat, dyspnea, and chills. The patient may feel anxious and report a "pounding heart." A detectable friction rub, or grating sound, in phase with the heartbeat can be heard on *auscultation* with a stethoscope. Tachycardia may be present. Pericarditis can occur in different forms. It can be a benign or isolated process or can be secondary to infection elsewhere in the body, so the clinical signs vary.

PATIENT SCREENING
Patients complaining of chest pain are advised to seek immediate medical attention.

ETIOLOGY
Pericarditis is idiopathic or a consequence of inflammation or infection elsewhere in the body. Other causative agents are viruses, bacteria (producing a suppurative pericarditis), trauma, rheumatic fever, and malignant *neoplastic* disease. The condition may occur secondary to myocardial infarction. Acute inflammation of the pericardium can cause adhesions (scarring) to form between the pericardium and the heart, or it can cause a loss of elasticity, producing a constrictive pericarditis. Conversely, chronic pericarditis can incite fibrous calcification of the visceral membrane, which comes in direct contact with the myocardium. A scarred and rigid pericardium interferes with the heart's ability to contract normally, with a subsequent drop in cardiac output (Fig. 10–24).

DIAGNOSIS
Blood studies may lead to the identification of a causative organism. They also may reveal elevated *white blood cell (WBC) count, erythrocyte sedimentation rate (ESR),* and cardiac enzyme levels. Changes are noted on ECG. Echocardiogram confirms the presence of pericardial fluid and reveals a thickened pericardium. In constrictive pericarditis, cardiac catheterization shows elevated pressures in the cardiac chambers.

TREATMENT
Treatment is directed at managing the underlying systemic disease and at reducing inflammation and pain. Therapy for infectious pericarditis requires antibiotic drugs and possibly surgical drainage or

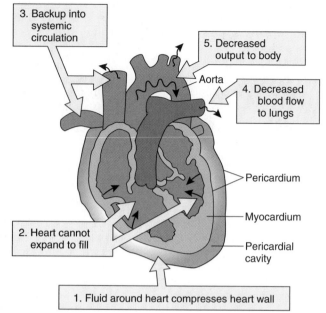

3. Backup into systemic circulation

5. Decreased output to body

Aorta

4. Decreased blood flow to lungs

Pericardium

Myocardium

Pericardial cavity

2. Heart cannot expand to fill

1. Fluid around heart compresses heart wall

FIGURE 10–24 Effects of pericardial effusion. (From Gould B: *Pathophysiology for the health professions,* ed 2, Philadelphia, 2002, Saunders.)

aspiration. Complete bed rest and the administration of *analgesics, antipyretics,* and nonsteroidal anti-inflammatory drugs (NSAIDs) are prescribed. Corticosteroids may be prescribed.

PROGNOSIS

Acute pericarditis usually resolves with complete recovery. Extensive adhesions or calcification resulting from chronic pericarditis may necessitate resection of pericardium.

PREVENTION

Prompt treatment of infections is a preventive measure for pericarditis.

PATIENT TEACHING

Encourage the patient to seek prompt treatment for infections. Emphasize the importance of completing the antibiotic regimen.

Myocarditis

DESCRIPTION

Myocarditis is inflammation of the muscular walls of the heart.

■ **ICD-9-CM Code** **429.0** *(Unspecified)*

SYMPTOMS AND SIGNS

Myocarditis involves damage to the myocardium by pathogenic invasion or **toxic** insult. The condition may be acute or chronic, may involve a small part of the myocardium or be diffuse, and can occur at any age. The patient may report palpitations, fatigue, and dyspnea. Physical examination may reveal fever, arrhythmia, and tenderness in the chest.

PATIENT SCREENING

Patients complaining of dyspnea and palpitations are advised to seek immediate medical attention.

ETIOLOGY

Myocarditis is frequently a viral, bacterial, fungal, or protozoal infection or a complication of other diseases such as influenza, diphtheria, mumps, and most significantly, rheumatic fever; it is occasionally idiopathic. It also may be associated with a myocardial infarction. Exposure to certain toxic agents, through lithium use, chronic use of cocaine, chronic alcoholism, radiation, and chemical poisoning, can cause inflammation of the myocardium. In addition, it may be a complication of a collagen disease.

DIAGNOSIS

Diagnostic findings may include an elevated WBC count, increased ESR, elevated cardiac enzyme levels, ventricular enlargement noted on radiographic

Endocarditis

chest film, and an abnormal ECG. Myocardial biopsy confirms the inflammation of cardiac muscle tissue and may identify the cause.

TREATMENT

When infection is the underlying cause, appropriate antiinfective agents are given. The patient is advised to rest and to reduce the heart's workload. Medications such as quinidine and procainamide may be required to stabilize arrhythmia. Analgesics, antiinflammatory agents, and oxygen are also prescribed.

PROGNOSIS

The prognosis for complete recovery is favorable, unless the condition is chronic and causes damage to the cardiac muscle.

PREVENTION

Depending on the underlying cause, prevention is not always possible. In some cases, early treatment of infections with a complete course of antimicrobial agents can prevent the onset of myocarditis.

PATIENT TEACHING

Emphasize the importance of rest and close monitoring by the physician through follow-up appointments during the recovery process. Give the patient a list of the complications that should be reported to the physician, such as difficulty breathing, weakness, and/or accumulation of fluid in the extremities.

Endocarditis

DESCRIPTION

Endocarditis is inflammation of the lining and the valves of the heart (Fig. 10–25).

■ **ICD-9-CM Code 424.90**
Endocarditis is coded by type and site. Refer to the physician's diagnosis and then to the current edition of the ICD-9-CM coding manual to ensure the greatest specificity of pathology and any appropriate modifiers.

SYMPTOMS AND SIGNS

Endocarditis is usually secondary to infection elsewhere in the body (Fig. 10–26), the result of pre-

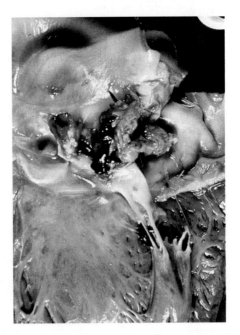

FIGURE 10–25 Bacterial endocarditis. The valves are covered with extensive vegetations. (From Damjanov I: *Pathology for the health related professions,* ed 2, Philadelphia, 2000, Saunders.)

existing heart disease, or the consequence of an abnormal immunologic reaction. The patient may have vague to pronounced symptoms of infection, including fever, chills, night sweats, weakness, *anorexia,* and fatigue.

The condition is characterized by vegetative growths on the cardiac valves that may be released into the blood stream in the form of emboli. These emboli can lodge in vessels and cause symptoms of ischemia. The sites of ischemia may be the heart, lungs, kidneys, brain, or extremities. Dysfunction of the valves, which may not close effectively, disrupts or obstructs blood flow through the chambers of the heart; this dysfunction of the valves usually produces a cardiac murmur heard on auscultation. Serious obstruction or regurgitation of blood flow through the heart affects the pumping effectiveness of the heart and causes complications.

PATIENT SCREENING

A patient complaining of persistent fatigue, night sweats, and/or fever requires prompt assessment by a physician.

ETIOLOGY

Bacteremia, or the presence of infectious agents in the blood stream, can lead to endocarditis. Common infecting organisms include *Staphylococcus aureus,* group A beta-hemolytic streptococci, and *Escherichia coli.* Intravenous drug users are at high risk for fungal endocarditis. Patients with damaged cardiac valves as a result of rheumatic disease are more prone to endocarditis. Septic emboli from endocarditis can be carried by the arterial circulation and then embed in major organs, resulting in infarcts and new places of bacterial infections (Fig. 10–27).

DIAGNOSIS

A complete blood count (CBC) may indicate leukocytosis, and an elevated ESR may be present. Blood cultures may reveal the causative organism. Echocardiogram shows valve involvement with vegetation or *abscesses.* ECG may indicate arrhythmia and conduction defects.

TREATMENT

Identification of the causative organism dictates the antiinfective therapy (usually intravenous antibiotics), which continues for several weeks. Other medications include antipyretics, anticoagulants, and drugs indicated to treat any complications.

Bed rest is recommended during the acute phase. Damaged cardiac valves may need surgical repair or replacement.

PROGNOSIS

Early diagnosis and treatment with antibiotics usually brings complete recovery. Untreated cases can have a poor prognosis.

PREVENTION

After recovery, the patient must understand the importance of taking *prophylactic* antibiotics before dental work, childbirth, or any invasive procedures associated with transient bacteremia.

PATIENT TEACHING

Instruct the patient to take the full course of antibiotics and to obtain plenty of rest.

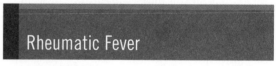

Rheumatic Fever

DESCRIPTION

Rheumatic fever is a systemic inflammatory and autoimmune disease involving the joints and cardiac tissue.

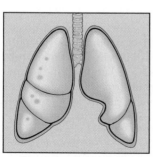
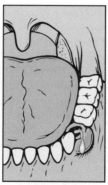
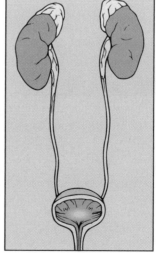
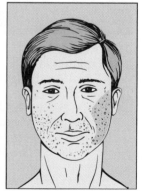

Respiratory tract infection   Dental infection   Urinary tract infection   Skin infection

FIGURE 10–26 Causative factors in endocarditis.

ICD-9-CM Code 390

Rheumatic fever is coded according to mention of heart involvement. Refer to the physician's diagnosis and then to the current edition of the ICD-9-CM coding manual to ensure the greatest specificity of pathology and any appropriate modifiers.

SYMPTOMS AND SIGNS

Rheumatic fever follows a sore throat caused by group A beta-hemolytic streptococcus. The patient, usually a child, experiences a fever and polyarthritis, including joint pain, edema, redness, and limited range of motion. Joints frequently involved include finger, knee, and ankle joints, with inflammation transient among these joints. In addition, the patient experiences carditis, cardiac murmurs, cardiomegaly, and even CHF. Other symptoms include weakness, malaise, anorexia, weight loss, a rash on the trunk, abdominal pain, and the development of small nodules on the tendon sheaths in the knees, knuckles, and elbows. The symptoms occur 1 to 5 weeks after the upper respiratory tract infection.

PATIENT SCREENING

Patients with vague symptoms of fatigue, joint pain, and fever after an episode of upper respiratory infection and sore throat require prompt assessment by a physician.

ETIOLOGY

After a sore throat caused by group A beta-hemolytic streptococcus, *antibodies* against the bacteria develop and cross-react with normal tissue. This autoimmune disease causes the antibodies to attack the body's own cells and to initiate an inflammatory reaction. The antibodies migrate to the endocardium and the mitral and sometimes the aortic valves, where vegetations form on the tissue. The carditis usually follows the joint pain and fever by a week and can affect all layers of the heart (Fig. 10–28).

DIAGNOSIS

The history of an upper respiratory tract infection in the preceding few weeks suggests rheumatic fever. No single diagnostic feature identifies the condition. The presence of carditis and polyarthritis adds to the evidence for the disease. The streptococcal antibody level, antistreptolysin O titer, is elevated in a series of tests. Increases in cardiac enzyme levels, WBC count, and ESR aid in the diagnosis.

TREATMENT

After the diagnosis of streptococcal pharyngitis (strep throat), which precedes rheumatic fever, treatment with a *complete* course of antibiotics prevents the onset of the fever and subsequent rheumatic heart disease. The administration of antibiotics (penicillin) is necessary to eradicate the streptococcal infection. Antipyretics are given for

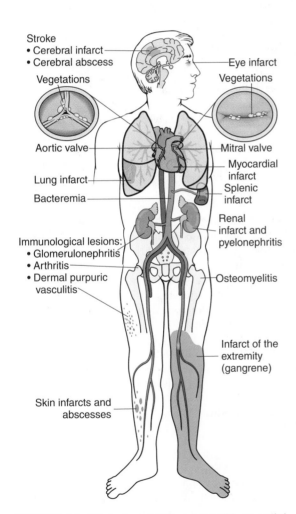

FIGURE 10–27 Septic emboli from endocarditis are carried by the arterial circulation and may lodge in major organs, causing infarcts and new sites of bacterial infection. (From Damjanov I: *Pathology for the health related professions,* ed 2, Philadelphia, 2000, Saunders.)

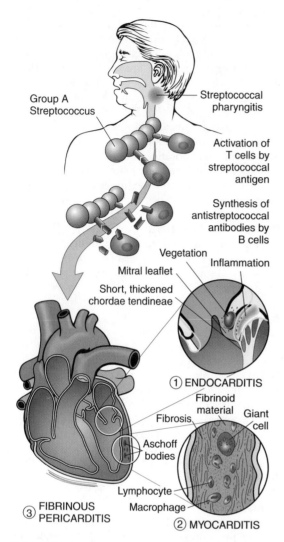

Group A Streptococcus

Streptococcal pharyngitis

Activation of T cells by streptococcal antigen

Synthesis of antistreptococcal antibodies by B cells

Vegetation

Inflammation

Mitral leaflet

Short, thickened chordae tendineae

① ENDOCARDITIS

Fibrinoid material

Fibrosis

Giant cell

Aschoff bodies

Lymphocyte

Macrophage

③ FIBRINOUS PERICARDITIS

② MYOCARDITIS

FIGURE 10–28 Pathogenesis of rheumatic fever. After infection, (with "strep throat"), an immune response elicited by the streptococci acts on the heart and several other organs, most notably the joints, skin, and central nervous system. In the heart, it causes endocarditis, myocarditis, and pericarditis. (From Damjanov I: *Pathology for the health related professions,* ed 2, Philadelphia, 2000, Saunders.)

fever, and antiinflammatory agents are given for relief of the arthritic symptoms. Bed rest is indicated, as is prophylactic administration of antibiotics.

PROGNOSIS
The prognosis is good with treatment.

PREVENTION
The prevention is prophylactic administration of antibiotics for a diagnosed episode of strep throat.

PATIENT TEACHING
Emphasize the importance of completing the full course of the antibiotic therapy. Reassure the parents of the child with rheumatic fever that recovery usually follows medical treatment. Encourage parents to seek medical attention for a child's sore throats and to include a Beta strep screen.

Rheumatic Heart Disease
DESCRIPTION
Rheumatic heart disease refers to cardiac manifestations that follow rheumatic fever.

ICD-9-CM Code 391
Rheumatic heart disease is coded according to type and tissue involvement. Refer to the physician's diagnosis and then to the current edition of the ICD-9-CM coding manual to ensure the greatest specificity of pathology and any appropriate modifiers.

SYMPTOMS AND SIGNS
The acute endocarditis, which leads to chronic cardiac involvement, includes valvular damage because the vegetations cause stenosis of the valves, particularly the mitral and aortic valves (Fig. 10–29). Congestive heart failure causes dyspnea, tachycardia, edema, a nonproductive cough, and cardiac murmurs.

PATIENT SCREENING
Patients with vague symptoms of fatigue, joint pain, and fever after an episode of upper respiratory infection and sore throat require prompt assessment by a physician.

ETIOLOGY
After rheumatic fever, the vegetations may become enlarged or the valves may scar, causing stenosis of the openings. The frequency of rheumatic heart disease is decreasing as a result of diagnosis and aggressive antibiotic treatment of streptococcal pharyngitis (strep throat). Patients who experienced rheumatic fever and rheumatic heart disease before the advent of penicillin may have damaged cardiac valves (Fig. 10–30).

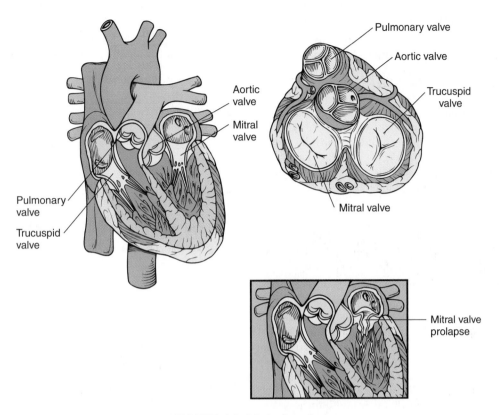

Pulmonary valve

Aortic valve

Trucuspid valve

Mitral valve

Aortic valve

Mitral valve

Pulmonary valve

Trucuspid valve

Mitral valve prolapse

FIGURE 10–29 Cardiac valves.

DIAGNOSIS

The diagnosis is based on the history of rheumatic fever and cardiac murmurs. An echocardiogram shows the vegetations or resulting damage to the valves.

TREATMENT

Treatment is aimed at reducing the stenosis of the valves and preventing further damage. Surgery to relieve the stenosis or to replace the valve may be necessary. Good dental hygiene is important to prevent gingival infection, which would cause further bloodborne infection and damage the valves. Prophylactic antibiotics are given to the patient before any dental procedures.

PROGNOSIS

The prognosis varies according to the extent of the damage to the valves. Recurrences are likely. Valve replacement may give the patient a better outlook.

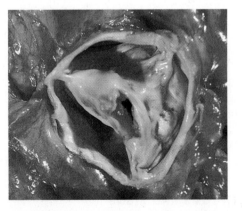

FIGURE 10–30 Chronic rheumatic endocarditis of the aortic valve. The valves are deformed, and the orifice is stenosed. (From Damjanov I, Linder J: *Pathology: a color atlas,* St. Louis, 1999, Mosby.)

PREVENTION

The prevention is prophylactic administration of antibiotics for a diagnosed episode of strep throat.

PATIENT TEACHING

Emphasize the importance of completing the full course of antibiotic therapy. Encourage parents to seek medical attention for a child's sore throats and to include a Beta strep screen. Give information on incision care to patients who have had valve replacement surgery. Encourage the patient to comply with prescribed rehabilitation therapy and activity level.

Valvular Heart Disease

Valvular heart disease is an acquired or congenital disorder that can involve any of the four valves of the heart (see Fig. 10–29). This condition can occur in the form of either insufficiency or stenosis. Insufficiency, the failure of the valves to close completely, allows blood to be forced back into the previous chamber as the heart contracts. This exerts added pressure on that chamber and increases the heart's workload. Stenosis, a hardening of the cusps of the valves that prevents complete opening of the valves, impedes the blood flow into the next chamber (Fig. 10–31). The mitral valve is involved most often. The diagnosis of valvular heart disease requires ECG, radiographic chest studies, echocardiogram, and cardiac catheterization. Treatment entails the administration of digitalis or quinidine for arrhythmias and antibiotic prophylaxis.

Mitral Stenosis

DESCRIPTION

Mitral stenosis is a hardening of the cusps of the mitral valve that prevents complete and normal opening for the passage of blood from the left atrium into the left ventricle.

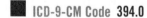 ICD-9-CM Code **394.0**

SYMPTOMS AND SIGNS

The mitral, or bicuspid, valve lies between the left atrium and the left ventricle. Mitral stenosis causes patients to have exertional dyspnea and fatigue. In

A. NORMAL VALVE

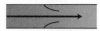
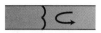

Blood flows freely forward | No backflow of blood

B. STENOSIS

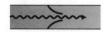
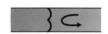

Less blood flows through narrowed opening | No backflow of blood

C. INCOMPETENT VALVE

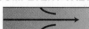
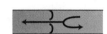

Blood flows freely forward | Blood regurgitates backward through "leaky" valve

D. EFFECT OF AORTIC STENOSIS

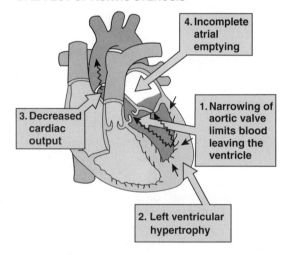

4. Incomplete atrial emptying

3. Decreased cardiac output

1. Narrowing of aortic valve limits blood leaving the ventricle

2. Left ventricular hypertrophy

FIGURE 10–31 Effects of heart valve defects. (From Gould B: *Pathophysiology for the health professions,* ed 2, Philadelphia, 2002, Saunders.)

addition, they may experience cough and palpitations followed by *hemoptysis.* In severe cases, patients may become cyanotic.

PATIENT SCREENING

Patients reporting exertional dyspnea and fatigue that may be accompanied by palpitations require prompt assessment by a physician.

ETIOLOGY

Rheumatic heart disease is the cause of most cases of mitral stenosis. The group A beta-hemolytic streptococcus stimulates antibody production, and the antibodies often attack the body tissue in an autoimmune response.

DIAGNOSIS

Symptoms of mitral stenosis may have an insidious or an acute onset. A cardiac murmur is heard, including a diastolic murmur. Echocardiogram confirms diagnostic suspicions.

TREATMENT

Limitation of sodium intake, along with the administration of diuretics, helps reduce the workload on the heart. Anticoagulants prevent the formation of thrombi. If atrial fibrillation results from stenosis, digoxin often is given to slow the rapid heart rate. Surgical intervention in the form of a *commissurotomy* may be needed to free up the valve and to allow adequate blood flow. Valve replacement is a final option.

PROGNOSIS

The prognosis improves with surgical intervention.

PREVENTION

Prevention of rheumatic fever and subsequent rheumatic heart disease is a major factor in preventing mitral stenosis.

PATIENT TEACHING

When possible, use visual aids to demonstrate the effect valvular disease has on blood circulation through the heart. Explain the medical regimen and how medications can improve the condition. Explain the procedure for surgical reconstruction of the valve if appropriate.

Mitral Insufficiency

DESCRIPTION

In mitral valve insufficiency, the mitral valve fails to close completely and allows blood from the left ventricle to flow back into the left atrium

■ **ICD-9-CM Code** **394.1** *(Rheumatic mitral insufficiency)*
394.2 *(Mitral stenosis with insufficiency)*

SYMPTOMS AND SIGNS

The patient with mitral insufficiency experiences dyspnea and fatigue. A heart murmur can be heard as the blood leaks back into the left atrium as a result of the valve's failure to close completely.

PATIENT SCREENING

These individuals often will call reporting that they are simply very tired and having some difficulty breathing. Anyone complaining of difficulty breathing requires prompt assessment by a physician. Those complaining of generalized fatigue should be scheduled for the next available appointment.

ETIOLOGY

The valve often fails to close because of scar tissue resulting from inflammation and vegetations, a consequence of rheumatic fever. Mitral valve prolapse also may be the culprit.

DIAGNOSIS

The diagnosis is based on a thorough patient history, especially a history of a sore throat or rheumatic fever. Physical examination reveals a murmur, and echocardiogram discloses the insufficiency. Cardiac status also is assessed with an ECG, radiographic chest film, and cardiac catheterization.

TREATMENT

Treatment includes bed rest, oxygen therapy, and the administration of antibiotics for any infectious process. When the condition is complicated by CHF, fluid restrictions and diuretic therapy are implemented.

PROGNOSIS

The prognosis generally is good, but the condition can lead to right ventricular hypertrophy.

PREVENTION

Preventing rheumatic fever and the resulting scarring of the mitral valve helps prevent mitral insufficiency.

PATIENT TEACHING

When possible, use visual aids to demonstrate the effect valvular disease has on blood circulation through the heart. Explain the medical regimen and how medications can improve the condition. Explain the procedure for surgical reconstruction of the valve if appropriate.

Mitral Valve Prolapse

DESCRIPTION
Mitral valve prolapse, usually a benign condition, occurs when one or more of the cusps of the mitral valve protrudes back into the left atrium during ventricular contraction.

ICD-9-CM Code 424.0

SYMPTOMS AND SIGNS
Mitral valve prolapse (MVP), usually a benign condition, occurs when the valve cusps do not close completely (see Fig. 10–29). Most patients are asymptomatic, and the condition usually is discovered during a routine examination. The few patients who experience symptoms report chest pain, dyspnea, dizziness, fatigue, and syncope. These patients may experience severe anxiety. This fairly common condition can affect all age groups.

PATIENT SCREENING
Most individuals with mitral valve prolapse are unaware of any problem. The condition is usually diagnosed incidental to a physical examination. Those who report chest pain require prompt assessment by a physician.

ETIOLOGY
Abnormally long or short chordae tendineae may be the cause of the valve's inability to close properly. Malfunctioning papillary muscles may increase the severity of the condition. Regurgitation of blood occurs during left ventricular systole and results in the rushing, gurgling cardiac murmur characteristic of the prolapse.

DIAGNOSIS
The typical click-murmur syndrome is heard on auscultation of the heart. Echocardiogram confirms the failure of the valve to close. The premature ventricular contractions (PVCs) that are detected on ECG are not considered harmful and are not an indication of insult to the myocardium.

TREATMENT
Treatment generally is not required for asymptomatic patients. Those who experience discomfort and anxiety often are treated with beta-blockers, and they are advised to avoid caffeine, smoking, and large, heavy meals.

PROGNOSIS
The prognosis is good.

PREVENTION
No prevention is known for this condition.

PATIENT TEACHING
Reassure patients that this is usually a benign condition. Emphasize the importance of avoiding caffeine and big meals.

Arrhythmias

DESCRIPTION
Cardiac arrhythmias are any deviation from the normal heartbeat, that is, the normal sinus rhythm. They are often called irregular heartbeats.

ICD-9-CM Code 427

Arrhythmias or dysrhythmias are coded by type and point of origin. Refer to the physician's diagnosis and then to the current edition of the ICD-9-CM coding manual to ensure the greatest specificity of pathology and any appropriate modifiers.

SYMPTOMS AND SIGNS
Arrhythmias result when there is interference with the conduction system of the heart, resulting in an abnormality of the heartbeat. Symptoms include palpitations, rapid heartbeat (tachycardia), skipped heartbeats, slow heart rate (bradycardia), syncope, and fatigue.

PATIENT SCREENING
Patients who report feeling abnormal heartbeats, usually as missed beats, palpitation, or rapid heartbeats, require prompt assessment by a physician.

ETIOLOGY
Arrhythmias can arise from disturbances in the normal conduction system of the heart, including the pacemaker (the sinoatrial [SA] node), the atrioventricular (AV) node, the bundle branches, and the Purkinje fibers (Fig. 10–32). Ischemia and

drugs cause many arrhythmias. Failure of the SA node may be responsible. Table 10-1 lists the causes of arrhythmias.

DIAGNOSIS

The diagnosis is made from a 12-lead ECG. Various arrhythmias are evident to the physician. Echocardiography may help confirm a particular arrhythmia (Fig. 10–33). The patient may wear a Holter monitor (ambulatory ECG) to capture any arrhythmic event.

TREATMENT

Treatment depends on the cause (see Table 10–1). Drug-induced arrhythmias usually resolve with cessation of the drug administration. Anticoagulants, especially Coumadin, are given to prevent a thromboembolism and resulting agun. Ischemia should respond to oxygen administration and increased blood flow to the tissue. If the arrhythmia is not too unstable or too serious, cardioversion

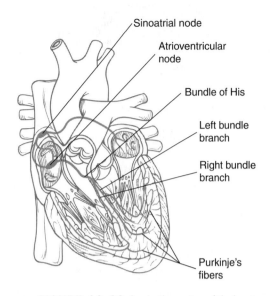

FIGURE 10–32 Conduction system of the heart.

	TABLE 10–1			
	Arrhythmias			
TYPES	**SYMPTOMS AND SIGNS**	**ETIOLOGY**	**DIAGNOSIS**	**TREATMENT**
Normal sinus rhythm	Rate of 60-100 bpm, regular, P wave uniform	Impulse originates in SA node, conduction normal	Normal	None indicated
Sinus tachycardia	Rate >100 bpm, regular, P wave uniform	Rapid impulse originates in SA node, conduction normal	Rapid rate	Beta blockers, calcium channel blockers
Sinus bradycardia	Rate <60 bpm, regular, P wave uniform	Slow impulse originates in SA node, conduction normal	Slow rate	Atropine
Premature atrial contraction	Rate depends on underlying rhythm, usually normal P wave, morphology different from other P waves	Irritable atrium, single ectopic beat that arises prematurely, conduction through ventricle normal	Irregular heartbeat, diagnosis by ECG	Treatment usually unnecessary; if needed, antiarrhythmic drugs
Atrial tachycardia	Rate of 150-250 bpm, rhythm normal, sudden onset	Irritable atrium, firing at rapid rates, normal conduction	Rapid rate with atrial and ventricular rates identical, diagnosis by ECG	Reflex vagal stimulation, calcium channel–blocking drugs (verapamil), cardioversion

AV, Atrioventricular; *bpm,* beats per minute; *ECG,* electrocardiogram; *IV,* intravenous; *PR,* pulse rate; *PVC,* premature ventricular contraction; *SA,* sinoatrial.

Continued

TABLE 10–1
Arrhythmias—cont'd

TYPES	SYMPTOMS AND SIGNS	ETIOLOGY	DIAGNOSIS	TREATMENT
Atrial fibrillation	Atrial rate >350 bpm, ventricular rate <100 bpm (controlled) or <100 bpm (rapid ventricular response)	Atrial ectopic foci discharging at too rapid and chaotic rate for muscles to respond and contract, resulting in quivering of atrium; AV node blocks some impulses and ventricle responds irregularly	ECG shows no P waves, grossly irregular ventricular rate	IV verapamil; if unsuccessful, procainamide; if unsuccessful, cardioversion
First-degree heart block	Rate depends on rate of underlying rhythm, PR interval >0.20 second	Delay at AV node, impulse eventually conducted	ECG shows PR interval >0.20 second	Atropine; if unsuccessful, artificial pacemaker insertion
Second-degree heart block, Wenckebach block	Intermittent block with progressively longer delay in conduction until one beat is blocked; atrial rate normal, ventricular rate slower than normal, rhythm irregular	SA node initiates impulse, conduction through AV node is blocked intermittently	ECG shows normal P waves, some P waves not followed by QRS complex; PR interval progressively longer, followed by block of impulse	Mild forms, no treatment; severe, insertion of artificial pacemaker
Classic second-degree heart block	Ventricular rate slow (½, ⅓, or ¼ of atrial rate); rhythm, regular; P waves normal, QRS complex dropped every 2nd, 3rd, or 4th beat	SA node initiates impulse, conduction through AV node is blocked	ECG shows P waves present, QRS complex blocked every 2nd, 3rd, or 4th impulse	Artificial pacemaker is inserted
Third-degree heart block	Atrial rate normal, ventricular rate 20-40 or 40-60 bpm; no relationship between P wave and QRS complex	SA node initiates impulse, which is completely blocked from conduction, causing atria and ventricles to beat independently	ECG shows P waves and QRS complexes with no relationship to each other, rhythms are regular but independent of each other	Insertion of artificial pacemaker is necessary
Premature ventricular contraction (single focus)	Single ectopic beat, arising from ventricle, followed by compensatory pause	Ectopic beat originates in irritable ventricle	ECG shows a wide, bizarre QRS complex >0.12 second usually followed by a compensatory pause	Usually no treatment if <6 per minute and single focus

AV, Atrioventricular; *bpm,* beats per minute; *ECG,* electrocardiogram; *IV,* intravenous; *PR,* pulse rate; *PVC,* premature ventricular contraction; *SA,* sinoatrial.

TABLE 10–1
Arrhythmias—cont'd

TYPES	SYMPTOMS AND SIGNS	ETIOLOGY	DIAGNOSIS	TREATMENT
Multifocal arrhythmia Coupling, 2 in a row Bigeminy, every other beat Trigeminy, every 3rd beat Quadrigeminy, every 4th beat	Rate dependent on underlying rhythm; rhythm regular or irregular; P wave absent before ectopic beat	Same as single focus	Same as single focus	Same as single focus
Ventricular tachycardia	Rate of 150-250 bpm, rhythm usually regular; focus of pacemaker normally single, patient experiences palpitations, dyspnea, and anxiety followed by chest pain	Four or more consecutive PVCs at a rapid rate due to advanced irritability of myocardium, indicating ventricular command of heart rate	ECG shows runs of four or more PVCs, P wave buried in QRS complex	Often forerunner of ventricular fibrillation; immediate intervention necessary; IV lidocaine; if unsuccessful, follow by cardioversion; procainamide or bretylium may be used
Ventricular fibrillation (a lethal arrhythmia)	Patient loses consciousness immediately after onset; no peripheral pulses palpable, no heart sounds, no blood pressure	Ventricular fibers twitch rather than contract, reason unknown	Pulseless, unconscious patient; ECG shows rapid, repetitive, chaotic waves originating in ventricle	Recognize and terminate rhythm; precordial shock (defibrillation)

AV, Atrioventricular; *bpm,* beats per minute; *ECG,* electrocardiogram; *IV,* intravenous; *PR,* pulse rate; *PVC,* premature ventricular contraction; *SA,* sinoatrial.

may be performed by electric shock to the heart to restore normal heart rhythm. This mild shock interrupts the arrhythmia pattern by resetting the heart rhythm and may enable the patient's heart to be normal enough to allow discontinuation of antiarrhythmic medications. Occasionally, the heart rhythm does not stabilize, and the arrhythmia can be fatal.

PROGNOSIS
The prognosis varies depending on the type and cause of the arrhythmia.

PREVENTION
Preventing drug-induced arrhythmias requires stopping the intake of the offending drug substances. Avoiding the identified causative activities

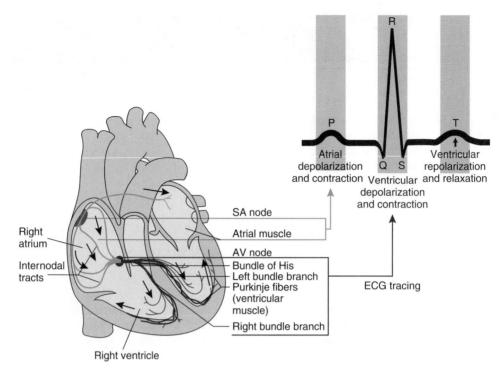

FIGURE 10–33 Conduction system in the heart and relationship to electrocardiogram. (From Gould B: *Pathophysiology for the health professions,* ed 2, Philadelphia, 2002, Saunders.)

helps prevent certain arrhythmias. Certain types of arrhythmias may have no prevention.

PATIENT TEACHING

Give patients information about the causes of arrhythmias. Emphasize the importance of complying with prescribed drug therapy. Encourage patients to comply with scheduled appointments. Emphasize the symptoms that require prompt medical intervention.

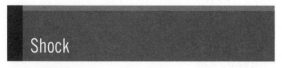

DESCRIPTION

Shock is the collapse of the cardiovascular system, including vasodilation and fluid shift accompanied by inefficient cardiac output.

ICD-9-CM Code   **785.50** *(Shock unspecified, failure of peripheral circulation)*
    785.51 *(Cardiogenic shock)*
    785.59 *(Other)*
Refer to the physician's diagnosis and then to the current edition of the ICD-9-CM coding manual to ensure the greatest specificity of pathology and any appropriate modifiers.

SYMPTOMS AND SIGNS

Shock causes inadequate perfusion of organs and tissues. The patient has pale, cold, and clammy skin; a rapid, weak, and thready pulse; rapid breathing; and an altered level of consciousness. The blood pressure drops, and the patient may be anxious, irritable, or restless and often expresses a feeling of impending doom. The patient may experience dizziness, extreme thirst, and profuse sweating. In late stages, the pupils dilate, the eyes become dull and lusterless, and the patient experiences shaking and trembling.

PATIENT SCREENING
Shock is a life-threatening condition requiring the patient's immediate entry into the emergency medical system. Instruct or assist the caller in contacting EMS.

ETIOLOGY
This life-threatening emergency can be caused by *anaphylaxis,* hemorrhage, sepsis, respiratory distress, heart failure, neurologic failure, emotional catastrophe, or severe metabolic insult. Regardless of the cause, the amount of blood that is effectively circulating in the body is reduced. The final effect is that the vital organs (heart, brain, lungs, and kidneys) do not receive sufficient oxygen and nutrients to sustain life. Rapid blood loss or significant fluid loss with subsequent **hypovolemia** precipitates shock. Failure of the heart to pump adequately is another cause of shock. Vascular collapse with subsequent massive dilation or constriction of the vessels can cause blood to pool away from vital areas. Insufficient oxygen supply to the circulating system can generate shock (Fig. 10–34).

DIAGNOSIS
The clinical picture, along with a history of a precipitating event, leads to the diagnosis of shock resulting from inadequate cellular perfusion. The altered level of consciousness and respiratory distress suggest shock. Immediate intervention is needed to halt the progression of the condition.

TREATMENT
Because of the severity and rapid progression of the condition, aggressive intervention is undertaken at the earliest possible opportunity. The ABCs (airway, breathing, and circulation) of emergency care require maintaining an open airway and establishing ventilation to supply the vital organs with oxygen. Any visible bleeding is controlled, and surgical intervention may be needed to halt internal bleeding. The patient should be placed in a *supine* position, with the feet and legs elevated, and should be kept warm but not overheated. If the patient is not in an inpatient facility, contact with the emergency medical service (EMS) for immediate transport to an emergency facility is indicated. Vital signs are monitored, and volume replacement is instituted with intravenous fluids. When supplemental oxygen is available, it is administered.

PROGNOSIS
Immediate assessment and intervention improves the prognosis for complete or near-complete recovery. When the condition is not addressed promptly, shock may become unstoppable and the consequences may be irreversible, resulting in an unfavorable outcome.

PREVENTION
Most occurrences of shock are not preventable. Immediate intervention helps prevent rapid progression of the condition into a fatal occurrence.

PATIENT TEACHING
Give patients and family members information about causes and emergency intervention measures for patients with known allergic reactions. Encourage community education in first aid and CPR to help reduce damaging outcomes of shock.

Cardiogenic Shock
DESCRIPTION
Cardiogenic shock is the inadequate output of blood by the heart.

 ICD-9-CM Code 785.51

SYMPTOMS AND SIGNS
In cardiogenic shock (shock resulting from inadequate cardiac output), the myocardium fails to pump effectively. The patient exhibits the previously mentioned symptoms and signs of shock. The event usually is preceded by MI or severe heart failure, certain arrhythmias, or acute valve failure.

PATIENT SCREENING
These patients have a life-threatening condition. Enter them promptly into the emergency medical system.

ETIOLOGY
Any insult that disturbs the heart's ability to pump blood can cause cardiogenic shock. MI, severe heart failure, certain arrhythmias, or valve failure can lead to cardiogenic shock (Fig. 10–35).

Shock

DIAGNOSIS

The clinical picture and a history of a major cardiac insult lead to the suspicion of cardiogenic shock. An ECG is another diagnostic tool, as are radiographic chest studies. A hypotensive state that continues to worsen also indicates the diagnosis.

TREATMENT

Treatment consists of general measures for shock, along with the administration of medications that increase the efficiency of the myocardium. Blood supply to vital organs must be improved, and the oxygen demands of myocardial tissue must be

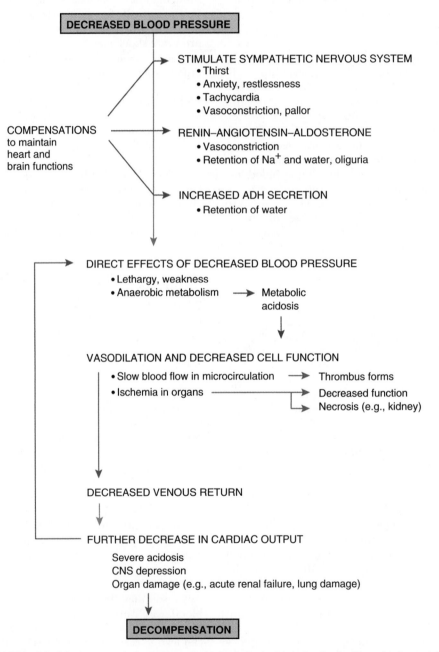

FIGURE 10–34 Progress of shock. (From Gould B: *Pathophysiology for the health professions,* ed 2, Philadelphia, 2002, Saunders.)

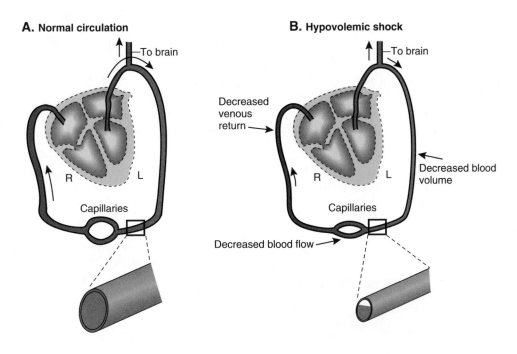

FIGURE 10–35 Causes of shock. (From Gould B: *Pathophysiology for the health professions,* ed 2, Philadelphia, 2002, Saunders.)

reduced. Blood volume assessment determines whether drugs are given to dilate or constrict cardiac vessels.

PROGNOSIS

The prognosis varies but in many cases is unfavorable.

PREVENTION

Prevention in most cases is unlikely. An important factor in preventing a fatal outcome is immediate assessment and intervention when symptoms and signs are identified.

PATIENT TEACHING

Emphasize the importance of immediate emergency intervention when symptoms are detected. Promote community awareness of the benefits of first aid and CPR training in increasing survival rates in the community.

Cardiac Tamponade

DESCRIPTION

Cardiac tamponade is the compression of the heart muscle and restriction of heart movement caused by blood or fluid trapped in the pericardial sac. It may be called cardiac compression.

■ **ICD-9-CM Code** **423.9**

SYMPTOMS AND SIGNS

Cardiac tamponade occurs when a coronary, epicardial, or pericardial vessel breaks and blood is trapped in the pericardial sac. In addition, the myocardium may rupture, also sending blood into the pericardial sac. The blood constricts the heart, thus restricting heart movement, and less blood can enter the heart chambers per beat. The patient with cardiac tamponade experiences sudden severe dyspnea and rapidly falling blood pressure. The pulse becomes weak, thready, and rapid. The patient is in shock and becomes cyanotic above the nipple line. The level of consciousness falls.

PATIENT SCREENING

These patients have a life-threatening condition. Enter them promptly into the emergency medical system.

ETIOLOGY

Cardiac tamponade results from an insult to the integrity of a vessel in the pericardium, allowing blood to fill the pericardial space. The pressure of the blood causes the heart to beat inappropriately, leading to cardiac arrest.

DIAGNOSIS

The diagnosis is based on the clinical picture and a history of a traumatic event. Heart sounds become muffled or distant, but breath sounds remain normal.

TREATMENT

Treatment consists of inserting a needle into the pericardial space and withdrawing the offending blood. Surgery usually is indicated to repair the leak.

PROGNOSIS

The prognosis varies and depends on the causative factor, the success of the intervention, and the health status of the patient. Surgical repair usually has a positive outcome.

PREVENTION

Because of the etiology of this condition, prevention usually is not possible.

PATIENT TEACHING

Give the patient and family information about the mechanism and results of the insult. Explain care of the incision and emphasize the importance of following postoperative orders.

Vascular Conditions

The vascular system, a closed transport system composed of arteries, arterioles, capillaries, venules, and veins, is responsible for supplying blood tissues with blood containing oxygen and nutrients. This system also conveys waste products and carbon dioxide to the appropriate organs for excretion. Arteries carry blood away from the heart (Fig. 10–36, *A*), veins transport blood back to the heart (Fig. 10–36, *B*), and capillaries are the point of exchange at the cellular level (Fig. 10–36, *C*).

Blood vessel walls, other than one-cell–walled capillaries, are composed of three coats: the tunica

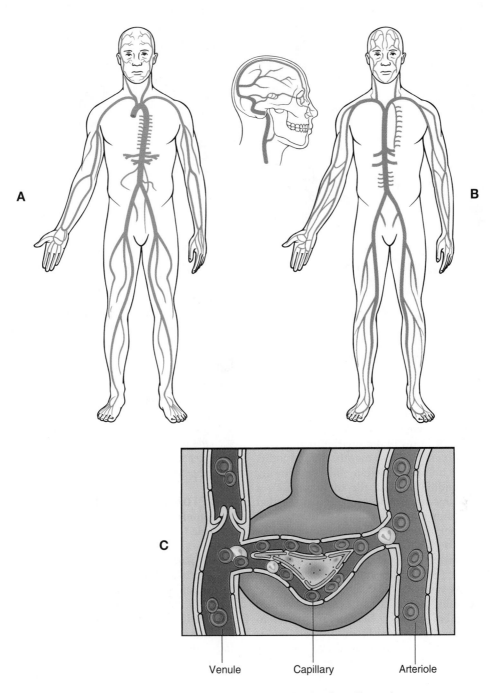

Venule   Capillary   Arteriole

FIGURE 10–36 Vascular system. **A,** Arteries; **B,** veins; **C,** capillary exchange.

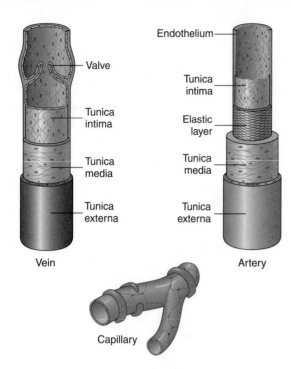

FIGURE 10–37 Vessel wall structure.

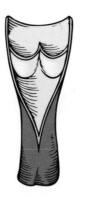 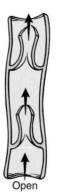 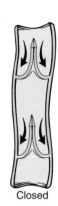

Open Closed

FIGURE 10–38 Venous valves.

intima, the tunica media, and the tunica externa (Fig. 10–37). The lining of the vessel lumen, the tunica intima, is composed of smooth, thin endothelium, allowing minimal friction with the flowing blood. The middle portion, the tunica media, is composed of smooth muscle and elastic tissue that is under the control of the sympathetic nervous system. This innervation allows constriction or dilation of the vessel walls and changes in blood pressure. Connective tissue composes the outermost layer, the tunica externa, creating support and protection for the vessels.

Arterial walls are much thicker than venous walls. The tunica media is heavier in arteries to compensate for the stronger blood pressure under which the arteries must function. Veins, with their lower blood pressure, contain valves to prevent backflow and to assist the return of blood to the heart (Fig. 10–38).

Vascular conditions include emboli, arteriosclerosis, atherosclerosis, aneurysms, phlebitis, thrombophlebitis, varicose veins, thromboangiitis obliterans (Buerger disease), and Raynaud disease.

Emboli

DESCRIPTION

Emboli are clots of aggregated material (usually blood). They can lodge in a blood vessel and inhibit the blood flow.

ICD-9-CM Code 444

Emboli are coded according to location of involvement in the arterial system. Refer to the physician's diagnosis for the location of arterial involvement and then to the current edition of the ICD-9-CM coding manual to ensure the greatest specificity of pathology and any appropriate modifiers.

SYMPTOMS AND SIGNS

Symptoms of emboli depend on the location of the occluded vessel and the magnitude of the area of tissue served by the vessel. The initial symptom is severe pain in the area of the embolus. Emboli lodging in arteries of the extremities cause the area to become pale, numb, and cold to the touch. In addition, arterial pulses are absent below the occlusion if it is arterial. When a large artery is involved, the patient also experiences nausea, vomiting, fainting, and eventually shock. Pulmonary obstructions are discussed in Chapter 9. Cerebral obstructions and CVAs are discussed in Chapter 13.

PATIENT SCREENING

A patient reporting severe pain in an extremity that is accompanied by paleness, numbness, and coolness in the area requires prompt assessment by a

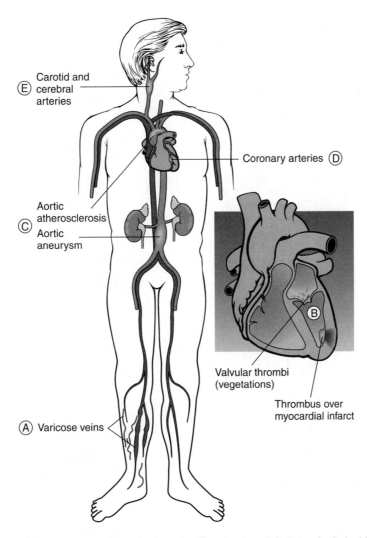

E Carotid and cerebral arteries

Coronary arteries D

C Aortic atherosclerosis
Aortic aneurysm

B

A Varicose veins

Valvular thrombi (vegetations)

Thrombus over myocardial infarct

FIGURE 10–39 Common sites of thrombus formation. (From Damjanov I: *Pathology for the health related professions,* ed 2, Philadelphia, 2000, Saunders.)

physician. In addition, those experiencing nausea, vomiting, fainting, and shock are in an emergency state and require immediate entrance into the emergency medical system.

ETIOLOGY

Emboli are usually blood clots, but the offending embolus also may be composed of air bubbles, fat globules, bacterial clumps, or pieces of tissue, including placenta. The most common offender is a venous thrombosis, a blood clot that has formed in

the deep veins of the legs as a result of venous stasis (Figs. 10–39, 10–40, and 10–41). A portion of the thrombus breaks loose from the clot and travels through the venous system until it becomes lodged in a vessel that is too narrow to allow passage, often in the lungs. Cardiac arrhythmias also can cause thrombi to form in the heart. Those that travel from the left ventricle can enter the coronary arteries, resulting in an MI, or can enter the carotid and cerebral arteries, compromising blood supply and resulting in CVAs.

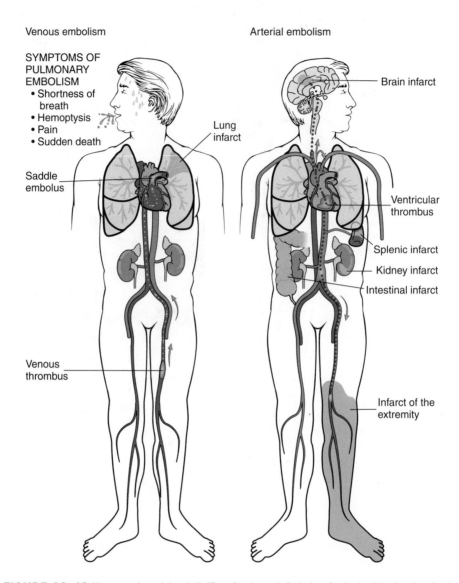

Venous embolism

SYMPTOMS OF
PULMONARY
EMBOLISM
• Shortness of
  breath
• Hemoptysis
• Pain
• Sudden death

Saddle
embolus

Venous
thrombus

Arterial embolism

Brain infarct

Lung
infarct

Ventricular
thrombus

Splenic infarct

Kidney infarct

Intestinal infarct

Infarct of the
extremity

FIGURE 10–40 Venous and arterial emboli. (From Damjanov I: *Pathology for the health related professions,*
ed 2, Philadelphia, 2000, Saunders.)

DIAGNOSIS

The clinical picture and a history of bed rest, physical inactivity, heart failure, arrhythmias, and any condition that has put pressure on or decreased flow in the veins of the legs or pelvis alert the physician to the possibility of an embolus. Pain in the calf of the leg in a patient who has any of the aforementioned predispositions is another clue.

TREATMENT

Treatment depends on the area of involvement. Treatment of pulmonary **embolism** (see Chapter 9), myocardial infarction, and CVA (see Chapter 13) is aggressive and immediate if the patient is to survive. The treatment of a patient with an arterial embolus in an extremity is also aggressive and immediate to prevent the death of tissue and eventual

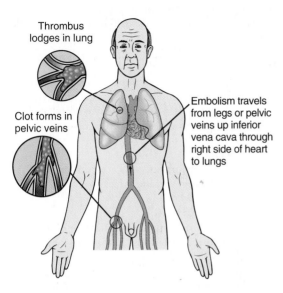

Thrombus lodges in lung

Clot forms in pelvic veins

Embolism travels from legs or pelvic veins up inferior vena cava through right side of heart to lungs

FIGURE 10–41 Venous thrombosis.

gangrene. Blood flow is re-established to the affected part by lowering the limb, wrapping it to maintain warmth to the area, and treating any constriction of blood vessels. Heparin or enoxaparin (Lovenox) are administered to deter further clot formation, and antispasmodic drugs are given for vascular spasms. If this therapy is not successful, surgical intervention may be indicated to remove the obstruction and to restore circulation. In another option, a thrombolytic drug, such as urokinase, can be administered via a central catheter directly into the spot of the coronary embolism to break down the emboli.

PROGNOSIS
The prognosis varies and depends on the location of the emboli. When the embolus is in an extremity, aggressive treatment and/or surgical intervention usually is successful.

PREVENTION
Preventing the formation of deep vein thrombosis during periods of immobilization or reduced physical activity is essential.

PATIENT TEACHING
Encourage those who will be traveling and sitting for long periods of time to get up and walk every hour for a few minutes. If this is not possible, suggest exercises that stimulate contraction of the calf muscles.

Arteriosclerosis

DESCRIPTION
Arteriosclerosis is a group of diseases characterized by hardening of the arteries. Arteriosclerosis has three forms: atherosclerosis, Mönckeberg arteriosclerosis, and arteriolosclerosis. Atherosclerosis occurs when plaques of fatty deposits form within the arterial tunica intima. Mönckeberg arteriosclerosis, medial calcific sclerosis, involves the arterial tunica media; there is destruction of muscle and elastic fibers along with calcium deposits. Arteriolosclerosis occurs when the walls of the arterioles thicken, with loss of elasticity and contractility.

Atherosclerosis

DESCRIPTION
Atherosclerosis, a thickening and hardening of the arteries, occurs when plaques of cholesterol and lipids form in the arterial tunica intima.

ICD-9-CM Code 440
Atherosclerosis is coded according to site. Refer to the physician's diagnosis and then to the current edition of the ICD-9-CM coding manual to ensure the greatest specificity of pathology and any appropriate modifiers.

SYMPTOMS AND SIGNS
Atherosclerosis is responsible for most myocardial and cerebral infarctions. The patient with atherosclerosis often is asymptomatic. The first symptoms may be angina pectoris, dizziness, elevated blood pressure, and shortness of breath.

PATIENT SCREENING
Patients reporting symptoms of angina pectoris, dizziness, elevated blood pressure, and shortness of breath require prompt assessment by a physician. Those who are asymptomatic may report just not feeling well; after careful questioning, these patients should be scheduled as soon as possible or referred to a facility where they can be seen quickly.

ETIOLOGY
The etiology of atherosclerosis is multifactorial and complicated, but there are risk factors that appear to increase the risk that the condition will develop. Heredity seems to increase the occurrence, as do a sedentary lifestyle, a diet rich in lipids and

cholesterol-producing foods, cigarette smoking, diabetes mellitus, hypertension, and obesity. The lipids and cholesterol in the blood form thick, stiff, and hardened lesions in the medium-size and large arteries. The lesions are eccentric and eventually expand to occlude the artery (Fig. 10–42). A fatty streak forms in the arterial wall and migrates to the tunica intima. Plaque forms and thickens the arterial wall. A sequela is an *ulceration,* crack, or fissure in the plaque where platelets can aggregate and form a thrombosis. Ischemia results from reduced blood supply to the dependent tissue, with resulting pain. Infarct occurs with advanced occlusion of the artery and is followed by tissue *necrosis.*

DIAGNOSIS

The diagnosis often is made during a routine physical examination or screening process. Blood studies indicate elevated cholesterol, triglyceride, and lipid levels. Hypertension may be noted. *Doppler* studies of major vessels show reduced blood flow.

TREATMENT

Treatment consists of dietary changes to reduce saturated fats and foods high in cholesterol and lipids. Cigarette smokers are encouraged to stop smoking. Hypertension and diabetes mellitus are treated and controlled. Hyperlipidemic drugs such as lovastatin (Mevacor) and simvastatin (Zocor) are prescribed. Recent additions to the recommended drug therapy include a niacin and lovastatin combination (Advicor) and azetimibe (Zetia), a drug that inhibits the absorption of cholesterol in the intestine. Research is being conducted to confirm claims that

hyperlipidemic drug therapy can bring about regression of the condition and actually reverse the plaque buildup.

PROGNOSIS

The prognosis varies and depends on patient compliance with prescribed drug therapy, exercise, and dietary changes. It is possible with good compliance to prevent progression of the disease.

PREVENTION

Prevention is important, as is education about risk factors and changes in lifestyle.

PATIENT TEACHING

Emphasize the importance of following dietary and exercise recommendations. If the patient is a diabetic, explain the need to keep blood glucose levels in normal range. Inform smokers of the dangers that smoking poses to their health. Give details about agencies that offer patients additional information about the condition as well as support groups in the community.

Aneurysms

DESCRIPTION

An aneurysm is a weakening and resulting local dilation of the wall of an artery (Fig. 10–43).

■ **ICD-9-CM Code 442.9** *(Of unspecified site)*
Aneurysms are coded according to site and type. Refer to the physician's diagnosis for site and type of aneurysm and then to the current

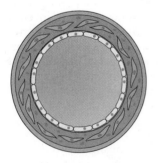

Normal arterial
lumen

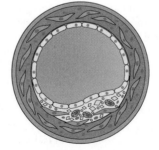

Atherosclerotic
plaque deposit

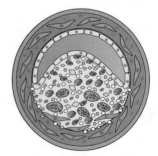

Advanced arterial
atherosclerotic
disease

FIGURE 10–42 Atherosclerosis.

edition of the ICD-9-CM coding manual to ensure the greatest specificity of pathology and any appropriate modifiers.

SYMPTOMS AND SIGNS

The symptoms of an aneurysm may have either an insidious or a sudden, acute onset. Symptoms depend on the location and size of the aneurysm and the extent of the dilation. Abdominal aortic aneurysm is the most common form. An asymptomatic aneurysm of the aorta often is discovered during a routine physical examination when the abdomen is being palpated or as the result of an abdominal radiographic study conducted for another reason. As the aortic aneurysm enlarges, the patient may experience abdominal or back pain, and a pulsating mass is observed in the abdomen.

A complication of any aneurysm is leakage from the wall of the artery or sudden rupture of the weak area. When this occurs, the patient exhibits symptoms and signs of hemorrhagic shock. Rupture of a cerebral aneurysm mimics signs of a CVA, with unilateral neurologic deficits being noted.

PATIENT SCREENING

Patients reporting a pulsating mass in the abdomen require prompt physician assessment. Those with symptoms of impending or evolving rupture require immediate entry into the emergency medical system.

ETIOLOGY

A common cause of aneurysms is a buildup of atherosclerotic plaque that weakens the vessel wall. Trauma, infection or inflammation, and congenital tendencies are additional causative factors.

DIAGNOSIS

The aortic mass is noted mid abdomen, and pulsation is observed. A **bruit** heard on auscultation is another sign of the arterial dilation. Cerebral aneurysms usually are discovered when they rupture with catastrophic consequences. Radiographic studies, ultrasonography, computed tomography (CT), and magnetic resonance imaging (MRI) all help to confirm the diagnosis. The ruptured aneurysm precipitates symptoms and signs of shock.

TREATMENT

Treatment depends on the size, location, and likelihood of rupture of the defect. Most diagnosed aortic aneurysms should be treated with surgical repair before they leak or rupture. After the aorta wall's integrity has been breached, immediate surgical intervention is required to repair the rupture, usually with a synthetic graft, if the patient is to survive. Watchful waiting often is employed when the aneurysm itself is small or is in a small vessel.

PROGNOSIS

The prognosis varies depending on the location and extent of the aneurysm. Surgical intervention before rupture or severe leakage of the vessel creates a better prognosis than when the aneurysm has ruptured or is leaking large amounts of blood. The speed of emergency intervention also affects the prognosis.

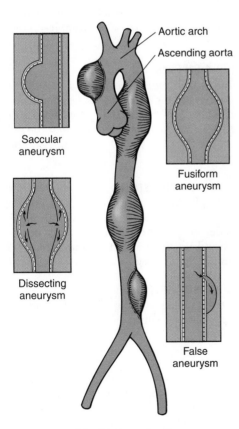

Saccular aneurysm

Aortic arch

Ascending aorta

Fusiform aneurysm

Dissecting aneurysm

False aneurysm

FIGURE 10–43 Types of aortic aneurysms.

PREVENTION

Prevention is unlikely as the condition is the result of many uncontrollable factors.

PATIENT TEACHING

Instruct those who have had surgery about postoperative care of the incision. Encourage compliance with any prescribed drug therapy, dietary modifications, and exercise regimens.

Phlebitis

DESCRIPTION

Phlebitis, an inflammation of a vein, occurs most often in the lower legs, but any vein, including cranial veins, may be affected.

> **ICD-9-CM Code 451**
> *Phlebitis is coded by site. Refer to the physician's diagnosis for location of phlebitis and then to the current edition of the ICD-9-CM coding manual to ensure the greatest specificity of pathology and any appropriate modifiers.*

SYMPTOMS AND SIGNS

Superficial vein involvement results in pain and tenderness in the affected area and becomes more severe as the condition progresses. Swelling, redness, and warmth are noted, followed by the development of a tender cordlike mass under the skin.

Deep venous inflammation affects the tunica intima, allowing the formation of clots (thrombophlebitis).

PATIENT SCREENING

Patients reporting swelling, redness, warmth, and pain in a limb require prompt assessment by a physician.

ETIOLOGY

The cause is uncertain, and the condition may appear for no apparent reason. Possible causes include venous stasis, obesity, blood disorders, injury, and surgery.

DIAGNOSIS

The clinical picture and history of a preceding event help establish the diagnosis.

TREATMENT

Treatment of superficial phlebitis is symptomatic, with analgesics given for pain. Caution must be taken not to massage the affected tender area because this manipulation may stimulate the formation of clots or the release of formed clots as emboli.

PROGNOSIS

The prognosis is usually positive with treatment.

PREVENTION

Because the cause is uncertain, prevention is probably not possible.

PATIENT TEACHING

Give patients and family members information warning against massaging the affected area.

Thrombophlebitis

DESCRIPTION

Thrombophlebitis is the result of inflammation of a vein with the formation of a thrombus on the vessel wall.

> **ICD-9-CM Code 451**
> *Thrombophlebitis is coded by site. Refer to the physician's diagnosis for location of phlebitis and then to the current edition of the ICD-9-CM coding manual to ensure the greatest specificity of pathology and any appropriate modifiers.*

SYMPTOMS AND SIGNS

Thrombophlebitis causes an interference with blood flow and resulting edema. As with phlebitis, the patient experiences pain, swelling, heaviness, and warmth in the affected area along with chills and fever. The involved area is tender to palpation.

PATIENT SCREENING

Patients reporting swelling, redness, warmth, and pain in a limb require prompt assessment by a physician.

ETIOLOGY

Venous stasis, blood disorders that cause a *hypercoagulable* state, and injury to the venous wall play important roles in the occurrence of thrombophlebitis. The deep venous inflammation of phlebitis affects the tunica intima, allowing the formation of clots (thrombophlebitis).

DIAGNOSIS

The clinical picture of gross edema in one leg, resulting in a measurable difference in the circumference of the legs, suggests thrombophlebitis. The affected area is tender to palpation. Imaging of the vessel with radiographic venography and ultrasonography confirms the diagnosis.

TREATMENT

Immediate intervention is necessary. The affected part is immobilized to prevent the thrombus from spreading and dislodging to become an embolus. Heparin is administered to prevent the clot from enlarging, and antibiotics are given to prevent infection.

PROGNOSIS

Prompt intervention usually leads to a positive outcome. The condition usually resolves, and no further treatment is indicated. If the condition does not resolve, surgical intervention may be needed to ligate the affected vessel. Collateral circulation develops. As with emboli, preventing the formation of deep vein thrombosis during periods of immobilization or reduced physical activity is essential.

PATIENT TEACHING

Encourage those who will be traveling and sitting for long periods of time to get up and walk every hour for a few minutes. If this is not possible, suggest exercises that stimulate contraction of the calf muscles. Emphasize the importance of immediate attention should the patient experience a recurrence of the symptoms.

Varicose Veins

DESCRIPTION

Varicose veins are swollen, tortuous, and knotted veins that usually occur in the lower legs (Fig. 10–44).

■ **ICD-9-CM Code 454**
Varicose veins are coded by type. Refer to the physician's diagnosis for specific site and then to the current edition of the ICD-9-CM coding manual to ensure the greatest specificity of pathology and any appropriate modifiers.

SYMPTOMS AND SIGNS

Symptoms of varicose veins develop gradually, with a feeling of fatigue in the legs, followed by a continuous dull ache. Leg cramps may be experienced at night, and the ankles may swell. As the condition progresses, the veins thicken and feel hard to the touch. Pain worsens and can have a dull or stabbing quality.

PATIENT SCREENING

These patients usually are not in acute distress and can be scheduled for the next available appointment. Should they report swelling accompanied by pain and redness in the area, prompt assessment by a physician is suggested.

ETIOLOGY

Varicose veins have no clearly identifiable cause. However, defective or absent valves may be suspected. Prolonged standing or sitting causes pressure on the valves in the superficial veins of the lower legs. Normal movement of the legs causes the muscles to contract and relax, thus "milking" the blood upward. When the person stands or sits for extended periods, gravity pushes the blood downward, with resulting pressure on the valves.

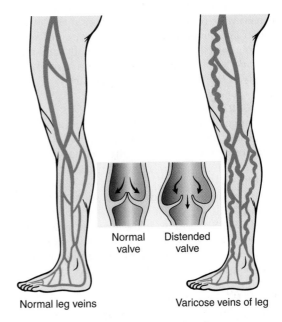

Normal valve   Distended valve

Normal leg veins   Varicose veins of leg

FIGURE 10–44 Varicose veins.

Without the normal muscular contractions, the venous walls distend, reaching a point at which they and the valves are no longer competent. Stasis of blood follows, causing the swelling of the veins. The enlarging uterus during pregnancy increases the pressure on the leg veins and pelvic veins, compromising the free flow of the venous blood.

DIAGNOSIS

The presence of the twisted, swollen, knotted veins of the lower legs on clinical inspection and a history of prolonged standing, prolonged sitting, or pregnancy are usually all that is needed to make the diagnosis. Advanced varicosities cause the skin around the affected areas to take on a brown discoloration.

TREATMENT

Rest periods throughout the day, with the patient lying down and elevating the feet higher than the heart, afford relief in mild cases. Engaging in exercise and submerging the legs in warm water increase the flow of blood. The patient may wear support stockings that encourage the return flow of blood. Those who have to stand for long periods are instructed to move the legs at frequent intervals to stimulate the muscular milking of the veins.

Painful, twisted, and swollen veins that have progressed beyond the treatment of rest and exercise usually require surgical intervention in the form of a vein ligation and stripping or injection of *sclerosing* solutions that harden and eventually *atrophy* the affected veins. Collateral circulation develops to augment the blood return to the heart.

PROGNOSIS

Treatment including venous ligation or injection of sclerosing solutions usually affords relief for the symptoms and resolution to the condition.

PREVENTION

Wearing support stockings and moving the legs during long periods of standing help prevent this condition. Some individuals, however, may be predisposed to the condition, especially during pregnancy. Weight loss that relieves abdominal pressure also helps.

PATIENT TEACHING

Give patients information about preventing stasis of blood flow in the legs. Give information on care of postoperative incisions.

Thromboangiitis Obliterans (Buerger Disease)

DESCRIPTION

Thromboangiitis obliterans (Buerger disease) is an inflammation of the peripheral arteries and veins of the extremities with clot formation (Fig. 10–45).

 ICD-9-CM Code 443.1

SYMPTOMS AND SIGNS

The patient experiences intense pain in the affected area, usually the legs or the instep of the foot, that is aggravated by exercise and relieved by rest. If the condition is not resolved and circulation is not restored to the affected area, atrophy, ulcers, and even gangrene can develop.

PATIENT SCREENING

Patients, especially males, reporting intense pain in the limbs that is aggravated by exercise and relieved by rest usually are scheduled for the next available appointment. Those complaining of breakdown of skin tissue require prompt assessment by a physician.

ETIOLOGY

The primary cause of Buerger disease is long-term smoking of tobacco. The inflammation and resulting clot formation in the vessels continue to ad-

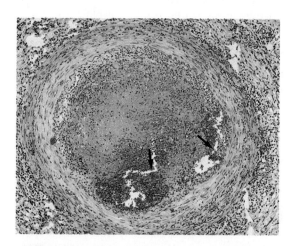

FIGURE 10–45 Thromboangiitis obliterans (Buerger disease). The lumen is occluded by a thrombus containing two abscesses. The vessel wall is infiltrated by leukocytes. (From Kumar V, Cotran RS, Robbins SL: *Robbins basic pathology*, ed 7, Philadelphia, 2003, Saunders.)

vance until the entire vessel is obliterated and circulation to the area is completely compromised. The ischemic tissue dies, and gangrene follows. This condition affects primarily males, most often those of Jewish descent.

DIAGNOSIS
The diagnosis follows reports of intense pain, usually in the legs or the instep. An arteriogram and other studies such as an ultrasonogram identify the site of the clot or obliteration. The ulcers on the skin are another indication of the disease and its severity. The history of long-term smoking of tobacco products suggests the diagnosis.

TREATMENT
The first step in treatment is the immediate and complete cessation of smoking. This often reduces the inflammation and restores partial circulation to the area. Buerger-Allen exercises also help to improve circulation to the area. In these exercises, the patient elevates the feet and legs 45 degrees to 90 degrees until they blanch and then lowers them below the rest of the body until they redden. The patient then rests in a supine position. If these steps do not restore circulation, surgical intervention to establish detours or to bore a pathway through the clot itself may be needed. Amputation of gangrenous tissue is imperative.

PROGNOSIS
No cure is known for this condition, but cessation of smoking relieves symptoms. Surgical intervention may help. When treatment fails, amputation may be necessary.

PREVENTION
Because the primary cause is smoking of tobacco products, prevention requires not smoking or cessation of smoking.

PATIENT TEACHING
Give information about the care of foot injuries and instructions about avoiding constrictions around the affected limb.

Raynaud Disease

DESCRIPTION
Raynaud disease is a vasospastic condition of the fingers, hands, or feet. It causes pain, numbness, and sometimes discoloration in these areas.

ICD-9-CM Code 443.0

SYMPTOMS AND SIGNS
This bilateral condition is precipitated by cold and causes a blanching (white) discoloration, followed by blue as venous blood remains, and finally red or purple when circulation is restored. The attacks occasionally are triggered by stressful events. Raynaud disease is much more common in women than in men. When the disorder is primary, it is called Raynaud disease; when it is secondary to another disease, it is called Raynaud's phenomenon. In severe cases, the digits may ulcerate and become very painful. In most cases, the prognosis is good.

PATIENT SCREENING
Those who have been diagnosed usually know they need to warm the area gently. Those experiencing the condition for the first time and experiencing the severe pain of the condition require prompt intervention.

ETIOLOGY
The small peripheral arteries and arterioles supplying the fingers, hands, and feet spasm and constrict, compromising the circulation to these appendages. The spasm follows exposure to cold or possibly results from a stressful occurrence. The episode usually resolves spontaneously after the application of warmth. The condition also is made worse by smoking tobacco.

DIAGNOSIS
The diagnosis is based on the clinical picture and a history of numbness and paleness of the areas. Normal arterial pulses are present. The condition most often affects women between puberty and the age of 40 years, especially those who smoke. In severe cases, the compromise in circulation can lead to tissue necrosis and even amputation.

TREATMENT
Treatment of the episode involves the application of warmth to the affected areas. Patients are encouraged to stop smoking, to avoid exposure to cold, and to avoid stressful situations that bring on the attacks. Drug therapy to dilate vessels and to increase blood flow includes vasodilators, alpha-adrenergic blockers, and calcium channel blockers. The side effects of the drug therapy often are worse than the condition.

PROGNOSIS

The painful event resolves with application of warmth to the affected area. The condition will continue to recur, however, with exposure to cold and as long as the individual continues to smoke.

PREVENTION

Preventing the attacks requires avoiding exposure to cold and wearing gloves and heavy socks and shoes for protection from the extreme cold. Cessation of smoking also helps prevent recurrences of the condition.

PATIENT TEACHING

Give patients information about the effect of smoking on their blood vessels. Encourage them to avoid direct skin exposure to extreme cold and to wear gloves and heavy socks and warm shoes to protect the fingers, hands, feet, and toes.

Blood Dyscrasias

Blood is composed of formed elements, red blood cells (erythrocytes), white blood cells (leukocytes), platelets (thrombocytes), and a liquid portion (plasma). It is responsible for transporting vital elements, including oxygen, nutrients, and hormones, to the body cells. It also plays a part in the removal of waste products, in the inflammatory response, and in the function of the immune system. In addition, blood helps to maintain *hemostasis*, acid–base and fluid balance, and body temperature.

Blood is synthesized by the *hematopoietic* system in the bone marrow (myeloid) and lymphoid tissue found in the lymph nodes, spleen, thymus, bone marrow, and gastrointestinal tract (Fig. 10–46). The *reticulo-endothelial* system is found in the spleen, liver, lymph nodes, and bone marrow. It is responsible for removing worn-out blood cells from the bloodstream and breaking down the blood cell components for recycling or elimination from the body.

Stem cells in the bone marrow form blast cells, including erythroblasts (rubriblasts), which eventually become erythrocytes, and myeloblasts, which eventually become leukocytes (Fig. 10–47).

Deviation or malfunctioning in this system results in various blood **dyscrasias,** either by impairment in the formation of the blood components or by unusual destruction of the cells. Dyscrasias involving erythrocytes and platelets are anemias, thrombocytoses, thrombocytopenias, and polycythemias. Leukocyte dyscrasias include leukemias, lymphomas, and leukopenias. Bleeding and clotting problems arise from alterations affecting thrombocytes and plasma-clotting factors. Normal values of blood components are measured by specific laboratory testing.

Anemias

DESCRIPTION

Anemia is defined as a condition in which there is a reduction in the quantity of either RBCs or hemoglobin in a measured volume of blood, reducing the blood's ability to carry oxygen to the cells.

Depending on the severity of the anemia, one or many symptoms may occur, including pallor, fatigue, dizziness, shortness of breath, and irregular heartbeats. The treatment varies with the cause. Several possible causes are acute or chronic blood loss, impaired production of RBCs (including aplastic anemia, iron-deficiency anemia, anemias of chronic disease, or megaloblastic anemia), inherited or acquired hemolytic conditions, anorexia nervosa, and hemolytic–hemoglobin disorders. Hemoglobin in RBCs is needed to transport oxygen to all cells, and any condition that reduces the amount of hemoglobin results in anemia. Iron and other components are needed to synthesize the hemoglobin.

Types of anemias include iron deficiency, folic acid deficiency, pernicious, aplastic, sickle cell, hemorrhagic, and **hemolytic.**

Important presenting symptoms that tend to recur in patients with anemia and need further investigation include:

- Fatigue
- Dyspnea (difficulty in breathing)
- Headache
- Loss of appetite
- Heartburn
- Edema, especially of the ankles
- Numbness and tingling sensations
- Syncope (fainting)
- Pallor

ICD-9-CM Code 280-289

Anemias are coded by type. Refer to the physician's diagnosis for specific type of anemia and then to the current edition of the ICD-9-CM coding manual to ensure the greatest specificity of pathology and any appropriate modifiers.

SYMPTOMS AND SIGNS

Regardless of the cause, anemic patients experience fatigue. Most appear pale. As the disease progresses, the symptoms become more pronounced, and the patient may have dyspnea, tachycardia, and a pounding of the heart. Pallor is noted on the palmar surface of the hands and in the nail beds, conjunctiva, and mucous membranes of the mouth.

PATIENT SCREENING

Anemias often are diagnosed incident to a physical examination or during evaluation of other disorders. The individual reporting dyspnea, tachycardia, and a "pounding" heart requires prompt assessment by a physician. Those reporting they are pale and "just plain tired" should be scheduled at the next available appointment.

ETIOLOGY

Anemias are classified by the color and size of the RBC as hypochromic, normochromic, or hyperchromic (spherocytosis), and as microcytic, normocytic, or macrocytic (Fig. 10–48). They also are classified by the causative factor, as previously mentioned.

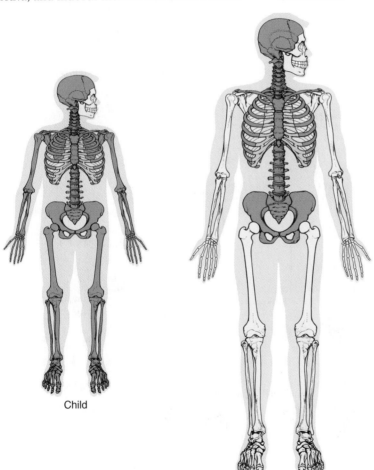

Child

Adult

FIGURE 10–46 Sites of blood cell formation.

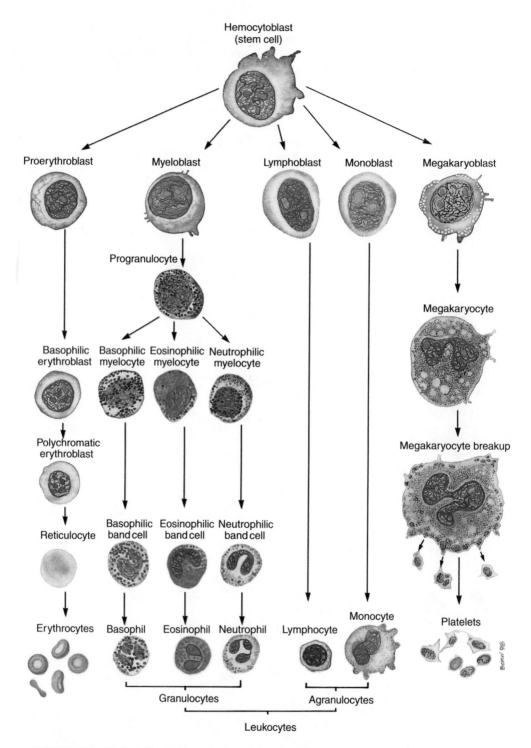

FIGURE 10–47 Formation of blood cells. (From Patton KT, Thibodeau GA: *Mosby's handbook of anatomy and physiology,* St. Louis, 2000, Mosby.)

Iron-deficiency anemia may be secondary to blood loss through hemorrhage, a slow insidious bleed such as bleeding hemorrhoids, and even heavy menstrual flow, or because of insufficient intake of dietary iron.

Folic acid deficiency anemia results when insufficient amounts of folic acid are available for DNA (deoxyribonucleic acid) synthesis, thus preventing the maturation of the blood cells. This can be the consequence of a dietary deficiency and is clinically similar to pernicious anemia.

Pernicious anemia is considered a macrocytic anemia, in which immature RBCs are larger than normal. The hemoglobin volume is reduced, with subsequent reduction in oxygen-carrying capacity. This anemia is considered the result of an autoimmune response and is discussed in Chapter 3.

Autoimmune hemolytic anemia also is considered an autoimmune response and is discussed in Chapter 3.

Aplastic anemia results from an insult to the hematopoietic cells (stem cells) in the bone marrow. Erythrocyte, leukocyte, and thrombocyte production is reduced because of exposure to myelotoxins, such as benzene, alkylating agents, antimetabolites, certain drugs and insecticides, and radiation.

Sickle cell anemia, a chronic hereditary hemolytic form of anemia, is found predominately in those of the black race. The presence of hemoglobin S along with hemoglobin A is noted in erythrocytes, causing them to acquire a sickle or elongated shape on deoxygenation (Fig. 10–49). These rigid misshapen cells obstruct capillary flow and lead to tissue hypoxia and further sickling; this in turn causes further obstruction and eventually infarction. When the sickled cells are reoxygenated, they resume the natural round disk shape of a normal erythrocyte. In addition, hemoglobin S has reduced oxygen-carrying capacity.

Hemorrhagic anemia results from the loss of large amounts of blood volume (hypovolemia) in a short time.

Hemolytic anemia is caused by abnormal destruction of the RBCs. Heredity plays a role in some hemolytic anemias, but exposure to chemical toxins and certain bacterial toxins or autoimmunity also may be the cause.

DIAGNOSIS

Blood studies show reduced RBC numbers, reduced hemoglobin levels and *hematocrit*, and changes in the morphology of the corpuscles (Table 10–2). Bone marrow studies may be ordered to detect any aberrations.

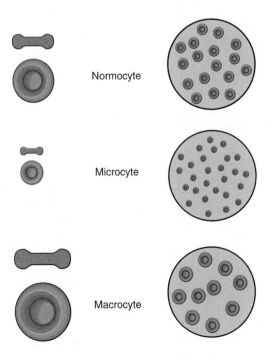

FIGURE 10–48 Sizes of erythrocytes.

Normocyte

Microcyte

Macrocyte

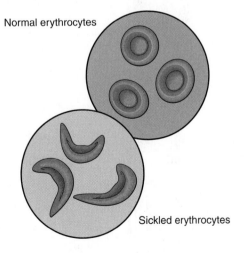

Normal erythrocytes

Sickled erythrocytes

FIGURE 10–49 Sickled erythrocytes.

TABLE 10–2
Blood Values in Anemia

	RBC (PER mm³)	Hb (g/dl)	Hct (%)	MCV (PER µm³)	MCH (pg)	MCHC (g/dl)	WBC (PER mm³)	RETICULOCYTE COUNT (PER mm³)	PLATELET COUNT (PER mm³)
Normal	Male: 4.7-6.1; female: 4.2-5.4	Male: 14-18; female: 12-16	Male: 42-52; female: 37-47	80-90	27-31	32-36	5000-10,000	0.5-2	150,000-400,000
Acute hemorrhagic anemia	Initial increase, latent decrease	Initial decrease, latent decrease	Initially normal, latent decrease	Increase	Decrease	Normal	Increase	Increase	Decrease
Chronic hemorrhagic anemia	Decrease	Decrease	Decrease	Slight decrease	Slight decrease	Slight decrease	Normal	Decrease	Normal
Iron-deficiency anemia	Decrease	Decrease	Decrease	Decrease	Decrease	Decrease	Normal	Decrease	Normal to increase
Aplastic anemia	Gross decrease	Gross decrease	Gross decrease	Moderate decrease	Gross decrease	Gross decrease	Gross decrease	Decrease	Gross decrease
Pernicious anemia	Decrease	Gross decrease	Gross decrease	Increase	Increase	Increase	Slight decrease	Decrease	Slight decrease
Folic acid deficiency anemia	Decrease	Gross decrease	Gross decrease	Increase	Increase	Increase	Slight decrease	Decrease	Slight decrease
Sickle cell anemia	Decrease	Decrease	Decrease	Decrease	Normal	Normal	Increase	Increase	Normal
Hemolytic anemia	Decrease	Decrease	Decrease	Increase	Slight decrease	Normal	Normal	Increase	Normal to increase

Hb, Hemoglobin; *Hct*, hematocrit; *MCH*, mean corpuscular hemoglobin; *MCHC*, mean corpuscular hemoglobin concentration; *MCV*, mean corpuscular volume; *RBC*, red blood cell; *WBC*, white blood cell.

TREATMENT

Treatment is directed at the cause of the anemia. Dietary or supplemental iron administration is beneficial in iron-deficiency anemias. If anemia is the result of a slow insidious bleed, the underlying cause must be found and treated. Folic acid replacement is indicated in folic acid deficiency anemia. Vitamin B_{12} injections are the treatment of choice for pernicious anemia. The causative factor must be uncovered in hemolytic and aplastic anemias and, if possible, eliminated. No cure is known for sickle cell anemia, so treatment is symptomatic. Rest, increased fluid intake, and the administration of analgesics are helpful. When the condition is exacerbated, the patient requires hospitalization for oxygen administration, intravenous therapy, the use of narcotic analgesics, and packed RBC transfusion. In all forms of anemia, blood replacement may be needed when other measures fail to restore the RBC numbers and hemoglobin levels.

PROGNOSIS

The prognosis varies and depends on the cause and type of anemia as well as the patient's response to prescribed therapy.

PREVENTION

Prevention also depends on the type and cause of the anemia. Most are not preventable. Proper nutrition may play a role in preventing anemia caused by low iron intake.

PATIENT TEACHING

Give patients information about proper nutrition. Emphasize the importance of complying with prescribed drug therapy.

Agranulocytosis

DESCRIPTION

Agranulocytosis (also called neutropenia) is a blood dyscrasia in which leukocyte levels become extremely low.

 ICD-9-CM Code 288.0

SYMPTOMS AND SIGNS

This condition can have a rapid onset. The patient experiences severe fatigue and weakness, followed by a sore throat, ulcerations on the oral mucosa, *dysphagia,* elevated body temperature, weak and rapid pulse, and chills.

PATIENT SCREENING

Patients reporting severe fatigue and weakness followed by a sore throat, ulcerations on the oral mucosa, dysphagia, an elevated body temperature, weak and rapid pulse, and chills require prompt assessment by a physician.

ETIOLOGY

Agranulocytosis usually is caused by drug toxicity or hypersensitivity. For example, cancer chemotherapy with chemotoxic agents can be a cause. Benzene is another chemical agent that causes neutropenia. Agranulocytosis, or neutropenia, is an acute insult to the body's immune system and drastically reduces the body's response to bacterial infection. The infectious agents usually invade the body through the oral or pharyngeal mucosa and often are already present but are no longer held in check by the now-absent granulocytes. Patients occasionally are sensitive to a particular drug, such as chlorpromazine, propylthiouracil, phenytoin, chloramphenicol, and phenylbutazone. Agranulocytosis also can accompany aplastic or megaloblastic anemia, tuberculosis, *uremia,* or malaria. This condition occurs most often in the female population.

DIAGNOSIS

Blood studies show leukopenia, with a marked decrease in the number of polymorphonuclear cells. Bone marrow studies reveal a lack of granulocytes, and the developing WBCs are not mature and are reduced in number. History may reveal exposure to the offending infectious agents; blood, urine, and oral cultures may be positive for bacteria; and toxins may be present.

TREATMENT

The primary thrust of treatment is to eliminate any offending microorganism through aggressive antimicrobial therapy. Cultures are repeated several times and are monitored for the growth of microbes. If the cause of the toxicity is identified as a drug or chemical, exposure to the toxic agent must be halted. Aggressive therapy is indicated because the condition can be fatal within a week if left untreated.

PROGNOSIS

The prognosis varies and depends on the etiology of the condition. Cessation of exposure to a toxic substance often produces improvement. As previously mentioned, some cases of this condition may be fatal within a week if left untreated.

PREVENTION

Prevention involves avoiding the toxic substance after it has been identified. Prevention is not always possible.

PATIENT TEACHING

Give the patient information about exposure to the toxic substance. Help the patient and family find information about exposure to hazardous materials.

Polycythemia

DESCRIPTION

Polycythemia (polycythemia vera) is an abnormal increase in the amount of hemoglobin, the RBC count, or the hematocrit, causing an absolute increase in RBC mass.

 ICD-9-CM Code 238.4

SYMPTOMS AND SIGNS

Symptoms of polycythemia are related to the increased RBC mass and include headaches, dyspnea, irritability, mental sluggishness, dizziness, syncope, night sweats, and weight loss. Circulatory stagnation, thrombus, and increased blood viscosity may be noted. *Splenomegaly* and clubbing of the fingers along with cyanosis may be observed.

PATIENT SCREENING

Patients reporting headaches, dyspnea, irritability, mental sluggishness, dizziness, syncope, night sweats, and weight loss require prompt assessment. Schedule an appointment as soon as possible. If a prompt appointment is not possible, refer the patient to a facility where assessment can be performed quickly.

ETIOLOGY

It is not known why a sustained increase in the **hematopoiesis** of the bone marrow causes absolute, or primary, polycythemia. Relative polycythemia results when the plasma volume is reduced by dehydration, plasma loss, fluid and electrolyte imbalances, or burns. Reduced oxygen supply to the tis-

sues results in a compensation by the body as it manufactures additional hemoglobin to carry additional oxygen. The body uses this compensatory process when patients have chronic pulmonary and cardiac diseases or live at high altitudes, where the oxygen concentration is reduced.

DIAGNOSIS

An abnormal increase in RBC numbers, hemoglobin levels, and hematocrit suggests the condition. Leukocyte and thrombocyte counts also are elevated, and the spleen may be enlarged. The clinical picture aids in the diagnosis. The total RBC mass evaluation is also diagnostic.

TREATMENT

Periodic phlebotomy is employed to reduce the blood volume. Myelosuppressive drugs and radiation also improve the blood count. Relative polycythemia usually subsides when the causative factors are eliminated.

PROGNOSIS

The periodic phlebotomies help to reduce the red blood cell count and hematocrit. This treatment is a required lifelong protocol for many patients. Some cases will resolve, as previously mentioned.

PREVENTION

With no known etiology, no prevention is known.

PATIENT TEACHING

Emphasize the importance of routine blood cell counts and the need for continued phlebotomy. Encourage patients to keep routine appointments.

Thrombocytopenia

Idiopathic thrombocytopenic **purpura** is considered an autoimmune response. This dyscrasia involving reduced clotting capabilities of the blood is discussed in Chapter 3.

Leukemias

Leukemias are malignant neoplasms of the blood-forming organs (bone marrow, spleen, and lymph nodes) that produce an abnormal, uncontrolled, clonal proliferation of one specific type of blood cell in the lymphoid or myeloid cell lines. The large number of leukemic cells leads to bone marrow overcrowding, resulting in reduced production and function of normal blood cells. The reduced numbers of functional neutrophils, erythrocytes, and platelets result in frequent infections, anemia, and clotting problems.

Leukemias are classified by the cell type and the degree of differentiation of the neoplastic cells. Acute leukemias are composed of immature-appearing, large hematopoietic cells (blasts). Chronic leukemias produce more mature-appearing, yet hypofunctional, cells. Acute disease has a rapid progression and can be quickly fatal (with a natural history of 1 to 5 months), while chronic leukemias have a slower progression measured in years rather than months. The leukemic cell type refers to whether the neoplastic cells derive from the lymphoid or the myeloid lineage. Common types of leukemia include acute lymphocytic leukemia, chronic lymphocytic leukemia, acute myelogenous leukemia, and chronic myelogenous leukemia.

Acute Lymphocytic Leukemia

DESCRIPTION

Acute lymphocytic leukemia (ALL) is characterized by an overproduction of immature lymphoid cells (lymphoblasts) in the bone marrow and lymph nodes.

> ■ **ICD-9-CM Code 204.0** *(Acute lymphoid leukemia)*
> *Refer to the physician's diagnosis for specific type of lymphoid leukemia and then to the current edition of the ICD-9-CM coding manual to ensure the greatest specificity of pathology and any appropriate modifiers.*

SYMPTOMS AND SIGNS

The patient appears pale and may report bone pain, weight loss, sore throat, fatigue, night sweats, and weakness. Bleeding of the gingiva may be noted. There is a tendency toward increased bruising and recurrent infections. As the leukemic cells infiltrate the spleen, liver, lymph nodes, and nervous system, they interfere with the normal functioning of these organs. Lymphadenopathy and splenomegaly are common at presentation. Symptoms of CNS involvement include headache, blurred vision, nausea, vomiting, and cranial nerve palsies.

PATIENT SCREENING

Patients complaining of bone pain, weight loss, sore throat, fatigue, night sweats, weakness, bleeding of the gingiva, a tendency toward increased bruising and recurrent infections, headache, blurred vision, nausea, vomiting, and/or cranial nerve palsies require prompt assessment by a physician.

ETIOLOGY

ALL tends to affect children and those older than 65. It accounts for 20% of adult leukemias and is the most common childhood leukemia. Childhood ALL is covered in more detail in Chapter 2. The exact cause is unknown. Prolonged exposure to radiation, certain chemicals and drugs, smoking, viruses, and genetic factors (Down syndrome and other chromosomal abnormalities) are considered contributing factors.

DIAGNOSIS

A peripheral blood smear shows increased numbers of immature lymphocytes and reduced numbers of erythrocytes and platelets. Microscopic examination of a bone marrow aspiration or biopsy is necessary for definitive diagnosis. Blast cells should make up more than 30% of all nucleated cells in the bone marrow to diagnose ALL. Cerebral spinal fluid (CSF) may be withdrawn and examined for leukemic cells. A karyotype is performed to look for any abnormalities that may help determine prognosis and treatment options.

TREATMENT

Treatment for ALL includes aggressive systemic chemotherapy, usually with vincristine, prednisone, L-asparaginase, and daunorubicin. Even after chemotherapy has induced remission, additional treatments of chemotherapy (methotrexate and 6-mercaptopurine) are administered periodically for 2 to 3 years to kill any leukemic cells that may have survived the first round. In addition, because CNS invasion is common in ALL, the CNS is treated prophylactically with intrathecally administered methotrexate and intracranial radiation therapy. Allogenic bone marrow transplantation is an option for patients who have relapsed or for adults with poor prognostic features. Complete remission is defined as normal peripheral blood cell counts and less than 5% lymphoblasts in the bone marrow aspirate.

PROGNOSIS

The overall 5-year survival rate is 63% for adults and 85% for children. Adults often have cytogenetic abnormalities that carry a worse prognosis than the ones found in children. In addition, children often can tolerate relatively higher doses of the drugs currently used to treat ALL than adults can. Poor prognostic indicators include age of less than 1 year or greater than 10 years, leukocyte counts of greater than 50,000/ml, CNS invasion, presence of the Philadelphia chromosome, and failure to achieve remission after 4 weeks of chemotherapy treatment.

PREVENTION

No prevention methods are known for ALL.

PATIENT TEACHING

Give patients and parents of children information about the chemotherapy. Help them find and contact community support groups.

Chronic Lymphocytic Leukemia

DESCRIPTION

Chronic lymphocytic leukemia (CLL) is a neoplasm that usually involves the B lymphocytes. It is a slowly progressing disease that results in the accumulation of mature-appearing, but hypofunctional, lymphocytes.

ICD-9-CM Code 204.1 *(Chronic lymphoidleukemia)*
Refer to the physician's diagnosis for specific type of lymphoid leukemia and then to the current edition of the ICD-9-CM coding manual to ensure the greatest specificity of pathology and any appropriate modifiers.

SYMPTOMS AND SIGNS

Patients often have no symptoms when a routine CBC reveals lymphocytosis, thrombocytopenia, anemia, or a low hemoglobin level. Symptoms may include weight loss, fever, night sweats, extreme fatigue, splenomegaly, hepatomegaly, and painless swelling of cervical, supraclavicular, or axillary lymph nodes that spontaneously waxes and wanes. Patients are susceptible to frequent viral and fungal infections.

PATIENT SCREENING

Patients complaining of weight loss, fever, night sweats, extreme fatigue, and noticeable swelling of cervical, supraclavicular, or axillary lymph nodes require prompt assessment by a physician.

ETIOLOGY

No single chromosomal change is specific for CLL. Certain patterns, such as trisomy of chromosomes 12, 3, or 16 or a deletion of chromosome 13, may be seen. The median age at diagnosis is 60 years, and most patients are males. During the initial asymptomatic phase, patients often can maintain their normal lifestyle, but performance levels during the terminal phase are poor, and frequent causes of death include systemic infection, bleeding, and cachexia.

DIAGNOSIS

Nearly 95% of cases are discovered incidentally during routine blood work. Peripheral blood smear and bone marrow studies are performed and reveal an increased number of mature-appearing lymphocytes. The lymphocytes are more mature and more differentiated than in ALL. In most cases of CLL, the absolute lymphocyte count is greater than $10,000/\mu l$ and the bone marrow is hypercellular with lymphocytes accounting for 30% to 40% of all nucleated cells. "Smudge cells" (broken lymphocytes) may be seen on the peripheral blood smear. Because CLL most often involves the B-lymphocytes, screening for the presence of certain B cell markers may be performed. Radiographic studies are not required for diagnosis, but a chest x-ray and CT scans may help in evaluating the extent of disease.

Many staging systems for CLL have been proposed, but the Rai system is the most common in the United States. The stage is important in determining appropriate treatment and the prognosis. The Rai system stratifies patients into risk groups according to their symptoms and assigns an average survival time to those groups. Patients usually move through the risk groups during the course of their disease.

Stage 0: Patients have lymphocytosis and bone marrow infiltration of greater than 30% blasts. Median survival time is 12 years.
Stage I: Patients have lymphadenopathy. Median survival time is 10 years.
Stage II: Patients have splenomegaly and/or hepatomegaly. Median survival time is 8 years.
Stage III: Patients have anemia. Median survival time is 2 years.
Stage IV: Patients have thrombocytopenia. Median survival time is 2 years.

TREATMENT

Treatment often is withheld until the patient is symptomatic and has evidence of hemolytic anemia, painful lymphadenopathy, symptomatic organomegaly, or cytopenia; or prolonged fever, chills, or weight loss. Early-stage CLL may be treated with a chemotherapy agent (usually fludarabine), a corticosteroid to control the leukocytosis, or radiation therapy to reduce symptoms caused by lymphadenopathy and splenomegaly. More advanced stages are treated with systemic combination chemotherapy. Newer therapies include the use of monoclonal antibodies directed against B lymphocyte surface antigens such as rituximab (Rituxan) (directed against CD20) or alemtuzumab (Campath) (directed against CD52). Bone marrow transplantation is generally not an option for CLL patients, although the newly developed non-myeloablative transplants show promise as a potential treatment for CLL.

PROGNOSIS

CLL has a variable natural course of disease. Survival times from diagnosis range from 2 to 20 years. The overall 5-year survival rate is 73%. Poor prognostic indicators are low platelet count and low hemoglobin level at the time of diagnosis.

PREVENTION

No methods for prevention of CLL are known.

PATIENT TEACHING

Give patients and parents of children information about the chemotherapy. Help them find and contact community support groups.

Acute Myelogenous Leukemia

DESCRIPTION

Acute myelogenous leukemia (AML) (also known as acute myeloid, myelocytic, or granulocytic leukemia) is a rapidly progressive neoplasm of cells committed to the myeloid line of development. Leukemic cells accumulate in the bone marrow, peripheral blood, and other tissues.

ICD-9-CM Code   205.0 *(Acute promyelocytic leukemia)*
Refer to the physician's diagnosis for specific type of myeloid leukemia and then to the current edition of the ICD-9-CM coding manual to ensure the greatest specificity of pathology and any appropriate modifiers.

SYMPTOMS AND SIGNS

A rapid accumulation of myeloblasts (myeloid precursors) leads to pancytopenia and the resulting symptoms of anemia, easy bleeding and bruising, and increased risk of infection. Bleeding symptoms include gingival bleeding, epistaxis, and menorrhagia. Weight loss, fatigue, and pallor are common.

ETIOLOGY

Acute myelocytic leukemia (AML) is the most common adult leukemia and accounts for about 20% of childhood leukemia as well. Risk factors include a positive family history for AML or other leukemias; prior therapeutic treatment with ionizing radiation; prior aggressive chemotherapy treatment for Hodgkin disease, non-Hodgkin lymphoma, ovarian cancer, or breast cancer; chronic exposure to benzene (a toxic liquid found in gasoline, rubber cement, and cleaning solvents); and cigarette smoking. About 10% to 15% of AML cases are treatment-related (with prior radiation or chemotherapy). Many cases of AML occurred among Japanese survivors of the atomic bomb attack.

DIAGNOSIS

The diagnosis is suggested by the clinical picture and peripheral blood smear. Bone marrow aspiration and biopsy is needed for definitive diagnosis. The bone marrow usually is hypercellular with greater than 20% to 30% myeloblasts. Half of the patients will have an Auer rod (abnormal lysosomal granules) visible inside the leukemic cell (Fig. 10–50). The presence of an Auer rod is diagnostic for AML. After diagnosis, a morphologic classification and cytogenetic analysis must be performed to determine the treatment selection. Cases are grouped into seven subtypes using the French-American-British (FAB) classification system based on the predominant morphologic cell type.

TREATMENT

Routine laboratory testing (e.g., CBC, liver function tests, coagulation studies), as well as chest x-ray, ECG, and HSV (herpes simplex virus) and CMV (cytomegalovirus) serology are obtained to identify potential complications of therapy. Chemotherapy is the first approach to treating AML. Cytosine arabinoside and daunorubicin are given to induce remission, followed by high-dose cytosine arabinoside to kill the small number of remaining leukemic cells. Bone marrow transplantation during the first remission may improve

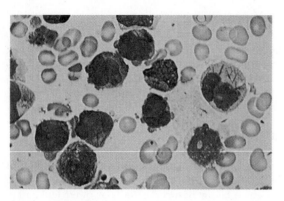

FIGURE 10–50 Auer rod cells. (From Wiernik et al: *Neoplastic diseases of the blood,* ed 3, New York, 1996, Churchill Livingstone.)

survival. Allopurinol is often given to treat the hyperuricemia found in many patients with AML. Complete remission is defined as having normal peripheral blood cell counts and less than 5% blasts in the bone marrow.

Acute promyelocytic leukemia (APL), FAB type M3, is a form of AML that is distinct from the other subtypes. It is characterized by a translocation between the long arms of chromosomes 15 and 17, t(15;17), creating a fusion gene, PML/RAR-α. The gene product impairs differentiation and apoptosis of promyelocytes. The impairment can be overcome by administration of all-trans retinoic acid (ATRA), a derivative of vitamin A, often in conjunction with cytotoxic chemotherapy (cytarabine and daunorubicin). The patient should be monitored for signs of disseminated intravascular coagulation (DIC) and retinoic acid syndrome (such as fever, peripheral edema, respiratory distress, and renal and hepatic dysfunction).

PROGNOSIS

The overall 5-year survival rate for AML in adults is 19%. For children, 5-year survival is 46%. Adverse prognostic indicators are advanced age, history of a prior hematologic disorder, and poor performance status at diagnosis. Some cytogenetic abnormalities, such as the translocations t(8;21) and t(15;17), have a more favorable prognosis. The t(15;17) translocation is considered favorable because of the excellent treatment response of APL to ATRA and chemotherapy. The 5-year survival rate for APL can approach 70% with appropriate treatment.

PREVENTION

No methods of preventing AML are known.

PATIENT TEACHING

Give patients and parents of children information about the chemotherapy. Help them find and contact community support groups.

Chronic Myelogenous Leukemia

DESCRIPTION

Chronic myelogenous leukemia (CML) (also known as chronic myeloid or myelocytic leukemia) accounts for 15% to 20% of leukemia cases in adults. It is a slowly progressing neoplasm that arises in a hematopoietic stem cell or early progenitor cell, resulting in an excess of mature-appearing, but hypofunctional, neutrophils.

> **ICD-9-CM Code 205.1** *(Chronic myeloid leukemia)*
> *Refer to the physician's diagnosis for specific type of myeloid leukemia and then to the current edition of the ICD-9-CM coding manual to ensure the greatest specificity of pathology and any appropriate modifiers.*

SYMPTOMS AND SIGNS

About 50% of patients are asymptomatic at diagnosis, with the disease being suspected from abnormalities, such as leukocytosis and thrombocytosis, on routine blood tests. Symptomatic patients may exhibit fatigue, weight loss, excessive sweating, bleeding episodes, upper left quadrant pain, acute gouty arthritis, and tenderness of the lower sternum. Anemia and splenomegaly also are common.

ETIOLOGY

CML occurs most often in adults over the age of 40. Exposure to ionizing radiation is the only known risk factor. CML is almost invariably associated with an abnormal chromosome 22-, the Philadelphia chromosome (see the Enrichment box). The disease has a triphasic course: a chronic phase, an accelerated phase, and a blast crisis. Most patients are diagnosed in the chronic phase, where abnormal proliferation of white blood cells has begun. Splenomegaly is common, but symptoms are mild. In the accelerated phase, leukocytosis increases and neutrophil differentiation becomes further impaired. The patient may experience bone pain,

ENRICHMENT
THE PHILADELPHIA CHROMOSOME

THE PHILADELPHIA CHROMOSOME (named after the city in which it was discovered) is the hallmark of chronic myelogenous leukemia (CML). It results from a reciprocal translocation between the region of chromosome 9 that carries the abl proto-oncogene and the breakpoint cluster region (bcr) on chromosome 22. The term *Philadelphia chromosome* (also written Ph' or Ph+) refers to the truncated chromosome 22 that carries the bcr/abl fusion. This translocation is written t(9;22) and results in the formation of a novel protein that displays a much greater amount of tyrosine kinase activity than the normal abl protein. This active kinase is believed to be involved in the neoplastic transformation seen in CML. Routine cytogenetic testing detects Ph' in 90% of patients with CML, and Southern blot or PCR analyses will show the bcr/abl rearrangement in nearly all of the remaining patients with CML. Although acquiring the Ph' translocation is thought to be the initiating event for CML, accumulation of other mutations leads disease progression into the accelerated phase and blast crisis. Complete remission in patients with CML requires the eradication of the Ph'. Ph' also may be seen in some patients with ALL and indicates poor prognosis for these patients.

---

fever, night sweats, and other systemic symptoms. The blast crisis resembles AML and is defined by the presence of 30% or more blasts in the peripheral blood or bone marrow. Symptoms worsen, and new chromosomal abnormalities are acquired. CML progresses to blast crisis an average of 3 to 5 years after diagnosis and 3 to 18 months after initiation of the accelerated phase. Average survival after blast crisis is 3 months.

DIAGNOSIS
The diagnosis is suggested by the clinical picture and blood and bone marrow studies. A CBC reveals anemia, leukocytosis, and thrombocytosis. A bone marrow biopsy shows hyperplasia, but the cells appear more mature than the leukemic cells in AML. Definitive diagnosis requires demonstrating the presence of the Philadelphia chromosome or the bcr/abl fusion gene product by cytogenetic analysis, Southern blot, or RT-PCR. The presence of the Philadelphia chromosome distinguishes CML from other disorders that may resemble CML clinically.

TREATMENT
Bone marrow transplantation (BMT) is the only chance for a complete cure for CML. However, BMT is a viable option for only about 25% of patients. Transplantation during the chronic phase of the disease offers the best results, so patients who have progressed are treated with chemotherapy to induce a return to the chronic phase. Among patients for whom BMT is not an option, chemotherapy (usually with hydroxyurea or interferon-alfa) is used to keep the disease under control for as long as possible. A new drug that specifically inhibits the abl tyrosine kinase, imatinib mesylate (Gleevec), was recently approved for the treatment of CML and has shown promising results. Complete remission is defined as ablation of the Philadelphia chromosome and its gene product.

PROGNOSIS
The overall 5-year survival rate is 35%. Indicators of poorer prognosis include large spleen size, older age of the patient, higher percentage of blast cells, and a platelet count above 700,000/μl.

PREVENTION
No methods are known to prevent CML.

PATIENT TEACHING
Give patients and parents of children information about the chemotherapy. Help them find and contact community support groups.

Lymphatic Diseases

BONE MARROW TRANSPLANTATION

MANY PATIENTS WITH LEUKEMIAS and lymphomas cannot be cured with conventional chemotherapy treatments alone. The very large doses of chemotherapy or radiation that would be required to fully destroy all the neoplastic cells in patients with relapsed disease or disease refractory to conventional treatment make people very sick and destroy the bone marrow. Few people could survive this severe treatment.

Bone marrow transplantation (BMT) was developed to treat these people. In the traditional BMT protocol, the patient first receives high-dose chemotherapy and/or radiation therapy to eradicate all malignant cells in the body and to suppress the body's immune system so it is less likely to attack the donor marrow. Next, stem cells obtained from a donor's bone marrow are infused into the recipient. The stem cells find their way into the marrow space of the recipient and restore marrow functioning in 2 to 4 weeks.

A newer method of BMT has been developed in recent years. Studies have shown that stem cells may be harvested directly from the donor's peripheral blood after hematopoietic growth factors have been administered to the donor to mobilize stem cells from the marrow to the blood stream. The stem cells are collected using a pheresis machine and then infused into the recipient. These peripheral blood cells can restore neutrophil and platelet production several days faster than stem cells derived from bone marrow. Therefore this peripheral-blood stem-cell transplantation is preferred to the traditional BMT for many patients.

An investigational approach called a non-myeloablative transplantation, or "mini-transplantation," has shown some promise in treating the elderly and other patients who are unable to tolerate the high initial doses of chemotherapy in conventional BMT. It uses mild chemotherapy and low-dose radiation before transplantation of the donor stem cells. The donor cells gradually replace the host marrow and kill neoplastic cells by an immunologic "graft vs. tumor" effect.

All of these transplantations carry the risk of severe infections and bleeding, serious damage to vital organs caused by initial chemotherapy and radiation therapy, and graft rejection by the host's cells. Graft-versus-host disease (GVHD), an immunologic reaction in which the donor T lymphocytes see the host tissue, especially the skin, liver, and GI tract, as foreign and attack it, is not uncommon. Relapse may also occur and is seen most often with ALL and CML transplanted during blast crisis.

Definitions of some terms commonly used in conjunction with BMT are:

Autologous transplant: Transplant in which the patient serves as his or her own donor for stem cells.

Allogeneic transplant: Transplant in which the donor is HLA-identical to the patient (usually a sibling).

HLA type: The identity of the leukocyte surface antigens, the human leukocyte antigens (HLA), which is determined for the patient and donor to determine the degree of compatibility. The closer the match is, the lower is risk of transplant-related complications.

Syngeneic transplant: Transplant in which the patient's identical twin serves as the stem cell donor.

Unrelated donor/mismatched transplant: Transplant in which the donor does not match all of the key HLA antigens. This type of transplant is associated with the greatest risk of complications such as GVHD.

Lymphatic Diseases

The lymphatic system is composed of lymphatic vessels, lymphatic tissue (lymph nodes, tonsils, thymus, and spleen), and *lymph*. The lymphatic vessels originate at the capillary level and, along with the venous system, progress to empty into the right and left subclavian veins (Fig. 10–51). This system has no pump. Lymph nodes, collections of lymphatic tissue, filter foreign material such as bacteria and viruses from the lymphatic circulation (Fig. 10–52). Lymphocytes are produced mainly in the lymph nodes as part of the body's defense mechanism. The lymphatic vessels are thin walled, and the larger vessels contain valves. Similar to the case for the venous system, the muscles exert intermittent pressure on the vessels, causing the lymph to flow by a milking action. Smooth muscle in the vessel wall contracts to aid the return of lymph to the cardiovascular system. Swollen lymph nodes or glands may indicate trapping of microbes during an infectious process.

Lymphedema

DESCRIPTION
Lymphedema is an abnormal collection of lymph, usually in the extremities.

■ **ICD-9-CM Code** **457.1** *(Other lymphedema)*
457.0 *(Postmastectomy lymph-edema syndrome)*

SYMPTOMS AND SIGNS
Lymphedema results in a swelling of the extremity. The patient experiences no pain. The extremity becomes swollen and grossly distended (Fig. 10–53).

PATIENT SCREENING
Patients reporting unilateral limb swelling require prompt assessment. Schedule these patients to be seen as soon as possible or refer them to a facility where they can be assessed quickly.

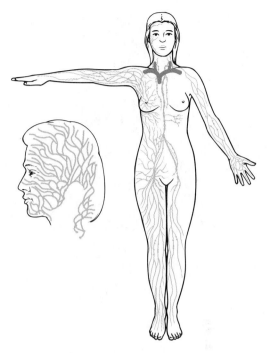

FIGURE 10–51 Lymphatic system.

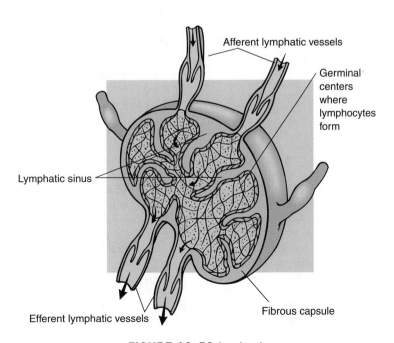

FIGURE 10–52 Lymph node.

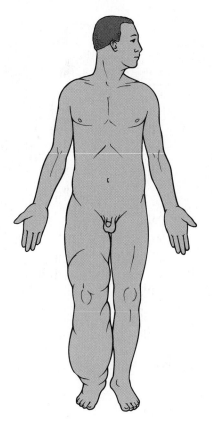

FIGURE 10–53 Lymphedema.

DIAGNOSIS

Painless swelling in an extremity suggests lymphedema. Imaging procedures, including lymphangiography and radioactive isotope studies, are means of confirming the diagnosis and ascertaining the site of obstruction.

TREATMENT

Treatment is aimed at reducing the swelling. The affected limb is elevated above the heart to encourage drainage of the lymph. Elastic bandages or stockings are applied when the affected part is elevated to compress the area, also encouraging lymph drainage. Diuretics may be administered to reduce fluid volume. Surgical intervention may be attempted to relieve a mechanical obstruction. Antibiotics may be administered if infection is present.

PROGNOSIS

The prognosis varies and depends on the cause of the lymphedema as well as the patient response to therapeutic intervention. When conservative measures fail to reduce the swelling, surgical intervention to remove the cause of the obstruction usually has a positive outcome. When lymphedema is left untreated, the connective tissues can lose their elasticity, resulting in the edema becoming permanent.

Lymphedema is not in itself life threatening, but it carries a danger that uncontrolled infection can develop in the affected tissue. The essentially stagnant interstitial fluids are a breeding ground for infections and their resulting toxins (poisons). Local defenses are overwhelmed, and the normal systemic defense system is not activated.

ETIOLOGY

The obstruction of the lymph vessel or node may be inflammatory or mechanical. If lymphedema is left untreated, the connective tissues lose their elasticity and the edema becomes permanent. The lymphatic circulation may be compromised by infections, neoplasms, or thrombus. Allergic reactions also may be implicated, along with trauma or surgery involving the affected part. Tight clothing that constricts the lymphatic vessels can cause temporary lymphedema. Removing the constriction usually resolves the swelling. Women who have had mastectomies may experience lymphedema in the adjacent arm. Prolonged lymphedema rarely is associated with the development of lymphosarcoma (a cancer).

PREVENTION

Many cases are not preventable. Wearing of tight clothing that can restrict lymphatic flow is discouraged.

PATIENT TEACHING

Give patients information about preventable causes of lymphedema. Encourage postmastectomy patients to follow prescribed rehabilitation exercises to help reduce the incidence of lymphedema.

Lymphangitis

DESCRIPTION

Lymphangitis is an inflammation of the lymph vessels.

■ **ICD-9-CM Code 457.2**

SYMPTOMS AND SIGNS

Lymphangitis usually is manifested by a red streak at the site of entry of the infective organism. The redness extends to the regional lymph node, which is swollen and tender. **Cellulitis** may develop in surrounding tissue. Manifestations of generalized infection, including fever, chills, and malaise, are present.

PATIENT SCREENING

Patients reporting fever, chills, and generalized malaise accompanied by tenderness and redness in the region of a lymph node require prompt assessment by a physician.

ETIOLOGY

Bacterial invasion into the lymph vessels at the site of local trauma or ulceration is a frequent cause of lymphangitis. Occasionally, no portal of entry is detectable. The bacteria travel to the regional lymph nodes and stimulate inflammation.

DIAGNOSIS

Visual inspection of the involved area and observance of typical systemic manifestations of bacterial invasion are usually sufficient for diagnosis. Blood studies indicate leukocytosis. Final confirmation is made by cultures of the infected tissue.

TREATMENT

Treatment includes the administration of systemic antibiotics. The affected area is elevated and rested, and warm and wet dressings are applied locally. Surgical drainage of *purulent* material is indicated.

PROGNOSIS

The prognosis varies depending on the amount of tissue involved as well as the nature of the causative organism. The patient response to antibiotics also plays a role in recovery. Surgical intervention usually contributes to a more positive outcome.

PREVENTION

This condition usually cannot be prevented. Good hand washing always helps prevent any infectious process.

PATIENT TEACHING

Give patients information about care of postoperative incision sites. Emphasize the importance of complying with, and completing, any prescribed antibiotic therapy.

Lymphoma

Lymphomas are malignant neoplasms that arise from uncontrolled proliferation of the cellular components of the lymph system. The dysfunctional cells may be B cells, T cells, or, rarely, both. The neoplastic lymphocytes are migratory and can be found not only in the lymph structures, but also in the bloodstream, bone marrow, and, later in the disease, non-lymph organs (e.g., liver, lung). Lymphomas are divided into two main categories: Hodgkin disease and the other types that are grouped as non-Hodgkin lymphoma.

Treatment selection is determined by the cell type and the stage of the disease. Both kinds of lymphoma are staged using the Ann Arbor-Cotswolds staging system, which considers the neoplastic involvement of lymph structures (lymph nodes, spleen, thymus), extranodal tumor sites, and the presence or absence of the systemic B symptoms of lymphoma (unexplained weight loss of more than 10% of body weight in the past 6 months, persistent or recurrent fevers above 38° C during the previous month, and recurrent, drenching night sweats during the previous month).

> **Stage I:** A single lymph structure or region is involved.
> **Stage II:** Two or more lymph structures are involved, with the involvement being on the same side of the diaphragm.
> **Stage III:** Lymph regions on both sides of the diaphragm are involved.
> **Stage IV:** There is widespread involvement of extranodal tissue above and below the diaphragm.

Each stage designation carries either an "A" or a "B" after the stage number, indicating whether any of the B symptoms are absent (A) or present (B).

Hodgkin Disease

DESCRIPTION

Hodgkin disease (also called Hodgkin lymphoma) is a cancer of the body's lymphatic system, in which the involved cells proliferate and interfere with normal functioning by collecting in masses in various parts of the body. Tumors arise in the tissue of the lymph nodes and spread to other lymph nodes, the spleen, the liver, and the bone marrow.

■ **ICD-9-CM Code 201.90** *(Unspecified)*
Hodgkin disease is coded by type. Refer to the physician's diagnosis and then to the current edition of the ICD-9-CM coding manual to ensure the greatest specificity of pathology and any appropriate modifiers.

SYMPTOMS AND SIGNS

The initial symptoms of Hodgkin disease are painless enlargement of the lymph nodes in the neck or mediastinum, fatigue, alcohol-induced pain, and pruritus (Fig. 10–54). As the disease progresses, the patient may experience the systemic "B" symptoms of fever, night sweats, and weight loss. Hodgkin disease is differentiated from other lymphomas by the presence in the lymphatic tissue of a Reed-Sternberg cell, a large cell with two or more mirror-image nuclei, each with a single nucleolus (Fig. 10–55).

PATIENT SCREENING

Patients reporting a painless enlargement of cervical lymph nodes, fatigue, and pruritus should be scheduled as soon as possible. When the complaints include fever, night sweats, and weight loss, prompt assessment by a physician is required.

ETIOLOGY

Hodgkin disease represents 15% of all lymphomas. There are two peaks of incidence: one in patients in their 20s and the other in those over the age of 50. Risk factors for the development of Hodgkin disease include previous history of malignancy, prior treatment with chemotherapy or radiation therapy, family history of Hodgkin disease or other lymphomas, immunosuppression, and exposure to infectious agents, especially the Epstein-Barr virus.

DIAGNOSIS

A history of painless lymphadenopathy and the typical symptoms of Hodgkin disease lead to an excisional lymph node biopsy for definitive diagnosis. The node biopsy shows the presence of Reed-Sternberg cells. Blood studies indicate a mild normochromic, normocytic anemia; neutrophilic

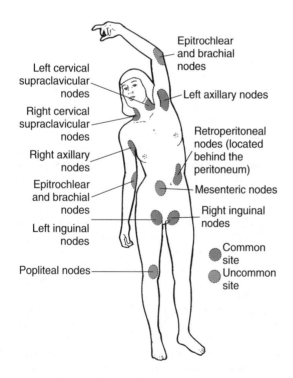

FIGURE 10–54 Lymph node sites for Hodgkin disease. (From Huether SE, McCance KL: *Understanding pathophysiology*, ed 3, St. Louis, 2004, Mosby.)

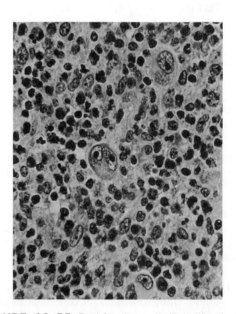

FIGURE 10–55 Reed-Sternberg cell. (From Wiernik et al: *Neoplastic diseases of the blood*, ed 3, New York, 1996, Churchill Livingstone.)

leukocytosis; lymphopenia; and eosinophilia. The ESR is elevated, as is the serum alkaline phosphatase level. Bone marrow biopsy is performed only on select patients and may show abnormal cells. Staging laparotomy is no longer a required procedure, but it may be performed in some cases. CT scans of the chest, abdomen, and pelvis help evaluate the extent of disease. Ultrasonography may detect spleen involvement. Liver and kidney function tests are performed.

TREATMENT

Patients with stage I and II disease and a favorable prognosis may be treated with radiation therapy alone. Combined chemoradiotherapy is preferred for the remainder of patients in stages I and II and some patients in stage III. Patients in stage IIIB and stage IV often are treated with chemotherapy alone. The preferred regimen is ABVD (doxorubicin, bleomycin, vinblastine, dacarbazine) therapy. Relapses usually are treated with additional chemotherapy. Bone marrow transplantation may be used to treat patients with multiple relapses.

PROGNOSIS

Hodgkin disease is one of the most treatable forms of cancer and can be cured. The overall 5-year survival rate is 83%. Death may result from Hodgkin disease itself, or from secondary cancers or cardiovascular disease, side effects of treatment that often are not apparent until years after therapy. Important indicators of poor prognosis include the presence of B symptoms, low serum albumin and hemoglobin levels, male gender, age over 45 years, low lymphocyte count, and a high ESR.

PREVENTION

No ways of preventing Hodgkin disease are known.

PATIENT TEACHING

Give patients information about chemotherapy and radiation therapy. Help them find and contact community support groups.

Non-Hodgkin Lymphoma

DESCRIPTION

Non-Hodgkin lymphoma (NHL) describes a number of heterogeneous neoplasms of the lymphoid cells that exhibit a wide variety of clinical signs and symptoms, ranging from slow, indolent growth to rapidly fatal progression. Some can be cured with appropriate treatment, but for others, treatment does not prolong survival.

 ICD-9-CM Code 202.8

SYMPTOMS AND SIGNS

As with Hodgkin disease, symptoms include painless lymphadenopathy, fatigue, pruritus, bone pain, and GI symptoms. Other lymphatic tissue, such as tonsils and adenoids, may be enlarged, and the patient can experience the "B" symptoms of fever, night sweats, and weight loss.

PATIENT SCREENING

As with Hodgkin disease, patients reporting a painless enlargement of cervical lymph nodes, fatigue, and pruritus should be scheduled as soon as possible. When the complaints include fever, night sweats, and weight loss, prompt assessment by a physician is required.

ETIOLOGY

The incidence of NHL reaches a peak in preadolescents, drops in incidence, and then increases again with increasing age. Risk factors include a personal or family history of prior malignancy; previous treatment with radiation therapy, immunotherapy, or chemotherapy; infection with HIV, human T-cell lymphotropic virus (HTLV), Epstein-Barr virus, or hepatitis C virus; and connective tissue disorders such as lupus and rheumatoid arthritis. GI lymphoma may be seen in patients with Crohn disease, celiac disease, and *H. pylori*-associated chronic gastritis.

NHL is grouped into three main categories based on how aggressively each neoplasm in the group behaves. The indolent lymphomas represent 35% to 40% of NHLs. The most common subtypes are follicular lymphoma (grades I and II behave as indolent; grade III behaves as aggressive), small lymphocytic lymphoma, mantle cell lymphoma, and marginal zone lymphoma. They may arise from any B-cell, T-cell, or NK (natural killer)-cell line. Aggressive lymphomas represent 50% of NHLs. The most common subtypes are diffuse large B-cell lymphoma and peripheral T-cell lymphoma. Highly aggressive lymphomas are more rare, representing 5% of all NHLs. These include Burkitt's lymphoma (thought to be caused in part by the Epstein-Barr virus) and adult T-cell lymphoma (caused by HTLV).

DIAGNOSIS

The patient evaluation must include determination of the histologic subtype, extent of disease, and performance status of the patient, because treatment and prognosis greatly depend on this information. All potentially involved lymphoid sites should be physically examined. Excisional biopsy of an intact, involved lymph node is necessary for accurate histopathologic identification of the disease. Immunologic, cytogenetic, and molecular studies may be performed to further aid in therapeutic decisions and determination of prognosis. Bone marrow aspiration and biopsy are performed to determine the extent of disease. If the marrow is involved, the patient is placed at stage IV. Lab tests after diagnosis generally include CBC, peripheral blood smear, and studies of renal and liver function. Staging laparotomy usually is not needed. Chest radiographs and CT scans of the abdomen and pelvis are performed to determine the extent of disease. GI endoscopy may detect GI involvement (seen in 10% to 60% of patients). An MRI of the CNS may be performed if neurologic signs are present in the patient.

TREATMENT

Stage I and II indolent lymphomas are treated with radiation therapy. The treatment plan for stages III and IV usually involves watchful waiting until the symptoms necessitate starting chemotherapy or local radiation for palliation because the later stage indolent lymphomas are generally not curable with conventional therapies. The more aggressive lymphomas have a rapid progression but may be cured with appropriate treatment. They are treated with CHOP chemotherapy (cyclophosphamide, doxorubicin, vincristine, and prednisone) with or without radiation therapy. The chemotherapy may be administered with rituximab for some patients. Relapses may be treated by high-dose chemotherapy followed by bone marrow transplantation or by chemotherapy alone.

PROGNOSIS

The 5-year overall survival rate is 53%. Histopathology is the most important prognostic indicator, followed by patient age, presence of extranodal disease, presence of "B" symptoms, and stage at the time of diagnosis. The indolent lymphomas generally are associated with a survival measured in years even if left untreated. However, they generally are not curable with treatment. In contrast, the aggressive lymphomas are curable but are rapidly fatal if left untreated or if they are unresponsive to therapy.

PREVENTION

No methods of prevention for NHL are known.

PATIENT TEACHING

Give patients information about chemotherapy and radiation therapy. Help them find and contact community support groups.

Transfusion Incompatibility Reaction

DESCRIPTION

Transfusion incompatibility results when the blood or blood product transfused has antibodies to the recipient's RBCs or the recipient has antibodies to the donor's RBCs.

ICD-9-CM Code **999.6** *(ABO incompatibility)*
999.7 *(Rh incompatibility reaction)*
999.8 *(Other transfusion reaction)*

SYMPTOMS AND SIGNS

This hypersensitivity reaction can range from mild to fatal. Most severe transfusion reactions are incompatibility-related and are characterized by hemolysis or **agglutination.** Other forms include bacterial, allergic, and circulatory-overload transfusion reactions. The severity of the reaction depends on the amount of incompatible blood that is transfused and prior transfusion reactions of the patient.

The patient with incompatibility reaction who is receiving the blood transfusion experiences chills, fever, and tachycardia. The patient with a more severe reaction has severe back pain, vomiting, diarrhea, hives or rash, a substernal tightness, and dyspnea. The patient becomes hypotensive and progresses to a state of circulatory collapse. As the condition worsens, there is bleeding from the puncture site, blood in the urine, and eventually renal failure.

The most frequent transfusion reaction is associated with WBCs or WBC remnants in donor blood. It is febrile and short lived, ceasing when the transfusion is halted, and there is no hemolysis or allergic response.

The patient experiencing an allergic reaction exhibits hives and itching and possibly bronchial spasms and *anaphylaxis.*

PATIENT SCREENING

Patients receiving blood transfusions will be in a clinic or hospital environment. The trained professionals observing the patient will immediately institute intervention and care to reverse or modify the reaction. Those who have survived the reaction as well as family members may request additional information about the reaction. Schedule an appointment as soon as possible for the discussion. Family members may be included in the discussion as long as HIPAA guidelines are followed.

ETIOLOGY

ABO- and Rh-incompatible blood causes an antigen—antibody reaction that produces hemolysis (destruction of RBCs) or agglutination (clumping of RBCs that obstructs the flow of blood through capillaries). Histamine and serotonin are released from mast cells and platelets. Disseminated intravascular coagulation (DIC) usually is triggered (see Disseminated Intravascular Coagulation), with resulting coagulation problems.

DIAGNOSIS

Any sign of chills, fever, hives, back pain, or dyspnea during the transfusion alerts the health-care professional attending the patient to a possible reaction. Blood and urine specimens are examined, along with the used blood, to confirm an incompatibility and the presence of hemolysis or activated coagulation.

TREATMENT

Transfusion protocol mandates that a set of baseline patient vital signs be taken before the start of a transfusion. During the first 15 minutes, the patient is observed closely, and assessment of vital signs is repeated. This monitoring of vital signs and observation of the patient continue at designated intervals until the procedure is completed. At the first indication of any symptoms or signs of reaction, the blood transfusion is stopped immediately. Blood and urine samples are obtained from the patient and sent to the laboratory, along with the remaining untransfused blood. Mild reactions are treated with antihistamines, and anaphylaxis is treated aggressively according to institutional protocol.

PROGNOSIS

The prognosis varies depending on the amount of blood infused, the cause of the reaction, and the speed of the intervention.

PREVENTION

Prevention is the best form of treatment. Careful typing and crossmatching of the blood product is mandatory. Two attendants must compare the patient information with that on the blood bag and orders before starting the transfusion.

PATIENT TEACHING

Instruct the patient to report any untoward symptoms or unusual sensations during the transfusion process immediately, especially early in the transfusion.

Clotting Disorders

Classic Hemophilia

DESCRIPTION

Classic hemophilia is a hereditary bleeding disorder resulting from deficiency of clotting factors.

 ICD-9-CM Code **286.0** *(Congenital factor VIII disorder)*

SYMPTOMS AND SIGNS

The condition can be mild, moderate, or severe. Any unusually prolonged bleeding episode, easy bruising, hematomas, or excessive nosebleeds in a male child suggest hemophilia. The first sign of hemophilia may be **ecchymosis** at birth or bleeding from a circumcision. Joint swelling and pain suggest bleeding in the joints.

PATIENT SCREENING

When parents report that a male infant, toddler, or child has experienced unexplained prolonged bleeding, noticeable hematomas, easy bruising, and/or excessive nose bleeds, the physician should promptly assess the child. The condition often is diagnosed during the neonatal period of hospitalization. These parents may request an appointment to learn about the disorder. Schedule as soon as possible and for the next available appointment.

ETIOLOGY

An X-linked genetic disorder in males, hemophilia is transmitted by the asymptomatic carrier mother to her son. Factor VIII, a clotting factor in the intrinsic clotting cascade, is functionally inactive. Any minor trauma can initiate the bleeding episode.

DIAGNOSIS

The diagnosis is based on the clinical picture and a thorough history. Clotting studies indicate normal platelet count, bleeding time, and prothrombin time (PT); prolonged partial thromboplastin time (PTT); and a factor VIII assay of 0% to 30%.

TREATMENT

Hemophilia cannot be cured, but treatment prevents crippling deformities. Concentrated factor VIII (antihemophilic factor [AHF]) is administered to stop the bleeding. Transfusions of whole blood may be necessary. The patients are encouraged to avoid situations that initiate bleeding episodes. Cases have been documented of human immunodeficiency virus (HIV) infection resulting from transfusion with contaminated or infected blood products.

PROGNOSIS

No cure for hemophilia is known. Transfusions of blood or blood products may be a life-long intervention. Blood-borne infections may complicate the condition and place the patient at higher risk for other disease entities.

PREVENTION

No prevention is known for this condition. Genetic counseling may help in exploring the probability of the disorder being transferred to offspring.

PATIENT TEACHING

Give parents information about X-linked genetic disorders.

Disseminated Intravascular Coagulation

DESCRIPTION

Disseminated intravascular coagulation is a condition of simultaneous hemorrhage and thrombosis. It is a syndrome that occurs secondary to other diseases.

 ICD-9-CM Code 286.6

Refer to the physician's diagnosis and then to the current edition of the ICD-9-CM coding manual to ensure the greatest specificity of pathology and any appropriate modifiers.

SYMPTOMS AND SIGNS

Oozing of blood from needle puncture sites, mucous membranes, or incisions may be noted, as may bleeding in the form of *purpura,* wound hematomas, or **petechiae.** *Hematemesis, hematuria,* and bloody stools may be present. The patient is weak, reports headaches, and experiences air hunger and tachycardia. Disseminated intravascular coagulation follows a major event, such as obstetric complications, septicemia, trauma, burns, hypothermia, and extensive tissue destruction.

PATIENT SCREENING

Most of these individuals will be in an in-patient facility, and immediate response is indicated. If they suffer the condition at home after a major precipitating event, they must be entered into the emergency medical system for prompt assessment. Family members requesting an appointment after the event for information should be scheduled as soon as possible according to HIPAA guidelines.

ETIOLOGY

Thrombin activates the production of fibrin, causing clots to form where they are not needed (i.e., in the microcirculation). The thrombin also causes platelet **aggregation,** forming more clots. In addition, the fibrinolytic system is activated by the presence of thrombin in the plasma; thrombin causes excessive fibrinolysis and additional bleeding. Predisposing factors include hypotension, hypoxemia, acidosis, and stasis of capillary blood. Any of these factors may be the result of the aforementioned major precipitating events (Fig. 10–56).

DIAGNOSIS

The diagnosis is based on the clinical picture; a thorough history, including a probable precipitating event; and laboratory studies. Platelet count and fibrinogen levels are reduced, whereas PT is prolonged.

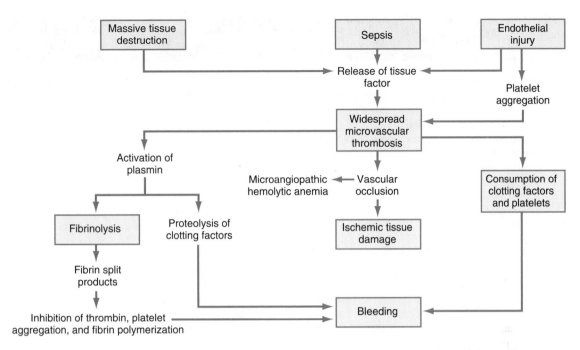

FIGURE 10–56 Pathophysiology of disseminated intravascular coagulation. (From Kumar V, Cotran RS, Robbins SL: *Robbins basic pathology,* ed 7, Philadelphia, 2003, Saunders.)

TREATMENT
Administration of intravenous heparin inhibits the formation of additional microthrombi and prevents the aggregation of platelets. Platelet replacement and plasma-clotting factors are administered when serious hemorrhage is present. The condition is life-threatening and often fatal.

PROGNOSIS
The prognosis is guarded.

PREVENTION
Because this condition is a sequela to a major systemic insult, prevention is unlikely.

PATIENT TEACHING
If the patient survives the event, teaching may include an explanation of the incident. Help family members to find and contact support groups in the community.

REVIEW CHALLENGE

Answer the following questions:

1. What are the common symptoms of cardiovascular disease?
2. How would you describe the pathology in coronary artery disease?
3. How is the patient likely to describe the pain in angina pectoris?
4. How do the symptoms of myocardial infarction differ from those of angina pectoris?
5. Why is angioplasty used for myocardial infarction?
6. What conditions can cause cardiac arrest? What is the time frame in which cardiopulmonary resuscitation (CPR) may be successfully initiated?
7. What are the diagnostic criteria for essential hypertension?

Continued

REVIEW
CHALLENGE—cont'd

8. What happens when the pumping action of the heart is inadequate? How can congestive heart failure be treated?

9. Which conditions may lead to cor pulmonale?

10. How is pulmonary edema treated?

11. To what does cardiomyopathy refer, and how is it treated?

12. How does endocarditis affect the cardiac valves?

13. Why is rheumatic fever described as a systemic disease? What infection often precedes it?

14. What is the relationship between rheumatic fever and valvular heart disease?

15. What are the sources of cardiac arrhythmias? How are they diagnosed?

16. Why is shock considered a life-threatening emergency? What are the signs and symptoms?

17. What is cardiac tamponade?

18. What is the relationship between venous thrombosis and pulmonary emboli?

19. What is the difference between arteriosclerosis and atherosclerosis? Why are both conditions a threat to health?

20. How might an aneurysm be detected? When are they a serious threat?

21. What is the relationship of phlebitis to thrombophlebitis? Why should the clinician avoid massage of the affected area?

22. What medical intervention is available for severe varicose veins?

23. Which conditions may precipitate an episode of Raynaud disease?

24. What are the presenting symptoms of anemia?

25. What are some possible causes of anemia?

26. How are the following anemias differentiated: aplastic, sickle cell, hemolytic, iron-deficiency, hemorrhagic, and pernicious?

27. What are some usual causes of agranulocytosis?

28. What are typical symptoms in all types of leukemia?

29. Which leukemia is considered more a disease of later life?

30. How does lymphedema differ from lymphangitis?

31. Which lymphoma is characterized by the presence of Reed-Sternberg cells in lymphatic tissue?

32. What symptoms does a patient experience with a transfusion incompatibility reaction?

33. How is classic hemophilia treated?

REAL-LIFE
CHALLENGE

Essential Hypertension

A 46-year-old man reports intermittent headaches and lightheadedness for about 3 months. In the past 2 weeks he has had several episodes of epistaxis. Vital signs are temperature, 98.6° F, pulse, 106; respirations, 20; and blood pressure, 168/98. His weight is 265 lbs, and his height is 5 feet, 11 inches.

The history reveals that the patient has a highly stressful job requiring extensive travel with overnight stays. He regards himself as a high achiever. A family history discloses that his father died at 53 years of age of a CVA and that his mother at 69 years of age has CHF and hypertension. His brother has a history of hypertension, and his two sisters are alive and well. The patient smokes one pack of cigarettes a day and has for 30 years.

The patient is advised to stop smoking or at least cut down on the number smoked per day. In addition, he is advised to begin a weight-reduction and exercise program and to reduce sodium intake. If possible, he also should reduce stressful situations. Medications ordered are a beta-blocker, atenolol, and an ACE inhibitor, ramipril. The patient is instructed to return in 1 week for reevaluation. Essential hypertension is a suspected diagnosis.

QUESTIONS

1. What factors contribute to the symptoms and signs of essential hypertension that this patient is experiencing?

2. Why would his onset of symptoms be considered insidious?

3. Why could the diagnosis of essential hypertension not be confirmed on the initial encounter?

4. Why might a diuretic be ordered?

5. What is the significance of the family history?

6. What is the action of calcium channel blockers in the treatment of essential hypertension?

7. If essential hypertension is not controlled, what complications may evolve from the condition?

8. How important in the diagnosis was the symptom of epistaxis?

REAL-LIFE CHALLENGE

Anemia

A 32-year-old woman reports feeling tired all the time, having an excessively fast heartbeat, having difficulty catching her breath, and experiencing some lightheadedness. She appears quite pale. Vital signs are temperature, 98.4° F; pulse, 118; respirations, 26; and blood pressure, 100/69.

The patient is married, has three children ages 7 years, 4 years, and 6 months, and is employed outside the home. She says she can scarcely get out of bed in the morning and can barely make it through the day. She has had four episodes of syncope in the past week. Menstrual periods have been regular but heavy. She denies experiencing any observable blood in the urine or stools. A CBC with differential is ordered. The RBC is below normal and normocytic, hemoglobin is 9, hematocrit is 27, and WBC and platelet counts are normal. The patient is diagnosed with iron-deficiency anemia and encouraged to rest and to increase her dietary intake of red meat, liver, and egg yolks. Supplementary iron is prescribed in the form of ferrous sulfate tablets, and the patient is instructed to return to the office in 1 week for follow up.

QUESTIONS

1. What might have been the cause of the iron-deficiency anemia in this patient?
2. What causes RBCs to be microcytic? Macrocytic?
3. What is the importance of the absence of blood in the stool and urine?
4. What might be the connection with the previous pregnancy?
5. What type of food in addition to the red meat, liver, and egg yolks would help increase the hemoglobin?
6. What might blood tests show if this were sickle cell anemia?
7. Compare hemolytic anemia with iron-deficiency anemia.
8. As the hemoglobin improves, what changes might be expected in the vital signs?

INTERNET ASSIGNMENTS

1. Research suggested treatment interventions for congestive heart failure from the American Heart Association. In particular, research and list drug interventions and patient teaching about administration of these drugs.
2. Research suggested treatment interventions for cardiac arrhythmias from the American Heart Association. Use the arrhythmia chart in the chapter to identify the arrhythmias that are considered potentially lethal arrhythmias. Record findings from the website about treatment interventions.
3. Research the incidence of hypertension at the American Heart Association website. Record the ages and sex of patients and the seriousness of their condition. Verify and record any drug therapy suggested.
4. Research the incidence of hemophilia in the U.S. population in the past 10 years at the National Hemophilia Association website. Also research suggested drug treatments along with side effects.

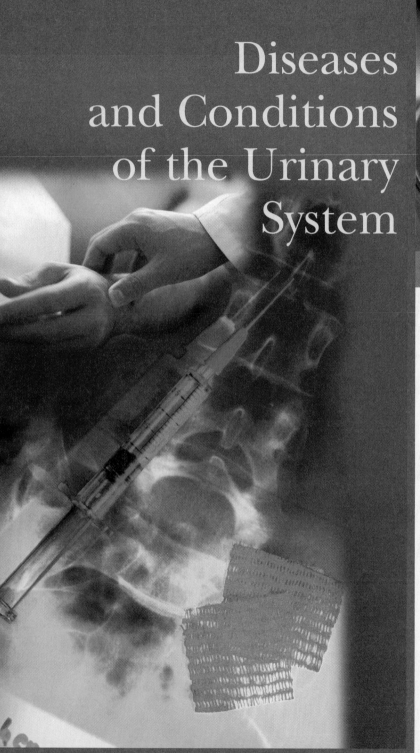
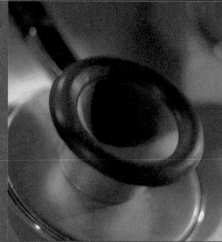

CHAPTER 11

Diseases and Conditions of the Urinary System

Chapter Outline

Learning Objectives

After studying Chapter 11, you should be able to:

1. Explain how pathologic conditions of the urinary system threaten homeostasis and result in illness.
2. Explain the diagnostic value of urinalysis.
3. Relate the symptoms and signs of acute glomerulonephritis.
4. Describe how immune mechanisms are suspected to be a causative factor of acute and chronic glomerulonephritis.
5. Distinguish between hemodialysis and peritoneal dialysis.
6. Identify the hallmark sign of nephrosis.
7. List some nephrotoxic agents.
8. Explain why acute renal failure is considered a clinical emergency.
9. Discuss treatment measures for prolonging life of the patient with chronic renal failure.
10. Identify the etiology and diagnosis of pyelonephritis.
11. Describe hydronephrosis.
12. Describe the common symptoms of renal calculi, and list possible complications.
13. List causes of infectious cystitis and urethritis.
14. Describe diabetic nephropathy.
15. Contrast neurogenic bladder with stress incontinence.
16. Describe the polycystic kidney, and discuss the treatment options.
17. Identify those most at risk for renal cell carcinoma and bladder tumors.
18. List and describe symptoms of renal cell and bladder carcinoma.

Key Terms

azotemia (**ah**–zoh–**TEE**–me–ah)
catheterization (**kath**–eh–ter–eye–**ZAY**–shun)
creatinine (kree–**AT**–in–in)
cystoscopy (sis–**TOSS**–ko–pee)
dialysate (dye–**AHL**–ih–sate)
glomeruli (gloh–**MER**–you–lye)
glomerulonephritis (gloh–**mer**–you–low–neh–**FRY**–tis)
glomerulosclerosis (gloh–**mer**–you–low–sklee–**ROW**–sis)
hemodialysis (**he**–moh–dye–**AHL**–ih–sis)
hydronephrosis (**high**–droh–neff–**ROW**–sis)

immunosuppressive (**im**–you–noh–sue–**PRESS**–ihv)
lithotripsy (**LITH**–oh–**trip**–see)
nephrectomy (neh–**FRECK**–toh–me)
nephropathy (neh–**FROP**–ah–thee)
nephrotoxic (**neff**–row–**TOCKS**–ick)
oliguria (ohl–ih–**GOO**–rhee–ah)
peritoneal dialysis (**per**–ih–toe–**NEE**–al dye–**AHL**–ih–sis)
pyelonephritis (**pye**–eh–low–neh–**FRY**–tis)

ORDERLY FUNCTION OF THE URINARY SYSTEM

THE URINARY SYSTEM is responsible for producing, storing, and excreting urine; these processes prevent the body from becoming **toxic.** This cleansing the blood of the waste products of metabolism and regulating the water, salts, and acids in the body fluids ensure homeostasis. The urinary system includes the kidneys, which manufacture the urine and play a role in the regulation of systemic blood pressure, and the accessory structures, which transport and store urine in the bladder until it is excreted voluntarily through the urethra. The organs of the urinary system consist of two kidneys, two ureters, the urinary bladder, and the urethra (Fig. 11–1).

Each kidney (Fig. 11–2) is composed of about 1 million microstructures called **nephrons** (Fig. 11–3). The nephrons, the units of function in the kidney, are responsible for filtration, reabsorption, and secretion of urine. Figure 11–4 depicts the formation of urine. The urine is transported from the nephron to the renal pelvis and then to the ureters. The kidney has many other

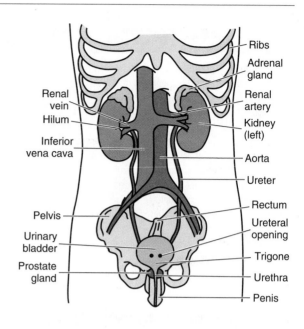

FIGURE 11–1 Gross anatomy of the urinary system (male). (From Gould B: *Pathophysiology for the health professions,* ed 2, Philadelphia, 2002, Saunders.)

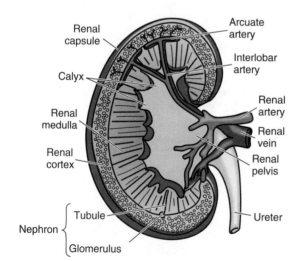

FIGURE 11–2 Anatomy of the kidney. (From Gould B: *Pathophysiology for the health professions,* ed 2, Philadelphia, 2002, Saunders.)

functions, including the secretion of *renin,* a hormone that raises blood pressure, and *erythropoietin,* which acts as a stimulus for red blood cell (RBC) production. It also has a role in the activation of vitamin D.

Infection, scarring, toxic *necrosis,* or trauma of the urinary tract can result in disturbances of renal function that allow urea (the nitrogenous waste of metabolism in urine) or extracellular fluid and electrolytes to accumulate in the blood. Con-

genital or acquired structural defects and tumors cause obstructive diseases of the urinary system. Other important diseases of the urinary tract are immunologic disorders, circulatory disturbances, cystic disease, and metabolic disorders (e.g., diabetes mellitus).

The function of the urinary system often is evaluated by urinalysis (Table 11–1) and blood tests (Table 11–2). Normal results demonstrate proper filtration, absorption, and elimination of metabolic

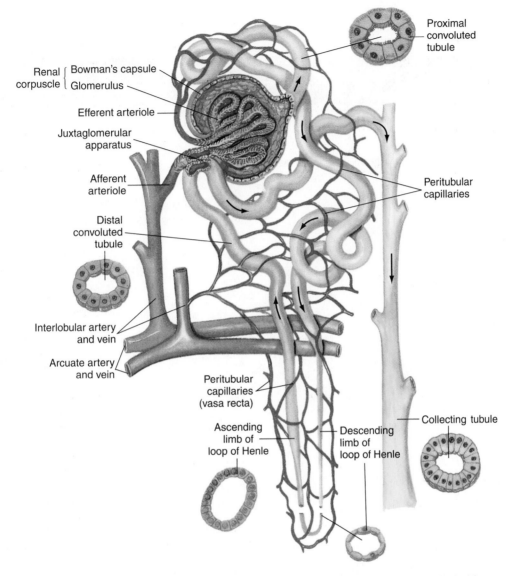

FIGURE 11–3 The nephron. (From Patton KT, Thibodeau GA: *Mosby's handbook of anatomy & physiology,* St. Louis, Mosby, 2000.)

waste and precise fluid and electrolyte balance. Other tests for urinary tract disorders include culture and sensitivity tests to determine appropriate antibiotic therapy, radiologic tests that visualize structural abnormalities, **cystoscopy** (see Fig. 11–4), and biopsy of lesions.

Usually symptoms of urinary diseases reflect an accumulation of waste products in the blood and cause electrolyte imbalances in the body. Common symptoms include the following:

Nausea
Loss of appetite
Fever
Headache and body aches
Flank or low back pain
Bloody urine
Edema
Decreased urinary output
Hypertension
Pruritus

TABLE 11–1
Routine Urinalysis*

	NORMAL	ABNORMAL	PATHOLOGY
CHARACTERISTICS			
Color and clarity	Pale to darker yellow, and clear	Very pale	Excessive water
		Cloudy, milky, white blood cells	Pus, urinary tract infection
		Hematuria, red blood cells, reddish to reddish brown	Bleeding in infection, calculi, or cancer
Odor	Aromatic	Fishy	Cystitis
		Fruity	Diabetes mellitus
		Foul	Urinary tract infection
Chemical nature	pH is generally slightly acidic, 6.5	Alkaline	Infections cause ammonia to form
Specific gravity	1.003-1.030—reflects amount of waste, minerals, and solids in urine	Higher—causes precipitation of solutes	Kidney stones, diabetes mellitus
		Lower—polyuria	Diabetes insipidus
CONSTITUENT COMPOUNDS			
Protein	None, or small amount	Albuminuria	Nephritis, renal failure, infection
Glucose	None	Glycosuria	Faulty carbohydrate metabolism, as in diabetes mellitus
Ketone bodies	None	Ketonuria	Diabetic acidosis
Bile and bilirubin	None	Bilirubinuria	Hepatic or gallbladder disease
Casts	None—or small number of hyaline casts	Urinary casts composed of red or white blood cells, fat, or pus	Nephritis, renal diseases, inflammation, metal poisoning
Nitrogenous wastes	Ammonia, creatinine, urea, and uric acid	Azoturia, creatinine, and urea clearance tests disproportionate to normal BUN/creatinine ratio	Hepatic disease, renal disease
Crystals	None to trace	Acidic urine, alkaline urine, hypercalcemia, metabolism error	Not significant unless the crystals are large (stones); certain types interpreted by physician
Fat droplets	None	Lipoiduria	Nephrosis

BUN, Blood urea nitrogen.
*Routine urinalysis is a physical, chemical, and microscopic examination of urine for abnormal elements that may help to estimate renal function and provide clues of systemic disease. This table includes some important characteristics and elements screened for in basic urinalysis. Other normal constituents of urine that are studied routinely for diagnosis include calcium, potassium, sodium, phosphorus, creatinine, and volume in a 24-hour period.

TABLE 11-2
Some Renal Diagnostic Tests

TEST	DESIGNED TO EVALUATE
Clearance test	Rate of glomerular filtration
Concentration and dilution tests	Functional capacity of renal tubular cells to adaptively retain and/or eliminate water
Serum creatinine and BUN	Capacity to eliminate end products of protein metabolism
Protein in urine	Permeability of glomerular membrane

BUN, Blood urea nitrogen.
From Miller M: *Pathophysiology: principles of disease,* Philadelphia, 1983, Saunders.

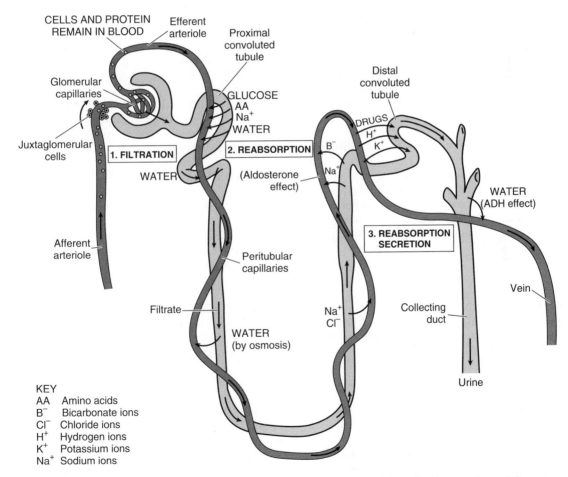

FIGURE 11-4 Formation of urine. (From Gould B: *Pathophysiology for the health professions,* ed 2, Philadelphia, 2002, Saunders.)

Acute Glomerulonephritis

DESCRIPTION

Acute **glomerulonephritis** is an inflammation and swelling of the **glomeruli** (see Fig. 11–3) of the kidneys. It can be a primary disease of the kidney or may develop secondary to a systemic disease. This condition usually follows a streptococcal bacterial infection of the throat or skin.

ICD-9-CM Code 580

Acute glomerulonephritis is coded according to sites and types of lesions. Refer to the physician's diagnosis for site and type of lesion and to the current edition of the ICD-9-CM coding manual for specific code modifiers.

SYMPTOMS AND SIGNS

Acute glomerulonephritis is marked by proteinuria (protein in the urine), edema, and decreased urine volume. *Hematuria* can range from insignificant to a sudden onset of urine that is grossly bloody (gross hematuria). The urine may appear dark or may be described as coffee colored. Occurring most often in children and adolescents, this disease process usually follows a streptococcal infection by 1 to 2 weeks (poststreptococcal glomerulonephritis). Hypertension related to altered renal function and fluid retention is possible, accompanied by headaches, and visual disturbances, *malaise, anorexia,* and a low-grade fever. Flank or back pain develops as a result of swelling of the kidney tissue.

PATIENT SCREENING

Patients complaining of bloody urine accompanied by edema, headache, and flank or pelvic pain require prompt medical attention.

ETIOLOGY

This condition usually follows an infection caused by group A beta-hemolytic streptococcus. It also can be *idiopathic* or may result from an immune reaction that causes circulating antigen–antibody complexes to become trapped within the network of capillaries of a glomerulus. In some cases, the antigen is endogenous (arising from within) as an accompaniment of tumors. The injury to the glomeruli results in a decrease in the rate of filtration of the blood, and consequently retention of water and salts in the body.

DIAGNOSIS

The diagnosis is made by the clinical findings, clinical history, and urinalysis. The urine shows gross blood and the presence of RBCs, *white blood cells* (WBCs), renal tubular cells, and **casts.** Proteinuria may be present because of increased permeability of the glomerular membrane. Blood tests show elevated *blood urea nitrogen (BUN), hypoalbuminemia,* and an elevated *erythrocyte sedimentation rate (ESR).* Kidney-ureter-bladder (KUB) radiographic films and ultrasonography may reveal bilateral enlargement of the kidneys. Renal *biopsy* may confirm the diagnosis (Fig. 11–5).

TREATMENT

No specialized therapy is available for the poststreptococcal type of glomerulonephritis other than antibiotic therapy, if infection is still present, and rest. *Diuretics* help control edema and hypertension. Sodium intake is restricted to prevent circulatory overload and convulsions. Occasionally, corticosteroids are used if an immune reaction is the suspected cause.

PROGNOSIS

Most cases resolve within 2 weeks, and the patient experiences a spontaneous recovery.

PREVENTION

Prevention depends on the cause of the condition. Streptococcus type infections require medical intervention with antibiotics.

PATIENT TEACHING

Explain the underlying cause to patients and their families. Patients are instructed to take medications as prescribed, especially antibiotics, until all are gone. During the acute stage, bed rest should be instituted along with sodium intake restriction. It is helpful to review the symptoms to be reported to the physician. These symptoms include weight gain, decreased urinary output, changes in urine color, and an increase in blood pressure. Pregnant women with a history of acute glomerulonephritis require frequent medical evaluation.

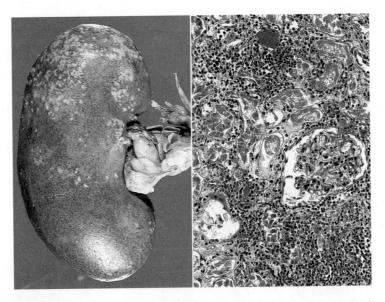

FIGURE 11–5 Acute pyelonephritis. (From Stevens A, Lowe J: *Pathology: illustrated review in color,* ed 2, London, 2000, Mosby.)

Chronic Glomerulonephritis

DESCRIPTION

Chronic glomerulonephritis (CGN) is a slowly progressive, noninfectious disease that can lead to irreversible renal damage and renal failure. As an advanced stage of many kidney disorders, CGN results in inflammation followed by progressive destruction of the glomeruli. This progressive destruction causes a reduction in glomerular filtration with resulting retention of uremic poisons.

ICD-9-CM Code 582

Chronic glomerulonephritis is coded according to sites and types of lesions. Refer to the physician's diagnosis for site and type of lesion and to the current edition of the ICD-9-CM coding manual for specific code modifiers.

SYMPTOMS AND SIGNS

At first, chronic glomerulonephritis is *asymptomatic;* then subclinical progression of the disease leads to hypertension, hematuria, proteinuria, **oliguria,** and edema. In the later stages with increasing renal failure, the hypertension becomes severe and **azotemia** develops. When the kidneys fail to remove urea from the blood (the condition of azotemia), the body compensates by attempting to excrete urea through the sweat glands. Tiny crystals of urea appear on the skin; this condition is termed *uremic frost.* The patient experiences fatigue, malaise, nausea, vomiting, *pruritus,* and *dyspnea.*

PATIENT SCREENING

Patients with CGN probably will already have been diagnosed and scheduled for routine follow-up visits. New patients may be referrals and will require scheduling as soon as possible. Any patient complaining of hematuria should be scheduled for an appointment as soon as possible. Often, hypertension symptoms along with malaise and edema are

Chronic Glomerulonephritis

the reported symptoms and that indicates the need for prompt attention.

ETIOLOGY

Immune mechanisms are suspected to be a major cause of chronic glomerulonephritis; antigen–antibody complexes lodge in the glomerular capsular membrane, triggering an inflammatory response and glomerular injury. Primary renal disorders and multisystem diseases such as systemic lupus erythematosus are other possible causes.

DIAGNOSIS

The diagnostic studies used to detect CGN are the same as those used for acute glomerulonephritis:

urinalysis, blood tests, radiographic studies, ultrasonography, and renal biopsy. The findings include signs of advanced renal insufficiency, rising BUN and serum **creatinine** levels, and grossly abnormal findings on urinalysis. Renal biopsy and the use of sophisticated tools such as electron microscopy and immunofluorescence are valuable in determining the optimal treatment and the prognosis.

TREATMENT

The goals of treatment are to control edema, treat the hypertension, and prevent congestive heart failure and *uremia*. The patient is given supportive measures for comfort. Medical treatment includes the administration of antihypertensives, diuretics,

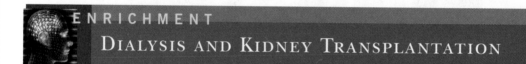

ENRICHMENT

DIALYSIS AND KIDNEY TRANSPLANTATION

IN THE UNITED STATES, end-stage renal disease (ESRD) develops in an average of 1.3 in 10,000 people each year. In renal failure, the kidneys no longer can process blood and form urine. Therapy should begin before the development of ultimately fatal uremic symptoms. Dialysis or kidney transplantation, if successful, offers rehabilitation and extended life to patients with ESRD.

DIALYSIS

Dialysis filters out unwanted elements from the blood by diffusion across a semipermeable membrane; the healthy kidneys usually remove these wastes. Thus the proper fluid, electrolyte, and acid–base balances are maintained in the body. Two methods used to dialyze the blood are hemodialysis and peritoneal dialysis (Fig. 11–6). Even though these procedures do not cure renal failure, many patients are stabilized after 10 to 15 years of treatment.

Hemodialysis. Hemodialysis can take place in the home or at a hospital. It removes impurities or wastes from the patient's blood by using an artificial kidney (hemodialyzer). Access to the blood stream is created surgically in the arm or leg with an internal fistula, which allows the blood to pass from the patient's body to the semipermeable membrane in the machine. The cleaned blood then returns to the patient in a procedure that takes 8 to 12 hours, divided into several sessions a week.

Peritoneal Dialysis. Peritoneal dialysis is carried out in the patient's own body by using a **dialysate** solution and the peritoneal membrane to filter out the harmful toxins and excessive

fluid. The clean dialyzing fluid passes into the peritoneal cavity through a permanent indwelling peritoneal catheter, and wastes diffuse across the peritoneal membrane into the fluid. The contaminated fluid then is drained and replaced with fresh fluid.

- Continuous ambulatory peritoneal dialysis (CAPD) takes place without a machine by allowing the solution to drain by gravity into a dialysis bag worn around the waist. This procedure takes about 15 minutes and is repeated 3 to 4 times a day and once at night.
- Continuous cycling peritoneal dialysis (CCPD) takes place while the patient sleeps, using a cycling machine.
- Intermittent peritoneal dialysis (IPD) takes several hours, 3 to 5 times a week, and usually is done in a clinic.

KIDNEY TRANSPLANTATION

Kidney transplantation is a surgical placement of a donor kidney into a patient with irreversible renal failure. Used synergistically with clinical dialysis, kidney transplantation is one of medicine's success stories. Kidney transplantation leads the field of organ replacement, with many patients being on waiting lists. **Immunosuppressive** agents are used to prevent or treat rejection syndrome. Sophisticated evaluation of the donor and the recipient to find a good human leukocyte antigen (HLA) match offers the best chance for a good prognosis.

Of the 10,000 kidney transplants done annually in the United States, 75% are performed on patients with diabetes adrenal failure, hypertensive renal disease, and glomerulonephritis.

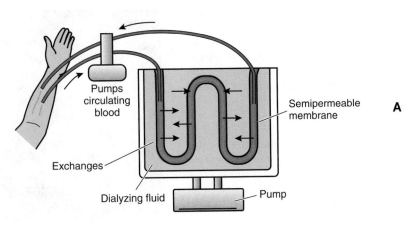

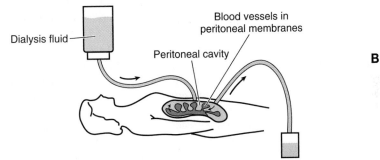

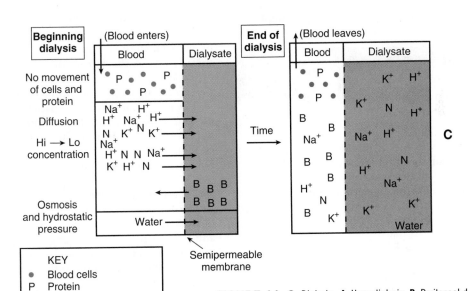

FIGURE 11–6 Dialysis. **A,** Hemodialysis. **B,** Peritoneal dialysis. **C,** Principles of dialysis. (From Gould B: *Pathophysiology for the health professions,* ed 2, Philadelphia, 2002, Saunders.)

and antibiotics if urinary tract infection (UTI) develops. Protein, salt (Na$^+$ and phosphate), and fluid intake may be limited in the diet. Ace inhibitors are often used in the reduction of excess protein in the urine. The patient may require *dialysis* (see Fig. 11–6) or may be a candidate for kidney transplantation.

PROGNOSIS

Prognosis is variable according to the extent of the destruction and the patient response to therapy. Eventually chronic glomerulonephritis will lead to end-stage renal disease (Fig. 11–7). Dialysis may help the patient until a kidney transplant can be performed.

PREVENTION

Prompt treatment of acute glomerulonephritis can help in the prevention of CGN.

PATIENT TEACHING

Compliance with treatment regimens to reduce hypertension should be stressed to the patient. Prompt attention to infections is an important factor also to be stressed. When dialysis is necessary, encourage the patient and family to seek out support groups as well as available community resources. Advise patients to take diuretics in the morning to avoid disruption of sleep at night.

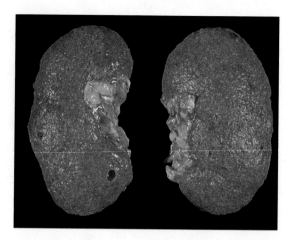

FIGURE 11–7 Chronic glomerulonephritis. (From Damjanov I, Linder J: *Pathology: a color atlas,* St. Louis, 1999, Mosby.)

Nephrotic Syndrome (Nephrosis)

DESCRIPTION

Nephrotic syndrome, a disease of the basement membrane of the glomerulus, is secondary to a number of renal diseases and a variety of systemic disorders. Nephrotic syndrome encompasses a group of symptoms sometimes referred to as the protein-losing kidney.

ICD-9-CM Code 581
Nephrotic syndrome is coded according to sites and types of lesions. Refer to the physician's diagnosis for site and type of lesion and to the current edition of the ICD-9-CM coding manual for specific code modifiers.

SYMPTOMS AND SIGNS

The patient with nephrotic syndrome loses excessive amounts of protein, mainly albumin, in the urine (proteinuria). The excessive loss of protein in the urine results in depressed plasma protein levels (hypoalbuminemia). Glomerular filtration becomes diminished and water and sodium are retained, resulting in edema and hypertension. The syndrome includes microscopic or gross hematuria. Plasma lipid levels are elevated, but the reason for this is not understood. Sloughed-off fat bodies can be found in the urine. The patients are especially susceptible to infections.

The syndrome causes the patient to feel lethargic and depressed, with loss of appetite. He or she appears pale and puffy around the eyes, has swollen ankles (pitting edema), and gains weight. Skin irritation related to edema may be present.

PATIENT SCREENING

As previously mentioned, patients complaining of bloody urine accompanied by edema, headache, and flank or pelvic pain require prompt medical attention. The additional complaints of lethargy and sudden weight gain indicate the need for prompt attention as well.

ETIOLOGY

Nephrotic syndrome is caused by increased permeability of the glomerulus, indicating renal damage.

This condition may follow an attack of glomerulonephritis or it may be the result of exposure to certain toxins or drugs (Box 11–1), pregnancy, or kidney transplants. Metabolic diseases such as diabetes mellitus, certain infections, and allergic reactions are conditions that may lead to nephrotic syndrome.

DIAGNOSIS

The diagnosis is based on the clinical findings and the presence of gross proteinuria and lipiduria (the presence of fatty casts) in a 24-hour urine specimen. Abnormal blood study serum values, including hypoalbuminemia and *hyperlipidemia,* support the diagnosis. If renal tumor is suspected, a renal biopsy with histologic study is indicated.

TREATMENT

Effective treatment begins by addressing the underlying cause. Dietary intake of protein is adjusted to the glomerular filtration rate (GFR), and sodium intake is lowered to control edema as well as the use of diuretics. A course of corticosteroids, such as prednisone, may have the positive effect of controlling the proteinuria for some patients. Urine output must be monitored. If the condition does not improve with treatment, the syndrome can progress to end-stage renal disease.

PROGNOSIS

Prognosis is variable according to the extent of the destruction and patient response to therapy. Eventually nephrotic syndrome that is non-responsive to treatment leads to end stage renal disease.

PREVENTION

Prompt treatment of glomerulonephritis is important in prevention of this condition. Avoiding exposure to certain toxins or drugs (see Box 11–1) helps prevent the syndrome as does prompt treatment after exposure to these toxins. Monitoring the kidney function of women during pregnancy and of any patients with metabolic diseases such as diabetes mellitus, certain infections, and allergic reactions may assist the physician in detecting malfunction early on, and therefore treatment can be instituted early on.

PATIENT TEACHING

Advise patients and families to contact the physician immediately if any exacerbation of symptoms is noted. Encourage patients to remain active, to

---

BOX 11–1
Nephrotoxic Agents

SOLVENTS
Carbon tetrachloride
Methanol
Ethylene glycol

HEAVY METALS
Lead
Arsenic
Mercury

PESTICIDES

ANTIBIOTICS
Kanamycin
Gentamicin
Polymyxin B
Amphotericin B
Colistin
Neomycin
Phenazopyridine

NONSTEROIDAL ANTI-INFLAMMATORY DRUGS

IODINATED RADIOGRAPHIC CONTRAST MEDIA

ANTINEOPLASTIC AGENTS

MISCELLANEOUS COMPOUNDS
Acetaminophen
Amphetamines
Heroin
Silicon
Cyclosporine

POISONOUS MUSHROOMS

Modified from Phipps WJ et al, eds: *Medical–surgical nursing, health and illness perspectives,* ed 7, St. Louis, 2003, Mosby.

---

exercise, and to practice good skin care. Additionally, encourage them to seek out support groups and resource agencies in the community. Refer patients to a dietician for instruction on planning a high-protein, low-sodium diet as prescribed.

Nephrotic Syndrome (Nephrosis)

Acute Renal Failure

DESCRIPTION

Acute renal failure (ARF), a sudden and severe reduction in renal function, is a common clinical emergency because nitrogenous waste products begin to accumulate in the blood quickly, thereby causing an acute uremic episode.

ICD-9-CM Code 584

Acute renal failure is coded according to sites and types of lesions. Refer to the physician's diagnosis for site and type of lesion and to the current edition of the ICD-9-CM coding manual for specific code modifiers.

SYMPTOMS AND SIGNS

Initially, symptoms of acute renal failure include oliguria, gastrointestinal disturbances, headache, drowsiness, and other alterations in the level of consciousness. A host of other symptoms can occur, depending on the underlying cause, the degree of impairment, and the BUN.

PATIENT SCREENING

Many times patients that develop acute renal failure are already under a physician's care or may even be receiving treatment as inpatients when initial symptoms occur. If not, anyone reporting sudden onset of these symptoms requires prompt attention. Follow office protocol as to scheduling an immediate appointment in the office or referring the individual to an emergency facility for observation and treatment intervention.

ETIOLOGY

The causes of acute renal failure are classified as those that result in diminished blood flow to the kidney (e.g., circulatory shock or heart failure), those that involve intrarenal damage or disease (e.g., glomerulonephritis), and those that result from mechanical obstruction of urine flow. Of special concern is intrarenal damage, which can be prevented by control of exposure to substances known to be **nephrotoxic,** including drugs, insecticides, organic solvents, and cleaning agents (see Box 11–1). Whatever the cause, sudden renal dysfunction disrupts other body systems and, if left untreated, can lead to death. Certain antibiotics (i.e., gentamycin, streptomycin) can cause ARF in patients who have predisposing factors (i.e., existing kidney problems, elderly) (Fig. 11–8).

DIAGNOSIS

Blood tests and urinalysis will reveal many abnormal findings associated with oliguria and the retention of nitrogenous wastes. The BUN, serum creatinine, and potassium levels are elevated in the blood. Other diagnostic studies include kidney scans, ultrasonograms, radiographic films, and *intravenous pyelograms.* Monitoring the equality of fluid intake and output also is important in determining kidney function.

TREATMENT

Determining the cause of acute renal failure, if possible, is crucial in the course of medical management to reduce the risk of permanent kidney damage. However, the ultimate goal is to reverse the decreased renal perfusion. All body systems are monitored and supported as needed through the uremic crisis. The patient may be evaluated for dialysis. Fluid intake and output are balanced to avoid overload. It is important to carefully manage nutritional support to ensure that protein is being replaced in the right proportions to avoid *metabolic acidosis.* Initiating a high carbohydrate/low protein diet will accomplish this. Sodium and potassium intake is controlled as well. Drug therapy may include antihypertensives, diuretics, and antiinfective agents because infection is a common complication in acute renal failure.

PROGNOSIS

In many cases, with prompt treatment ARF is reversible and recovery is rapid and complete. Prognosis is variable as related to cause and response to treatment. Regardless of the cause, sudden renal dysfunction disrupts other body systems and, if left untreated, can lead to death.

PREVENTION

Prevention is variable depending on the causative factors. Promptly treating circulatory shock or heart failure, identifying conditions involving intrarenal damage or disease and those that result from mechanical obstruction of urine flow, and controlling exposure to substances known to be

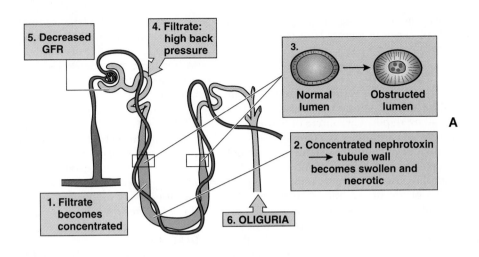

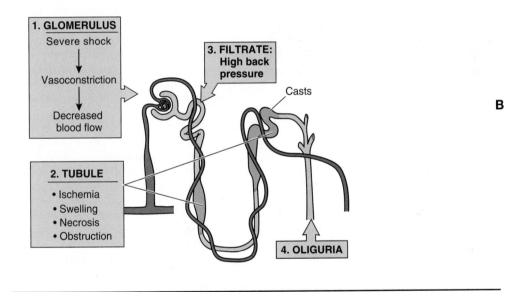

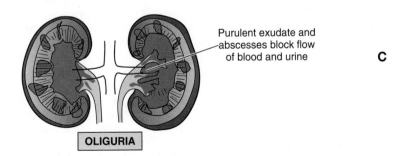

FIGURE 11–8 Causes of acute renal failure. **A,** Nephrotoxins. **B,** Ischemia. **C,** Pyelonephritis. (From Gould B: *Pathophysiology for the health professions,* ed 2, Philadelphia, 2002, Saunders.)

nephrotoxic, including drugs, insecticides, organic solvents, and cleaning agents help prevent acute renal failure.

PATIENT TEACHING

Encourage patients who have recovered from acute renal failure to be cognizant of causative factors and to be aware of possible sources of toxins. Warn them of signs and symptoms of complications such as decreased urine output, weight gain, muscle weakness, palpitations, shortness of breath, and excessive bruising. Instruct them to report such symptoms to the physician. Additional instructions on the topics of eating a modified diet as tolerated, good skin care and oral hygiene, and a review of the prescribed diet should be given. Assist those who have residual effects to seek out community resource agencies and support groups.

Chronic Renal Failure

DESCRIPTION

Chronic renal failure (CRF) results from the gradual and progressive loss of nephrons (see Fig. 11–3), with irreversible loss of renal function and gradual onset of uremia. The systemic effects eventually can be manifested in any and all body systems.

ICD-9-CM Code 585
Referral to the current edition of the ICD-9-CM coding manual is recommended for modifiers to identify the manifestations of this disorder.

SYMPTOMS AND SIGNS

The patient with chronic renal failure feels weak, tired, and lethargic. Hypertension and edema result from the retention of fluids in the body as the condition progresses. As the uremic syndrome worsens, many other symptoms and signs are generated: *arrhythmias,* muscle weakness, dyspnea, metabolic acidosis, *ulceration* of the gastrointestinal mucosa, and hair and skin changes.

PATIENT SCREENING

Patients with chronic renal failure probably have already been diagnosed and are scheduled for routine follow-up visits. New patients may be referrals

and require scheduling as soon as possible. Any patient complaining of hematuria requires prompt attention. Often, hypertension symptoms along with malaise and edema are the relayed symptoms and these symptoms indicate the need for prompt attention.

ETIOLOGY

There are numerous causes of CRF, including primary diseases or infections of the kidney such as glomerulonephritis, **pyelonephritis,** and polycsytic kidneys. Often CRF is the end stage of chronic renal diseases or of chronic obstruction of the outflow of urine.

DIAGNOSIS

Blood studies show elevated BUN, serum creatinine, and potassium levels, along with decreased hemoglobin level and *hematocrit.* Urinalysis is grossly abnormal, with excessive protein, glucose, leukocytes, and casts; the 24-hour urine volume is greatly decreased. Diagnostic studies include radiographic KUB films, renal ultrasonograms, kidney scans, intravenous pyelograms, and renal arteriograms.

TREATMENT

The underlying cause, if known, must be treated. The patient is evaluated for dialysis or kidney transplantation to prolong life. Diet and nutritional modifications control protein and sodium intake to reduce the work of the diseased kidney. Fluid intake and output are monitored and regulated. Drug therapy includes the administration of diuretics, antihypertensives, antiinfective agents, and *antiemetics.* The symptoms of nausea, vomiting, and loss of appetite may be reduced by a change in diet that includes more carbohydrate and fat calories and fewer protein calories. Severe anemia can occur with CRF and often the administration of erythropoietin, a protein, can help form new red blood cells. Bone degeneration also can result from CRF and Calcitriol, a form of Vitamin D, can be given to help prevent the bones from weakening. The patient is given supportive care and kept as comfortable as possible. Many different complications are possible, so the prognosis is uncertain.

PROGNOSIS

Prognosis is variable for chronic renal failure depending on the etiology. No total cure for this condition is known. Preventing complications and providing supportive care are important.

PREVENTION

Prevention is variable depending on the causative factors. Promptly treating acute renal failure and recognizing and treating the cause of the intrarenal damage or those diseases that result from mechanical obstruction of urine flow will help prevent further damage. Additionally controlling exposure to substances known to be nephrotoxic, including drugs, insecticides, organic solvents, and cleaning agents, can help prevent acute renal failure and subsequent chronic failure.

PATIENT TEACHING

Provide a list of support groups and encourage patients and their families to seek out support groups and resource agencies in the community. Help them become aware of sources of possible toxic exposures that contribute to renal disease.

Pyelonephritis

DESCRIPTION

Pyelonephritis, the most common type of renal disease, is an inflammation of the renal pelvis and connective tissues of one or both kidneys.

■ **ICD-9-CM Code 590.80** *(Unspecified)*
Pyelonephritis is coded according to site and type of lesion. Refer to the physician's diagnosis for site and type of lesion and to the current edition of the ICD-9-CM coding manual for specific code modifiers.

SYMPTOMS AND SIGNS

Pyelonephritis usually is caused by infection, pregnancy, or renal *calculi*. Pus collects in the renal pelvis, with the formation of *abscesses*. The patient experiences rapid onset of fever, chills, nausea and vomiting, and flank (lumbar) pain. This usually is preceded by a UTI with urinary frequency and urgency. The patient may report a foul odor to the urine with hematuria and *pyuria*. Tenderness is noted in the suprapubic region, the abdomen be-

comes rigid, and a tender enlarged kidney may be palpated. Urinalysis results show abnormal constituents, including urinary casts.

PATIENT SCREENING

Patients complaining of bloody or foul smelling urine accompanied by fever, chills, nausea, vomiting, and pelvic and flank pain require prompt medical attention.

ETIOLOGY

Bacteria that ascend from the lower urinary tract to the kidneys usually cause pyelonephritis; it is less commonly caused by hematogenous or lymphatic spread of bacteria. Obstruction and stasis of urine by *renal calculi* (kidney stones), tumors, and benign prostatic *hypertrophy* predispose the kidneys to infection. Stasis of urine allows invading bacteria, usually *Escherichia coli*, to cause the infectious process. Women are more at risk because sexual activity or poor perineal hygiene can introduce bacterial contamination into the urinary tract. **Catheterization** or diagnostic procedures such as endoscopic (cystoscopic) examination can directly introduce organisms into the urinary bladder. The infection then moves upward in the urinary tract (ascending infection) to one or both kidneys (Fig. 11–9).

DIAGNOSIS

The diagnosis is made by assessing the clinical findings and by a urinalysis of a *clean-catch urine specimen* that shows increased WBCs and RBCs with the presence of bacteria, pus, protein, and casts. Blood cultures and urine cultures can identify the causative organism. Radiographic studies reveal kidneys that appear swollen or enlarged.

TREATMENT

The treatment of choice consists of intravenous or oral antibiotics, usually penicillin or cephalosporin, given for a full 7 to 10 days. At the present time, common antibiotic treatment is a 10- to 14-day regimen of fluoroquinolones (Cipro, Levaquin) or second or third generation cephalosporins also given for 7 to 10 days. Increased fluid intake to dilute the urine and bed rest are urged. Unless patients are at high risk for UTI, they respond well to treatment without recurrences. When pyelonephritis reoccurs, then certain tests such as an IVP (intravenous pyelography) and a renal ultrasound need to be performed to determine whether a renal abnormality such as

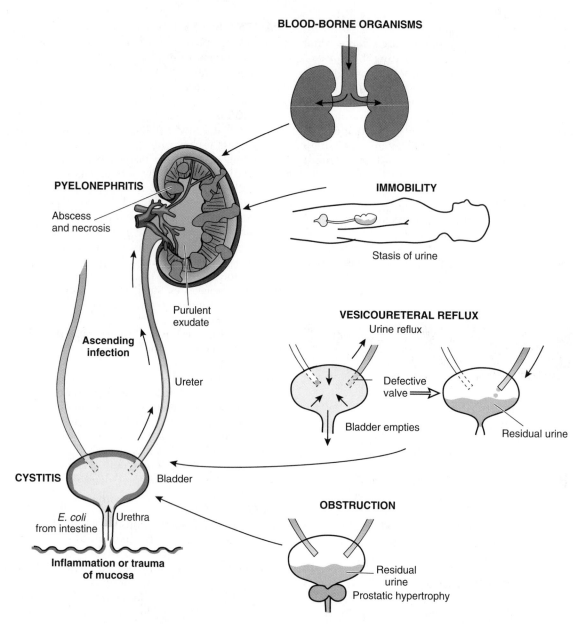

FIGURE 11–9 Causes of infection in the urinary tract. (From Gould B: *Pathophysiology for the health professions,* ed 2, Philadelphia, 2002, Saunders.)

vesicoureteral reflux is present. In more complicated cases, surgery may be indicated to relieve obstruction or to correct an anomaly.

PROGNOSIS

Early detection and prompt treatment usually result in a good prognosis. However, untreated and recurrent pyelonephritis may be the cause of hypertension, bacteremia, and chronic pyelonephritis leading to permanent kidney damage.

PREVENTION

Prevention includes drinking eight glasses of water a day. Those who have a history of pyelonephritis are advised to void frequently. Proper use of toilet tissue when wiping is important in the prevention of infection.

PATIENT TEACHING

Advise females to void after engaging in sexual intercourse. Also, patients who begin to experience symptoms should increase fluid intake, especially water. Females should be encouraged to wipe the perineum from the front to the back to avoid spreading fecal matter from the rectum to the urinary meatus.

Hydronephrosis

DESCRIPTION

Hydronephrosis is an abnormal dilation of the renal pelvis caused by pressure from urine that cannot flow past an obstruction in the urinary tract (Figs. 11–10 and 11–11).

■ **ICD-9-CM Code 591**

SYMPTOMS AND SIGNS

When the obstruction is severe and prolonged, *fibrotic* changes and loss of function of the involved nephrons occurs. Hydronephrosis is usually a chronic condition, with destruction of the kidneys that transpires without pain or symptoms. Its detection often is accidental, occurring during

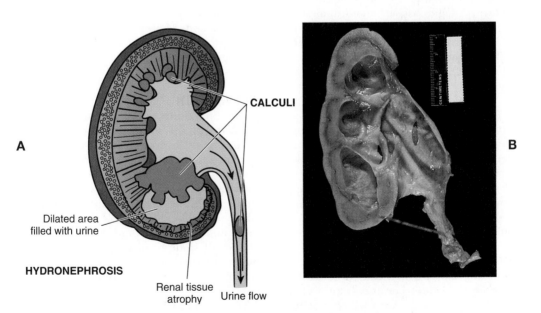

FIGURE 11–10 A, Renal calculi and hydronephrosis. **B,** Hydronephrosis with dilation of the renal pelvis and calyces and atrophy of renal tissue. (**A** from Gould B: *Pathophysiology for the health professions,* ed 2, Philadelphia, 2002, Saunders; **B** from Cotran RS, Kumar V, Collins T: *Robbins pathologic basis of disease,* ed 6, Philadelphia, 1999, Saunders.)

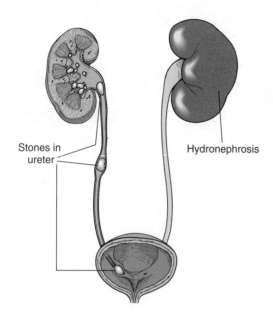

Stones in ureter

Hydronephrosis

FIGURE 11–11 Renal calculi.

radiographic examination or ultrasonography of the abdomen. A vague backache and diminished urine output might be the only symptoms that the patient can identify. If an infection accompanies the condition, the patient may experience fever, chills, hematuria, and pyuria, and the kidney may be palpable.

PATIENT SCREENING

Many patients with hydronephrosis will be asymptomatic for some time and request an appointment only when they began to feel sick. A history of kidney stones or other possible obstruction of the ureter may be mentioned by the patient making an appointment request. As with many other kidney disorders, prompt medical attention is required for these patients.

ETIOLOGY

Dilation of the renal pelvis is caused by buildup of pressure in the kidney because of an obstruction. Usually the right kidney is affected, but both can be involved. The cause of the obstruction could be renal calculi, tumors, inflammation caused by infections, prostatic hyperplasia (enlargement), bladder tumors, or congenital ab-

normalities. During pregnancy the enlarged uterus can cause hydronephrosis.

DIAGNOSIS

The first indication of hydronephrosis is usually the result of investigation of other abdominal structures. Follow-up contrast studies of the ureters and the kidneys need to be done. A retrograde pyelogram is necessary. Cystoscopy (Fig. 11–12 in the Enrichment box on Cystoscopy) to rule out an obstruction by a tumor of the bladder or prostate is helpful.

TREATMENT

The treatment of hydronephrosis depends on the underlying cause of the obstruction and the duration of the condition. When obstruction is discovered early, the source can be identified and removed by surgical intervention. Usually after 2 months the kidney is no longer functional; therefore, surgical intervention is not indicated. Concurrent infection necessitates antibiotic therapy. When surgical intervention is not an option and/or the obstruction cannot be relieved, a nephrostomy tube may be inserted.

PROGNOSIS

Once the obstruction causing the hydronephrosis has been resolved, the kidneys may return to normal function. However, when the condition has been present for an extended period, permanent damage may result. Prolonged hydronephrosis causes permanent damage.

PREVENTION

Preventing kidney stones and the subsequent obstruction of the urine flow they can cause also helps prevent hydronephrosis. As previously mentioned, urine and blood chemistry measurements and stone analysis provide clues that can help determine which preventative measures are likely to help prevent recurring kidney stone formation. Additionally, modification of diet, increased exercise, and adequate fluid intake minimize the chance of stone formation. Prompt treatment of an enlarged prostate may prevent an obstruction with resulting hydronephrosis.

PATIENT TEACHING

Encourage patients to follow a suggested diet and fluid regimen to prevent kidney stones. If a nephrostomy tube is in place, care instructions may be necessary.

CYSTOSCOPY

CYSTOSCOPY ALLOWS direct examination and treatment of the urinary tract. A cystoscope is inserted through the urethra (see Fig. 11–12); this instrument has its own lighting system, a viewing scope, and a passage for catheters and surgical devices. Cystoscopy is used to obtain biopsy specimens for diagnosis and to remove stones or tumors.

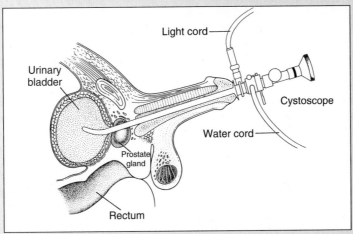

FIGURE 11–12 Cystoscopy. (From Chabner D: *The language of medicine,* ed 5, Philadelphia, 1996, Saunders.)

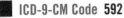

Renal Calculi

DESCRIPTION
Renal calculi are stones in the kidney or elsewhere in the urinary tract formed by the concentration of various mineral salts (see Figs. 11–10 to 11–12).

ICD-9-CM Code 592
Renal calculi are coded according to location. Refer to the physician's diagnosis for location of the calculus and to the current edition of the ICD-9-CM coding manual for specific code modifiers.

SYMPTOMS AND SIGNS
Kidney stones can be solitary or multiple and vary in size; a larger stone formed in the shape of the re- nal pelvis is known as a stag horn calculus (Fig. 11–13). Small stones can be passed spontaneously, unnoticed. The patient's symptoms vary with the degree of obstruction. If infection or blockage caused by the calculi are present, the patient experiences sudden severe pain in the flank area, known as renal colic, with urinary urgency and other urinary abnormalities. Other symptoms include nausea and vomiting, hematuria, fever, chills, and abdominal distention. Blood in the urine can be the result of trauma caused by the presence of small stones, which may be gravel-like or sand-like in consistency, or larger stones, such as staghorn calculi. Hydronephrosis can develop if urine is prevented from flowing past the calculi.

PATIENT SCREENING
The patient experiencing pain from a kidney stone should be considered an emergency situation. If

such patients cannot be seen in the office as soon as possible, they should be referred to an emergency care facility where they can receive analgesic intervention. The patient experiencing sudden onset of severe flank pain and pelvic pressure and pain that is accompanied by nausea and vomiting requires immediate observation and treatment.

ETIOLOGY

Often the cause of calculi is unknown, although an hereditary tendency for development of certain types of stones has been noted. Kidney stones are formed when there is an excessive amount of calcium or uric acid is present in the blood. Males are more prone to kidney stones than females, and the occurrences increase from the age of 30 years up to and including the 50s. Calculi form when sources of crystals are found in the urine, along with the absence of crystalline inhibitors, and the urine is supersaturated with poorly soluble substances.

Risk factors include prolonged dehydration, prolonged immobilization, infection, urinary stasis from obstruction, long-term ingestion of certain medications, and metabolic factors such as *hyperparathyroidism* and gout. (Gout is discussed in Chapter 7.)

DIAGNOSIS

The diagnosis of renal calculi is made based on the family history, clinical findings, urinalysis, radiographic KUB studies, *intravenous urogram,* renal ultrasonogram, and computed tomography (CT) scans. The patient is encouraged to strain the urine to capture any stones that are passed during urination so that they can be analyzed in the laboratory. The possible existence of metabolic disorders can be investigated using blood tests.

TREATMENT

The goals of medical care are to remove the calculi, treat pain and infection, and resolve causative factors. These measures should prevent permanent kidney damage and recurrence of calculi.

The treatment begins with analgesic therapy during the evaluation. Location and size of the calculi indicate the course of treatment. Small calculi (less than 3 mm) may be treated by observation and with fluid hydration in the hope that the stone will pass naturally. Large calculi can be removed by any of several surgical procedures. Attempts are made to crush stones that are (1) too large to pass down the ureter, (2) lodged in the pelvis of the kid-

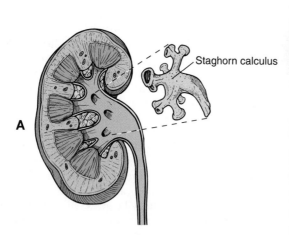
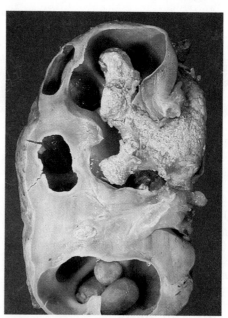

FIGURE 11–13 Staghorn calculi. (**B** from Stevens A, Lowe J: *Pathology: illustrated review in color,* ed 2, London, 2000, Mosby.)

ney, or (3) trapped in the proximal portion of the ureter. Extracorporeal shock wave **lithotripsy** (ESWL) is a procedure that breaks apart (crushes) the stones, thus allowing the small particles to flush out of the body naturally.

A surgical procedure using an ureteroscope to capture the stone in a basket and remove it is attempted for stones trapped in the distal aspect of a ureter. If the attempt to capture the stone is unsuccessful, electrohydraulic lithotripsy (EHL) or laser lithotripsy is used in an attempt to break the stone apart into small particles that can be flushed out of the system. This procedure usually is done with the patient under general anesthesia and with the aid of fluoroscopy. After removal of the calculus, the ureter is visualized via the ureteroscope, and often the pelvis of the kidney also is inspected for any scarring, damage, or pathology. A stent that extends into the urinary bladder is placed in the pelvis of the kidney as a means of preventing edema and spasms of the ureter and subsequent occlusion of the ureter. The stent is removed in 2 to 5 days.

Stones in the urinary bladder often pass spontaneously. When this does not happen, an attempt to remove bladder stones is done during cystoscopy. When previously mentioned procedures are unsuccessful in removing the calculi, surgical intervention in the form of percutaneous nephro-lithotomy may be indicated to remove the stones before permanent damage is caused. A small incision is made into the kidney, and the stone is shattered by ultrasound or EHL. Rarely, when the aforementioned procedures are unsuccessful, surgical incision of the kidney is performed to remove the stone.

Depending on the chemical composition, some kidney stones can be dissolved or prevented from forming with medication. Often the patient may pass small or microscopic stones naturally and without pain. The patient is encouraged to drink 8 to 12 glasses of water a day and may be given diuretics to prevent urinary stasis. Patients are encouraged to strain their urine to catch any stones or particles of stones that may be passed spontaneously. In that way, analysis of the calculi composition is made possible, which can help direct preventive measures.

PROGNOSIS
Prognosis is good after successful removal or spontaneous passage of the stone. However, additional stone formation is possible.

PREVENTION
Urine and blood chemistry measurements and stone analysis provide clues as to which preventative

---

BOX 11–2
Food Containing Oxalates, Purines, and Phosphorus

CONTAINING OXALATES
Chocolate
Coffee
Cola
Nuts
Red beets
Spinach
Strawberries
Tea
Wheat bran

CONTAINING PURINES
Anchovies
Beer
Brains
Gravies
Herring

Kidneys
Liver
Mackerel
Sardines
Shellfish
Sweetbreads

CONTAINING PHOSPHORUS
Beef
Cheese
Cottage cheese
Dairy products
Ice cream
Liver
Milk
Other meats

measures are likely to help. Prevention includes modification of diet, increased exercise, and adequate fluid intake to minimize the chance of stone formation in the future.

PATIENT TEACHING

Encourage patients to strain urine for stones making sure they have an appropriate strainer to use. Instruct them in the proper way of straining the urine. Encourage intake of at least 8 glasses of water a day. Explain risk factors such as UTI, stasis of urine, prolonged dehydration, prolonged immobilization, and long-term ingestion of certain medications. Patients should avoid foods high in oxalates, purine, and phosphorus (Box 11–2 on previous page). Referral to a dietician for advice on dietary control is helpful. Some physicians prefer limiting the intake of calcium, whereas others place no restrictions on calcium intake.

Infectious Cystitis and Urethritis

DESCRIPTION

Cystitis, inflammation of the urinary bladder, and urethritis, inflammation of the urethra, are two common forms of lower UTI.

ICD-9-CM Code **595.9** *(Cystitis unspecified)*
597.80 *(Urethritis unspecified)*
Cystitis and urethritis are coded according to type of infectious process. Refer to the physician's diagnosis for type of infectious process and to the current edition of the ICD-9-CM coding manual for specific code modifiers.

SYMPTOMS AND SIGNS

The inflammation and infection cause the patient to experience urinary urgency, frequency, and possibly even incontinence. Additionally, the patient may have pain in the pelvic region and low back, spasm of the bladder, fever and chills, and a burning sensation with urination. The color of the urine may be dark yellow, or pink or red if blood is present.

PATIENT SCREENING

Patients experiencing pelvic and low back pain accompanied by fever and chills, along with the classic symptoms of frequency and urgency require prompt attention. Advise them they will need to provide a urine specimen upon arrival at the office.

ETIOLOGY

The usual cause of cystitis and urethritis is an ascending bacterial invasion of the urinary tract. The most common causative microorganism is *E. coli*, followed by *Klebsiella, Enterobacter, Proteus,* and *Pseudomonas* species. Sexually transmitted diseases can cause cystitis and urethritis. Other sources of the conditions are viruses, fungi, parasites, and inflammation caused by chemotherapy or radiation. Lesions can develop in the bladder secondary to inflammation, thereby intensifying the symptoms.

DIAGNOSIS

The diagnosis is determined by evaluating the clinical findings, urinalysis of a clean-catch urine specimen, urine culture, and cystoscopy. Urinalysis shows dark yellow, pink, or red urine with abnormal urinary sediment and possibly blood and pus. Microscopic examination of the urine shows RBCs (occult blood), increased numbers of epithelial cells or leukocytes, and bacteria. The urine may have a foul odor. The urine culture grows the causative agent for identification. Cystoscopy shows a reddened inflamed bladder wall (Fig. 11–14). Tenderness in the suprapubic region and pain in the lower back may be elicited on palpation.

TREATMENT

Treatment consists of organism-specific antibiotic or urinary antiseptic therapy such as amoxicillin (Amoxil), and trimethoprim-sulfamethoxazole (Bactrim DS, Septra DS). Ciprofloxacin (Cipro) and levomethadyl (Levaquin), along with Bactrim DS, are both first-line agents. Penicillin derivatives are used to treat complicated cystitis, which tends to recur often. Treatment is a minimum 3 to 5 days of medication for uncomplicated infections and 7 to 10 days for reoccurring infections. Phenazopyridine (Pyridium), a urinary analgesic also can be given to stop dysuria, or painful urination.

Increased fluid intake is encouraged, as is regular complete evacuation of the bladder.

PROGNOSIS

Most lower urinary tract infections respond well to antiinfective drug therapy.

PREVENTION

Prevention includes drinking eight glasses of water a day. Those who have a history of lower urinary tract infections are advised to void frequently. Proper use of toilet tissue when wiping is important in preventing infection. Women with frequent cystitis and urethritis are advised to use prophylactic antibiotic therapy (i.e., nitrofurantion [Macrobid]) either consistently or directly after intercourse.

PATIENT TEACHING

Advise females to void after engaging in sexual intercourse. Also, patients who begin to experience symptoms should increase fluid intake, especially water. Females should be encouraged to wipe the perineum from the front to the back to avoid spreading fecal matter from the rectum to the urinary meatus. Many patients will need to be taught proper procedure for performing a clean-catch mid-stream urine sample.

Diabetic Nephropathy

DESCRIPTION

Diabetic **nephropathy** refers to the renal changes resulting from diabetes mellitus, a systemic endocrine disease caused by failure of the pancreas to release enough insulin into the body (see Diabetes Mellitus in Chapter 4). These changes, called **glomerulosclerosis,** can be expected eventually in all patients with insulin-dependent (type I) diabetes, which increases their morbidity and mortality. Additionally many patients with non-insulin dependent (type II) diabetes also can develop this kidney disorder.

ICD-9-CM Code **250.4** *(Diabetes with renal manifestations)*
583.81 *(Nephrotic syndrome in diseases classified elsewhere)*

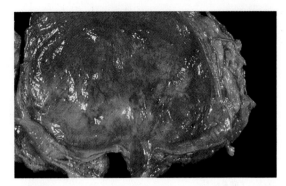

FIGURE 11–14 Acute cystitis. The mucosa of the bladder is red and swollen. (From Damjanov I: *Pathology for the health-related professions,* ed 2, Philadelphia, 2000, Saunders.)

It is important to code diabetes with renal manifestations first and then list the nephrotic syndrome.

SYMPTOMS AND SIGNS

Clinical manifestations, once they begin, include urinary retention, hypertension, nausea, and protein in the urine. UTI and pyelonephritis are common complications. Although those afflicted with insulin-dependent diabetes mellitus have a greater likelihood of developing nephropathy, all patients with diabetes whose blood glucose levels and blood pressure are not controlled are at risk for this irreversible disorder.

PATIENT SCREENING

Those diagnosed with diabetes usually are scheduled for routine assessments. Patients with diabetes who report urinary tract symptoms require prompt assessment.

ETIOLOGY

Diabetic glomerulosclerosis is a complication of diabetes mellitus; lesions of the glomeruli eventually cause the filtration rate to decrease. Insufficient control of blood glucose levels and blood pressure in the patient with diabetes may hasten the deterioration of renal function.

DIAGNOSIS

Blood tests reveal an elevated BUN level and an increase in cholesterol level. Urinalysis shows protein and pus in the urine. Urinary microalbumin will signal the presence of urinary albumin, an indication of nephropathy. Hypertension is another factor to be noted. The diagnosis is confirmed by radiographic studies of the kidneys and renal biopsy.

TREATMENT

Patients with diabetes vary in their susceptibility to renal failure, so the treatment plan must be individualized. Medical control of the diabetes and blood pressure is important, as is prompt treatment of infection. Drug intervention includes an ACE inhibitor for blood pressure control and the prolongation of proper kidney function. Fluid intake and output should be balanced; diuretics may be prescribed if needed. For patients with diabetes, a diet with low-protein and low-fat modifications may be recommended. Dialysis or evaluation for kidney transplantation may be part of the long-term management of ESRD.

PROGNOSIS

Prognosis is varied based on stage at which intervention begins. Early detection and treatment leads to the best outcome. There is no cure for diabetic nephropathy known. When blood glucose and blood pressure are not kept under control, the outcome becomes bleaker. End-stage renal disease is the final outcome, which necessitates dialysis. Kidney transplant is the final option for treatment.

PREVENTION

Close monitoring of both blood glucose levels and blood pressure with appropriate treatment intervention is helpful for all patients with diabetes. The sooner these are brought under control, the better the outcome.

PATIENT TEACHING

Make patients with diabetes aware of the importance of maintaining blood glucose at appropriate levels. They also should be advised about the importance of monitoring their blood pressure and keeping it at acceptable levels. Compliance with prescribed drug therapy is also important.

Polycystic Kidney Disease

DESCRIPTION

Polycystic kidney disease is a slowly progressive and irreversible disorder in which normal renal tissue is replaced with multiple grape-like cysts (Fig. 11–15). The condition is bilateral, with cysts that form from dilated nephrons and collecting ducts. Eventually, the kidneys become grossly enlarged, with compression of surrounding tissue leading to impaired renal function and renal failure.

 ICD-9-CM Code **753.12** *(Congenital)*
753.13 *(Polycystic kidney, autosomal dominant)*
753.14 *(Polycystic kidney, autosomal recessive)*

SYMPTOMS AND SIGNS

As the kidneys become dilated, they are palpable on physical examination. The patient experiences lumbar pain, hematuria, and systemic hypertension, and is more prone to renal infections and renal calculi.

PATIENT SCREENING

Patients complaining of bloody urine accompanied by edema, headache, and flank or pelvic pain require prompt medical attention

ETIOLOGY

Polycystic kidney disease is inherited, but may not be manifested until adolescence or adulthood. It is not clearly understood why the cysts form. Acquired cystic kidney disease (non-inherited) is a sequela of long-term kidney disease and/or long-term dialysis.

DIAGNOSIS

The diagnosis is made by evaluating the clinical findings and renal function tests such as urinalysis, which shows gross blood, proteinuria, and pus. Radiographic films and intravenous pyelogram show enlarged kidneys with irregular outlines and a spidery appearance throughout.

TREATMENT

Because polycystic disease cannot be cured, treatment of this ESRD consists of dialysis and kidney

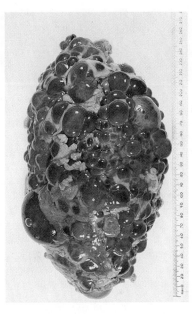

FIGURE 11–15 Adult polycystic disease. (From Stevens A, Lowe J: *Pathology: illustrated review in color,* ed 2, London, 2000, Mosby.)

transplantation. Management of UTIs is necessary, as is management of hypertension.

PROGNOSIS
At the present time, no cure for polycystic disease is known.

PREVENTION
The majority of cases are inherited; therefore, there is no prevention of inherited polycystic kidney disease. Acquired polycystic kidney disease, as a sequela to long-term kidney disease and/or dialysis, also has no means of prevention.

PATIENT TEACHING
Suggest to patients and their families that they seek out community resources for those with kidney disease. Encourage them to locate support groups and possibly interact with those families who are dealing with a similar situation. Be prepared to answer questions about the disease process and outcomes. Advise patients that emptying the bladder

regularly is helpful in preventing UTIs. Also remind them to monitor urinary output, blood pressure, and weight and to take frequent rest breaks and to avoid fatigue.

Neurogenic Bladder

DESCRIPTION
Neurogenic bladder is a dysfunction of urinary bladder control that consists of difficulty in emptying the bladder or urinary incontinence.

◼ **ICD-9-CM Code 596.54** *(NOS)*

SYMPTOMS AND SIGNS
Symptoms and signs of neurogenic bladder may vary depending on the cause of the condition. Some patients with sensory-related problems experience hesitancy and decreased volume of the urinary stream. Others may experience urinary retention resulting from decreased or absent stimuli to void. If the condition is the result of motor paralysis, the patient has the sensation of a full bladder but is unable to initiate the stream to empty. The patient with uninhibited neurogenic bladder is not able to control the voiding pattern and is persistently incontinent of small amounts of urine. In reflex neurogenic bladder, normal sensation is absent, with uncontrolled bladder contractions occurring, which results in spontaneous voiding of spurts of urine. With autonomous neurogenic bladder, all sensations and contraction capabilities are absent, resulting in inability to void without applying pressure to the suprapubic area (*Valsalva* and *Credé maneuvers*).

PATIENT SCREENING
In most circumstances, inability to empty the bladder as well as urinary incontinence is stressful for the patient. Prompt assessment should be considered.

ETIOLOGY
An insult to the brain, spinal cord, or the nerves supplying the lower urinary tract, whether by trauma or disease process, may result in the inability to empty the bladder of urine or to maintain continence. Damage may be caused by cerebrovascular accident, spinal cord trauma, tumors, neuropathies,

ENRICHMENT
URINARY INCONTINENCE

ORMALLY, AS THE BLADDER distends with urine, a reflex is stimulated to initiate voluntary urination (micturition); the sphincters of the bladder and the pelvic diaphragm relax, the bladder muscles contract, and the bladder empties. Urinary incontinence is partial or total loss of voluntary control of the bladder with inability to retain urine. The causes vary from muscle or sphincter impairment to nerve damage or structural abnormalities.

This condition is very prevalent in the elderly, commonly because of overactivity of the bladder musculature, resulting in urgency and incontinence with an inappropriately small volume of urine. Incontinence sometimes is experienced temporarily after the stretching of muscles during childbirth. Children may experience a form termed *enuresis,* or bedwetting. Older women may experience "stress incontinence" resulting from postmenopausal changes in the pelvic musculature that allow intraabdominal pressure to surpass intraurethral pressure. Other types of overactive bladder—or frequency and urge incontinence—are the subject of much-noted current research. Neurologic damage such as brain damage or spinal cord injury may result in permanent incontinence.

Incontinence is treated or managed according to the degree, the type, and the cause. Antispasmodic agents, adult diapers, "bladder training," estrogen therapy for women, and pelvic muscle exercises are some of the therapeutic measures that may be tried. Chronic indwelling catheters are avoided in the management of incontinence because of the prevalence of infection.

---

herniated lumbar disks, poliomyelitis, spinal cord lesions, or myelomeningocele.

DIAGNOSIS
The diagnosis is based on a history of trauma or a disease process, the clinical findings, and urodynamic studies that assess bladder function. Urine flow rate may be evaluated by an uroflowmeter, a device for continuous recording of urine flow in milliliters per second.

TREATMENT
The treatment is directed toward prevention of UTIs and attempts to restore some normalcy in function. Providing a means of storing urine and of bladder emptying are of primary importance. Catheterization (see Fig. 11–16 in the Enrichment box on Urinary Catheterization), whether intermittent or indwelling, is necessary to help the patient maintain an acceptable quality of life. Drug therapy with parasympathomimetic agents may be indicated in some cases. Surgery and the use of external collection devices are other alternatives. Possible complications include hydronephrosis and renal failure.

PROGNOSIS
Usually, no cure for the neurologic deficit that caused the bladder dysfunction is possible. Drug therapy may be helpful. Oxybutynin (Ditrapan XL) and toleradine (Detrol XL) are both used in cases of urinary incontinence due to muscle spasms of the bladder.

PREVENTION
Prevention varies depending on the cause.

PATIENT TEACHING
Patients may require instructions for self-catheterization or other techniques for emptying the bladder. Assist patients and family in finding community resources available to them. Provide the names and phone numbers of support groups and encourage patients to contact these groups.

ENRICHMENT

URINARY CATHETERIZATION

URINARY CATHETERIZATION involves the insertion of a catheter into the urinary bladder through the urethra for the withdrawal of urine (see Fig. 11–16) or for irrigation of the bladder with a therapeutic solution. Strict sterile technique is necessary to prevent cystitis. Urinary catheterization is indicated to empty the bladder before surgery, to obtain a sterile urine specimen, to relieve urinary retention, and to treat incontinence (an indwelling catheter is attached to a drainage bag when the patient is incontinent).

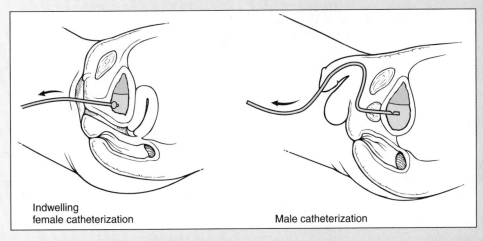

Indwelling
female catheterization

Male catheterization

FIGURE 11–16 Urinary catheterization.

Stress Incontinence

Referral to the current edition of the ICD-9-CM coding manual is recommended to confirm the appropriate code.

DESCRIPTION
Stress incontinence is the uncontrollable leakage of small amounts of urine from the urinary bladder during physical exertion or actions that stress the pelvic muscles, such as laughing, sneezing, coughing, lifting, stretching, or running.

■ **ICD-9-CM Code** **625.6** *(Female)*
788.32 *(Male)*
788.33 *(Mixed)*

SYMPTOMS AND SIGNS
Stress incontinence is a symptom, a sign, and a diagnosis. It occurs when increased abdominal pressure forces urine through the bladder sphincter. The patient (usually female) experiences leakage of urine on coughing, sneezing, laughing, lifting, or running, without feeling prior urgency. The patient is unable to control the leakage during physical exertion.

PATIENT SCREENING

Although not a urologic emergency, stress incontinence can seem like an emergency for the individual experiencing it. Therefore, when possible, the patient should be scheduled for an appointment as soon as possible.

ETIOLOGY

Weakening of the pelvic floor muscles and the urethral structure causes this embarrassing disorder. Trauma to the area resulting from childbirth is the most common cause. Pressure from an existing pregnancy also may be the cause. The hormonal changes of aging and menopause make the condition more common in older women. Certain medications and obesity can precipitate the disorder.

DIAGNOSIS

The symptoms clearly point to the diagnosis. Endoscopy and voiding cystourethrogram (VCUG) reveal abnormal bladder position, with leakage provoked by coughing or straining, *urodynamics.*

TREATMENT

The treatment consists of exercises (*Kegel exercises,* or pelvic floor muscle tightening), estrogen replacement (most effective when estrogen cream is inserted vaginally), drug therapy, surgical repair, or collagen injections.

PROGNOSIS

Prognosis varies depending on the etiology.

PREVENTION

Strengthening pelvic and perineal muscles is helpful. Some females experience stress incontinence as a result of the aging process and normal reduction in the amounts of estrogen produced in their bodies. Medication can control the symptoms in some women; for others there is no prevention.

PATIENT TEACHING

Patient teaching involves providing information on **Kegel exercises** and other exercises to strengthen pelvic and perineal muscles. Diet and fluid intake modifications may be discussed. Assistance with locating community resources or other agencies and information is helpful. Suggest locating support groups.

Renal Cell Carcinoma

DESCRIPTION

Renal cancer is a condition in which one or more malignant tumors develop in one or both kidneys. The most common primary tumor of the kidney is termed *renal cell carcinoma.* Less common tumors include Wilms tumor, a congenital renal tumor of childhood, and cancer of the renal pelvis, an urothelial tumor that closely resembles an urothelial bladder carcinoma.

 ICD-9-CM Code 189.0
Referral to the current edition of the ICD-9-CM coding manual is recommended to determine appropriate code and modifiers according to the site and type of the carcinoma.

SYMPTOMS AND SIGNS

The classic triad of symptoms of renal cell carcinoma is hematuria, abdominal mass, and flank pain. Less than 10% of patients have all three findings, however, and those that do are likely to have advanced disease. Other less common signs and symptoms are weight loss, anemia, fever, and hypercalcemia. Still, many patients with renal cell carcinoma experience no symptoms until the disease is advanced.

PATIENT SCREENING

Patients experiencing hematuria require prompt assessment, as do those reporting an abdominal mass and/or flank pain.

ETIOLOGY

Around 95% of cases of renal cell carcinoma are sporadic, but some familial forms are known. The most common is a component of the von Hippel-Lindau (VHL) syndrome. Patients with this disorder are predisposed to develop multiple bilateral renal cysts and carcinomas as well as tumors in other locations (Fig. 11–17). Risk factors for sporadic renal cell carcinoma are smoking, obesity, dialysis patients with acquired cystic kidney disease, and prolonged exposure to chemicals such as asbestos and cadmium. Incidence varies geographically, with the highest rates found in Scandinavia

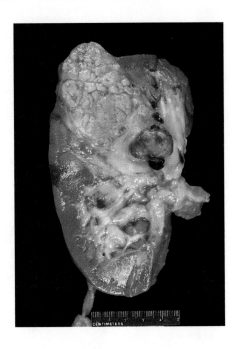

FIGURE 11–17 Renal cell carcinoma: typical cross-section of yellowish, spherical neoplasm in one pole of the kidney. Note the tumor in the dilated, thrombosed renal vein. (From Kumar V et al: *Robbins basic pathology,* ed 7, Philadelphia, 2003, Saunders.)

and North America. It is more common in men and in patients who are 50 to 70 years of age.

DIAGNOSIS

Increasing numbers of renal cell carcinomas are being detected incidentally by radiology exams done in the course of working up some other unrelated disease. Procedures used to diagnose suspected neoplasms are abdominal CT scan, abdominal ultrasound, and intravenous pyelogram (IVP). Once a diagnosis is made, the clinician must look for metastasis using CT scans of the abdomen and chest and a bone scan. A biopsy of the tumor is generally not required. Two staging systems are used for renal cell carcinoma: the TNM (Tumor, Node, Metastasis) system developed by the American Joint Committee on Cancer, and the Flocks and Kadesky system which is based on the gross physical characteristics of the tumor and the degree of vascular involvement.

TREATMENT

The treatment of choice for renal cell carcinoma is surgical removal. Depending on the stage, the patient can be treated with partial **nephrectomy** (for small tumors and for patients with only one functional kidney) or radical nephrectomy. Metastatic renal cell carcinoma is usually resistant to surgical cure and to chemotherapy. However, it may be sensitive to immunotherapy with interferon-alpha or interleukin-2.

PROGNOSIS

The single most important determinant of prognosis is the pathologic stage at diagnosis. This is usually determined by histologic evaluation of the resected tumor by a pathologist. The overall 5-year survival rate is 40%, with early stage tumors having a 5-year survival of 79% to 94%, and metastatic tumors having a less than 5% survival rate at 5 years.

PREVENTION

Large-scale screening of asymptomatic individuals is not recommended. However, individuals at high risk (those with von Hippel-Lindau [VHL] syndrome, history of kidney irradiation, end-stage renal disease and 3 to 5 years on dialysis, or a strong family history of renal cell carcinoma) should undergo periodic screening of urine cytology and abdominal ultrasound to detect early disease. Cessation of smoking is recommended.

PATIENT TEACHING

Encourage patients to seek out support groups and resource agencies in the community. Encourage regular check-ups for other family members when a family history of cancer is known.

Bladder Tumors

DESCRIPTION

Bladder neoplasms usually involve the transitional epithelium *(urothelium)* that lines the surface of the bladder, although a minority are squamous cell carcinomas. The urothelium also lines the entire urinary tract from the renal pelvis to the urethra. Although the bladder is the most common site for a tumor to occur, they can develop—and bladder tumors can recur—at any site in the urothelium-lined urinary tract (Fig. 11–18).

ICD-9-CM Code **239.4** *(Malignant)*
188.9 *(Bladder part unspecified)*
As with other carcinomas, refer to the physician's diagnosis for specific type and site of carcinoma and to the current edition of the ICD-9-CM coding manual for appropriate code and modifiers.

SYMPTOMS AND SIGNS

The most common symptom of a bladder tumor is gross, intermittent, painless hematuria. Pain in the flank or suprapubic area may occur as the carcinoma becomes locally advanced or metastatic. Voiding symptoms such as dysuria, urgency, and increased frequency are sometimes experienced. Symptoms of advanced disease include fatigue, weight loss, and anorexia.

ETIOLOGY

Environmental exposures are thought to account for most cases of bladder cancer because the surface epithelium is exposed to potential carcinogens excreted in the urine (Fig. 11–19). Several risk factors are known: occupational exposure to aniline dyes or diesel exhaust, cigarette smoking, and history of prior bladder cancer. Schistosomiasis (infection with the parasitic worm *Schistosoma haemotobium*) leads to the development of squamous cell carcinoma in endemic areas such as Egypt. Over 80% of cases are diagnosed in patients over the age of 60. White males are affected most often.

DIAGNOSIS

The presence of otherwise unexplained hematuria in a person over the age of 40 denotes cancer in the urinary tract until proven otherwise. A full uro-

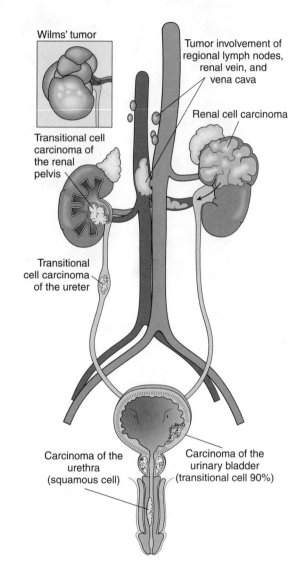

FIGURE 11–18 Neoplasms of the urinary tract. (From Damjanov I: *Pathology for the health-related professions,* ed 2, Philadelphia, 2000, Saunders.)

logic evaluation of the entire urinary tract is indicated. This consists of cystoscopy, urinary cytology (examination of transitional cells in the patient's voided urine), and intravenous pyelogram (IVP). Once the diagnosis is known, ultrasonongraphy or a CT scan may be used to evaluate for extravesical extension and for metastatic disease. The most

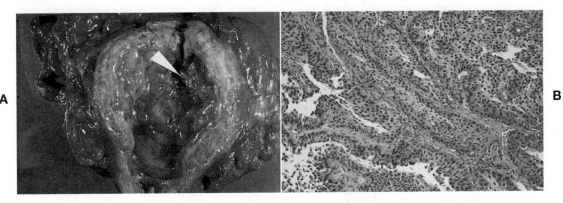

FIGURE 11–19 Bladder cancer. **A,** Gross appearance of an intraluminal mass *(arrow);* **B,** histologic examination reveals that the mass is a papillary transitional cell carcinoma. (From Damjanov I: *Pathology for the health-related professions,* ed 2, Philadelphia, 2000, Saunders.)

commonly used staging system is the TNM (Tumor, Node, Metastasis) system proposed by the American Joint Committee on Cancer, where T indicates the degree of invasion of the bladder wall. A transurethral resection of bladder tumor (TURB) is usually necessary to stage the cancer. This procedure involves a complete cystoscopic resection of any visible tumors and selected biopsies of bladder mucosa. Accurate staging is necessary to direct treatment and predict prognosis.

TREATMENT
The treatment of bladder cancer has three main goals: to eradicate the disease, to prevent recurrence, and to avoid development of invasive disease. The standard initial treatment is tumor resection via TURB. Despite a complete TURB, however, up to 80% of tumors will recur within 12 months. For noninvasive carcinoma, post-TURB follow-up includes urine cytology and cystoscopy at 6-month intervals for 3 to 5 years. An annual IVP for 5 years is also recommended. Recurrent tumors are removed by TURB. If the patient is at high risk for recurrence, bacillus Calmette-Guerin (BCG) is administered into the bladder. BCG is a mycobacterium modified to a less pathologic state, which induces a local immune reaction that suppresses tumor growth. These patients are followed up with urine cytology and cystoscopy at 3- to 6-month intervals for 4 years. For patients with many recurrences and resistance to this intravesical therapy, cystectomy is indicated.

Invasive carcinoma confined to the bladder is treated by either radical cystectomy or partial cystectomy with adjuvant chemoradiotherapy. Postsurgery follow-up is similar to that for noninvasive carcinoma. For patients with metastatic carcinoma, multidrug chemotherapy (currently methotrexate, vinblastine, doxorubicin, and cisplatin, or gemcitabine and cisplatin) may result in tumor shrinkage and moderately increased survival, but it does not result in a cure.

PROGNOSIS
Stage is the most important independent prognostic indicator for disease progression and overall survival. Once invasion outside the bladder or nodal disease is detected, outcomes without systemic therapy are poor. However, recurrence is a more common problem than progression. The grade of the tumor, the degree of cell differentiation, is often used to predict the speed of recurrence. Lower grade, more well-differentiated tumors have a slower growth rate and a better prognosis.

PREVENTION
Efforts should be made to reduce occupational exposures and to cease cigarette smoking.

PATIENT TEACHING
Encourage patients to seek out support groups and resource agencies in the community. Encourage regular check-ups for other family members when a family history of cancer is noted.

REVIEW CHALLENGE

Answer the following questions:

1. Specifically, how does the urinary system work to maintain homeostasis?
2. What are some of the common symptoms of urinary system diseases?
3. What are the etiologic factors of acute glomerulonephritis? Chronic glomerulonephritis?
4. What are some examples of abnormal findings in a urinalysis?
5. Which individuals may require dialysis? Kidney transplant?
6. What are the classic clinical symptoms and signs of nephrosis? What causes nephrosis?
7. Why is acute renal failure considered a clinical emergency?
8. When is renal failure irreversible?
9. How would a patient with pyelonephritis describe his or her symptoms?
10. How might organisms be introduced into the urinary tract and cause pyelonephritis?
11. Which condition is a complication of urinary tract obstruction? What are some causes of urinary tract obstruction?
12. What are the risk factors for renal calculi?
13. What are the etiologic sources of infectious cystitis and urethritis?
14. How does diabetes mellitus contribute to diabetic nephropathy?
15. How would you describe the polycystic kidney?
16. How would you compare the pathology of neurogenic bladder to that of stress incontinence?
17. When may catheterization be indicated?
18. What is the treatment and prognosis for renal cell carcinoma? For bladder tumors?

REAL-LIFE CHALLENGE

Cystitis

A 35-year-old woman reports pain in the pelvic region and lower back, frequency and urgency of urination, and burning on urination. The onset of symptoms was about 4 hours before the office visit.

Vital signs are temperature, 100.5° F; pulse, 96; respirations, 18; and blood pressure, 130/88. A clean-catch urine specimen is obtained, and it is pink in color and has a foul odor. The urine specimen is sent to the laboratory for a urinalysis and culture and sensitivity. The examination reveals tenderness over the bladder. Microscopic examination of the specimen revealed blood, pus, leukocytes, and bacteria.

A diagnosis of cystitis was made and trimethoprim-sulfamethoxazole (Bactrim DS) was prescribed. The patient was encouraged to force fluids and was instructed to call the office the next day to report her progress.

QUESTIONS

1. What is another term for cystitis?
2. What additional symptoms might a patient with cystitis exhibit?
3. What is the usual cause of cystitis?
4. Why is a urinalysis important in diagnosing cystitis?
5. Why would the urine have a foul odor?
6. Why would a culture and sensitivity be important in the treatment of cystitis?
7. What alternative drug therapy is available to treat cystitis?
8. Why would the patient be encouraged to force fluids?

REAL-LIFE CHALLENGE

Renal Calculus

The wife of a 42-year-old man called the office stating that within the last hour her husband had a sudden onset of severe pain in his left side and back. He also has experienced nausea and vomiting. Questioning revealed the pain to be in the left flank area and quite severe. She also reported that the pain radiated down toward the scrotum and that he was experiencing pressure in the perineal area and the frequent urge to urinate. A renal calculus was suspected, and the patient's wife was advised to transport him to an emergency facility.

Vital signs were temperature, 99.6° F; pulse, 96; respirations, 20; and blood pressure, 124/88. A urine specimen was obtained, and the dipstick indicated blood in the urine. The abdomen was slightly distended, the left flank area exhibited tenderness on palpation, and tenderness was noted over the bladder. A renal calculus was suspected, and a KUB, intravenous pyelogram (IVP), and ultrasound of the kidneys were ordered. An intravenous (IV) line was started, and the patient was given 2 mg of morphine sulfate IV push.

The KUB revealed a suspicious area 8 cm distal to the origin of the left ureter. The IVP confirmed the presence of a 3.5 mm calculus distal to the ureteral origin. The renal ultrasound indicated hydronephrosis of the left kidney. The patient was admitted for observation and for pain management.

QUESTIONS

1. What causes renal calculi to form?
2. Why would patients' symptoms vary?
3. What would be the significant symptom or symptoms leading to suspicion of renal calculi?
4. What is renal colic?
5. What would cause blood in the urine?
6. What is the cause of hydronephrosis?
7. Why would the patient be instructed to strain all urine?
8. What are the treatment options for the patient with renal calculi?
9. Why would IV morphine be given?

INTERNET ASSIGNMENTS

1. Research the incidence and treatment of urinary incontinence at the websites of the National Kidney Foundation and the American Urological Association. Compare information found on both sites.
2. Research the incidence, types of stones, and treatment of renal calculi at the websites of the National Kidney Foundation and the American Urological Association. Compare information found on both sites.
3. Research transplant donations using both live and cadaver donors at the websites of the National Kidney Foundation and the American Urological Association. Include information about expenses associated with the transplant, including possible third-party payment for the procedure.

CHAPTER 12

Diseases and Conditions of the Reproductive System

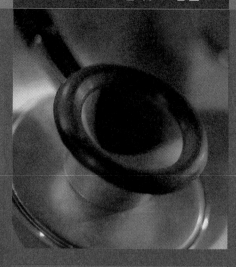

Chapter Outline

Chapter Outline—Cont'd

Learning Objectives

After studying Chapter 12, you should be able to:

1. Identify risk factors for sexually transmitted diseases (STDs).
2. Explain what a silent STD is, and give an example.
3. Name the complications of untreated gonorrhea.
4. Recall how trichomoniasis is diagnosed.
5. Explain how genital herpes is transmitted.
6. Explain why women with genital herpes are advised to have regular Pap (Papanicolaou) smears.
7. Describe the stages of untreated syphilis.
8. Explain why hepatitis B is classified as sexually transmitted.
9. List the possible causes of dyspareunia in men and women.
10. Name drugs that can contribute to impotence.
11. Name a common causative factor in male and female infertility.
12. Explain the value of prostate-specific antigen (PSA) as a screening test.
13. Discuss the medical interventions for prostatic cancer.
14. Explain how varicocele may contribute to male infertility.
15. Explain why physicians encourage monthly testicular self-examinations for younger men.
16. Explain what causes the dysmenorrhea associated with endometriosis.
17. Discuss the importance of early diagnosis and prompt treatment of pelvic inflammatory disease.
18. Discuss the advantages and possible risks of hormone replacement therapy for the postmenopausal woman.
19. Explain how uterine prolapse, cystocele, and rectocele may be corrected surgically.
20. List the risk factors for cervical cancer.
21. Name the leading cause of deaths attributed to female reproductive system disorders.
22. List some possible causes of ectopic pregnancy.
23. Explain how a pregnant woman is monitored for toxemia.
24. Describe abruptio placentae.
25. List the factors that place women at higher risk for breast cancer.

Key Terms

amenorrhea (ah–**men**–o–**REE**–ah)
autoinoculation (**aw**–toh–in–**ock**–u–**LAY**–shun)
chancre (**SHANG**–ker)
colporrhaphy (kol–**POUR**–ah–fee)
curettage (**ku**–reh–**TAHZH**)

dysmenorrhea (**dis**–men–oh–**REE**–ah)
dyspareunia (**dis**–pah–**RUE**–nee–ah)
dysuria (dis–**YOU**–ree–ah)
genitourinary (**jen**–ih–toe–**YU**–rih–nar–ee)
hysterosalpingography (**hiss**–ter–oh–**sal**–pin–**GOG**–rah–fee)

Continued

Key Terms—Cont'd

laparoscopy (lap–ar–**OS**–ko–pee)
leiomyoma (**lye**–o–my–**OH**–ma)
menorrhagia (**men**–oh–**RAY**–jee–ah)
metrorrhagia (**met**–roh–**RAY**–jee–ah)
multiparous (mul–**TIP**–ar–us)
orchitis (or–**KYE**–tis)
pessary (**PESS**–ah–ree)
primipara (pry–**MIP**–ah–rah)
prolapse (pro–**LAPS**)
prostatectomy (**pros**–tah–**TECK**–toh–me)

psychosexual (**sigh**–ko–**SEKS**–you–al)
salpingo-oophorectomy
 (sal–**ping**–go–oh–ouf–oh–**RECK**–toh–me)
septicemia (sep–tih–**SEE**–me–ah)
spermicidal (**spur**–mih–**SIGH**–dal)
ultrasonography (uhl–tra–son–**OGG**–rah–fee)
urethritis (**you**–ree–**THRYE**–tis)
vaginismus (vaj–in–**IZ**–mus)
varicocele (**VAR**–ih–ko–seel)

THE NORMALLY FUNCTIONING REPRODUCTIVE SYSTEMS

THE REPRODUCTIVE PROCESS in humans is sexual and involves the union of two sex cells, one male and one female. In early embryonic development the sex organs are not differentiated, and therefore gender is difficult to identify. As the fetus develops, male or female definition becomes evident. The organs of the reproductive system usually are classified into two groups: the gonads (testes and ovaries), which produce germ cells and hormones, and the series of ducts necessary for the transportation of the germ cells.

The male reproductive system functions to transfer the sperm cells to the female for fertilization of the ovum. The testes produce the sperm and the hormones necessary for the development and maintenance of the secondary sex characteristics. The sperm is transported through the series of ducts beginning with the epididymis, the ductus deferens, and the ejaculatory ducts. The seminal vesicles, the prostate gland, the bulbourethral glands, and the penis are accessory organs that help to propel the sperm on its journey to meet the egg (Fig. 12–1).

The female reproductive system nourishes and enables the development of the fertilized ovum. The ovaries (which contain the woman's lifetime supply of eggs) produce and release the egg and the hormones necessary for the development of secondary sex characteristics and for maintenance of a pregnancy. The ductal system for transport,

nourishment, and growth of the fertilized ovum includes the fallopian tubes and the uterus. Other principal parts of the female reproductive system include the cervix, the vagina, and the external genitalia (Fig. 12–2).

The breasts are accessory organs of reproduction and are two milk-producing glands (Fig. 12–3). When a woman is pregnant, the breast tissue is stimulated by both ovarian and placental hormones to prepare for lactation. After delivery, lactating hormones further stimulate the breast tissue to produce and release milk to nourish the infant.

The process of reproduction requires that the sperm fertilize the egg. After release from the ovary, the egg progresses down the fallopian tube. In a typical pregnancy, the egg is met, about a third of the way down the fallopian tube, by the sperm cell. After the sperm cell fertilizes the egg, the *zygote* continues to travel down the fallopian tube to the uterus, where it eventually attaches to the uterine lining *(endometrium)* to be nourished and to grow. The placenta forms within the uterine wall and provides a mechanism for the exchange of nourishment and waste products between the mother and the developing fetus. A normal gestational period is 38 weeks after conception, at which time the birth process begins with labor and subsequently, the infant is delivered.

The anterior pituitary gland produces gonadotropic hormones that cause the ovaries to

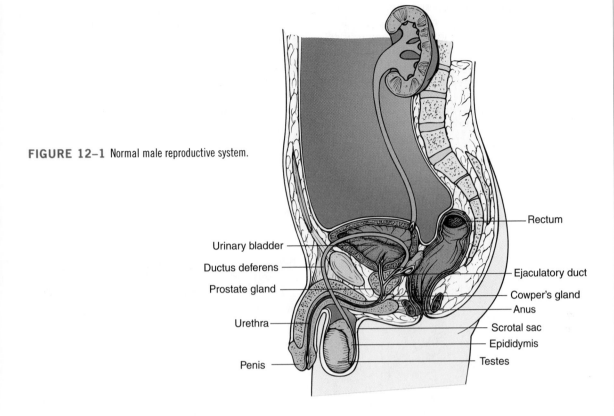

FIGURE 12–1 Normal male reproductive system.

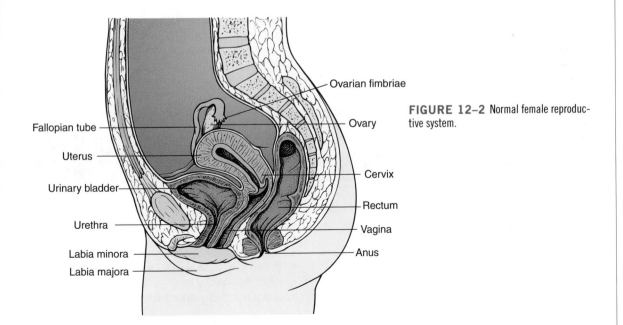

FIGURE 12–2 Normal female reproductive system.

produce estrogen and progesterone, which regulate the menstrual cycle. During menstruation, the endometrium (the disintegrated endometrial cells along with secretions and blood cells) is shed via the vagina. This is followed by the ovarian production of estrogen, causing the ovum to mature and to be released from the ovary. The corpus luteum then develops, and progesterone and additional estrogen are secreted into the bloodstream to stimu-

late the growth of the endometrium to prepare for implantation of the fertilized ovum. If pregnancy does not occur, the endometrium again is shed through menses in anticipation of the next cycle and a possible pregnancy.

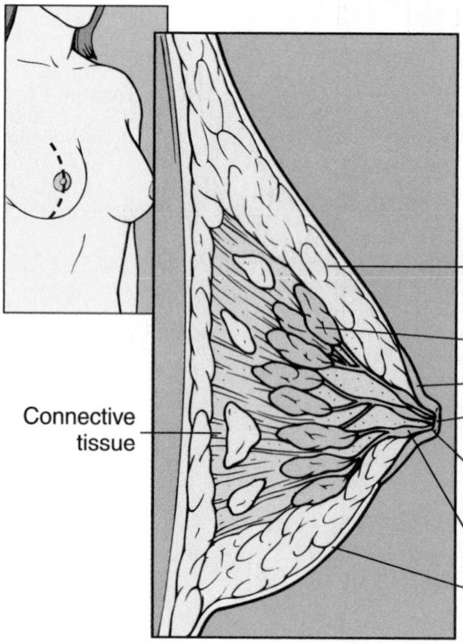

Both the male and female reproductive systems are vulnerable to many diseases, including sexually transmitted diseases (STDs), malignancies, benign growths, and chemical imbalances. Abnormal function of the reproductive system sometimes results from functional, structural, or emotional causes. Complications often develop during pregnancy, some severe and some merely aggravating. This chapter explores the most common disease entities, conditions, and complications of both male and female reproductive systems.

FIGURE 12–3 Normal female breast.

Sexually Transmitted Diseases

More than 20 infectious diseases are spread by sexual contact, all of which can damage health or even threaten life. Sexually transmitted diseases (STDs), formerly called venereal diseases, are among the most common contagious diseases in the United States. In some cases STDs are asymptomatic and are spread by people unaware that they are infected. These diseases represent a "silent epidemic." No one is immune, and one can have more than one STD at a time. Recurrent infections are common. The infections are transmitted from one person to another through bodily

ALERT

RISK FACTORS FOR SEXUALLY TRANSMITTED DISEASES

- Sex with someone whose sexual history one does not know
- Drug use with sharing of needles
- Sex with many people
- Sexual intimacy with someone who has been diagnosed with an STD or one who is being treated for an STD
- Exposure with skin-to-skin contact in the presence of any open lesion, such as a chancre or a wart

- Use of alcohol or other drugs that may cloud one's judgment about a sexual encounter
- Hemophilia
- Transfusion of blood or blood products
- Babies being carried by an HIV-positive mother
- Breast-fed infants of an HIV-positive mother
- Lack of education or concern about risky sexual behavior

fluids such as blood, semen, and vaginal secretions during vaginal, anal, or oral sex; some are spread by direct contact with infected skin. Most STDs are treatable, but there is no cure for viral STDs such as herpes and human immunodeficiency virus (HIV). Among the many concerns about STDs is the possible transmission by an infected mother to a fetus or newborn, sometimes with dire consequences to the baby.

STD rates in the United States are among the highest in the world and are growing; syphilis is rising in the United States for the first time in many years. Recent statistics show 1 in 4 teenagers get sexually transmitted diseases. Attempts to control this rampant public health problem are focusing on research studies, education, and prevention campaigns. Prevention messages point out high-risk sexual behavior patterns and lifestyles, and warn of possible predisposing health problems. There are four STDs that, when diagnosed, must be reported to state health departments and the CDC for statistical purposes: chlamydia, gonorrhea, syphilis, and hepatitis B. (See Chapter 8 for a discussion of hepatitis B.)

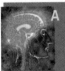

A L E R T

INFECTION CONTROL AND STANDARD PRECAUTIONS

Guidelines: Treat body fluids as if infected and remember to use the following precautions:

1. Practice frequent and thorough hand washing.
2. Report any accidental needle sticks.
3. Wear protective equipment, including mask, gown, gloves, and goggles.
4. Use caution with laboratory specimens.

5. Dispose of contaminated sharps in designated biohazard containers. *Caution:* Do not recap or break needles.
6. Use proper linen disposal containers.
7. Use clean mouthpieces and resuscitation bags.
8. Obtain hepatitis B vaccination for occupational exposure to blood.
9. Use proper decontamination techniques.

A L E R T

MALE LATEX CONDOMS AND SEXUALLY TRANSMITTED DISEASES

The surest way to avoid transmission of sexually transmitted diseases is to abstain from sexual intercourse, or to be in a long-term mutually monogamous relationship with a partner who has been tested and whom you know is uninfected.

For people whose sexual behaviors place them at risk for STDs, correct and consistent use of the male latex condom can reduce the risk of STD transmission. No protective method is 100% effective, however, and condom use cannot guarantee absolute protection against any STD. Furthermore, condoms lubricated with spermicides are no more effective than other lubricated condoms in protecting against the transmission of HIV and other STDs. To achieve the protective effect of condoms, they must be used correctly and consistently. Incorrect use can lead to condom slippage or breakage, thus reducing their protective effect. Inconsistent use (e.g., failure to use condoms with every act of intercourse) can lead to STD transmission because transmission can occur with a single act of intercourse.

Condom use has been associated with a reduced risk of cervical cancer, but the use of condoms should not be a substitute for routine Pap smears to detect and prevent cervical cancer.

Source: CDC Fact Sheet for Public Health Personnel: National Center for HIV, STD, and TB Prevention.

Chlamydia

DESCRIPTION
Chlamydia, one of the most frequently reported infectious diseases in the United States, causes **urethritis** in men and urethritis and cervicitis in women.

 ICD-9-CM Code 079.98

SYMPTOMS AND SIGNS
Chlamydia sometimes is called the silent STD because it often has no symptoms and thus it is sexually transmitted unknowingly. A high percentage of women have no symptoms before dangerous complications start. More common than gonorrhea and the leading cause of *pelvic inflammatory disease (PID)*, chlamydia is a major cause of female sterility. Conversely, 75% of men have symptoms 1 to 3 weeks after exposure.

Early female symptoms include a thick vaginal discharge with a burning sensation, itching, abdominal pain, and **dyspareunia.** Infected men experience discharge from the penis, with a burning sensation and itching, and a burning sensation when urinating, the latter caused by urethritis. The scrotum may be swollen. The inguinal lymph nodes often are enlarged in either sex. A small transient lesion and skin irritation may be noticed. Newborns can acquire chlamydia from the infected mother during birth, resulting in conjunctivitis, blindness, arthritis, or overwhelming infection.

PATIENT SCREENING
Symptoms usually start 1 or 2 weeks after exposure; they are likely to be mild, such as burning with urination and a genital discharge in both men and women. Schedule an early appointment to confirm diagnosis and begin treatment.

ETIOLOGY
Chlamydia trachomatis, an intracellular bacterium, is the cause of chlamydia and usually is transmitted by sexual contact. The site of primary infection is usually around the genitals, but it can be oral or anal, depending on sexual practice. The organism can be transmitted unknowingly.

DIAGNOSIS
In the laboratory, swab cultures specifically reveal the parasite *C. trachomatis* in the infected person's body fluids. A *Giemsa stain* of cell scrapings is performed to test for the presence of *antibodies,* and *antigen*-specific *serologic* studies are performed. Newer nucleic acid probes are available.

TREATMENT
Antibiotic therapy is given to both partners, beginning with a single injection, and followed with a course of oral antibiotics, such as azithromycin, erythromycin, or a 7-day regimen of doxycycline. Prompt treatment can cure the infection and prevent complications such as PID and problem pregnancy. Follow-up testing is recommended.

PROGNOSIS
Chlamydial infection can be cured with a complete course of antibiotics, taken as directed, even after symptoms subside.

PREVENTION
Use standard precautions when caring for a patient with chlamydial infection. Infected patients should inform sexual contacts of their infection. See the risk factors for sexually transmitted disease. Some states require reporting cases of chlamydia to the public health department.

PATIENT TEACHING
Emphasize the importance of taking the complete course of antibiotic therapy as prescribed. Recommend that patients abstain from intercourse until both partners are cured. Inform patients that meticulous personal hygiene and frequent hand washing are necessary to avoid spreading the infection to the eyes.

Gonorrhea

DESCRIPTION
Gonorrhea, a common STD, is an infection of the **genitourinary** tract.

 ICD-9-CM Code 098.0

SYMPTOMS AND SIGNS
Gonorrhea, also a common infection of the genitourinary tract, causes symptoms and complications similar to those of chlamydia in male and female patients. A *purulent* discharge from the male or female genitourinary tract and **dysuria** are often present but can vary in severity. Up to 50% of men are *asymptomatic,* so they may unknowingly continue to spread the infection, making transmission

difficult to control. The disease also can infect the eyes and throat or become systemic.

PATIENT SCREENING

Males develop symptoms, if any, after an incubation period of 3 to 6 days. Symptoms in females vary. Early treatment is indicated because untreated gonorrhea can spread.

ETIOLOGY

Infection with the common bacterium *Neisseria gonorrhoeae* usually results from sexual transmission. Because transmission is also possible during birth, newborns must be protected from eye infections that can lead to blindness (Fig. 12–4). Therefore prophylactic erythromycin salve is administered routinely at birth.

DIAGNOSIS

Laboratory cultures of infectious body secretions and microscopic examination of exudate with a *Gram stain* are performed to identify the *N. gonorrhoeae* organism.

TREATMENT

Treatment is recommended for the infected individual and any sexual partners as well. Ciprofloxacin, ceftriaxone, or doxycycline administration is started as soon as the diagnosis is made. Many strains of *N. gonorrhoeae* have become resistant to tetracycline and penicillin. After the antibiotic therapy, follow-up culture studies are ordered to ensure a complete cure because some strains are antibiotic-resistant. Neglecting treatment of a

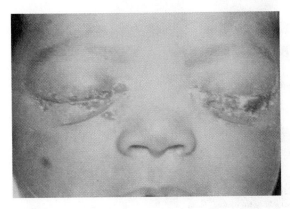

FIGURE 12–4 Gonorrhea ophthalmia. (From Grimes D: *Infectious diseases—Mosby's clinical nursing series*, St. Louis, 1991, Mosby.)

gonococcal infection can lead to complications, including PID, **septicemia,** and septic arthritis.

PROGNOSIS

With early and complete treatment the prognosis is excellent, even when there are complications.

PREVENTION

Use standard precautions when caring for a patient with gonorrhea. Report all cases to the local public health department. Routine instillation of erythromycin or 1% silver nitrate drops into the eyes of newborns is practiced. Abstinence from sexual contact is maintained until treatment is complete and follow-up cultures prove negative.

PATIENT TEACHING

Emphasize the importance of complying with a complete treatment plan and follow-up testing to ensure a cure. Inform the patient of the risk factors. (See the Alert box.)

Trichomoniasis

DESCRIPTION

Trichomoniasis is a protozoal infection of the lower genitourinary tract.

 ICD-9-CM Code 131.9 *(Unspecified)*
The above code may be valid as a principal diagnosis. Refer to the physician's diagnosis and then to the current edition of the ICD-9-CM coding manual to ensure the greatest specificity of pathology and any appropriate modifiers.

SYMPTOMS AND SIGNS

About 15% of people who are sexually active have trichomoniasis. Most infected men and women, however, are asymptomatic. This contributes to spreading of the unrecognized infection as well as delays in treatment.

The initial symptoms for male and female patients include urethritis with dysuria and itching. In addition, women may notice a profuse greenish yellow discharge from the vagina. The discharge may subside without treatment, but the infection remains, and it can become chronic.

PATIENT SCREENING

Discomfort associated with the irritating discharge usually prompts a request for an appointment for an examination.

ETIOLOGY

Trichomoniasis is a protozoal infection caused by *Trichomonas vaginalis* and usually is transmitted through sexual contact.

DIAGNOSIS

A wet preparation of vaginal secretions or discharge from the male urethra is studied for the microorganism *T. vaginalis.* Urinalysis also may reveal the organism. The cervix is examined for the presence of small hemorrhages with a strawberry-like appearance.

TREATMENT

If the laboratory culture is positive, antiinfective drugs are given orally (such as metronidazole [flagyl] for 7 days) or vaginally.

PROGNOSIS

The prognosis is good if both partners receive medical treatment, including a follow-up examination that ensures that the infection is cured completely. Failure to treat both partners causes reinfection, called a "ping-pong" vaginitis.

PREVENTION

Because this disease is transmitted primarily by sexual contact, prevention requires avoiding sex with someone whose sexual history one does not know.

PATIENT TEACHING

See remarks under Prevention and Prognosis.

Genital Herpes

DESCRIPTION

Genital herpes is an infection of the skin of the genital area, with *ulcerations* spread by direct skin-to-skin contact, causing painful genital sores similar to cold sores (Fig. 12–5).

> ◼ **ICD-9-CM Code 054.10** *(Unspecified)*
> *Genital herpes is coded according to the site of the lesion(s). Refer to the physician's diagnosis and then to the current edition of the ICD-9-CM coding manual to ensure the greatest specificity of pathology and any appropriate modifiers.*

SYMPTOMS AND SIGNS

Genital herpes is caused by herpes simplex virus type 2 (HSV-2) and is a recurrent, incurable viral disease. A large percentage of infections are subclinical, so the initial episode may go unnoticed. More often, one or more blister-like lesions are noted somewhere on the genitals or around the anus. The painful ulcers and blisters usually occur 2 to 30 days after sexual contact with an infected person. Systemic influenza symptoms, swollen glands, fever, headache, and painful urination also

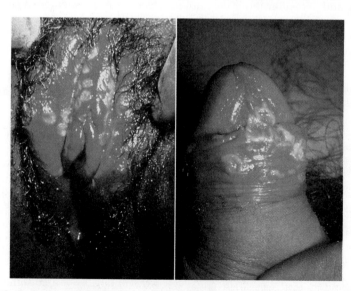

FIGURE 12–5 Genital herpes in the female (left) and the male (right). (From Behrman RE, Kliegman RM, Arvin AM: Slide set, *Nelson textbook of pediatrics,* ed 15, Philadelphia, 1996, Saunders.)

may be present. The condition is infectious when sores are present, but some people, called "shedders," can transmit the virus without symptoms. Subsequent outbreaks can occur for months or years because the virus hides in the nervous system and lies dormant between flare-ups.

PATIENT SCREENING

Systemic symptoms may be present during the acute stage. When fever, headache, muscle aches, and swollen glands are present the individual is scheduled for investigative medical evaluation.

ETIOLOGY

One in six adults carries the highly contagious HSV-2; it usually is transmitted sexually with skin-to-skin contact. Cross-infection may result from oral-genital sex.

The presence of open lesions increases the risk of contracting acquired immunodeficiency syndrome (AIDS) during sexual acts between persons infected with HSV-2 and those who are positive for human immunodeficiency virus (HIV).

DIAGNOSIS

The presence of the characteristic lesions on the male or female genitalia is noted during physical examination. An antigen test or tissue culture laboratory techniques are used to identify the HSV-2 virus and to confirm the diagnosis.

TREATMENT

There is no cure, but prescription drugs currently are available to reduce the duration and frequency of outbreaks. These drugs include acyclovir (Zovirax), famciclovir (Famvir), and valacyclovir (Valtrex). In some cases, the body's own immunity makes the episodes less severe. The presence of sores in the genital area and the fear of transmitting or acquiring herpes contribute to emotional stress and social embarrassment. In addition, women with genital herpes must be watched more carefully for cervical cancer. A Pap (Papanicolaou) smear every 6 months is recommended. Finally, a cesarean section may be indicated because the virus is dangerous to the newborn.

PROGNOSIS

Recurrent herpes usually has prodromal symptoms such as tingling, itching, or burning 1 to 5 days before the lesion(s) appear. Recurrent episodes tend to be milder and often are triggered by fatigue and stress.

PREVENTION

Sexual abstinence and mutual monogamy are the only absolute prevention. Condoms do not necessarily provide a complete barrier against skin-to-skin contact. After years of research, a recent report states that a new vaccine has been developed and has been shown to significantly reduce the incidence of genital herpes in women.

PATIENT TEACHING

Counsel the patient about the preventive measures and prognosis mentioned above. Recommend frequent and thorough hand washing; the infection possibly can spread into the eyes or other areas of the skin.

Genital Warts (Condylomata Acuminata)

DESCRIPTION

Condyloma acuminatum is a genital infection that causes raised cauliflower-like growths in or near the vagina or rectum or along the penis (Fig. 12–6).

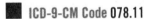 **ICD-9-CM Code 078.11**

SYMPTOMS AND SIGNS

These genital warts are usually painless, but they may itch or burn. These contagious lesions appear several weeks to several months after direct skin-to-skin contact during sexual intercourse with an infected person. The discomfort experienced varies with the size, number, and location of the warts.

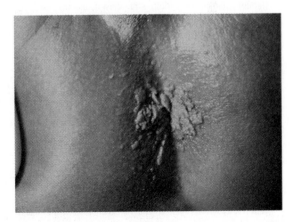

FIGURE 12–6 Genital warts. (From Behrman RE, Kliegman RM, Arvin AM: Slide set, *Nelson textbook of pediatrics*, ed 15, Philadelphia, 1996, Saunders.)

PATIENT SCREENING

Schedule the male or female patient for a pelvic examination.

ETIOLOGY

A virus called the human papillomavirus (HPV) is the cause of genital warts and usually is transmitted sexually. It has a prolonged incubation period of 1 to 6 months.

DIAGNOSIS

Genital warts can be identified by their appearance, but a biopsy sometimes is suggested to rule out carcinoma. The wart must be differentiated from a syphilitic lesion.

TREATMENT

The treatment is chemical or surgical removal of the warts, but recurrence is common. Topical drug therapy to remove the warts includes a keratolytic agent such as podofilox and trichloroacetic acid. Imiquimod, an antiviral cream, also is widely used to stop new genital warts from forming. Surgical procedures for wart removal include cryosurgery, which involves the freezing and re-moval of affected tissue. Electrodesiccation is a process that uses lasers to remove larger warts and is also very effective. Some genital warts go away without treatment.

Studies show that women with genital HPV infection are at greater risk for cervical cancer. Because the warts spread more rapidly during pregnancy, a cesarean section may be necessary if the warts occlude the birth canal.

PROGNOSIS

Genital warts have no complications, but the disease tends to recur. Pregnancy promotes the growth and spread of the lesions.

PREVENTION

Avoid sexual contact with an infected individual, and do not have sexual contact with someone whose sexual history you do not know. The long incubation period introduces added risk of infecting others or in contracting the disease.

PATIENT TEACHING

Counseling about all aspects of prevention and transmission of genital warts is important.

ALERT

HUMAN PAPILLOMAVIRUS AND CANCER

Human papillomavirus (HPV) is the most commonly diagnosed STD in the United States. It is often associated with genital warts (condylomata acuminata) but also has been linked to the development of many different types of cancer. The biology of HPV has been widely studied because of its link to malignancy. More than 70 types of HPV have been described. They are differentiated based on their DNA sequence and placed into groups based on the likelihood to cause cancer in the infected individual. For example, the group that includes HPV types 6, 11, 42, 43, and 44 usually causes genital warts and low-grade cervical intraepithelial neoplasia (CIN), but it only rarely leads to invasive tumors.

HPV infection is most often associated with cervical cancer. It also has been implicated in most anal, vulvar, and vaginal cancers, as well as some oropharyngeal cancers. HPV types 16 and 18 make up the group carrying the highest risk for development of invasive cancer at most of these sites. Coinfection with HIV causes a further increase in HPV-related cancer risk, and intermediate and low-risk HPV groups often cause invasive cancer in these individuals.

Although most people infected with HPV will not go on to develop an invasive neoplasm, it is important to reduce one's risk of infection. The virus may be spread not only by unprotected intercourse, but also by close physical contact with an infected area, and probably through digital/anal, oral/anal, and digital/vaginal contact as well. Using barrier contraception and limiting one's number of sexual partners are recommended to reduce risk of infection. No antiviral drugs currently are available to treat HPV. Those who are infected should know the risk of cancer development and should follow up periodically with their physician to monitor for premalignant neoplastic changes.

Early phase trials and studies of a vaccine against HPV have proven somewhat effective in young women vaccinated before first intercourse. The vaccine's usefulness is limited by the fact that it offers protection only against one type of HPV.

Syphilis

DESCRIPTION

Syphilis is a chronic, systemic, sexually transmitted infection that consists of four stages.

■ **ICD-9-CM Code** **091.0** *(Genital syphilis, primary)*
091.9 *(Unspecified secondary syphilis)*
097.1 *(Latent syphilis, unspecified)*
Refer to the physician's diagnosis and then to the current edition of the ICD-9-CM coding manual to ensure the greatest specificity of pathology and any appropriate modifiers.

SYMPTOMS AND SIGNS

Syphilis begins with the presence of a painless but highly contagious local lesion called a **chancre** on the male or female genitalia (Fig. 12–7). Without early treatment during the primary stage, it becomes a systemic, chronic disease that can involve any organ or tissue. In 1 to 2 months, when the primary lesion heals, the causative organism (the *Treponema pallidum* spirochete) has disseminated throughout the body and multiplied, producing lesions wherever the organisms are most prevalent, including the skin, lymph nodes, cardiovascular system, brain, and spinal cord.

The disease continues to be contagious during the secondary stage, when there is systemic manifestation. This stage can present many symptoms, including fever, headaches, aching of the joints, mouth sores, and rashes on the palms of the hands and soles of the feet (Fig. 12–8). Then a latent period, lasting from 1 to 40 years, may follow, during which the infection is generally subclinical or asymptomatic. In the late stage, the lesions, called gummas, have invaded body organs and systems, causing widespread damage to the point of being disabling and life-threatening.

When a fetus is infected, the child may die in utero or be born with congenital syphilis and multiple abnormalities.

PATIENT SCREENING

It is important to treat syphilis in the early stage. NOTE: Syphilis is on the rise in the United States for the first time in many years.

ETIOLOGY

Syphilis is caused by infection with the *T. pallidum* spirochete through sexual contact or other direct contact with infected lesions or infected body fluids. Congenital transmission can occur during pregnancy.

DIAGNOSIS

A smear taken from the primary lesion is examined microscopically for the spiral bacteria *T. pallidum*. Antibodies can be detected in the patient's serum, and this is the most common means of recognition.

TREATMENT

Syphilis can be cured with a course of antibiotic therapy using penicillin G. If the patient is allergic to penicillin, other antibiotics such as doxycycline or tetracycline are used. The disease is best treated in the early stage, before it causes irreversible damage to the body. Patients are monitored with follow-up blood tests for the presence of *T. pallidum* for up to a year.

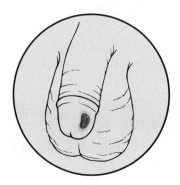

FIGURE 12–7 Chancre of primary syphilis.

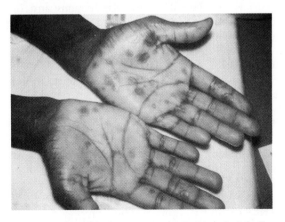

FIGURE 12–8 Secondary syphilis. (From Grimes D: *Infectious diseases—Mosby's clinical nursing series,* St. Louis, 1991, Mosby.)

PROGNOSIS

Treatment for syphilis can cure the disease. Untreated syphilis progresses to severe systemic complications.

PREVENTION

Health-care providers should practice standard precautions. Avoid sexual contact with an infected individual, and avoid contact with body fluids. Syphilis can be transmitted in the first few years of the latent stage as well as in the first two stages. When in doubt, a VDRL test should be performed to detect infection. See the list of risk factors for STDs. Syphilis cases are reportable to the local department of health.

PATIENT TEACHING

Emphasize the importance of finishing the course of medication, even if symptoms improve. Urge the patient to inform sexual partners of the infection so they can seek treatment if needed. Instruct the patient to avoid all risk factors for STDs.

Chancroid

DESCRIPTION

Chancroid, also called soft chancre, is a bacterial infection of the genitalia that causes a necrotizing ulceration and lymphadenopathy.

 ICD-9-CM Code 099.0

SYMPTOMS AND SIGNS

The shallow and painless lesion appears on the skin or mucous membrane, at the site of entry, 7 to 10 days after sexual contact with an infected person (Fig. 12–9). The ulcer usually deepens and becomes purulent and can be spread to other areas of the body by **autoinoculation.**

ETIOLOGY

The causative agent of chancroid is the bacterium *Haemophilus ducreyi.*

DIAGNOSIS

The diagnosis is based on the clinical appearance of the lesions. In the laboratory, Gram stain smears of the *exudate* are performed to confirm the cause of the infection.

TREATMENT

The patient usually responds well to antibiotic therapy (i.e., azithromycin, clarithromycin, or ceftriax-

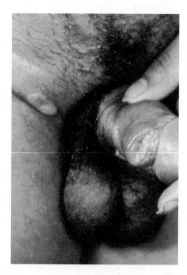

FIGURE 12–9 Chancroid: male. (From Grimes D: *Infectious diseases—Mosby's clinical nursing series,* St. Louis, 1991, Mosby.)

one). The lesions sometimes must be drained surgically. Good personal hygiene is advised. The patient is told to keep the infected areas clean and dry and to refrain from sexual contact during the entire time of treatment.

PROGNOSIS

Antibiotic therapy is usually curative.

PREVENTION

No vaccine is available. Use of a condom helps prevent spread of the infection.

PATIENT TEACHING

All regular sexual partners should be examined and treated if needed. Serologic testing for HIV is recommended for patients treated for chancroid.

Hepatitis B

(See Chapter 8 for discussion on Hepatitis B.)

Sexual Dysfunction

The most common male and female sexual dysfunctions are discussed briefly. Sexual health and proper sexual functioning are important to human beings for the pleasure they provide, for the intimacy they nurture in a relationship, and for reproduction. To fulfill these purposes, the individuals must be free from organic disease and **psychosexual** disorders.

Ideally, the human sexual response cycle progresses from a state of desire or arousal, through orgasm, to resolution or a feeling of well-being and relaxation. This cycle depends on a balance and interplay among the mind, the nervous system, and biogenic physical factors.

Dyspareunia

DESCRIPTION
Dyspareunia refers to recurrent painful or difficult sexual intercourse.

 ICD-9-CM Code 608.89 *(Male)*
625.0 *(Female)*

SYMPTOMS AND SIGNS
Both men and women can experience dyspareunia, but it is more common in women. The nature of the pain (superficial or deep), the amount of pain, and the conditions under which it occurs are significant because the possible causes are diverse for men and women.

PATIENT SCREENING
A male or female may seek consultation because of the pain or discomfort associated with sexual intercourse. The consultation may be scheduled at the patient's convenience.

ETIOLOGY
In a woman, organic causes such as an intact *hymen,* insufficient lubrication, the presence of an STD, or the use of a spermicide may cause superficial pain during sexual intercourse. Other conditions that cause deeper pelvic pain during intercourse include *endometriosis,* PID, and the presence of cysts or tumors in the genitourinary tract or pelvis.

The condition can have a psychological basis resulting from past trauma, sexual abuse, or fears, including a fear of pregnancy. Anxiety alone can be sufficient to cause *vaginismus.* Allergic reactions to **spermicidal** creams and jellies or even to semen can cause irritation, itching, and burning.

In a man, causes of dyspareunia may include anatomic abnormalities, such as a "bowed" erection, a tight foreskin, or prostatitis. Lesions on the penis and urethritis secondary to an STD are other causes. Anxiety or guilt often point to psychosexual dysfunction as the root of the problem.

DIAGNOSIS
A careful history of the type and nature of the pain experienced during intercourse is significant. A physical examination, with laboratory tests depending on the possible causes, helps to determine the basis of the dyspareunia.

TREATMENT
Treatment of male or female dyspareunia is based on the cause. The use of lubricants during intercourse or a gentle stretching of the vaginal opening helps in some cases. Underlying conditions such as infection are treated. In more complex situations, corrective surgery may be required. The patient may be advised to address any psychosexual dysfunctions through counseling.

PROGNOSIS
The prognosis is highly variable. Eliminating functional and psychological causes is effective in improving dyspareunia.

PREVENTION
Early intervention may shorten the duration of the condition.

PATIENT TEACHING
The course of treatment determines the type of information offered to the patient.

Erectile Dysfunction/Impotence

DESCRIPTION
Erectile dysfunction/impotence is a consistent inability to achieve or maintain penile erection.

ICD-9-CM Code 607.84 *(Impotence of organic origin)*
302.72 *(Inhibited sexual excitement)*
Impotence is coded by specific disorders. Refer to the physician's diagnosis and then to the current edition of the ICD-9-CM coding manual to ensure the greatest specificity of pathology and any appropriate modifiers.

SYMPTOMS AND SIGNS
Erectile dysfunction (ED/impotence) is the inability of a man to perform sexual intercourse, usually because he is unable to attain or maintain an erection

of the penis sufficient for satisfactory sexual activity. It is a common disorder, affecting most men at some time during their lives. The condition can be temporary or may become chronic.

PATIENT SCREENING

A complete physical examination or a private consultation may be scheduled.

ETIOLOGY

Sexual arousal causes the arteries in the penis to relax and dilate, thus allowing an increased blood flow to the penis. The expansion and hardening of the penis cause a compression of the veins carrying blood away from the penis, resulting in an erection. Anything that impedes the nerve response or that alters the necessary pattern of blood flow results in failure of an erection.

ED/impotence often has a psychological basis in depression, unconscious guilt, or some kind of anxiety about sex. Sexual trauma, repressed inhibitions, depression, stress, and discordant relationships are other possible contributing factors. Chronic fatigue and stress also can impair sexual function.

Many physical or medical conditions can play a significant role in ED. Medical conditions affecting the blood vessels and restricting blood flow to the penis include diabetes mellitus, hypertension, heart disease, and hypercholesterolemia. Neurologic elements, such as nerve insult resulting from prostate surgery and spinal cord, pelvic, or perineal trauma, may interrupt the impulse transmission between the central nervous system and the penis. Medications prescribed to treat hypertension and depression can have a side effect of ED. Other common offenders are alcohol, recreational drugs, antihistamines, and diuretics.

DIAGNOSIS

A medical history and physical examination to reveal any underlying medical causative factors are necessary. The history should include the disease history of the patient and his family members, including diabetes mellitus, hypertension, heart disease, cerebral vascular accidents, spinal cord injuries, and vascular or renal disease; any surgery or trauma to the pelvic area; medications that the patient currently is or previously has taken; lifestyle, including smoking habits and alcohol consumption; stress levels; and relationship with sexual part-

ner. Laboratory tests to rule out organic disease help the physician make the diagnosis.

TREATMENT

The treatment sometimes is as simple as changing or discontinuing medications being taken. Testosterone therapy is used for men with androgen deficiency. Other courses of remedies are more complex and take time, such as programs for substance abuse or psychological counseling. Interventions such as psychoanalysis, discussion, behavioral modification, and sensate exercises are aimed at restoring the patient's ability to complete the entire sexual response cycle. Other approaches include penile implants, external vacuum devices, and penile injection therapy.

A more recent approach is oral drug therapy with sildenafil citrate (Viagra). During sexual stimulation, nitric oxide is released in the corpus cavernosum, initiating an enzymatic cascade, ultimately resulting in relaxation of the smooth muscle of the corpus cavernosum and an inflow of blood. Sildenafil citrate increases the effect of nitrous oxide, consequently helping the male to have an erection satisfactory for desired sexual activity. Sexual stimulation is needed for sildenafil citrate to assist with the erection, and at the recommended dosage, it has no effect in the absence of sexual stimulation.

PROGNOSIS

The prognosis varies greatly with the cause. Effective therapy is available in many cases. The prevalence increases with advancing age.

PREVENTION

Impotence is usually secondary to one of many diseases and conditions.

PATIENT TEACHING

If the cause is psychogenic, refer the patient to counseling. Other patient teaching is directed toward treating the organic cause.

Frigidity

DESCRIPTION

Frigidity is the lack of sexual desire or response in a woman. It is viewed as a dysfunction if the woman is dissatisfied or frustrated.

■ **ICD-9-CM Code 302.72**

SYMPTOMS AND SIGNS

Some women experience symptoms of mild to severe depression. The patient may report an inability to experience sexual arousal and excitement or to achieve orgasm.

PATIENT SCREENING

Schedule a private consultation with the healthcare provider.

ETIOLOGY

Underlying medical problems rarely can cause nerve damage that results in frigidity. More common contributing factors include specific medications being taken, chronic fatigue, stress, and depression. More complicated psychological causes such as rape and past sexual abuse are possible.

DIAGNOSIS

A physical examination with a medical and sexual history should help to identify any physical or psychological causes.

TREATMENT

When the dysfunction is primary, proper stimulation or the use of sensate focus exercises may be all that is required to solve the problem. Inhibited female orgasm can stem from a psychological obstacle, such as a troubled relationship between the partners. In this case, a behaviorist approach of counseling both partners may bring positive results and fulfillment. Drug therapy for loss of sexual interest involves the use of testosterone cream, which helps increase libido.

PROGNOSIS

After any causes have been addressed and treated, good results are expected.

PREVENTION

There is no specific prevention.

PATIENT TEACHING

Assure the patient that behavior modification helps many women with psychological sexual dysfunction.

Premature Ejaculation

DESCRIPTION

Premature ejaculation is a condition in which ejaculation occurs before a suitable time.

 ICD-9-CM Code 302.75

SYMPTOMS AND SIGNS

When a man regularly ejaculates during foreplay or after only a minimal amount of stimulation, he may be unable to satisfy his partner or impregnate a woman. The problem is fairly common in young men and is not serious.

PATIENT SCREENING

Advise the patient to make an appointment for a consultation with the physician.

 A L E R T

PRECAUTIONS CONCERNING SILDENAFIL CITRATE (VIAGRA)

Men in whom underlying cardiovascular disease has made sexual activity inadvisable should not take sildenafil citrate (Viagra). In addition, men who have had a heart attack, stroke, or life-threatening arrhythmia in the past 6 months also are warned not to take this drug. Other factors that preclude the use of sildenafil citrate include a history of hypotension, hypertension, unstable angina, or retinitis pigmentosa, and any anatomic deformity of the penis.

Side effects may include headache, flushing, stomach pain, or mild temporary vision changes, including changes in color perception and blurred vision. Men are advised to take the smallest possible dose to achieve an erection. In addition, experiencing a prolonged erection (more than 4 hours) is an indication to notify a physician.

Any male experiencing chest pain after taking sildenafil citrate should seek immediate emergency medical assistance and should advise emergency personnel of the use of sildenafil citrate. Furthermore, concurrent use of any form of nitrate drug therapy or short-acting nitrate drug may initiate life-threatening hypotension.

ETIOLOGY

Premature ejaculation often has a psychological basis that may stem from guilt or anxiety. A troubled or negative relationship with the sex partner could contribute. Certain diseases such as infections and degenerative neurologic conditions are possible causes.

DIAGNOSIS

The diagnosis is based on the patient history and a medical evaluation with a physical examination and laboratory tests to rule out pathologic conditions. All factors that affect stimulation during foreplay and ejaculation are considered.

TREATMENT

Any underlying physical causes are treated, and psychological factors are addressed. Certain techniques that help delay ejaculation or control male stimulation during lovemaking are suggested to the female partner. This allows more time for the woman to reach orgasm and enables ejaculation to occur after penetration of the vagina.

PROGNOSIS

The prognosis is usually good with behavior modification and when the underlying condition, if any, is treated.

PREVENTION

No specific prevention is known.

PATIENT TEACHING

The treatment plan may require referral for counseling, behavior modification, or treatment for any organic condition.

Male and Female Infertility

DESCRIPTION

Infertility may be defined as the involuntary inability to conceive.

 ICD-9-CM Code **606.9** *(Male infertility)*
628.9 *(Female infertility)*

SIGNS AND SYMPTOMS

With regular, unprotected intercourse, about 90% of couples conceive within 1 year. The inability of a couple to conceive can originate from female fac-

tors, male factors, or both. In about 40% of cases the male causes infertility; in remaining cases various female factors are found to be the cause, with less than 10% of cases unexplained.

PATIENT SCREENING

Both partners should be scheduled for a complete medical evaluation.

ETIOLOGY

In a man, insufficient number or motility of sperm can cause infertility. The presence of an STD or any infection or blockage in the genitourinary tract is another familiar cause. Less often, structural anomalies, genetic diseases, and endocrine disorders result in sterility. The presence of a **varicocele** can reduce the sperm count. Finally, other causes include injuries that affect the blood or nerve supply, radiation exposure, exposure to pollutants, chronic stress, and hormonal imbalances.

In a woman, the causes include:

- STDs or other infections of the reproductive organs
- Ovulatory dysfunction or failure to ovulate
- Blocked fallopian tubes
- Congenital structural or chromosomal disorders
- Scar tissue from infection, ectopic pregnancy, or surgery
- Tumors
- Endometriosis
- Antisperm antibodies in the female vaginal secretions
- Medications that compromise fertility

DIAGNOSIS

After a physical examination and an interview of both partners, specific testing procedures are chosen. The cause of infertility sometimes is identified quickly and easily. If not, the clinical observation and therapeutic approaches can become time-consuming and expensive.

In men, a complete history, with special attention to childhood diseases, is followed by a thorough physical examination for any structural abnormalities. Semen analysis is essential. Genetic and endocrine disorders are ruled out.

In women, ovulatory function is established by charting of the menstrual cycle. Hormone levels are studied through blood tests. The fallopian tubes and uterine cavity are visualized through

hysterosalpingography to determine tubal patency. In some cases, **laparoscopy** may be necessary to rule out endometriosis or chronic infection.

TREATMENT

Each treatment plan is individual, depending on the problems that surface in the medical and psychological evaluation. Unless the condition is untreatable, the course of action to achieve pregnancy may include treatment of infection, surgery to remove blockage, and the use of fertility drugs (e.g., clomiphene, follitropin) or artificial insemination.

PROGNOSIS

About half of the couples who seek treatment for infertility do achieve pregnancy. Some have untreatable causes or take as long as 3 years to achieve pregnancy.

PREVENTION

When possible, preventing the causative factors that lead to sterility is preferable. Methods of preventing male infertility include regular physical examinations and protection of the testicles during athletics. Early and complete treatment of any sexually transmitted disease is important for men and women.

PATIENT TEACHING

Much of the patient teaching involves answering questions about the complexity of the medical evaluation and the selected therapeutic approach.

Male Reproductive Diseases

The most common diseases of the male reproductive system are those affecting the prostate gland. The gland can become inflamed or enlarged as a result of bacteria and cause urinary problems. Common symptoms are:

- Any urinary symptoms, such as frequency, urgency, incontinence, and dysuria
- Pain, swelling, or enlargement of any of the reproductive organs
- Any sexual dysfunction, such as erectile dysfunction (ED/impotence)

Epididymitis

DESCRIPTION

Epididymitis is inflammation of the epididymis, the excretory duct of the testicles.

 ICD-9-CM Code 604.90 *(Unspecified)*
The above code may be valid as a principal diagnosis. Use an additional code to identify the causative organism. Refer to the physician's diagnosis and then to the current edition of the ICD-9-CM coding manual to ensure the greatest specificity of pathology and any appropriate modifiers.

SYMPTOMS AND SIGNS

Symptoms of inflammation of the epididymis can include fever, *malaise,* and pain. The epididymis may become enlarged, tender, and hard. The patient may have groin and scrotal tenderness with severe pain in the testes. Walking may be difficult for the patient, as he tries to protect a painful scrotum.

PATIENT SCREENING

The patient often experiences great discomfort during the acute phase, requiring a same-day appointment if possible.

ETIOLOGY

N. gonorrhoeae and *C. trachomatis* are the most common causes of epididymitis. *Escherichia coli, Staphylococcus,* and *Streptococcus* are other bacterial causes of this condition. Epididymitis also can result from a urinary tract infection, prostatitis, and STDs such as gonorrhea and syphilis. Tuberculosis, mumps, removal of the prostate gland (**prostatectomy**), trauma, and the prolonged use of an indwelling catheter also may predispose the patient to epididymitis.

DIAGNOSIS

Physical examination, urinalysis, and urine cultures are used to make the diagnosis of epididymitis. The patient also may have an elevated *white blood cell (WBC) count.*

TREATMENT

Antibiotic treatment combined with the administration of *analgesics,* rest, and the avoidance of alcohol and spicy foods is beneficial. Use of a scrotal support also may help. Epididymitis usually responds well to treatment. Scarring may occur, which can lead to sterility, if treatment is delayed. This is especially true if the disease is bilateral.

PROGNOSIS
The prognosis is usually good with early treatment. The possible complications include sterility.

PREVENTION
The best prevention for epididymitis is the early treatment of urinary tract infections. Condom use during sexual intercourse also is recommended.

PATIENT TEACHING
Advise the use of comfort measures including ice packs, scrotal support, lightweight clothing, and elevation of the scrotum while at rest. List warning signs of complications: increased pain, swelling, or discharge.

Orchitis

DESCRIPTION
Orchitis is infection of the testis.

 ICD-9-CM Code 604.90 *(Unspecified)*
The above code may be valid as a principal diagnosis. Use an additional code to identify the causative organism. Refer to the physician's diagnosis and then to the current edition of the ICD-9-CM coding manual to ensure the greatest specificity of pathology and the appropriate modifiers.

SYMPTOMS AND SIGNS
Inflammation of the testes is caused by viral or bacterial infection or injury. It may affect one or both testes, causing swelling, tenderness, and acute pain. The patient also may experience chills, fever, nausea, vomiting, and general malaise.

PATIENT SCREENING
Prompt treatment is indicated to alleviate pain and begin appropriate antibiotic therapy.

ETIOLOGY
Orchitis may be a consequence of infection from the mumps virus. Other viruses and bacteria also can cause this condition, and it may follow epididymitis. Acute infection is frequently associ-

ated with a sexually transmitted disease. About one half of severe cases result in atrophy of the affected testicle. If both sides are affected, sterility results.

DIAGNOSIS
Urinalysis, *serologic* study, or throat cultures may be used to isolate or identify causative agents, such as the mumps virus. Taking a clinical history to determine the patient's exposure to mumps or other related disease may be beneficial.

TREATMENT
If the orchitis is bacterial, appropriate antibiotic treatment should be started immediately. The mumps virus–induced orchitis has no specific treatment. Bed rest usually is prescribed, along with certain adrenal steroid drugs to reduce fever and swelling in severe cases. The use of a scrotal support also may help.

PROGNOSIS
Healing follows successful treatment with antibiotics, but scarring may compromise fertility.

PREVENTION
Risk factors for sexually transmitted disease should be avoided. To prevent orchitis related to mumps virus, all adult men who have not had a clinical case of mumps should be vaccinated.

PATIENT TEACHING
Emphasize the importance of finishing the entire course of antibiotics as prescribed. Suggest comfort measures such as scrotal support and the use of ice packs.

Torsion of the Testicle

DESCRIPTION
Torsion of the testicle is a condition in which one testicle is twisted out of its normal position (Fig. 12–10, *A*).

 ICD-9-CM Code 608.2

SYMPTOMS AND SIGNS
The primary symptom is a sudden, severe pain in one testicle. The pain can be so severe that it causes nausea and even vomiting. When the torsion occurs, the scrotum becomes swollen, red, and tender. Torsion can cause the blood vessels supplying

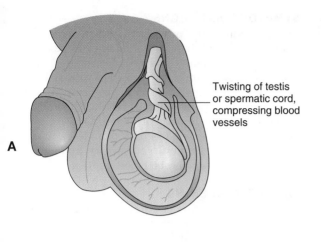

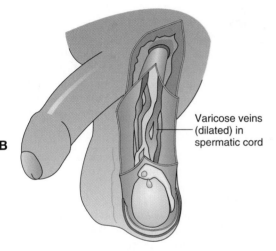

Twisting of testis
or spermatic cord,
compressing blood
vessels

A

Varicose veins
(dilated) in
spermatic cord

B

FIGURE 12-10 A, Torsion of testis. **B,** Varicocele. (From Gould B: *Pathophysiology for the health professions,* ed 2, Philadelphia, 2002, Saunders.)

the testicle to become kinked, which in turn prevents blood flow to and from the affected testicle.

PATIENT SCREENING
Emergency treatment is required.

ETIOLOGY
This condition occurs when the testis rotates on the spermatic cord, causing a sudden, extreme twist or torsion. It can happen spontaneously or as a result of trauma. The arteries and veins are compressed, ischemia develops, and the scrotum swells.

DIAGNOSIS
Diagnosis is based on the patient history and a gentle physical examination by the physician. Because symptoms of testicular torsion and epididymitis are similar, an ultrasound may be performed to determine whether testicular torsion is the cause of the pain and swelling.

TREATMENT
Gentle manipulation may be tried to untwist the testicle. No treatment is needed if the testicle can somehow untwist itself. Immediate relief from the pain and swelling follows. If this does not occur, surgery is necessary. Delaying surgery can result in permanent damage to the testicle.

PROGNOSIS
The prognosis is good if treatment is received promptly when the torsion does not correct itself. Even if the condition corrects itself, and pain is relieved, the torsion may recur. With surgery, the testicle is untwisted and stitched into position so that the problem cannot recur.

PREVENTION
No prevention is known.

PATIENT TEACHING
Surgical intervention, if necessary, is on an emergency basis. Give as much preoperative help as possible by answering questions and giving direction to the patient or family. The patient also will need information about postoperative care.

Varicocele

DESCRIPTION
In varicocele, the veins of one of the testicles become abnormally distended, causing swelling around the testicle that expands within the scrotal sac (Fig.12–10, *B*).

 ICD-9-CM Code 456.4

SYMPTOMS AND SIGNS
This is a rather mild disorder that is more uncomfortable than painful. A varicocele may be especially uncomfortable in hot weather or after exercise and may be relieved temporarily by lying down. Because the increased presence of venous blood raises the temperature within the scrotum, varicocele may contribute to a lower sperm count.

PATIENT SCREENING

The condition often is asymptomatic. If a vein ruptures as a result of local injury, pain and swelling in the scrotum cause the patient to seek prompt medical intervention.

ETIOLOGY

Varicocele has no apparent cause or prevention. It may be congenital and usually occurs in the 15- to 25-year-old age group.

DIAGNOSIS

The patient history, physical symptoms, and an examination by the physician confirm the diagnosis.

TREATMENT

Treatment consists of measures to relieve the symptoms. These can include the wearing of tight-fitting underwear or the use of an athletic supporter. If the varicocele affects fertility, surgery can remove the distended veins, but the results may not justify the risks of the surgery. Results vary and depend on the severity of the distention.

PROGNOSIS

In some cases surgical repair has been reported to improve fertility.

PREVENTION

No prevention is known.

PATIENT TEACHING

Encourage the patient to use comfort measures to relieve the symptoms. If the patient undergoes surgical repair, review the postoperative care.

Prostatitis

DESCRIPTION

Prostatitis is acute or chronic inflammation of the prostate gland.

> ICD-9-CM Code **601.0** *(Acute)*
> **601.1** *(Chronic)*
> *Refer to the physician's diagnosis and then to the current edition of the ICD-9-CM coding manual to ensure the greatest specificity of pathology and any appropriate modifiers for the causative organism, such as Staphylococcus (041.1) or Streptococcus (041.0).*

SYMPTOMS AND SIGNS

Inflammation of the prostate gland is more common in men older than 50 years. The prostate may be enlarged and tender, and in some instances, pus may be seen at the tip of the penis. The patient may be asymptomatic or may experience acute symptoms in mild or sporadic forms. He has pain and a burning sensation during urination. Other common symptoms include low back pain, fever, muscular pain or tenderness, and urinary frequency with urgency. There may be blood in the urine.

PATIENT SCREENING

When a patient presents with acute symptoms of pain and other urinary symptoms, prompt medical evaluation is indicated.

ETIOLOGY

The cause of inflammation of the prostate is usually infection but is not always known. Infection may be either bacterial or nonbacterial. Bacterial causes may include gonococci from a patient with gonorrhea, *E. coli* that has caused a urinary tract infection, *Staphylococcus, Streptococcus,* or *Pseudomonas.*

DIAGNOSIS

Urinalysis, urine culture, and a rectal examination are used to diagnose prostatitis.

TREATMENT

The usual treatment is *antimicrobial* penicillin therapy. Other medications used are Bactrim DS, levofloxacin (Levaquin), and ciprofloxacin (Cipro) for chronic prostatitis. The physician also may order sitz baths, rest, an increase in fluid intake, and the administration of analgesics.

Chronic prostatitis has the potential to develop from recurrent urinary tract infection, urethral obstruction, and acute urinary retention.

PROGNOSIS

The prognosis for acute prostatitis is good because it responds well to treatment. The outlook for chronic prostatitis is not as favorable. Complications such as epididymitis, cystitis, and urethritis can occur.

PREVENTION

The best prevention for prostatitis is the early treatment of urinary tract infections with the prescribed antibiotics.

PATIENT TEACHING

Emphasize the need for strict adherence to the prescribed medications. Encourage the practice of comfort measures ordered by the physician. (See Treatment.)

Benign Prostatic Hyperplasia (BPH)

DESCRIPTION

BPH is nonmalignant, noninflammatory hypertrophy of the prostrate gland.

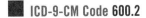 **ICD-9-CM Code 600.2**

SYMPTOMS AND SIGNS

Enlargement of the prostate gland is a common condition in men older than 50 years, and the frequency increases with age. BPH usually progresses to the point of causing compression of the urethra with urinary obstruction (Fig. 12–11). Common signs and symptoms may include difficulty in starting urination, a weak stream of urine, or inability to empty the bladder completely. Urinary frequency, including nocturia, or fecal incontinence, and in severe cases, inflammation and symptoms of renal disease, have been seen.

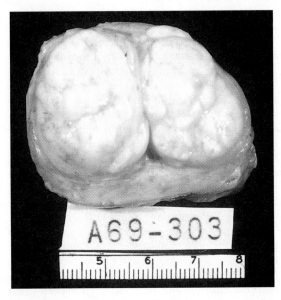

FIGURE 12–11 Benign prostatic hyperplasia. (From Kumar V, Cotran RS, et al: *Robbins basic pathology,* ed 7, Philadelphia, 2003, Saunders.)

PATIENT SCREENING

A routine physical examination is appropriate to evaluate the BPH.

ETIOLOGY

The cause of benign prostatic hyperplasia (BPH) is not completely understood, but the condition seems to be associated with the aging process and hormonal and metabolic changes. As the prostate gland enlarges, it compresses either the neck of the bladder or the urethra, causing obstruction of the urinary flow.

DIAGNOSIS

The usual diagnosis is based on the patient history and a rectal examination by a physician. To confirm the diagnosis, the physician may order a urinalysis, urine culture, *intravenous pyelogram* (IVP), or a cystoscopy.

TREATMENT

Treatment of BPH may be symptomatic and include sitz baths, catheterization, and massage of the prostate gland. Drug therapy with alpha-adrenergic blockers, including tamsulosin hydrochloride (Flomax), doxazosin mesylate (Cardura), and terazosin hydrochloride (Hytrin), may be prescribed to relax the tightened muscles inside the prostate and relieve symptoms; finasteride (Proscar), which has been claimed to shrink the enlarged prostate gland, may be prescribed in some cases. A surgical treatment, transurethral resection, may be performed to remove any urinary tract obstruction.

PROGNOSIS

The prognosis for BPH is good with intervention. If it is left untreated, however, infection may reach the kidneys. Complications of this condition may include cystitis, dilation of the ureters, *pyelonephritis, hydronephrosis,* and uremia.

PREVENTION

Prevention of benign prostatic hyperplasia is unknown. Physicians highly recommend that older men have regular prostate examinations to detect any enlargement.

PATIENT TEACHING

Inform the patient that ingestion of decongestants, antidepressants, tranquilizers, alcohol, and *anticholinergics* tends to increase urinary obstruction.

If a prostatectomy is scheduled, review the physician's explanation of the procedure, and give the patient appropriate information about presurgical and postsurgical care.

Prostate Cancer

DESCRIPTION

Prostate cancer is a malignancy of the small gland located below the bladder and anterior to the rectum in males, known as the prostate gland. Although this is a very common cancer, it grows so slowly that only 3% of men with prostate cancer will die from it. Nonetheless, prostate cancer is the second-leading cause of cancer death in men (Fig. 12–12).

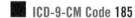 **ICD-9-CM Code 185**

SYMPTOMS AND SIGNS

Prostate cancer is often asymptomatic at diagnosis and is detected clinically by abnormalities on routine digital rectal exam (DRE) or by a high concentration of *prostate specific antigen* (PSA) in the serum. Asymmetric areas of induration and nodules felt on DRE suggest prostate cancer, and malignant prostate tissue generates more PSA than normal or hyperplastic tissue do. (Refer to Table 12–1 for PSA Values.) The usual symptoms, when

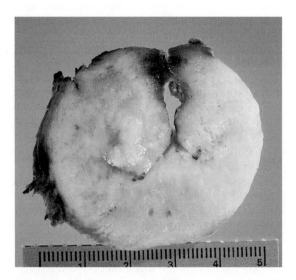

FIGURE 12–12 Cancer of the prostate. (From Kumar V, Cotran RS, et al: *Robbins basic pathology,* ed 7, Philadelphia, 2003, Saunders.)

present, are those associated with urinary obstruction. These include weak or interrupted urine flow, urinary frequency, difficulty starting or stopping urine flow, urinary retention, dysuria, and hematuria. However, these symptoms also often are common to BPH or an infection or inflammation of the prostate gland. New onset of erectile dysfunction also should raise suspicion for prostate cancer.

PATIENT SCREENING

Schedule a physical examination with screening for prostate cancer, annually, at age 50 or over or when a patient reports dysuria or blood in the urine.

ETIOLOGY

Risk factors for prostate cancer include age, heredity, and lifestyle. Prostate cancer is more common in older men and rarely occurs before age 45. Ethnicity is also important, as prostate tumors are much more common in black men than in white or Hispanic men. This may be because black men generally have a higher serum testosterone level than men of other races. Risk is also higher in men who have a particular, heritable mutation in the BRCA1 or BRCA2 genes (breast cancer susceptibility genes). Dietary risk factors include a diet high in animal fat, low in vegetables, or low in selenium.

DIAGNOSIS

Although abnormally high PSA level and abnormal DRE are highly suggestive findings, prostate biopsy is necessary for a cancer diagnosis. A biopsy is advised if the PSA level is greater than 10 ng/ml. A transrectal ultrasound-guided biopsy that takes samples from suspicious areas, as well as six core tissue specimens, is usually performed. If the biopsy is negative but the PSA level remains high, a repeat biopsy is performed 6 to 8 weeks later. Up to 25% of prostate cancers are missed on initial biopsy. If a biopsy specimen is found to contain carcinoma, further evaluation and clinical staging is needed to select the appropriate treatment strategy. The TNM (Tumor, Node, Metastasis) staging system proposed by the American Joint Committee on Cancer is the most popular method used for staging. Clinical staging uses a DRE, a PSA measurement, a radionuclide bone scan (not performed unless extension beyond the prostate is suspected), abdominal and pelvic CT scans, and an intravenous pyelogram (IVP). Analysis of the tumor histology (the Gleason grade) leads to a scoring system based on the degree of glandular differentiation and structural architecture. The Gleason score produces an index of prognosis and may also guide local therapy.

TREATMENT

Treatment of prostate cancer depends on the stage of the disease, the Gleason score, the PSA level, the age and physical condition of the patient, and risks and benefits of each treatment option. Surgical interventions include radical prostatectomy and transurethral resection of the prostate (TURP). Radical prostatectomy has potential complications of ED/impotence and urinary incontinence. Hormone therapy describes any treatment that reduces the amount of androgen hormones in the body or prevents the body from responding to them as a method to inhibit growth of cancer cells. Methods used include *orchiectomy* (surgical removal of a testicle) or use of drugs such as luteinizing hormone releasing hormone (LHRH) antagonists, which act to stop the production of testosterone. Radiation therapy may be tried to kill cancer cells and shrink tumors. Watchful waiting and careful observation without aggressive intervention is sometimes considered for men older than 70 years, those with significant coexisting illnesses, and those who fear the side effects of the more aggressive approaches. For patients with metastatic prostate cancer, hormone therapy is the primary mode of treatment. Eventually most men will stop responding to hormone therapy, and a second type of hormone therapy or chemotherapy usually is tried. Regardless of the therapy selected and the disease stage, patients should be followed up with a PSA measurement and DRE every 6 to 12 months to monitor the efficacy of treatment and to detect recurrences.

PROGNOSIS

The most important predictors of disease progression are TNM stage, Gleason score of the biopsy specimen, and serum PSA level. For early-stage tumors, radiation therapy and prostatectomy offer similar 10-year survival rates. Watchful waiting is less successful unless the patient is over the age of 70 or 75 and has a low Gleason score. The overall 5-year survival rate is 96% because many prostate cancers are diagnosed in early stages as a result of current screening procedures. The survival rate declines, however, with longer follow-up. The 10-year survival rate of men with cancer confined to the prostate gland is 75%; with locally advanced disease, 55%; and with metastatic disease, 15%.

PREVENTION

Widespread screening of PSA has led to the increased detection of prostate cancer while it is still confined to the capsule and therefore curable. Clinicians should explain to male patients the benefits of early detection of prostate cancer, the risk of false-positive and false-negative results, and the significant risks associated with aggressive treatment should prostate cancer be detected. Screening consists of annual DRE and serum PSA measurement, followed by transrectal ultrasound-guided prostate biopsy if either test is positive. Screening should be offered annually, beginning at age 50, to men who have a life expectancy of at least 10 years. Men considered to be at high risk for prostate cancer (African-American males and men with two or more first-degree relatives with prostate cancer) should begin screening at age 45. Primary chemoprevention, the use of drugs to reduce hormone levels in the body to reduce the likelihood of cancer development, may be an option for men at very high risk.

TABLE 12-1	
Prostate Specific Antigen (PSA) Values—Acceptable Levels by Age*	
AGE (YR)	**ACCEPTABLE LEVELS**
Up to 40	0-2 ng/ml
40-50	0-4 ng/ml
50-60	0-5 ng/ml
60-70	0-6 ng/ml

* PSA blood tests are reported as ng/ml.
PSA is considered a marker in the screening for prostatic cancer. Zero to 4 ng/ml usually is considered to be in the normal range; 4-10 ng/ml is considered borderline; and values >10 ng/ml are considered high. Increasing age makes slightly higher values acceptable.
Any increase of 20% or more in the PSA value in 1 year is suspicious and requires further investigation.
The PSA screening is to be completed before the digital rectal examination. A constant increase in the PSA leads to suspicion of prostate cancer. PSA levels that fluctuate up and down usually do not indicate cancer but an inflammatory process in the prostate or benign prostatic hypertrophy. PSA is a screening tool and must be combined with a digital rectal examination for a more accurate screen. Men older than 50 are encouraged to have prostate screening annually.

PATIENT TEACHING

Emphasize the importance of annual screening for prostate cancer after age 50. Describe and explain diagnostic procedures. Review the information given by the physician about the mode of treatment and likely side effects. Explain the warning signs of complications that should be reported to the physician. Encourage the patient to ask questions and voice concerns about sexual function and prognosis.

Testicular Cancer

DESCRIPTION

The testicles are the male gonads that produce sperm and are the primary source of male hormones. Cancer of the testicle is one of the most curable solid neoplasms, but it still has a significant effect on the economic and emotional status of the young population it usually affects. Nearly all testicular tumors are germ cell tumors (GCT), equally distributed between two main types: seminomas and all others, termed nonseminomatous germ cell tumors (NSGCT).

■ ICD-9-CM Code **186.9**

SYMPTOMS AND SIGNS

The most common presentation is a nodule or painless swelling of one testicle. Some patients complain of a dull ache or a heavy sensation in the abdomen, perianal area, or scrotum. Fewer patients have acute pain or *gynecomastia*. The tumor may cause *oligospermia* leading to infertility. Symptoms of advanced disease include neck mass, dyspnea, anorexia, bone pain, and lower-extremity swelling.

PATIENT SCREENING

When a patient reports any nodule or swelling of a testicle, schedule him for a medical evaluation at the next available appointment.

ETIOLOGY

Testicular neoplasms are most common in males between the ages of 20 and 35 (Fig. 12–13). The incidence of testicular cancer varies geographically, with the highest incidence in Scandinavia, Germany, Switzerland, and New Zealand, and the lowest incidence in Africa and Asia. Risk factors include *cryptorchidism* (undescended testicle), a personal family history of testicular cancer, previous GCT, infertility, and HIV infection. Down syndrome and Klinefelter syndrome may predispose affected males to development of testicular cancer.

DIAGNOSIS

Diagnosis begins with physical examination of the testes and palpation for nodal involvement. Any firm, hard area in the affected testis is cause for concern. The diagnostic evaluation of suspected testicular cancer continues with scrotal ultrasound, CT scan of the abdomen and pelvis, chest radiograph, and measurement of serum tumor markers. Radical orchiectomy also is performed to create a histologic evaluation of the tumor. Biopsy is not attempted because of the risk of causing tumor spread. In young men for whom future fertility is an issue, efforts should be made to perform a baseline sperm count and sperm banking before radiographic procedures so that radiation does not damage the sperm. Serum tumor markers that are elevated in many testicular cancers are alpha fetoprotein (AFP), the beta subunit of human chorionic gonadotropin (alpha-hCG), and lactate dehydrogenase (LDH). These markers help in initial diagnosis, but they are more useful for subsequent disease follow-up.

A TNM (Tumor, Node, Metastasis) staging system for testicular cancer was recently developed by the American Joint Committee on Cancer. It considers the primary tumor, nodal involvement, and distant metastases as well as the serum tumor

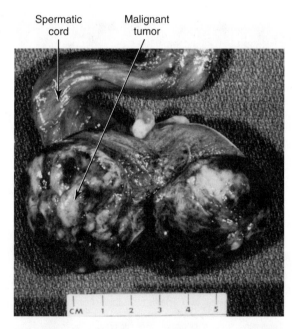

FIGURE 12–13 Cancer of the testes. (Courtesy of Shaw RW, North York General Hospital, Toronto, Ontario, Canada. In Gould B: *Pathophysiology for the health professions*, ed 2, Philadelphia, 2002, Saunders.)

marker values for AFP, alpha-hCG, and LDH. These parameters define stage groupings from I to III that define good, intermediate, and poor prognosis, respectively. The staging system applies to both seminomas and NSGCTs.

TREATMENT

Radical orchiectomy of the affected testicle is performed to aid in diagnosis and staging. Testicular germ cell tumors are highly chemosensitive. Cisplatin-based combination chemotherapy can cure up to 80% of patients, even those with distant metastases. For those with advanced disease, residual masses may remain after chemotherapy. Surgical resection may be performed to excise the masses, remove any histologically malignant elements, and prevent compression of adjacent structures. Seminomas often are radiosensitive, so the patient may be treated with radiation therapy. For men with elevated levels of a serum tumor marker, monitoring the level throughout treatment often produces the best indicator of treatment effectiveness.

As a result of the high cure rate for testicular cancer, posttreatment follow-up is an important part of the care for these patients. Periodic follow-up includes history and physical exam, serum tumor marker measurement, and radiographic studies for a minimum of 5 years after orchiectomy. The optimal surveillance schedule is determined by tumor type and pretreatment disease stage.

PROGNOSIS

Patients with good (60% of GCTs), intermediate (26% of GCTs), and poor (14% of GCTs) prognosis are defined by the stage groupings. Good prognosis carries a 5-year survival rate of 91%, intermediate carries a rate of 79%, and poor carries a 5-year survival rate of 48%. Factors that affect the prognosis include initial serum concentration of tumor markers, time between diagnosis and treatment, age of the patient, extent of visceral organ involvement, and number of distant metastases.

PREVENTION

Males with unilateral postpubertal abdominal cryptorchidism are urged to undergo prophylactic orchiectomy. Men with a history of cryptorchidism should undergo a biopsy of both testes at age 18 to 20 years to test for carcinoma in situ. Monthly testicular self-exam is the most reliable screening method for detecting a testicular tumor. Males at high risk for testicular cancer, especially those with a previous history of a germ-cell tumor, should perform a monthly testicular self-exam to look for abnormal growth or nodules.

PATIENT TEACHING

Review appropriate preventive measures listed previously, and emphasize the importance of monthly self-examination. Explain all diagnostic and treatment procedures. Review the physician's explanations and encourage questions. Give the patient information about fertility and sexual potency. Emphasize the importance of the long-term surveillance schedule.

Female Reproductive Diseases

The female reproductive organs are affected by disease in several ways. First, microorganisms can invade the organs, allowing infections to develop. Second, tumors, both benign and malignant, and cysts can develop in the reproductive organs. Common symptoms are:

- Any abnormal vaginal discharge or itching
- Lower pelvic or abdominal pain
- Menstrual symptoms, such as pain (**dysmenorrhea**), absence of menstruation (**amenorrhea**), scanty menstruation (oligomenorrhea), irregular menstruation (**metrorrhagia**), and heavy menstrual flow (**menorrhagia**)
- Fever
- Pain during sexual intercourse (dyspareunia) or any sexual dysfunction

Premenstrual Syndrome

DESCRIPTION

Premenstrual syndrome (PMS) is a syndrome of physical and emotional symptoms that appear during the days immediately before the menstrual flow begins and that subside with its onset.

 ICD-9-CM Code 625.4

SYMPTOMS AND SIGNS

The female patient may notice changes that are related to the hormone levels that fluctuate monthly to prepare her for ovulation and pregnancy. Some changes, such as increased energy and sexual desire, are positive. Other symptoms, which can range from mild to severe, may be troublesome.

The most common include tension and irritability, headache, fatigue, restlessness, feelings of sadness, breast tenderness, and joint pain. Some women experience edema, a bloated feeling, and abdominal pain as well.

PATIENT SCREENING

Consultation with a physician and a pelvic examination are scheduled.

ETIOLOGY

The cause is not certain, but the disorder seems to be related to fluctuations in estrogen and progesterone. Sodium and fluid are retained. PMS occurs only in ovulating females.

DIAGNOSIS

The patient may be asked to observe and record her menstrual symptoms monthly. There are no specific medical tests to diagnose PMS, but blood testing may be performed to rule out general medical problems. Symptoms subside within 2 to 3 hours after the onset of menses. PMS can be confused with depression.

TREATMENT

The treatment of PMS is directed toward the relief of symptoms. Reduced dietary intake of sodium, moderate exercise, the administration of mild analgesics and **diuretics,** and emotional support all help. In addition, some women notice less breast tenderness when they eliminate caffeine from their diet. In severe cases, antidepressant medication or hormone therapy (which is usually an estrogen/progesterone combination) may be indicated. Conditions such as thyroid disease, endometriosis, or a psychiatric disorder must be ruled out.

PROGNOSIS

Some cases of premenstrual syndrome tend to worsen as the woman ages and continue until after menopause. Antisocial behavior that is potentially dangerous is a possible complication of PMS.

PREVENTION

No prevention is known, apart from therapeutic intervention.

PATIENT TEACHING

Some women benefit from a stress-reduction program or counseling to better cope with symptoms. Assure the patient that an estimated 50% of menstruating women experience PMS in some form.

Amenorrhea

DESCRIPTION

The absence of menstrual periods, whether temporary or permanent, is known as amenorrhea.

 ICD-9-CM Code 626.0

SYMPTOMS AND SIGNS

This condition is classified as either primary, if menstruation has not occurred by the age of 18 years, or secondary, if a woman who has been having regular menses has a delay or absence of menstruation for a period of 6 months. Amenorrhea is normal before sexual maturity, during pregnancy, during lactation, and after menopause.

PATIENT SCREENING

A medical consultation and physical examination are indicated for a female presenting with amenorrhea.

ETIOLOGY

In primary amenorrhea, the cause is generally a late onset of puberty. It also can be caused by an abnormality in the reproductive system or hormonal imbalances. These conditions usually are not suspected unless the girl has reached 18 years of age and still is not having periods. The causes of secondary amenorrhea are mainly hormone-related. Pregnancy is one cause, but emotional factors, illness, a condition such as anorexia nervosa, malnutrition, sudden weight loss or gain, athletic training, and ovarian or pituitary tumors also may cause amenorrhea. Failure to resume menstruation at the appropriate time after childbirth can be due to postpartum pituitary necrosis, which is a failure of the pituitary gland to produce hormones.

DIAGNOSIS

The physician diagnoses amenorrhea after a thorough pelvic examination and diagnostic procedures. The pelvic examination rules out physical abnormalities and pregnancy. Blood and urine samples detect any hormonal problems, and radiographic studies, laparoscopy, and biopsy detect tumors.

TREATMENT

For primary amenorrhea, no treatment may be needed if all test results indicate that no physical abnormalities are present. If periods do not begin spontaneously, hormone therapy is used to stimulate the menstrual cycle. Secondary amenorrhea may necessitate long-term hormone therapy, when pregnancy has been ruled out.

PROGNOSIS

Neither primary nor secondary amenorrhea presents any health risks when the underlying cause can be determined and corrected.

PREVENTION

Certain preventive measures can reduce the risk of primary amenorrhea. These measures include the reduction of emotional problems, control of weight, and a balanced exercise program.

PATIENT TEACHING

Reinforce any medical regimen as prescribed and review any adverse effects of hormonal therapy that should be reported to the physician.

Dysmenorrhea

DESCRIPTION

Dysmenorrhea is pain associated with menstruation.

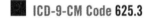 **ICD-9-CM Code 625.3**

SYMPTOMS AND SIGNS

Painful periods are one of the most frequent gynecologic problems. Primary dysmenorrhea results from factors inherent to the uterus and the process of menstruation; it is not associated with a pathologic disorder. In secondary dysmenorrhea, the woman has been having periods for longer than 3 years before she begins having pain. Symptoms range from a dull pain in the abdomen or back to sharp abdominal cramping. Pain also may radiate to the thighs and genitalia. Painful bowel or bladder function may be experienced. The symptoms are generally worse at the beginning of a period.

PATIENT SCREENING

Severe pain associated with menstruation can result in loss of time at work or inability to perform usual daily activities. The patient should be scheduled for an initial evaluation to diagnose the chief cause and select an analgesic.

ETIOLOGY

In primary dysmenorrhea, the cause is thought to be the normal hormonal changes associated with menstruation. Secondary dysmenorrhea is more likely to be caused by an underlying disorder or disease condition, including pelvic infections, fibroids, endometriosis, and cervical *stenosis*.

DIAGNOSIS

The physician makes the diagnosis after a complete patient history and pelvic examination. **Ultrasonography,** laparoscopy, and a dilation and **curettage** (D and C) also may be used to confirm the diagnosis.

TREATMENT

Nonsteroidal antiinflammatory drugs (NSAIDs), whether prescription or over the counter, are generally all that is needed for pain relief. Using a heating pad on the abdomen also may help.

Other treatment is directed toward any organic disease that is found, such as endometriosis. Fibroids and cervical stenosis may necessitate surgery. In the absence of specific pathologic conditions, the best remedy for dysmenorrhea is the use of oral contraceptives, which usually produce lighter and more regular periods.

PROGNOSIS

The prognosis for dysmenorrhea is good when the underlying causes are corrected. Primary dysmenorrhea often abates after a woman gives birth.

PREVENTION

Secondary dysmenorrhea is not preventable; brief episodes of primary dysmenorrhea are considered normal.

PATIENT TEACHING

Comfort measures are individualized in mild cases. Help the patient understand the most effective use of analgesics. When surgical repair of underlying causes is required, preoperative and postoperative instructions are explained.

Ovarian Cysts

DESCRIPTION

Ovarian cysts are fluid-filled or semi–fluid-filled sacs that form on or near the ovaries (Fig. 12–14).

 ICD-9-CM Code 620.2
Refer to the physician's diagnosis and then to the current edition of the ICD-9-CM coding manual to ensure the greatest specificity of pathology, any appropriate modifiers, and any exclusions.

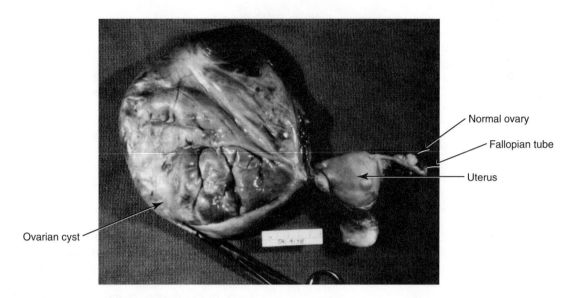

Normal ovary

Fallopian tube

Uterus

Ovarian cyst

FIGURE 12–14 Ovarian cyst. (Courtesy of Shaw RW, North York General Hospital, Toronto, Ontario, Canada. In Gould B: *Pathophysiology for the health professions,* ed 2, Philadelphia, 2002, Saunders.)

SYMPTOMS AND SIGNS

These cysts can become large before any symptoms appear. The patient may notice a painless swelling in the lower abdomen that feels firm to the touch or may experience pain during sexual intercourse. The patient may report prolonged, excessive, or irregular menses. Urinary retention can result when a large cyst presses on the area near the bladder. Vaginal bleeding or an increase in hair growth on the body may occur if a cyst affects hormone production. A cyst also can cause an ovary to twist on its blood supply, which causes severe abdominal pain, nausea, and even a fever. The risk from a torsion of an ovary is that it may rupture and cause *peritonitis.*

PATIENT SCREENING

The pain and other symptoms associated with an ovarian cyst, or possible complications, prompt the call for urgent medical intervention.

ETIOLOGY

There are two basic types of ovarian cysts: physiologic cysts (those caused by normal functioning of the ovary) and neoplastic cysts. Neoplastic cysts are either benign or malignant and are not directly related to structures normally present in the ovary.

Most ovarian cysts are physiologic, resulting from ovarian follicle growth or a corpus luteum that persists too long. They are most likely to occur from puberty to menopause. Inflammatory cysts may result from sexually transmitted diseases or after an acute infection.

DIAGNOSIS

A pelvic mass may be noted during a pelvic and rectal examination. An ultrasonogram is performed to view the ovaries indirectly. Laparoscopy with direct vision of the ovaries or even surgical removal may be appropriate if cysts are not physiologic because cancer must be ruled out.

TREATMENT

Benign physiologic cysts are common, and small cysts seldom require any treatment. Large cysts sometimes can be drained during laparoscopy or can even be removed. This often can be performed without affecting the ovary. Cysts that are drained are more likely to recur than those that are removed. Small physiologic cysts usually disappear spontaneously. Several months of oral contraceptive therapy (birth control pills) often resolve larger physiologic cysts without surgery.

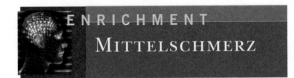

ENRICHMENT
MITTELSCHMERZ

MITTELSCHMERZ IS THE TERM applied to unilateral pain occurring in the region of an ovary during ovulation, usually midway through the menstrual cycle. This dull pain has a duration of a few minutes to a few hours and can indicate the time of ovulation for couples attempting to conceive.

Although the etiology is unknown, a leakage of follicular fluid into the abdomen during ovulation may be the cause. The pain occasionally is severe enough for the woman to seek medical care. A history of occurrence at the midpoint of the menstrual cycle and the elimination of other pelvic or abdominal causes lead to the diagnosis of mittelschmerz. Mild analgesics provide pain relief.

PROGNOSIS

Ovarian cysts that require therapeutic management are monitored for position and size. The prognosis for cysts that are not related to malignancy is excellent.

PREVENTION

No prevention is known.

PATIENT TEACHING

Explain the nature of the cyst. Encourage the patient to use the analgesic medication as prescribed for comfort. Offer appropriate assurance about the prognosis. Give preoperative and postoperative instructions when curative surgery is scheduled.

Endometriosis

DESCRIPTION

Endometriosis is a condition in which endometrial tissue implants outside the uterus in the pelvic cavity or in the abdominal wall (Fig. 12–15).

ICD-9-CM Code 617.9 *(Site unspecified)*
Endometriosis may be coded by site and the pathology. Refer to the physician's diagnosis and then to the current edition of the ICD-9-CM coding manual to ensure the greatest specificity of pathology and any appropriate modifiers.

SYMPTOMS AND SIGNS

Although endometriosis is considered a benign condition, its severe symptoms are painful and chronic. Acquired dysmenorrhea, beginning before and extending several days after menstruation, is a classic symptom. The patient has constant pain and cramping in the lower abdomen, the vagina, and the back. The patient, usually of childbearing age, also may experience heavy menses, pelvic pain during intercourse, and even painful defecation. The cyclical inflammation and scarring eventually can lead to symptoms even when a woman is not menstruating. Complications include infertility, *ectopic* pregnancy, and spontaneous abortion.

PATIENT SCREENING

When a patient presents with extremely painful menstruation, she should be scheduled for a physical examination, including a pelvic examination for evaluation. In some cases the initial complaint may be infertility.

ETIOLOGY

When functioning endometrial tissue grows outside the uterine cavity, it responds to the ovarian hormones as the endometrium (lining of the uterus) does during the normal menstrual cycle. These misplaced islands of endometrial tissue usually implant on other pelvic organs, where they imitate the menstrual cycle, irritating the surrounding tissues. The thickening and sloughing (bleeding) in unnatural areas and the ensuing cysts, scar tissue, and adhesions are the cause of much pain and discomfort. What causes the lining tissue of the uterus to break away and travel to other parts of the body is not known. The use of tampons may foster displacement of endometrial tissue up through the fallopian tubes during menstruation, so their use is discouraged. Risk factors include a family history of the disease, menstrual cycles shorter than every 28 days, and periods lasting longer than a week.

DIAGNOSIS

During the pelvic examination, the physician may be able to detect multiple tender nodules, as well as the presence of ovarian cysts. Laparoscopy may confirm the diagnosis and help to stage the extent of endometrial implant or adhesions according to size, character, and location (Fig. 12–16). The treatment then can be determined, depending on

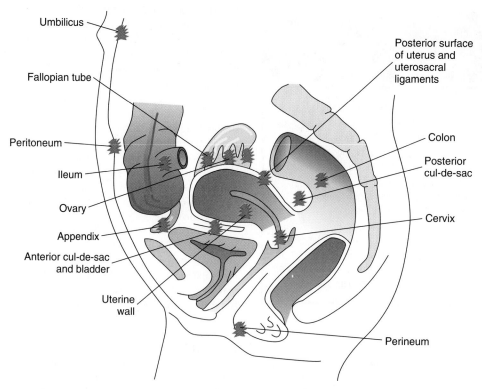

FIGURE 12–15 Endometriosis (ectopic sites). (From Gould B: *Pathophysiology for the health professions,* ed 2, Philadelphia, 2002, Saunders.)

the woman's age, general health, and severity of her symptoms.

TREATMENT

Conservative treatment with various hormones is indicated for younger patients who wish to have children. Specific hormones used in treatment include danazol (a testosterone derivative) or a GRH (gonadotropin-releasing hormone) agonist. Although there is no cure, pregnancy, nursing a baby, or menopause brings remission of symptoms because the aberrant tissue tends to shrink under these conditions. Surgery can be used to remove or destroy endometrial growths. In severe cases or in the presence of ovarian masses, a total hysterectomy with bilateral **salpingo-oophorectomy** may be indicated.

PROGNOSIS

Although no cure for endometriosis is known, a variety of treatment options are available. Com-plications include reduced fertility and sponta-neous abortion.

PREVENTION

The mechanisms that cause the disease are not clear, so no effective prevention is known.

PATIENT TEACHING

Advise adolescents to use sanitary napkins in place of tampons. Review the physician's advice not to postpone childbearing, and offer appropriate re-ferrals. Review any drug therapy as prescribed by the physician.

Pelvic Inflammatory Disease (PID)

DESCRIPTION

PID is a mild to serious infection that involves some or all of the female reproductive organs.

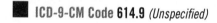

ICD-9-CM Code 614.9 *(Unspecified)*

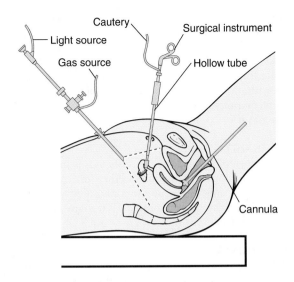

FIGURE 12–16 Laparoscopy.

SYMPTOMS AND SIGNS

The infection can occur after miscarriage, childbirth, or abortion, but it is most common in young nulliparous females and is not necessarily related to a pregnancy. The symptoms are those of an active infection: fever, chills, malaise, a foul-smelling vaginal discharge, backache, and a painful, tender abdomen. If an abscess has developed, a soft, tender pelvic mass may be palpated. The white blood cell (WBC) count is elevated.

PATIENT SCREENING

The patient with fulminating PID reports constitutional symptoms and has significant pain. When symptoms are severe, arrange for immediate medical intervention.

ETIOLOGY

The causative organism, one that is sexually transmitted or a common vaginal bacterium, can enter the body through the vagina and travel up through the cervix into the pelvic cavity. Young, sexually active women and those who use intrauterine devices (IUDs) for contraception are at higher risk.

DIAGNOSIS

The vaginal examination is painful because of the swelling and inflammation. A specimen is taken for Gram stain and sensitivity studies. This allows the physician to prescribe an antibiotic that is specific in action against the bacteria that are found. A laparoscopy can be performed to look for an *abscess* or hepatic involvement, or even to confirm the diagnosis if cervicovaginal cultures are negative. Ultrasonography also can be useful by showing a mass (possible abscess) or fluid in the *cul-de-sac*.

TREATMENT

Early diagnosis and prompt treatment lessen the damage to the reproductive system. The treatment plan begins with aggressive antibiotic therapy, the administration of analgesics, and bed rest. Follow-up includes education about measures to minimize the risks and the importance of early treatment to prevent complications.

The inflammation of the female reproductive organs can cause scar tissue (adhesions) to form. If an adhesion forms in the fallopian tubes, it can cause infertility or increase the risk of ectopic pregnancy. In addition, adhesions can develop rapidly between any of the pelvic organs and structures.

PROGNOSIS

Without effective treatment, serious and life-threatening complications can develop. Peritonitis can spread the infection throughout the abdominal cavity, or, if the infection becomes blood borne, septicemia and even death may result. Recurrent or severe PID can cause scarring of the fallopian tubes, obstruction, and infertility. Antibiotic therapy can abate the infection.

PREVENTION

Risk factors for sexually transmitted disease should be avoided. If infection is due to an STD, the women's sexual partners also are treated with antibiotics. Frequent vaginal douching is contraindicated, especially with a history of previous PID. Unsanitary conditions during childbirth or elective abortion can allow pathogens to be introduced into the pelvic cavity. Those who have a history of immunological or renal disorders especially should seek prompt treatment of infection.

PATIENT TEACHING

Inform the patient that infection typically begins intravaginally and ascends through the entire genital tract. Review all risk factors. Sexually active women with multiple partners should be told that PID is frequently associated with sexually transmitted disease. Insertion of an intrauterine device (IUD) is also a risk factor.

Leiomyomas and Fibroids

DESCRIPTION

Leiomyomas are noncancerous (benign) tumors of the smooth muscle within the uterus. Fibroids are also benign tumors but are composed of fibrous tissue. They may vary in number, size, and location within the uterus (Fig. 12–17).

■ **ICD-9-CM Code 218.9** *(Unspecified)*
Leiomyomas are coded according to site. Refer to the physician's diagnosis and then to the current edition of the ICD-9-CM coding manual to ensure the greatest specificity of pathology and any appropriate modifiers.

SYMPTOMS AND SIGNS

Leiomyomas and fibroids are the most common tumors of the female reproductive system, and they tend to calcify after menopause. They occur in about 30% of women over 35 years of age. These tumors may not cause any symptoms at all. If symptoms do occur, they may include pelvic pain and pressure, constipation, urinary frequency, abnormal bleeding, and heavy or prolonged periods. The latter symptom is the most common. The severity of symptoms is related to the number, size, and location of the tumors.

PATIENT SCREENING

Schedule a gynecologic examination and medical consultation for a woman experiencing the symptoms mentioned previously. Ask the woman if she is pregnant or could be pregnant.

ETIOLOGY

The cause of leiomyomas and fibroids is unknown. Their development is stimulated by estrogen, and they occur only in the premenopausal woman and sometimes the postmenopausal woman on hormone replacement therapy.

DIAGNOSIS

The diagnosis is based on pelvic examination and the patient history. Definitive diagnosis can be based on ultrasonography; small fibroids occasionally are discovered incidentally at laparoscopy. In the case of abnormal bleeding in the nonpregnant women, a D & C procedure or endometrial biopsy usually is performed to rule out *adenocarcinoma* of the uterus.

TREATMENT

Treatment generally depends on the severity of the symptoms, the patient's age, and her desire to have children. In women of childbearing age, surgery can be performed to remove the tumors. If bleeding continues, surgical removal of the uterus (hysterectomy) is recommended. Hysterectomy is the only procedure for definitive relief of symptoms and prevention of recurrence. Only rarely do leiomyomas become malignant.

PROGNOSIS

Ongoing gynecologic examinations are recommended to monitor fibroids. Surgical resection is sometimes indicated. Fibroids return after removal in about 10% of patients who have undergone surgery.

PREVENTION

No method for the prevention of either leiomyomas or fibroids is known.

PATIENT TEACHING

Teach the patient the signs of complications, such as hemorrhage or sudden onset of pain and fever.

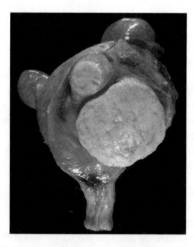

FIGURE 12–17 Leiomyomas. (From Cotran RS, Kumar V, Collins T: *Robbins pathologic basis of disease,* ed 6, Philadelphia, 1999, Saunders.)

Vaginitis

DESCRIPTION

Vaginitis is inflammation and/or infection of the vaginal tissues.

 ICD-9-CM Code 616.10 *(Vaginitis and vulvovaginitis, unspecified)*
Refer to the physician's diagnosis and then to the current edition of the ICD-9-CM coding manual for an additional code to identify causative organism.

SYMPTOMS AND SIGNS

Inflammation of the vagina is common, and all age groups are at risk. It is generally not perilous, but it can be irritating and painful. Vaginal discharge is the principal symptom. Depending on the causative agent, the discharge varies from clear and odorless to copious, greenish yellow, and foul smelling. The discharge causes itching, burning, and soreness of the vulva. Fever may be present.

PATIENT SCREENING

The discomfort and irritation secondary to vaginal infection prompt the earliest possible appointment for a pelvic examination, diagnosis, and treatment.

ETIOLOGY

Vaginitis can be caused by a variety of organisms, but an organism called *Trichomonas,* which usually is transmitted through sexual intercourse, often causes it. The sex partner probably also will have the infection. The infection may not cause any symptoms in the man, but if he is carrying the organism, he can reinfect the woman. Other causative organisms are bacterial, viral, or fungal. Mechanical irritation, irritating chemicals, latex condoms, and nonabsorbent underwear are causative agents. Atrophic vaginitis can occur after menopause. With the loss of estrogen, the vaginal lining changes and becomes thinner and more susceptible to infections.

DIAGNOSIS

After taking a medical history, the physician performs a pelvic examination and swabs the vagina. Specimens from the vagina and cervix are analyzed for the presence of the *Trichomonas* organism.

TREATMENT

Depending on the results of cultures and wet preparation examination, treatment can consist of hormonal therapy, the administration of antibiotics, a vaginal antifungal such as clotrimazole (Gyne-Lotrimin), or the use of steroid creams. If the vaginitis has been transmitted sexually, both partners must be treated.

PROGNOSIS

With proper treatment, the inflammation usually clears up in about a week. However, vaginitis is a recurring problem for many women.

PREVENTION

Preventive measures are directed toward known causes: avoidance of sexually transmitted disease, good hygiene, avoidance of known chemical irritants, and recognition of risk factors for postmenopausal women.

PATIENT TEACHING

The information to be given to the patient is determined by the etiology. The importance of complying with the antibiotic therapy exactly as directed is emphasized when infection is identified. Review the risk factors for STDs, if appropriate. Mechanical or chemical irritants are to be avoided. These may include irritants found in douches, deodorant sprays, spermicide, latex condoms, detergents, or bubble bath products. Tight, nonporous underclothing and poor personal hygiene can promote bacterial growth. The use of a nonirritating vaginal lubricant during intercourse may help the postmenopausal woman.

Toxic Shock Syndrome

DESCRIPTION

Toxic shock syndrome is an acute, systemic infection with exotoxin-producing strains of *Staphylococcus aureus.* The syndrome often has been associated with menstruating females who use tampons.

ICD-9-CM Code 040.82
Refer to the physician's diagnosis and then to the current edition of the ICD-9-CM coding manual for an additional code to identify the bacterial agent.

SYMPTOMS AND SIGNS

Super-absorbent tampon use may predispose the woman to a *S. aureus* infection. The sudden onset is characterized by high fever, headache, sore throat, and rash. The syndrome progresses rapidly to hypotension and shock. Other symptoms and signs that the patient might experience are gastrointestinal symptoms, neuromuscular disturbances, and an elevation of the liver enzyme levels. Without treatment, the disease may become life-threatening within 48 hours.

PATIENT SCREENING

Immediate medical treatment is indicated.

ETIOLOGY

The cause of TSS is thought to be an increase in staphylococcal toxin production in the presence of the synthetic fibers found in super-absorbent tampons. These fibers remove magnesium from the vagina. This then creates an ideal environment for the bacteria to produce the toxins. Since the composition of tampons was changed and because women are warned about their use, the incidence of TSS has declined. The synthetic fibers also have been found in surgical dressings. This may explain why some cases of TSS in nonusers of tampons have been reported. TSS also has been seen in newborns and men, but only rarely.

DIAGNOSIS

A diagnosis of TSS is based on clinical evaluation and laboratory tests. The Centers for Disease Control has listed specific diagnostic criteria.

TREATMENT

Therapy for TSS includes the replacement of fluids to counteract shock and the use of prescribed antibiotics to treat the infection. Vancomycin is used for drug-resistant staphylococcal infection. If treatment is delayed, death can result from overwhelming shock. NOTE: Use of universal precautions for all body secretions is necessary.

PROGNOSIS

Prompt diagnosis followed by antibiotic treatment offers the best prognosis. However, toxic shock syndrome can result in neurologic, renal, and respiratory complications, and death.

PREVENTION

Although the synthetic fiber composition of tampons has changed, physicians advise women who use tampons to avoid the super-absorbent type, to use them only during the daytime, and to change them frequently.

PATIENT TEACHING

Review the preventive measures mentioned previously and other advice given by the health-care provider. Explain the importance of taking the entire course of antibiotics as prescribed.

Menopause

DESCRIPTION

Menopause (change of life or climacteric) is the cessation of menstrual periods.

 ICD-9-CM Code 627.2

SYMPTOMS AND SIGNS

Many women experience the onset of menopause between age 45 and 55. Fluctuation in the menstrual cycle and flow is noted, with periods becoming lighter and less frequent. Hot flashes and night sweats often are reported as a mild to intolerable nuisance; vaginal dryness and skin changes appear. Many women experience transient to troublesome psychological symptoms, including depression, poor memory, anxiety, sleep disorders, and loss of interest in sex.

PATIENT SCREENING

Schedule the patient for a medical examination and consultation with the physician. Inform the patient that a pelvic examination may be required.

ETIOLOGY

Between 45 and 55 years of age, a woman's ovaries gradually produce less estrogen, resulting in the cessation of ovulation and menstruation. This change and changes in the pituitary hormone levels result in physical and psychological changes. This natural process can be induced artificially by a bilateral oophorectomy, removal of both ovaries.

DIAGNOSIS

A patient history suggests menopause. The blood serum levels of follicle-stimulating hormone are elevated, and the estrogen levels are low.

TREATMENT

Hormonal changes can be noted in blood serum levels, and these chemical changes increase the incidence of cardiac disease and osteoporosis in the postmenopausal female. Until recently many doctors routinely recommended hormone replacement therapy to menopausal and postmenopausal women to help protect against certain age-related diseases and to relieve the other aforementioned symptoms. Medical opinion has changed, however, because of the findings of clinical trials that link HRT with increased breast cancer, heart disease, stroke, and blood clots in women taking the drugs. HRT has many benefits, but the risks are greater than previously thought for some women. Some physicians suggest short-term use of HRT for 2 to 5 years.

Each woman should consult her doctor or nurse practitioner and weigh the side effects and risks against the benefits of HRT. Alternative approaches to protecting against age-related diseases can be considered for high-risk women. A more natural approach to the treatment of hot flashes associated with menopause is the use of soy products, which contain isoflavones. Medications are available that strengthen bones, lower cholesterol, and help relieve vaginal dryness. Alendronate sodium (Fosamax) and risedronate sodium (Actonel) are two medications that are used in the prevention of osteoporosis, along with the recommended daily dose of calcium and vitamin D.

PROGNOSIS

Menopause is a normal, temporary condition with a variable course.

PREVENTION

Menopause cannot be prevented, and the prognosis is generally good.

PATIENT TEACHING

Give the patient informative brochures about menopause, the pros and cons of hormone replacement therapy, and alternatives to HRT. Encourage questions about symptoms being experienced. Recommend a healthy lifestyle as a first line of defense against aging.

Uterine Prolapse

DESCRIPTION

Prolapse of the uterus is a downward displacement of the uterus from its normal location in the body.

■ **ICD-9-CM Code 618.1**

SYMPTOMS AND SIGNS

The uterus becomes prolapsed when the pelvic floor muscles and ligaments become extremely overstretched or weakened. Feelings of heaviness, discomfort, and backache are common symptoms. In some women, *stress incontinence* develops; in other women, prolapse has the opposite effect of urinary retention, and urination becomes more difficult. Bowel movements also may become more difficult.

PATIENT SCREENING

Schedule the patient for a routine appointment and a pelvic examination.

ETIOLOGY

Uterine prolapse results when the pelvic floor muscles weaken from childbirth or old age. As the muscles and ligaments become overstretched, they no longer can hold the uterus in place, so it falls or sags downward. This causes a lump or bulge on the vaginal wall. The prolapse occasionally is so severe that the cervix bulges out of the vagina (Fig. 12–18). This is called a complete prolapse. This condition can be uncomfortable and inconvenient, but it carries no risk to general health unless the prolapsing organ ulcerates or bleeds or the urethra becomes completely obstructed.

DIAGNOSIS

The prolapse is visible upon pelvic examination or by visual inspection if it is protruding from the vagina. A speculum examination can reveal the descent of the rectum or bladder.

TREATMENT

Treatment consists of Kegel exercises, a technique for strengthening the muscles of the pelvic floor, of weight loss if the woman is overweight, and of a high-fiber diet to prevent bowel straining. If there is no improvement, the woman may be fitted with a **pessary.** This device is inserted into the vagina to support the uterus. Surgery usually is necessary to correct serious prolapse.

PROGNOSIS

The prognosis is good even if surgery is required.

PREVENTION

Exercises that strengthen the muscles of the pelvic floor after childbirth are recommended.

PATIENT TEACHING

Review the anatomy and nature of the condition and make sure the patient understands how to do

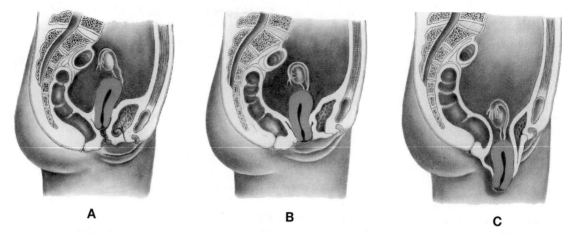

A   **B**   **C**

FIGURE 12–18 Uterine prolapse. **A,** First degree. **B,** Second degree. **C,** Complete prolapse. (From Seidel HM et al: *Mosby's guide to physical examination,* ed 5, St. Louis, 2003, Mosby.)

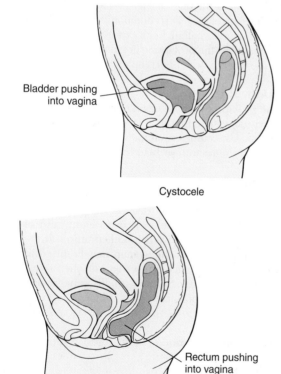

Bladder pushing into vagina

Cystocele

Rectum pushing into vagina

Rectocele

FIGURE 12–19 Cystocele and rectocele.

the exercises (Kegel exercises). If applicable, answer questions about surgical correction of the condition.

Cystocele

DESCRIPTION
Cystocele is a downward displacement and protrusion of the urinary bladder into the anterior wall of the vagina (Fig. 12–19).

■ **ICD-9-CM Code 618.0** *(Female)*

SYMPTOMS AND SIGNS
This disorder causes the female patient to experience pelvic pressure, frequency, urgency, and incontinence of urine, including stress incontinence. The bladder cannot be emptied completely, predisposing the woman to cystitis.

PATIENT SCREENING
Schedule the patient for a routine appointment and a pelvic examination. Symptoms of cystitis such as painful and frequent urination may require an earlier appointment.

ETIOLOGY
This condition results from trauma to the fascia, muscle, and pelvic ligaments during pregnancy and delivery or from atrophy of the muscles of the pelvic floor with age.

DIAGNOSIS
Diagnosis is based on the clinical picture and findings of the physical examination.

TREATMENT
Treatment consists of exercises to strengthen the pelvic floor muscles (Kegel exercises), which involve voluntary isometric tightening of the pelvic-floor muscles, including stopping of the flow of urine midstream. Surgical repair is anterior vaginal **colporrhaphy.**

PROGNOSIS
The prognosis is good.

PREVENTION
Exercise to strengthen the pelvic floor muscles after childbirth may help; the tissue changes associated with aging cannot be prevented

PATIENT TEACHING
Review the prescribed exercises. Give preoperative and postoperative instructions to candidates for colporrhaphy.

Rectocele

DESCRIPTION
A rectocele is the protrusion of the rectum into the posterior aspect of the vagina.

 ICD-9-CM Code 618.0 *(Female)*

SYMPTOMS AND SIGNS
The rectocele causes the female patient to experience a bearing-down feeling and constipation (see Fig. 12-19). She also may have incontinence of gas and feces or may experience difficulty in fecal evacuation.

PATIENT SCREENING
Schedule the patient for a routine appointment and a pelvic examination as soon as possible.

ETIOLOGY
Similar to a cystocele, a rectocele occurs when the posterior wall of the vagina is weakened, allowing a protrusion of the rectum into the vagina. This also can result from trauma to the area during childbirth, although the patient may not exhibit symptoms until years after the pregnancy.

DIAGNOSIS
Diagnosis is based on the clinical picture and findings of the physical examination.

TREATMENT
Treatment consists of surgical repair of the posterior wall of the vagina (posterior colporrhaphy). If both the cystocele and the rectocele are repaired at the same time, the procedure frequently is called an anterior and posterior (A & P) repair.

PROGNOSIS
The prognosis is good with surgical repair.

PREVENTION
No prevention is known. Efforts are made to prevent maternal birth trauma.

PATIENT TEACHING
Appropriate preoperative and postoperative instructions are given. Anticipate questions and reassure the patient about how the procedure may affect sexual intercourse.

Cervical Cancer

DESCRIPTION
The cervix is the lower part of the uterus, extending from the uterine isthmus into the vagina. It functions to allow sperm into the uterine cavity and the infant to pass into the birth canal. Most cervical cancers are squamous cell carcinomas that arise in the transitional zone between the different epithelial types of the uterus corpus and the vagina, but adenocarcinoma may also occur (Fig. 12-20).

ICD-9-CM Code 180.9/M8000

SYMPTOMS AND SIGNS
The two main symptoms of cervical cancer are a watery, bloody vaginal discharge that may be heavy and foul smelling, and bleeding between menstrual periods, after intercourse, or after menopause. The most common sign is the abnormal Pap smear test result. The appearance of the cervical lesion varies, but it is often a mass or an ulcer on the surface of the cervix. Signs and symptoms of advanced disease include pelvic or lower back pain, hematuria, dysuria, or rectal bleeding.

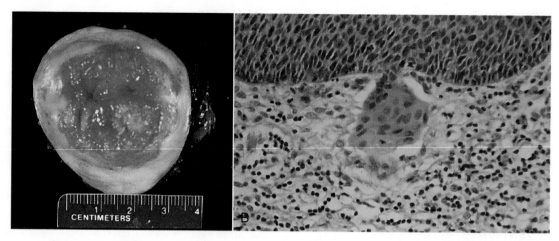

FIGURE 12–20 Cancer of the cervix. (From Cotran RS, Kumar V, Collins T: *Robbins pathologic basis of disease,* ed 6, Philadelphia, 1999, Saunders.)

PATIENT SCREENING

Encourage females to have regular cervical Pap smear screening. Schedule a gynecologic examination for the female experiencing abnormal vaginal bleeding, prolonged or intermittent periods, or bleeding after intercourse.

ETIOLOGY

Invasive cervical cancer is often considered a preventable disease because it has a long premalignant stage (often 10 years or longer) and an effective screening program, and because treatment of preinvasive disease is effective. Therefore the biggest risk factor for development of invasive cervical carcinoma is lack of regular cervical Pap smear screening. The other major risk factor is exposure to oncogenic types of human papilloma virus (HPV), such as 16, 18, 31, and 45. These are more common in individuals who have had early and frequent unprotected sexual activity with multiple partners. HPV DNA is detected in more than 90% of invasive cervical cancers. HPV infection alone is probably not sufficient to cause cervical neoplasia, however, and it is often found with other risk factors such as smoking, low socioeconomic status, early and multiple parity, use of oral contraceptives, and other venereal diseases. The most common age for diagnosis is 45 to 55 years, but it is also a significant problem in women over age 65, who are less likely to get a Pap smear. The premalignant lesion for cervical cancer is called cervical intraepithelial neoplasia (CIN), and it involves dysplasia or atypical changes in the cervical epithelium.

DIAGNOSIS

The Pap smear test was developed specifically to detect cervical cancer. By obtaining scrapings from the cervix and cervical os and examining them microscopically, one can detect cellular abnormalities. The diagnosis of cancer is then confirmed through biopsy of the cervical lesion. The stage is determined clinically through physical examination of the patient, chest x-ray, intravenous pyelogram, *colposcopy,* cystoscopy, and proctoscopy. Lymph node sampling also may be performed. The International Federation of Gynecologists and Obstetricians developed the staging system that is used. It differs from the commonly used TNM system in that it relies on the clinical evaluation rather than the pathologic features of the tumor. This is because cervical cancer is most common in developing countries where more modern techniques are not available for staging of the tumor.

TREATMENT

Treatment is determined by stage. Low-grade CIN is treated with laser therapy, *cryoablation,* or electrocoagulation. Simple hysterectomy is sufficient for high-grade CIN. Radical hysterectomy (removal of ovaries, oviducts, lymph nodes, lymph channels, uterus, and cervix) is performed to treat invasive stages. For carcinomas that have invaded the pelvic wall or have distant metastases, radiation therapy is included in the treatment. Cisplatin-based chemotherapy often is used in conjunction with the radiotherapy. Patients should be followed-up with periodic physical examination and Pap smear to detect recurrences.

PROGNOSIS

Stage is the most important determinant of prognosis, followed by lymph node status, tumor volume, and depth of tumor invasion. HPV subtype also may affect the prognosis, with HPV 18 having a poorer prognosis than the other subtypes. The 5-year survival rate ranges from 92% for women with stage-I cancer to 15% for those with stage-IV neoplasms. Recurrence is usually local (e.g., cervix, uterus, vagina) and carries the very poor prognosis of a 10% to 15% 1-year survival rate.

PREVENTION

All sexually active women should undergo an annual Pap smear and pelvic examination. After three or more consecutive normal Pap smears, screening can be performed less often at the discretion of the physician. Women with a Pap smear suggesting CIN should be evaluated with colposcopy and possible endometrial biopsy, and CIN should be treated. Unfortunately, developing countries often lack screening programs. Other risk-reducing methods include use of barrier contraception, limiting one's number of sexual partners, and smoking cessation.

PATIENT TEACHING

Emphasize that, with early diagnosis, the survival rate for cervical cancer is excellent. Review the recommendations listed under Prevention. Women diagnosed with invasive stages of cervical cancer require information about treatment and possible complications. Explain preoperative and postoperative instructions for hysterectomy, radiation therapy, and/or chemotherapy. Encourage the patient to express feelings associated with a loss of body image, changes in sexual functioning, and changes in fertility. Furnish a referral to a support group.

Vaginal Cancer

DESCRIPTION

Primary cancer of the vagina is rare, and malignancy usually results from the involvement of neoplasms of adjacent structures. Most primary tumors are squamous cell carcinomas, but other types such as melanoma or adenocarcinoma may be seen.

 ICD-9-CM Code 184.0

SYMPTOMS AND SIGNS

Most patients present with vaginal bleeding, usually postcoital or postmenopausal. Other symptoms include a malodorous vaginal discharge, urinary symptoms such as dysuria or frequency, constipation, melena, or vaginal mass. The tumor itself presents as a mass, plaque, or ulcer on the vaginal wall.

PATIENT SCREENING

Unusual vaginal bleeding, pelvic pain, or the symptoms mentioned above require diagnostic evaluation. Suggest the patient be prepared for a gynecologic examination.

ETIOLOGY

Little information is available on the etiology of vaginal cancer, but risk factors are thought to include HPV infection, prior history of gynecologic malignancy, advanced age, multiple lifetime sexual partners, early age at first intercourse, low socioeconomic status, and cigarette smoking. Vaginal intraepithelial neoplasia (VAIN), atypical squamous cells without invasion, may be a premalignant lesion for vaginal cancer. It is usually asymptomatic but can be associated with postcoital spotting or vaginal discharge.

For squamous cell carcinoma, the mean age at diagnosis is 60 years. Adenocarcinomas usually occur in women under the age of 20 and have been linked to the synthetic hormone diethylstilbestrol (DES). DES has been used in the past to prevent spontaneous abortions and manage diabetic pregnancies. The cancer tends to develop in the daughters of mothers who received DES during their pregnancies.

DIAGNOSIS

Diagnosis is difficult because the malignant lesion may be small and missed on gynecologic exam. Pap smear may discover malignant cells of the vagina incidentally when screening for cervical cancer. Definitive diagnosis is accomplished through colposcopic exam and direct biopsy of the lesion. Cervical biopsies also must be taken to rule out primary cervical cancer. Carcinomas are staged by means of physical and pelvic examination, cystoscopy, proctoscopy, chest x-ray, and bone scan. A TNM (Tumor, Node, Metastasis) staging system is used, where T reflects the extent of tumor penetration through the vaginal wall.

TREATMENT

Treatment is based on location, size, and clinical stage of the tumor. Surgery usually includes hysterectomy, upper vaginectomy, and bilateral pelvic lymphectomy and may be performed with adjuvant radiation therapy. Radiotherapy alone may be sufficient to treat early-stage vaginal cancers.

PROGNOSIS

The major indicator of prognosis is stage at the time of diagnosis, although lymph node status, age, and lesion location also are important. Because many vaginal cancers are diagnosed at an advanced stage, and because a high percentage of locally advanced cancers recur within 6 months of initial treatment, the overall 5-year survival rate for squamous cell vaginal cancer is only 44%. The 5-year survival rate for adenocarcinoma is 75%, largely because women exposed to DES are followed closely, and many cancers are diagnosed at an early stage.

PREVENTION

Obtaining a regular Pap smear, using barrier contraceptives, and limiting one's number of sexual partners reduce the risk of developing vaginal cancer. Diagnosis and treatment of VAIN by surgical excision, *laser ablation,* or topical 5-fluorouracil may prevent progression to invasive disease. Periodic follow-up should be performed to look for recurrent VAIN or invasive disease.

PATIENT TEACHING

Emphasize the importance of early diagnosis and treatment. Enforce the physician's recommendation for a screening schedule, based on the patient's history of risk factors. If treatment is required, review the physician's explanation of procedures and possible complications of therapy. Help the patient with referrals to care and support groups.

Labial or Vulvar Cancer

DESCRIPTION

The vulva is the area of the female external genitalia. Any condition that can affect skin on other parts of the body can affect the vulva. More than 90% of vulvar malignancies are squamous cell carcinomas.

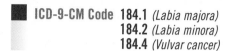

ICD-9-CM Code   **184.1** *(Labia majora)*
                    184.2 *(Labia minora)*
                    184.4 *(Vulvar cancer)*

SYMPTOMS AND SIGNS

Most patients present with a nodule or ulcer, usually on the labia majora, labia minora, or clitoris. The lesion may be multifocal or associated with pruritis or burning. Less common symptoms and signs include vulvar bleeding, discharge, dysuria, and enlarged lymph node in the groin.

PATIENT SCREENING

The patient may complain of a sore or nodule of the labia causing discomfort; schedule a gynecologic examination.

ETIOLOGY

Vulvar neoplasms are encountered most often in postmenopausal women. The mean age at diagnosis is 65 years. Risk factors include cigarette smoking; HPV, HIV, or HSV2 (herpes simplex virus type 2) infection; multiple sexual partners; prior history of cervical, endometrial, or breast cancer; and northern European ancestry. Vulvar intraepithelial neoplasia (VIN), noninvasive epithelial dysplasia of the vulva, is thought to be a premalignant lesion for invasive carcinoma.

DIAGNOSIS

Diagnosis requires excision biopsy of the lesion. Colposcopy may be used to define areas to biopsy. After the diagnosis of cancer is confirmed, examination for involvement of regional lymph nodes is mandatory. Evaluation for metastasis includes a chest radiograph, cystoscopy, proctoscopy, and intravenous pyelogram. A Pap smear is performed to check for cervical cancer. The stage is evaluated according to a TNM (Tumor, Node, Metastasis) staging system.

TREATMENT

The usual treatment of vulvar carcinoma is either surgical removal of the growth and surrounding skin or removal of all or part of the vulva itself. The latter procedure is known as a vulvectomy. Radiation therapy sometimes is used in combination with the surgery. Patients with distant metastases or recurrences may be treated with systemic chemotherapy, but the rate of response to this treatment is typically low, and the prognosis for these patients is poor.

PROGNOSIS

Inguinofemoral lymph node status is the most important indicator of prognosis, regardless of stage. The overall 5-year survival rate is 70% to 75%.

PREVENTION

The risk for development of vulvar carcinoma is reduced by the use of barrier contraceptives, by regular gynecologic examinations, and by treatment of VIN with excision, laser vaporization, or topical 5-fluorouracil. Close follow-up is necessary after a diagnosis of VIN because of the high risk of recurrence.

PATIENT TEACHING

Inform the patient of the purpose of biopsy and when to expect the results. Explain the medical treatment, when indicated; this may include preoperative and postoperative instruction, the use of analgesics, and the side effects to expect from radiation therapy or chemotherapy. Explain sitz baths as directed and the application of sanitary napkins as needed. Support the patient in any expressions of anxiety or concerns about sexuality and body image. Emphasize the importance of follow-up care.

Ovarian Cancer

DESCRIPTION

Ovarian cancer accounts for more deaths than any other gynecologic malignancy. Because of the location of the ovaries deep within the pelvis, disease is often asymptomatic until the more advanced stages. Primary ovarian tumors usually derive from epithelial cells.

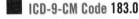 **ICD-9-CM Code 183.0**

SYMPTOMS AND SIGNS

Ovarian neoplasms may cause such nonspecific symptoms as lower abdominal discomfort, bloating, constipation, lower back pain, irregular menstrual cycles, urinary frequency, or dyspareunia. The most common sign is enlargement of the abdomen caused by accumulation of fluid (ascites), but this usually indicates advanced disease. Persistent, vague digestive disturbances such as discomfort, gas, or distention that cannot be explained by any other cause should be evaluated for ovarian cancer.

PATIENT SCREENING

Schedule a woman experiencing the nonspecific symptoms listed previously for a physical examination including a pelvic exam. Women who are at high risk need regular gynecologic examinations.

ETIOLOGY

The incidence varies geographically, with the highest incidences in industrialized countries except Japan. Most ovarian cancers occur in women between the ages of 40 and 65. The etiology is largely unknown, but multiple risk factors have been identified. Pregnancy, prolonged use of oral contraceptives, and tubal ligation may reduce the risk of development of ovarian cancer. Women who have had breast cancer or who have a family history of breast or ovarian cancer have an increased risk. This history may be due to mutations in BRCA1 or BRCA2, the breast cancer susceptibility genes. People with hereditary nonpolyposis colon cancer (HNPCC) also have an increased risk for ovarian cancer.

DIAGNOSIS

Early-stage ovarian cancer is sometimes diagnosed on palpation of an abnormal *adnexal* mass during a routine pelvic examination. Because of the deep anatomic location of the ovary, however, early-stage tumors often are not discovered. The finding of a pelvic mass usually leads to laparoscopic surgery to confirm the diagnosis, although transvaginal ultrasound and the use of serum tumor markers may help distinguish malignant from benign masses. If not clinically suggestive of malignancy, the mass should be followed for 2 months to see whether it resolves. Serum CA125, a glycoprotein tumor marker that is elevated in more than 80% of ovarian cancers, should be measured. Tumors are staged using a TNM (Tumor, Node, Metastasis) system. The stage is based on surgical evaluation during the laparoscopic surgical diagnostic procedure. Therapeutic cytoreduction (surgical reduction of tumor volume) also is performed at this time. Abdominal or pelvic CT scan may be used to identify distant metastases.

TREATMENT

Optimal therapy for ovarian cancer is determined by the extent of disease at the time of diagnosis and by the size and location of any residual tumor after the surgical staging procedure. Early stage disease (I and II) is treated by surgical removal of the ovaries and fallopian tubes (bilateral salpingo-oophorectomy) and the uterus (hysterectomy), although if the cancer is diagnosed in a very early stage and the woman still wishes to have children, only one ovary may be removed. The risk of relapse is reduced by adjuvant chemotherapy with platinum-based compounds (carboplatin plus paclitaxel). Treatment for advanced disease is aggressive surgical *cytoreduction* in combination with chemotherapy. The efficacy of treatment is evaluated through radiographic testing and is indicated by a decline in serum CA125 level. After a full course of chemotherapy, a second-look surgery may be performed on women with a complete clinical response. The surgery checks for any residual tumor and offers another method to assess the response to treatment.

PROGNOSIS

The overall 5-year survival rate for epithelial ovarian cancer is about 50% because more than 75% of cancers have spread beyond the ovary at the time of diagnosis. The stage at diagnosis guides prognosis, with women diagnosed in stage I having a 95% 5-year survival rate, and those with metastatic disease having a 29% 5-year survival rate.

PREVENTION

Periodic pelvic exams are very important for women. Screening is recommended only for women with known BRCA1 or BRCA2 gene mutations after consultation about the benefits and risks of screening with their physicians. These women should be screened with transvaginal ultrasound and serum CA125 measurement every 6 to 12 months beginning at the age of 25 to 35. Alternately, women at high risk for ovarian cancer may choose to have a prophylactic oophorectomy by the age of 35.

PATIENT TEACHING

Emphasize the importance of regular gynecologic examinations. If a pelvic mass is found, completely explain the procedures for diagnosis. Explain presurgical and postsurgical instructions, and explain the terminology particular to staging and grading of cancer, when appropriate. Refer all questions about the prognosis to the physician. Make referrals as needed for psychological support.

Endometrial Cancer

DESCRIPTION

Endometrial cancer involves the lining of the uterus, which undergoes cyclic changes as a result of hormonal stimulation. It is the most common gynecologic malignancy (Fig. 12–21).

■ **ICD-9-CM Code 182.0**

SYMPTOMS AND SIGNS

The disease usually begins with endometrial thickening (hyperplasia), abnormal tissue development (dysplasia), and carcinoma in situ. Ulcerations of the endometrium develop, and as blood vessels erode, vaginal spotting or bleeding occurs. The most common presenting symptom is abnormal perimenopausal or postmenopausal uterine bleeding. This occurs even in the early stages of the disease. Late manifestations of this cancer include pain and systemic symptoms. The disease may be revealed by atypical endometrial cells on a routine Pap smear.

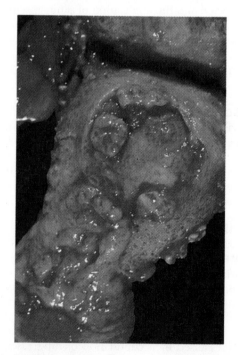

FIGURE 12–21 Endometrial cancer. (From Cotran RS, Kumar V, Collins T: *Robbins pathologic basis of disease,* ed 6, Philadelphia, 1999, Saunders.)

PATIENT SCREENING

Schedule a gynecologic examination and a Pap smear for the woman presenting with abnormal uterine bleeding.

ETIOLOGY

There are two types of endometrial cancer. The most common type is related to high cumulative exposure to estrogen and usually presents as a low-grade adenocarcinoma. Excess estrogen may come from sources such as estrogen replacement therapy for postmenopausal women, tamoxifen therapy for breast cancer, obesity, early onset of menarche, late menopause, never having children, and chronic anovulation. Endometrial hyperplasia with cellular atypia caused by endometrial exposure to continuous estrogen unopposed by progesterone is a precursor lesion for this type of carcinoma. The second type is unrelated to estrogen exposure or hyperplasia and often presents as a high-grade papillary serous or clear cell carcinoma with poorer prognosis.

Endometrial cancer is a disease of primarily postmenopausal women. The median age at diagnosis is 61 years. Women with hereditary nonpolyposis colorectal cancer syndrome are at high risk for development of endometrial cancer. Pregnancy and the use of oral contraceptives for at least 12 months appear to offer a protective effect.

DIAGNOSIS

Endometrial biopsy should be performed on all women with abnormal uterine bleeding or abnormal cells on a Pap smear. Diagnosis is often based on an office endometrial biopsy, but dilation and curettage remains the gold standard and is usually performed when the endometrial biopsy is nondiagnostic. After the diagnosis is made, preoperative evaluation includes a CBC, renal and liver function tests, urinalysis, chest x-ray, and ECG. The staging system developed for endometrial cancer correlates with the TNM (Tumor, Node, Metastasis) system. Staging requires a total hysterectomy with bilateral salpingo-oophorectomy to fully evaluate the extent of disease. The serum tumor marker CA125 also may be measured to predict the spread of disease beyond the uterus.

TREATMENT

Very-early-stage endometrial cancer is treated with surgery alone, while adjuvant radiation therapy is recommended for those with more advanced disease. A radioactive implant can be inserted into the uterus and left in place for the duration of treatment while the patient is in the hospital. Combined chemoradiotherapy is beginning to be explored for possible improvement of survival. For patients with advanced disease, a combination of chemotherapy and hormone therapy (progestin and/or tamoxifen therapy) is the optimal treatment regime. The risk of recurrent disease is greatest within the first 3 years of diagnosis. Follow-up tests to detect recurrence are physical exam, measurement of serum CA125, and vaginal cytology.

PROGNOSIS

The prognosis is determined by the stage of the disease and the tumor grade. Early-stage tumors carry a 5-year survival rate of 96%; regionally advanced tumors carry a rate of 63%; and metastatic tumors, 26%.

PREVENTION

Routine screening is not recommended for most women because no sensitive or specific test is available. An endometrial biopsy is recommended at menopause and before beginning hormone replacement therapy or tamoxifen therapy. For those at risk for HNPCC, however, annual endometrial biopsy is recommended starting at age 35. These women also should be counseled about prophylactic hysterectomy at completion of childbearing.

PATIENT TEACHING

Women should be counseled about the symptoms of endometrial cancer and should be instructed to report any abnormal bleeding or spotting to their health-care provider. After endometrial cancer is diagnosed, preoperative and postoperative instructions are given. Patients with more advanced disease who are receiving adjunctive radiation therapy require additional information about procedures. Explain the purpose, duration, and possible side effects of any therapeutic regimen. Offer referrals for every possible avenue of support, especially in more advanced cases.

Conditions and Complications of Pregnancy

Most pregnancies progress to term uneventfully (Fig. 12–22). Complications ranging from worrisome or annoying conditions to life-threatening condi-

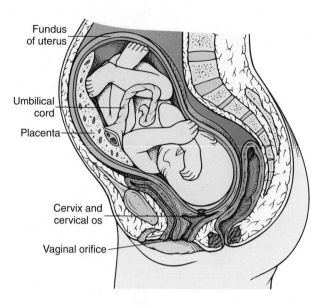

Fundus of uterus

Umbilical cord

Placenta

Cervix and cervical os

Vaginal orifice

FIGURE 12–22 Normal uterine pregnancy.

tions affecting the mother or the fetus occasionally occur. Complications can develop at any point in the gestational period, emphasizing the importance of early and continual prenatal care and patient education.

Morning Sickness

DESCRIPTION
Morning sickness is transient nausea or vomiting experienced in the first trimester of pregnancy.

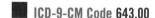 **ICD-9-CM Code 643.00**

SYMPTOMS AND SIGNS
The patient with morning sickness experiences transient nausea or vomiting, usually on arising. This generally occurs between the sixth and twelfth weeks in the pregnancy, often as the first sign of pregnancy.

PATIENT SCREENING
Follow office policy for scheduling an examination for possible pregnancy. If the patient is experiencing excessive nausea and vomiting, make a prompt appointment for a regular pregnancy checkup.

ETIOLOGY
Elevated estrogen, progesterone, and *human chorionic gonadotropin (hCG)* levels are believed to be responsible for the nausea and vomiting. In some cases, emotions may trigger the episodes.

DIAGNOSIS
The diagnosis is based on symptoms and a positive pregnancy test result.

TREATMENT
The nausea and vomiting usually subside by the end of the first trimester. The patient is encouraged to eat small amounts of food at frequent intervals. She also is advised that eating soda crackers before getting up may help. A drug-free remedy with clearance of the U.S. Food and Drug Administration (FDA) to treat nausea and vomiting associated with pregnancy is the Relief Band, a watch-like device that is battery operated and worn on the wrist. When turned on it emits a low-level electrical pulse across 2 small electrodes. *No* medication has been approved by the FDA for this condition, but several medications are used universally. Vitamins B_6, B_{12}, and folic acid are used to reduce morning sickness if a vitamin deficiency is suspected.

PROGNOSIS

The condition usually is self-limiting and gradually resolves. If the condition becomes severe, it is called hyperemesis gravidarum.

PREVENTION

No prevention is known.

PATIENT TEACHING

Instruct the pregnant woman to keep her scheduled appointments and to notify the nurse or physician of any worsening of nausea and vomiting.

Hyperemesis Gravidarum

DESCRIPTION

Hyperemesis gravidarum is severe nausea and excessive vomiting that cause starvation during pregnancy.

 ICD-9-CM Code 764.2 *(Fetus)*
643.10 *(Mother)*

SYMPTOMS AND SIGNS

Hyperemesis gravidarum, excessive vomiting in pregnancy, occurs when the pregnant patient experiences frequent, severe episodes of nausea and vomiting, weight loss, and dehydration, and is unable to keep either food or liquid in the stomach. If it is left untreated, fluid and electrolyte imbalances can cause acid–base disturbances in the baby as well as in the mother.

PATIENT SCREENING

Severe nausea and vomiting during pregnancy require prompt medical evaluation.

ETIOLOGY

The etiology is unknown. As with morning sickness, elevated estrogen and progesterone levels are believed responsible for this condition. Again, emotions may play a big part in the onset and severity of the vomiting. The patient is unable to ingest any food or liquid without vomiting.

DIAGNOSIS

The diagnosis is based on the symptoms, weight loss, and signs of dehydration, which disturb the serum electrolyte balance. Serum electrolyte levels are monitored to detect any potassium depletion or *acidosis*.

TREATMENT

In severe cases, the hospitalized patient usually is treated with intravenous fluid and electrolyte replacement, and all food and fluids are withheld. The acidosis must be corrected through intravenous fluid and electrolyte replacement. Sedatives or *antiemetics* are administered to control nausea and vomiting. Hyperemesis gravidarum can be treated in the hospital but more often is treated through home nursing services.

PROGNOSIS

Severe vomiting can cause complications including rupture and bleeding of the liver or bleeding in the retina of the eye caused by the increased pressure during vomiting. The condition usually subsides as the pregnancy progresses into the second trimester.

PREVENTION

Timely medical intervention can prevent complications from affecting the mother and her fetus.

PATIENT TEACHING

After the patient becomes stable, she is instructed to eat small, frequent meals of bland food. Portions are increased as tolerated. Warn the mother to report signs of dehydration or recurrence of symptoms.

Spontaneous Abortion (Miscarriage)

DESCRIPTION

A spontaneous abortion is a naturally occurring loss of the nonviable fetus.

 ICD-9-CM Code 634
Coding spontaneous abortion requires modifiers to identify stage. Refer to the physician's diagnosis and then to the current edition of the ICD-9-CM coding manual to ensure the greatest specificity of pathology and the appropriate modifiers.

SYMPTOMS AND SIGNS

The pregnant patient presents with vaginal bleeding and cramping pelvic pain. When the pulse rate is increased and blood pressure is reduced, the vital signs indicate shock. The patient usually has missed at least one menstrual period and has positive results of hCG testing. Vaginal examination reveals bleeding from the mouth of the cervix, an enlarged uterus, and dilation of the cervix (Fig. 12–23).

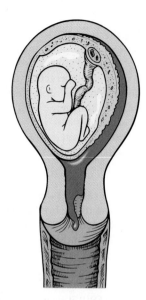

FIGURE 12–23 Miscarriage.

These symptoms occur at any time during the first trimester of pregnancy. If miscarriage occurs early in the second trimester, *amniotic fluid* can leak from the vagina. The term *abortion* means that the fetus is less than 20 weeks' gestation and weighs less than 500 g.

PATIENT SCREENING

Vaginal bleeding and cramping during pregnancy should be reported to the attending physician immediately, and the patient should be directed to prompt medical care.

ETIOLOGY

The etiology is unknown, but about 10% to 15% of all pregnancies terminate in spontaneous abortion. Many spontaneous abortions are believed to be the result of a maldeveloped or genetically abnormal fetus. Occasionally the cervix is incompetent and begins to dilate. Other causes may be infection, injury, drug ingestion (especially crack cocaine), hormonal imbalance, an immunologic response against the fetus, and blood-group incompatibility.

DIAGNOSIS

The diagnosis is based on the clinical picture and pelvic ultrasonography (see Fig. 12–24 and the Enrichment box on Ultrasonography). Ultrasound can determine whether the fetus is still alive.

TREATMENT

If bleeding is not severe, the mother is treated conservatively with bed rest. Although not a routine treatment, cervical *cerclage* may be attempted in the form of a purse-string suture to keep the cervix closed. This procedure is performed on only the patient in the second trimester with a history of habitually incompetent cervix. If bleeding is severe or the expulsion of the contents of the uterus is incomplete, surgical intervention (D & C) is indicated after negative results of hCG testing. Blood replacement may be indicated in these cases.

PROGNOSIS

The prognosis for the mother and fetus is guarded. In many cases, the pregnancy terminates, and the products of conception are expelled spontaneously. Aggressive medical intervention controls bleeding and infection in the mother, even when the infant does not survive.

PREVENTION

The cause often is not certain, but good prenatal care is recommended.

PATIENT TEACHING

Any increased vaginal discharge, bleeding, or progressive cramping should be reported to the nurse or physician. In mild cases bed rest and abstinence from sexual intercourse are advised. After a spontaneous abortion, alert the patient to the signs of infection; these should be reported immediately. A referral for grief counseling may help.

Ectopic Pregnancy

DESCRIPTION

An ectopic pregnancy occurs when the fertilized ovum implants and grows in a structure outside the uterus, most often the fallopian tube (Fig. 12–25).

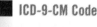 **ICD-9-CM Code**   **761.4** *(Fetus)*
                                       633.90 *(Mother)*

SYMPTOMS AND SIGNS

The first sign of this type of problem pregnancy sometimes appears when the patient experiences a sudden onset of severe lower abdominal pain, which may be accompanied by vaginal bleeding. If blood vessels are ruptured, vital signs may indicate shock. Testing for hCG, the hormone of pregnancy, is positive. HCG levels begin to fall with fetal *demise*.

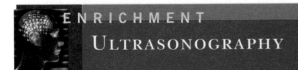

ENRICHMENT

ULTRASONOGRAPHY

ULTRASONOGRAPHY IS A TECHNIQUE in which high-frequency intermittent sound waves are reflected off tissue and read by scanners. The various densities of the tissue then are displayed on a screen, and still pictures can be taken to record the real-time image.

Pelvic ultrasonography is specific for the lower abdominal tissue, including the uterus, adnexa, and fetus. This noninvasive, nonradiating, painless technique helps in diagnosing fe-

tal anomalies, fetal age and size (Fig. 12–24, *A*), fetal position, the condition and placement of the placenta, and many other conditions of the female reproductive system.

A more recent advance is three-dimensional (3-D) prenatal ultrasound, which produces 3-D, crystal-clear images of the baby that are as detailed as a photograph. (Fig. 12–24, *B*). Ultrasonography is considered harmless for both mother and baby and is of particular value in high-risk obstetrics.

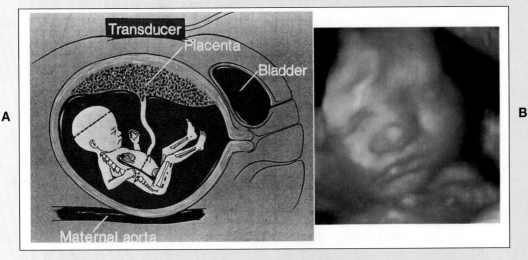

FIGURE 12–24 A, Ultrasonography. **B,** 28-week 3-D ultrasound. Note distortion of the right forehead, which is caused by the uterine wall. (**A** from Hadlock FP: The role of fetal biometry in obstetric sonography. In Putman CE, Ravin CE: *Diagnostic imaging,* Philadelphia, 1988, Saunders. **B** courtesy Carli Reed.)

PATIENT SCREENING

The sudden onset of severe lower abdominal pain accompanied by vaginal bleeding signals the need for prompt medical evaluation. Defer to the physician or nurse for instructions.

ETIOLOGY

Ectopic pregnancies have been known to develop on an ovary, the intestine, or the outer wall of the uterus and even in the vaginal canal. The fertilized ovum often cannot follow the normal progression to the uterus because of blockage in the fallopian tube resulting from adhesions, pelvic in-

flammatory disease (PID), recurrent infections, or congenital conditions. A failed tubal ligation or previous ectopic pregnancy increases the risk of ectopic pregnancy.

DIAGNOSIS

Diagnosis is made by evaluating the clinical picture. Pelvic examination may reveal a tender pelvic mass, which then is scrutinized further through endovaginal ultrasonography. The uterus may be enlarged but smaller than expected for the date of the last menstrual period.

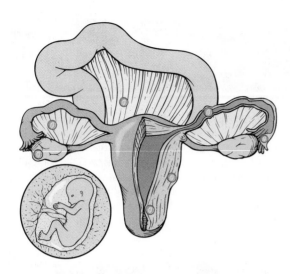

FIGURE 12–25 Sites of ectopic (tubal) pregnancy.

TREATMENT

The usual treatment is laparoscopic surgery to terminate the pregnancy by removal of the fetus and placenta. Prompt diagnosis and intervention are essential to save the mother's life. Lost blood often must be replaced. Attempts are made to preserve the ovary and tube, but this is not always successful, and the patient may be unable to conceive at a later date. In some instances during early ectopic pregnancy, and without evidence of fetal heartbeat, the drug methotrexate is used rather than surgery to precipitate a therapeutic abortion.

PROGNOSIS

The prognosis is good with prompt medical intervention. If the fetus dies at an early stage and the fallopian tube is not damaged, future fertility and pregnancy may not be affected. Complications like massive bleeding in the abdomen are life-threatening. The possibility of recurrence of ectopic pregnancy is 10% after the first instance and 50% after two ectopic pregnancies.

PREVENTION

Avoiding pelvic inflammatory disease and sexually transmitted disease can reduce the risk. Causes frequently are not preventable.

PATIENT TEACHING

During emergency medical care, the patient in pain and distress needs reassurance; this is provided through frequent updates and explanations of the procedures being performed and the reasons. Give analgesics as prescribed. Anticipate the normal emotional response to a problem pregnancy that has terminated.

Premature Labor

DESCRIPTION

Premature labor occurs before the thirty-seventh or thirty-eighth week of gestation or before the fetus has reached a viable weight.

■ **ICD-9-CM Code 644.00** *(Threatened premature labor)*

SYMPTOMS AND SIGNS

Premature labor occurs when the pregnant woman in the late second or early third trimester begins experiencing contractions, spotting, or leakage of amniotic fluid. A vaginal examination may reveal cervical dilation or *effacement;* pelvic ultrasonography also may demonstrate dilation or effacement.

PATIENT SCREENING

A patient with premature contractions must be brought to the attention of the physician or nurse for immediate instructions for medical intervention.

ETIOLOGY

In many cases the onset of preterm labor is spontaneous, and the cause is unknown. The condition also may be iatrogenic, that is, caused by a medical procedure or surgery. Predisposing conditions include maternal infection, uterine abnormalities, uterine bleeding, and incompetent cervix. Maternal age, weight, and socioeconomic status, and inadequate prenatal care are thought to increase the risk.

DIAGNOSIS

Uterine contractions, cervical effacement and dilation, and/or rupture of the amniotic membranes (bag of waters [BOW]) before the expected date of confinement (EDC) signal the onset of premature labor.

TREATMENT

The treatment consists of monitoring of the patient, fetal heart tones (FHTs), and fetal movement (see Fig. 12–26 in the Enrichment box on Fetal Movement). Drug therapy includes the administration of terbutaline sulfate (Brethine) or magnesium sulfate. Calcium channel blockers along with indomethacin, and atosiban (an oxytocin antagonist) also are used. Ideally, labor can be postponed until the fetus can develop to maturity.

PROGNOSIS

In some pregnancies, preterm labor results in a good outcome. The prognosis generally is guarded for the mother and infant, depending on underlying conditions of both; significant complications can be associated with preterm babies.

PREVENTION

The causes of premature labor are not clearly understood; good prenatal care is the best deterrence.

PATIENT TEACHING

All elements of good prenatal care with attention to individual needs and the medical history are clearly presented with as many teaching aids as possible. Help the patient set goals for a healthy outcome for mother and infant. Give written instructions about signs of possible complications or early onset of labor to report.

Preeclampsia (Toxemia) and Eclampsia

DESCRIPTION

Preeclampsia describes a serious disease of pregnancy characterized by the classic triad of hypertension, edema, and proteinuria.

Eclampsia is the ultimate manifestation of preeclampsia and is characterized by grand mal seizure, coma, hypertension, proteinuria, and edema.

■ **ICD-9-CM Code** **642.40** *(Preeclampsia)*
    642.6 *(Eclampsia)*

SYMPTOMS AND SIGNS

Pregnancy-induced hypertension can be associated with the potentially life-threatening disorder preeclampsia (toxemia). The pregnant patient, usually in the third trimester, experiences sudden weight gain with edema, primarily in the face, hands, and feet. Headaches, dizziness, spots before the eyes, and nausea and vomiting may occur. The blood pressure is elevated, and protein is found in the urine. Both mother and fetus can be in danger. The disease usually occurs after the thirty-second week of pregnancy. Impending eclampsia is characterized by fever, restlessness, persistent extremely high blood pressure, and clonus (exaggerated reflexes); this may be followed by seizure and coma.

PATIENT SCREENING

The woman who is pregnant or suspects pregnancy, who reports the onset of edema, sudden weight gain, headaches, or sudden elevation of blood pressure, should be evaluated by the physician promptly. The onset of seizures requires emergency intervention.

ETIOLOGY

The etiology of preeclampsia, which is unique to pregnant females, remains unknown. Poor nu-

ENRICHMENT
FETAL MOVEMENT

FETAL MOVEMENT is an indicator of fetal well-being. Some physicians have the expectant mother chart fetal kicks (see Fig. 12–26) to record fetal activity. Kick-counting methods vary; the attending physician or nurse midwife provides the guidelines. For example, the mother may be instructed to drink a glass of juice, lie down on her left side, and count fetal movements over a certain period of time (up to 2 hours). She records the weeks of gestation and the date and time she starts, she then counts the movements until the baby moves 10 times, and then she records the time again. The expected number of movements varies from patient to patient, but the mother becomes familiar with her baby's pattern and can notice any reduction in movement. If fetal movement remains absent or reduced from the norm, she is to notify her physician, who can investigate and further evaluate the fetal status.

Figure 12–26 shows a sample kick count chart.

* Personal kick count chart *

Name_____ **Due date**_____

Care provider_____ **Hospital**_____

Week 25

Date _____ Time _____ 10 Kicks in _____Mins
Date _____ Time _____ 10 Kicks in _____Mins
Date _____ Time _____ 10 Kicks in _____Mins
Date _____ Time _____ 10 Kicks in _____Mins
Date _____ Time _____ 10 Kicks in _____Mins
Date _____ Time _____ 10 Kicks in _____Mins
Date _____ Time _____ 10 Kicks in _____Mins

Week 26

Date _____ Time _____ 10 Kicks in _____Mins
Date _____ Time _____ 10 Kicks in _____Mins
Date _____ Time _____ 10 Kicks in _____Mins
Date _____ Time _____ 10 Kicks in _____Mins
Date _____ Time _____ 10 Kicks in _____Mins
Date _____ Time _____ 10 Kicks in _____Mins
Date _____ Time _____ 10 Kicks in _____Mins

Week 27

Date _____ Time _____ 10 Kicks in _____Mins
Date _____ Time _____ 10 Kicks in _____Mins
Date _____ Time _____ 10 Kicks in _____Mins
Date _____ Time _____ 10 Kicks in _____Mins
Date _____ Time _____ 10 Kicks in _____Mins
Date _____ Time _____ 10 Kicks in _____Mins
Date _____ Time _____ 10 Kicks in _____Mins

Week 28

Date _____ Time _____ 10 Kicks in _____Mins
Date _____ Time _____ 10 Kicks in _____Mins
Date _____ Time _____ 10 Kicks in _____Mins
Date _____ Time _____ 10 Kicks in _____Mins
Date _____ Time _____ 10 Kicks in _____Mins
Date _____ Time _____ 10 Kicks in _____Mins
Date _____ Time _____ 10 Kicks in _____Mins

Week 29

Date _____ Time _____ 10 Kicks in _____Mins
Date _____ Time _____ 10 Kicks in _____Mins
Date _____ Time _____ 10 Kicks in _____Mins
Date _____ Time _____ 10 Kicks in _____Mins
Date _____ Time _____ 10 Kicks in _____Mins
Date _____ Time _____ 10 Kicks in _____Mins
Date _____ Time _____ 10 Kicks in _____Mins

Week 30

Date _____ Time _____ 10 Kicks in _____Mins
Date _____ Time _____ 10 Kicks in _____Mins
Date _____ Time _____ 10 Kicks in _____Mins
Date _____ Time _____ 10 Kicks in _____Mins
Date _____ Time _____ 10 Kicks in _____Mins
Date _____ Time _____ 10 Kicks in _____Mins

Week 31

Date _____ Time _____ 10 Kicks in _____Mins
Date _____ Time _____ 10 Kicks in _____Mins
Date _____ Time _____ 10 Kicks in _____Mins
Date _____ Time _____ 10 Kicks in _____Mins
Date _____ Time _____ 10 Kicks in _____Mins
Date _____ Time _____ 10 Kicks in _____Mins
Date _____ Time _____ 10 Kicks in _____Mins

Week 32

Date _____ Time _____ 10 Kicks in _____Mins
Date _____ Time _____ 10 Kicks in _____Mins
Date _____ Time _____ 10 Kicks in _____Mins
Date _____ Time _____ 10 Kicks in _____Mins
Date _____ Time _____ 10 Kicks in _____Mins
Date _____ Time _____ 10 Kicks in _____Mins
Date _____ Time _____ 10 Kicks in _____Mins

FIGURE 12–26 Fetal movement.

Week 33

Date _____ Time _____ 10 Kicks in _____ Mins
Date _____ Time _____ 10 Kicks in _____ Mins
Date _____ Time _____ 10 Kicks in _____ Mins
Date _____ Time _____ 10 Kicks in _____ Mins
Date _____ Time _____ 10 Kicks in _____ Mins
Date _____ Time _____ 10 Kicks in _____ Mins
Date _____ Time _____ 10 Kicks in _____ Mins

Week 34

Date _____ Time _____ 10 Kicks in _____ Mins
Date _____ Time _____ 10 Kicks in _____ Mins
Date _____ Time _____ 10 Kicks in _____ Mins
Date _____ Time _____ 10 Kicks in _____ Mins
Date _____ Time _____ 10 Kicks in _____ Mins
Date _____ Time _____ 10 Kicks in _____ Mins

Week 35

Date _____ Time _____ 10 Kicks in _____ Mins
Date _____ Time _____ 10 Kicks in _____ Mins
Date _____ Time _____ 10 Kicks in _____ Mins
Date _____ Time _____ 10 Kicks in _____ Mins
Date _____ Time _____ 10 Kicks in _____ Mins
Date _____ Time _____ 10 Kicks in _____ Mins
Date _____ Time _____ 10 Kicks in _____ Mins

Week 36

Date _____ Time _____ 10 Kicks in _____ Mins
Date _____ Time _____ 10 Kicks in _____ Mins
Date _____ Time _____ 10 Kicks in _____ Mins
Date _____ Time _____ 10 Kicks in _____ Mins
Date _____ Time _____ 10 Kicks in _____ Mins
Date _____ Time _____ 10 Kicks in _____ Mins
Date _____ Time _____ 10 Kicks in _____ Mins

Week 37

Date _____ Time _____ 10 Kicks in _____ Mins
Date _____ Time _____ 10 Kicks in _____ Mins
Date _____ Time _____ 10 Kicks in _____ Mins
Date _____ Time _____ 10 Kicks in _____ Mins
Date _____ Time _____ 10 Kicks in _____ Mins
Date _____ Time _____ 10 Kicks in _____ Mins
Date _____ Time _____ 10 Kicks in _____ Mins

Week 38

Date _____ Time _____ 10 Kicks in _____ Mins
Date _____ Time _____ 10 Kicks in _____ Mins
Date _____ Time _____ 10 Kicks in _____ Mins
Date _____ Time _____ 10 Kicks in _____ Mins
Date _____ Time _____ 10 Kicks in _____ Mins
Date _____ Time _____ 10 Kicks in _____ Mins
Date _____ Time _____ 10 Kicks in _____ Mins

Week 39

Date _____ Time _____ 10 Kicks in _____ Mins
Date _____ Time _____ 10 Kicks in _____ Mins
Date _____ Time _____ 10 Kicks in _____ Mins
Date _____ Time _____ 10 Kicks in _____ Mins
Date _____ Time _____ 10 Kicks in _____ Mins
Date _____ Time _____ 10 Kicks in _____ Mins

Week 40

Date _____ Time _____ 10 Kicks in _____ Mins
Date _____ Time _____ 10 Kicks in _____ Mins
Date _____ Time _____ 10 Kicks in _____ Mins
Date _____ Time _____ 10 Kicks in _____ Mins
Date _____ Time _____ 10 Kicks in _____ Mins
Date _____ Time _____ 10 Kicks in _____ Mins
Date _____ Time _____ 10 Kicks in _____ Mins

Week 41

Date _____ Time _____ 10 Kicks in _____ Mins
Date _____ Time _____ 10 Kicks in _____ Mins
Date _____ Time _____ 10 Kicks in _____ Mins
Date _____ Time _____ 10 Kicks in _____ Mins
Date _____ Time _____ 10 Kicks in _____ Mins
Date _____ Time _____ 10 Kicks in _____ Mins
Date _____ Time _____ 10 Kicks in _____ Mins

Week 42

Date _____ Time _____ 10 Kicks in _____ Mins
Date _____ Time _____ 10 Kicks in _____ Mins
Date _____ Time _____ 10 Kicks in _____ Mins
Date _____ Time _____ 10 Kicks in _____ Mins
Date _____ Time _____ 10 Kicks in _____ Mins
Date _____ Time _____ 10 Kicks in _____ Mins
Date _____ Time _____ 10 Kicks in _____ Mins

FIGURE 12–26, cont'd Fetal movement. (Courtesy Hood P, Babyworks Ltd., www.babyworksltd.com.)

trition and abnormally high sodium intake are possible contributing factors. It occurs in about 7% of pregnant women in the United States and most often in **primiparas** who are 12 to 18 years old or older than 35 years. Symptoms may appear earlier in patients with underlying renal disease or may be associated with hydatidiform mole.

If the preeclampsia is allowed to progress to eclampsia, the patient experiences convulsions, which may result in *abruptio placentae* (separation of the placenta from the uterine wall) and fetal or maternal demise. Many other serious multisystem complications can occur.

DIAGNOSIS

The diagnosis is based on the clinical picture, the history, the serum electrolyte levels, an elevated blood albumin level, and exaggerated reflexes.

TREATMENT

The patient's blood pressure, weight, and urine protein level customarily are monitored in prenatal care. As the pregnancy progresses, the monitoring becomes more frequent. At the first indication of signs and symptoms of toxemia, the patient is encouraged to add no salt to the diet. If the symptoms become more severe (e.g., spots before the eyes, headache, and higher blood pressure), the patient may be hospitalized and monitored. The room is kept dark and quiet to reduce stimuli in an effort to prevent convulsions. FHTs and fetal movement are monitored closely. Medications are given to reduce blood pressure. The condition is resolved by inducing labor if the child is viable or by terminating the pregnancy. Within 24 to 48 hours, the patient's blood pressure usually returns to normal levels, edema subsides, and protein is no longer present in the urine.

PROGNOSIS

Early diagnosis and treatment of preeclampsia offer the best prognosis for mother and baby. For eclampsia, the mortality rate is 10%; the fetal mortality rate is 25%.

PREVENTION

Good prenatal care and diet help substantially in reducing the frequency and severity of toxemia. Other possible preventive steps being explored are calcium supplementation and low-dose aspirin therapy.

PATIENT TEACHING

Teach the advantages of early and regular prenatal care to monitor weight, blood pressure, and urinalysis. If a pregnant woman is considered at risk for eclampsia, teach the warning signs to report: sudden weight gain, edema, headache, and increased blood pressure. Early signs can be managed to help prevent hospitalization and the onset of complications.

Abruptio Placentae

DESCRIPTION

Abruptio placentae is premature detachment of a normally positioned placenta occurring during pregnancy.

 ICD-9-CM Code **762.1** *(Affecting fetus or newborn)*
641.20 *(Affecting mother)*

SYMPTOMS AND SIGNS

When the placenta separates from the uterine wall too early during pregnancy, it causes the mother to hemorrhage, and the fetus is deprived of oxygen. The pregnant patient, generally in the third trimester, experiences sudden, severe abdominal pain with board-like rigidity and a large amount of bright vaginal bleeding. Vital signs indicate shock, with an increased pulse rate that is weak and thready, falling blood pressure, and cool, clammy, moist, pale skin. The patient is apprehensive. FHTs decrease and have no variability, indicating impending fetal demise. Fetal activity or movement is reduced.

PATIENT SCREENING

The signs of abruptio placentae represent a medical emergency for mother and fetus. The physician is contacted immediately, and the patient is directed to the emergency room.

ETIOLOGY

Abruptio placentae is a complete or partial separation of the placenta from the uterine wall (Fig. 12–27). Marginal or complete cases have massive bright bleeding, whereas concealed cases have no visible bleeding but have extreme abdominal pain with board-like rigidity.

Trauma or seizures can cause the separation. In many cases, the cause is unknown. Women with hypertension or preeclampsia and women who use cocaine are at higher risk for this condition.

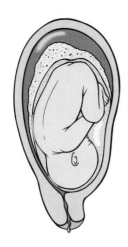

FIGURE 12–27 Abruptio placentae.

DIAGNOSIS

The diagnosis, if time permits, is made by pelvic ultrasonography along with the clinical picture. The abruptio placentae often is so severe and sudden that the clinical picture is the only basis for treatment.

TREATMENT

The patient with partial separation is hospitalized, placed on bed rest, and monitored watchfully. Labor may be induced if pregnancy is near term and bleeding persists. When indicated, a falling fetal heart rate and maternal shock demand immediate surgical intervention. Blood replacement may be indicated.

PROGNOSIS

The maternal or fetal mortality rate depends on the severity of the abruptio placentae and prompt intervention. Severe hemorrhage is a significant cause of maternal and fetal mortality.

PREVENTION

Good prenatal care with individualized attention to risk factors may help prevent some occurrences.

PATIENT TEACHING

Reinforce the principles of prenatal care and instruct the patient to report unexpected symptoms, such as sudden bleeding or abdominal pain, immediately.

Placenta Previa

DESCRIPTION

Placenta previa is a condition in which the placenta that is implanted in the lower uterine segment encroaches on the internal cervical os, causing bleeding.

 ICD-9-CM Code 641.00

SYMPTOMS AND SIGNS

The patient experiences painless, bright vaginal bleeding, usually in the last trimester of pregnancy. Occasionally, the patient has experienced painless vaginal bleeding earlier in the pregnancy. The abdomen is soft and nontender. Vital signs may indicate shock, with the pulse being rapid and thready and the blood pressure falling. The fetal heart rate may indicate that the blood supply to the fetus is compromised.

PATIENT SCREENING

The onset of bright red vaginal bleeding during pregnancy requires immediate attention, close observation, and diagnostic evaluation. The attending physician is notified.

ETIOLOGY

The etiology is unknown, but the incidence appears to be increased in women who have a history of breech presentation or who have had multiple pregnancies (**multiparous**).

DIAGNOSIS

The diagnosis is based on a pelvic ultrasonogram that shows the placenta implanted over the cervical os. In a complete placenta previa, the placenta totally overlies the os (Fig. 12–28). In a partial placenta previa, the placenta is implanted low in the uterus but does not entirely overlie the os. As the cervix begins to dilate, the vessels tear loose and the placenta bleeds. *It is of utmost importance that nothing be placed in the vagina and that no vaginal examination be performed.*

TREATMENT

To control the mother's hemorrhaging and to save the baby, treatment of complete placenta previa is immediate surgical termination of the pregnancy with delivery of the infant by cesarean section. Blood transfusion may be required for profuse

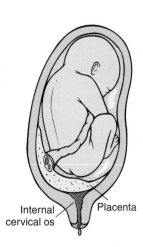

FIGURE 12–28 Placenta previa.

blood loss. Partial placenta previa of nonterm pregnancies may be treated conservatively with observation of the mother in a hospital. Surgical intervention is employed when the fetus is nearer to term or if the bleeding becomes profuse.

PROGNOSIS

The prognosis is guarded depending on the degree of impingement on the cervix as pregnancy progresses.

PREVENTION

No prevention is known.

PATIENT TEACHING

Conditions requiring surgical intervention to save the life of the mother and/or the infant conjure strong emotional responses that require recognition and care by the medical team. Explain all procedures and offer reassurance throughout. Conservative treatment may require bed rest and lifestyle modification for an extended period during pregnancy; reinforce the purpose of the treatment and address the need for home-care referrals. Vaginal intercourse may be contraindicated.

Hydatidiform Mole

DESCRIPTION

Hydatidiform mole is an intrauterine tumorous growth resulting from a pathologic ovum.

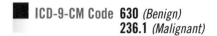

■ **ICD-9-CM Code 630** *(Benign)*
236.1 *(Malignant)*

SYMPTOMS AND SIGNS

The patient with a hydatidiform mole, a developmental anomaly of conception, experiences symptoms that mimic those of pregnancy. Toward the end of the third month of gestation, she begins to experience bright red or brownish vaginal bleeding. The bleeding may be spotty or continuous. The uterus increases in size out of proportion to the gestational age. The patient also may experience severe nausea and vomiting. The hCG levels are elevated, but no FHTs are present. The signs and symptoms of toxemia may be present as early as 20 weeks of gestation.

PATIENT SCREENING

The patient may report symptoms of a spontaneous abortion; in this case immediate medical care is given. A pregnant woman reporting any exaggerated symptoms of pregnancy needs a prompt appointment for evaluation.

ETIOLOGY

This developmental anomaly of conception occurs when the chorionic villi develop into a mass of clear grapelike vesicles (see Fig. 12–31 on p. 591). Usually, no fetus is present. There may be a paternal genetic link. For some unknown reason it is much more common in Asian women.

DIAGNOSIS

The diagnosis is based on the clinical picture, the absence of FHTs, abnormally elevated hCG levels, ultrasonogram, and *amniography*.

TREATMENT

The mole normally is not expelled spontaneously, so surgical intervention is definitely indicated, with the usual treatment being evacuation of the uterus by D & C. Observation for hemorrhage is important. If the mole is found to be cancerous, patients may receive chemotherapy in the form of antimetabolite drugs.

PROGNOSIS

Most hydatidiform moles are not cancerous, and the prognosis is good with early treatment. Complications like infection, bleeding, and preeclampsia can occur. This condition can be a precursor to choriocarcinoma, and the patient

Usual and Unusual Presentations

MOST FETUSES PRESENT in the *cephalic,* or *vertex* (head first), presentation; however, some present in other manners, such as footling *breech* (feet first), frank breech (buttocks), or transverse lie (across the uterus) (Fig. 12–29). Even some of the cephalic presentations (brow or chin) cause complications that may prevent a normal vaginal delivery. In the abnormal presentations, delivery is accomplished by cesarean section.

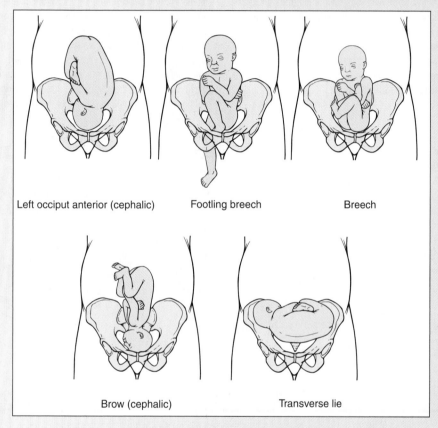

Left occiput anterior (cephalic)   Footling breech   Breech

Brow (cephalic)   Transverse lie

FIGURE 12–29 Fetal presentations.

must be instructed to have frequent follow-up examinations.

PREVENTION
No prevention is known. It occurs in about 1 in 1500 pregnancies in the United States.

PATIENT TEACHING
Explain the surgical procedure. Anticipate the emotional responses to "false pregnancy." Emphasize the importance of follow-up care. The condition usually does not affect fertility, but the patient is advised not to become pregnant for 1 year.

ENRICHMENT
MULTIPLE PREGNANCIES

MULTIPLE PREGNANCIES are occurring more often (Fig. 12–30). Infertility treatment contributes to this increase, because drugs such as clomiphene citrate (Clomid) are given to stimulate ovulation. These drugs often cause several ova to be released at ovulation, thus giving the sperm multiple opportunities for fertilization. During the process of in vitro fertilization, several fertilized ova are implanted in the hope that at least one successful pregnancy will result. The ovaries sometimes release more than one ovum in a natural course of events. Finally, a fertilized zygote sometimes divides to produce identical twins.

Problems associated with multiple pregnancies are many. The mother is at greater risk for toxemia. She experiences dyspnea, urinary frequency, constipation, edema of the feet and legs, and heartburn earlier in the pregnancy than does the mother with a single fetus. The expectant mother of triplets, quadruplets, quintuplets, or sextuplets often is hospitalized by the beginning of the third trimester and restricted to bed rest. The fetuses are monitored frequently and usually must be delivered by cesarean section. The size of the multiple pregnancy generally prevents the pregnancy from continuing to term. This may result in very small, immature infants who need intensive nursing care and monitoring. See Chapter 2 for conjoined twins.

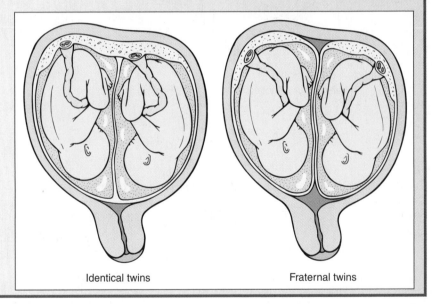

FIGURE 12–30 Multiple pregnancies.

Identical twins   Fraternal twins

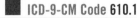

Diseases of the Breast

Ranging from mild to fatal, diseases of the breast necessitate frequent screening, including monthly self-examinations and routine mammograms as prescribed by the physician. Although diseases of the breast are most common in women, men do experience diseases of the breast. Any changes in the breast tissue, such as lumps, indentations, nipple crusting, or leaking, should be cause for concern and investigation.

Cystic Disease of the Breast

DESCRIPTION
Cystic disease of the breast is a common, benign breast disorder.

■ ICD-9-CM Code 610.1

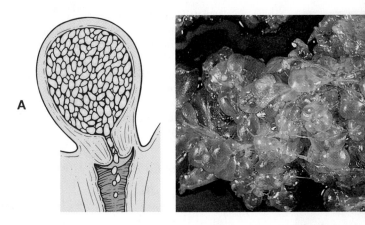

FIGURE 12–31 Hydatidiform mole. (**B** from Damjanov I, Linder J: *Pathology: a color atlas*, St. Louis, 1999, Mosby.)

SYMPTOMS AND SIGNS

The female patient with mammary fibroplasia experiences an uncomfortable feeling in the breasts. Lumps and cysts, single or multiple, smooth and rounded, can be palpated in one or both breasts. The breasts are tender on palpation, and the patient may experience shooting pains in the breast tissue. Tenderness is usually more intense premenstrually.

PATIENT SCREENING

A female who discovers one or more breast lumps is scheduled for a breast examination.

ETIOLOGY

The etiology is unknown. There is an increase in the formation of fibrous tissue and a hyperplasia of the epithelial cells of the ducts and glands, resulting in a dilation of the ducts. Cystic disease is the most common disease of the female breast, usually occurring between the ages of 35 and 50 years, and is possibly endocrine related.

DIAGNOSIS

Prompt diagnosis is based on palpation and mammogram (Fig. 12–32) to differentiate cystic disease from malignant neoplasm. Ultrasonography may be performed to determine whether the lump is solid or hollow. This can help to distinguish between cysts and tumors of the breasts.

TREATMENT

No specific treatment of this condition is known. Some physicians aspirate the cysts with a needle.

The patient is advised to wear a firm, supporting bra and avoid caffeine intake and smoking.

PROGNOSIS

The condition is benign, but the symptoms are not easily mitigated.

PREVENTION

No universal means of prevention is known. Some women report improvement by eliminating caffeine from the diet.

PATIENT TEACHING

The patient must be taught the importance of breast self-examination and of annual mammograms. The lumps and cysts of the disease can mask malignant lumps.

Mastitis

DESCRIPTION

Mastitis is inflammation of the breast.

 ICD-9-CM Code 611.0

SYMPTOMS AND SIGNS

Acute puerperal mastitis is the inflammation of breast tissue during lactation postpartum. The nursing mother experiences sudden pain, redness, and heat in the breasts at either the beginning or end of the lactation period. The breasts are hot and feel doughy and tough, and the axillary lymph nodes may be enlarged. There is a discharge from the nipple. Other symptoms are fever and malaise.

Diseases of the Breast

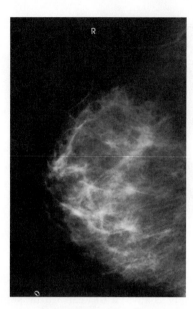

FIGURE 12–32 Mammogram. (From *Mosby's medical, nursing, & allied health dictionary,* ed 6, St. Louis, 2002, Mosby.)

PATIENT SCREENING
Schedule a same-day appointment for a woman experiencing symptoms of mastitis.

ETIOLOGY
Mastitis often is caused by a streptococcal or staphylococcal infection. Bacteria invade the milk ducts and cause inflammation and occlusion. Milk stagnates in the lobules, producing a dull pain. The baby, the nursing staff, or even the mother's own body may be the source of the infection.

DIAGNOSIS
The diagnosis is based on the clinical picture.

TREATMENT
A firm, supportive bra should be worn, heat may be applied to the area, progesterone may be prescribed, and drug therapy in the form of antibiotics is implemented. Palliative care includes rest, analgesia, and warm soaks. Breast feeding need not be discontinued if the patient improves.

PROGNOSIS
The prognosis for this benign condition is good with treatment. Abscesses may form with inadequate treatment.

PREVENTION
Anyone in contact with a nursing mother should practice infection-prevention techniques.

PATIENT TEACHING
The mother is instructed in good personal hygiene, especially in hand-washing techniques. Emphasize the importance of taking antibiotics as prescribed until all are taken.

Fibroadenoma of the Breast
DESCRIPTION
Fibroadenoma is a nontender benign tumor of the breast (Fig. 12–33).

 ICD-9-CM Code 217

SYMPTOMS AND SIGNS
The female patient in her late teens or early 20s feels a firm, round, encapsulated, movable mass in the breast. She experiences no pain or tenderness.

PATIENT SCREENING
Schedule an appointment for a breast examination to evaluate a breast mass.

ETIOLOGY
The etiology is unknown, but fibroadenomas are hormonally responsive, growing in size during the late phases of the menstrual cycle.

DIAGNOSIS
The diagnosis is based on palpation, the clinical picture, and mammogram.

TREATMENT
Treatment of this benign tumor of the breast is surgical removal under local anesthesia. A pathology report can confirm the diagnosis.

PROGNOSIS
The tumors tend to recur.

PREVENTION
No prevention is known.

PATIENT TEACHING
Discuss the surgical course of action with the patient. Assure the patient that the physician or nurse will tell her the results of the pathology report as soon as possible.

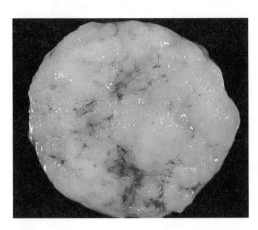

FIGURE 12–33 Fibroadenoma of the breast. (From Damjanov I, Linder J: *Pathology: a color atlas,* St. Louis, 1999, Mosby.)

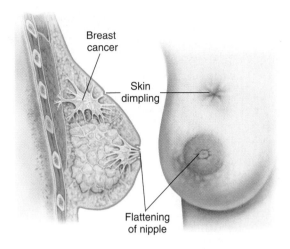

FIGURE 12–34 Clinical signs of breast cancer. (From Seidel HM et al: *Mosby's guide to physical examination,* ed 5, St. Louis, 2003, Mosby.)

Cancer of the Breast

DESCRIPTION

Breast cancer usually arises from the terminal ductal lobular unit (TDLU) of the breast, the functional unit of the breast tissue, which is very hormonally responsive.

ICD-9-CM Code	**174.9** *(Female)*
	175.9 *(Male)*

SYMPTOMS AND SIGNS

Physical symptoms and signs of breast cancer include a lump, swelling, or tenderness of the breast; irritation or dimpling of the breast skin *(peau d'orange);* and pain, ulceration, or retraction of the nipple (Fig. 12–34). Visual examination may reveal that the breasts are asymmetric. The earliest sign, however, is an abnormality on a mammogram, which usually appears before the woman or her physician can feel a lump. In advanced stages of untreated lesions, the nodule becomes fixed to the chest wall, and axillary masses and ulceration develop (Fig. 12–35). Breast pain is not a common factor in early breast cancer.

PATIENT SCREENING

A woman (or man) presenting with any lump, nodule, dimpling, abnormal nipple discharge, or change in breast shape, with or without pain, requires the first available appointment for diagnostic evaluation. The same applies for a patient with abnormal screening mammogram findings.

ETIOLOGY

Breast cancer is the most common cancer and the second leading cause of cancer death among women. The highest incidence rates are in North America and Northern Europe, whereas Asia and Africa have the lowest rates. Mortality rates are highest in those younger than 35 (because of more aggressive tumors) and older than 75 (because their bodies are less able to fight cancer and handle treatment side effects). The two greatest risk factors for the development of breast cancer are increased age and female gender. Breast cancer is 100 times more common in women than men.

Other risk factors have to do with hormonal, reproductive, and genetic factors. Prolonged exposure to and higher concentrations of endogenous estrogen increase the risk of breast cancer. Therefore younger age at menarche, older age at first full-term pregnancy, and older age at menopause are risk factors. Long-term (greater than 5-year) use of combined estrogen/progesterone hormone replacement therapy modestly increases the risk of breast cancer, whereas the use of tamoxifen reduces it. The presence of benign breast disease such as atypical ductal hyperplasia increases risk, as does prior personal history of breast cancer. The use of alcohol increases risk. Family history is important in

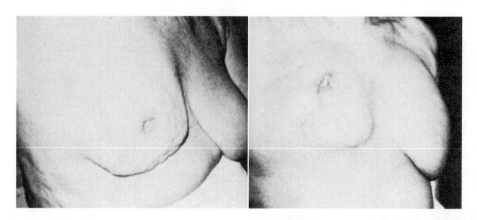

FIGURE 12–35 Locally advanced cancer of the breast. (From Gallagher SH, Leis HP Jr, Snyderman RK, et al: *The breast,* St. Louis, 1978, Mosby.)

determining risk, but only 10% of women diagnosed with breast cancer have a positive family history. About 5% of breast cancers are associated with a specific gene mutation such as BRCA1 or BRCA2, the inherited breast cancer susceptibility genes.

Ductal carcinoma in situ (DCIS), defined as a malignant population of cells that lack the capacity to invade through the basement membrane, is a precursor lesion for breast cancer. These cells can spread through the duct system to involve an entire sector of the breast, or they can even migrate up to involve the nipple skin, possibly leading to Paget disease of the breast. The presence of DCIS multiplies the risk of invasive carcinoma by 8 to 10 times.

The risk of breast cancer is lower in the male because the breast is much less sensitive to hormonal influences. In addition, the normal male breast does not have lobules; thus it has no TDLU. Risk factors for male breast cancer are Klinefelter syndrome, gynecomastia, testicular dysfunction, and BRCA2 gene mutation.

DIAGNOSIS

More than 90% of breast cancers are diagnosed through abnormal mammogram findings, with the remainder being detected solely through physical examination. Because not all mammographic findings represent cancer, further evaluation such as diagnostic mammography and ultrasound are used to determine the need for biopsy. Ultrasound is used to differentiate solid from cystic masses and to determine whether malig-

nant features are present, although a contrast-enhanced MRI may need to be used in women with dense breasts. All suspicious lumps should be biopsied for a definitive diagnosis. Breast cancer is staged according to the TNM (Tumor, Node, Metastasis) system. After the diagnosis of breast cancer, the work-up should include physical examination and blood tests. Staging mammography of both breasts is important for patients considering breast-conserving treatment. If advanced stage is expected, a chest x-ray, CT scan of the abdomen and pelvis, and bone scan should be performed. Tumor estrogen receptor and progesterone receptor status, as well as expression of the oncogene c-erbB-2 and its protein product HER2/neu, should be measured because they have predictive and prognostic value.

TREATMENT

DCIS should be treated by local excision, radiation, and/or tamoxifen to prevent progression to invasive neoplasm. Treatment of invasive breast cancer takes stage and patient preferences into account. Possible modalities include *lumpectomy* or *mastectomy* with removal of axillary lymph nodes, radiation therapy, hormone therapy (depending on the estrogen/progesterone receptor status of the tumor), or chemotherapy. Trastuzumab (Herceptin) is a humanized monoclonal antibody directed against c-erbB-2 that may be effective against tumors that overexpress this oncogene. More than one treatment method usually is used.

PROGNOSIS

Axillary lymph node positivity is the most important prognostic indicator. The presence of estrogen and progesterone receptors is associated with a better prognosis and tumor responsiveness to hormone therapy, while expression of c-erbB-2 is associated with a poorer prognosis. Other factors associated with prognosis are tumor size, grade, and proliferative rate. Localized breast cancer has a 5-year survival rate of 96%. Regional spread reduces the rate to 78%, and distant metastasis results in a 5-year survival rate of 21%.

PREVENTION

Some lifestyle changes may reduce the risk of breast cancer, such as having a child before the age of 25, breast feeding for at least 6 months, avoiding weight gain, and limiting alcohol consumption. Women at very high risk may reduce their risk by 50% by taking tamoxifen for 5 years. Tamoxifen is the only drug approved by the U.S. Food and Drug Administration for the prevention of breast cancer. General screening of the population for BRCA1 or 2 mutations is not recommended.

Regular mammography screening can reduce the risk of death from breast cancer. Mammography can identify breast cancer at an early stage, before physical symptoms develop. The screening recommendation from the American Cancer Society is for women age 40 and older to have an annual mammogram and an annual clinical breast exam by a health professional (preferably before the scheduled mammogram), and to perform monthly breast self-examination. The recommendation for women aged 20 to 39 is to have a clinical breast examination every 3 years and to perform breast self-examination each month.

PATIENT TEACHING

Review and reinforce the preventive measures mentioned above. Women diagnosed with localized tumors need information about the procedure of local resection and the importance of follow-up care, including mammogram and/or ultrasound, breast self-exam, and clinical breast examination by a health professional.

More aggressive therapy for invasive or metastatic disease requires a great deal of teaching. Explain the purpose of the procedures and any discomfort they normally may experience as a result of surgery, radiation, chemotherapy, or hormone therapy. Psychological concerns about loss of the breast and the entire recovery process are best placed in the hands of volunteers from cancer survival support groups. Most patients express great concern about their prognosis; this issue is always referred to the attending physician, as are questions about breast reconstruction.

Paget Disease of the Breast

DESCRIPTION

Paget disease of the breast is a characteristic breast lesion that signifies the presence of malignant adenocarcinoma cells. Underlying carcinoma of the breast is present in 97% of cases.

 ICD-9-CM Code 174.0

SYMPTOMS AND SIGNS

The skin of the nipple develops an erythematous, eczematous, scaly, or ulcerated lesion. The lesion, often unilateral, may heal spontaneously, or topical treatments may mask the inflammation, but this does not mean that Paget disease is not present. Signs of more advanced disease include crusting, serous or bloody discharge from the nipple, and nipple retraction. Some patients may present with only persistent pain or pruritis of the nipple. The patient also may have a breast mass or abnormality on mammogram.

PATIENT SCREENING

Schedule a breast examination for any patient reporting redness, scaling, or lesions of the nipple, discharge from the nipple, or changes in the shape of the nipple; this is important even when the patient reports an eventual improvement in the condition.

ETIOLOGY

It is unknown whether the Paget cells arise from underlying mammary adenocarcinoma (the most widely accepted theory) or whether they represent a carcinoma in situ that is independent of any underlying carcinoma. The peak age of disease onset is 50 to 60.

DIAGNOSIS

The diagnosis can be established by means of a biopsy or by nipple scrape cytology. Any breast masses or mammogram abnormalities should be evaluated to aid in treatment decisions.

TREATMENT

Treatment historically has consisted of simple mastectomy, but the breast-conserving surgeries used to treat breast cancer are now being used to treat Paget disease as well. Whole-breast irradiation may be performed in addition to surgery.

PROGNOSIS

The prognosis is affected by the presence of a palpable breast mass and by metastasis to the axillary nodes. Women with a palpable mass have a 5-year survival rate ranging from 20% to 60%, and those without a mass have a survival rate of 90% to 100%.

PREVENTION

Monthly breast self-examination may aid in detecting nipple lesions in the early stages of the disease.

PATIENT TEACHING

Review the value of regular breast examination, especially for women between ages 50 and 60. Clarify the procedure and purpose of biopsy of the nipple lesion. Additional teaching explains the treatment decision; this could include patient preparations for breast surgery and radiation therapy. The value of woman-to-woman support is again emphasized.

REVIEW CHALLENGE

Answer the following questions:

1. What are the risk factors for sexually transmitted diseases (STDs)?
2. Why is chlamydia called the silent STD?
3. What are the possible complications of untreated gonorrhea?
4. What is meant by the term "ping-pong" vaginitis?
5. What is the pathologic course of genital herpes? How is it treated? Can it be cured?
6. How is genital herpes contracted?
7. Why is early diagnosis and treatment of syphilis important?
8. What are some of the diverse causes of dyspareunia in men and women?
9. Which drugs may contribute to male impotence?
10. What are the possible causes of male and female infertility? Are any preventable?
11. How is benign prostatic hyperplasia treated? What are the possible complications?
12. What are the possible causes of epididymitis? Of orchitis?
13. What are the symptoms and signs of torsion of the testicle?
14. What is a varicocele? How may it be a factor in male infertility?
15. Why is PSA screening valuable? Why is early detection of prostatic cancer vital?
16. What is often the first sign of testicular cancer?
17. What are some of the common symptoms of female reproductive diseases?
18. What are some possible causes of primary and secondary dysmenorrhea?
19. How is mittelschmerz related to ovulation?
20. What is the pathology associated with endometriosis?
21. Why is pelvic inflammatory disease (PID) a serious condition? What is the etiology?
22. What are the most common tumors of the female reproductive system?
23. What organism is commonly the cause of vaginitis?
24. What is toxic shock syndrome (TSS)?
25. How has medical opinion changed recently regarding the use of hormone replacement therapy during menopause?
26. Which etiologic factor do uterine prolapse, cystocele, and rectocele have in common?
27. What are the risk factors for cervical cancer? How is cervical cancer detected by the Papanicolaou (Pap) smear?
28. What is the leading cause of death attributed to female reproductive system disorders? Why is it called a "silent" cancer?
29. What are the possible causes of ectopic pregnancy?
30. What are the clinical indications of toxemia?
31. What is the life-threatening complication that may occur in abruptio placentae? In placenta previa?
32. What are the factors that place women at a higher risk for cancer of the breast?

REAL-LIFE CHALLENGE

Benign Prostatic Hyperplasia

A 60-year-old man reports urinary frequency and nocturia three to four times a night. On questioning, he reveals having difficulty starting urination and a weak stream of urine. He also reports that he thinks he is not completely emptying his bladder. The symptoms have had an insidious onset.

The examination reveals a well-nourished 60-year-old man with vital signs as follows: temperature, 98.6° F; pulse, 72; respirations, 14; and blood pressure, 116/78. His skin is warm, dry, and pink. A PSA test is ordered, and results return at 5 ng/ml. The subsequent digital rectal exam (DRE) reveals an enlarged prostate gland with no nodules or depressions. The urinalysis results are normal, and the urine cultures are negative.

Drug therapy with tamsulosin hydrochloride (Flomax) is ordered. The patient is instructed to have a repeat PSA test in 6 weeks and to return for follow-up DRE. The diagnosis is possible BPH.

QUESTIONS

1. What is the underlying reason for the urinary symptoms?
2. What are normal results for PSA?
3. What causes the prostate to enlarge?
4. Why is the PSA drawn before the DRE?
5. What are treatment options other than drug therapy?
6. What are possible side effects of drug therapy?
7. What might be the side effects of surgical treatment of BPH?
8. What symptoms of BPH are similar to symptoms of prostate cancer?

REAL-LIFE CHALLENGE

Endometriosis

A 35-year-old woman presents with dysmenorrhea, often having onset of pain the day before onset of menses. The pain occasionally continues a few days after menses have ceased. She describes the pain as constant cramping-type pain in the lower abdomen, vagina, and back. The patient describes her menstrual flow to be unusually heavy and also states that she has pain with defecation.

The patient is a gravida III, para II, with a history of a miscarriage 5 years ago. Her living children are 7 and 11 years of age. The patient also states that she has been unable to conceive after 3 years of unprotected intercourse. She also reveals a history of tampon use during the past 10 years.

The pelvic examination reveals generalized tenderness throughout the pelvis. Vital signs are: temperature, 98.8° F; pulse, 88; respirations, 16; and blood pressure, 106/74. Endometriosis is suspected, and the patient is given the choice of conservative treatment with hormones or a laparoscopy to visualize the condition of the reproductive organs. The Pap smear result is negative.

QUESTIONS

1. What is the cause of endometriosis?
2. What is the significance of the obstetric history?
3. Why would the patient experience pain before menses?
4. What other pelvic organs might be involved?
5. Why would hormone therapy be prescribed?
6. What other types of treatment may be used?
7. What is the significance of the patient being unable to conceive?

INTERNET ASSIGNMENTS

1. Explore a medical website to research the latest findings on hormone replacement therapy for women experiencing menopause or perimenopause.
2. Visit the Women's National Health Resource Center website and select a health topic of interest to you and research it. Report a summary of your findings to the class.
3. Visit the National Centers for Disease Control and Prevention website and research the latest campaign to stop the spread of genital herpes through an STD awareness outreach.
4. Visit the American Society for Reproductive Medicine website and go to *Headlines in Reproductive Medicine* to research a topic of current interest, such as the risks of midlife motherhood.

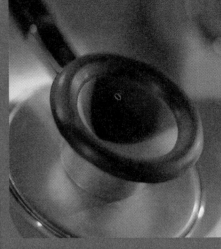

Neurologic Diseases and Conditions

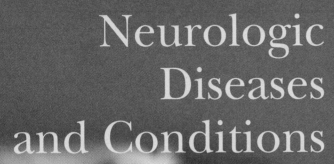

Continued

Chapter Outline—Cont'd

Learning Objectives

After studying Chapter 13, you should be able to:

1. Name the main components of the nervous system.
2. List some of the problems to which the nervous system is susceptible.
3. Describe how data are collected during a neurologic assessment.
4. Name the common symptoms and signs of a cerebrovascular accident (CVA).
5. Name the three vascular disorders that may cause a CVA.
6. Define a transient ischemic attack (TIA).
7. Distinguish between (a) epidural and subdural hematomas and (b) cerebral concussion and cerebral contusion.
8. Describe three mechanisms of spinal injuries.
9. Name the goals of treatment of spinal cord injuries.
10. Explain the neurologic consequences of the deterioration or rupture of an intervertebral disk.
11. Describe the symptoms of migraine.
12. Explain why cephalalgia sometimes is considered a symptom of underlying disease.
13. Describe first aid for seizures.
14. Explain how the symptoms of Parkinson disease are controlled.
15. Describe the progression of amyotrophic lateral sclerosis (ALS).
16. Discuss transient global amnesia.
17. Distinguish between trigeminal neuralgia and Bell palsy.
18. List the diagnostic tests used for meningitis and explain how the causative organism is identified.
19. Name the common causes of encephalitis.
20. Explain the pathologic course of Guillain-Barré syndrome.
21. Explain what is meant by postpolio syndrome.

Key Terms

aphasia (ah–**FAY**–zee–ah)
aura (**AW**–rah)
autonomic (aw–toe–**NOM**–ic)
cephalalgia (sef–ah–**LAL**–jee–ah)
chorea (ko–**REE**–ah)
concussion (kon–**KUSH**–un)
contusion (kon–**TOO**–zhun)
craniotomy (**kray**–nee–**OTT**–toe–me)
demyelination (dee–**my**–eh–lih–**NAY**–shun)
diplopia (dip–**LOW**–pee–ah)

epidural (ep–ih–**DUR**–al)
fasciculation (fa–**sik**–you–**LAY**–shun)
hematoma (hem–ah–**TOE**–mah)
hemiparesis (**hem**–ee–**PAR**–ee–sis)
hemiplegia (**hem**–ee–**PLEE**–jee–ah)
neurotransmitter (**new**–roh–**TRANS**–mit–er)
paraplegia (par–ah–**PLEE**–jee–ah)
parasympathetic (**par**–ah–**sim**–pa–**THET**–ik)
paresis (pah–**REE**–sis)
quadriplegia (kwod–rih–**PLEE**–jee–ah)

ORDERLY FUNCTION
OF THE NERVOUS SYSTEM

THE NERVOUS SYSTEM is a complex, sophisticated, and elaborate network of many interlaced nerve cells (neurons) that make up the brain (Fig. 13–1, *A*), the spinal cord (Fig 13–1, *B*), and the nerves. Electrical impulses are carried throughout the body by the neurons (Fig. 13–1, *C*, and Fig. 13–2). This entire system regulates and coordinates the body's activities and produces responses to stimuli, which help the body adjust to changes in its environment, both internal and external.

The nervous system is composed of two divisions, the central nervous system (CNS) and the peripheral nervous system (PNS). The CNS includes the brain and spinal cord. Its function is to process and store sensory and motor information and to govern the state of consciousness. For example, the structures of the brain that control the intellectual functions of thinking, willing, remembering, and deciding, as well as those that control personality, are located in the frontal lobe of the cerebrum. Coordination, equilibrium, and posture are coordinated in the cerebellum area of the brain. The hypothalamus regulates the secretion of hormones from the pituitary gland and regulates many visceral activities. Five pairs of the 12 cranial nerves originate in the medulla oblongata, an extension of the spinal cord; the medulla also contains vital centers that help regulate heart rate, blood pressure, and respiration. All the sensory and motor nerve fibers pass through the medulla oblongata, connecting the brain and the spinal cord. The spinal cord, a continuation of the medulla oblongata, extends to the first lumbar vertebra. It is divided into 31 segments, each giving rise to a pair of spinal nerves that act like a telephone switchboard, or reflex center, carrying impulses to and from the brain (Fig. 13–1, *D*).

The vast network of nerves throughout the rest of the body is part of the PNS (Fig. 13–3, *A*). Peripheral nerves connect with the spinal cord at many levels, and the information (impulses) they carry travels to and from the brain and spinal cord. Sensory (afferent) nerves transmit impulses from parts of the body (e.g., skin, eye, ear, and nose) to the spinal cord and brain. Motor (efferent) nerves transmit impulses away from the CNS and produce responses in muscles and glands. The PNS contains 12 pairs of cranial nerves (Fig. 13–3, *B*), 31 pairs of spinal nerves (Fig. 13–3 *C*), and the sympathetic and parasympathetic nerves. The sympathetic and **parasympathetic** nerves make up the **autonomic** nervous system (ANS), which regulates the involuntary muscle movements and glandular actions of the body. The PNS also controls all conscious activities, which greatly affect unconscious processes such as the heart rate and bowel functions.

Four major blood vessels on each side of the head supply the brain with essential oxygen and nutrients. The carotid arteries (two internal and two external) originate from the two common carotid arteries and are located in the anterior portion of the neck; the two vertebral arteries, located within the vertebral column (Fig. 13–4), join with the two anterior and posterior cerebral arteries and the two anterior and posterior communicating arteries to form the brain's vascular system in a roughly circular configuration of arteries known as the *circle of Willis*. Branches from the circle of Willis supply blood to all portions of the brain (Fig. 13–5). Areas of the brain that depend on a single branch for survival are especially vulnerable to any disruption in the blood flow (e.g., thrombus or *embolus*). (See Vascular Disorders.)

Like the rest of the body, the nervous system is susceptible to a variety of problems. Defects in the circulatory system of the brain can lead to vascular disorders and damaged brain cells. The brain also can be damaged by injuries, infections, metabolic derangement, inherited defects, congenital defects, degeneration, and tumors. Because of the complex nature of the CNS and the PNS, damage to either of the systems can cause extremely diverse symptoms.

Common problems within the nervous system that necessitate attention from health-care providers include the following:

- Headaches
- Dizziness
- Muscle weakness
- Tremors
- Motor disturbances, other disturbances of movement, or paralysis
- Radiating pain
- Memory impairment
- Altered levels of consciousness
- Drowsiness
- Sensory disturbances or numbness
- Speech disturbances
- Visual disturbances

Text continued on p. 606

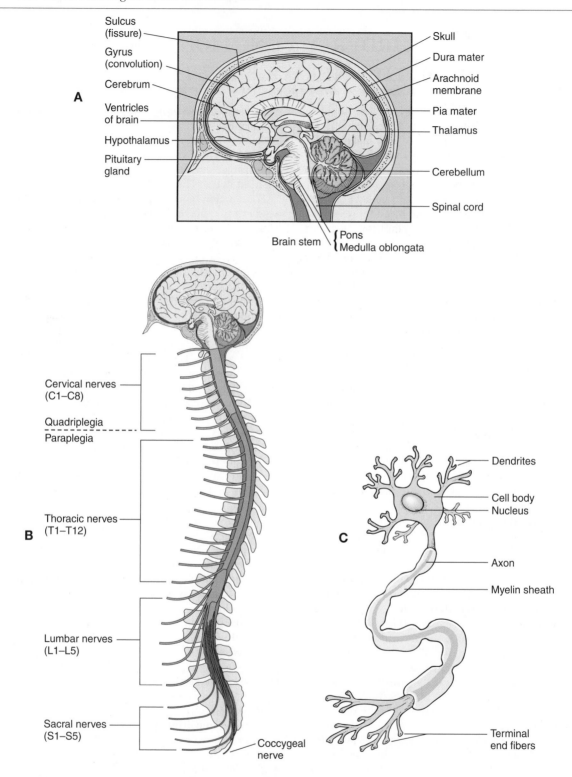

A

Sulcus (fissure)
Gyrus (convolution)
Cerebrum
Ventricles of brain
Hypothalamus
Pituitary gland

Skull
Dura mater
Arachnoid membrane
Pia mater
Thalamus
Cerebellum
Spinal cord

Brain stem { Pons
Medulla oblongata

B

Cervical nerves (C1–C8)
Quadriplegia
Paraplegia
Thoracic nerves (T1–T12)
Lumbar nerves (L1–L5)
Sacral nerves (S1–S5)
Coccygeal nerve

C

Dendrites
Cell body
Nucleus
Axon
Myelin sheath
Terminal end fibers

FIGURE 13–1 **A,** Normal brain. **B,** Spinal cord. **C,** Neuron.

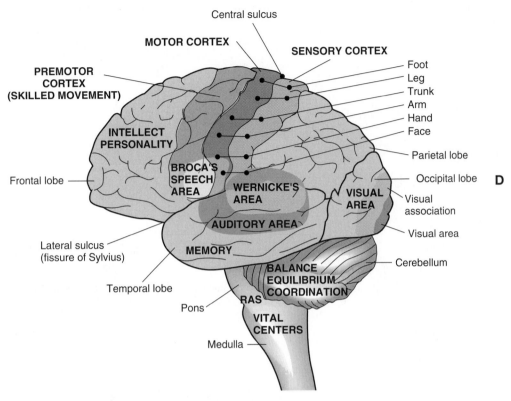

FIGURE 13–1, cont'd D, Functional areas of the brain. (**D** from Gould BE: *Pathophysiology for the health-related professions*, ed 2, Philadelphia, 2002, Saunders.)

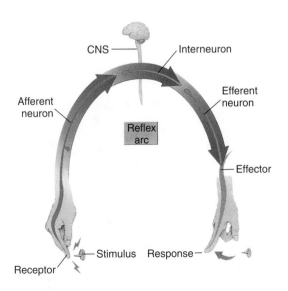

FIGURE 13–2 Functional classification of neurons. Neurons can be classified according to the direction in which they conduct impulses. The most basic route of signal conduction follows a pattern called *reflex arc*. (From Patton K, Thibodeau G: *Mosby's handbook of anatomy & physiology*, St. Louis, 2000, Mosby.).

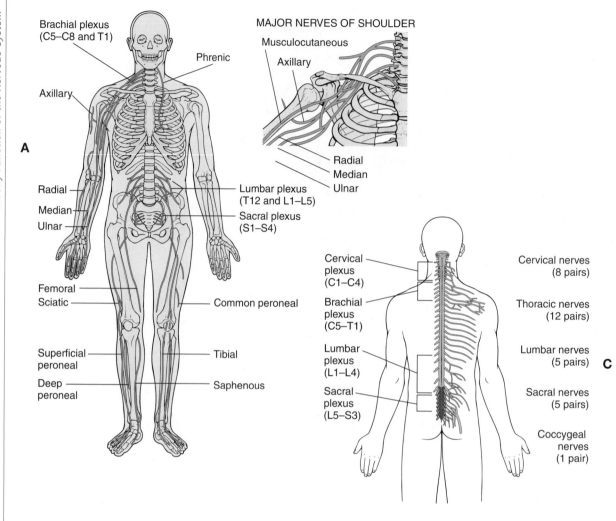

A

Brachial plexus
(C5–C8 and T1)

Phrenic

Axillary

Radial

Median

Ulnar

Femoral

Sciatic

Superficial
peroneal

Deep
peroneal

Lumbar plexus
(T12 and L1–L5)

Sacral plexus
(S1–S4)

Common peroneal

Tibial

Saphenous

MAJOR NERVES OF SHOULDER

Musculocutaneous

Axillary

Radial
Median
Ulnar

C

Cervical
plexus
(C1–C4)

Brachial
plexus
(C5–T1)

Lumbar
plexus
(L1–L4)

Sacral
plexus
(L5–S3)

Cervical nerves
(8 pairs)

Thoracic nerves
(12 pairs)

Lumbar nerves
(5 pairs)

Sacral nerves
(5 pairs)

Coccygeal
nerves
(1 pair)

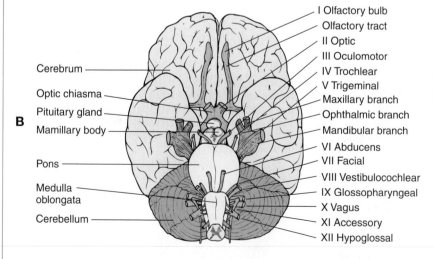

B

Cerebrum

Optic chiasma

Pituitary gland

Mamillary body

Pons

Medulla
oblongata

Cerebellum

I Olfactory bulb
Olfactory tract
II Optic
III Oculomotor
IV Trochlear
V Trigeminal
Maxillary branch
Ophthalmic branch
Mandibular branch
VI Abducens
VII Facial
VIII Vestibulocochlear
IX Glossopharyngeal
X Vagus
XI Accessory
XII Hypoglossal

FIGURE 13–3 A, Peripheral nervous system. **B,** Cranial nerves. **C,** Spinal nerves.

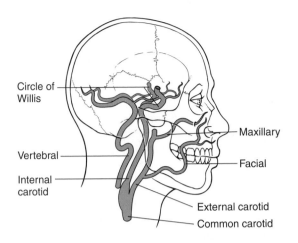

FIGURE 13-4 Cerebral circulation: major arteries of the head and neck.

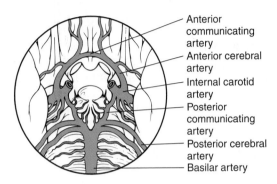

FIGURE 13-5 Circle of Willis.

ENRICHMENT

NEUROLOGIC ASSESSMENT

NEUROLOGIC ASSESSMENT relies on a step-by-step collection of data to evaluate the neurologic status and cognitive function of a person. The examination is appropriate after head trauma occurs or cranial surgery is performed or when a neurologic disorder, such as a brain tumor, is suspected. Observations and findings are graded on a scale and documented. The assessment is done within the constraints of circumstances (e.g., the location [the scene of an accident or a physician's office] and the patient's state of consciousness).

Neurologic assessment begins with a thorough medical history, noting past and current problems, and a record of medications being taken. The patient's comprehension and judgment are noted during the examination.

The patient's mental status may be graded with the Glasgow coma scale, which is a standardized system for assessing the response to stimuli.

Next, more sophisticated mental functions are tested, including speech, language, and writing skills. Is the patient having difficulty in putting words together, or is speech slurred? Do the patient's ideas and thoughts make sense? Behavior, emotional state, long-term and recent memory, and attention span are observed.

The cranial nerves are assessed by testing the patient's sense of smell, visual acuity, and eye movements, muscles of mastication, taste perception, facial muscles, hearing, and tongue movements and swallowing.

Motor function is evaluated by testing muscle tone and strength. Asymmetry in size, shape, or strength of corresponding muscles may be significant. Changes in extension and flexion of muscles and spasticity or flaccidity of muscles are noted.

Coordination and balance are assessed by watching for unsteadiness or a shuffling gait or the dragging of a foot. The patient is asked to perform rapid alternating movements and tasks to demonstrate fine motor coordination. A reflex hammer is used to test deep tendon reflexes in the arms and legs; and any depression or hyperactivity is recorded.

Sensory examination determines diminished or abnormal sensation. A cotton ball is brushed against the skin at different points. A slight pin stick tests for superficial pain. Temperature and vibration tests also are done.

Findings lead the clinician to begin focusing on any problem area. The need for further testing also is indicated as abnormal assessment findings emerge.

Vascular Disorders

Cerebrovascular Accident (Stroke)

DESCRIPTION

A cerebrovascular accident (CVA), or stroke, occurs when the brain is damaged by a sudden disruption in the flow of blood to a part of the brain or by bleeding inside the head.

■ **ICD-9-CM Code 436**

SYMPTOMS AND SIGNS

CVAs are the number one cause of adult disability. Because of the inadequate blood supply, the physical and mental functions controlled by the affected area fail to operate properly. The brain tissue in the affected area becomes bloodless (Fig. 13–6, *A*).

The symptoms and signs of a stroke reflect the portion of the brain affected (Fig. 13–6, *B*). Common stroke symptoms include the following:

- Sudden severe headache
- Sudden **aphasia,** *dysphasia,* or difficulty understanding language
- Sudden weakness, numbness, or paralysis of the face, or **hemiparesis** including one-sided drooping mouth and eyelid
- Sudden confusion or impaired consciousness
- Sudden loss of vision, blurred vision, unequal pupils, or **diplopia**
- Sudden onset of dizziness, loss of balance, or loss of coordination

A severe stroke can result in coma and death. Early recognition of symptoms and prompt medical intervention can help reduce the chances of disability and death.

PATIENT SCREENING

Any individual experiencing *sudden* onset of weakness, numbness or paralysis, difficulty speaking or understanding language, confusion or loss of consciousness, loss of vision or double vision, loss of balance or coordination, and dizziness requires immediate assessment and aggressive intervention. These individuals should be immediately entered into the emergency medical system (EMS) by the medical office or a family member.

ETIOLOGY

A CVA is usually the result of one of three types of vascular disorders: cerebral thrombosis (clot), cerebral hemorrhage, or cerebral embolism (moving clot). These vascular disorders most often are caused by atherosclerosis (see Atherosclerosis in Chapter 10) and hypertension (high blood pressure). Strokes also can result from blood disorders, *arrhythmias,* systemic diseases (e.g., diabetes mellitus and syphilis), *hyperlipidemia,* rheumatic heart disease, or head trauma. A high-fat diet, lack of exercise, cigarette smoking, obesity, and a family history of atherosclerotic disease are contributing factors.

CVAs caused by an embolus or hemorrhage often have a sudden onset, whereas strokes caused by a thrombus usually appear more gradually. A cerebral thrombosis occurs if one of the cerebral arteries becomes narrowed because of *plaque* buildup from atherosclerotic disease. This thrombus, or clot, can enlarge until it partially or completely blocks blood flow to the artery, thereby starving the tissue it feeds of oxygen.

A cerebral embolism is also a blockage, but it is caused by a foreign object, or embolus. This embolus can be a piece of arterial wall, a small blood clot from a diseased heart, or a bacterial clot; usually, platelet *fibrin* from an ulcerated arterial wall of the heart or valve of the heart is the causative factor. It is carried in the bloodstream until it becomes wedged in a blood vessel and obstructs the flow of blood to an area of the brain.

With a cerebral hemorrhage, the cerebral artery is not blocked but instead ruptures, flooding the surrounding brain tissue with blood. The initial effects of a hemorrhage may be more severe than those of a thrombosis or embolism, and the long-term effects are much more serious (Fig. 13–6, *C*). (Refer to the Enrichment box on Arteriovenous Malformations [AVM].).

DIAGNOSIS

Physical examination of the patient leads the physician to suspect a CVA and to gauge impairments on a functional scale. It can be confirmed by *magnetic resonance imaging (MRI), computed tomography (CT),* cerebral angiography, or electroencephalography (EEG). Blood tests for bleeding and clotting disorders may be performed.

TREATMENT

Immediate appropriate medical intervention (within 3 hours) from onset of stroke symptoms

ENRICHMENT

ARTERIOVENOUS MALFORMATIONS

FORMED DURING FETAL DEVELOPMENT, arteriovenous malformations (AVM) are abnormal structures of the blood vessels (Fig. 13–6, *C*). Etiology of this congenital condition that is rarely discovered before the age of 20 years is unknown. Although usually found in the brain, AVMs may be located in any vascular structure. Blood normally flows from the artery through capillaries to veins. In arteriovenous malformations, an abnormal connection is noted in which the capillaries are lacking. As a result, arterial blood moves directly into the veins, giving the blood vessels the appearance of a tangled mass of arteries and veins. These fragile vascular structures have a tendency to bleed and often result in hemorrhage. When located in the brain, symptoms of the bleeding are similar to those of a stroke. The patient complains of generalized or region-specific headache. Vomiting, stiff neck, confusion, lethargy, generalized weakness, visual problems, and irritability may be noted. As the bleeding progresses, speech may become impaired, muscle weakness and paralysis may be noted in the face, ringing in the ears may be reported, and dizziness and syncope may follow. Some patients may lose consciousness.

Diagnosis is made by assessment of the clinical signs and imaging studies including CT scans and MRIs of the brain. Prompt treatment is required and includes surgical intervention, radiation therapy, or embolization of the involved vessel. Cerebral AVMs have a mortality rate of approximately 10%. Additionally, it is possible for residual conditions caused by the insult of oxygen and nutrition deprivation of the brain tissue. Seizure activity and other neurologic problems may follow. No method of prevention is known for this condition.

---

may limit brain damage and thereby improve the prognosis. *Anticoagulants* (warfarin sodium [Coumadin]), thrombolytic agents, and antiplatelet medications (aspirin) may be given. A recently introduced protocol includes having the individual immediately chew an aspirin if possible. Surgery to improve circulation within the cerebral arteries or to remove clots is considered. Other therapeutic measures include surgery to repair broken or bleeding blood vessels and drugs to prevent or reverse brain swelling. Long-term treatment for CVA depends on the size and location of the stroke and the presence and severity of impairments. The goal of medical treatment is to restore lost functions and treat underlying disorders. A team approach to rehabilitation includes help from family members and a medical team of speech, physical, and occupational therapists; nurses; and doctors.

PROGNOSIS

Recovery varies in rate of improvement and degree of rehabilitation; some permanent disability may remain even after rehabilitation efforts. Brain cells destroyed do not recover and are not replaced; patients can learn new ways of functioning and use other undamaged brain cells.

PREVENTION

Prevention of stroke includes positive lifestyle changes to reduce controllable risk factors such as smoking, excesses in diet and alcohol consumption, untreated high blood pressure, and uncontrolled diabetes. Other risk factors over which the individual has no control include family history of stroke and age.

PATIENT TEACHING

Review warning signs of a stroke with the patient and family and instruct them concerning the importance of quickly seeking medical intervention for any signs of impending stroke. Assist the family in finding appropriate medical equipment for home use that will facilitate the home care and safety of the patient. Talk with the family about achievable goals. Assist the family by providing referrals to support groups and encouraging them to seek available help in the community.

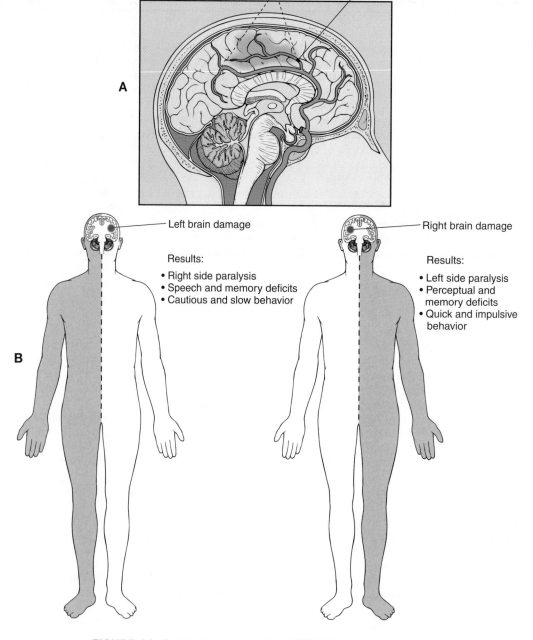

Affected area   Blockage

A

Left brain damage

Results:
• Right side paralysis
• Speech and memory deficits
• Cautious and slow behavior

Right brain damage

Results:
• Left side paralysis
• Perceptual and memory deficits
• Quick and impulsive behavior

B

FIGURE 13–6 **A,** Cerebrovascular accident (CVA). **B,** Areas of the body affected by CVA.

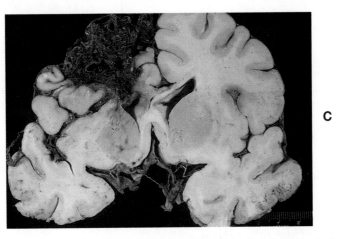

FIGURE 13–6, cont'd C, Arteriovenous malformation. (**C** from Kumar V et al: *Robbins basic pathology,* ed 7, Philadelphia, 2003, Saunders.)

Transient Ischemic Attack

DESCRIPTION

Transient ischemic attacks (TIAs) are temporary episodes of impaired neurologic functioning caused by an inadequate flow of blood to a portion of the brain.

■ ICD-9-CM Code **435** *(Transient cerebral ischemia, unspecified)*
435.09 *(Transient cerebral ischemia)*
Transient cerebral ischemia can occur in various sites and therefore various diagnostic codes are used. After the physician has diagnosed the site of the ischemia, refer to the current edition of the ICD-9-CM coding manual to confirm the appropriate code for transient cerebral ischemia.

SYMPTOMS AND SIGNS

TIAs often are referred to as "little strokes" or "mini strokes" because they resemble a stroke caused by an embolism. The individual may report sudden weakness and numbness down one side of the body, dizziness, dysphagia, or confusion. Usually, TIAs do not cause unconsciousness. These little strokes are often manifested as recurring episodes, lasting from just seconds to possibly hours, with symptoms gradually subsiding. The symptoms of a true stroke (or CVA) last longer than 24 hours, but TIAs should not be discounted as a minor condition because often they are important signals of an impending stroke (CVA). The symptoms, like those of a stroke, depend on which part of the brain is affected.

PATIENT SCREENING

As with individuals complaining of CVA-type symptoms, these individuals require immediate assessment and intervention to reduce residual effects. Instruct them or their families to contact EMS or to be transported immediately to an emergency facility.

ETIOLOGY

The most common cause of TIA is a piece of plaque, formed by atherosclerosis, that breaks away from the wall of an artery or heart valve and travels to the brain (Fig. 13–7). This is known as an *embolus* or moving clot. Platelet fibrin emboli from an arterial *ulcer* are often the causative factor. Arterial vascular spasms and minute blood clots also may be etiologic factors.

DIAGNOSIS

A physical examination and history are the first steps in diagnosing the problem. Next is determining the source of a possible embolus. A likely source of emboli is the carotid arteries. Cranial MRI scan, CT scan, and an EEG are all helpful in confirming the diagnosis; however, all can appear normal.

TREATMENT

Treatment depends on the location of the TIA and the underlying cause. Anticoagulants commonly are used during an episode to lessen the frequency or chance of recurrences. Recent protocol is to have the patient chew an aspirin tablet as soon as symptoms appear. In certain cases, surgery may be attempted to increase the blood flow to the affected area.

PROGNOSIS

Prognosis varies according to extent and duration of the ischemia. Most attacks resolve with minimal residual effects. TIAs should be considered as warning signals for future CVAs. Stress reduction and lifestyle changes to reduce risk factors should be implemented.

PREVENTION

As with CVA, prevention includes positive lifestyle changes to reduce controllable risk factors such as smoking, excesses in diet and alcohol consumption, untreated high blood pressure, and uncontrolled diabetes. Other risk factors over which the individual has no control include family history of stroke and age.

PATIENT TEACHING

As with patients who have suffered a stroke, instructions should be given concerning possible symptoms of an impending stroke. The family members should be encouraged to seek medical intervention for the patient at the first sign of a stroke. Give instructions for monitoring blood pressure and emphasize the importance of complying with the prescribed drug therapy.

Head Trauma

Epidural and Subdural Hematomas

DESCRIPTION

An **epidural** hematoma is a collection or mass of blood that forms between the skull and the dura mater, the outermost of the three meningeal layers covering the brain. With a subdural hematoma, the blood collects or pools between the dura mater and the arachnoid membrane, the second meningeal membrane (Fig. 13–8).

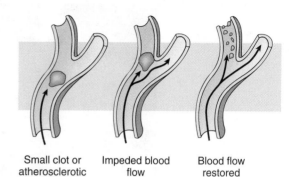

Small clot or atherosclerotic plaque embolus | Impeded blood flow | Blood flow restored

FIGURE 13–7 Embolus causing transient ischemic attack.

ICD-9-CM Code **852** *(Subarachnoid, subdural and extradural hemorrhage, following injury)*
852.4 *(Epidural hematoma)*
852.2 *(Subdural hematoma)*
Intracranial injuries are coded according to site, type of wound, state of consciousness, or length of unconsciousness. The fifth-digit subclassification refers to the level of consciousness as well as its duration and is a required digit in these codes. Refer to the current edition of the ICD-9-CM coding manual for verification of the appropriate code once the diagnosis has been confirmed.

SYMPTOMS AND SIGNS

Pressure on the brain resulting from either of these **hematomas** can result in impaired functioning of the brain, or possible death.

Symptoms of an epidural hematoma typically appear within a few hours of head trauma. They include sudden headache, dilated pupils, nausea and often vomiting, increased drowsiness, and perhaps hemiparesis. If the hematoma is not treated promptly, unconsciousness, coma, and death occur. Deterioration of the patient's condition can be rapid. This is a neurologic emergency.

Subdural hematomas often exhibit symptoms similar to those of an epidural hematoma, except that the onset is delayed because of a slower accumulation of blood. This delayed onset may mimic the symptoms of a TIA, stroke, or dementia. Diplopia is a common occurrence in patients with a subdural hematoma.

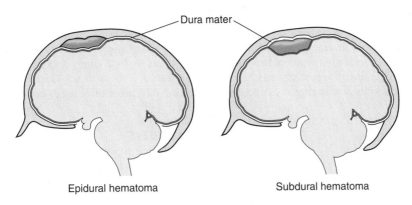

FIGURE 13–8 Hematomas (two types).

PATIENT SCREENING

Most trauma victims with closed and open head injuries will be transported to an emergency facility for treatment. When a head injury is not obvious, the onset of symptoms may be insidious. When a family member, or possibly the injured individual himself, calls in complaining of head pain and onset of other neurologic symptoms after head trauma, instruct the family member to have the victim of the trauma transported to an emergency facility for immediate assessment. Emphasize that the victim should not drive. The victim of any acceleration-deceleration type injury such as motor vehicle accidents or falls requires prompt assessment and follow-up intervention.

ETIOLOGY

Both types of hematomas can result when blood from ruptured vessels seeps into and around the meningeal layers. Head trauma is the usual cause; a blow to the head can cause an epidural hematoma, or the head striking an immovable object can cause a subdural hematoma. Subdural hematomas often occur among the elderly as a result of falls. Cerebral hematoma often follows a skull fracture.

DIAGNOSIS

The clinical findings noted upon examination of the patient, along with a history of recent head trauma, suggests to the physician the possibility of either an epidural or a subdural hematoma. Cranial radiographic films, CT scans, and cere-

bral arteriograms locate the hematoma and rule out other causes of the symptoms. Prompt investigation of the condition is vital. Obtaining the history of the mechanism of injury and time of the initial insult is an additional aid in determining the diagnosis.

TREATMENT

If the person loses consciousness because of head trauma, rapid medical attention is needed. A **craniotomy,** cranial trephination (bur hole, a hole made in the skull with a drill to relieve pressure by draining off the blood that has accumulated), may be necessary. This procedure is performed to remove the accumulated blood and to cauterize the bleeding vessels if increasing intracranial pressure indicates a life-threatening situation. When this procedure is performed promptly, a complete recovery is possible. A patient not losing consciousness but displaying symptoms, either immediately or delayed, should be seen by a physician as soon as possible for evaluation.

PROGNOSIS

Unchecked bleeding enlarges the hematoma and increases pressure on the blood vessels supplying the brain tissue, depriving them of oxygen. Prompt assessment and intervention are the keys to a good prognosis.

PREVENTION

Safety measures that deter head trauma are the best prevention (as mentioned in Patient Teaching).

PATIENT TEACHING

Provide postsurgical instructions for care of the incision. Instruct caregivers to assess for indications of neurologic changes and other signs of increased intracranial pressure. Encourage the use of seat belts, child restraint seats, and helmets for contact sports and cycling.

Cerebral Concussion

DESCRIPTION

A cerebral **concussion** is a bruising of the cerebral tissue that is caused by violent back and forth movement of the head, as in an acceleration-deceleration insult. This injury is also termed a *contra-coup insult*. Blunt force trauma also may result in a cerebral concussion.

■ **ICD-9-CM Code 850.9** *(Cerebral concussion, unspecified)*
Cerebral concussions have various codes according to the level of consciousness and duration of any periods of unconsciousness and are designated by the fourth-digit modifier. Refer to the current edition of the ICD-9-CM coding manual to determine the appropriate code.

SYMPTOMS AND SIGNS

With a cerebral concussion, an immediate loss of consciousness occurs. It often is referred to as being "knocked out." This state may last from a few seconds to several minutes and may be followed by a varying period of *amnesia*, lasting from 12 to 24 hours. Respirations become shallow, pulse rate is depressed, and muscle tone is flaccid. Symptoms appearing after the person has regained consciousness may include headache, nausea, vomiting, diplopia or blurred vision, and photophobia (sensitivity to light). Persons with this injury may exhibit irritability, decreased levels of concentration, and amnesia.

PATIENT SCREENING

Individuals who have suffered a head injury and have loss of consciousness are in need of immediate assessment and intervention. In most cases, treatment at an emergency care facility is the optimal choice. The unconscious individual should be transferred to the EMS for immediate assessment and transport to an emergency facility.

ETIOLOGY

A concussion is an injury resulting from impact with a blunt object, either by receiving a blow to the head or by falling. A concussion causes a disruption of the normal electrical activity in the brain, but the brain itself usually is not injured (Fig. 13-9).

DIAGNOSIS

A complete neurologic examination, along with a history of the injury, is required. CT scan indicates no evidence of damage to the brain tissues. History from others (e.g., relative, friend, observer, and ambulance staff) is vital.

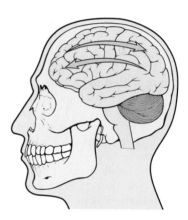

Concussion

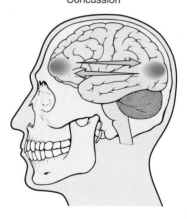

Contusion

FIGURE 13-9 Head injuries.

TREATMENT

The usual treatment of a concussion is quiet bed rest with observation of the patient for signs of behavioral changes. Recently developed concepts suggest it is acceptable to allow the patient to sleep, but make sure the patient is fully awake when aroused. Any changes noted, including changes in the level of consciousness, could indicate a progressive brain injury.

PROGNOSIS

Prognosis is unpredictable and depends on the extent of the insult and any additional trauma. Many people recover with no residual damage.

PREVENTION

Cerebral concussions are difficult to prevent. The consistent use of seat belts, child restraint seats, and the wearing of helmets may help reduce the severity of the injury.

PATIENT TEACHING

Encourage all patients to consistently use seat belts, secure children in child restraint seats, and wear helmets for contact sports or cycle riding. Provide family or caregivers with written information about care of a victim with a closed head injury.

Cerebral Contusion

DESCRIPTION

A cerebral contusion is more serious than a concussion. This injury to the brain involves bruising of tissues along or just beneath the surface of the brain.

ICD-9-CM Code 851 *(Cerebral lacerations and contusions)*
Cerebral lacerations and contusions are coded according to site, type of wound, state of consciousness, or length of unconsciousness. Additionally various codes relating to the level of consciousness and duration of any periods of unconsciousness are designated by the fourth-digit modifier. The fifth-digit subclassification refers to the level of consciousness as well as its duration and is a required digit in these codes. Once the diagnosis has been confirmed, refer to the current edition of the ICD-9-CM coding manual for assistance in verifying the appropriate code.

SYMPTOMS AND SIGNS

The symptoms and signs of a contusion vary, according to the site and extent of the injury, and persist for longer than 24 hours. They may range from temporary loss of consciousness to coma. When conscious, the person may report a severe headache and hemiparesis. Symptoms may be progressive in nature. The person may appear drowsy and lethargic or hostile and combative.

Permanent damage to the brain may result from a contusion caused by subdural and epidural hematomas (see Epidural and Subdural Hematomas), causing impaired intellect, dysphasia, paralysis, epilepsy, impaired gait, and continuing stupor.

PATIENT SCREENING

Individuals who have suffered a head injury and complain of severe headache develop one-sided paralysis and experience a period of unconsciousness and are in need of immediate assessment and intervention. In most cases, treatment at an emergency care facility is the optimal choice. The unconscious individual should be transferred to the EMS for immediate assessment and transport to an emergency facility.

ETIOLOGY

A contusion of the brain is caused by a blow to the head or impacting against a hard surface, as occurs in an automobile accident. The twisting or shearing force against the two hemispheres of the brain that occurs when colliding with the cranial bones may damage structures deep within the brain (see Fig. 13–9). A contusion often is associated with a skull fracture.

DIAGNOSIS

A thorough neurologic examination is necessary, as well as obtaining the history of the mechanism of the injury. CT scans reveal the location and extent of brain damage (Fig. 13–10). Cranial radiographic films rule out a possible skull fracture.

TREATMENT

Patients with a cerebral contusion need to be hospitalized so their vital signs can be monitored and rapid medical intervention will be available if required. Specific treatment is provided according to the site and severity of the contusion.

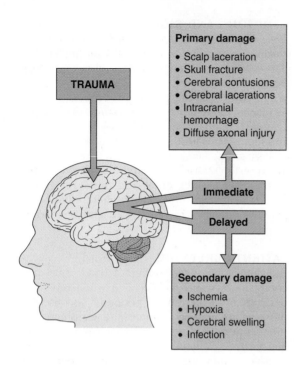

Primary damage
- Scalp laceration
- Skull fracture
- Cerebral contusions
- Cerebral lacerations
- Intracranial hemorrhage
- Diffuse axonal injury

TRAUMA

Immediate

Delayed

Secondary damage
- Ischemia
- Hypoxia
- Cerebral swelling
- Infection

FIGURE 13–10 Closed head injury (From Stevens A, Lowe J: *Pathology: illustrated review in color,* ed 2, St. Louis, 2000, Mosby.)

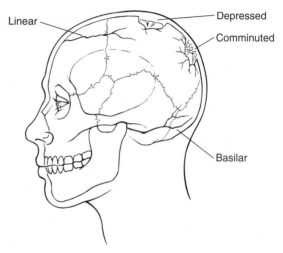

Linear — Depressed
— Comminuted
— Basilar

FIGURE 13–11 Skull fractures.

PROGNOSIS

Prognosis is unpredictable and depends on additional trauma and the health of the individual. Underlying pathology may compromise the possibility of a favorable outcome. Increased intracranial pressure and possible herniations are complications that may follow the injury.

PREVENTION

As with cerebral concussions, cerebral contusions are difficult to prevent. The consistent use of seat belts, child restraint seats, and helmets may help reduce the severity of the injury.

PATIENT TEACHING

As with cerebral concussions, all patients should be encouraged to consistently use seat belts and secure children in child restraint seats when traveling by car and wear helmets when engaging in contact sports or cycle riding. Provide family members or caregivers with written information about the care of a victim with closed head injury.

Depressed Skull Fracture

DESCRIPTION

A fractured skull occurs when a break or fracture occurs in one of the bones of the cranium (Fig. 13–11). When the skull bones are depressed or torn loose, they are pushed below the normal surface of the skull.

■ **ICD-9-CM Code** **803.00**
Once diagnosis has been made specifying site and type of skull fracture, refer to the current edition of the ICD-9-CM coding manual to confirm the appropriate diagnostic code.

SYMPTOMS AND SIGNS

When a portion of the skull is broken and is pushed in on the brain, causing injury, it is said to be a depressed skull fracture (see Fig. 13-11). The symptoms depend on the site of the fracture. For example, a bone fragment pressing on the motor area of the brain may cause **hemiplegia** (Fig. 13–12). Characteristically, symptoms from a depressed fracture are not progressive. They tend to remain static until the depressed bone is elevated

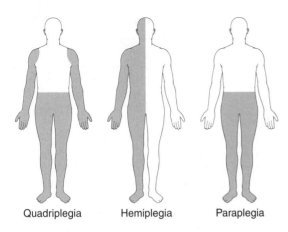

Quadriplegia   Hemiplegia   Paraplegia

FIGURE 13–12 Types of paralysis.

and the pressure is relieved. Epilepsy is a common complication of depressed skull fractures. (See Fig. 13–11 for additional types of skull fractures.)

PATIENT SCREENING

Patients with head injuries are in need of prompt intervention. Immediate transfer to the EMS for transportation to an emergency facility is recommended. Head injuries should always be considered life threatening until ruled otherwise.

ETIOLOGY

Direct impact on the skull with a blunt object is the most common cause of depressed fractures. Industrial injuries and automobile accidents are two of the many possible causes. The fractured bone may cut an artery or vein, causing hemorrhage in the brain.

DIAGNOSIS

Physical examination of the patient most likely reveals a defect in the skull. Cranial radiographic films indicate whether and where the brain is being crushed. CT scans show the presence of life-threatening cerebral edema.

TREATMENT

Treatment is aimed at relieving the intracranial pressure. A craniotomy is performed, and the depressed bone is elevated back into place. Head protection is worn until the fracture has at least partially healed.

PROGNOSIS

Prognosis is unpredictable; it depends on the extent of the insult, timely intervention, possible complications, additional trauma, and any underlying medical conditions. Successful surgical intervention in which intracranial pressure is relieved and bleeding is arrested usually has a positive outcome.

PREVENTION

Prevention is difficult because of the accidental nature of the fracture. Consistent use of seat belts and child restraint seats when riding in motor vehicles and wearing helmets for cycling and contact sports are helpful measures that can reduce the extent of damage in a head injury.

PATIENT TEACHING

Reinforce the potential dangers of head injuries in children to parents and remind them of the importance of children wearing helmets while cycling and playing contact sports. Advise parents and others to seek professional emergency intervention in the event of a head injury.

Spinal Cord Injuries

Paraplegia and Quadriplegia

DESCRIPTION

Injuries to the spinal cord affect the innervation of any spinal nerves distal to the point of insult. The extent of the injury and consequential edema often results in the failure of spinal nerve functioning with resulting loss of motor and sensory function. **Paraplegia** is loss of nerve function below the waist and paralysis of the lower trunk and legs. **Quadriplegia** is loss of nerve function below the cervical region resulting in paralysis of the arms, hands, trunk, and legs.

ICD-9-CM Code 344.1 *(Paraplegia)*
                344.0 *(Quadriplegia)*
Quadriplegia is coded by site and type. Once diagnosis confirms site and type, refer to the current edition of the ICD-9-CM coding manual for the appropriate code.

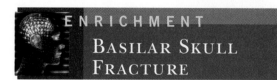

ENRICHMENT

BASILAR SKULL FRACTURE

A BASILAR SKULL FRACTURE is a fracture of the bones of the floor of the cranial vault (see Fig. 13–11). This injury usually results from a massive insult to the cranium during a motor vehicle accident or other violent trauma in which the head is struck anteriorly or laterally in the mid-portion. As with other head injuries, symptoms, signs, and treatment depend on the area involved and the extent of the fracture. *Raccoon eyes* and *Battle sign* are manifestations of basilar skull fracture, and these signs alert the physician to order imaging of the cranial vault for further investigation. Cerebrospinal fluid (CSF) flowing from the ears or nares may be associated with a skull fracture. The level of consciousness is assessed, as are other neurologic signs. Treatment is similar to that of head injuries, including surgical intervention to relieve intracranial pressure. Occasionally, the severity of the fracture causes severing of the pituitary stalk, resulting in *panhypopituitarism.*

SYMPTOMS AND SIGNS

When the spinal cord is injured, a part or parts of the body inferior to the point of injury may be affected. The damage to the cord may be only temporary, but it usually leads to some degree of permanent disability because nerve pathways control many bodily functions and actions. Paraplegia results in the loss of motor and sensory control of the trunk of the body and lower extremities. Loss of bowel, bladder, and sexual function is also common. Quadriplegia results in paralysis of the lower extremities and usually the trunk, with either partial or total paralysis in the upper limbs. Hypotension, hypothermia, bradycardia, and respiratory problems also may be present. In some patients, respiration is maintained or assisted by mechanical ventilation.

PATIENT SCREENING

Individuals that sustain the acceleration-deceleration type of injury require stabilization for transportation to an emergency care facility. Families of injured persons who are requesting information from the physician concerning the condition of their loved ones will be experiencing extensive anxiety and should be scheduled to see the physician at the next available appointment. Recovering patients will be scheduled for follow-up appointments as necessary.

ETIOLOGY

Generally, spinal cord injuries that cause paraplegia and quadriplegia are the result of vertebral fractures or vertebral dislocation. The site of the injury, the type of trauma to the cord, and the severity of the trauma determine whether the person becomes paraplegic or quadriplegic (see Fig. 13–12).

Trauma to the thoracic and lumbar regions of the spine (T1 and below) usually results in paraplegia (see Fig. 13–1, *B*). Vertical compression and hyperflexion of the spine usually produce this injury. Trauma to the cervical vertebrae (C5 or above) may result in quadriplegia. Injuries between C5 and C7 in the cervical vertebrae may produce varying degrees of **paresis** to the shoulders and arms. Damage occurring above C3 is usually fatal. The usual cause of this fatal injury is hyperextension or flexion of that portion of the spine. Mechanisms of spinal cord injury are presented in Figure 13–13.

DIAGNOSIS

A complete assessment of neurologic functioning is needed. Spinal radiographic films, MRI scans, and CT scans are ordered to determine the type and extent of injury. Figure 13–14, *A* and *B,* show the effects of spinal cord damage.

TREATMENT

The goals of treatment for all spinal cord injuries include restoration of the normal alignment and stability of the spine; decompression of the spinal cord, nerves, and vertebrae; and early rehabilitation of the patient. These goals may involve surgery or using specialized medications and procedures.

PROGNOSIS

The prognosis for a person with a spinal cord injury always is guarded. However, the earlier treatment is begun, the better the prognosis. Research focused on improving outcomes for spinal cord injuries is ongoing. Partial or total severing of the spinal cord results in permanent, irreversible damage and paralysis below the insult.

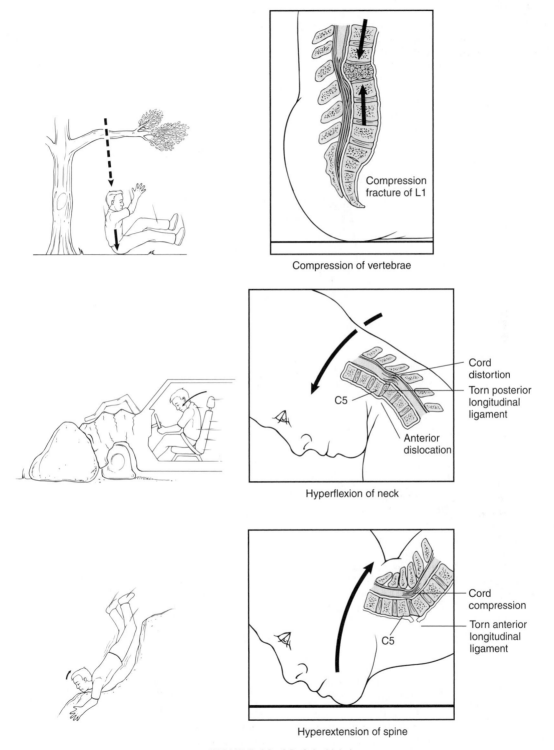

Compression fracture of L1

Compression of vertebrae

Cord distortion

Torn posterior longitudinal ligament

C5

Anterior dislocation

Hyperflexion of neck

Cord compression

Torn anterior longitudinal ligament

C5

Hyperextension of spine

FIGURE 13–13 Spinal injuries.

PREVENTION

Absolute prevention of spinal cord injury is not possible. Preventing injury beyond the initial insult is helped by immediate stabilization of injured persons before any form of movement is attempted.

PATIENT TEACHING

Assist patients and family in locating and contacting available community resources. Encourage patients to continue with recommended therapy.

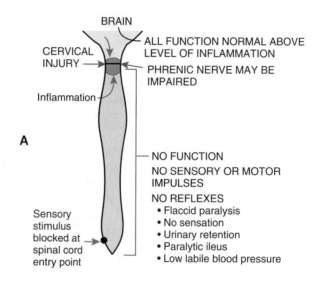

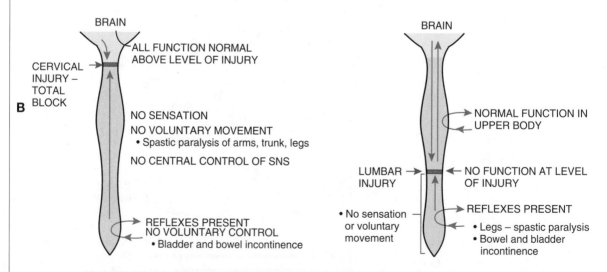

FIGURE 13–14 Effects of spinal cord damage. **A,** During spinal shock (period immediately following injury). **B,** Overview of permanent effects (postspinal shock). (From Gould B: *Pathophysiology for the health professions,* ed 2, Philadelphia, 2002, Saunders.)

Intervertebral Disk Disorders

Degenerative Disk Disease

DESCRIPTION

The degeneration or deterioration of an intervertebral disk results in pain in the areas served by the spinal nerves of the involved disk space.

ICD-9-CM Code 722.6 *(Site unspecified)*
Degenerative disk disease is coded by site. Once the site is confirmed by diagnosis, refer to the current edition of the ICD-9-CM coding manual for the appropriate code.

SYMPTOMS AND SIGNS

The pain radiates down the nerve path, is burning and constant, and can become *intractable.* The constant back pain and the severe pain that radiates down one or both legs may be accompanied by loss of some motor functions in the legs.

PATIENT SCREENING

Patients complaining of severe back pain require prompt assessment. Schedule an appointment for as soon as possible. A report of loss of motor function in the legs requires prompt assessment. Refer the patient to an emergency treatment facility.

ETIOLOGY

The degeneration usually is mechanical and is the result of constant wearing on the disk. A misalignment of the vertebrae causes a continual rubbing on the disk involved, resulting in inflammation and gradual destruction of the disk. The inflammation eventually involves the spinal nerve roots and causes scarring. A sequela is spinal *stenosis,* in which the nerve roots become trapped in the *foramen* as they leave the spinal canal.

DIAGNOSIS

The clinical findings and a history of previous back involvement leads to investigation with various types of imaging, including radiographic films, CT scan, MRI scan, and myelogram with contrast to show the disk status. The narrowing of the intervertebral spaces is consistent with the condi-

tion. *Electromyogram* (EMG) and neurologic testing demonstrate the involvement of dependent nerves and also measure the nerve conduction. The observation of neurologic deficits, including footdrop and the dragging of a leg when walking, adds to suspicion of the degeneration.

TREATMENT

Conservative treatment involves resting the back and lower extremities. Bracing the back is helpful. Analgesics and nonsteroidal antiinflammatory drugs (NSAIDs) are prescribed for pain relief. Surgical intervention includes spinal fusion and freeing of the spinal nerve roots from entrapment. In severe cases, nerve blocks, the use of *transcutaneous electrical nerve stimulation (TENS)* units, or a continuous infusion of morphine, by pump, into the epidural space may be employed to treat intractable pain.

PROGNOSIS

Prognosis varies depending on the extent of the degenerative process and the response of the patient to treatment.

PREVENTION

Prevention is difficult because this is a degenerative process and common in aging.

PATIENT TEACHING

Encourage patients to be compliant with physical therapy prescribed. Provide them with information about pain control measures. When a surgical procedure is involved, discuss wound care.

Herniated and Bulging Disk

DESCRIPTION

A herniated disk, also known as a *ruptured* or *slipped disk,* is the rupture of the nucleus pulposus through the annular wall of the disk and into the spinal canal (Fig. 13–15, *A* and *C*).

ICD-9-CM Code 722.2 *(Displacement of intervertebral disk, site unspecified without myelopathy)*
Herniated intervertebral disk disorders are coded according to sites and involvement of myelopathy. Once diagnosis has been confirmed, refer to the current edition of the ICD-9-CM coding manual for the appropriate code.

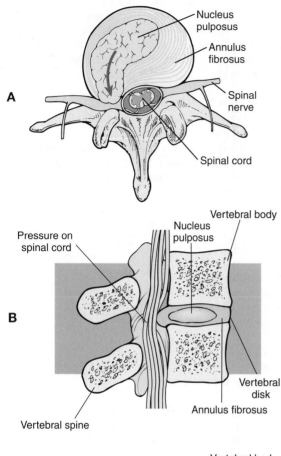

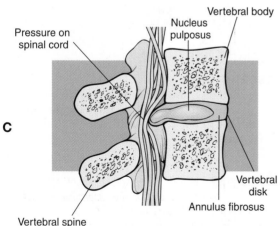

FIGURE 13–15 A, Herniated disk. Nucleus pulposus protrudes through annulus fibrosus, putting pressure on spinal cord and spinal nerve. **B,** Bulging disk (lateral view). Nucleus pulposus contained in annulus fibrosus. **C,** Herniated disk (lateral view). Nucleus pulposus through annular wall (annulus fibrosus) and pressure on the spinal cord.

SYMPTOMS AND SIGNS

Intervertebral disks are soft pads of cartilage located between each of the vertebrae that make up the spine. Each disk acts as a shock-absorbing cushion for the vertebrae and gives the back its flexibility for movement. Within each of these disks is a gelatinous center called the *nucleus pulposus,* which is surrounded by a circular wall-like structure, an annulus. The nucleus pulposus is contained within the annular wall in a bulging disk (see Fig. 13–15, *B*), thus the protrusion into the spinal canal is not as severe. The rupture can cause severe back pain and even disability if it presses against or pinches the spinal nerves. Sudden, sharp pain that worsens with movement results. It may radiate from the back to the buttocks, thigh, and leg following the course of the impinged nerve and causing paresthesia and muscle weakness in the leg. When this pain results from pinching of the sciatic nerve, it is known as *sciatica* (Fig. 13–16). Most herniated disks occur in the lower back, between the fourth and fifth lumbar vertebrae or the fifth lumbar and first sacral vertebrae (lumbosacral area). Ruptured disks in the cervical region of the spine often produce pain and weakness in the arms and neck. Pain from injury to a disk can be either unilateral or bilateral.

PATIENT SCREENING

A herniated disk is a painful and serious condition and necessitates immediate medical attention. It occurs more often in men than in women.

ETIOLOGY

Herniated and bulging intervertebral disks usually result from accumulated trauma (e.g., improper body mechanics when lifting) or sudden impact. Poor posture and the aging process can cause the disks to degenerate. The rupture may occur at the time of the trauma or shortly thereafter.

DIAGNOSIS

A thorough history of the back pain is important. Physical examination of the back is performed to rule out other possible causes of the patient's symptoms. The diagnosis of lumbar disk herniation can be considered if the patient has sciatic pain when the physician performs a straight leg raising test. The physician may order a CT scan, an MRI study, or a myelogram to help confirm the diagnosis.

In a bulging or contained disk herniation, the disk material is herniated through the inner annulus but not the outer annulus, so the contained material can still distort the path of the nerve with re-

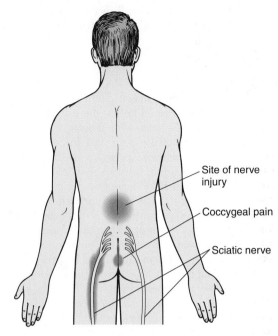

Site of nerve injury

Coccygeal pain

Sciatic nerve

FIGURE 13–16 Radiation of sciatic nerve pain.

sulting pain. In more severe herniation, which is considered noncontained, the nucleus pulposus penetrates both the inner and outer layers of the annulus.

TREATMENT
Conservative treatment consists of bed rest for 24 to 48 hours, traction, the use of hot or cold packs, and the administration of muscle relaxants and analgesics, such as aspirin and ibuprofen. A back brace for a herniated lumbosacral disk or a cervical collar for a herniated cervical disk may prove beneficial in relieving some of the discomfort.

When conservative treatment is not successful, surgical excision of the herniated disk may be needed. Procedures include percutaneous diskectomy, in which a needle is introduced into the intravertebral space and the encroaching portion of the nucleus pulposus is aspirated (for uncomplicated disk herniation); microdiskectomy, involving a small surgical incision, allowing the offending material to be aspirated; diskectomy as a surgical procedure combined with laser ablation and evaporation of the disk; or removal of the disk along with a laminectomy with fusion of the vertebrae.

Some patients may be treated with an enzyme called *chymopapain*. It is injected directly into the disk with the hope that it will dissolve the nucleus pulposus. This process is called *chemonucleolysis* and is considered controversial because of potentially serious complications, namely paralysis of a leg or arm, or death from anaphylactic shock. Often pain from bulging disks resolves with rest and drug therapy.

PROGNOSIS
Prognosis varies and depends on the extent and duration of the herniation. Many herniated disks resolve with rest. When surgical intervention is necessary, the outcome usually is favorable.

PREVENTION
Use of good and proper body mechanics is helpful in prevention; however, accidental slips and falls cannot always be prevented.

PATIENT TEACHING
Provide these patients with information about good and proper body mechanics. Encourage those for whom rest and physical therapy is prescribed to be compliant.

Sciatic Nerve Injury—Spinal Stenosis

DESCRIPTION
Sciatic nerve injury is a pathologic condition. It is brought about by trauma, degeneration, or rupture of the nucleus pulposus within intervertebral disks L4 through S1. Spinal stenosis, a narrowing of the spinal canal, often is termed *sciatica* because of the compression on the spinal cord and spinal nerve roots.

■ **ICD-9-CM Code 956.0** *(Sciatic nerve injury)*
 724.00 *(Spinal stenosis, unspecified region)*
Spinal stenosis is coded by region. Once the diagnosis has confirmed the affected region, refer to the current edition of the ICD-9-CM coding manual for the appropriate code.

SYMPTOMS AND SIGNS
The degeneration or rupture of the nucleus pulposus exerts pressure directly on the sciatic nerve, or on other closely positioned spinal nerves, sending impulses down the sciatic nerve. Rupture of one or more disks or their nuclei produces severe, sharp pain radiating from the sciatic nerve down the leg and to the foot (see Fig. 13–16). The pain may be

continuous or intermittent, and areas of the skin supplied by the affected nerves may feel numb. A rupture of the nucleus pulposus posteriorly, toward the neural canal, results in pressure on the sciatic nerve and causes low back pain. Anterior or lateral ruptures may or may not produce symptoms. Resulting symptoms depend on the extent of the rupture, the proximity of the nerves to the site, and the strength of the muscles and ligaments surrounding the spine. Nerve injury can produce severe disability, which may be temporary or permanent. Persons with sciatic nerve involvement may be so uncomfortable that they are unable to sit or stand.

Patients with spinal stenosis also report back pain and pain radiating down the legs and in the buttocks, thighs, or calves, which increases with walking or exercise. Additionally, they may experience numbness in these same areas that is worse when standing, walking, or exercising. A weakness in the legs may be noted. Reflexes in the lower extremities often are asymmetric, and sensation may be decreased.

PATIENT SCREENING

Patients reporting lower back pain that radiates down the leg require prompt assessment for pain relief and to prevent further exasperation of the condition. If an appointment is not available on the day of request, refer the patient to an emergency facility for evaluation and treatment.

ETIOLOGY

Trauma to the sciatic nerve may result from a fall, poor body mechanics, or gunshot or stab wounds. The aging process can lead to the degeneration of the disk or the nucleus pulposus. An inflammatory autoimmune response may prompt more rapid degeneration within a disk. The aging process, along with arthritic changes, may cause a narrowing of the spinal canal and the foramen where the spinal nerves exit the vertebrae. Formation of osteophytes on the foramen where the spinal nerves exit also can cause pain that radiates down the leg. A congenital narrowing of the spinal canal may be involved as well.

DIAGNOSIS

After a medical history is obtained and physical examination is performed, the physician may order several diagnostic tests. These tests can include spinal radiographic films, MRI scan, CT scan, myelogram or diskogram, and blood serum studies.

Vascular integrity is assessed and insufficiency is ruled out. Often a radiograph of the spine shows degenerative changes along with a narrowed spinal canal. EMG studies may show neurologic changes.

TREATMENT

Conservative treatment may include bed rest on a firm mattress for 24 to 48 hours, the use of a back brace, *ultrasound diathermy* with massage, and *iontophoresis.* After the acute pain and inflammation have subsided, an exercise program to strengthen the back and abdominal muscles may be ordered. Drug therapy consists of analgesics (e.g., aspirin [acetylsalicylic acid, ASA] and acetaminophen [Tylenol]), muscle relaxants (e.g., diazepam [Valium] and methocarbamol [Robaxin]), and antiinflammatory medications (e.g., piroxicam [Feldene], ibuprofen [Motrin, Advil, and Nuprin], and naproxen [Naprosyn]). For severe pain not controlled by the aforementioned medications, narcotic drugs (e.g., meperidine [Demerol], codeine, morphine, and oxycodone–aspirin [Percodan]) may be necessary.

Physical therapy, including applications of heat and cold or gentle massage (myofascial release), may help relieve acute pain. Corticosteroid injections may relieve pain too; however, they will not cure the spinal stenosis or sciatica. Often, leaning forward while sitting relieves the pain in the back.

Disabling pain or increasing weakness may necessitate surgical intervention. If a disk is causing the pain, then removal of part or all of the disk or nucleus pulposus (diskectomy or microdiskectomy), spinal fusion, or chemical dissolving, by an enzyme, of the nucleus pulposus (chemonucleolysis) may be helpful. Surgery may not relieve low back pain caused by underlying conditions such as osteoarthritis.

PROGNOSIS

Prognosis varies and depends on the extent of the degeneration and traumatic insult. Surgical intervention may provide relief from pain.

PREVENTION

Preventing injury associated with traumatic insults is difficult. Degeneration of disks is unavoidable.

PATIENT TEACHING

Provide instructions for good and proper body mechanics. Encourage compliance with prescribed physical and drug therapy.

Functional Disorders

Headache

DESCRIPTION
A headache (**cephalalgia**) is pain in the head that is not confined to any one specific nerve distribution area.

■ ICD-9-CM Code **784.0**

SYMPTOMS AND SIGNS
Headaches may be acute or chronic and located in the frontal, temporal, or occipital regions of the head. Cephalalgia also may be confined to only one side of the head or may be over one or both eyes. The type of pain may vary from dull and aching to almost unbearable. It can be an intense intermittent pain, throbbing pain, pressure pain, or penetrating pain driving through the head. Brain tissues themselves never ache because they do not contain sensory nerves; however, meninges do have pain receptors. Sensitivity in this area exists in only the meninges, the skin and muscles covering the skull, and many nerves that travel from the brain to the head and face.

Headaches are commonly experienced and usually are self-limiting. Cephalalgia is sometimes a symptom of an underlying disorder or disease (e.g., hypertension, stroke, brain tumor, and *encephalitis*). In most cases, however, headaches are caused by nothing more serious than fatigue or tension.

Some types of headaches are not symptoms of underlying disorders but are considered a specific disease. One of these is the cluster headache in which the pain is generally severe, developing around or behind one eye. The affected eye may tear. Cluster headaches usually occur at night and continue occurring for several weeks or months, then disappear for some time, even years. Another example of a severe type of headache is the migraine (see Migraine).

PATIENT SCREENING
Patients complaining of intractable head pain require prompt assessment. Schedule the patient for an appointment as soon as possible. If unable to schedule a same-day appointment, refer the patient to an emergency treatment facility. Other reports of headache type pain should be scheduled for an appointment as soon as possible.

ETIOLOGY
Many factors can irritate the pain-sensitive tissues or structures in the head, either alone or in combination, and produce headaches. Examples are stress, too little or too much sleep, overeating or drinking, a stuffy or noisy environment, and heavy physical labor, either indoors or outdoors. From a physiologic standpoint, however, there are actually only two causes of headaches. The first cause is strain on facial, neck, and scalp muscles resulting from tension. This is called a *tension headache*. The second cause is edema within the blood vessels of the head, which results in change in arterial size. This is called a *vascular headache*.

DIAGNOSIS
The medical history is vitally important in identifying a pattern to the headaches and is helpful in detecting any underlying causes. Physical examination and neurologic testing are necessary if a recurring pattern of headaches is revealed. Cranial and spinal radiographic films, an EEG, and a cranial CT scan may be ordered to rule out organic causes.

TREATMENT
The cause of the headache determines the type of treatment chosen. If the physician does not find an underlying cause of the headache, the use of *analgesics* (e.g., aspirin, acetaminophen, and NSAIDs), muscle relaxants, minor tranquilizers, and muscle massages, and relaxation with a warm bath are effective in providing temporary relief from a headache.

PROGNOSIS
Prognosis for the typical headache is good. Prognosis for intractable head pain is variable depending on the cause. Drug therapy often helps relieve the pain. Stress reduction and relaxation techniques may lead to a positive outcome.

PREVENTION
Prevention involves avoiding known or suspected trigger factors.

PATIENT TEACHING
Provide patients with information on relaxation techniques and stress reduction.

Migraine

DESCRIPTION

Periodic severe headaches that may be completely incapacitating and almost always are accompanied by other symptoms, such as nausea and vomiting, *anorexia*, intense hemicranial or bilateral throbbing pain, and visual signs and symptoms, are known as *migraine headaches.*

> **ICD-9-CM Code 346.9** *(Migraine unspecified)*
> *Migraine headaches are coded in the fourth digit by type or form of migraine. A fifth-digit modifier is required according to intractability of the migraine. Once the diagnosis has been confirmed, refer to the current edition of the ICD-9-CM coding manual for the appropriate code.*

SYMPTOMS AND SIGNS

Before the onset of the headache, many persons who experience migraine headaches have visual **auras:** flashing lights, zigzagging lines, or areas of total darkness. Photophobia is another warning sign. The nature of each attack varies from person to person, but usually a warning period during which the person feels abnormally fatigued and irritable is experienced. Other less common symptoms that occur occasionally are numbness or tingling in one arm or on one side of the body, dizziness, and temporary mental confusion.

These headaches may begin in adolescence or early adulthood, become less frequent and intense with age, and affect women nearly twice as often as men.

PATIENT SCREENING

Patients known to experience migraine headaches, as well as those reporting typical migraine headache symptoms, require prompt treatment. If an office appointment is not immediately available, refer the patient to an emergency treatment facility.

ETIOLOGY

Despite much medical research, it is not known why some people are subject to migraines or what triggers them. Certain factors do appear to be involved in many cases. Susceptibility to migraines, for instance, tends to appear in families, leading to a strong suspicion of inherited or genetic aspects of the disorder. In some cases, certain foods (e.g., aged cheese, chocolate, and red wine) have been found to provoke an attack.

The biologic cause of migraines may be changes in the cerebral blood flow. This is presumably attributable to vasoconstriction followed by vasodilation of the cerebral and cranial arteries.

DIAGNOSIS

A medical history of recurring, severe headaches, preceded by any combination of the aforementioned symptoms or signs, suggests the diagnosis. An EEG, a CT scan, and possibly an MRI scan may be ordered to rule out any organic conditions.

TREATMENT

In some cases, the treatment is simply bed rest in a quiet, darkened room and the administration of analgesics at the first sign of attack. For other patients, drug therapy in the form of vasoconstrictors, to constrict dilated blood vessels, and *antiemetics,* to control vomiting, may be needed. The use of *ergot* preparations has been effective for some patients in forestalling an impending attack or lessening the symptoms of an ongoing attack. Beta-blocking drugs and tricyclic antidepressant drugs can be prescribed. Sumatriptan succinate (Imitrex) is used for pain relief. Relaxation therapy or biofeedback has been used successfully to lessen the number of migraines for some people.

PROGNOSIS

Prognosis is usually favorable when the patient complies with drug therapy and rest.

PREVENTION

Encourage patients to avoid "trigger" factors if possible. Stress the value of implementing drug therapy and relaxation techniques at the first sign of onset of headache. If additional drug therapy is required for pain relief, it should be employed as soon as possible.

PATIENT TEACHING

Provide patients with information on stress reduction. Advise them on the importance of taking the preventive medications on a regular basis.

Epilepsy

DESCRIPTION

Epilepsy is a chronic brain disorder, characterized by sudden episodes of abnormal intense electrical activity in the brain, which result in seizure activity.

■ **ICD-9-CM Code** **345.90** *(Unspecified without mention of intractable epilepsy)*
Epilepsy is coded according to type. Both fourth- and fifth-digit modifiers are required. Once the diagnosis has been confirmed, refer to the current edition of the ICD-9-CM coding manual for the appropriate code.

SYMPTOMS AND SIGNS

The recurring seizures may entail involuntary contractions of muscles (convulsions) with disturbances of consciousness and sensory phenomena. Epilepsy takes many forms and has a variety of manifestations; more than 30 types of seizures are known, and it is possible for a person to have more than one type. Epileptic seizures are classified as partial or generalized. Status epilepticus is a complication of prolonged seizure activity.

Partial seizures do not involve the entire brain but arise from a localized area in the brain. The effects may involve the hand or face, with motor signs such as a rhythmic twitching of a group of muscles or compulsive lip smacking or picking at clothing. Behavioral, psychic, and sensory manifestations (auras) can occur. The patient usually experiences amnesia of the attack. However, no loss of consciousness occurs.

Generalized seizures cause a diffuse electrical abnormality within the brain and include absence (petit mal) and tonic–clonic (grand mal) attacks. Absence seizures, also called *petit mal epilepsy,* consist of a brief change in the level of consciousness indicated by staring, blinking, or blankly staring, with loss of awareness of surroundings. The episodes last only a few seconds and can occur many times a day, if not treated. Absence seizures occur most often in children and young adults.

Tonic–clonic seizures (grand mal epilepsy) may begin with a loud cry, followed by falling to the ground and loss of consciousness. During the tonic phase, the body stiffens and the tongue may be bitten. Prolonged contraction of the respiratory muscles causes the patient to become **cyanotic.** Then generalized rhythmic muscle spasms occur, followed by relaxation, the clonic phase. The patient may be incontinent of urine and feces. The seizure subsides in 1 to 2 minutes, but consciousness may be regained slowly. The person may be drowsy, confused, and weak; report headache; and have no memory of the event afterward.

Status epilepticus occurs when one seizure follows another with no recovery of consciousness between attacks. This is considered a medical emergency that requires immediate anticonvulsant therapy to prevent cerebral anoxia, hyperpyrexia, vascular collapse, and even death.

PATIENT SCREENING

Patients experiencing any form of seizure activity are in need of immediate assessment and intervention.

ETIOLOGY

In idiopathic epilepsy, no apparent cause for the abnormal electrical discharge is found, although a greater frequency may be found in some families.

In symptomatic epilepsy, a known abnormality in the brain resulting from a pathologic process, genetic or acquired, seems to trigger seizures. Pathologic conditions associated with seizure disorder include scar tissue on the cerebral cortex from infection or trauma, cortical *neoplasms,* cerebral edema, and CVAs (strokes). Other possible causes are birth trauma (cerebral palsy), drug toxicity (e.g., alcohol), diabetes, hypoglycemia, and other conditions that deprive the brain of oxygen.

DIAGNOSIS

Not all seizures imply epilepsy; thus a medical history is essential for determining diagnosis. An EEG shows semispecific brain activity, suggesting epilepsy; MRI also may be helpful. Classification of epilepsy is based on the location of the abnormal activity and its duration. CT scan shows structural changes in the brain, such as tumors, scars, and malformations. Cerebral angiography may identify vascular changes in the brain. A skull radiographic film may reveal evidence of fracture, separation of cranial sutures, or movement of the pineal gland. Blood serum chemistry changes may indicate metabolic disease, drug toxicity, or hypoglycemia.

TREATMENT

Anticonvulsant medications are the treatment of choice for epilepsy; more commonly used drugs include phenytoin (Dilantin), carbamazepine (Tegretol), primidone (Mysoline), and valproic acid. Close monitoring and adjustments of dosage to attain good therapeutic control are essential. In rare cases, surgical intervention may be necessary to excise an identified lesion in the brain. Certain restrictions may be necessary. For instance, depending on state regulations, a license to drive a motor vehicle may not be issued unless the person has been seizure free, with treatment, for a specific period. Emotional support for the patient and the family is made available.

PROGNOSIS

Prognosis varies. Drug therapy often can control seizure activity. Status epilepticus is a life-threatening event. Immediate intervention may afford a positive outcome.

PREVENTION

Prevention of the initial onset of seizure activity is impossible. Compliance with drug therapy has a positive affect on the ultimate outcome of epilepsy.

PATIENT TEACHING

Because this disease often is feared and misunderstood, education is necessary to dispel myths. First aid instructions are available that can teach family members how to care for the patient in the event of

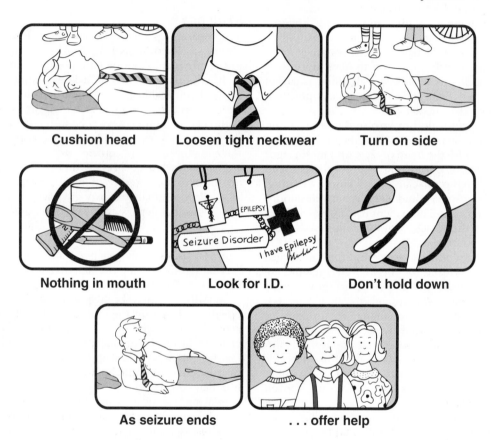

Cushion head   **Loosen tight neckwear**   **Turn on side**

Nothing in mouth   **Look for I.D.**   **Don't hold down**

As seizure ends   **. . . offer help**

Most seizures in people with epilepsy are not medical emergencies. They end after a minute or two without harm and usually do not require a trip to the emergency room.

But sometimes there are good reasons to call for emergency help. A seizure in someone who does not have epilepsy could be a sign of serious illness.

Other reasons to call an ambulance include:

• A seizure that lasts more than 5 minutes

• No "epilepsy" or "seizure disorder" I.D.

• Slow recovery, a second seizure, or difficult breathing afterward

• Pregnancy or other medical I.D.

• Any signs of injury or sickness

FIGURE 13–17 First aid for seizures. (From Epilepsy Foundation of America, Landover, MD, 1990.)

grand mal seizures (Fig. 13–17). Emphasize local restrictions about driving a motor vehicle. Additionally, stress the importance of drug therapy compliance. Assist the patient and family in locating and contacting support groups in the community.

Parkinson Disease

DESCRIPTION
Parkinson disease is a common, slowly progressive neurologic disorder characterized by the onset of recognizable disturbances: a "pill-rolling" tremor of the thumb and forefinger, muscular rigidity, slowness of movement, and postural instability.

 ICD-9-CM Code 32.0

SYMPTOMS AND SIGNS
Usually *insidious* in onset, the Parkinson symptoms, which vary from person to person, may be associated with aging until the recognizable paradigm of Parkinson disease emerges. The posture is stooped, and the patient moves with a peculiar shuffling gait: the head is bowed, the body is flexed forward, the knees are slightly bent, and the patient has a tendency to fall (Fig. 13–18). The face takes on a mask-like or expressionless appearance, speech is muffled, and swallowing is difficult. Gradual changes in behavior and mental activity are noted in some patients as the disease progresses. The mean age of onset is 60 years, but many cases appear in younger persons. Parkinson disease afflicts more men than women, and the usual life span after diagnosis is 10 years.

PATIENT SCREENING
Because of the insidious onset of Parkinson disease, patients and family members may contact the office for an appointment because of vague neurologic symptoms. Schedule these individuals for the next available appointment. Individuals already identified as having the disease will be scheduled for routine follow-up care.

ETIOLOGY
What causes the degeneration of nerves in the motor system of the brain stem is not known. A deficiency of dopamine, a **neurotransmitter** manufactured in the midbrain, has been clinically demonstrated in patients with Parkinson disease. Parkinsonism (as a syndrome) also can occur after ingestion of poison, after encephalitis, and after taking certain major tranquilizers and certain anti-

hypertensive drugs (Fig. 13–19). Degenerative diseases of the brain involve preferentially various parts of the brain.

DIAGNOSIS
The diagnosis is based on the characteristic history and careful neurologic examination. Decreased dopamine levels may be noted in the urine.

TREATMENT
Parkinson disease cannot be cured; therefore, medical management consists of supportive measures and control of symptoms with the administration of drugs such as levodopa, carbidopa, antidepressants, and anticholinergics for tremor and rigidity. Many patients report improvement when taking deprenyl. Physical therapy helps the patient maximize his or her mobility within the limitations of the disease. The patient is given every possible supportive measure to encourage independence and self-care.

PROGNOSIS
At the present time, no cure for Parkinson disease is known. Research continues in the hope of finding a cure.

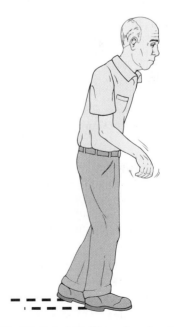

FIGURE 13–18 Typical shuffling gait and posture of patients with Parkinson disease.

Functional Disorders

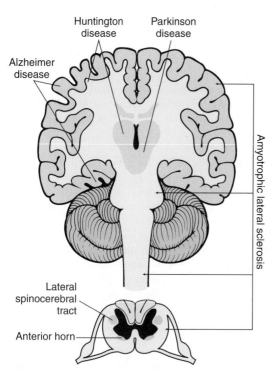

Huntington disease

Parkinson disease

Alzheimer disease

Amyotrophic lateral sclerosis

Lateral spinocerebral tract

Anterior horn

FIGURE 13–19 Degenerative diseases of the brain involve preferentially various parts of the brain. Alzheimer disease causes atrophy of the frontal and occipital cortical gyri. Huntington disease affects the frontal cortex and basil ganglia. Parkinson disease is marked by changes in the substantia nigra. Amyotrophic lateral sclerosis affects the motor neurons in the anterior horn of the spinal cord, brain stem, and the frontal cortex of the brain. (From Damjanov I: *Pathology for the health-related professions,* ed 2, Philadelphia, 2000, Saunders.)

PREVENTION

No method of preventing Parkinson disease is known.

PATIENT TEACHING

Assist the patient and family in locating and contacting available community resources. Encourage family members to be supportive of therapy prescribed to help the patient remain independent as long as possible.

Huntington Chorea

DESCRIPTION

Huntington **chorea** (Huntington disease) is a hereditary degenerative disease of the cerebral cor-

tex and basal ganglia; progressive atrophy of the brain occurs.

 ICD-9-CM Code 333.4

SYMPTOMS AND SIGNS

The chronic, progressive chorea (ceaseless, uncontrolled, involuntary movements) has an insidious onset, with the loss of musculoskeletal control exhibited by subtle, semipurposeful movements. Typically, the arms and face are the first areas to be involved, with movements ranging from mild fidgets to tongue smacking. Speech difficulties are experienced and the emotional state deteriorates, followed by dementia. Disruption of the personality is displayed by the untidy and careless appearance of the individual. Personality changes noted are described as apathetic, moody behavior, a loss of memory, and onset of paranoia. The onset of symptoms typically begins in early middle age.

PATIENT SCREENING

The insidious onset of Huntington chorea results in vague symptoms; therefore, the condition inadvertently may be exposed during a routine visit. Because it is a familial type disease, patients with a family history of the disease may be aware of the progression of symptoms and request an appointment. Although not considered an emergency, the occurrence of symptoms can create high anxiety levels in patients, so they should be scheduled for the next available appointment.

ETIOLOGY

Although the exact etiology of this condition is uncertain, it is transmitted by an *autosomal*-dominant trait that can be inherited by either sex.

DIAGNOSIS

No definitive method of diagnosis is known, except by careful neurologic appraisal and by detection of the defective gene through DNA analysis. A history of progressive chorea and dementia, along with a familial trait for the disease, leads to further investigation. A cerebral CT scan shows brain atrophy.

TREATMENT

No cure for this progressively deteriorating condition is known; therefore, treatment is supportive, symptomatic, and protective. Haloperidol lactate

(Haldol) and fluphenazine hydrochloride (Prolixin) are prescribed in an attempt to control choreic movements and to reduce agitation.

PROGNOSIS

At the present time, no cure for Huntington chorea is known. Drug therapy may help control agitated behavior. Eventually, institutionalization may be necessary to provide the care required to manage the deteriorating condition of the patient.

PREVENTION

Being an inherited familial type disorder, no method of prevention is known.

PATIENT TEACHING

Provide the patient and family with information about the disease. Assist them in locating and contacting community resources.

Amyotrophic Lateral Sclerosis

DESCRIPTION

Amyotrophic lateral sclerosis (ALS), also known as *Lou Gehrig disease,* is a progressive, destructive motor neuron disease that results in muscular atrophy.

 ICD-9-CM Code 335.20

SYMPTOMS AND SIGNS

Fasciculations (small local involuntary muscular contractions) and accompanying atrophy and weakness are noted in the forearms and hands. These patients progress to having difficulties in speech, chewing, swallowing, and breathing; eventually, a ventilator is required. No sensory neuron involvement is noted, and functioning of the mind is not affected. ALS characteristically affects men slightly more often than women, with onset occurring after the age of 50 to 60 years.

PATIENT SCREENING

Patients complaining of weakness and involuntary muscular contractions of the hands and arms should be assessed promptly. Anyone complaining of difficulty breathing and swallowing requires immediate assessment.

ETIOLOGY

Although the etiology of ALS is uncertain, some cases may be caused by autosomal inherited traits.

DIAGNOSIS

The clinical findings of upper and lower motor neuron involvement without any sensory neuron involvement will lead to further investigation. EMG and muscle *biopsy* are employed to confirm nerve, not muscle, involvement. Over a period of several months, the diagnosis is confirmed by the typical progression of the disease.

TREATMENT

Because no cure for the condition is known, treatment involving a team of caregivers consists of supportive measures and therapy directed at controlling symptoms. Death usually occurs within 6 to 10 years after onset. Pulmonary management is vital.

PROGNOSIS

No cure for ALS is known, and death usually follows within 6 to 10 years after diagnosis.

PREVENTION

No method of prevention is known; the disease is thought to be caused by autosomal inherited traits.

PATIENT TEACHING

Provide the patient and family with information about the disease. Assist them in locating and contacting community resources.

Transient Global Amnesia

DESCRIPTION

Transient global amnesia, although frightening and anxiety provoking, usually is a benign event. As the name implies, the event is transient or temporary, having a duration of 1 to 6 (maybe even up to 12) hours. It is considered to be global in nature because it encompasses the entire memory of current events. The amnesia manifests as total loss of recent memory; the learning process is completely blocked. Memory disturbances are involved.

 ICD-9-CM Code 437.7

SYMPTOMS AND SIGNS

The individual experiencing the onset of transient global amnesia has a sudden onset of memory loss, primarily of both current and recent events. Repetitive asking of questions such as, "Where are we going?" "Why are we going there?" "Where am I?" and "Why did we do that?" is typical. Confusion is apparent; nevertheless, the individual has recall of personal identity as well as orientation to place as long as the place is a normal environment. Memory loss may encompass the preceding 3 to 5 years and specific events. Usual tasks, including those requiring mechanical abilities, often are performed without difficulty. Neurologic signs are normal; no numbness, tingling, or weakness (unilateral or total) is noted; pupils are equal and react to light and accommodation (PERLE) and vocalization is normal. Communication skills concerning current events and status suffer from the amnesic event that begins and ends abruptly. Memory usually returns within 6 to 12 hours; however, the period of amnesic experience will remain unavailable to any recall; this also may be true of events that occurred a few hours to a few days before the amnesic event. Some will complain of headache.

PATIENT SCREENING

The patient should be seen as soon as possible if the office schedule will allow. This will permit observation of the symptoms and help reduce anxiety of both patient and family. Neurologic signs need to be observed, evaluated, and recorded. If working the patient into the schedule is not possible, refer the patient to an emergency facility for prompt observation and to rule out TIA and cerebral accident.

ETIOLOGY

Etiology is unknown; however, evidence points to the precursors of experiencing stress or emotional events, swimming or immersion in cold water, driving a motor vehicle, or having sexual intercourse. The individual may have experienced migraine headaches on previous occasions, usually without nausea, vomiting, or photosensitivity.

DIAGNOSIS

Diagnosis is made by observing the symptoms and signs and establishing a negative neurologic examination. TIA, cerebral accident, and seizure activity is to be ruled out first.

TREATMENT

Treatment is supportive; the patient is given reassurance during and after the episode.

PROGNOSIS

Prognosis is good; recurrence is very unlikely. The individual probably will never regain memory of

events that occurred during the episode or during the hours or days immediately preceding the episode.

PREVENTION

No method of prevention is known. All patients are encouraged to reduce stress factors in their lives.

PATIENT TEACHING

Provide patient and family with reassurance that this event is transient in nature and in all likelihood will not occur again. Additionally, instructions should be provided to the family to return if symptoms do reoccur.

Peripheral Nerve Disorders

Peripheral Neuritis

DESCRIPTION

Peripheral neuritis is a degeneration of the peripheral nerves.

 ICD-9-CM Code 356.9 *(Unspecified)*

SYMPTOMS AND SIGNS

Peripheral neuritis, the degeneration of peripheral nerves, affects the distal muscles of the extremities. Unless the precipitating factors are severe infection or chronic alcohol intoxication, the onset is insidious. Clumsiness and loss of sensation in the hands and feet are followed by a flaccid paralysis and a wasting of muscles in these areas. Deep tendon reflexes become diminished, and tenderness is noted in the atrophied muscles. The skin may take on a glossy, red appearance, and sweating is decreased. With leg and foot involvement, footdrop may be experienced. Some patients have pain in the affected regions.

PATIENT SCREENING

Patients reporting loss of sensation in hands and feet should be promptly assessed. Schedule an appointment for the soonest possible time.

ETIOLOGY

Chronic alcohol intoxication; toxicity from arsenic, lead, carbon disulfide, benzene, or phosphorus; infectious diseases, including mumps, pneumonia, and diphtheria; metabolic or inflammatory disorders, including diabetes, rheumatoid arthritis, gout, and systemic lupus erythematosus; and certain nutritional deficiency diseases are all causative factors. The nerve degeneration leads to muscle weakness and sensory loss.

DIAGNOSIS

The history, combined with the clinical findings characteristic of motor and sensory involvement, leads to additional investigation. Motor and sensory nerve impairment usually is detected by EMG.

TREATMENT

The first step in effective treatment is to ascertain the cause and, if possible, to correct or eliminate the condition. *Toxic* substances need to be removed, if possible, and vitamin and nutritional deficits corrected. Underlying disease processes are treated or controlled. When chronic alcoholism is the cause, the patient must avoid all alcohol in any form. Supportive measures, such as the administration of anticonvulsants and tricyclic antidepressants and getting rest and physical therapy, are employed to relieve pain.

PROGNOSIS

Control of underlying causes may provide relief of symptoms. Proper nutrition is helpful.

PREVENTION

Prevention is difficult when the etiology is based on a preceding disease process or exposure to toxic substances. Avoidance of alcohol may help prevent recurrence of the neuritis.

PATIENT TEACHING

Encourage patients to be compliant with drug and physical therapy as prescribed.

Trigeminal Neuralgia (Tic Douloureux)

DESCRIPTION

Trigeminal neuralgia, or tic douloureux, is pain of the area innervated by the fifth cranial nerve, the trigeminal nerve.

ICD-9-CM Code 350.1

SYMPTOMS AND SIGNS

The transient, excruciating pain of trigeminal neuralgia radiates along the fifth cranial nerve distribution and can affect any of the three fifth cranial nerve branches (Fig. 13–20). When the ophthalmic branch is affected, pain is experienced in the eye and forehead. The maxillary branch involves the nose, upper lip, and cheek. The mandibular branch involves the lower lip, the outer portion of the tongue, and the area of the cheek close to the ear. Additionally, several branches may be involved. The pain is always unilateral and does not cross midline because only one side of the face is involved. The abrupt and sudden onset of pain is triggered by mechanical or thermal stimulation. These persons sleep poorly and may be undernourished and dehydrated because chewing, swallowing, or any touching of the area may set off the pain.

PATIENT SCREENING

The pain of trigeminal neuralgia is so severe that these individuals require immediate pain relief. When an immediate appointment is not available, refer the patient to an emergency facility for assessment and medication for pain relief.

ETIOLOGY

The cause is uncertain, although some cases have been found to be related to compression of a nerve

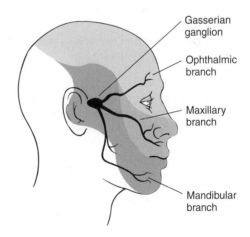

FIGURE 13–20 Trigeminal nerve (fifth cranial nerve) and branches.

root by a tumor or vascular lesion. Occasionally, trigeminal neuralgia is a sequela to multiple sclerosis or herpes zoster. Most cases have no identified cause.

DIAGNOSIS

The reports of an excruciating pain that has an abrupt onset and a duration of seconds to minutes on one side of the face suggest trigeminal neuralgia. Observation of the patient, both during an attack and at normal times, demonstrates the presence of pain. The patient avoids touching the face to prevent triggering an attack. Because even a draft or gentle breeze may set off the pain, the face is protected and temperature extremes are avoided. No impairment of sensory or motor function is noted. The episodes may last from months to years and then subside. Infection of a sinus or tooth and tumors must be ruled out.

TREATMENT

Analgesics are prescribed for pain. When relief cannot be obtained, surgical intervention to dissect the nerve roots is performed. Patients who smoke are advised to cease smoking.

PROGNOSIS

Prognosis varies depending on the underlying causative factors. Some incidents will resolve spontaneously whereas others may respond to drug therapy. Surgical intervention, as a last resort, will afford pain relief; however, nerve function of the affected nerve may be compromised as a result.

PREVENTION

No method of prevention is known. Smokers are encouraged to stop smoking.

PATIENT TEACHING

Provide information about the condition to the patient and family. Assist them in locating and contacting community support groups.

Bell Palsy

DESCRIPTION

Bell palsy is a disorder of the facial nerve (seventh cranial nerve) that causes a sudden onset of weakness or paralysis of facial muscles.

▇ **ICD-9-CM Code** **351.0**

SYMPTOMS AND SIGNS

The severity of paralysis in Bell palsy varies widely. The patient may be aware of pain or a drawing sensation behind the ear, followed by an inability to open or close the eye and drooping of the mouth and drooling of saliva. Often the disorder is first noticed in the morning, having developed overnight. Initially, the patient is unable to smile, whistle, or grimace, and the facial expression is distorted (Fig. 13–21). Taste perception may be diminished, contributing to loss of appetite. The condition is usually unilateral. It may be transient or permanent and usually occurs between 20 and 60 years of age, in men and women alike.

PATIENT SCREENING

The individual reporting sudden onset of one-sided facial paralysis requires prompt assessment to rule out a cerebral vascular accident. Referral is usually to an emergency facility for diagnosis. Anxiety will be high in the individuals and their families so any requests for appointments to discuss the condition after diagnosis should be scheduled for the next available opening.

ETIOLOGY

The cause of Bell palsy is not always certain. The symptoms result from blockage of impulses from the facial nerve (cranial nerve VII) caused by com-

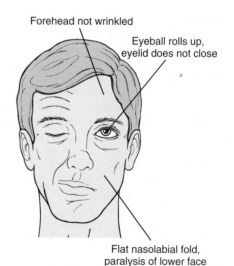

Forehead not wrinkled

Eyeball rolls up, eyelid does not close

Flat nasolabial fold, paralysis of lower face

FIGURE 13–21 Bell palsy. (From Lewis SM, Heitkemper MM, Dirksen SR: *Medical-surgical nursing: assessment and management of clinical problems,* ed. 6, St. Louis, 2004, Mosby.)

pression of the nerve in the bony canal. Bilateral facial paralysis has been noted in a small percentage of people with Lyme disease.

DIAGNOSIS

Bell palsy is diagnosed from symptoms and signs and the characteristic history. The differential diagnosis includes CVA (stroke) and autoimmune disease.

TREATMENT

Early treatment is critical. The application of warm moist heat, gentle massage, and facial exercises to stimulate muscle tone are recommended. Prednisone may be prescribed to reduce edema of the facial nerve. Analgesics also may be required. Inability to close the eye may result in dry, sore eyes; artificial tears and an eye patch for protection from outside elements may be needed unless the case is mild. Electrotherapy stimulates the nerve and prevents atrophy of muscles.

PROGNOSIS

Complete recovery is possible if the disease is treated early, and recovery often occurs spontaneously, especially in younger individuals. Nevertheless, residual effects may remain for an undetermined period of time. Patients who smoke are advised to cease smoking.

PREVENTION

No method of prevention is known.

PATIENT TEACHING

Provide information about the condition to the patient and family. Assist them in locating and contacting community support groups.

Infectious Disorders

Meningitis

DESCRIPTION

Meningitis is an inflammation of the meninges, the membranous coverings of the brain, and spinal cord.

ICD-9-CM Code 322.9 *(Unspecified)*

Meningitis is coded according to cause or type. Once the diagnosis has confirmed the cause and type, refer to the current edition of the ICD-9-CM coding manual for the appropriate code.

SYMPTOMS AND SIGNS

Early symptoms of meningitis include vomiting and a headache that increases in intensity with movement or shaking of the head. Attempts of the examiner to move the head reveal *nuchal rigidity*, a stiffness of the neck that resists any sideways or flexion–extension movements of the head; this is a classic sign. Positive Kernig sign (resistance to leg extension after flexing the thigh on the body) and Brudzinski sign (neck flexion causes flexion of the hips from a supine position) indicate meningeal irritation. Deep tendon reflexes increase, and the patient exhibits irritability, photophobia, and a hypersensitivity of the skin. Seizures caused by cortical irritation can be late manifestations of the process. Drowsiness may progress to stupor and coma.

PATIENT SCREENING

Early symptoms of meningitis are easily overlooked and may not appear severe enough to demand immediate assessment at first. As the symptoms and signs increase in nature, prompt assessment and intervention is necessary. Refer the patient to an emergency facility without delay.

ETIOLOGY

The infection can originate directly from the brain, spinal cord, or sinuses. Open head injuries are additional portals of entry for the offending bacteria. *Haemophilus influenzae, Neisseria meningitidis,* and *Streptococcus pneumoniae* are the bacteria responsible for most meningeal infections; however, the causative microorganism can be either bacterial or viral (Fig. 13–22).

DIAGNOSIS

The clinical findings alert the physician to the possibility of meningitis. A diagnostic *lumbar puncture* reveals increased cerebrospinal fluid (CSF) pressure and the presence of *white blood cells* (WBCs), protein, and glucose in the CSF. Culture of the CSF with resulting growth of microbes confirms the diagnosis. The CSF may appear cloudy because of the presence of the WBCs.

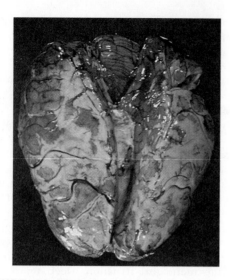

FIGURE 13–22 Bacterial meningitis. The surface of the brain is covered with pus. (From Damjanov I: *Pathology for the health-related professions,* ed 2, Philadelphia, 2000, Saunders. Courtesy Dr. John J. Kepes, Kansas City, Kan.)

TREATMENT

Meningitis is treated aggressively with intravenous antibiotic therapy. Anticonvulsive drugs are administered to control seizure activity. Aspirin or acetaminophen are given for the headache. Stimuli are kept at a minimum; the room is kept dark and quiet.

PROGNOSIS

Prognosis is unpredictable and depends on the source of the infection and response to drug therapy. Bacterial forms respond well to aggressive antibiotic therapy. Most viral forms run their course. The degree of residual damage, if any is noted, also depends on the response to drug intervention.

PREVENTION

Prevention is difficult. Persons who have had contact with known cases are often prescribed prophylactic antibiotics. Good hand washing techniques are always helpful in preventing the spread of any bacterial or viral infection.

PATIENT TEACHING

Stress the importance of completing a prescribed regimen of antibiotics.

Encephalitis

DESCRIPTION

Encephalitis is inflammation of brain tissue.

■ **ICD-9-CM Code 323.9** *(Unspecified cause of encephalitis)*
Once the diagnosis has confirmed the cause and type, refer to the current edition of the ICD-9-CM coding manual for the appropriate code.

SYMPTOMS AND SIGNS

Encephalitis, an inflammation of the brain tissue, may have an insidious or sudden onset. Primary symptoms include a headache and elevated temperature. The patient experiences a stiffness in the neck and back, muscular weakness, restlessness, visual disturbances, and lethargy. Mental confusion progresses to disorientation and even coma.

PATIENT SCREENING

Individuals reporting stiffness in the neck and back, muscle weakness, accompanied by headache, fever, restlessness, visual disturbances, and lethargy should be referred to an emergency facility without delay.

ETIOLOGY

The inflammation leads to cerebral edema and subsequent cell destruction. It is caused by viruses or the toxins from chickenpox, measles, or mumps. Most cases are the result of a bite from an infected mosquito. Eastern equine, western equine, and Venezuelan equine encephalomyelitis and St. Louis encephalitis are forms of encephalitis encountered in the United States. Recently West Nile viral encephalitis, a form of encephalitis that is not **endemic** to the United States, has evolved and is spreading across the country.

DIAGNOSIS

The clinical findings lead the physician to further investigation, including a lumbar puncture; the CSF pressure is elevated. Blood and CSF studies reveal the virus. The EEG is abnormal.

TREATMENT

Antiviral agents are effective against only the herpes simplex encephalitis. Otherwise, treatment is symptomatic, with mild analgesics for pain, *antipyretic* drugs for elevated temperature, anticonvulsants for seizure activity, and antibiotics for any intercurrent infection.

PROGNOSIS
Prognosis is unpredictable and depends on the type of infection and response to drug therapy. Most viral forms run their course. Residual damage to the brain tissue may result.

PREVENTION
Prevention is difficult. Avoiding environments heavily populated with mosquitoes may prevent the bites. Use of mosquito spray and wearing long sleeved shirts and long pants may prevent bites. Preventing mosquito breeding sites by eliminating standing water helps control the mosquito population. Community Boards of Health monitor the mosquito population and that of *vectors* such as the birds that carry the West Nile virus.

PATIENT TEACHING
Prevention is important. Stress the use of mosquito repellant when in an outdoor environment. Encourage patients and their families to be aware of encephalitis outbreaks in the community.

Guillain-Barré Syndrome

DESCRIPTION
Guillain-Barré syndrome is an acute, rapidly progressive disease of the spinal nerves.

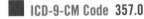 **ICD-9-CM Code 357.0**

SYMPTOMS AND SIGNS
The individual with Guillain-Barré syndrome experiences numbness and tingling of the feet and hands at the onset of the disease, followed by increasing muscle pain and tenderness. Progressive muscle weakness and paralysis usually start in the lower extremities and move up the body in 24 to 72 hours. Although most patients experience an ascending paralysis occasionally, some patients have a descending weakness and paralysis. Respiratory insufficiency is possible, as is difficulty swallowing.

PATIENT SCREENING
Individuals reporting numbness and tingling of the feet and hands, followed by increasing muscle pain and tenderness and subsequent progressive muscle weakness and paralysis are in need of immediate assessment and intervention. Refer the patient to an emergency facility for prompt care.

ETIOLOGY
Knowledge of the etiology is limited, but the syndrome is thought to have an autoimmune basis. The condition has been known to follow a respiratory infection or gastroenteritis in 10 to 21 days. **Demyelination** of the nerves occurs with the syndrome.

DIAGNOSIS
Confirmation is made by the finding of elevated protein level in the CSF, which peaks in 4 to 6 weeks after onset. Leukocyte count is normal, as is CSF pressure.

TREATMENT
Hospitalization usually is required for observation. Treatment is supportive. *Plasmapheresis* washes the plasma to remove antibodies, thereby shortening the time required for recovery. Intravenous human immunoglobulin may be beneficial.

PROGNOSIS
Prognosis varies, but recovery is usually complete.

PREVENTION
No method of prevention is known.

PATIENT TEACHING
Encourage patients to keep follow-up appointments as scheduled.

Brain Abscess

DESCRIPTION
A brain abscess, a collection of pus, can occur anywhere in the brain tissue (Fig. 13–23).

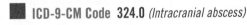 **ICD-9-CM Code 324.0** *(Intracranial abscess)*

SYMPTOMS AND SIGNS
The primary symptom of a brain abscess is a headache. Other symptoms and signs depend on the location and extent of the abscess. Generally, the patient exhibits symptoms and signs of increased intracranial pressure, including nausea and vomiting, visual disturbances, unequal pupil size, and seizures. Many times, the eyes look toward the insult, moving to the side of the head where the abscess is located. Nuchal rigidity may be noted.

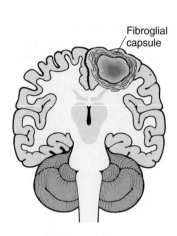

FIGURE 13–23 Brain abscess.

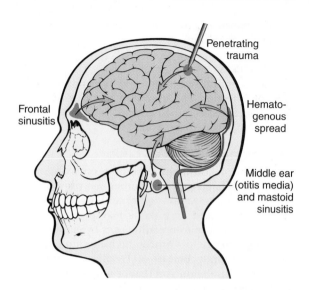

FIGURE 13–24 Bacterial infections of the central nervous system. Infectious organisms may reach the brain through several routes: hematogenously; by direct entry because of penetrating trauma; or by direct spread from adjacent structures, such as the inner ear or the nasal sinuses. (From Damjanov I: *Pathology for the health-related professions,* ed 2, Philadelphia, 2000, Saunders.)

PATIENT SCREENING

Individuals who complain of an unusual headache should be scheduled for an appointment as soon as possible. When reports of nausea, vomiting, visual disturbances, unequal pupil size, and possible seizures are relayed, the situation has progressed to a state that requires prompt assessment and intervention. Refer the patient to an emergency facility or advise the individual or family to call 911 and enter the individual into the EMS.

ETIOLOGY

CNS abscesses may be the result of a local infection or may be secondary to infections elsewhere in the body. Common causative organisms are staphylococci, streptococci, or pneumococci. Any occurrence that breaches the integrity of the CNS, including head trauma and a craniotomy wound, may be the portal of entry for the microorganisms. The abscess may be secondary to another infectious process, including sinusitis, otitis, dental abscess, subdural empyema, and bacterial endocarditis (Fig. 13–24).

DIAGNOSIS

A history of infection, especially of the sinuses or ear, or an insult to the CNS coupled with the characteristic clinical features of increased intracranial pressure suggests an abscess. An EEG and CT scans are used to verify the diagnosis. *Lumbar puncture* **is**

contraindicated because the resulting increased intracranial pressure may cause the brain stem to herniate, with the consequence of death.

TREATMENT

Intravenous antibiotics are administered to resolve the infection. Mannitol or steroids are prescribed to reduce cerebral edema. Surgical drainage of the abscess may be necessary to relieve intracranial pressure and to culture the offending organism. Additional treatment is supportive.

PROGNOSIS

Prognosis varies depending on the location, size, and causative agent of the abscess. Underlying pathology and the health status of the patient also affect the recovery process. When intracranial pressure cannot be controlled, death may result.

PREVENTION

Prevention is difficult because of the numerous possible sources of the infection. Prompt treatment of potential secondary sources or another infectious process, including sinusitis, otitis, dental abscess, subdural empyema, and bacterial endocarditis, helps in prevention.

PATIENT TEACHING

Encourage prompt reporting of infectious processes involving the head so treatment can resolve these potential sources of the abscess in a timely manner.

Poliomyelitis and Postpolio Syndrome

DESCRIPTION

Poliomyelitis is a viral infection of the anterior horn cells of the gray matter of the spinal cord and causes a selective destruction of the motor neurons.

■ **ICD-9-CM Code** **045.90** *(Unspecified)*
138 *(Postpolio syndrome [old with deformity])*
Poliomyelitis is coded according to type and paralytic involvement. Once the diagnosis has been confirmed, refer to the current edition of the ICD-9-CM coding manual for the appropriate code and fourth- and fifth-digit modifiers.

SYMPTOMS AND SIGNS

This highly contagious disease is no longer the threat to humankind that it was before the 1960s. The Salk and Sabin vaccines have virtually eliminated poliomyelitis in the Western world.

The patient with poliomyelitis has a low-grade fever, a profuse discharge from the nose, and *malaise.* These symptoms are followed by a progressive muscle weakness, stiff neck, nausea and vomiting, and a flaccid paralysis of the muscles involved. Atrophy of the muscles follows, with decreased tendon reflexes, then muscle and joint deterioration.

Poliomyelitis that involves the muscles supplied by spinal nerves is termed *spinal,* whereas involvement of the muscles supplied by cranial nerves (gray matter of the medulla) is termed *bulbar.*

PATIENT SCREENING

Any individual complaining of progressive muscle weakness, stiff neck, nausea and vomiting, and a flaccid paralysis of the muscles involved requires prompt assessment. Refer the patient to an emergency facility. Individuals who are known to have previously contracted polio (usually 30 years before) and report the onset of progressive weakness in the already affected muscles should be scheduled for the next available appointment.

ETIOLOGY

The poliovirus enters the body through the nose and throat and crosses into the gastrointestinal tract. Traveling by way of the bloodstream, the virus progresses to the CNS. The incubation period is 7 to 21 days. Poliovirus is transmitted from person to person by infected oropharyngeal secretions or feces that contain the virus.

DIAGNOSIS

The clinical symptoms along with possible exposure to an infected person are the primary tools of diagnosis. Isolation of the poliovirus from throat washings or from feces confirms the diagnosis. When the CNS is involved, cultures of CSF are positive for poliovirus.

TREATMENT

Treatment is supportive. Analgesics are administered for pain relief, along with moist heat applications. Bed rest is indicated until the acute stage is resolved. Physical therapy, including the use of braces, may be necessary. When difficulty with respiration is involved, respiratory support with mechanical ventilation may be necessary. Prevention by means of Sabin and Salk vaccines has rendered poliomyelitis almost nonexistent in the world.

Three distinct serotypes of poliovirus exist: types 1, 2, and 3. All three types can be found worldwide, and immunization with the Sabin trivalent oral vaccine affords immunity to all three forms. A monovalent Sabin vaccine also is available, which grants immunity to only one form, as does the Salk vaccine. Persons with *immunosuppressive* conditions should not be given the trivalent vaccine because they are at risk for contracting poliomyelitis. Additionally, any immunosuppressed person should not come in contact with feces or nasal secretions of a recently vaccinated person. Two poliovirus vaccines currently are licensed in the United States: inactivated poliovirus vaccine (IPV) and oral poliovirus vaccine (OPV).

Postpolio syndrome occurs later in life in persons who have previously experienced the disease. Functional deterioration of muscles is accompanied by loss of strength. The progressive weakness begins 30 years or more after the initial attack and involves already affected muscles. Fasciculations and muscular atrophy may accompany the weakness. Treatment is supportive, and generally the prognosis is good.

PROGNOSIS

Prognosis is fair and depends on which muscles are involved. Muscles involved in respiration may require intervention to maintain ventilation. Muscles in the arms and legs require intensive rehabilitation with physical therapy. Prognosis for those with postpolio syndrome is good.

PREVENTION

Administration of the polio vaccines has helped to significantly reduce the incidence of polio.

PATIENT TEACHING

Encourage all parents to have their children vaccinated according to the recommended inoculation schedule.

Intracranial Tumors (Brain Tumors)

DESCRIPTION

Brain tumors can be primary tumors, neoplasms that originate in the brain itself, or secondary tumors, cancer that has metastasized from another area of the body such as the lung, liver, kidney, or skin. Primary tumors can arise from any cell within the cranium (Fig. 13–25). They are named according to the tissues from which they originate.

■ **ICD-9-CM Code** **239.6**

SYMPTOMS AND SIGNS

Regardless of the tumor cell type, symptoms and signs result from displacement and compression of normal brain tissue by the tumor, causing progressive neurologic deficits, expansion of the brain (cerebral edema), and increased intracranial pressure (ICP) (Fig. 13–26), and possible herniation. Common symptoms include headache (usually dull, constant, and worse at night or in the morning), focal or generalized seizures (common in gliomas and secondary tumors), nausea and vomiting, loss of consciousness, cognitive dysfunction (including memory problems and personality changes), muscle weakness, sensory loss, aphasia, gait disturbance, and visual dysfunction. Cerebellar tumors such as medulloblastoma often present with the classic symptoms of gait disturbance, nystagmus, lethargy, dysarthric

speech pattern, clumsiness, and balance difficulty. Elevated ICP may result in cranial nerve defects. Edema of the optic nerve (papilledema) can be seen with an ophthalmoscope. If the pressure becomes too high within the cranial compartment, herniation of brain tissue will occur—a life-threatening condition.

PATIENT SCREENING

Symptoms of early brain tumors are somewhat vague. Individuals complaining of constant headaches with increasing severity and worsening at night require prompt assessment. Reports of seizures, loss of consciousness, and reduced cognitive functioning require prompt assessment. Refer the patient to an emergency facility.

ETIOLOGY

Primary brain tumors are classified histologically according to the predominant cell type. Gliomas, tumors derived from glial cells; meningiomas, tumors arising from the arachnoid membrane; and embryonal tumors, neoplasms that arise in children, together account for 95% of all primary brain tumors. Incidence of gliomas and meningiomas increases after the age of 45, whereas embryonal tumors rarely occur after the age of 20. For children under age 15, brain tumors are the most common solid malignancy.

The incidence of brain tumors is greater in developed, industrialized countries such as the United States, Western Europe, and Australia. Whites are

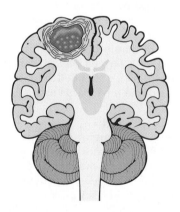

FIGURE 13–25 Brain tumor.

affected more often than any other race. Although many risk factors for brain tumor development are under investigation, only therapeutic ionizing radiation and genetic predisposition through inherited cancer syndromes such as neurofibromatosis and von Hippel-Lindau syndrome are established risk factors. However, these account for only a fraction of cases.

DIAGNOSIS

The evaluation of a patient with a suspected brain tumor includes a detailed history, a neurologic examination, and diagnostic neuroimaging studies. Neurologic examination findings are associated with particular regions affected by destruction of neural tissue. Cranial MRI is the diagnostic imaging modality of choice. A functional MRI, which measures blood flow through regions of the brain during various activities, can be helpful for preoperative planning. CSF cytology may be obtained by lumbar puncture to check for neoplastic cells, indicating metastasis to the spinal cord. Tissue obtained during surgery or from a stereotactic biopsy is necessary for correct histologic diagnosis of the tumor type. Staging of most brain tumors uses a modified TNM (Tumor, Node, Metastasis) system. The N component of the staging system is not very informative because the CNS does not contain lymphatic structures. Only tumor grade and histologic classification are taken into account to estimate the malignant potential of the tumor. (Refer to Chapter 1 for staging and grading of cancer.)

Although brain tumors can be malignant or benign, the distinction is blurred in the brain. Unlike benign neoplasms in other locations of the body, benign brain tumors may present with the same symptoms as malignant cancers, and distinguishing between benign and malignant on clinical grounds can be very difficult. Even a benign tumor with little to no metastatic potential can be lethal if it occurs in a region of the brain that precludes full surgical resection.

TREATMENT

Benign and malignant neoplasms are often treated similarly. Patients with primary brain tumors must be treated for their symptoms as well as for their neoplasm. Symptomatic treatment includes use of anticonvulsants to treat seizures, corticosteroids to help decrease ICP, and use of anticoagulants to prevent venous thromboembolic disease. Surgery is the initial treatment for most tumors. It provides tissue samples for definitive diagnosis and relieves symptoms by reducing tumor bulk. The extent of surgery is limited by the goal of not inflicting incapacitating neurologic damage on the patient. Surgery is usually followed by radiotherapy and/or chemotherapy, depending on the tumor type and stage. Although still experimental, immunotherapy is showing promise as an additional modality to treat brain tumors.

Treatment of secondary brain tumors focuses on relief of neurologic symptoms and long-term tumor control. Treatment choice is based upon location, size, and number of metastases; patient age; neurologic status; and extent of systemic cancer. In general, patients with solitary brain lesions and no other sites of metastasis are candidates for treatment with surgery and whole brain radiation therapy (WBRT). Although the patient may still be affected

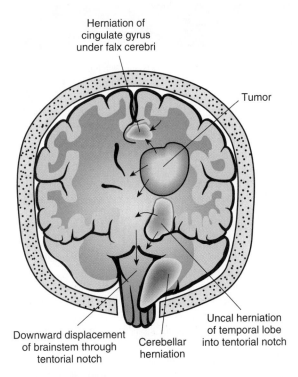

Herniation of cingulate gyrus under falx cerebri

Tumor

Downward displacement of brainstem through tentorial notch

Cerebellar herniation

Uncal herniation of temporal lobe into tentorial notch

FIGURE 13-26 Increased intracranial pressure and possible herniations. (From Gould B: *Pathophysiology for the health professions,* ed 2, Philadelphia, 2002, Saunders.)

by extracranial disease, this treatment improves quality of life and reduces the likelihood of death resulting from neurologic causes. Patients with multiple metastases generally undergo WBRT without surgery. Recurrent brain metastases are treated with surgery or radiation with palliative intent.

It is important to remember that patients may be affected by the long-term complications of surgery, radiation, and chemotherapy in the years following treatment, especially children. Problems include neurocognitive defects, growth hormone deficiency, learning disability, loss of vision, and second malignancies.

PROGNOSIS

The overall 5-year survival rate for all types of brain tumors combined is 32%. This ranks among the lowest survival rates for all types of cancer. Poor prognostic indicators include older age of the patient, a high tumor grade, presence of mental changes at the time of diagnosis, large tumor size, CSF cytology positive for neoplastic cells, and inability to fully resect the tumor during surgery.

PREVENTION

No methods are known to prevent intracranial neoplasms and no screening programs are available for early detection.

PATIENT TEACHING

Assist patient and family members in locating and contacting available community resources. Discuss that insults to the brain may result in neurocognitive functional deficits; in children, growth delay and learning disabilities may occur. Encourage compliance with any prescribed drug or physical therapy.

REVIEW CHALLENGE

Answer the following questions:

1. What does the central nervous system comprise? The peripheral nervous system?
2. What are some possible causes of disease of the nervous system?
3. How is the nervous system evaluated during a diagnostic examination?
4. What are the three vascular disorders that may result in a cerebrovascular accident (CVA)?
5. How does a transient ischemic attack (TIA) differ from a CVA?
6. What are some of the likely causes of epidural and subdural hematomas? Which condition is more likely to have a delayed onset of symptoms?
7. Which condition is more serious, a cerebral concussion or cerebral contusion? Why?
8. What is the relationship between the location of a spinal cord injury and the signs and symptoms?
9. Which diagnostic findings may indicate a degeneration or rupture of an intervertebral disk?
10. How does spinal stenosis contribute to sciatic pain?
11. Are headaches always a symptom of an underlying disease? What are some causative factors of cephalalgia?
12. What are the classic signs and symptoms of migraine?
13. What are the different types of epileptic seizures? What are the first aid guidelines?
14. What are the characteristic signs and symptoms of (a) Parkinson disease, (b) Huntington chorea, and (c) amyotrophic lateral sclerosis (ALS)?
15. What are suggested causes of and treatment interventions for transient global amnesia?
16. What are some causative factors of peripheral neuritis?
17. How does a patient with trigeminal neuralgia typically describe the pain?
18. What is the clinical appearance of a person with Bell palsy?
19. What is the diagnostic significance of nuchal rigidity in the presence of headache and photophobia?
20. What are the possible etiologic agents of encephalitis?
21. What is the pathologic progression of Guillain-Barré syndrome?
22. How do infectious organisms reach the brain? How is a brain abscess treated?
23. What is postpolio syndrome?
24. How are intracranial tumors classified, and what determines the symptomatology?

REAL-LIFE CHALLENGE

Epilepsy

A 26-year-old man was previously (2 weeks prior) in a motor vehicle accident (MVA) with closed head injury. Recovery was uneventful, and the patient was dismissed from the hospital. The patient returned to work 2 days ago. The patient's wife called the office to state that she awakened this morning to find her husband having seizure-type activity. The patient was responsive but appeared confused.

The patient was transported to a hospital. Vital signs were T—98.4° F, P—72, R—18, and BP—116/78. The patient was responsive but not oriented to time, place, or person, appearing postictal. An EEG was ordered, as was a cerebral CT scan. The patient was diagnosed with seizure activity (epilepsy) secondary to the cerebral trauma received in the previous MVA. The patient was placed on antiseizure medication and admitted for observation.

QUESTIONS

1. What patient or family teaching regarding patient activity is indicated?
2. What is the significance of the cerebral trauma to the onset of seizure activity?
3. As what type of epilepsy is this seizure activity classified?
4. Compare the three types of epilepsy as per seizure activity, treatment, and predisposing factors.
5. Which other diagnostic tests might be ordered?
6. Describe appropriate first aid intervention for a grand mal seizure patient.
7. Explain status epilepticus.

REAL-LIFE CHALLENGE

Transient Ischemic Attack (TIA)

The wife of a 67-year-old man called the office and reported that her husband awoke this morning with weakness and numbness of the right side. He had difficulty getting out of bed and complained of intermittent episodes of dizziness. He also was experiencing difficulty speaking. The patient has a history of hypertension and is taking enalapril maleate (Vasotec) and propranolol hydrochloride (Inderal). The wife was advised that her husband should be seen in an emergency care facility, and an ambulance was called for transport.

On examination in the emergency facility, the patient was found to have diminished strength in the right hand and foot, diminished movement in the right arm and leg and had slurred speech. Vitals signs were T—98.6° F, P—106 and irregular, R—22, and BP—172/96. Oxygen therapy was started. Reflexes were diminished, as was pain response on the right side, including the extremities.

A cerebral MRI scan, CT scans, an EEG, skull radiographs, and an ECG were ordered. The ECG showed atrial fibrillation. Approximately 6 hours postonset, the symptoms began to resolve, with improvement in feeling and movement of the right extremities. Speech slowly became less slurred. The patient was diagnosed as having a TIA and was scheduled for follow-up evaluation. He was started on anticoagulant therapy.

QUESTIONS

1. What is the importance of the right-side involvement and slurring of speech?
2. Why would ambulance transportation to an emergency facility be recommended?
3. What is the significance of the elevated blood pressure?
4. Explain the differences between a TIA and a CVA.
5. In what area of the brain would the diminished circulation and subsequent reduced oxygenation be anticipated?
6. Why would anticoagulant therapy be prescribed?
7. Research the importance of the ECG results indicating atrial fibrillation.

INTERNET ASSIGNMENTS

1. Go to The National Spinal Cord Injury Association to research advances in the treatment of spinal cord injuries.
2. Go to The National Parkinson Foundation to research latest developments in treatment interventions for Parkinson disease.
3. Research diagnostic tests used by neurosurgeons at the American Association of Neurological Surgeons. What other procedures are used to treat head trauma and CVAs?
4. Investigate the American Neurological Association and write a report on a disease entity or condition you find discussed there. (Suggestions: pain management, headache treatment, cancers of the neurological system, encephalitis, and West Nile encephalitis.)

Mental Disorders

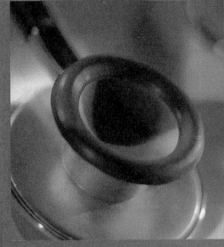

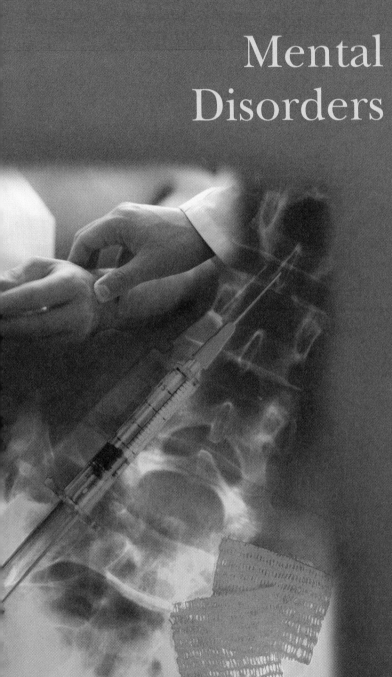

Chapter Outline

Learning Objectives

After studying Chapter 14, you should be able to:
1. Name some contributing factors to mental disorders.
2. List some of the many causes of mental retardation.
3. Describe the characteristic manifestations of autism.
4. List some examples of tic disorders.
5. Describe the progressive degenerative changes in an individual with Alzheimer disease.
6. Explain important factors in the treatment of Alzheimer disease.
7. Explain the cause of vascular dementia.
8. Relate treatment options for alcohol abuse.
9. Name the classic signs and symptoms of schizophrenia. Explain what is included in the multidimensional treatment plan.
10. Explain why bipolar disorder is considered a major affective disorder. Describe the treatment approach.
11. Explain the difference between reactive depression and a major depressive disorder.
12. Name the distinguishing characteristics of personality disorders.
13. Discuss how each type of anxiety disorder prevents a person from leading a normal life.
14. Explain how post-traumatic stress disorder differs from other anxiety disorders.
15. Explain how a somatization disorder is diagnosed.
16. Discuss the relationship between anxiety and conversion disorder.
17. Describe Munchausen syndrome.
18. Contrast insomnia to narcolepsy.

Key Terms

affect (**AF**–feckt)
amyloid (**AM**–ih–loyd)
autism (**AW**–tism)
catatonic (kat–ah–**TOH**–nic)
circadian (sir–**KAY**–dee–an)
cognitive (**KOG**–nih–tive)
deficit (**DEAF**–ih–sit)
delusion (dee–**LOO**–zhun)
endarterectomy (**end**–ar–ter–**EK**–toh–me)

hallucination (ha–loo–sih–**NAY**–shun)
hypoxia (hi–**POX**–ee–ah)
ischemia (is–**KEY**–me–ah)
mutism (**MYOO**–tizm)
narcissistic (nar–sis–**SIST**–ik)
paranoid (**PAR**–ah–noid)
psychotic (sigh–**KOT**–ik)
schizoid (**SKIZ**–oyd)

MENTAL WELLNESS AND MENTAL ILLNESS

A T SOME TIME IN LIFE, almost everyone is affected by mental disorders, either personally or by the involvement of a family member or friend. Stress is considered a contributing factor of mental disorders. Other factors are hereditary or congenital, accidental, traumatic, or related to drug toxicity. Chemical imbalances in the brain and its neurotransmitters also are postulated to be causative factors. The specific causes of mental illness remain unclear in many cases.

Mental illness has been linked to the patient's inability to cope with stress imposed by modern society. Pressures imposed by life circumstances can be a source of personal pain and distress. The definition of mental wellness, or being in a good state of mental health, varies and is a relative state of mind. When healthy people have the capacity to cope and adjust in a reasonable manner to the ongoing stresses of everyday life, they are considered to be in a state of mental wellness.

Psychological pain is real and intense and can affect physical health. Subsequently, impaired or pathologic coping skills emerge in people's behavior. Some coping behaviors are conscious, and some are not easily controlled because they are unconscious. Certain disorders in thinking, perceiving, and behaving can be organized into clusters of signs and symptoms. These clusters become diagnostic criteria and a part of a total physical and psychological evaluation. The American Psychiatric Association's *Diagnostic and Statistical Manual of Mental Disorders,* fourth edition (DSM-IV) (Fig. 14–1), is the accepted reference that offers guidelines for criteria to be used in the clinical setting when diagnosing a mental disorder. In addition to diagnostic criteria, the DSM-IV gives the practitioner a standardized diagnostic code, similar to the ICD-9-CM (International Classification of Diseases, ninth revision, Clinical Modification) coding system.

Mental disorders include those of congenital and hereditary origins. Other categories such as maladaptive disorders, phobias, anxiety, depression, addiction, and **psychotic** disorders have uncertain or unknown causes and possibly more than one contributing factor. Mental disorders cause mild to severe disruption in a person's ability to

function in interpersonal relationships, self-care, and occupational settings. In some disorders, the person may experience incapacitating psychotic symptoms. The DSM-IV includes sleep disorders

In some mental disorders, oxygen and nutrient deprivation with necrosis result in the death of brain cells; these disorders are permanent and cannot be reversed. Supportive therapy and custodial care often are the only available interventions.

Modern therapeutic approaches include control of symptoms with *psychotropic drugs,* including antipsychotic drugs, antidepressants, anxiolytics (antianxiety agents), central nervous system (CNS) stimulants, and antimanic agents; hospitalization during acute episodes; psychotherapy; electroconvulsive therapy; and group therapy. Outpatient treatment is available and preferred in many cases (Fig. 14–2). Play therapy is included in counseling sessions for some children. (See the Enrichment box on play therapy.) Patients with mental illnesses and conditions need established routines as well as consistency in treatment and daily living activities.

Mental illnesses are categorized by axis. The process of diagnosing a mental illness in DSM-IV

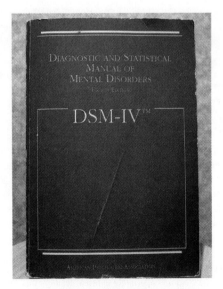

FIGURE 14–1 DSM-IV manual. (Courtesy Mark Boswell, 2003.)

format uses a five-axis system. Each axis represents a different part of the diagnosis, as follows:

Axis I: Mood and thought disorders, which often respond to medication and psychotherapy.

Axis II: Mental retardation and personality disorders, which often do not respond to medication. Many third-party providers currently

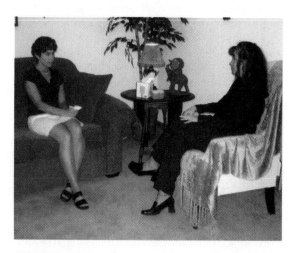

FIGURE 14-2 Counseling session in progress. (Courtesy Mark Boswell, 2003.)

do not reimburse for Axis-II disorders. The patient usually shows little or no response to psychotherapy as the condition is very much a part of the person.

Axis III: Medical conditions that contribute to the psychological condition.

Axis IV: Stressors that contribute to the psychological condition.

Axis V: GAF (Global Assessment of Functioning). This is a number, 0 to 100, that indicates level of functioning.

Many patients with an Axis-II diagnosis can function at a level that maintains normal daily living. Patients with these conditions are unresponsive to treatment with medications and usually do not heal because Axis-II conditions currently have no cure.

Mental Retardation

DESCRIPTION

Mental retardation, or developmental disability, is not a disease but a wide range of conditions with many causes. A causative factor interferes with the

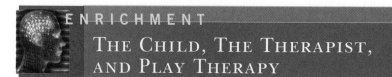

ENRICHMENT
THE CHILD, THE THERAPIST, AND PLAY THERAPY

THERAPISTS WORKING WITH CHILDREN use play therapy in assessment and treatment interventions. Children often cannot verbalize their thoughts and feelings, and play therapy becomes a nonverbal avenue for them to communicate with the therapist. This type of therapy creates a nonthreatening atmosphere for the children. Play therapy may be employed on a one-to-one basis or in the group setting. Children are allowed, and occasionally encouraged, to act out or express feelings and experiences. During play therapy sessions, the therapist establishes rapport with the child and encourages the child to act out any feelings of anxiety and tension he or she may be experiencing. The therapist's goals are to give the child an opportunity to reveal feelings that he or she cannot verbalize, to understand the child's interactions and relationships with important people in his or her life, and to teach

the child appropriate coping mechanisms and adaptive socialization skills.

Children who have been exposed to abuse often will respond to the therapist in the nonthreatening environment of play therapy. The use of dolls and various toys gives the child a means of acting out the abuse as well as offering an avenue for positive interaction.

Therapists may use objects and toys during play therapy. All kinds of dolls, a doll house, stuffed animals, puppets, soft balls and foam bats, toy vehicles, punching toys, a sand box, and paper and markers or crayons may be used during the play therapy. During these play sessions, family interactions and dynamics may become apparent. Sand therapy may include small plastic animals or people and allows the child to act out feelings (see Fig. 14-3, *A* and *B*).

developmental processes, resulting in changes in the acquisition of intellectual skills and adaptive functioning in a variety of areas, including social and interpersonal skills, self-care, communication, self-direction, health, and safety. In addition, the level of behavioral performance is reduced. General intellectual functioning is subaverage, and the individual has noticeable **deficits** in adaptive behavior. This condition is manifested during the developmental period and before the age of 18 years.

■ **ICD-9-CM Code** **317** *(Mild)*
318.0 *(Moderate)*
318.1 *(Severe)*
318.2 *(Profound)*
319 *(Severity unspecified)*

SYMPTOMS AND SIGNS

During early childhood, those with mild intellectual impairment often appear normal because they have no obvious physical defects. The first indication may be observed at school, where the individual fails to progress intellectually and socially at a normal rate. Those who have an underlying condition that is responsible for the impairment usually exhibit early symptoms of the underlying condition. Certain anomalies (e.g., Down syndrome) are found at birth. Occasionally, delayed development of communication and motor skills is suspected, but the disability is not confirmed until the child enters school. Delayed adaptive behavior, coupled with difficulties with schoolwork, lead to further evaluation and the diagnosis of mental retardation.

PATIENT SCREENING

Signs of mental retardation may appear on well-baby examinations or during preschool routine check-ups. The first significant indications of mental retardation sometimes appear when the child begins school or pre-school. When these parents contact the office, an appointment should be made for the earliest possible date when schedules will allow sufficient time for the physician to conduct a thorough assessment. The parents possibly will be feeling great anxiety, and the child should be assessed as soon as possible.

ETIOLOGY

Mental retardation has a variety of causes, many of which are unidentifiable. The predisposing factors include heredity (inborn errors of metabolism, genetic disorders, or chromosomal abnormalities); early alterations of embryonic development (Down syndrome or damage from *toxins*); prenatal, perinatal, or postnatal conditions (prematurity, **hypoxia,** viral infections, or trauma); general medical conditions (infections, trauma, or poisoning); and environmental influences. Any condition that compromises the blood supply to the developing brain, depriving it of oxygen and nutrients, can result in neurologic damage and mental retardation. Some examples are placental insufficiency, cord or head compression during the perinatal period, failure to breathe at birth, prematurity, and viral infections of the mother in the prenatal period or of the infant or child after birth. Trauma of any type that causes hypoxia or anoxia also may contribute to the deficit. Fetal alcohol syndrome also may result in mental retardation.

DIAGNOSIS

Diagnosis requires observation and confirmation of the intellectual capabilities and adaptive behavior of the child. A lack of control of emotions and reduced socialization skills are noted. Intellectual testing with standardized tests, such as Wechsler Intelligence Scales for Children—Revised, Stanford-Binet, and Kaufman Assessment Battery for Children, to develop an intelligence quotient (IQ) also is considered. Acceptable terms to describe intelligence based on the IQ determined by the Stanford-Binet test are:

110 to 90—average
90-70—below average
70 to 50—mild retardation
50 to 35—moderate retardation
35 to 20—severe retardation
Below 20—profound retardation

The IQ measurement is only one factor to be considered, and slight error can occur in testing, so allowances should be made for borderline scores, and possible testing with other instruments should be considered before a diagnosis is made.

Criteria for the diagnosis of mental retardation include subaverage general intellectual functioning accompanied by significant limitations in adaptive functioning. The diagnosis requires limitations in at least two of the following areas: communication, home living, self-care, social or interpersonal skills, self-direction, and health and safety. Onset **must be before 18 years of age.**

TREATMENT

When the deficit occurs, the brain cells die and cannot be restored. The child can be trained, however, and, in some cases, even educated to perform tasks of various levels. Underlying causes should be treated, and intervention may prevent or delay progression of the condition.

Many mildly to moderately retarded people can function in society. Patients whose retardation is severe or profound may be institutionalized to ensure the needed daily care. Mental retardation has no cure, and no drug therapy is available.

PROGNOSIS

The prognosis varies depending on identifiable etiology and adaptive skills.

PREVENTION

Preventing all mental retardation might not be possible, but early and good prenatal care and nutrition are encouraged for all pregnant women to reduce the occurrence. Fetal monitoring during labor may signal the labor and delivery staff when the fetus is deprived of adequate oxygen. In such a case, immediate intervention is necessary. Prompt attention to head injuries in children may prevent the onset of mental retardation during childhood.

PATIENT TEACHING

Parents require encouragement to recognize that there is no cure. Some retarded individuals may be educable or trainable. Routines and consistency are important in enabling the individual to function at the highest possible level.

Learning Disorders

DESCRIPTION

Learning disorders are conditions that cause children to learn in a manner that is not normal. Performance on standardized tests is lower than expected for age, schooling, and intelligence level.

■ **ICD-9-CM Code 315.2**

SYMPTOMS AND SIGNS

The person with a learning disorder exhibits difficulty in acquiring a skill in a specific area of learning, such as reading, writing, and mathematics.

This lower level of achievement occurs despite the child's normal (sometimes above normal) intelligence and adequate schooling. Many of these individuals become school dropouts, have low self-esteem, and feel demoralized. They also may exhibit deficits in social skills.

PATIENT SCREENING

Most learning disorders are noted as the child begins the formal education process. At that point, the parent usually contacts the physician's office for an evaluation and a treatment plan. The parents possibly will be feeling a high level of anxiety, and the child should be assessed as soon as possible.

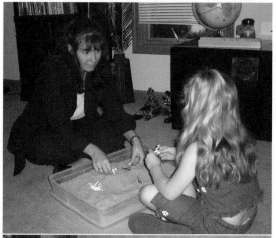

A

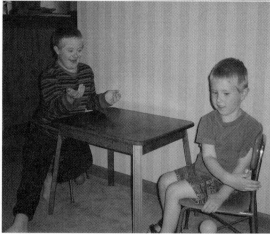

B

FIGURE 14–3 Play therapy sessions with children. (Courtesy David L. Frazier, 2003.)

ETIOLOGY

The etiology of this condition is uncertain, but there may be underlying abnormalities in **cognitive** processing. Deficits in visual perception, language processes, attention, or memory may contribute to the problem.

DIAGNOSIS

When the physician has established that the child has met all the diagnostic criteria listed in the DSM-IV, further evaluation is performed. In addition to ruling out normal variations in academic attainment, the physician eliminates inadequate schooling, language barriers, lack of opportunity, and poor teaching as causes. Hearing and vision must be tested. Other mental disorders are ruled out.

TREATMENT

Some children who are learning disabled also may be diagnosed with hyperactivity and therefore may respond to drug therapy, usually with stimulants. Other children may respond favorably to special instructional techniques (Figs. 14–3 and 14–4). Continuing research is attempting to help develop additional treatments for children with learning disabilities.

PROGNOSIS

The prognosis varies depending on the etiology and support of the community, school system, and family.

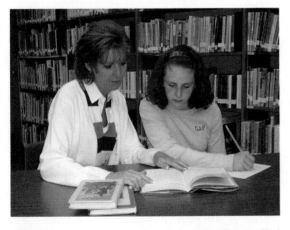

FIGURE 14–4 Tutoring session in progress. (Courtesy Mark Boswell, 2003.)

PREVENTION

Other than good prenatal care and close monitoring during labor, no specific prevention for learning disorders is known.

PATIENT TEACHING

Parents are encouraged to seek out community and educational resources as well as support groups in the community. Help parents to learn about special services provided by the state through the school systems.

Communication Disorders

Children often exhibit difficulties in communication. These disorders may be psychologically based and are listed in the DSM-IV. There are a variety of expressive language disorders, including mixed receptive or expressive language disorders.

Stuttering

DESCRIPTION

Stuttering, a *phonological* or communication disorder, is defined as frequent repetitions or prolongations of sounds or syllables.

ICD-9-CM Code 307.0

SYMPTOMS AND SIGNS

The frequent repetition or prolongation of sounds or syllables constitutes a disturbance of the pattern and fluency of speech, a disturbance that is inappropriate for the child's age. There also may be broken words, filled or unfilled pauses in speech, word substitutions, or word repetitions. The onset usually occurs between 2 and 7 years of age.

PATIENT SCREENING

Although this is not an emergency, a parent who calls for an appointment for a child who is stuttering should be given the next available regular appointment. The family's anxiety will be high, and they should be seen as soon as is convenient.

ETIOLOGY

Although the etiology is uncertain, genetic factors may be involved. Stuttering appears to have a familial tendency, with the condition occurring more often in males. Parents also may unwittingly cause anxiety in their child by overreacting to mild speech limitation. Anxiety appears to be a major factor that creates and maintains stuttering.

DIAGNOSIS

Observation of the speech pattern usually is all that is needed for the diagnosis. Hearing should be assessed, however, and any hearing difficulty should be ruled out.

TREATMENT

Speech therapy helps in the treatment. The condition may resolve spontaneously.

PROGNOSIS

The prognosis is good with intervention.

PREVENTION

No prevention is known.

PATIENT TEACHING

Parents should be supportive and non-critical of the child. In addition, they should be encouraged to seek out support groups in their community.

Pervasive Development Disorders

A primary characteristic of pervasive development disorders is severe impairment in several areas of development, including communication and social interaction skills. The disorders can include particular behaviors that cause failure to develop peer relationships and interactions with others, including lack of nonverbal communication and lack of reciprocation of emotions. This impairment is related directly to the person's developmental level or mental age. **Autism** is a pervasive development disorder.

Autistic Disorder

DESCRIPTION

Autistic disorder (autism) is a syndrome of extreme withdrawal and obsessive behavior. It has its onset in infancy, and manifestations are apparent by the second or third year of age. Infant autism is also called pervasive developmental disorder.

 ICD-9-CM Code 299.0 *(Infantile and childhood autism)*
Autism is coded by active or residual status. When the activity status of the autism has been determined by diagnosis, refer to the physician's diagnosis and then to the current edition of the ICD-9-CM coding manual to ensure the greatest specificity of pathology and the appropriate fifth-digit modifier.

SYMPTOMS AND SIGNS

The autistic child will exhibit a marked impairment in socialization, communication, activities, and other interests. The impairment is noted in nonverbal behaviors, such as eye-to-eye gaze, facial expressions, and other forms of nonverbal communication. Seizures may occur. In addition, the child fails to establish normal peer relationships and to seek shared enjoyment. Communication impairments include delayed or absent verbal communication, inability to initiate a conversation, and repetitive use of inappropriate language. The child does not initiate age-appropriate play activities. Repetitive motions, often self-destructive, may be noted, along with an inflexibility toward change and a compulsion for sameness. These youngsters display a persistent preoccupation with objects and may have a memory for certain lists or facts.

Four symptoms that are nearly always present are social isolation, cognitive impairment, language deficits, and repetitive naturalistic motions. Aversion to physical contact or cuddling also can be a sign. The autistic child resists any change.

PATIENT SCREENING

The parent of the child with autistic behavior often is aware of problems that are developing. Often this issue will be discussed on regular well-child (toddler) visits. When the parents first become aware of a problem, an appointment should be scheduled as soon as schedules will allow for an extensive examination and history.

ETIOLOGY

The etiology is uncertain, but evidence indicates a possible organic factor or possible predisposing factors that may include maternal rubella, encephalitis, and phenylketonuria. The occurrence is more common in males.

DIAGNOSIS

Observation of the behavior usually is all that is needed for the diagnosis. The child exhibits impairment in social interaction and communication; restricted, repetitive patterns of behavior; and delayed or abnormal patterns of symbolic or imaginative play.

TREATMENT

Behavioral therapy and self-instructed training have helped some autistic children. This therapy is most beneficial when parents also are trained in behavioral techniques and have the goal of helping these children to learn some adaptive responses, enabling the children to function outside of custodial care. Although not widely used, mirtazipine (Remeron), an antidepressant, is an option for treating agitation and sleeplessness in autistic children.

PROGNOSIS

The prognosis depends on the severity of the disorder. Children with Asperger syndrome, a milder form of autism, seem to adjust better as they get older. Research is ongoing, but currently there is no specific drug therapy for this disorder. Greater public awareness is being generated to support additional research.

PREVENTION

No prevention for this disorder currently is known.

PATIENT TEACHING

Encourage parents to investigate community and educational resources and to seek out support groups.

Attention-Deficit Hyperactivity Disorder

DESCRIPTION

Attention-deficit hyperactivity disorder (ADHD) is a condition of persistent inattention leading to hyperactivity and impulsivity. ADHD is traditionally considered a hyperactivity issue, but many children and adults simply have difficulty maintaining attention and have no hyperactivity problems. Therefore ADHD has been broken down into subtypes: ADHD combined type, ADHD predominately inattentive type, and predominately hyperactivity-impulsive type.

ICD-9-CM Code 314.01 *(Attention-deficit disorder with hyperactivity)*

SYMPTOMS AND SIGNS

Typical ADHD behavior can be observed at any age, but symptoms are usually present before the age of 7 years. Failure to give close attention to details; careless mistakes; messy work, performed carelessly; and difficulty in sustaining attention and completing tasks are manifestations of the condition. The child avoids activities that require sustained attention, effort, concentration, and organization. An inability to sit quietly without fidgeting or squirming, or even to remain seated, denotes hyperactivity. Inappropriate running and climbing, difficulty in playing, and excessive talking are other signs of the condition.

A display of impatience, difficulty in waiting for one's turn, frequent interruptions, and failure to listen to directions are manifestations of impulsivity. The inability to organize activities and define goals creates difficulty in performing simple tasks, such as picking up toys. Sexual and relationship problems may occur as the child ages.

Any aspect of this behavior may be displayed at home, school, work, or social occasions. The behavior seems to be exaggerated in group situations.

PATIENT SCREENING

Similar to learning disorders, most attention-deficit hyperactivity disorders are first noted as the child begins the formal education process. At that time the parent usually contacts the physician's office for an evaluation and a treatment plan. The appointment should be scheduled as soon as schedules will allow enough time for the physician to conduct a thorough assessment. The parents may be feeling a great deal of anxiety, and the child should be assessed as soon as possible.

ETIOLOGY

The cause is uncertain, but there appears to be a familial pattern. Observers now postulate that this condition is genetic with definite brain malfunction.

DIAGNOSIS

The diagnosis is based on observation of behavior and an evaluation concluding that the inattention is not age-appropriate. The inattention must last for longer than 6 months and appear in at least two of the following settings: home, school, work, and social activities. Persistent hyperactivity and impulsivity also must meet the aforementioned criteria. Some of the symptoms are present before the age of 7 years. The behavior severely impairs functioning.

TREATMENT

An effective treatment for some children is the use of amphetamines, such as dextroamphetamine sulfate (Dexedrine), methylphenidate hydrochloride (Ritalin), and mixed salts of a single-entity amphetamine product (Adderall). The most commonly used stimulants now are extended-release methylphenidate (Concerta), extended-release amphetamine salts (Adderall XR), and a new drug that is becoming very popular, atomoxetine (Stratterra), which is not a **controlled drug.** Other successful treatments have used behavioral therapy, rewarding appropriate behavior to extinguish inappropriate behavior.

PROGNOSIS

Prompt diagnosis with appropriate management via medication leads to an excellent prognosis. Compliance with the medication dosage and frequency, however, is imperative. Effective parenting skills improve the prognosis.

PREVENTION

ADHD is genetic and therefore has no prevention.

PATIENT TEACHING

Parents who use effective discipline and consistent routines are most successful in managing the condition. In addition, when medical treatment calls for drug therapy to treat the disorder, compliance is imperative. Proper nutrition with low amounts of sugar and red dye are helpful.

Oppositional Defiant Disorder

DESCRIPTION

Oppositional defiant disorder (ODD) is a behavior disorder in which children demonstrate behaviors that are oppositional toward adults. This is the most common referral complaint to counselors and a major source of family stress, as ODD behaviors occur hundreds of times per week. Comorbid conditions include ADHD (incidence increases with age), conduct disorder, post-traumatic stress disorder (PTSD), learning disabilities, school underperformance, poor social skills, dysthymia, and major depression. ODD is a strong predictor of poor outcomes (i.e., school underachievement, poor peer relations, delinquency, major depression, early substance initiation and abuse, and school expulsion and drop out.

 ICD-9-CM Code 313.81

SYMPTOMS AND SIGNS

Children with ODD often demonstrate behaviors such as losing their tempers, arguing with adults, defying or refusing to comply with the adult's requests or rules, deliberately annoying others, and blaming others for mistakes and behaviors. In addition, they are irritable and easily annoyed, are angry and resentful, and are spiteful and vindictive.

PATIENT SCREENING

The appointment should be scheduled as soon as schedules will allow time for a thorough assessment by the physician. The parents may be experiencing great anxiety, and the child should be as assessed as soon as possible.

ETIOLOGY

ODD has four main causes. These are negative child temperament and ADHD, negative parent temperament, ineffective child management, and parent and family stress events.

DIAGNOSIS

Many parents report that their child never came out of the "terrible twos." Thus some symptoms may appear as early as age 3. Patients generally present at about the ages of 8 to 10 years. Patients must often (at least three times per week) demonstrate at least one of the eight symptoms listed above, for at least 6 months.

TREATMENT

Mood stabilizers such as risperidone (Risperdal) and olanzapine (Zyprexa) are often prescribed and helpful for these patients. The most effective form of treatment is parent training and individual psychotherapy for the child.

PROGNOSIS

Treatment is effective for children who demonstrate behaviors of ODD. If the child begins to demonstrate conduct disorder (a more severe disorder), outcome is poor.

PREVENTION

Reducing family chaos and improving parenting skills helps to control the onset of ODD.

PATIENT TEACHING

Parent training courses and education are encouraged. The lack of responsibility the child accepts for behaviors is somewhat indicative of this disorder.

Tic Disorders

Tic disorders appear as sudden, rapid, recurrent motor movement or vocalization that is nonrhythmic. The tics are irresistible, but they may be suppressed for varying lengths of time and diminish during sleep. Eye blinking, facial grimacing, coughing, and neck jerking are examples of simple motor tics. Making facial gestures, jumping, touching, and stamping are examples of complex motor tics. Simple vocal tics include throat clearing, sniffing, snorting, and grunting. The repetition of words out of context, the use of socially unacceptable words, and the repetition of one's own words or of the last sound heard are examples of complex vocal tics. Tic disorders may be motor or vocal and may be chronic.

Tourette Disorder

DESCRIPTION

Tourette disorder, also known as Gilles de la Tourette syndrome, is a syndrome of multiple motor tics coupled with one or more vocal tics, which may appear simultaneously or at different times.

ICD-9-CM Code 307.23

SYMPTOMS AND SIGNS

The location, nature, and number of tics tend to change over time. The head typically is involved. Other body parts such as the torso or upper and lower limbs may be involved. Clicks, grunts, yelps, barks, and snorts are examples of vocal tics. The vocal tics also may include the uttering of obscenities.

PATIENT SCREENING

The appointment should be scheduled for the earliest date that schedules will allow sufficient time for a thorough assessment by the physician. The parents possibly will be feeling great anxiety, and the child should be assessed as soon as possible.

ETIOLOGY

The etiology is uncertain, but some observers postulate that Tourette is inherited. The incidence is higher in males.

DIAGNOSIS

The observation of symptoms is usually enough for diagnosis. The onset may be as early as 2 years of age and is before 18 years of age. Remissions may occur, but the syndrome is of lifelong duration. The severity of the symptoms usually diminishes, and the symptoms may even disappear by early adulthood.

To meet diagnostic criteria, both motor and vocal tics must occur, although not necessarily at the same time. They occur several times a day over a period of a year without a tic-free period of longer than 3 months. The patient has significant impairment in functioning at work or in socialization, and the condition is not the result of substance use or a general medical condition.

TREATMENT

Some patients with Tourette disorder have improved with the administration of haloperidol lactate (Haldol). Other treatment options include clonidine or clonazepam for their calming effects.

PROGNOSIS

Although there is no cure for Tourette, some patients experience a lessening of symptoms as they reach maturity. However, this usually is a lifelong, chronic condition.

PREVENTION

No prevention is known for this disorder.

PATIENT TEACHING

Encourage the patient and family to seek out support groups and to access information from community health organizations. All those involved should work with the educational system to help the youth exhibiting Tourette syndrome to obtain all possible educational assistance.

Dementia

DESCRIPTION

Dementia brings a progressive, general deterioration of mental faculties, including deterioration of perceiving, thinking, and remembering. Cognitive functioning declines abnormally. The irreversible brain damage may be the result of compromised blood flow to the brain resulting from atherosclerosis, thrombi, or trauma. In addition, toxins, metabolic conditions, organic disorders, infections, tumors, or Alzheimer disease may be responsible for the deterioration (refer to Fig. 13–19 in Chapter 13). The onset may be slow and insidious or may be sudden, depending on the cause.

Alzheimer Disease

DESCRIPTION

Alzheimer disease is a progressive degenerative disease of the brain that produces a typical profile of loss of mental and physical functioning. It is the most common cause of deterioration in intellectual capacity, or dementia. It is most common in people older than 65, and its incidence increases in people older than 80.

 ICD-9-CM Code 331.0

SYMPTOMS AND SIGNS

The onset of Alzheimer disease is gradual and insidious, with early signs including loss of short-term memory, inability to concentrate, incapacity to learn new information, impairment of reasoning, and subtle changes in personality. As its course continues, communication skills decline, and the patient struggles to find the right words, uses meaningless words, or interjects nonsensical phrases. Over a span of 5 to 10 years, there is profound deterioration of intellectual and physical ability. The patient becomes increasingly dependent on a caretaker. The response to stimulation by the outside world diminishes, and the patient seems emotionally detached. The patient may exhibit restlessness, sleep disturbances, disorientation, hostility, or combativeness. The patient eventually is bedridden and ultimately dies of undercurrent infection or other complications.

PATIENT SCREENING

The onset is insidious, and symptoms may be uncovered during routine office visits. When a family member notices obvious signs and calls for an appointment, the appointment should be scheduled as soon as schedules will allow for a thorough assessment. Anxiety will be high, so the next available appointment should be suggested.

ETIOLOGY

The cause of Alzheimer disease is not known, but the disease is age related and may have a genetic basis in some families. Research has focused on an abnormality found on chromosome 21 as a genetic link. Patients with Down syndrome (a syndrome also linked to an abnormality on chromosome 21) show the same brain changes as patients with Alzheimer disease. In later life, people with Down syndrome have the clinical symptoms of Alzheimer disease. Other theories for the cause of Alzheimer disease include biochemical changes in brain growth, an autoimmune reaction, infection with a slow virus, toxic chemical excess, chemical deficiency, blood vessel defects, and a deficiency of neurochemical factors in the brain. Research shows a higher rate of occurrence in people with history of head trauma.

DIAGNOSIS

Obtaining direct evidence of Alzheimer disease is difficult. When other causes of organic brain disease have been ruled out, diagnostic criteria for Alzheimer disease include evidence of memory and cognitive disturbances. As the disease progresses, neurologic examination reveals sensory and motor deficits. In later stages, diagnostic studies include brain scans, which may detect brain atrophy, widened sulci, and enlarged cerebral ventricles. Positive diagnosis is possible after death, when evidence of brain atrophy and characteristic lesions in the cerebral cortex can be found on pathologic examination of the brain (Fig. 14–5). The brain shows loss of neurons and the presence of *senile plaques,* which include microscopic deposits of **amyloid** material. Neurofibrillary tangles also are evident (Fig. 14–6). Some of the same postmortem anomalies may be found, however, in people who never were diagnosed with or exhibited symptoms of Alzheimer disease. Alzheimer disease is one of the most overdiagnosed or misdiagnosed mental-functioning disorders of older adults because it is not easily distinguished from other dementias that result from excessive use of medication, depression, brain tumors, subdural hematomas, and certain other metabolic diseases.

TREATMENT

No cure is known for Alzheimer disease, so the treatment is supportive and is geared to helping alleviate symptoms. Drug therapy to help alleviate cognitive symptoms includes the use of cholinesterase inhibitors, with the primary drug being donepezil hydrochloride (Aricept). Galantamine (Reminyl) is another option but is not prescribed as often as Aricept. Tacrine (Cognex) is not prescribed as often as it used to be. Antipsychotic or neuroleptic agents including haloperidol; antianxiety agents including alprazolam (Xanax), lorazepam (Ativan), and buspirone hydrochloride (BuSpar); and selective serotonin reuptake inhibitor (SSRI) antidepressants including paroxetine hydrochloride (Paxil) are used to manage behavioral symptoms. Ativan has a longer duration of action than Xanax.

Other drugs used for agitation associated with AD are risperidone (Risperdal) and olanzapine (Zyprexa) for those who start to have delusional symptoms caused by Alzheimer progression. Valproate sodium (Depakote) and gabapentin (Neurontin) are used as mood stabilizers as well as SSRIs. Trazadone sometimes is used for "sundowning," a condition associated with AD in which patients become confused and disoriented after dark.

In addition to reducing symptoms and suffering, treatment aims to increase the patient's ability to cope and to reduce the patient's frustration level. As the patient's ability for self-care declines, general management of fluid intake, adequate nutrition, and personal hygiene is necessary. Treatment gives the patient opportunities to be mobile and to maintain his or her remaining mental abilities for as long as possible. Provisions are employed to protect the patient from injury. Finally, emotional support for the patient and the family or caregiver is vital because the disease forces them to make enormous adjustments.

Research continues to delve into the etiology of Alzheimer disease. Researchers hope that identifying the cause may lead to prevention, because currently there is no way to reverse the neurologic damage created by the disease. Early diagnosis and drug therapy may help to slow the course of the disease.

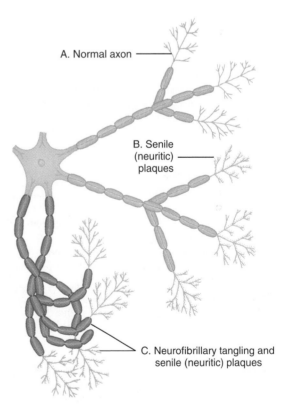

FIGURE 14–6 Neurofibrillary tangles and senile plaques found in patient with Alzheimer's disease. (From Black JM, Matassarin-Jacobs E: *Medical-surgical nursing,* ed 6, Philadelphia, 2000, Saunders.)

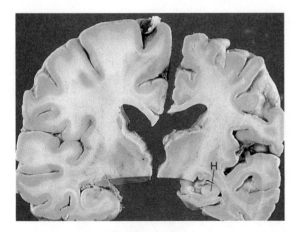

FIGURE 14–5 Alzheimer disease. The diseased brain tissue *(H)* shows loss of cortex and white matter. (From Stevens A, Lowe J: *Pathology—illustrated review in color,* ed 2, St. Louis, 2000, Mosby.)

PROGNOSIS

No cure is known for Alzheimer disease. Drug therapy may help to delay the progression of the disorder. Cholinesterase inhibitors should be discontinued when patients can no longer care for themselves. Advanced status of the disease usually indicates custodial care.

PREVENTION

No prevention for Alzheimer disease is currently known.

PATIENT TEACHING

Advise the caregiver to be consistent in planning daily activities for the patient and to keep activities simple. Emphasize the importance of complying with the prescribed drug therapy regimen. Encourage the family to use community resources and local support groups.

Vascular Dementia

DESCRIPTION

A reduction in blood flow to the brain can result from narrowed and stenosed arteries. Functional areas of the cerebrum are pictured in Figure 14–7. The resulting hypoxia and reduced nourishment to the brain cells cause a general loss in intellectual abilities.

> ■ **ICD-9-CM Code**   **290.40** *(Arteriosclerotic dementia, uncomplicated)*
>   **437.0** *(Atherosclerosis)*
>   **290.0** *(Senile dementia, uncomplicated)*
> *Refer to the physician's diagnosis and then to the current edition of the ICD-9-CM coding manual to ensure the greatest specificity of pathology and any appropriate modifiers.*

SYMPTOMS AND SIGNS

Along with general loss of intellectual abilities, the examiner notes changes in memory, judgment, abstract thinking, and personality. A disregard for personal hygiene is observed, along with apathy, disorientation, and inappropriate responses. Depression, anxiety, and irritability often are noted. Restlessness, sleeplessness, **hallucinations,** and psychotic tendencies appear as the condition advances. Stupor and coma are final stages (Fig. 14–8).

PATIENT SCREENING

Similar to the onset of Alzheimer disease, the onset of vascular dementia is insidious, and symptoms may be uncovered during routine office visits. When a family member notices obvious signs and calls for an appointment, allow enough time

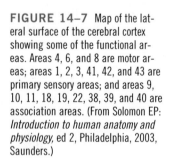

FIGURE 14–7 Map of the lateral surface of the cerebral cortex showing some of the functional areas. Areas 4, 6, and 8 are motor areas; areas 1, 2, 3, 41, 42, and 43 are primary sensory areas; and areas 9, 10, 11, 18, 19, 22, 38, 39, and 40 are association areas. (From Solomon EP: *Introduction to human anatomy and physiology,* ed 2, Philadelphia, 2003, Saunders.)

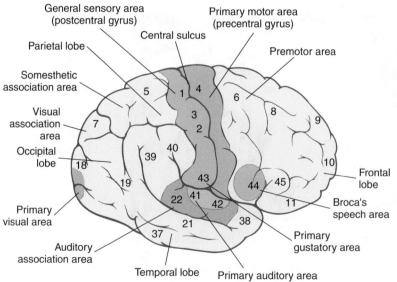

for a thorough assessment. Anxiety levels will be high, so the next available appointment should be suggested.

ETIOLOGY

As atherosclerotic plaque grows in the carotid and cerebral arteries, blood flow to brain tissue is reduced. Prolonged hypoxia with resulting **ischemia** leads to irreversible *necrosis* and death of the brain cells. When an embolism causes the blockage, the hypoxia is sudden and complete. Small aneurysms may be responsible for minute cerebral bleeds. When the cerebral cortex is involved, cognitive capabilities are compromised. (See Cerebrovascular Accident [Stroke] in Chapter 13.)

DIAGNOSIS

Because symptoms of atherosclerotic involvement have an insidious onset, the family often does not notice the subtle changes taking place. When the patient's personal hygiene deteriorates, along with memory and judgment, family members may notice a problem. A thorough history with physical and neurologic examination is necessary to rule out other causes of the altered behavior. Vascular assessment of the carotid and cerebral arteries may yield information about compromised blood flow.

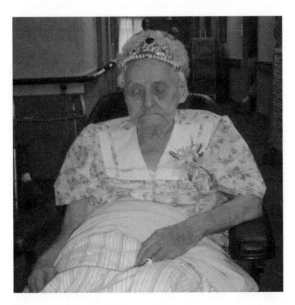

FIGURE 14–8 A 103-year-old female after several "ministrokes." (Courtesy David L. Frazier, 2003.)

Cerebral arteriograms or magnetic resonance imaging (MRI) arteriograms confirm the presence of the condition.

TREATMENT

Treatment aims to increase the blood supply to the brain. Low-dose aspirin, clopidogrel (Plavix), and cilostazol (Pletal) all are used for their antiplatelet effect in preventing stroke or its recurrence, especially with patients who are hypertensive or have had a myocardial infarction. Drug therapy may help increase the blood flow. When the carotid arteries are compromised, surgical intervention in the form of carotid **endarterectomy** may limit the progress of the condition. Brain cell death is irreversible. As the condition progresses, the patient may need to be institutionalized to ensure his or her safety and care.

PROGNOSIS

Improvement is guarded and depends on the extent of the cerebral insult. Many of these patients are trainable with rehabilitation and can function in the community.

PREVENTION

Very little is known about preventing this condition. Early diagnosis and treatment may slow the progress of the dementia.

PATIENT TEACHING

As previously mentioned in the discussion about patient teaching for the Alzheimer patient, consistency in patient activities and therapy is necessary. The caregivers should encourage patients to do what they can do for themselves. Advise the family that improvement is not likely and they should prepare themselves and the patient for that possibility.

Dementia Caused by Head Trauma

DESCRIPTION

A traumatic insult causing reduced blood flow to the cerebrum may result in dementia. Deprivation of oxygen and nutrition (ischemia) results in death of brain cells. Both closed and open head injuries, hematomas, and skull fractures are examples of insults that cause reduced blood flow to the cells (Figs. 14–9 and 14–10).

■ **ICD-9-CM Code 959.01** *(Head injury, unspecified)*
 294.10 *(Dementia)*

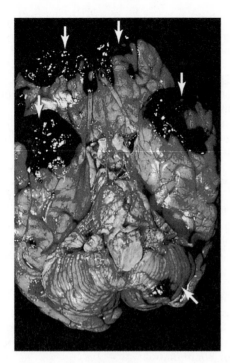

FIGURE 14-9 Contusion. Contrecoup lesion in the frontal and temporal poles *(arrows)* are located opposite to a small coup lesion over the cerebellum *(bottom right arrow)*. (From Damjanov I, Linder J: *Pathology: a color atlas,* St. Louis, 1999, Mosby.)

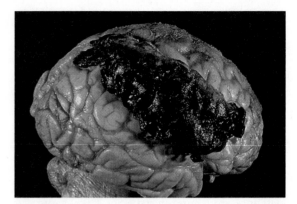

FIGURE 14-10 Acute subdural hematomas. (From Damjanov I, Linder J: *Pathology: a color atlas,* St. Louis, 1999, Mosby.)

SYMPTOMS AND SIGNS

Reductions in intellectual capabilities and cognitive functioning may result from trauma to the head. After a head injury, the patient exhibits reduced mental status and is unable to perform many of the cognitive tasks that were possible before the injury. Intelligence testing shows reduced capabilities.

PATIENT SCREENING

The patient probably will be in an inpatient facility because of the head trauma. After discharge, when the patient needs outpatient medical assessment and treatment, an appointment should be arranged as soon as both schedules allow time for complete assessment.

ETIOLOGY

Trauma to the head causes an insult to the brain as a result of edema, increased intracranial pressure, or damage to the vessel walls. The insult results in compromise of the cerebral blood supply. The hy-poxia is followed by ischemia and eventually irreversible necrosis of brain cells. (See Head Trauma in Chapter 13.)

DIAGNOSIS

The history of head trauma with reduced level of mental functioning is augmented by a thorough physical and neurologic examination. Imaging studies may include skull radiographic films, computed tomography (CT) scan of the brain, and MRI scan of the brain and cerebral vessels. Subdural or epidural hematomas may be noted, as may any type of skull fracture.

Ventricular shift indicates increasing intracranial pressure. Any neurologic deficit, such as unequal pupils, unequal grips, hemiparesis, and posturing, indicates insult to the brain tissue. As the condition progresses, reduced intellectual functioning is noted.

TREATMENT

Treatment includes correcting the insult to the brain to prevent further damage. After the necrosis has evolved, the damaged tissues cannot be repaired. Therapy and training to maintain the remaining functions are attempted.

PROGNOSIS

Similar to the prognosis for vascular dementia, improvement is guarded and depends on the extent of the cerebral insult. Many of these patients are trainable with rehabilitation and can function in the community. When the damage is severe, the patient may need to be institutionalized for care and safety.

PREVENTION

Prevention depends on the causative factors as well as the extent and type of the injury. Consistent use of seat belts in motor vehicles is known to reduce the severity of head injuries. Using helmets when cycling and in contact sports has a similar benefit.

PATIENT TEACHING

As previously mentioned in the discussion of patient teaching for other dementias, consistency in patient activities and therapy is necessary. Urge caregivers to encourage patients to do what they can for themselves. Rehabilitation and therapy may lead to improvement in the condition. Families may need encouragement to recognize the fact that there is no cure. Some patients who have experienced dementia caused by head trauma may be educable or trainable. Routines and consistency are important in enabling the patient to function at the highest possible level. Advise the family that improvement is not likely and that they should prepare themselves and the patient for that possibility.

■ **ICD-9-CM Code** **305.0** *(Non-dependent abuse of drugs)*
304.90 *(Unspecified drug dependence)*

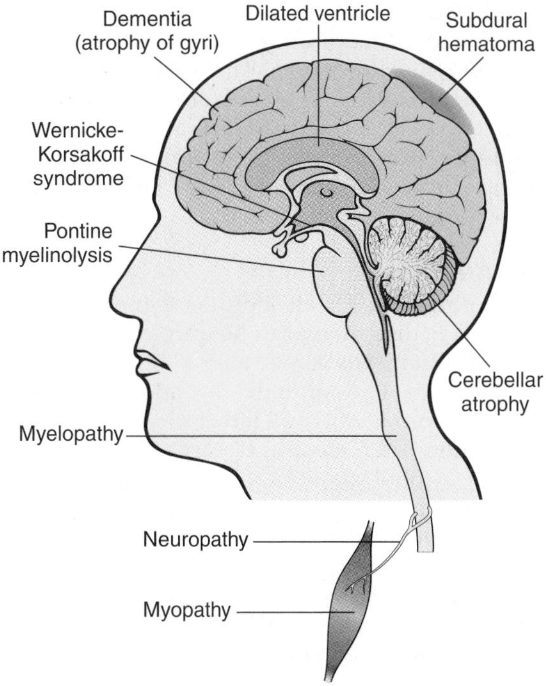

FIGURE 14–11 Pathological changes in the nervous system caused by chronic alcoholism. (From Damjanov I: *Pathology for the health related professions,* ed 2, Philadelphia, 2000, Saunders.)

Substance-Related Disorders

Alcohol Abuse

DESCRIPTION

Alcohol abuse is a disorder of physical and psychological dependence on daily or regular excessive intake of alcoholic beverages. The onset can be insidious or can be accelerated by an acute traumatic event.

■ **ICD-9 CM Code** **303.90**

SYMPTOMS AND SIGNS

Excessive use of alcohol often is associated with anxiety, depression, insomnia, impotence, and behavioral disorders both before and during intoxication. *Amnesia* often occurs after intoxication. Repeated heavy drinking of alcohol produces symptoms and signs in nearly every organ system (Fig. 14–11). Chronic alcoholism causes pathologic changes in the nervous system. Common physical findings include frequent infections, hypertension, and gastrointestinal (GI) problems. The patient may report unexplained seizure activity or symptoms of alcohol withdrawal. Prolonged heavy use of alcohol may cause cirrhosis of the liver, pancreatitis, and peripheral neuropathy, resulting in muscle weakness and *paresthesia*. The risk of cancer of the esophagus, stomach, and other parts of the GI system also is increased.

The consequences of chronic alcohol abuse include dysfunction within family and social relationships and disruption in occupational responsibilities. Some people are prone to aggressive or violent behavior, accidents, and threatened or attempted suicide. The patient often denies an inability to control or discontinue alcohol abuse.

PATIENT SCREENING

When the patients themselves call for the appointment, they require prompt assessment and intervention. When they state that they are in a crisis and are unable to be seen in the office right away, refer them to an emergency facility.

ETIOLOGY

Alcohol abuse has no single cause but a cluster of possible causative factors. The origin may include genetic or biologic factors, depression, emotional conflict, social factors, and cultural attitudes. Because the patient history frequently includes a familial pattern of alcohol abuse, genetic factors pose a recognized statistical risk.

DIAGNOSIS

Screening tests for alcohol abuse include questionnaires that attempt to identify pathologic behavior. Test results may be altered by the patient's attempts to deny or hide the addiction. Diagnostic information gathered during physical examination and a medical history may fit the profile of alcohol abuse. Laboratory findings may help to confirm the diagnosis. One sensitive indicator of heavy alcohol intake is a high gamma-glutamyltransferase (GGT) level in the blood. The amount of alcohol consumed may be calculated through the use of a chart, such as those used by law-enforcement agencies. Table 14–1 lists the effects of various levels of blood alcohol on the brain. Table 14–2 shows how an individual's weight and the amount of alcohol consumed determine blood alcohol content. Figure 14–12 compares the alcohol content of various forms of alcohol. Other abnormal laboratory findings emerge with organ system complications resulting from chronic alcohol abuse.

TREATMENT

Rehabilitation consists of a specialized treatment plan that meets the patient's physical and psychological needs and supports abstinence from alcohol. After detoxification, most patients benefit from psychotherapy or group therapy and participation in the 12-step program of Alcoholics Anonymous (AA). Ongoing therapy usually can continue on an outpatient basis. Willing participation in a recovery program on a sustained, as-needed basis usually offers a promising prognosis. Relapses are common and need not represent failure of treatment as long as the patient returns to a program of recovery and abstinence from alcohol. Only a small percentage of patients can ever become "social" or moderate drinkers again. (Some alcoholics volunteer to take a drug called disulfiram [Antabuse], which causes nausea and vomiting when alcohol is consumed. Other alcoholics are ordered by a court to use this drug.)

PROGNOSIS

The prognosis varies according to the duration of the alcoholism.

Text continues on p. 668

TABLE 14–1
Effects of Rising Blood Alcohol Level (BAL)*

BAL	EFFECTS
0.02	Mild euphoria, reduced inhibitions, slight body warmth, talkativeness
0.05	Noticeable relaxation, reduced alertness, increased self-confidence
0.08	**Legally drunk in 45 states,** impairment in coordination, judgment, memory, and comprehension
0.10	**Legally drunk in remaining states,** behavior becomes loud or embarrassing; mood swings are noticeable, and reaction time is reduced
0.15	Impaired balance and coordination; appears intoxicated
0.20	Disorientation, mental confusion, dizziness, lethargy, exaggerated emotional states
0.30	Staggering gait, slurred speech, visual disturbances, possible loss of consciousness
0.40	Inability to walk or stand, reduced response to stimuli, vomiting, incontinence, loss of consciousness, possible death ("dead drunk")
0.50	Respiratory effort depressed to point of ceasing, lack of reflexes, body temperature drops, impairment of circulation, possible death; immediate intervention and intense life-support measures required to sustain life
0.60	Death usually occurs or has occurred

*Blood alcohol level (BAL) is measured in milligrams of alcohol per 100 ml of blood and reported as a percentage. An individual with a BAL of 0.10 has 1/10 of 1% (1/1000) of total blood volume as alcohol. BAL depends on the blood volume (blood volume increases with weight) and the amount of alcohol consumed over a given time.

ENRICHMENT
BLOOD ALCOHOL LEVELS

AFTER ALCOHOL IS INGESTED, it is absorbed from the GI tract and distributed to all tissues. The rich blood supply to the brain results in a concentration of alcohol in the CNS proportional to blood alcohol concentration. The rate at which alcohol is metabolized in the liver is constant, and only 10 to 15 ml of pure alcohol can be metabolized in 1 hour. Figure 14–12 compares the amount of beer (12 oz), wine (6 oz), and 86-proof liquor (1 oz) that contains 10 to 15 ml of pure alcohol.

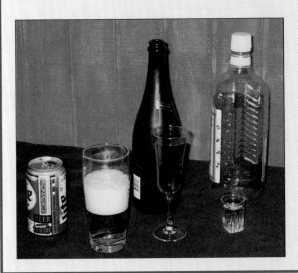

FIGURE 14–12 Comparison of the amounts of beer (12 oz), wine (6 oz), or 86-proof liquor (1 oz) that contain 10 to 15 ml of pure alcohol. (Courtesy David L. Frazier, 1999.)

TABLE 14–2
Blood Alcohol Content*

BODY WEIGHT (LB)	NO. OF DRINKS (1 OZ 86-PROOF LIQUOR, 3 OZ WINE, OR 12 OZ BEER)								
	1	2	3	4	5	6	7	8	9
100	0.032*	0.065†	0.097‡	0.129‡	0.162‡	0.194‡	0.226‡	0.258‡	0.291‡
120	0.027*	0.054†	0.081‡	0.108‡	0.135‡	0.161‡	0.188‡	0.215‡	0.242‡
140	0.023*	0.046*	0.069†	0.092‡	0.115‡	0.138‡	0.161‡	0.184‡	0.207‡
160	0.020*	0.040*	0.060†	0.080‡	0.101‡	0.121‡	0.141‡	0.161‡	0.181‡
180	0.018*	0.036*	0.054†	0.072†	0.090‡	0.108‡	0.126‡	0.144‡	0.162‡
200	0.016*	0.032*	0.048*	0.064†	0.080‡	0.097‡	0.113‡	0.129‡	0.145‡
220	0.015*	0.029*	0.044*	0.058†	0.073†	0.088‡	0.102‡	0.117‡	0.131‡
240	0.014*	0.027*	0.040*	0.053†	0.067†	0.081‡	0.095‡	0.108‡	0.121‡

*Blood alcohol content to 0.05%—Caution.
†Blood alcohol content 0.05%–0.079%—Driving impaired.
‡Blood alcohol content 0.08% and up—Presumed under the influence in most states.

ENRICHMENT

SUBSTANCE ABUSE

SUBSTANCE ABUSE is a significant social and medical concern. The altered behavior and medical complications of substance abuse are found in all social, economic, ethnic, racial, educational, and professional backgrounds. Some substances that are abused on a regular but episodic basis are alcohol, sedatives, stimulants, opioids, cannabis (marijuana), hallucinogens, inhalants, caffeine, nicotine, illicit synthetic (designer) drugs, and other chemical substances (Table 14–3). These substances, prescribed or illegal, give the user a stimulant or depressant effect. The overindulgence in or dependence on chemical substances often produces a detrimental effect on the user's physical and psychological well-being as well as on the welfare of others.

During substance abuse, tolerance to the chemical or drug often develops, necessitating increased amounts of the substance to achieve the desired effect. In addition to tolerance, both physical and psychological dependence can develop. Rapid withdrawal from certain drugs can cause life-threatening and even fatal reactions.

The individual under the influence of drugs often exhibits inappropriate behavior. Judgment often is impaired, and users are at risk for injury to themselves or others when driving or operating machinery while under the influence. They experience multiple social and interpersonal problems. While under the influence of

mood-altering drugs, some may appear intoxicated, but others may exhibit a fairly normal pattern of behavior. Over an extended time, performance and relationships deteriorate. Dependability decreases, legal problems develop, and desperation for more of the desired substance may lead to criminal behavior.

Many employers require applicants and employees to undergo drug screening. This type of drug screening usually is performed in one of two noninvasive methods. A urine sample can be analyzed for drug content. Urine drug screening typically reveals drug use only during the preceding 3 to 4 days. An individual may be able to abstain from the drug for 4 days and produce negative test results.

Another method is analysis of a hair sample (Fig. 14–13). Evidence of drug use stays in the hair shaft for about 90 days. Drugs are absorbed into the bloodstream and circulated in the blood, which nourishes the hair follicle, leaving trace amounts of residue entrapped in the core of the hair shaft. Washing, bleaching, or dying the hair does not remove the drug residue. Thus abstinence for a few days does not affect the results of the test. Finally, these tests do not reveal a pattern of use or the presence of dependence, so results should be interpreted and integrated into other clinical data.

Law enforcement officers use a breath analyzer to measure blood alcohol levels quickly. Qualitative or quantitative drug

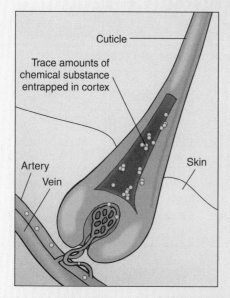

Cuticle

Trace amounts of chemical substance entrapped in cortex

Artery

Vein

Skin

FIGURE 14–13 The scientific principle behind hair analysis is that as drugs are ingested, they enter our bloodstream, which nourishes our hair follicles. In this way, trace amounts of drugs are deposited in the hair shaft that, when analyzed, can reveal a person's drug history. (With permission from Psychemedics Corp., Cambridge, Mass., 1998.)

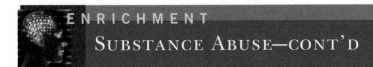

ENRICHMENT
SUBSTANCE ABUSE—CONT'D

assay tests (blood tests to detect the presence or level of specific drugs) also are performed. General toxicology drug screening determines only the presence or absence of a drug. Any identified drugs should be confirmed and their levels determined through a test specific for that drug. Blood screening for non-specific drugs usually is accompanied by urine drug screening.

DRUGS OF ABUSE
The misuse of various drugs that modify mood or behavior is called drug abuse. Many types of drugs, including depressants, stimulants, opiates, opiate-like drugs, hallucinogens, volatile

substances, cannabinoids, steroids, tobacco, and prescription drugs may be suspected in abuse and dependence (see Table 14–3). Some of these drugs have been used for centuries and often are called recreational drugs.

Peer pressure, a chaotic home environment, and poor coping skills can lead to drug abuse by individuals. The use of a prescription drug to treat illness and mental disorder often introduces the individual to the drug of abuse.

Table 14–3 presents popular drugs of abuse, their common names, and their many potential adverse effects.

TABLE 14–3
Drugs of Abuse

DRUG NAME	CLASSIFICATION	OTHER NAMES	HOW CONSUMED	EFFECTS
Alcohol	Depressant	Beer, wine, liquor, cooler, malt liquor, booze	Orally	Addiction (alcoholism), dizziness, slurred speech, disturbed sleep, nausea, vomiting, hangovers, impaired motor skills, violent behavior, impaired learning, fetal alcohol syndrome, respiratory depression and death (high doses)
Amphetamines	Stimulant	Speed, uppers, ups, hearts, black beauties, pep pills, copilots, bumble bees, Benzedrine, Dexedrine, footballs, biphetamine	Orally, injected, snorted, smoked	Addiction, anxiety, agitation, confusion, increased blood pressure, aggression, insomnia, dizziness, dilated pupils and blurred vision, loss of appetite, malnutrition, hyperthermia, rages, violent behavior, psychotic features withdrawal syndrome, progressive deterioration with heavy use

Continued

General principles of treatment for addiction to various drugs:
- A treatment plan must meet the individual's needs and be tailored to the drug of abuse.
- Identify the program or facility appropriate for the individual so it is available when needed.
- Effective treatment begins with a medical, psychological, and social assessment.
- Medical detoxification may be required.
- Treatment requires adequate time, individual and/or group counseling, support, and medication in some cases.
- Behavior therapy and a support program, such as a 12-step program, are crucial to recovery.
- Relapses can occur, so monitoring for drug use is important.
- NOTE: If the drugs of abuse have been injected, the patient has increased risk of exposure to HIV, hepatitis B and C, tuberculosis, and other infectious diseases.
- Education about drug abuse, the nature of addiction, and the importance of recovery as a long-term process is beneficial to family and friends, but essential to the recovering addict.

TABLE 14–3
Drugs of Abuse—cont'd

DRUG NAME	CLASSIFICATION	OTHER NAMES	HOW CONSUMED	EFFECTS
Meth-amphetamines	Stimulant	Speed, meth, crank, crystal, ice (street name for smokeable type), fire, croak, crypto, white cross, glass	Orally, injected, snorted, smoked	Addiction, irritability, anxiety, increased blood pressure, paranoia, psychosis, aggression, nervousness, hyperthermia, compulsive behavior, stroke, depression, convulsions, heart and blood vessel toxicity, insomnia, anorexia, hallucinations, formication (crawling sensation)
Ecstasy	Stimulant	XTC, Adam, MDMA; known as a "club drug"	Orally	Psychiatric disturbances including panic, anxiety, depression, and paranoia; muscle tension, nausea, blurred vision, sweating, tachycardia, hypertension, tremors, hallucinations, anorexia, sleep problems, marked hyperthermia, drug craving, fainting, chills, dehydration
Methylphenidate (Ritalin)	Stimulant	Speed, west coast (*NOTE:* used legally to treat Attention Deficit Disorder)	Tablet is crushed and is snorted or injected	Loss of appetite, fevers, convulsions, severe headaches, irregular heartbeat and respiration, paranoia, hallucinations, delusions, excessive repetition of movements and meaningless tasks, tremors, muscle twitching
Herbal ecstasy/ ephedrine	Stimulant	Cloud 9, Rave, Energy, Ultimate Xphoria, X	Orally	Increased heart rate, increased blood pressure, seizures, heart attacks, stroke, death (*NOTE:* active ingredients are caffeine and ephedrine)
Designer drugs (fentanyl-based)	Stimulant	Synthetic heroin, goodfella	Injected, sniffed, or smoked	Instant respiratory paralysis, potency creates strong possibility of overdose, many of same effects as heroin

General principles of treatment for addiction to various drugs:
- A treatment plan must meet the individual's needs and be tailored to the drug of abuse.
- Identify the program or facility appropriate for the individual so it is available when needed.
- Effective treatment begins with a medical, psychological, and social assessment.
- Medical detoxification may be required.
- Treatment requires adequate time, individual and/or group counseling, support, and medication in some cases.
- Behavior therapy and a support program, such as a 12-step program, are crucial to recovery.
- Relapses can occur, so monitoring for drug use is important.
- NOTE: If the drugs of abuse have been injected, the patient has increased risk of exposure to HIV, hepatitis B and C, tuberculosis, and other infectious diseases.
- Education about drug abuse, the nature of addiction, and the importance of recovery as a long-term process is beneficial to family and friends, but essential to the recovering addict.

TABLE 14-3
Drugs of Abuse—cont'd

DRUG NAME	CLASSIFICATION	OTHER NAMES	HOW CONSUMED	EFFECTS
GHB (gama hydroxybutyric acid)	Stimulant	Liquid ecstasy, somatomax, scoop, Grievous Bodily Harm, liquid x, Georgia Home Boy, goop	Snorted, orally in liquid form, smoked, or mixed into drinks	Liver failure, vomiting, tremors, seizures, coma, fatal respiratory problems
Cocaine	Stimulant	Coke, snow, nose candy, flake, blow, big C, lady, white, snowbirds; crack with heroin is a "speedball"	Snorted or dissolved in water and injected; freebase form (crack) is smokeable	Addiction, pupil dilation, elevated vital signs, paranoia, seizures, heart attack, respiratory failure, constricted peripheral blood vessels, restlessness, irritability, anxiety, loss of appetite, hallucinations, insomnia, hyperthermia, altered judgment, erratic behavior, death from overdose
Heroin (processed from morphine)	Opiate	Smack, horse, mud, brown sugar, junk, black tar, big H, dope	Injected, smoked, or snorted	Addiction, intense euphoria, slowed and slurred speech, slow gait, constricted pupils, droopy eyelids, impaired night vision, vomiting after first use and at very high doses, reduced sexual pleasure, reduced appetite, constipation, respiratory depression or failure, dry and itching skin, skin infections
Rohypnol (flunitrazepam)	Opiate-like	Roach, roofies, the forget pill, rope, rophies, ruffles, R2, roofenol, la roche, rib; known as the "date rape" drug	Orally in pill form, dissolved in a drink, or snorted	Blackouts with a complete loss of memory, sense of fearlessness and aggression, dizziness and disorientation, nausea, difficulty with motor movements and speaking, creates a drunk feeling
Ketamine hydrochloride	Opiate-like	Special K, Vitamin K, new ecstasy, psychedelic heroin, Ketalar, Ketaject, Super-K, breakfast cereal; used as rave drug	Snorted or smoked	Delirium, amnesia, impaired motor function, potentially fatal respiratory problems

Continued

TABLE 14–3
Drugs of Abuse—cont'd

DRUG NAME	CLASSIFICATION	OTHER NAMES	HOW CONSUMED	EFFECTS
LSD (lysergic acid diethyl-amide)	Hallucinogen	Acid, microdot, tabs, doses, trips, hits, sugar cubes	Tablets taken orally or gelatin/liquid put in eyes	Unpredictable effects, emotional swings (fear to euphoria), elevated body temperature and blood pressure, suppressed appetite, sleeplessness, tremors, flashbacks, drug-induced psychosis, chronic recurring hallucinations. (*NOTE:* LSD is the most common hallucinogen. LSD tabs are often decorated with colorful designs or cartoon characters.)
PCP (phencyclidine)	Dissociative drug	Angel dust, ozone, rocket fuel, peace pill, elephant tranquilizer, dust, boat, dummy dust, zombie	Snorted, smoked, taken orally, or injected	Out of body experience, impaired motor coordination, inability to feel pain, anxiety, disorientation, fear, panic, paranoia, altered perception of body image, mental turmoil, delusions, delirium, agitation, unpredictable violent outbursts, death. (*NOTE:* Marijuana joints can be dipped into PCP.)
Mushrooms (psilocybin)	Hallucinogen	Shrooms, caps, magic mushrooms	Eaten or brewed and drunk in tea	Increased blood pressure, sweating, nausea, hallucinations
Inhalants Vapors Aerosols	Volatile substances	Nitrous oxide, laughing gas, whispers, aerosol sprays, cleaning fluids, solvents; many household products	Sniffed, direct spray, bagging, huffing (from a soaked rag), inhaling	Intoxication similar to alcohol, headache, muscle weakness, abdominal pain, severe mood swings, violent behavior, numbness and tingling of hands and feet, nausea, nosebleeds, liver, lung, and kidney damage, dangerous chemical imbalances in the body, anorexia, fatigue, decreases in heart and respiratory rates, hepatitis or peripheral neuropathy

General principles of treatment for addiction to various drugs:
- A treatment plan must meet the individual's needs and be tailored to the drug of abuse.
- Identify the program or facility appropriate for the individual so it is available when needed.
- Effective treatment begins with a medical, psychological, and social assessment.
- Medical detoxification may be required.
- Treatment requires adequate time, individual and/or group counseling, support, and medication in some cases.
- Behavior therapy and a support program, such as a 12-step program, are crucial to recovery.
- Relapses can occur, so monitoring for drug use is important.
- NOTE: If the drugs of abuse have been injected, the patient has increased risk of exposure to HIV, hepatitis B and C, tuberculosis, and other infectious diseases.
- Education about drug abuse, the nature of addiction, and the importance of recovery as a long-term process is beneficial to family and friends, but essential to the recovering addict.

TABLE 14-3
Drugs of Abuse—cont'd

DRUG NAME	CLASSIFICATION	OTHER NAMES	HOW CONSUMED	EFFECTS
Marijuana/ Hash	Cannabinoid	Weed, pot, reefer, grass, dope, ganja, Mary Jane, sinsemilla, herb, Aunt Mary, skunk, boom, kif, gangster, chronic, 420	Smoked or eaten	Bloodshot eyes, dry mouth and throat, impaired comprehension, altered sense of time, reduced ability to perform tasks requiring concentration and coordination (such as driving a car), paranoia, intense anxiety or panic attacks, altered cognition; impaired learning, memory, thinking, perception, speaking, listening, problem solving, and forming of concepts
Steroids	Steroidal	Rhoids, juice	Orally or injected into muscle, gels or creams rubbed into the skin. May be "stacked" (by mixing oral and injectable types)	Mood swings ranging from euphoria to depression, acne, cardiovascular disease, liver tumors, liver cancer, irritability and aggression, sterility, increased energy, masculine traits in women and feminine traits in men
Tobacco	Others	Smoke, bone, butt, coffin nail, cancer stick	Cigarettes, cigars, pipes, smokeless tobacco (chew, dip, snuff)	Addiction, heart and cardiovascular disease, cancer of the lung, larynx, esophagus, bladder, pancreas, kidney, and mouth, emphysema and chronic bronchitis, spontaneous abortion, preterm delivery, low birth weight
Prescription drugs	Others	Opioids (narcotics), central nervous system depressants, stimulants	Orally, without the supervision of a physician	General types of effects from commonly abused prescription drugs may include: physical dependence, addiction, withdrawal symptoms, mood alteration, sleep disorders, seizures, psychological changes, cardiovascular failure, neurologic disorders

PREVENTION

No prevention is known for alcoholism.

PATIENT TEACHING

Encourage parents and family members to be aware of dangers related to ingestion of alcohol.

Schizophrenia

DESCRIPTION

Schizophrenia, a major psychiatric disturbance, is a group of disorders that may result in chronic mental dysfunction, producing varying degrees of impairment.

■ **ICD-9-CM Code 295.90**

SYMPTOMS AND SIGNS

Schizophrenia is a mental disorder characterized by the presence of either positive manifestations (an excess or distortion of normal functions) or negative manifestations (a loss of normal functions). Positive symptoms include **delusions,** hallucinations, disorganized speech, and grossly disorganized or **catatonic** behavior. Negative symptoms are affective flattening, alogia, and avolition.

Schizophrenia is very disabling for the affected individual. In most cases, a person with schizophrenia will have difficulty finishing their education, maintaining employment, and participating in relationships. Many experience trouble with activities of daily living. Schizophrenia is rarely seen in children. Most symptoms begin to manifest in the mid to late 20s. Careful consideration must go into the diagnosis of schizophrenia because some cultures and religions may regard some symptoms as normal. The onset of schizophrenia is usually insidious during adolescence or young adulthood.

Prodromal signs, such as withdrawal, odd behavior, disheveled appearance, and loss of interest in school or work may be noted. The patient may report feeling confused, isolated, anxious, and afraid. In the active phase of schizophrenia, a vast range of severe behavioral and perceptual manifestations is present, with marked social and occupational dysfunction.

One important feature is disorganized thinking, usually reflected by the patient's speech and by disturbances in language and communication. For example, the patient may switch from one topic to another, speak incoherently, give an unrelated answer to a question, or experience difficulty in speaking at all.

Distortions in perception called hallucinations are a common characteristic of schizophrenia. Hallucinations may be auditory, visual, olfactory, or sensory. The patient with auditory hallucinations acknowledges hearing voices that may be threatening, instructive, or conversational. Delusions, which are erroneous beliefs, represent exaggerations or distortions of perceptions or experiences. In persecutory delusion, for instance, people may believe that they are being mistreated, deceived, or stalked. More bizarre delusions may include belief that one's thoughts are controlled by an "alien."

Inappropriate **affect** (feeling) is another identifying characteristic of schizophrenia. Lack of emotional expression (flat affect) or unreasonable outbursts of emotions may be noted. Eye contact is minimal.

Behavior may be bizarre or grossly disorganized, unpredictable, agitated, or violent. The patient may assume rigid posturing (*catatonic posturing*), dress in an odd manner, and neglect self-care. Any of these behaviors can stem from the patient's delusional thinking. As the symptoms and signs persist, the patient's ability to function in interpersonal, social, or occupational relationships deteriorates.

Schizophrenia has subtypes, which are determined by a clustering of characteristics as follows:

■ **ICD-9-CM Code 295.30** *(Paranoid type)*
Paranoid schizophrenia features anger, hostility, violence, grandiose or persecutory delusions, or hallucinations. The patient may be intelligent and well informed.

295.10 *(Disorganized type)*
The patient is blatantly incoherent, with delusions that are not systematized into a theme. The patient's feelings are dull, inappropriate, or greatly exaggerated. Behavior may be odd or regressive. The patient has a history of extreme social impairment, poor functioning, and poor adaptation. The condition has a chronic course.

295.20 *(Catatonic type)*
Catatonic schizophrenia features either excitement or stupor with mutism, negativism, rigidity, and posturing.

295.90 *(Undifferentiated type)*

The behavior is grossly disorganized, and the patient is obviously incoherent, grossly delusional, and hallucinatory. Prominent symptoms of psychosis may fit more than one subtype.

295.60 *(Residual type)*

The patient has experienced at least one episode of schizophrenia but is currently without prominent symptoms. Continuing evidence of illness, such as illogical thinking and odd behavior, may prevent the patient from functioning in the workplace.

PATIENT SCREENING

Scheduling of the appointment for the schizophrenic patient varies depending on the situation. When the patient or family member reports a crisis, have them report to an emergency facility.

ETIOLOGY

The cause of schizophrenia is unknown, but evidence suggests that genetic factors play a substantial role. Close biologic relatives of patients with schizophrenia have a tenfold greater risk of schizophrenia. Vulnerability to stress and environmental factors are considered contributing catalysts.

DIAGNOSIS

The diagnosis of schizophrenia requires recognizing a group of psychotic signs and symptoms, including delusions, hallucinations, disorganized speech, grossly disorganized behavior, affective flattening, alogia, and avolition. According to the DSM-IV, "alogia or poverty of speech is manifested by brief, empty replies. Avolition is characterized by an inability to initiate and participate in goal-directed activities." Previously no laboratory findings have been identified as diagnostic of schizophrenia. Recent advances in medical imaging of the brain now provide images of brain activity. These include positron-emission tomography (PET), functional magnetic resonance (FMR), and magnetic encephalography (MEG). These tests, applied to schizophrenic patients by researchers, have produced an insight into the brain activity of schizophrenic patients and those without the disease.

Psychological tests that may help in diagnosis include the Rorschach (inkblot) test, the Thematic Apperception Test (TAT), and the Minnesota Multiphasic Personality Inventory (MMPI). Organic causes such as toxic psychosis associated with substance abuse, cerebral arteriosclerosis, and hyperthyroidism should be ruled out.

TREATMENT

During the acute phase of schizophrenia, antipsychotic drugs are used to control symptoms and to allow early release from the hospital. The minimal dose that produces remission of symptoms without troublesome side effects associated with antipsychotic medications is desirable. Subsequent long-term multidimensional treatment combines supportive psychotherapy, drugs, and family involvement. After the patient is stabilized, the goal of treatment is helping the patient to establish a better sense of self through personal, social, and vocational achievements.

Atypical antipsychotics are first-line therapy and include risperidone (Risperdal), olanzapine (Zyprexa), and, less often, ziprasidone (Geodon) and quetiapine (Seroquel). Older antipsychotic drugs are used for those who do not respond well to atypical drugs and in cases where the patient has been on the older drugs for a long time and reports no unmanageable side effects. These drugs include chlorpromazine (Thorazine), haloperidol (Haldol), perphenazine (Prolixin), and many more that are used less often. Intramuscular injections increase compliance because the medication can last for a month.

PROGNOSIS

The prognosis is moderate if the patient takes prescription drugs regularly and if the family is supportive and willing to participate in treatment. Treatment in a community support program also is beneficial. Responses to treatment vary, and relapses may occur.

PREVENTION

Schizophrenia is genetic, so no prevention is known. Compliance in taking medications reduces psychotic breaks, helping to prevent the illness from worsening. Each time a patient has a psychotic break, baseline functioning is reduced.

PATIENT TEACHING

Patients should be instructed to comply with the medication regimen despite the frequent unpleasant side effects. Because noncompliance can be an issue, involving the family is helpful. Advise family members and support persons that patients with schizophrenia are not bad people, but are simply people with a bad illness. In addition, family members are encouraged to help the patient with the activities of daily living.

Mood Disorders

In mood disorders, a person experiences a pathologic disturbance in mood that affects all aspects of his or her life. The terms affect and mood are used interchangeably to refer to the outward manifestation of a person's feeling or tone.

Bipolar Disorder

DESCRIPTION
Bipolar disorder is a major affective disorder with abnormally intense mood swings from a hyperactive, or manic, state to a depressive syndrome (Fig. 14–14). In some cases, symptoms of hyperactivity and depression may coexist. The patient may remain manic for days, weeks, or months before experiencing depression. Assessment findings vary with the type of episode (manic, depressive, or mixed) that the patient is experiencing at the time of medical evaluation.

■ **ICD-9-CM Code 296.7**

SYMPTOMS AND SIGNS
During a manic episode, the patient is excited, euphoric, and expansive. The person speaks rapidly with great certitude and conviction. Evidence of thought disorders, such as frequent changes of topic or flight of ideas, may be noted. Patients sleep little and seem to have excessive energy, which leads to overinvolvement in activities. Judgment is impaired, and they may spend money extravagantly. Behavior may appear bizarre, grandiose, or promiscuous. The patient may be delusional or experience auditory hallucinations.

During an episode of depression, the patient's mood becomes lowered, sad, or markedly indifferent (flat affect). Thoughts and speech are slow, and the patient may avoid communication. The patient becomes withdrawn and demonstrates loss of interest in life. Reports of sleep disturbance, loss of appetite, and feelings of guilt are common. The patient experiences a marked decrease in physical activity. Suicide may be threatened or attempted.

PATIENT SCREENING
Most often help will be sought during the depressive portion of the illness. Depressed individuals require immediate assessment.

ETIOLOGY
Bipolar disorder has no clear cause. Biochemical factors such as alterations of *neurotransmitter* levels in the brain, endocrine disorders, and electrolyte imbalances may play a role. The risk of mood disorders is higher among close relatives of the patient. Emotional or physical trauma may precipitate the onset of bipolar disorder in a predisposed person.

DIAGNOSIS
A thorough family history and patient history of symptoms is obtained. The patient may appear to be experiencing only depression.

Bipolar disorder is identified when certain prescribed diagnostic criteria can be documented during physical and psychological evaluation. The mood disturbance must be pervasive and persistent and cause marked impairment over a distinct

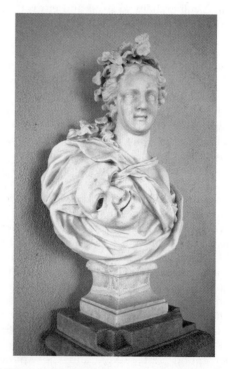

FIGURE 14–14 Representation of bipolar disorder. (Courtesy David L. Frazier, 2003.)

period of time. Other medical causes, such as organic diseases and psychiatric conditions, must be ruled out.

TREATMENT

After diagnosis, therapeutic treatment is dictated by the specific form of behavior the patient exhibits. Lithium carbonate is the drug of choice during an acute manic phase of bipolar disease. It may even abate a swing into the depressive phase. Valproate sodium (Depakote) and carbamazepine (Tegretol) are good drugs for add-on therapy in stabilizing manic episodes. During an episode of depression, antidepressants are used with caution because they may trigger a manic episode. Treatment includes a therapeutic milieu, or environment, that meets the patient's physical needs, encourages personal responsibility, and sets reasonable limits and goals for behavior. During this time, the patient may need to be protected from self-injury.

PROGNOSIS

The prognosis is good with treatment and drug therapy. Compliance is the key to successful treatment.

PREVENTION

No prevention is known.

PATIENT TEACHING

Encourage patients to take medications and to keep appointments with their therapist. Blood studies may be necessary depending on the medications prescribed and taken.

Major Depressive Disorder

DESCRIPTION

Major depressive disorder is a mood disorder characterized by one or more major depressive episodes. Persons with major depressive disorders have no history of a manic or hypomanic episode.

■ **ICD-9-CM Code 296.20**

SYMPTOMS AND SIGNS

Major depressive disorder is a serious alteration in mood that may be described as deep and persistent sadness, despair, and hopelessness (Fig. 14–15). Symptoms develop gradually over several days, during which an anxious or brooding appearance may be noted. The person may experience an empty or heavy feeling inside accompanied by a vague sense of loss. The person also may have an attitude of self-blame, remorse, guilt, or loss of self-esteem. Other symptoms include sleep disturbance (insomnia or hypersomnia), physical sluggishness or fatigue, loss of concentration, and inability to experience pleasure. In addition, a depressed person may have a variety of physical symptoms. Appetite disturbance produces a change in weight. The patient withdraws socially and may admit to having suicidal thoughts; suicidal behavior is common in major depression (Table 14–4).

PATIENT SCREENING

People experiencing symptoms of depression, often reported by family members, require immediate assessment. A risk of suicide requires immediate assessment and intervention.

ETIOLOGY

Major depressive disorder is thought to have a biologic basis and a familial pattern, but the precise cause is not understood. Psychosocial pressures, chronic physical illness, and alcohol dependence are considered predisposing factors. Although many patients blame their environment, it is not considered a cause of the disease.

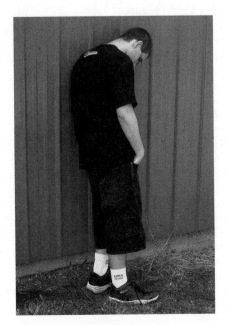

FIGURE 14–15 Depression. (Courtesy David L. Frazier, 2003.)

TABLE 14–4
Depression on a Continuum

MILD TO MODERATE	SEVERE
COMMUNICATION	
Slow speech; long pauses before answering; monotone	Slow in extreme; may be mute and not talk at all
AFFECT	
Crying and weeping, slumping in chair, drooping shoulders, look of gloom and pessimism	May appear without affect; may be experiencing "nothingness"; can sit for hours staring into space
Anxiety may or may not be manifested	
Anhedonia (inability to experience pleasure)	**Anhedonia**
THINKING	
No impairment in reality testing.	Grasp of reality may be tenuous.
Thinking is slow; concentration and memory are poor; interest narrows; perspective in situations is lost:	Thoughts may indicate delusional thinking, reflecting feelings of:
• "Everyone always lets me down."	• Low self-esteem
• "No one cares."	• Worthlessness
Thoughts reflect doubts and indecisions; thinking is often repetitive in negative cycle:	• Helplessness
• "Why was I born?"	• "I'm no good."
• "What's life all about?"	• "God is punishing me for my terrible sins."
Mild feelings of guilt and worthlessness	• "My insides are rotting."
	• "My heart has stopped beating."
	Concentration is extremely poor.
	Preoccupation with bodily symptoms.
May have suicidal ideation	**May have suicidal ideation**
PHYSICAL BEHAVIOR	
Fatigue and lethargy are hallmark symptoms. They do not prevent the person from working, but the person often works below potential. Initiative and creativity are impaired.	Severe and extreme chronic fatigue and lethargy markedly interfere with occupational functioning, social activities, or relationships with others.
Grooming and hygiene usually are neglected.	Client may show extreme neglect of personal grooming and hygiene.
VEGETATIVE SIGNS	
Sleep—middle or late insomnia, hypersomnia; EEG studies show shortened REM latency.	Sleep—usually insomnia; early morning waking at 3 or 4 AM.
Energy is often highest in AM, lowest in PM	Energy is often lowest in AM, highest in PM.
Eating—may have anorexia or overeat.	Eating—usually has anorexia; weight loss of more than 5% in 1 month.
Sexual appetite is diminished.	Loss of libido
Bowels—constipation if psychomotor retardation is present; may have diarrhea if psychomotor agitation is present.	Bowels—usually constipation
Psychomotor retardation (slow motor movements)—everything is an effort	Psychomotor retardation (most common)
or	*or*
Psychomotor agitation (agitated depression)—pacing up and down halls, wringing hands.	Psychomotor agitation

EEG, Electroencephalogram; *REM,* rapid eye movement.
From Varcarolis EM: *Foundations of psychiatric mental health nursing,* ed 3, Philadelphia, 1998, WB Saunders, p 560. Used with permission.

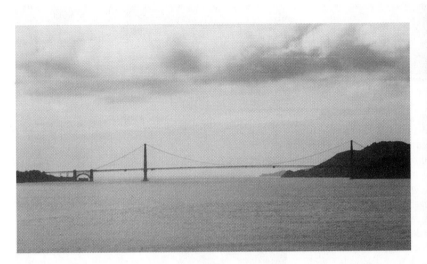

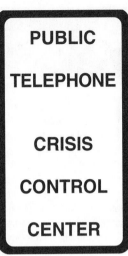

PUBLIC

TELEPHONE

CRISIS

CONTROL

CENTER

FIGURE 14–16 The Golden Gate Bridge, where many suicide jumps have been made. (Courtesy of David L. Frazier, 1999.)

DIAGNOSIS

Major depressive disorder must be differentiated from a reactive type of depression that results from a difficult or stressful life circumstance, such as a grief syndrome. Diagnostic criteria used in psychiatric evaluation include a prominent and persistent depressed mood lasting at least 2 weeks, with at least four of any of the aforementioned symptoms documented. A family history of depression is included in the patient assessment.

TREATMENT

The most effective treatment is a combination of medication and psychotherapy. Most patients have relief of symptoms and a good prognosis if they respond favorably to antidepressant therapy. SSRIs are first-line therapy, but many patients with major depression also may have been prescribed amitriptyline/nortriptyline along with the SSRI. Depression may occur as a single episode or may be recurrent. Electroconvulsive therapy (ECT) helps when a patient is severely incapacitated, has psychotic features, or does not respond to other therapeutic measures. Family support and education are considered important in the recovery process.

Patients who commit suicide have a high incidence of the hopelessness of acute depression. The suicidal patient often wishes to discuss suicidal fears and does not want to die but sees suicide as the only escape from an intolerable situation. A reluctance to discuss suicidal thoughts makes it important for the examiner to explore the patient's preoccupation with death or comments such as, "People would be better off without me" or "better off dead."

Suicide intervention is an attempt by medical, mental health, and community organizations to help the depressed individual through the crisis situation. Most telephone directories list crisis intervention centers. Hospital emergency departments and law enforcement agencies have professionals immediately available to offer support and personal contact to this individual. Mental health agencies routinely offer their clients a 24-hour "hot line" number for contacting a counselor. Structures that are often used as jumping points, such as bridges, have strategically placed signs that offer crisis intervention telephone numbers (Fig. 14–16).

ENRICHMENT
GRIEF RESPONSE

THE GRIEF RESPONSE is initiated primarily by the death of a loved one, but grieving also is a normal sequela to any loss, including loss of a function, body part, employment, or other important entity. The patient with a terminal illness faces the prospect of total separation and also must work through the various stages of grief.

The normal grieving process passes through several phases. The most recognized stages are those identified by Elisabeth Kübler-Ross. The first is denial: "No, I don't believe it." Second is anger: "Why did he or she do this to me?" or "Why is God letting this happen?" The third stage is bargaining: "If only this task can be accomplished or I can achieve this goal (live long enough), I will do this." Fourth is depression, in which people retreat within themselves and have little or no involvement with their environment. Finally, in the fifth stage, acceptance comes. Not everyone is able to move through these steps, and not everyone moves through them at the same pace or in the same order. Some people cannot express anger at the dead person or at God and do not move on. Many of these people never complete the grieving process, remain in a depressed state, and have reduced coping mechanisms. Medical intervention may help during depression, but most people recover with minimal treatment.

Different cultures grieve in different ways. Many groups grieve quietly and privately, whereas others cry, moan, rant, and even throw themselves on the funeral pyre. The important goal of funerals and the viewing of the remains is to allow closure of the relationship and to allow loved ones to say good-bye (Fig. 14–17 and Table 14–5).

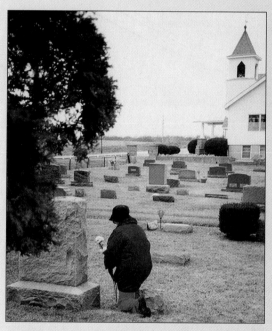

FIGURE 14-17 Grief response. (Courtesy David L. Frazier, 1999.)

ENRICHMENT
SEASONAL AFFECTIVE DISORDER

SEASONAL AFFECTIVE DISORDER (SAD), also known as seasonal pattern specifier, is a depressive condition that is manifested on a cycle at regular times of the year. The depression usually begins in the fall of the year, extends through the winter months, and then improves or goes into remission during the spring before returning in the fall. The individual may have an occasional summer episode. The episode pattern occurs over successive years. Symptoms include lack of energy, excessive sleeping, overeating, a craving for carbohydrates, and weight gain. The incidence of SAD is greater in women than in men, and younger people appear to be at higher risk than the elderly. The geographic latitude appears to be involved, with the occurrence increasing with higher latitudes and shorter daylight hours. In addition, a lack of sunshine and presence of snow and cloudy days tend to foster the condition (Fig. 14–18).

ENRICHMENT

SEASONAL AFFECTIVE DISORDER—CONT'D

The cause of SAD has been proposed to be an increase in the amount of the hormone melatonin secreted by the pineal gland. Melatonin is produced during dark hours, so observers speculate that an excessive amount affects certain people. The secretion of this hormone is suppressed by light. Increased amounts of melatonin are associated with lethargy and drowsiness. Drugs have been used to suppress melatonin secretion with some success. Another theory suggests that the body's **circadian** rhythm is delayed in people with SAD, causing the "vegetative" symptoms. This theory supports the use of light therapy, exposing the patient to artificially reproduced light for periods of time in the morning during the winter months. This treatment also has produced good results and improved the depressed state of people with SAD.

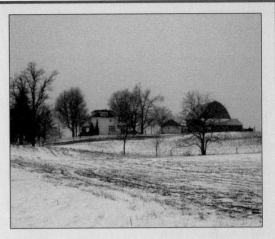

FIGURE 14–18 Desolate farm house during a snowstorm. (Courtesy David L. Frazier, 2003.)

ENRICHMENT

POSTPARTUM DEPRESSION

POSTPARTUM DEPRESSION, often labeled "Baby Blues," ranges from mild depression, to moderate depressive mood, to severe postpartum psychosis. Depressive symptoms after the birth of a baby have been recorded for centuries. Although no specific cause has been identified, abrupt changes in the levels of hormones, including estrogen and progesterone, have been proposed as the cause of this condition. In addition, changes in thyroid status may play a role in some cases. The responsibility of caring for a helpless newborn along with other demands of motherhood can be overwhelming. The frustration felt during feeding attempts along with the sleep disruption caused by the neonate add to the mother's despair. A previous history of depression or other mental-health conditions may increase the risk of PPD.

Symptoms usually begin within 24 to 48 hours after birth or during the first 6 weeks after giving birth. The symptoms may subside in a few days or a few weeks, or may last for several months. The new mother experiences fatigue, changes in normal appetite and sleep patterns, feelings of worthlessness and despair, crying episodes, poor personal hygiene, despair about her ability as a mother, feelings of anger, and recurrent thoughts of suicide. She also feels sad, has a flat affect, appears excessively angry, lacks interest in normal daily events, and experiences difficulty in concentrating and making decisions. She may express the desire to run away from everything, fears being alone, and expresses concern about potentially harming the baby. In the more severe cases of PPD, the mother may have thoughts of homicide, especially of killing the infant.

Maternal-child health-care providers must be alert for any symptoms of PPD. Prenatal teaching of both parents should include the typical symptoms of PPD and instructions to seek prompt medical intervention if and when they occur. Early intervention with medication and therapy helps to reduce symptoms and to prevent harm to the mother or child. The teaching also should urge parents not to feel any stigma for experiencing the condition, because it is a very common occurrence in most postpartum periods. Postpartum psychosis is considered a rare outcome, and when it does occur, it may bring serious events.

TABLE 14–5
Phenomena Experienced During Mourning

SYMPTOMS	EXAMPLES
SENSATION OF SOMATIC DISTRESS Tightness in throat, shortness of breath, sighing, "mental pain," exhaustion. Food tastes like sand; things feel unreal. Pain or discomfort may be identical to the symptoms experienced by the dead person. Symptoms normally are brief.	A woman whose husband died of a stroke complains of weakness and numbness on her left side.
PREOCCUPATION WITH THE IMAGE OF THE DECEASED The bereaved brings up, thinks, and talks about many memories of the deceased. The memories are positive. This process goes on with great sadness. The idealization of the deceased lets the bereaved relive the gratifications associated with the deceased and helps resolve any guilt the bereaved has toward the deceased. The bereaved also may take on many of the mannerisms of the deceased through identification. Identification serves the purpose of holding onto the deceased. Preoccupation with the dead person takes many months before it lessens.	A man whose wife just died states, "I just can't stop thinking about my wife. Everything I see reminds me of her. We picked up this seashell on our honeymoon. I remember every wonderful moment we had together. The pain is so great, but the memories just keep coming." His friends notice that when he talks, his hand gestures and expressions are very like those of his recently deceased wife.
GUILT The bereaved reproaches himself or herself for real or fancied acts of negligence or omissions in the relationship with the deceased.	"I should have made him go to the doctor sooner." "I should have paid more attention to her, been more thoughtful."
ANGER The anger the bereaved experiences may not be toward the object that gives rise to it. The anger often is displaced onto the medical or nursing staff. It is often directed toward the deceased. The anger is at its height during the first month but is often intermittent throughout the first year. The overflow of hostility disturbs the bereaved, resulting in the feeling that he or she is going "insane."	"The doctor didn't operate in time. If he had, Mary would be alive today." "How could he leave me like this...how could he?"
CHANGE IN BEHAVIOR (DEPRESSION, DISORGANIZATION, RESTLESSNESS) A person may exhibit marked restlessness and an inability to organize his or her behavior. Routine activities take a long time to do. Depressive mood is common as the year passes and as the intensity of the grief declines. Absence of depression is more abnormal than its presence. Loneliness and aimlessness are most pronounced 6 to 9 months after the death.	Six months after her husband died, Mrs. Faye stated, "I just can't seem to function. I have a hard time doing the simplest tasks. I can't be bothered with socializing." "I feel so down...so, so empty."
REORGANIZATION OF BEHAVIOR DIRECTED TOWARD A NEW OBJECT OR ACTIVITY The person gradually renews his or her interest in people and activities. The grieving thus releases the bereaved from one interpersonal relationship, and new ones are free to take its place.	Twenty months after her husband's death, Mrs. Faye tells a friend, "I'll be away this weekend. I am going fishing with my brother and his friend. This is the first time I've felt like doing anything since Harry died."

From Varcarolis EM: *Foundations of psychiatric mental health nursing*, ed 4, Philadelphia, 2002, WB Saunders, p 840. Used with permission.

Anxiety Disorders

DESCRIPTION

Anxiety is a common form of psychological disorder (Fig. 14–19). For most people, anxiety is just a temporary response to stress. For some people, however, anxiety becomes a chronic problem, and they regularly experience excessive levels of anxiety. They often exhibit anxiety that is inappropriate to the circumstance. Only when anxiety persists and prevents the person from leading a normal life does it become an illness. As a group, anxiety disorders represent the single largest mental health problem in the United States. They can lead to more severe disorders, such as depression and alcoholism.

Anxiety disorders, previously known as neuroses, include four specific disorders or syndromes that are different in behavioral manifestations but share the fact that the person's behavior is dominated by anxiety. The four disorders are generalized anxiety disorder, panic disorder, phobic disorder, and obsessive-compulsive disorder.

Anxiety Disorders: Stress Response

Posttraumatic Stress Response

1. The person experienced, witnessed, or was confronted with an event that involved actual, threatened death to self or others, responding in fear, helplessness, or horror

2. The event is persistently reexperienced by
   (a) Distressing dreams or images
   (b) Reliving the event through flashbacks, illusions, hallucinations

3. Persistent avoidance of stimuli associated with trauma:
   (a) Avoidance of thoughts, feelings, conversations
   (b) Avoidance of people, places, activities
   (c) Inability to recall aspects of trauma
   (d) Decreased interest in usual activities
   (e) Feelings of detachment, estrangement from others
   (f) Restriction in feelings (love, enthusiasm, joy)
   (g) Sense of shortened feelings

4. Persistent symptoms of increased arousal (two or more):
   (a) Difficulty falling/staying asleep
   (b) Irritability/outbursts of anger
   (c) Difficulty concentrating

5. Duration more than 1 month:
   • Acute: Duration less than 3 months
   • Chronic: Duration 3 months or more
   • Delayed: If onset of symptoms is at least 6 months after stress

Acute Stress Response

1. The person experienced, witnessed, or was confronted with an event that involved actual, threatened death to self or others, responding in fear, helplessness, or horror.

2. The event is associated with three or more of the following dissociative symptoms:
   (a) Sense of numbing, detachment, or absence of emotional response
   (b) Reduced awareness of surroundings (e.g., "in a daze")
   (c) Derealization
   (d) Depersonalization
   (e) Amnesia for an important aspect of the trauma

3. The event is persistently reexperienced by
   (a) Distressing dreams or images
   (b) Reliving the event through flashbacks, illusions, hallucinations

4. Marked avoidance of stimuli that arouse memory of trauma (thoughts, feelings, people, places, activities, conversations).

5. Marked symptoms of anxiety:
   (a) Difficulty falling/staying asleep
   (b) Irritability/outbursts of anger
   (c) Difficulty concentrating

6. Causes impairment in social, occupational, and other functioning, or impairs ability to complete some memory tasks.

7. Lasts from 2 days to 4 weeks and occurs within 4 weeks of the traumatic event.

FIGURE 14–19 Anxiety disorders. (Adapted from American Psychiatric Association, 2000. *Diagnostic and statistical manual of mental disorders,* ed 4, text revised. Washington DC: Author. Copyright 2000 American Psychiatric Association.)

SYMPTOMS AND SIGNS

Symptoms can range from worry and stress to extreme panic depending on which anxiety disorder the patient is experiencing. Mild to moderate levels of anxiety can easily be mistaken for depression because of the similarity in symptoms, such as irritability, difficulty concentrating, and disturbance in sleep patterns.

Some symptoms of anxiety disorders are observed behaviors such as nail biting, compulsive rituals such as hand washing and checking, and other nervous movements.

Generalized Anxiety Disorder and Panic Disorder

 ICD-9-CM Code 300.01 *(Panic disorder)*
300.02 *(Generalized anxiety)*

Patients with generalized anxiety disorder have a condition known as free-floating anxiety and live in a constant state of apparently causeless anxiety. They constantly worry about previous mistakes and future problems. These individuals dislike making decisions and worry about the decisions they have made. Their constant worrying often is accompanied by physiologic symptoms such as diarrhea, elevated blood pressure, and sustained muscular tension. Inability to sleep and nightmares are common. Some patients are even prone to panic attacks.

In panic disorder, the anxiety also is unfocused. With a panic attack, the anxiety begins suddenly and unexpectedly, reaching a peak within 10 minutes. The attack often is accompanied by a sense of impending doom and a feeling that the one is "going crazy," losing control, or dying. The world may seem unreal (derealization), or patients may seem unreal to themselves (depersonalization). In addition, these patients may experience palpitations, rapid pulse, pounding heart, sweating, trembling, shortness of breath, chest pain, nausea, paresthesia, dizziness, and chills or hot flashes.

The anxiety characteristic of a panic disorder can be differentiated from generalized anxiety by its sudden, intermittent nature and greater severity. A person is said to have panic disorder if he or she has four panic attacks within a month's time or if one or more attacks have been followed by a persistent fear of having another attack.

Phobic Disorder

DESCRIPTION

A phobic disorder is marked by excessive, persistent, and irrational fear and the avoidance of the phobic stimulus. In phobic disorders, the person's excessive anxiety has a specific focus (Fig. 14–20), some object or a situation that presents no real danger. Many people with phobias realize that their fears are irrational but feel powerless to control or prevent them. Phobic people must design their lives to avoid the things that they fear. When they confront an object or situation that causes them anxiety, they often have a severe attack of anxiety. Phobias can develop from or against almost anything (Table 14–6).

 ICD-9-CM Code 300.20 *(Unspecified phobia)*

Obsessive-Compulsive Disorder

DESCRIPTION

Obsessive-compulsive disorder is marked by the presence of obsessions (persistent unwanted thoughts) and compulsions (persistent urges to carry out specific actions).

ICD-9-CM Code 300.3

SYMPTOMS AND SIGNS

Obsessions are persistent intrusions of unwanted thoughts, and compulsions are uncontrollable urges to carry out certain actions. The two features of this disorder usually, but not always, occur together. People with obsessions often have thoughts of harming others, committing suicide, or performing sexual acts considered immoral. These people feel as though they have lost control of their minds, which causes them great anxiety. People with compulsions develop senseless actions or rituals that relieve their anxiety temporarily (e.g., excessive hand washing). Examples include an obsession with germs resulting in a compulsion to clean or wash one's hands, and an obsession with fire or theft that results in a compulsion to check doors, appliances, and outlets.

PATIENT SCREENING

Patients presenting with complaints of persistent intrusion of unwanted thoughts and compulsions and uncontrollable urges to carry out certain actions require prompt assessment.

ETIOLOGY

Many theories attempt to explain the causes of anxiety disorders. Some anxiety disorders are caused by severe stress. In people who are anxiety prone, only slight stress, or none at all, can be a cause. A physical condition such as hyperthyroidism (overactive thyroid gland) or a cerebrovascular disorder also can produce the symptoms of anxiety. The role of neurotransmitters and genetic factors has been studied. Obsessive-compulsive disorder also may be related to dysfunction in the frontal lobe of the brain.

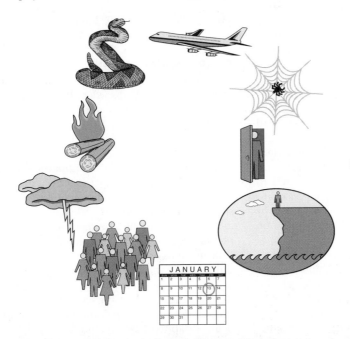

FIGURE 14–20 Phobias.

TABLE 14–6
Phobias

Acrophobia	Fear of high places	Olfactophobia	Fear of odor
Agoraphobia	Fear of open spaces	Ombrophobia	Fear of rain
Algophobia	Fear of pain	Ophidophobia	Fear of snakes
Androphobia	Fear of men	Pathophobia	Fear of disease
Arachnophobia	Fear of spiders	Pharmacophobia	Fear of drugs
Astrophobia	Fear of storms, thunder, and lightning	Phasmophobia	Fear of ghosts
Aviophobia	Fear of flying	Phobophobia	Fear of fear
Claustrophobia	Fear of closed or narrow spaces	Ponophobia	Fear of work
Hematophobia	Fear of blood	Pyrophobia	Fear of fire
Hodophobia	Fear of travel	Sitophobia	Fear of food
Hydrophobia	Fear of water	Thanatophobia	Fear of death
Iatrophobia	Fear of physicians	Toxophobia	Fear of being poisoned
Kainophobia	Fear of change	Traumatophobia	Fear of injury
Kakorrhaphiaphobia	Fear of failure	Triskaidekaphobia	Fear of the number 13
Lalophobia	Fear of speaking in public	Xenophobia	Fear of strangers
Monophobia	Fear of being alone	Zoophobia	Fear of animals
Ochlophobia	Fear of crowds		

DIAGNOSIS

Anxiety disorders are diagnosed after much investigation into the patient's symptoms and history, family history, and level of stress. In some cases, metabolic testing indicates abnormalities. *Positron-emission tomography (PET)* to detect chemical activity or metabolism of the brain and biochemical studies also have been used. Using the DSM-IV during assessment is important in arriving at a diagnosis; one must ask whether the individual meets the requirements for the diagnosis.

TREATMENT

If the anxiety prevents the person from living a normal life, a psychiatrist or a practitioner trained in treating psychological problems (e.g., psychologist or psychoanalyst) should be consulted. These therapists use many forms of treatment, depending on their perspective. Hypnosis sometimes is used to help the patient and the therapist to gain access to the subconscious mind. If the anxiety is caused by a specific stress (e.g., job related), steps should be taken to minimize or eliminate the problem.

Various methods of relaxation such as systematic desensitization, progressive relaxation, breathing exercises, and guided imagery can lessen the symptoms. Relaxation exercises (e.g., biofeedback) to relax tense muscles or a physical activity such as brisk walking, jogging, or swimming may be beneficial. In addition, or as an alternative, the physician may prescribe an *anxiolytic* drug. SSRIs are first-line therapy, but many patients with major depression also may have been prescribed amitriptyline/nortriptyline along with the SSRI and recommended psychotherapy. In severe cases of anxiety, a period of hospitalization also may be necessary. If severe anxiety is not treated, psychotic depression may develop.

PROGNOSIS

The prognosis is proportional to the patient's compliance with recommended medications and therapy interventions.

PREVENTION

No prevention is known.

PATIENT TEACHING

Encourage patients to attempt relaxation techniques. When drug therapy is prescribed, encourage compliance and follow-up with therapy as recommended.

Posttraumatic Stress Disorder

DESCRIPTION

Posttraumatic stress disorder is a delayed response to an external traumatic event that produces signs and symptoms of extreme distress.

 ICD-9-CM Code **308.3** *(Brief or acute)*
309.81 *(Prolonged)*

SYMPTOMS AND SIGNS

Posttraumatic stress disorders (PTSDs) are different from other anxiety disorders because the cause of the stress is an external event of an overwhelmingly painful nature (Fig. 14–21). The person may experience this disorder for weeks, months, or even years (transitory episode) after the event through painful recollections or nightmares. People with PTSD go out of their way to avoid being reminded of the painful event. They may be unable to respond to affection and have insomnia and irritability. These individuals also may exhibit strong physiologic responses to any reminder of the event.

Symptoms of PTSD usually appear within a short time of the event. In some cases, however, the person has a delayed response (onset). The person may be symptom-free for days or months after the event before signs of response to the painful event begin to appear. The symptoms disappear spontaneously, however, in about 6 months. Not all people exposed to severely traumatic events have such symptoms. The likelihood of developing PTSD appears to depend, to some degree, on the person's psychological strength before the event. The likelihood of this disorder also depends on the nature of the event.

PATIENT SCREENING

The patient experiencing PTSD suffers acute emotional pain and anxiety and requires prompt medical attention.

ETIOLOGY

PTSD caused by human actions (e.g., rape, acts of war, and continued abuse) tends to precipitate more severe reactions than PTSD caused by natural disasters (e.g., hurricanes, earthquakes, and floods). In the case of natural disasters, the greater the threat of death and the greater the number of people affected, the greater the likelihood of severe PTSD. The overwhelming experience of a threat to the individual's life is a causative factor.

Children also may be affected by experiencing or observing horror in their lives. Traumatic events include acts of war, in which they have observed family members killed or have been separated from the family unit. In addition, catastrophic events of nature, in which they have witnessed violent destruction of homes and surroundings, may make them fearful and withdrawn. Abuse also is known to cause PTSD, especially sexual abuse. Recognizing traumatic events in children's lives is essential, as is involving them in therapy.

DIAGNOSIS

The diagnosis is confirmed when the patient experiences intrusive symptoms and both recurrent and distressing recollections of the event, including re-current dreams and flashbacks of the event. An additional factor in the diagnosis is the individual's persistent avoidance of stimuli associated with the traumatic experience. The patient usually experiences hyperarousal in the form of rapid heartbeat, dyspnea, and panic.

Children often will reenact the event, have recurrent dreams or nightmares of the event, or have repetitive patterns of the event in their play.

TREATMENT

The goal of treatment of PTSD is to restore the individual's sense of control. Counseling and drug therapy are used in the treatment. The counseling therapy helps PTSD victims to accept the overwhelming memories without rearranging their lives to avoid the memories. They work to develop a

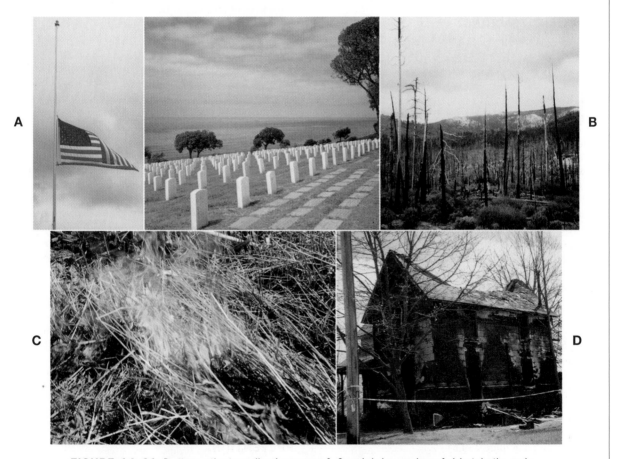

FIGURE 14-21 Posttraumatic stress disorder sources. **A,** Overwhelming numbers of violent deaths, as in wars; **B,** destruction by fire of one's environment, as in forest fires encroaching on communities; **C,** brush fires suddenly erupting on community property; **D,** fire destroying shelters and property. (Courtesy David L. Frazier, 1999.)

Somatoform Disorders

sense of safety and control. Feelings of guilt and self-blame need to be addressed. Cognitive behavior training to increase self-esteem and self-control is employed.

Sleep disturbances must be recognized and treated. Benzodiazepines may be prescribed to help the patient regain normal sleep patterns. In addition, antianxiety agents or selective serotonin reuptake inhibitors (SSRIs) may be used as drug therapy. Recovery may be complete in some individuals in a short time, whereas others may never completely recover.

PROGNOSIS
The prognosis is good with therapy and medications.

PREVENTION
No prevention is known.

PATIENT TEACHING
Encourage compliance with therapy and medication.

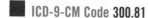
Somatoform Disorders

Somatoform disorders are a group of mental disorders in which the person experiences physical symptoms without the underlying organic cause. These symptoms are not under voluntary control and are real to the affected person. The opposite is true of factitious disorders (Munchausen syndrome) or malingering, in which the patient presents with feigned symptoms for personal or emotional gain. There is no confirmed, diagnosable, general medical condition that accounts for the symptoms of somatoform disorders.

Somatization Disorder

DESCRIPTION
Somatization disorder is also known as Briquet syndrome. This disorder is multisymptomatic, occurring before the age of 30. Extending over a period of years, it is typified by complaints of pain and GI, sexual, and neurotic symptoms without clinical basis.

■ **ICD-9-CM Code 300.81**

SYMPTOMS AND SIGNS
In somatization disorder, the patient experiences multiple, recurring somatic symptoms that have no underlying clinical pathologic basis. These symptoms appear before the age of 30 years and continue for several years. Symptoms include pain related to four or more areas or functions of the body. In addition, the patient reports GI symptoms (nausea, vomiting, and blood in the stool) other than pain, a symptom related to the reproductive system (e.g., for females, irregular or heavy menses, and for males, erectile or ejaculatory problems), and a neurologic symptom that is without clinical basis.

PATIENT SCREENING
Patients with initial complaints of severe pain and symptoms as mentioned above should be scheduled for the next available appointment. After the patient is determined to have somatization disorder, routine appointments can be scheduled. Patients demanding to be seen immediately should be referred to an emergency facility.

ETIOLOGY
The etiology is uncertain, but there appears to be a familial pattern. This nonspecific condition tends to have symptoms that intensify after a loss and during periods of severe stress.

DIAGNOSIS
The diagnosis is made after medical conditions are ruled out. Criteria include the presence of four pain symptoms, two GI symptoms, one sexual symptom, and one *pseudoneurologic* symptom. The onset is early in life, before the age of 30 years, and the condition is chronic, without a symptom-free period of longer than 1 year. There is no clinical pathologic change, and no laboratory findings support the symptoms.

TREATMENT
Treatment includes investigation of symptoms and ruling out of any underlying general medical condition. Psychotherapy including behavior modification is a helpful treatment option.

PROGNOSIS
The prognosis for cure is very poor. This chronic condition rarely has complete remission.

PREVENTION
With the etiology being unknown and a tendency for the disorder to be familial, no prevention is known. Encourage the patient to develop skills for dealing with stress.

PATIENT TEACHING

Encourage patients to keep regularly scheduled appointments. Support the patient and the condition. Explain any diagnostic test results.

Conversion Disorder

DESCRIPTION

Conversion disorders formerly were termed hysteria. Anxiety is changed (converted) to a physical or somatic symptom. The anxiety is too difficult to face, and as a defense mechanism, the physical symptoms allow the person to escape or avoid a stressful situation.

 ICD-9-CM Code 300.11

SYMPTOMS AND SIGNS

Symptoms include deficits in voluntary motor or sensory functions (paralysis) that are unintentional and preceded by conflicts or other stressors. Clinically significant social and occupational functioning is present.

Sensory symptoms may include *anesthesia, hyperesthesia, analgesia,* and *paresthesia.* Motor symptoms may include paralysis, tremors, tics, *contractures,* and ambulation disturbances. Speech disturbances may include *aphonia* and **mutism,** and visceral symptoms may include headaches, difficulty in swallowing and breathing, choking, coughing, nausea, vomiting, belching, cold and clammy extremities, weight loss, and *pseudocyesis.* Blindness and seizures also may be noted.

PATIENT SCREENING

Patients with initial symptomology as previously described demand prompt attention. Many of the complaints warrant referral to an emergency facility.

ETIOLOGY

The cause of this psychiatric syndrome is usually a highly stressful situation.

DIAGNOSIS

The diagnosis is based on a history of the preceding event and the classic pattern of acute onset of symptoms. A complete physical examination rules out underlying pathologic conditions.

TREATMENT

Treatment is supportive and symptomatic. The course of this disorder is usually short, with many cases resolving in a few weeks, especially when the stressful situation is eliminated. Recurrence is common. Psychotherapy and hypnosis are treatment options.

PROGNOSIS

The prognosis varies depending on the intensity of the stress. Most cases do resolve within a few weeks, but recurrence is common.

PREVENTION

Avoiding extremely stressful situations may prevent the condition.

PATIENT TEACHING

Encourage patients and families to find ways to reduce stressful situations. Help them to find support groups and encourage them to become involved in the groups.

Pain Disorder

DESCRIPTION

Pain disorder is manifested by pain that causes significant distress and physical and social impairment. This pain is very real to the patient and takes control of the patient's activities.

 ICD-9-CM Code 307.80

SYMPTOMS AND SIGNS

Pain disorders include the subtypes that are associated with psychological factors, those associated with both psychological factors and general medical conditions, and those associated with only general medical conditions. The pain is severe and lasting and may have a clinical basis. The response to pain depends on the patient's interpretation, but this type of pain interferes with life activities, including occupational, social, and other areas of functioning. The pain may be associated with musculoskeletal disorders (herniated disk, osteoporosis, and arthritis), neuropathies, and malignancies. Chronic pain often causes depression.

PATIENT SCREENING

Pain is very real in these patients. Underlying clinical factors should be assessed. These patients require prompt attention.

ETIOLOGY

The pain may be related to underlying clinical pathologic conditions. Psychological factors may play a role in the onset and severity of the pain.

Somatoform Disorders

Occasionally, both clinical pathologic and psychological factors contribute to the manifestation of the condition. This condition is not intentionally produced, as is malingering.

DIAGNOSIS

Diagnostic studies may reveal pathologic change. Because pain is subjective and pain disorder may or may not have a clinical basis, determining the extent of the pain and psychological involvement is difficult. Longstanding pain may cause depression and even lead to suicide.

TREATMENT

Any underlying identifiable pathologic change is treated. Patients with terminal disease may be given narcotics to relieve intractable pain. Psychotherapy may be of some help.

PROGNOSIS

The prognosis varies depending on underlying pathology. Pain of terminal disease may be treated, but the only relief is death.

PREVENTION

Because this condition is not intentionally produced, prevention depends on the underlying pathology.

PATIENT TEACHING

Patient teaching includes information about accepted methods of pain relief. Suggest to those with intractable pain that they take prescribed pain medication as scheduled, especially before the pain becomes severe. Relaxation techniques along with methods of psychological distraction may help. Pain-management clinics have been established to help patients with chronic pain to follow various forms of treatment. These include lifestyle adjustment, relaxation rooms, physical therapy, and group psychotherapy.

Hypochondriasis

DESCRIPTION

The patient with hypochondriasis is preoccupied with fear of having a serious disease. The patient has this excessive fear in spite of negative medical tests and reassurance that there is no clinical basis for the symptoms. Patients mistake body-system symptoms or aches and pains without clinical basis for serious illnesses.

 ICD-9-CM Code 300.7

SYMPTOMS AND SIGNS

Hypochondriasis is characterized by patients' reports and symptoms of possible physical illness without any identifiable evidence of the illness. These patients have a preoccupation with illness and an abnormal fear of disease. The patients provide a generalized history, their symptoms are vague, and they have difficulty with specifics. They do not consciously fake symptoms; these patients really do feel the conditions about which they complain.

PATIENT SCREENING

Until underlying clinical causes are eliminated, these patients require prompt attention.

ETIOLOGY

The etiology of hypochondriasis is uncertain.

DIAGNOSIS

The diagnosis is difficult because these people change physicians when a health-care provider does not affirm their illness. Laboratory and diagnostic studies often reveal no underlying condition. When a condition does exist, it may be overlooked. Social and occupational relationships suffer from the constant abnormal preoccupation with one's health. The complaints of the disorders will last more than 6 months.

TREATMENT

Treatment of any underlying conditions is necessary, but these conditions easily can be missed because of the vagueness of the symptoms reported and the changing of health-care providers. Some patients may benefit from psychotherapy.

PROGNOSIS

The prognosis varies according to the amenability of the patient to psychotherapy.

PREVENTION

Because the etiology is uncertain, no specific prevention is known.

PATIENT TEACHING

Encourage the patient to learn to live with the symptoms. A supportive attitude of the health-care provider builds confidence. Regular appointments should be scheduled, and the patient should be persuaded to keep these appointments.

Munchausen Syndrome and Munchausen Syndrome by Proxy

DESCRIPTION

Munchausen syndrome, or factitious disorder, occurs when the patient simulates symptoms of illness and presents for no apparent reason other than treatment.

■ ICD-9-CM Code **301.51**

SYMPTOMS AND SIGNS

Patients with Munchausen syndrome know that they are not ill but seek medical attention so they can draw attention to themselves. They believe they have no other way to get this type of attention. They feign symptoms and actually can make themselves ill by injecting foreign material to cause a fever. These patients generally have extensive knowledge of medical terminology and hospital routines.

Munchausen syndrome by proxy occurs when the parent projects the symptoms to the child, usually a preschooler. This parent often stimulates the illness in the child and then presents the child for treatment. The parent denies any knowledge of actual cause and relates the symptoms to be GI, genitourinary, or CNS in nature. As in Munchausen syndrome, the degree of the complaint is limited only by the parent's medical knowledge.

PATIENT SCREENING

Until underlying clinical causes are eliminated, these patients require prompt attention.

ETIOLOGY

The cause of this behavior is uncertain. The patient has no external motive other than to assume the sick role and draw attention to himself or herself.

DIAGNOSIS

These patients present at a hospital or physician's office with reports of fever, anemia, dermatitis, or seizure activity expecting to receive medical attention. The symptoms have an atypical clinical course, with laboratory findings that are inconsistent with the symptoms. They have a dramatic flair but give vague answers when questioned closely. When the initial workup indicates no particular disease entity, symptoms change. The patient eagerly undergoes multiple invasive procedures. The patient has a history of repeated hospitalizations with no firm evidence of an underlying disease process. In addition, the patient has no motive of financial gain, only that of attention.

TREATMENT

Eventually, the behavior is revealed, and when these patients are confronted with this fact, they seek attention at another facility. Some physicians believe this condition is untreatable.

PROGNOSIS

The prognosis varies according to the duration of the condition. Those who have experienced the condition on a long-term basis are the least amenable to treatment. Intervention is necessary in Munchausen by proxy, and in many situations the child is removed from the care of the adult inflicting the source of the illness.

PREVENTION

If one could detect the need for attention and then fulfill that need, the disorder might be prevented or at least reduced.

PATIENT TEACHING

A nonjudgmental attitude by the health-care provider may help to reduce the condition. Discuss the condition with the family and advise them that this disorder often requires therapeutic intervention.

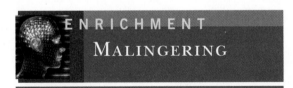

ENRICHMENT

MALINGERING

MALINGERING IS THE FEIGNING of symptoms for financial or personal gain. The action is deliberate and fraudulent, and the symptoms usually are exaggerated. The patient may report these symptoms to avoid or delay various undesirable events. The diagnosis is difficult because the symptoms often are subjective and cannot be disproved.

Gender Identity Disorders

DESCRIPTION

Gender identity disorders are conditions in which an individual feels a powerful connection with the opposite sex and wants to be the other sex.

 ICD-9-CM Code **302.6**
302.85 *(In adult)*

SYMPTOMS AND SIGNS

Gender identity is a person's inner sense of maleness or femaleness. In this disorder, the person feels as if she or he really should be the opposite sex. Evidence of a strong cross-gender identification is present, and the person has a discomfort about the assigned sex. These people also experience a sense of inappropriateness in their gender role.

Boys have a marked preoccupation with feminine activities, including dressing in feminine clothing and playing with traditionally girl toys. Competitive sports and typical boy activity and play are avoided. Some boys remark that they do not want their penis and would prefer to have a vagina.

Girls display a dislike for feminine attire and prefer boy-type clothing and short hair. They prefer boys as playmates and engage in typical boy sports and games. Many claim that they will grow a penis and do not want breast growth or menses.

During adulthood, these persons have a strong desire to adopt the role of the opposite sex and to seek out physical change through hormonal or surgical intervention. They are not comfortable in the gender role defined by society and prefer to act out as the opposite sex. They take on the characteristics of the other sex and dress accordingly.

Regardless of age, many of these patients experience social isolation and ostracism. They frequently have low self-esteem.

PATIENT SCREENING

Although not an emergency, a gender identity disorder becomes a very important issue in the individual's and his or her parent's life. When a parent recognizes that the child has a medical issue needing to be addressed and calls for an appointment, one should offer understanding and validation of the issue by scheduling an appointment at the earliest available time.

ETIOLOGY

The etiology of the syndrome is uncertain.

DIAGNOSIS

Observation of the behavioral patterns leads to suspicion of gender identity disorder, but there is no known diagnostic test for this syndrome. Psychological evaluation may reveal the tendency. A strong cross-gender identification persists, along with a discomfort with one's sex or a sense of inappropriate gender identification.

TREATMENT

Psychological counseling to recognize and acknowledge the feelings may be of value. Sex reassignment through hormone treatment and surgical intervention often helps these patients.

PROGNOSIS

The prognosis varies depending on the extent of the feeling and the extent of the action taken. Many sex-change surgical procedures are successful when accompanied by intense psychotherapy. Family and employment relationships may affect the success of treatment.

PREVENTION

No prevention is known.

PATIENT TEACHING

Help the patient to find support groups. Encourage family members to accept the condition as an illness and thereby accept the patient's choice, which will help the patient.

Sleep Disorders

Sleep disorders include insomnia, parasomnias, sleep *apnea,* and narcolepsy. Sleep disorders are assessed through polysomnography, which measures rapid eye movement (REM) and the four non–rapid eye movement (NREM) sleep stages, stages 1, 2, 3, and 4. Stage 1 NREM sleep is considered transitional and occupies 5% of normal sleep time. Stage 2 occupies about 50% of normal sleep time and is a deeper sleep. Stages 3 and 4 (slow-wave sleep) are the deepest states and occupy 10% to 20% of sleep time. Stages 3 and 4 lessen in duration with aging and even disappear in some people older than 55. The average adult requires 6 to 8 hours of continuous sleep, with younger people requiring more and the elderly needing less.

The disorders can be caused by functional or organic disorders, so underlying pathologic conditions must be ruled out or treated.

Insomnia

DESCRIPTION

The individual experiencing insomnia has difficulty in falling asleep and/or staying asleep.

 ICD-9-CM Code 780.52 *(Insomnia NOS)*

SYMPTOMS AND SIGNS

Insomnia, difficulty in falling asleep or staying asleep, tends to cause the individual to arise physically and mentally tired, groggy, tense, irritable, and anxious. In addition, some people experience extremely early morning awakening and report that their sleep was not restorative.

PATIENT SCREENING

Although not an emergency, chronic insomnia becomes a very important issue in the individual's life. When the patient recognizes that he or she has a medical issue needing to be addressed and calls for an appointment, the health-care provider understands and validates the issue by scheduling an appointment at the earliest available time.

ETIOLOGY

The cause may be related to a situation, a medical problem, or time zone changes, including jet lag, or the cause may be a change to high altitudes. Additional causes are pain, cardiovascular problems, thyroid conditions, and fever. Stimulants, including caffeine, amphetamines, steroids, alcohol, nicotine, and bronchodilators, tend to cause drug-related insomnia. Psychological causes include anxiety, stress, and even the fear of sleeplessness itself.

The older generation, shift workers, travelers experiencing jet lag, and those with chronic pain often experience periods of difficulty in sleeping. Other causative factors may be environmentally related and include room temperature that is too hot or too cold, noise, brightness or light, an uncomfortable bed, or a sleep partner who exhibits snoring, restlessness, or restless leg syndrome.

DIAGNOSIS

To be diagnosed as insomnia, the sleeplessness must have a duration of longer than 1 month and must interfere with normal functioning in social, occupational, or other areas. A study is conducted of the 24-hour sleep and wakefulness periods, along with an examination of any underlying factors. Polysomnography, a recording of several physiologic variables related to sleep made while the patient is sleeping, indicates poor sleep patterns, including increased stage 1 and reduced stage 3 and 4 periods, along with increased muscle tremors. The patient appears fatigued and exhibits no other abnormalities. The incidence of insomnia increases with age and is higher in females.

TREATMENT

The first step in treatment is to identify and remove the cause; this is followed by an attempt to improve sleep hygiene. Patients are counseled to change their lifestyle to relieve tension and reduce stress. They are encouraged to keep a regular sleep schedule, to consider the bedroom only for sleep, and not to worry about stressful situations. Noise and disruptions during the normal sleep time should be eliminated, and daily activities should be increased. Caffeine, nicotine, and stimulants should be avoided in late afternoon and evening. Strenuous physical exercise also should be avoided in the few hours before retiring. A darkened and quiet environment should help. The patient should keep a regular bedtime and a regular time for arising. Psychotherapy may be indicated to help relieve anxiety and stress. As a last resort, hypnotics of the benzodiazepine class may be prescribed. Although benzodiazepines are still used for this purpose, a newer class of hypnotics is used more often for sleep disorders. The two are zolpidem (Ambien) and zaleplon (Sonata). When these do not work, patients usually are referred to sleep-disorder clinics.

PROGNOSIS

The prognosis varies depending on the cause. Adjusting late-afternoon and early-evening activities and eliminating any drugs that interfere with sleep may relieve insomnia.

A favorable outcome depends on the patient's ability to modify the sleep environment and to reduce stressors.

PREVENTION

Eliminating the ingestion of caffeine, nicotine, and other stimulants during late afternoon and evening hours helps prevent insomnia. Developing good sleep habits, such as keeping regular hours to retire, also helps in prevention. Avoiding watching television or reading while in bed also may prevent insomnia.

PATIENT TEACHING

Instruct patients about normal sleep patterns and about avoiding caffeine, nicotine, and other stimulants in the late afternoon and evening hours. As previously mentioned, patients should be encouraged to avoid the habit of watching television or reading while in bed. Help them to identify environmental changes they could make to improve the sleep environment.

Parasomnias

DESCRIPTION

Parasomnias are a group of sleep disorders that include sleepwalking, night terrors, and nightmares.

■ **ICD-9-CM Code 780.50** *(Sleep disturbance, unspecified)*

SYMPTOMS AND SIGNS

Parasomnias usually occur in children early in the night. When they affect the elderly and have a late onset, a CNS pathologic process is responsible. People who sleepwalk generally have no memory of the event. They awake confused, with blank expressions on their faces, and are unaware of the environment. Those experiencing nightmares often have vivid recall and remember dreams of fear of attack, falling, and death. These dreams occur late at night.

PATIENT SCREENING

Although usually not an emergency, parasomnia becomes a very important issue in the individual's life. When the patient recognizes that he or she has a medical issue that needs to be addressed and calls for an appointment, the health-care provider should understand and validate the issue by scheduling an appointment at the earliest available time. When safety is an issue, prompt attention is essential.

ETIOLOGY

Several elements, including possible genetic, developmental, psychological, and organic factors, may precipitate the incidents. Febrile episodes or brain tumors may be causes. Lithium and certain drugs precipitate the condition. There is evidence that certain medications cause increased REM sleep periods and rebound REM sleep.

DIAGNOSIS

Reports of the episodes lead to further investigation. A thorough history should include any drug consumption. Any underlying cause in the elderly and mature adults should be investigated and diagnosed.

TREATMENT

Protection from injury is primary for the sleepwalking person. The sleepwalking person should not be interrupted or awakened. Minimizing the exposure to terror, especially from movies, videotapes, and television programs, reduces the occurrence of night terrors. Children usually outgrow these conditions. Adults often are treated initially with Ambien or Sonata, then benzodiazepines, because Ambien and Sonata do not leave patients feeling drugged when they wake up in the morning. When drugs are suspected as a contributing factor, alternative drug therapy is considered.

PROGNOSIS

The prognosis varies depending on the cause. Many children will outgrow parasomnia. When the etiology is drug related, eliminating the causative drug helps.

PREVENTION

Minimizing stimulating factors, such as exposure to frightening movies, helps prevent this condition. Additionally, having regular bedtime and a comfortable environment conducive to sleep and avoiding caffeine and other stimulants is helpful in prevention.

PATIENT TEACHING

Family members should be advised not to interrupt or attempt to awaken the sleepwalking person. Parents are advised to use caution when discussing terrorist activities or catastrophic events and to prevent children from hearing about such events.

Narcolepsy

DESCRIPTION

Narcolepsy, irresistible daytime sleep episodes, can have a duration of a few seconds to a half hour.

■ **ICD-9-CM Code 347**

SYMPTOMS AND SIGNS

Narcolepsy, a chronic neurologic condition, is an overwhelming recurring compulsion to fall asleep. Usually precipitated by sedentary, monotonous activity, narcolepsy attacks occur while driving, sitting in a lecture, or even eating. The onset normally is before the age of 25 years. A period of sleep paralysis lasts about 1 minute; the person is unable to move, but breathing continues.

PATIENT SCREENING

The patient experiencing episodes of narcolepsy requires prompt attention.

ETIOLOGY

The condition appears to have a familial incidence, and narcoleptics may have a genetic aberration of REM sleep time.

DIAGNOSIS

The history of repeated episodes suggests narcolepsy. Seizure activity and sleep apnea should be ruled out. The onset usually is during adolescence, producing disturbed night sleep. Sleep studies help in confirming the diagnosis.

TREATMENT

The patient should take therapeutic naps and establish a normal night sleep pattern. Drug therapy helps. Stimulants including methylphenidate and dextroamphetamine are prescribed. Modafinil (Provigil), a nonamphetamine stimulant and wakefulness-promoting drug, may be prescribed for excessive daytime sleepiness. These patients must be warned of the dangers of falling asleep while driving or operating machinery. This chronic disorder is not under voluntary control.

PROGNOSIS

The prognosis varies depending on the adaptation techniques the patient develops. The patient's response and tolerance to drug therapy also may dictate the outcome of this condition.

PREVENTION

No prevention is known.

PATIENT TEACHING

Patients and families should be told that this is a disease that may be treatable. They also need to understand the dangers that could arise, however, if the narcolepsy occurs while driving or operating machinery. Students are encouraged to discuss this condition with counselors and request special assistance in the classroom setting. Patients may be helped by scheduling classes for times when they are not sleepy. They should enlist the help of another student in note taking.

Those who are in the workplace should look for jobs that will keep them active and allow for interaction with others. Patients should avoid jobs that require them to make long drives or operate dangerous equipment. Encourage and help both patients and families to become involved in support groups.

Sleep Apnea

DESCRIPTION

Sleep apnea is intermittent short periods of breathing cessation during sleep.

 ICD-9-CM Code 780.57

SYMPTOMS AND SIGNS

Sleep apnea is considered a potentially life-threatening condition. During normal nocturnal sleep, the patient has periods in which breathing ceases, followed by snorting and gasping. This condition occurs more often in men than in women and may be associated with obesity, hypertension, or an airway-obstructive condition. The patient does not feel rested even after several hours of sleep.

Sleep apnea may be categorized as either obstructive or central. The more common type is obstructive, as air is unable to flow in or out of the upper airway. Attempts to breathe continue. During central episodes, the brain does not send appropriate messages to the intercostals and diaphragm to initiate the breathing process. The patient can experience 20 or more periods of apnea during an hour. The individual with sleep apnea occasionally will complain of choking episodes.

PATIENT SCREENING

The patient experiencing episodes of sleep apnea requires prompt attention.

ETIOLOGY

Patients appear to have an inherent predisposition to this condition. A nasal obstruction often is the cause. Alcohol ingestion, smoking-related bronchitis, and sleep deprivation are other causes. Obesity can cause extra tissue to develop in the throat,

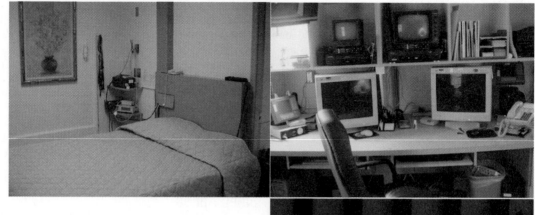

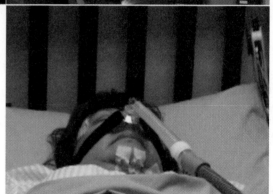

FIGURE 14–22 **A** and **B**, Sleep lab. **C**, Patient undergoing a sleep study. (**A** and **B** courtesy Saint Joseph's Hospital, Fort Wayne, Ind., 2003. **C** courtesy Cameron Memorial Community Hospital, Angola, Ind., 2003.)

creating a mechanical obstruction. As levels of O_2 drop and levels of CO_2 increase, the brain is alerted to stimulate the breathing process and the individual usually gasps for air.

DIAGNOSIS
The diagnosis begins with a sleep history. The onset usually occurs in middle age. Daytime sleepiness, sleep attacks, and snoring and snorting episodes also suggest sleep apnea. Sleep laboratory studies confirm the diagnosis by observing periods of breathing cessation while the patient is sleeping (Fig. 14–22).

TREATMENT
Weight loss is encouraged. Protriptyline is prescribed. Constant positive air pressure (CPAP) or dental appliances may be tried (Fig. 14–23). Any underlying pathologic condition should be diagnosed and corrected. The patient is advised to avoid the use of any drugs that depress the CNS. Uvulopalato-pharyngoplasty (UPPP), a surgical procedure to remove portions of the uvula, soft

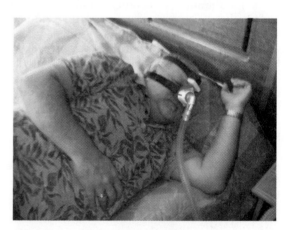

FIGURE 14–23 Patient using CPAP. (Courtesy David L. Frazier, 2003.)

palate, and posterior pharyngeal mucosa, is attempted as a last resort. Alcohol, tobacco, and sedatives tend to cause collapse of the upper airway passages during sleep and therefore should be avoided.

PROGNOSIS

The prognosis varies depending on the cause. When overweight patients lose weight, they often experience significant improvement. Use of CPAP usually relieves symptoms and reduces the danger of respiratory arrest.

PREVENTION

No prevention is known.

PATIENT TEACHING

Patients using CPAP will need instructions on the use of the equipment. If overweight, they should be encouraged to lose weight. Offer weight-reduction diets or help the patient find support groups.

Personality Disorders

DESCRIPTION

A personality disorder is a pattern of behavior that deviates from society's norms. In addition, a person with a personality disorder typically has thoughts about the self and the world that cause the inappropriate behavior. Signs of a personality disorder become evident in adolescence. There are 10 named personality disorders, categorized into three clusters. These clusters are: cluster A, patients who appear odd or eccentric; cluster B, patients who appear dramatic, emotional, or erratic; and cluster C, patients who appear anxious and fearful.

ICD-9-CM Code

Cluster A

301.0 *(Paranoid)*
301.20 *(Schizoid)*
301.22 *(Schizotypal)*

Cluster B

301.7 *(Antisocial)*
301.83 *(Borderline)*
301.50 *(Histrionic)*
301.81 *(Narcissistic)*

Cluster C

301.82 *(Avoidant)*
301.6 *(Dependent)*
301.4 *(OCPD)*
301.9 *(Unspecified personality disorder)*

SYMPTOMS AND SIGNS

Personality disorders influence the mental affect of a person and produce chronic, ingrained, maladaptive behavior. Disordered patterns of relating, thinking, and perceiving impair social and occupational performance. Personality disorders typically begin to appear in adolescence. PDOs should not be diagnosed until adulthood. A history of longstanding problems in interpersonal relationships and occupational difficulties is likely. Personality traits may give the person a reputation of arrogance or painful shyness and of rejecting responsibility for his or her behavior. The person tends to project negative feelings and blame others. Many types of personality disorders are recognized, each with unique distinguishing characteristics. Examples of personality disorders include **paranoid, schizoid,** antisocial, histrionic, and **narcissistic** disorders.

Antisocial Disorder

Behavior patterns of the antisocial personality cause frequent conflicts with societal values. Troublesome conduct usually emerges by 15 years of age, with truancy, fighting, stealing, a history of running away, or cruel behavior. Antisocial persons do not express guilt or learn from their mistakes. Other traits include a propensity for irresponsible and impulsive actions.

Cluster A

Cluster A personality disorders should be assessed and distinguished from delusional disorders and psychotic disorders.

Paranoid Personality Disorder

Those with paranoid personality disorder do not trust others and are suspicious of others. They assume others will exploit, harm, or deceive them. Individuals with PPD often misinterpret the meaning behind others' behaviors by thinking others are deliberately trying to exploit them.

Schizoid Personality Disorder

Individuals with SPD appear to lack, or show emotions of, pleasure or pain. They tend to be loners and do not enjoy relationships with others. They appear to be indifferent, flattened, or detached.

Schizotypal Personality Disorder

Persons with schizotypal personality disorder are similar to those with schizoid personality disorder wherein they have difficulty with social relationships. Individuals with schizotypal personality disorder, however, typically have ideas of reference; they may be superstitious or preoccupied with paranoid phenomena. In addition, they may believe they have magical control over others. More often, they seek treatment for associated symptoms of anxiety or depression.

Cluster B

Antisocial Personality Disorder

Individuals with APD have a disregard for, and tend to violate, the rights of others. They fail to conform to societal norms and often engage in behavior that could be grounds for arrest. These individuals are aggressive, manipulative, and reckless. They generally do not show remorse or make amends for their behavior.

Borderline Personality Disorder

A person with BPD has a pattern of unstable interpersonal relationships, self-image, and affects. Impending separation or rejection are central concerns for individuals with BPD. When those with BPD believe they are being rejected or abandoned, they often react with extreme emotions such as anger, panic, or despair. They may display extreme sarcasm and verbal outbursts. They are impulsive and manipulative with their behavior.

Histrionic Disorder

Histrionic individuals display overly dramatic and theatrical mannerisms. They have a conscious or unconscious pervasive need to be the center of attention. People with this disorder are immature and dependent, constantly seeking approval and reassurance. Behavior or appearance may be inappropriately seductive.

Narcissistic Disorder

The narcissistic personality demonstrates pathologic self-love or grandiose self-admiration. When criticized, the person reacts with rage or humiliation, based on an exaggerated sense of self-importance. These individuals lack empathy and tend to exploit others. They exhibit a preoccupation with fantasies of unlimited success.

Cluster C

Avoidant Personality Disorder

The avoidant personality avoids any social situation because of fears of criticism, disapproval, or rejection. Individuals with APD view themselves as socially inept, personally unappealing, and inferior to others. They are preoccupied with being judged or criticized by their peers.

Dependent Personality Disorder

Individuals with DPD have a pattern of excessively relying on others to make decisions for them. They are passive and have trouble disagreeing with others because they fear losing support or approval.

Obsessive Compulsive Personality Disorder

Individuals with obsessive compulsive personality disorder have an extreme pattern of preoccupation with orderliness, perfection, and mental and interpersonal control. They are preoccupied with details or lists to the point that they never finish a task.

PATIENT SCREENING

Individuals displaying this behavior or family members reporting the behavior and requesting an appointment should be scheduled for an appointment as soon as convenient.

ETIOLOGY

The cause of personality disorders has not been identified. Various theories include possible biologic, social, or psychodynamic origins.

DIAGNOSIS

The diagnosis of personality disorders is based on the documentation of diagnostic criteria defined in the American Psychiatric Association's DSM-IV (*Diagnostic and Statistical Manual of Mental Disorders,* fourth edition).

TREATMENT

The treatment of personality disorders depends on the symptoms and includes psychotherapy and, in some cases, drug therapy. Improved coping mechanisms and control of symptoms are the goals of therapy. A trusting relationship between patient and therapist is advantageous because some people with these disorders tend to be noncompliant and resist therapy. Hospitalization may be required during acute episodes that incapacitate the person. Family involvement in group therapy has proved beneficial for some patients. Treatment of *comorbid* conditions, such as anxiety and depression, with medications is essential. Personality disorders themselves do not respond to drug therapy.

PROGNOSIS

The prognosis for cure is very poor. Treatment of comorbid conditions improves outcome. Long-term treatment is necessary.

PREVENTION

Treatment in adolescence when symptoms first appear and ongoing treatment into adulthood seem to lessen the frequency of behaviors. No prevention is known.

PATIENT TEACHING

Compliance with continued treatment and drug therapy is an issue. Encourage the patient to continue with treatment and drug therapy.

REVIEW CHALLENGE

Answer the following questions:

1. What are the contributing factors to mental disorders?
2. What observations may indicate mental retardation?
3. What variants are considered in the diagnosis of a learning disorder?
4. What are the characteristics of a child with autism?
5. What is the diagnostic criteria for a tic disorder?
6. Under what conditions may dementia occur?
7. Why is Alzheimer disease so difficult to diagnose?
8. How may vascular dementia be related to atherosclerosis?
9. How might head trauma cause dementia?
10. How does repeated heavy alcohol abuse harm the body?
11. What are some effects of a rising blood alcohol level on the brain?
12. Why is schizophrenia termed a major psychiatric disturbance?
13. How do bipolar disorders affect an individual?
14. What is thought to cause a major depressive disorder?
15. What are the phases of the grief process?
16. What are some of the long-standing problems typical of personality disorders?
17. How are the major anxiety disorders classified? How do they differ from each other?
18. What condition may result as a delayed response to an external painful event?
19. What is a somatization disorder?
20. How is anxiety related to a conversion disorder?
21. What condition results from preoccupation with illness and abnormal fear of disease?
22. Can severe pain cause illness?
23. How is Munchausen syndrome diagnosed?
24. What is the typical pattern of sleep disorder in (1) insomnia, (2) narcolepsy, and (3) sleep apnea?

REAL-LIFE CHALLENGE

Alzheimer Disease

A 75-year-old man is diagnosed with Alzheimer disease. The retired businessman noticed many memory lapses, primarily in the area of short-term memory and the inability to concentrate. His family stated his verbalization appears somewhat diminished in that he has difficulty expressing his thoughts in an appropriate manner and interjects nonsensical phrases. He becomes agitated quite easily and has very little interest in grooming and self-appearance. The family has been advised they may have to have help in the future to care for the patient and that probably he will have to be institutionalized.

Since the patient exhibited both cognitive and behavioral symptoms of Alzheimer disease, he was treated with donepezil (Aricept) and alprazolam (Xanax).

QUESTIONS

1. Who is most likely to exhibit symptoms of Alzheimer disease?
2. List the typical symptoms.
3. What interventions may be taken?
4. What are some of the theories that have been advanced regarding the cause of Alzheimer disease?
5. How is Alzheimer disease diagnosed?
6. What is the anticipated prognosis for this patient?
7. What differentiates Alzheimer disease from senile dementia?
8. To what class of drugs does Xanax belong and what is the expected outcome of its administration?

REAL-LIFE CHALLENGE

Sleep Apnea

The wife of a 48-year-old man complains she cannot sleep due to the loud snoring of her husband. Questioning reveals she has noticed he has periods where he appears to stop breathing for about 30 seconds when sleeping. The patient has a history of mild alcohol consumption and also of smoking. He is approximately 30 pounds overweight.

Sleep studies are ordered since sleep apnea is suspected. He also says he does not feel rested after sleeping 8 to 9 hours a night.

QUESTIONS

1. What is the significance of the loud snoring?
2. Why is a history of social habits (smoking and alcohol consumption) important?
3. What are sleep studies?
4. What may happen if the sleep apnea is not diagnosed?
5. Which treatment may be prescribed?
6. What is the anticipated outcome of the treatment?

INTERNET ASSIGNMENTS

1. Ascertain what services are available to families of individuals diagnosed with Alzheimer disease at the Alzheimer's Association. Write a report listing and explaining these services as well as how the family may obtain the services.

2. Locate meeting sites for Alcoholics Anonymous in your community as well as the regular meeting times and days.

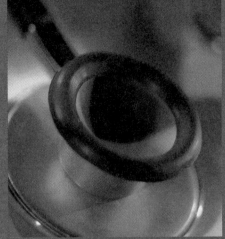

CHAPTER 15

Disorders and Conditions Resulting From Trauma

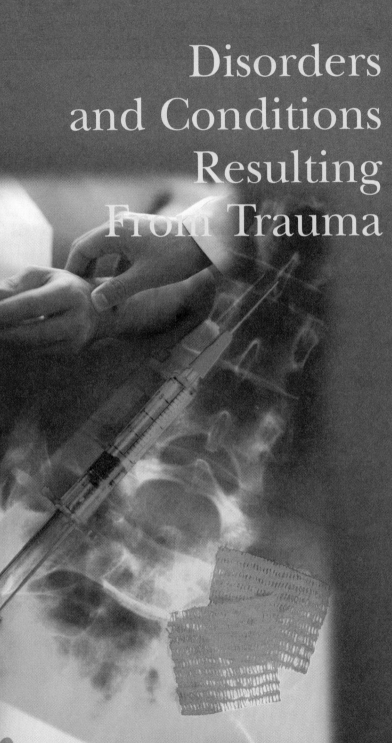

Continued

Chapter Outline—Cont'd

Learning Objectives

After studying Chapter 15, you should be able to:
1. List the major types of trauma.
2. List environmental factors that may result in trauma.
3. Name three factors that generally need to be addressed in open trauma.
4. Distinguish between an abrasion and an avulsion injury.
5. Describe conditions that require prophylaxis with tetanus toxoid.
6. Explain the risk to health-care workers of puncture wounds.
7. Describe management of foreign bodies in the ear, eye, and nose.
8. Name the conditions classified as thermal insults.
9. Explain the rule of nines in adults with burns and how it is used.
10. Describe the possible injuries caused by (a) electrical shock and (b) lightning.
11. Define hypothermia and list those most at risk.
12. Describe the guidelines for treating (a) frostbite, (b) insect bites, and (c) snake bites.
13. Explain the pathology that results in the pain and numbness of carpal tunnel syndrome.
14. Name the best treatment of child abuse and elder abuse.
15. Explain the importance of immediate intervention in shaken baby syndrome.
16. Discuss special concerns in the diagnosis of (a) battered spouse syndrome, (b) sexual abuse, and (c) rape.

Key Terms

abrasion (ah–**BRAY**–shun)
analgesic (**an**–ahl–**GEE**–sik)
antipyretic (an–tee–pye–**RET**–tic)
antiseptic (**an**–tih–**SEP**–tic)
avulsion (ah–**VUL**–shun)
cautery (**KAW**–ter–ee)
debride (day–**BREED**)
ergonomic (**er**–go–**NOM**–ic)

hyperabduction (**high**–per–ab–**DUCK**–shun)
hyperthermia (**high**–per–**THERM**–ee–ah)
hypothermia (**high**–poh–**THERM**–ee–ah)
laceration (lass–er–**AY**–shun)
prophylaxis (proh–fih–**LACK**–sis)
tendinitis (ten–deh–**NYE**–tis)
vector (**VECK**–tor)

TRAUMA

ALTHOUGH THEY ARE NOT SPECIFIC disease entities, traumatic occurrences do include physical and psychological injury that is derived from external force or violence; trauma may be self-inflicted, accidental, or the result of violence. Regardless of the cause, trauma can interfere with body functions or the homeostatic status of the body, it can inflict a permanent disability, or it may be life threatening. Major types are open trauma, assault trauma, thermal trauma, and psychological trauma. Whether physical or emotional, trauma, including abuse and sexual attack, is prevalent in current society. Physical trauma is the leading cause of death in young people in the United States.

Environmental factors sometimes result in traumatic circumstances. Weather-related conditions are often contributing factors in the occurrence of thermal insults and motor vehicle accidents, as well as accidents involving other types of machinery or accidents caused by natural elements (e.g., lightning strikes or tornadoes) Severe winds and changes in barometric pressure are responsible for trauma to tissue and to the respiratory system of those exposed to these elements. Poisons may result from contaminated ground water, toxins in the air, ingestion of seafood gathered from contaminated locations, or chemical spills. Bites from animals, insects, reptiles, or humans may occur under particular environmental circumstances. High altitudes also can affect body functions. Precaution and prevention are of primary concern whenever people are subjected to potentially traumatic circumstances.

Trauma centers can provide specialized critical care on a 24-hour basis for those seriously injured. Services include a specially trained medical team, medical devices to provide intensive care measures, and a facility equipped for surgical intervention if needed.

Open Trauma

Open trauma may involve only the skin surface or it may extend to the soft tissue and structures far below the skin. It may be in the form of an **abrasion,** in which the skin surface is scraped away, or it may be an **avulsion,** in which the tissue or an appendage is torn away. The injury can involve only a small area of the skin, as with a puncture wound, or encompass larger areas, as with crushing injuries. All incidents of open trauma have a commonality, the risk of infection if the wound is not appropriately cleansed and dressed. Pain also is usually involved in most open trauma.

Open wounds can be the source of tetanus infection; therefore, tetanus **prophylaxis** must be provided. Those who have completed the initial inoculation series for tetanus require a booster dose every 10 years. Those with no previous inoculation history are given tetanus immune globulin (human) and referred to a physician for the complete series of tetanus toxoid inoculations. When the patient has not had a booster injection within the past 10-year period, the booster injection is recommended.

Bleeding can be a factor in open trauma and must be addressed at once. Some injuries need only basic first aid, whereas others require medical intervention and surgical repair. Regardless of the severity of the injury, appropriate treatment aids healing and lessens scarring. Orthopedic and neurologic traumas are addressed in Chapters 7 and 13, respectively.

Abrasions

DESCRIPTION

Abrasions have occurred when the outer layers of the skin have been scraped away or roughed up.

> ■ **ICD-9-CM Code 919.0** *(Abrasion or friction burn without mention of infection)*
> *Open wounds are coded by site and type. Once the diagnosis has been confirmed, refer to the current edition of the ICD-9-CM coding manual for the appropriate code and modifier.*

SYMPTOMS AND SIGNS

The injured area appears raw and reddened, is painful, and has a small amount of bleeding (Fig. 15–1, *A* and *B*). The exposure of sensitive nerve endings causes a burning-type pain in the injured area; it may be embedded with small foreign particles.

PATIENT SCREENING

Abrasions require prompt cleansing. Current tetanus prophylaxis should be confirmed.

ETIOLOGY

Abrasions are caused by the friction created when a rough, hard surface comes in contact with skin as a consequence of a scrapping or sliding type of mo-

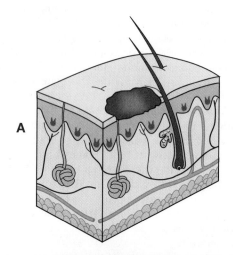

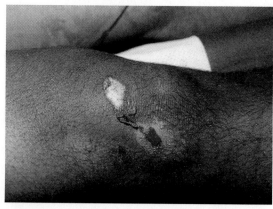

FIGURE 15–1 Abrasion. **A,** Outer layers of the skin are scraped away. **B,** Abrasion wounds of the kneecap caused by a fall to the ground after being struck by an automobile. (**B** from Henry MC, Stapleton ER: *EMT prehospital care,* ed 3, Philadelphia, 2004, Saunders.)

tion, often the result of a fall. Such injuries are often referred to as friction burns, floor burns, rug burns, or road rash.

DIAGNOSIS

Diagnosis is made by history and visual inspection.

TREATMENT

Treatment consists of gentle washing of the area with a germicidal soap and water. Any foreign particles such as gravel and dirt that have not been removed by cleansing should be removed carefully with forceps. A germicidal ointment or cream then may be applied. A nonadherent dressing may be applied as well, depending on the size and location of the abrasion. Prophylaxis with tetanus toxoid is confirmed or administered if necessary.

PROGNOSIS

The prognosis for healing is good once cleansing to remove any foreign bodies or bacteria is accomplished. The extent of scarring depends on the depth and extent of the insult.

PREVENTION

Prevention is difficult, especially for active individuals. Protective leather clothing worn sometimes by cyclists helps prevent extensive "road rash" abrasions.

PATIENT TEACHING

Instruct the patient regarding appropriate wound care and the importance of keeping the wound clean and dry. Reinforce the value of maintaining up-to-date tetanus prophylaxis.

Avulsion

DESCRIPTION

With avulsion injuries, a portion of the skin and possibly underlying tissue is torn away, either completely or partially (Fig. 15–2, *A* and *B*).

ICD-9-CM Code **879.8** *(Open wound[s] [multiple] of unspecified sites, without mention of complication)*
Open wounds are coded by site and type. Once the diagnosis has been confirmed, refer to the current edition of the ICD-9-CM coding manual for the appropriate code and modifier.

SYMPTOMS AND SIGNS

An avulsion injury can involve a limb, an appendage, or any soft tissue area anywhere on the surface of the body. The patient usually has severe pain in the area, and bleeding from the wound is common. When the avulsion is partial, the avulsed tissue is still partially attached to the injured area.

PATIENT SCREENING

Avulsion injuries require prompt cleansing and closure of the open wound. When the avulsed tissue is available (i.e., still partially attached to the body or retrieved from the accident site, as for example, in the case of a severed finger tip) and reattachment is possible, the surgical procedure is performed as quickly as possible. Current tetanus prophylaxis should be confirmed.

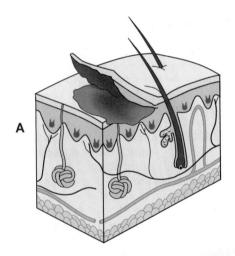

A

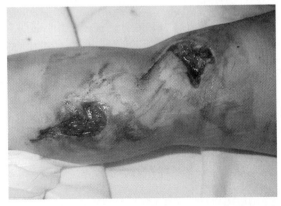

B

FIGURE 15–2 Avulsion. **A,** A flap of skin has been torn away. **B,** Avulsions over the knee and lower leg. (**B** from Henry MC, Stapleton ER: *EMT prehospital care,* ed 3, Philadelphia, 2004, Saunders.)

ETIOLOGY

The mechanism of this kind of injury is usually one in which the affected body part becomes entangled in machinery, clothing, or some other means of entrapment, causing the skin, tissue, and possibly bone to be torn and pulled away from the body. If the limb or appendage is severed completely from the body, it is termed an amputation.

DIAGNOSIS

Diagnosis is made by visual inspection of the affected part and by history of the mechanism of injury.

TREATMENT

Treatment consists of controlling the bleeding, cleansing the area, and surgically repairing the tissue. If an amputation has occurred, the stump or remaining area must be cleansed and surgically repaired. The patient probably will be treated prophylactically with antibiotics to prevent infection. A sterile dressing is applied to the repaired wound. Tetanus prophylaxis is confirmed or administered if necessary. Pain medication is prescribed and administered when necessary.

PROGNOSIS

Prognosis depends on the extent of the insult. Prompt intervention helps hasten the healing process.

PREVENTION

Prevention is difficult and the likelihood of injury is unpredictable. Following safety guidelines when operating machinery, especially that of not wearing loose clothing while operating machinery, is a prudent practice.

PATIENT TEACHING

Reinforce the importance of following safety guidelines. Instruct the patient on wound care and the importance of keeping the wound clean and dry. Reinforce the value of maintaining up-to-date tetanus prophylaxis. Encourage patients to keep any follow-up appointments as scheduled.

Crushing Injuries

DESCRIPTION

Crushing injuries occur when a part of the body is compressed with extreme force between two surfaces.

■ **ICD-9-CM Code 929.9**

SYMPTOMS AND SIGNS

A crushing injury may involve any body part, but most often, a finger, hand, toe, or foot is the involved part. The patient experiences pain and may not be able to move the injured part. Soft tissue is compressed, or crushed, and depending on the amount of pressure involved in the mechanism of injury, bone, nerves, and vessels also may be crushed.

PATIENT SCREENING

Crushing injuries require prompt assessment and intervention. Many individuals that sustain such as injury will be transported to an emergency facility. If not, schedule them to be seen as soon as possible on the day of the injury or refer them to an emergency facility.

ETIOLOGY

The crushing injury occurs when the affected body part becomes pressed between two hard surfaces. Examples of such injuries are fingers shut in doors, hands or fingers caught in presses, heavy objects being dropped on feet or toes, and compression of any body part as a result of a motor vehicle accident. Falling debris, such as building parts broken loose in a storm or earthquake, also can cause crushing injuries.

DIAGNOSIS

Diagnosis is made from history, visual inspection of the body area, and physical examination. Radiographic studies of the injured part also aid in the diagnosis.

TREATMENT

Treatment depends on the severity and location of the injury. When an open wound is present, the area is cleansed and **debrided** if necessary. Immobilization of the affected limb or appendage follows any surgical repair that is indicated. Sterile dressings will probably be applied to any open wound or surgical area. If the crushing injury involves the head or trunk of the body, appropriate monitoring of vital signs and surgical intervention is undertaken. Tetanus prophylaxis is confirmed or administered if necessary, and antibiotics may be prescribed as an additional prophylactic measure.

PROGNOSIS

Prognosis depends on the extent of the insult. Prompt intervention helps hasten the healing process.

PREVENTION

Prevention is difficult and the likelihood of injury is unpredictable. Following safety guidelines when operating machinery, especially that of not wearing loose clothing while operating machinery, is a prudent practice. Other such Occupational Safety and Health Administration (OSHA) guidelines should be followed whenever engaging in risky activities.

PATIENT TEACHING

Reinforce safety guidelines. Instruct the patient on wound care and the importance of keeping the wound clean and dry. Reinforce the value of maintaining up-to-date tetanus prophylaxis. Encourage patients to keep any follow-up appointments as scheduled.

Puncture Wounds

DESCRIPTION

Puncture wounds result when a pointed foreign object penetrates the soft tissue (Fig. 15–3, *A* and *B*). Animals bites, discussed later in this chapter, also may be considered puncture wounds.

ICD-9-CM Code **879.8** *(Open wound[s] [multiple] of unspecified sites without mention of complication)*
Open wounds are coded by site and type. Once the diagnosis has been confirmed, refer to the current edition of the ICD-9-CM coding manual for the appropriate code and modifier.

SYMPTOMS AND SIGNS

Puncture wounds cause pain and usually very little bleeding. Redness at the site may be noted, or there may be no indication of the wound other than the pain. If the foreign body that caused the injury is protruding out of the wound, it is described as an impaled object (Fig. 15–4).

PATIENT SCREENING

Puncture wounds require prompt assessment and cleansing. Tetanus prophylaxis needs to be confirmed. Impaled objects require stabilization until assessment and treatment are accomplished.

ETIOLOGY

A puncture wound occurs when a sharp, pointed object penetrates the skin and underlying soft tissue. The offending object may be a needle, a nail, a splinter of glass, wood, or metal, a knife, or even a bullet. The object first penetrates the skin and then the skin closes around the object or point of entry. As a result, bleeding is minimal. In some situations, bleeding will occur as the penetrating object is removed.

DIAGNOSIS

Diagnosis is made by visual examination, history, and sometimes radiographic studies (if the object can be visualized by imaging). An embedded organic object, such as a small twig, can be visualized only by using magnetic resonance imaging. An impaled object is easily observed because it protrudes from the injured site.

TREATMENT

Treatment involves removal of the foreign body, along with copious irrigation of the wound with sterile fluid. A sterile dressing is applied. Tetanus prophylaxis is confirmed or administered if necessary, and antibiotics may be prescribed as an additional prophylactic measure. Impaled objects are stabilized until they can be removed by the physician.

PROGNOSIS

Prognosis varies depending on the extent and depth of the puncture wound.

PREVENTION

Prevention is difficult. Health-care providers should practice OSHA guidelines when handling sharps and needles. Construction workers are encouraged to use air tools with great caution and wear recommended safety devices such as steel-toed safety shoes, hard hats, and safety goggles.

PATIENT TEACHING

Instruct the patient on wound care and on keeping the wound clean and dry. Reinforce the importance

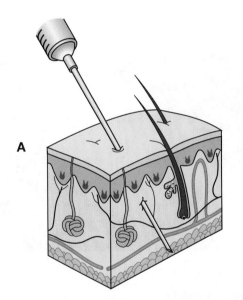

A

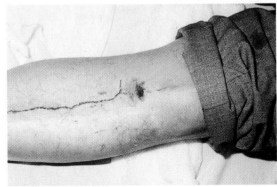

B

FIGURE 15-3 Puncture wound. **A,** A pointed object has punctured the skin. **B,** Puncture wound of the anterior lower leg. (**B** from Henry MC, Stapleton ER: *EMT prehospital care,* ed 3, Philadelphia, 2004, Saunders; Courtesy S. L. Wiener and J. Barrett.)

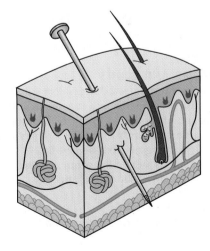

FIGURE 15-4   Impaled object. A nail is impaled in the skin.

ENRICHMENT
NEEDLESTICKS

HEALTH-CARE PROVIDERS are at risk for puncture wounds from contaminated needlesticks. United States Occupational Safety and Health Administration (OSHA) guidelines must be followed to lessen the risk of occurrence and to reduce the likelihood of transmitting acquired immunodeficiency syndrome (AIDS) or hepatitis B.

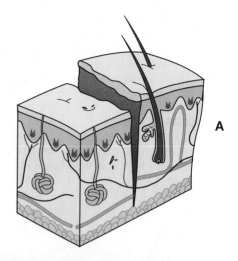

A

of tetanus prophylaxis. Encourage enforcement of OSHA guidelines when appropriate.

Lacerations

DESCRIPTION

Lacerations result when a sharp object cuts the skin and possibly underlying soft tissue.

> ■ **ICD-9-CM Code** **879.8** *(Open wound[s] [multiple] of unspecified sites without mention of complication)*
> *Open wounds are coded by site and type. Once the diagnosis has been confirmed, refer to the current edition of the ICD-9-CM coding manual for the appropriate code and modifier.*

SYMPTOMS AND SIGNS

Lacerations result when a sharp object cuts the skin and possibly the underlying soft tissue as well. They cause pain and moderate to severe bleeding. The edges of the cut may be smooth, or they may be jagged, depending on what object did the cutting. The bleeding is generally proportionate to the depth and length of the laceration.

PATIENT SCREENING

Lacerations require prompt cleansing and repair.

ETIOLOGY

Lacerations occur when a sharp instrument, such as a knife or sharp piece of glass or metal, cuts the skin and underlying soft tissue (Fig. 15–5, *A* and *B*).

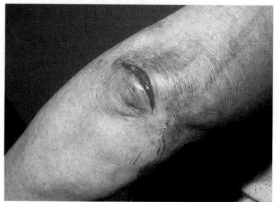

B

FIGURE 15–5 Laceration. **A,** Skin is cut by a sharp object. **B,** Laceration of the elbow caused by a fall on the street. (**B** from Henry MC, Stapleton ER: *EMT prehospital care,* ed 3, Philadelphia, 2004, Saunders.)

DIAGNOSIS

Diagnosis is made by visual examination. History may reveal the type of sharp object that caused the injury. A laceration with smooth edges that can be approximated cleanly is termed an *incision* (Fig. 15–6).

TREATMENT

Lacerations should be cleansed gently with a germicidal soap and water. If the laceration is not too deep and bleeding is controlled, approximating and securing the edges with tape, a butterfly dressing, or sterile adhesive strips *(Steri-Strips)* may be the only intervention necessary other than a sterile dressing application. In some cases, a new type of "glue" is used to hold the edges together, thereby eliminating the need for sutures. Lacerations that are deep, have jagged edges, or continue to bleed need to be debrided and have the edges trimmed to facilitate good approximation. Bleeding should be controlled by either *coagulation* or suture. Suturing of the wound will probably be necessary. If the laceration is over a movable joint, immobilization of the area is indicated. A sterile dressing should be applied. Tetanus prophylaxis is confirmed and administered if necessary, and antibiotics may be prescribed as an additional prophylactic measure.

PROGNOSIS
Prognosis varies depending on the location, length, depth, and condition of the laceration. The degree of approximation of the edges of the wound may determine the extent of the scarring.

PREVENTION
Prevention is difficult. Care when using knives should be stressed. Following OSHA guidelines when using power tools is a prudent practice.

PATIENT TEACHING
Instruct the patient on wound care and the importance of tetanus prophylaxis. When sutures have been used for closure, instruct the patient regarding when to return for suture removal.

Foreign Bodies

Anything that enters a portion of the body where it does not belong is considered a foreign body (FB). Common sites for entrapped foreign bodies include the ears, the eyes, and the nose, but any surface area of the body can be involved.

Foreign Bodies in the Ear
DESCRIPTION
Foreign bodies (FB) in the ear typically range from bugs, pebbles, and bits of cotton to anything small enough to fit in the ear canal.

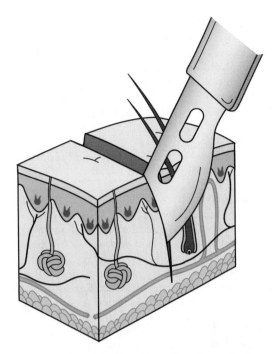

FIGURE 15–6 Incision. A laceration with smooth edges.

■ **ICD-9-CM Code 931**

SYMPTOMS AND SIGNS
The patient will present complaining of feeling a stuffiness and something in the ear. If the foreign object is a bug, the patient also may complain of a buzzing sound in the ear. Complaints of pain in the ear canal and decreased hearing capability may be expressed. Anything small enough to fit in the ear could be the offending foreign body. Visualization of the ear canal usually shows an apparent object.

PATIENT SCREENING
Although not a life-threatening condition, individuals with foreign bodies in the ear require prompt assessment and intervention.

ETIOLOGY
Flying insects may enter the ear canal accidentally in the course of flight, and instances of a bug crawling into the ear when an individual is lying down have been reported. Children have a tendency to place small objects in their ear canals. Small toys, cereal, grapes, peas, beans, and pebbles are examples

of some of the objects commonly found in the ear canals of children. Cotton from cotton-tipped applicators also may be the offending object; the cotton inadvertently comes off of the applicator stick during a cleaning process. Anything small enough to be placed into the ear canal could be the problem, especially in the case of children.

DIAGNOSIS

Diagnosis is made by history and visual and/or otoscopic inspection of the ear canal.

TREATMENT

The goal of treatment is removal of the offending object without damaging the ear canal or tympanic membrane. Many times the object simply may be grasped by forceps and removed. Food and cereal can absorb moisture from the ear canal and swell to the point of being compressed against the walls of the ear canal. Such objects may require removal by a physician using gentle controlled suctioning. The individual with a live bug in the ear should be placed in a dark room and have a flashlight shone in the ear. Bugs that are alive will crawl out of the ear toward the light. Bugs that are not responsive to the light technique may have to be washed out of the ear. In that case, the ear canal is gently irrigated with a warm solution of 50% water and 50% hydrogen peroxide; the bug usually flows out with the solution. If this is not successful, then gentle suction may be necessary to remove the FB. Caution is taken not to scratch or damage the ear canal or the tympanic membrane.

PROGNOSIS

Prognosis is good with prompt removal of the FB and no consequential damage to the ear canal or tympanic membrane.

PREVENTION

Prevention includes working with children to educate them about not putting anything in their ears. A good rule to teach them is "never place anything in your ears that is smaller than your elbow." Keep cotton-tipped applicators out of the reach of children and use extreme caution when attempting to cleanse the ears with them.

PATIENT TEACHING

Stress the dangers of putting small objects in the ears. Encourage parents to seek medical intervention when a child has a FB in the ear canal.

Foreign Bodies in the Eye

DESCRIPTION

Foreign bodies in the eye are objects that would not normally be found in the eye. Common offenders are bugs, rust, dust, sand, hair, small pieces of metal, or small pieces of brush or tree branches. Chemicals may be accidently splashed in the eye.

 ICD-9-CM Code 930.9 *(Unspecified site)*
Foreign bodies in the eye are coded by site. Once the diagnosis has been confirmed, refer to the current edition of the ICD-9-CM coding manual for the appropriate code and modifier.

SYMPTOMS AND SIGNS

The individual complains of scratching or irritation of the eye. The patient may experience pain in the eye and report blurred or compromised vision. Tearing is usually present.

PATIENT SCREENING

Foreign objects in the eye require prompt evaluation and intervention. If the injury involves splashed chemicals, advise immediate irrigation of the eye. If an immediate appointment is not available, refer the individual to an emergency facility. Encourage patients to have someone else provide their transportation because they should not attempt to drive. If the object is impaled and sticking out of the eye, the Emergency Medical System (EMS) is the recommended mode of transportation after stabilization of the impaled object has been accomplished.

ETIOLOGY

Foreign bodies in the eyes can result from a number of sources and routes of entry. A common source of rust and metal particles in the eye is the undercarriage of a car; the person working under a car may inadvertently knock loose rust particles or minute scraps of metal that then fall into the eye. Industrial accidents involving objects that have been propelled through the air, possibly as the result of an explosion, also can result in a foreign body entering the unprotected eye. Foreign objects also may be propelled into the eye as a result of a motor vehicle accident. Dust and other debris in the environment may be blown into open unprotected eyes. A bug flying into the eye is a common occurrence. Occasionally, just rubbing the eyes with dirty hands can be the source of entry for dirt or a chemical. Working with caustic liquids without wearing eye protection is another source of foreign substances in the eye resulting from splashing.

DIAGNOSIS
Diagnosis is made by visual and ophthalmoscopic examination of the eye. A history of feeling something in the eye combined with the circumstance of possible exposure to foreign bodies is helpful. Staining the eye with fluorescein to visualize a corneal abrasion will confirm the presence or previous presence of a foreign body. Refer to Chapter 5 for discussion on corneal abrasion.

TREATMENT
Treatment involves removal of the offending material. Many times gentle irrigation of the eye with normal saline will flush dust, bugs, or debris out of the eye. When the FB is embedded in the eye, the physician may attempt removal with surgical instruments or an eye spud. If these procedures are unsuccessful, immediate referral to an ophthalmologist is made. Ophthalmic antibacterial drops or ointments may be placed in the eye, and the eye is usually covered with a patch.

PROGNOSIS
Prognosis varies depending on the offending material and the depth and involvement of the eye structures. Many injuries caused by bugs and dust will resolve after cleansing irrigation. Extensive corneal abrasions may result in residual scarring and compromised vision. Chemical burns may result in blindness.

PREVENTION
The best prevention for occupational and other possible insults by foreign objects to the eye is wearing approved eye protection. Many accidental incidents can be prevented in that way.

PATIENT TEACHING
Encourage the use of eye protection whenever any possible hazard to the eye is anticipated. When a foreign object other than minute dust particles enters the eye and is not removed successfully by gentle irrigation, encourage the individual to seek professional treatment. When one eye is patched or covered with a bandage, make the patient aware that depth perception will be absent and encourage care in navigating steps.

Foreign Bodies in the Nose

DESCRIPTION
Any object or foreign material that is causing an obstruction in the nares should be considered a foreign body in the nose, and medical intervention for removal should be sought. Foreign bodies often found wedged in the nares of children are cereals, dried peas or beans, grapes, Styrofoam particles, pebbles, and cotton.

 ICD-9-CM Code 932

SYMPTOMS AND SIGNS
Children have the most occurrences of foreign bodies wedged or stuck in the nares. Parents usually note mucus running from one of the nares and congested breathing. Upon investigation they are able to confirm that one of the nares is constricted and air is not moving through the affected side.

PATIENT SCREENING
Foreign bodies in the nose require prompt assessment and treatment.

ETIOLOGY
Children have a tendency to insert foreign objects into their noses. These foreign bodies include but are not limited to cereals, dried peas or beans, grapes, Styrofoam particles, pebbles, toys, and anything else small enough to fit in the nares. Dry materials such as dried peas, beans, and cereal have a tendency to absorb moisture from the mucous membrane and then swell, creating an obstruction.

DIAGNOSIS
Diagnosis is made by history and visualization of the foreign body in the nares. Often mucus is dripping from the unobstructed nares.

TREATMENT
The child is encouraged to blow the nose, hopefully expelling the object. If the offending foreign substance is cereal, squeezing the nose usually will crush the cereal bit and permit it to be expelled by blowing the nose. A physician may need to grasp the object with forceps for removal.

PROGNOSIS
Prognosis is good when removal of the offending object is uncomplicated and complete.

PREVENTION

Prevention is difficult because children often have a tendency to insert small objects in their noses.

PATIENT TEACHING

Counsel children not to place any objects in their noses. Emphasize that dried objects will swell and that medical intervention may be needed to correct the situation.

Thermal Insults

Thermal insults can be caused by either heat or cold, which includes burns or frostbite. Extremes in temperatures cause conditions such as **hypothermia, hyperthermia,** heat stroke, and heat exhaustion. Regardless of the variance in temperature (hot or cold), most such conditions that result in a severely altered state can be life threatening if left untreated. However, hypothermia may be a protective factor in the case of cold-water near-drowning.

Burns

DESCRIPTION

Burns are the result of thermal insults to tissue. The insults may be caused by heat, chemical sources, electrical sources, or radiation. Heat sources that cause injury may be in the form of dry heat, steam, or hot substances; sun rays are also capable of causing a burn.

ICD-9-CM Code 949.0 *(Unspecified site, unspecified degree, unspecified body surface)*
Burns are coded by site, degree, and body surface involved. Once the diagnosis has been confirmed, refer to the current edition of the ICD-9-CM coding manual for the appropriate code and modifier.

SYMPTOMS AND SIGNS

The patient who has experienced a burn usually has pain. The extent of the burn, along with the percent of body surface involved, usually is related proportionately to the degree of pain. Depending on the depth and nature of the burn, the skin surface may be reddened, blistered, or charred (Fig. 15–7).

PATIENT SCREENING

Burns require prompt assessment and intervention. Patients with major burns are referred to burn centers for treatment. Knowing the mechanics of the injury are important in determining the type of treatment intervention required; this includes assessment of respiratory status, wound contamination, eye involvement, and fluid management.

ETIOLOGY

Burns can be caused by flame, dry heat, liquid scalds, radiation, chemicals, or electricity. The exposure of the skin to any of these sources can cause destruction of the skin. The injury to the underlying soft tissue is proportionate to the duration of the exposure and the intensity of the thermal source.

DIAGNOSIS

Diagnosis is made by visual examination and history. In a flame-type burn, it is necessary to determine whether the burn occurred inside an enclosed space or out in the open. The respiratory state of any patient with a flame-type burn must be assessed. The status of the eyebrows, eyelashes, and nasal hair must be determined. Any singeing of these hairs indicates that the patient inhaled the flame or superheated air and that the respiratory status may be in grave danger.

Determination of the depth (Fig. 15–8) and extent (Fig. 15–9) of a burn is important. Pain intensity depends on the amount of nerve tissue that is involved or destroyed. Superficial burns involve only the outer layers of the skin, which usually appear only reddened, and yet these burns are painful. Partial-thickness burns involve all layers of the skin; they produce blisters and are quite painful. Full-thickness burns involve both the skin and the underlying subcutaneous tissue. Resultant destruction of nerve endings often results in minimal pain in that particular area; however, pain may be reported in areas around the periphery of the burn site. Prompt assessment of the percent of skin surface area involved in the burn injury is achieved by applying the rule of nines. The rule of nines provides a fast and fairly accurate calculation of the body surface involved. Percentages used to ascertain the burned tissue area in the adult are as follows: head—9%; anterior trunk—18%; posterior trunk—18%; entire right arm—9%; entire left arm—9%; anterior surface right leg—9%; posterior surface right leg—9%; anterior surface left leg—9%; posterior surface left leg—9%; and perineum—1%. Percentages in children and infants are slightly different. Another method of designating a percentage of body surface involvement is used by the ICD-9-CM code book. Refer to the current edition of the ICD-9-CM code book for these percentages.

TREATMENT

Treatment depends on the source of the burns. Heat burns (from flame, liquid scalds, or superheated air) should be cooled with cool water and covered with dry sterile dressings until seen by a physician. Sunburns should be treated with the application of cool water, and the damaged skin may be sprayed with **antiseptic** and **analgesic** sprays (Fig. 15–10). Skin burned with chemicals other than lime, which must first be brushed away, should be flushed with cool water for at least 15 minutes, covered with a sterile dressing, and treated by a physician. Electrical burns should be examined for points of entry (rings, belts, necklaces) and exit (knees, toes) (Fig. 15–11). These areas should be covered with dry sterile dressings and treated by a physician.

A 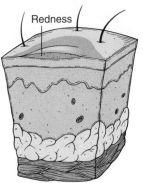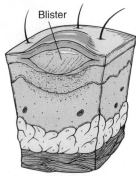 **B**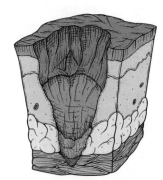

FIGURE 15–7 A, Examples of burns. Partial thickness burn, note the blisters. **B,** Full thickness burn, note the dark color. (Courtesy of Judy Knightton, Clinical Nurse Specialist, Ross Tilley Burn Center, Sunnybrook and Women's College Health Center, Toronto, Ontario, Canada.)

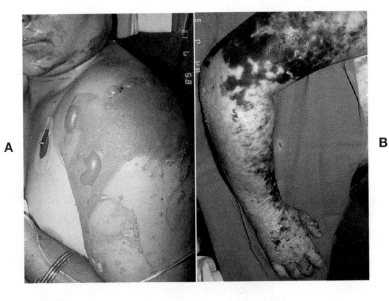

Superficial burn   Partial-thickness burn   Full-thickness burn

FIGURE 15–8 Depths of burns. The extent of involvement of layers of the skin.

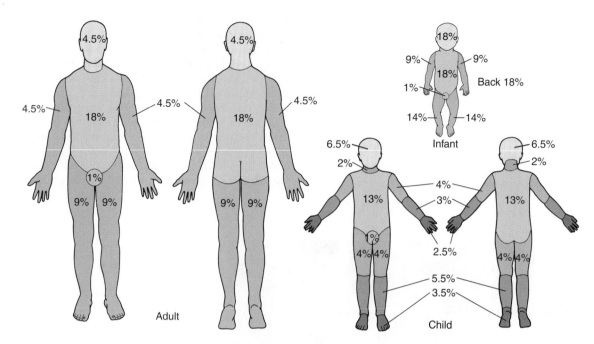

FIGURE 15–9 Rule of nines.

Analgesics are given to treat the pain. Minor burns usually are treated with an antibacterial cream or ointment. Severe burns require specialized treatment, with surgical debridement of the burned tissue and skin grafts if necessary.

Patients with severe large-area burns, the elderly and the very young, and those with severe burns to the face, hands, feet, or perineal area usually are admitted to a burn center, where they receive specialized burn care. Respiratory status (if the respiratory tract is involved), fluid and electrolyte balance, and vital signs are monitored. Pain control is accomplished with narcotic analgesics. Tetanus prophylaxis is confirmed or administered if necessary, and antibiotics may be prescribed as an additional prophylactic measure. Skin grafting, including the use of cloned skin as well as the use of autografts and adjacent tissue grafts, is used for treatment of extensive destruction of tissue.

PROGNOSIS

Prognosis varies depending on the cause and extent of the burned tissue and other organ or system involvement. Prompt intervention helps promote a positive outcome. Scarring is usual. (Refer to the Enrichment box on radiation.)

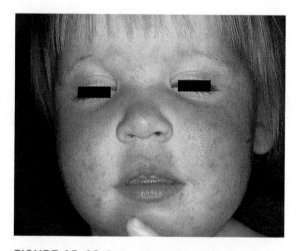

FIGURE 15–10 Sunburn on an infant's face. (From Weston WL, Lane AT, Morrelli JG: *Color textbook of pediatric dermatology,* ed 3, St. Louis, 2002, Mosby.)

PREVENTION

Prevention is difficult. Prudent use of fire or combustible materials is helpful. Being proactive to avoid situations where burns may occur is wise. Application of sunscreens when exposure to sun rays is anticipated is strongly recommended.

Text continued on p. 713

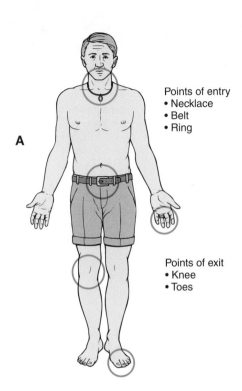

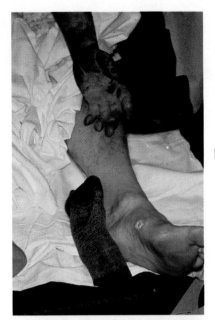

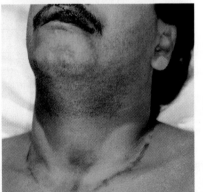

FIGURE 15–11 A, Points of entry and exit for electrical burns. **B,** Exit wound in the foot. **C,** Lightning burst a metal necklace chain on the patient, leaving a burn marking. (**B** and **C** from Henry MC, Stapleton ER: *EMT prehospital care,* ed 3, Philadelphia, 2004, Saunders.)

ENRICHMENT

SUNBURN

EXPOSURE TO THE ULTRAVIOLET ALPHA and beta rays from the sun can cause sunburn, ranging from mild to severe. The person who has experienced at least three severe sunburns with blistering is at risk for the development of skin cancer. Prevention of sunburn includes avoiding exposure from 10 AM to 2 PM, when the sun's rays are the strongest, applying a sunscreen to exposed skin areas, and wearing a hat to protect the scalp and eyes. Those at greatest risk have light or fair skin and freckles and blond or red hair (Fig. 15–12).

Sun protection factor (SPF) is the technical name for measurement of UVB protection provided by sunscreen. The numbers assigned to a product designate the length of time it takes to redden the skin as compared to no protection. SPFs of at least 15 are recommended by the Skin Cancer Foundation as a protection against the sun's harmful rays or UVB.

Continued

Thermal Insults

ENRICHMENT
SUNBURN—CONT'D

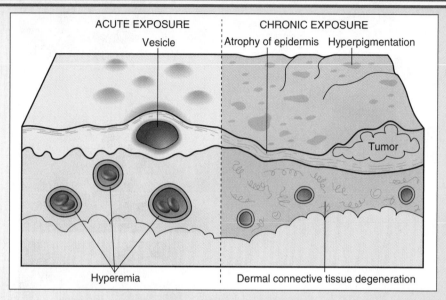

ACUTE EXPOSURE   CHRONIC EXPOSURE

Vesicle   Atrophy of epidermis   Hyperpigmentation

Tumor

Hyperemia   Dermal connective tissue degeneration

FIGURE 15–12 Short-term and long-term effects of sun bathing. Acute injury results in hyperemia of the dermis and blister formation. Long-term exposure may stimulate pigmentation but may also promote carcinogenesis and aging of the epidermis and dermis. (From Damjanov I: *Pathology for the health related professions,* ed 2, Philadelphia, 2000, Saunders.)

ENRICHMENT
RADIATION EXPOSURE

EXPOSURE TO RADIOACTIVE MATERIAL is another threat to society. "Dirty bombs" may contain radioactive particles that can be released into the environment upon explosion of the bomb. The three main types of exposure to ionizing radiation are slow, cumulative whole body exposure; sudden whole body exposure; and high-dose localized exposure. Sudden whole body exposure is the most likely form of ionizing radiation exposure for the general public in a terrorist-type event. The body's exposure to radiation may be external irradiation of all or part of the body from an external source including radiation therapy for cancer treatment, contamination by radioactive material in gases, liquids, or solids that have been released into the environment causing external, internal, or both types of contamination, or by incorporation of the radioactive material as a sequela to other contamination. Symptoms of radiation exposure include nausea, vomiting, and diarrhea; redness and blistering of skin burns; dehydration; weakness, fatigue, exhaustion, and fainting; hair loss, ulceration of oral mucosa, esophagus, and gastrointestinal (GI) tract; vomiting blood and experiencing bloody stools; bruising; sloughing of the skin; and bleeding from nose, mouth, and gums. The extent of the toxicity of ionizing radiation idepends on the dose, the distance from the source of radiation, and the length of time of the exposure. Body responses and long-term effects as an overview of major morphologic consequences are presented in Figures 15–13 and 15–14.

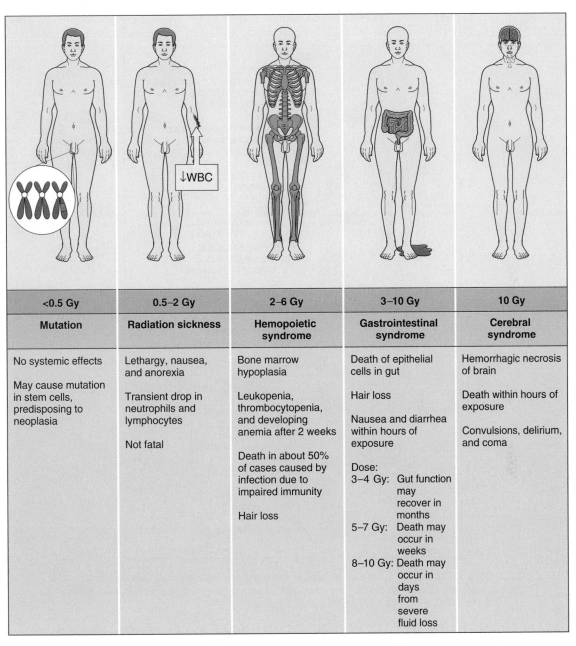

<0.5 Gy	0.5–2 Gy	2–6 Gy	3–10 Gy	10 Gy
Mutation	**Radiation sickness**	**Hemopoietic syndrome**	**Gastrointestinal syndrome**	**Cerebral syndrome**
No systemic effects May cause mutation in stem cells, predisposing to neoplasia	Lethargy, nausea, and anorexia Transient drop in neutrophils and lymphocytes Not fatal	Bone marrow hypoplasia Leukopenia, thrombocytopenia, and developing anemia after 2 weeks Death in about 50% of cases caused by infection due to impaired immunity Hair loss	Death of epithelial cells in gut Hair loss Nausea and diarrhea within hours of exposure Dose: 3–4 Gy: Gut function may recover in months 5–7 Gy: Death may occur in weeks 8–10 Gy: Death may occur in days from severe fluid loss	Hemorrhagic necrosis of brain Death within hours of exposure Convulsions, delirium, and coma

FIGURE 15–13 Responses to total body irradiation. (From Stevens A, Lowe J: *Pathology—illustrated review in color,* ed 2, London, 2000, Mosby.)

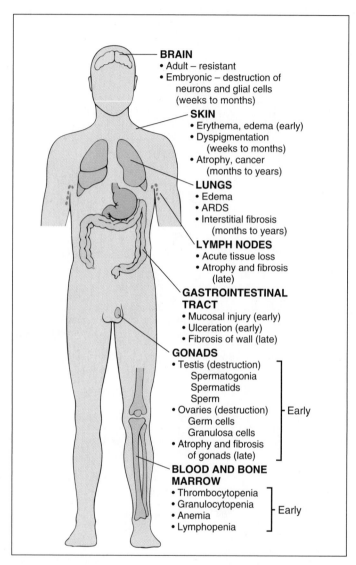

FIGURE 15–14 Overview of the major morphologic consequences of radiation injury. Early changes occur in hours to weeks; late changes occur in months to years. *ARDS,* Adult respiratory distress syndrome. (From Kumar V et al: *Robbins basic pathology,* ed 7, Philadelphia, 2003, Saunders.)

PATIENT TEACHING

Stress the importance of keeping follow-up appointments and compliance with prescribed therapy. Provide instruction on wound care. Emphasize the importance of current tetanus prophylaxis.

Electrical Shock

DESCRIPTION

Electrical shock is an injury that occurs as the result of exposure to or contact with electricity.

ICD-9-CM Code 994.8 *(Excluding electric burns)*
Burns are coded by site, degree, and body surface involved. Once the diagnosis of a burn has been confirmed, refer to the current edition of the ICD-9-CM coding manual for the appropriate code and modifier.

SYMPTOMS AND SIGNS

Patients who have experienced electrical shock may be in cardiac or respiratory failure. They have a visible burn at the entrance wound and at the exit wound. If conscious, they experience pain at these sites. Charred tissue may be noted.

PATIENT SCREENING

Individuals who have suffered electrical shock constitute a life-threatening emergency. They need to be entered into the *Emergency Medical System (EMS)* for transport to an emergency care facility. Resuscitation and life support may be required during transport.

ETIOLOGY

The person who has sustained electrical shock experiences tissue damage from the point of entry of the electricity to the point of exit. The electrical current follows the path of least resistance through the body, usually along nerve routes. The current enters the body at the point of contact with the electrical source and exits at the point of grounding (see Fig. 15–11). As the alternating current passes through the body, it may produce muscle contractions, causing the person to be thrown from the source. This can result in lacerations, fractures, or head trauma.

DIAGNOSIS

Diagnosis is made by visual examination and history.

TREATMENT

Treatment consists of maintaining the cardiac and respiratory status. If indicated, cardiopulmonary resuscitation (CPR) must be administered after the patient has been removed from the electrical source. The patient's neurologic and vascular status are assessed for the extent of tissue destruction. Any fractures, lacerations, and head injuries are treated. The burned areas are debrided and dressed with sterile dressings. Pain management is accomplished with narcotic analgesics. Tetanus prophylaxis is confirmed or administered if necessary, and antibiotics may be prescribed as an additional prophylactic measure.

PROGNOSIS

Prognosis varies depending on the extent of the insult and damage to organs and body systems. When cardiac arrest has occurred, prognosis may not be favorable, even with prompt resuscitative efforts. It is important to realize that electrical energy will follow nerves on its path through the body and therefore has the potential to cause damage in the peripheral nervous system (PNS).

PREVENTION

Extreme care should be taken in situations that involve repair of or close proximity to electrical power, and people should be alert for possible electrical accidents at all times. Use electrical outlet covers when the outlets are not in use. Avoid standing in water when it is possible that nearby electrical wires could come in contact with the water.

PATIENT TEACHING

Advise patients to follow OSHA guidelines when working with electricity. Encourage them to be aware of potential sources of electrocution in the workplace and home environment.

Lightning Injuries

DESCRIPTION

Lightning injuries occur when an individual is struck by lightning.

ICD-9-CM Code 994.0 *(Excludes burns)*
(Effects of lightning)
Burns are coded by type and site. Once the diagnosis of a burn has been confirmed, refer to the current edition of the ICD-9-CM coding manual for additional burn codes.

SYMPTOMS AND SIGNS

Lightning injuries can be classified by the severity of the injury or by the type of strike the person receives. Usually, the severity of the injury is in direct proportion to the intensity of the lightning strike.

The victim of a direct lightning strike is probably in a severely compromised state, unconscious and not breathing. A heartbeat may be present if the *apnea* has not caused cardiac arrest. Clothing may be literally "blown off" the victim, and the victim may have been propelled through the air by the jolt. Burns usually are noted in areas of the skin where moisture is normally found, such as the axillae and groin or where metal was touching the body (see Fig. 15–11). Motor and sensory disturbances are noted, along with possible ruptured *tympanic membranes.* The patient who has experienced moderate contact will have less severe symptoms, but with an altered level of consciousness and skin burns. The person with minor injuries exhibits fairly normal vital signs, some confusion, *amnesia* of preceding events, and some minor muscle or sensory nerve disturbances. All may experience some hearing or visual difficulties.

PATIENT SCREENING

Lightning strikes constitute a life threatening situation. Respiratory efforts of the patient may be compromised and providing immediate rescue breathing is imperative. If apnea has caused cardiac arrest, CPR must be instituted immediately. Call 911 to promptly enter the victim into the Emergency Medical System.

ETIOLOGY

Lightning can strike a person in five different ways. When the person is struck directly by a lightning discharge, it is termed a *direct strike.* When lightning strikes an object that the person is touching, resulting in a transference of the energy, it is termed a *contact strike.* If lightning strikes an object, travels a certain distance, then "jumps" through the air and strikes the person, it is termed a *side flash.* If the current enters the leg of the person, travels through the lower part of the body, and exits out the other leg, it is termed *stride potential.* Lastly, when the lightning bolt hits the ground and travels to the person by way of the ground, it is termed *ground current.*

Lightning tends to flow over the surface of the body, often sparing the deeper tissues.

DIAGNOSIS

Diagnosis is made by visual examination and a history of the person having been outdoors when lightning was present or inside a structure that was hit by lightning and in contact with a conductive or grounding source. A detailed neurologic assessment should be completed, as should a thorough examination of the surface of the body for burns. A classic fern-like pattern of burn may be noted on the skin. An eye examination should be conducted for retinal, optic nerve, or occipital lobe damage. Baseline visual acuity should be measured because *cataracts, corneal ulcers,* or hemorrhage may occur. The ears should be examined for ruptured tympanic membrane. Vital signs should be assessed, including screening for hypertension. The cervical spine and the entire musculoskeletal system should be evaluated for injury.

TREATMENT

Treatment consists of restoring or maintaining the patient's respiratory effort. If the person is apneic, cardiac function ceases in a few minutes. If the person is in cardiac arrest, CPR must be initiated and continued for an extended period. Cardiac monitoring is indicated, along with observation for cerebral edema and respiratory insult. Fractures and lacerations, burns, and other injuries need to be treated according to facility protocol. Tetanus prophylaxis must be confirmed or administered if necessary. Follow-up eye examinations should be conducted because cataracts may develop in the year after the lightning strike.

PROGNOSIS

Prognosis varies according to the extent of the insult. When respiratory efforts are maintained, survival may be possible. Prompt institution of CPR when respiratory efforts are found absent also may result in survival of the victim. Those who do not have respiratory or cardiac activity cessation usually survive but require follow-up examinations of eyes and ears for late-onset problems. Burn treatment of points of entry and exit, as well as treatment of any other skin burns, is required.

PREVENTION

Seeking shelter during a thunder and lightning storm is wise. It is best to avoid seeking shelter under a tree. When no shelter is available, positioning oneself as low as possible on the ground is a prudent action.

PATIENT TEACHING

Provide patients and family members with safety information regarding lightning and thunder storms. Emphasize the importance of having CPR training and of providing immediate intervention to a lightning strike victim when doing so is safe and possible.

Extreme Heat (Hyperthermia)

DESCRIPTION

Hyperthermia occurs when an individual's core body temperature is much higher than the normal body temperature of 98.6° F. Accidentally occurring hyperthermia is the consequence of prolonged exposure to extreme environmental heat.

> ■ **ICD-9-CM Code 992.9** *(Effects of heat, unspecified)*
> *Effects of heat are coded by type. Once the diagnosis has been confirmed, refer to the current edition of the ICD-9-CM coding manual for the appropriate code and modifier.*

SYMPTOMS AND SIGNS

The person with hyperthermia may be experiencing heat stroke or heat exhaustion as a result of prolonged exposure to extremely hot temperatures. Heat stroke occurs when the person has a body temperature of 105° F or greater. The skin is hot, red, and usually dry. The patient may have a dry mouth, headache, nausea or vomiting, dizziness and weakness, and shortness of breath. The pulse is rapid and strong at the onset, gradually becoming weak, and the blood pressure decreases. The pupils are constricted. Patients exhibit anxiety, mental confusion, irritability, aggression, and even hysterical behavior. In extreme cases, the person collapses and experiences altered levels of consciousness and may have seizure activity.

Heat exhaustion produces profuse sweating, fatigue, headache, weakness, nausea, dizziness, and possible heat or muscle cramps. The pulse is weak and rapid; the skin is pale, cool, and moist; and the body temperature is normal or subnormal. The pupils are dilated.

PATIENT SCREENING

Hyperthermia is a life threatening emergency. The individual should be entered into the Emergency Medical System without delay. Until emergency care arrives to transport the person to an emergency facility, encourage family, friends or co-workers to move the individual from the extremely hot environment to a colder environment. Instruct them to loosen clothing and place cool moist clothes on the individual's face, neck, arms, and hands.

ETIOLOGY

Heat stroke results when the body's heat-regulating systems are unable to cope with the exposure to severe external heat sources. As the body overheats, its temperature rises to 105° to 110° F. Approximately one half of patients in these circumstances fail to perspire. Because no effective cooling mechanism is taking place, the body stores the heat, which eventually results in damage to the brain cells and subsequently permanent brain damage or death. The aged, infants, children, and malnourished and debilitated people are the most susceptible to heat stroke. Others who experience heat stroke are those who work near furnaces and intense sources of heat, as well as athletes who are exposed to the combination of high temperatures and high humidity.

Heat exhaustion is the result of salt or water depletion. Generally, the person is involved in strenuous activity in a hot, humid environment. As a result, the person experiences prolonged and profuse sweating, causing the loss of excessive amounts of salt and water. This mimics a mild state of shock.

DIAGNOSIS

Diagnosis of heat stroke is made by the presence of symptoms, especially the elevated body temperature. The history of exposure to high temperatures and humidity, along with the altered level of consciousness, aids in the diagnosis.

Diagnosis of heat exhaustion is made from the history and clinical findings, specifically the moist, pale skin and normal or below-normal body temperature of the patient.

TREATMENT

Treatment of heat stroke, possibly a life-threatening condition, must be aggressive and instituted promptly. It consists of cooling the body down. The first step is to move the person to a cooler environment, to remove what clothing possible, and to cool the body by pouring cool water over it or soaking it with a cool wet cloth. If the person begins to shiver, the cooling process should be slowed. It is imperative to bring the core temperature of the body below 100° F. The person should be transported to an emergency facility where vital signs can be monitored.

Treatment of persons with heat exhaustion consists of moving them to a cool place and applying cool compresses. They should be lying down with the feet elevated. If the person is fully conscious, give 4 ounces of cool water every 10 to 15 minutes.

PROGNOSIS
Prognosis varies and depends on the duration of the exposure and any underlying pathology. Prompt intervention with effective cooling may afford a positive outcome.

PREVENTION
Encourage patients to avoid lengthy exposure to hot environments. Advise them of the importance of staying hydrated during hot weather or when working in hot environments.

PATIENT TEACHING
Provide printed material to the patient or family on precautions to take to avoid hyperthermia.

Extreme Cold (Hypothermia)

DESCRIPTION
Hypothermia is a generalized cooling of the body in which the core temperature of the body drops below 95° F.

 ICD-9-CM Code 991.6

SYMPTOMS AND SIGNS
Hypothermia, a generalized severe cooling of the body, causes the person to shiver and have a feeling of extreme cold or numbness. Fatigue is followed by loss of coordination, thick speech, and disorientation. The skin appears blue and puffy and ash-colored for dark-skinned people, with the pulse being slow and weak. Core body temperature drops below 95° F. Breathing is slow and shallow, and the pupils are dilated. As the body temperature drops, the person experiences confusion, stupor, and unconsciousness.

ETIOLOGY
Hypothermia can occur when a person is exposed to wind, a cold environment, or cold water for prolonged periods. The elderly, very young, exhausted, and physically debilitated persons have

the greatest risk of hypothermia. Lack of adequate clothing or becoming wet, as in a rain storm, can add to the risk. Sudden immersion in cold water can cause hypothermia.

DIAGNOSIS
Diagnosis is made by the history, the clinical picture, and the finding of below-normal body temperature.

TREATMENT
Treatment of hypothermia, a life-threatening condition, must be aggressive and immediate. Any wet clothing must be removed, and gradual rewarming of the body is begun by wrapping the person in warm blankets and keeping the body dry. If auxiliary sources of heat such as hot packs or warm stones are not available, the warmth from another person's body as he or she embraces the patient can help warm the patient too. If the person is conscious, warm liquids should be given orally in small quantities. The patient should be transported to an emergency facility where vital signs can be monitored.

PROGNOSIS
Prognosis varies and depends on the duration of the exposure to cold and any underlying pathology.

PREVENTION
Prevention involves avoiding extremely cold temperatures.

PATIENT TEACHING
Encourage patients to avoid situations in which they may experience long periods of exposure to extreme cold. Advise them to wear adequate layers of clothing when they must be in an extremely cold environment.

Frostbite

DESCRIPTION
Frozen or extremely cold tissue, usually on the face, ears, fingers, and toes, is termed *frostbite*.

 ICD-9-CM Code 991.3 *(Frostbite of other and unspecified sites)*
Frostbite is coded by site. Once the diagnosis has been confirmed, refer to the current edition of the ICD-9-CM coding manual for the appropriate code and modifier.

SYMPTOMS AND SIGNS

Frostbite, usually occurring on the face, fingers, toes, and ears, causes the affected skin area to become white, or ashen in the case of dark-skinned people (Fig. 15–15). The person does not realize that the condition is occurring because little or no pain is felt as the tissue freezes. As the freezing deepens, the underlying tissue becomes firm, and the skin takes on a waxy appearance (Fig. 15–16).

PATIENT SCREENING

Frostbite requires prompt assessment and intervention. Most individuals will be seen in an emergency facility and assessed for additional hypothermal insults.

ETIOLOGY

Frostbite occurs when tissue is exposed to cold air, water, or objects. Ice crystals form between the cells of the skin. As the freezing continues, fluid that is drawn from the cells subsequently freezes. People who have undergone trauma, the elderly, newborns, and those wearing wet clothing or tightly laced footwear are at greatest risk when exposed to cold temperatures.

DIAGNOSIS

Diagnosis is made by visual examination and a history of exposure to cold. The depth or degree of the frostbite is determined by the color and appearance of the skin.

TREATMENT

Treatment consists of removing the patient from the cold environment. People suffering from superficial frostbite should be warmed with an external source of even heat. The temperature of the heat source should not be above 105° F. The affected skin area should *never* be rubbed. Patients suffering from frostbite should be treated by a physician if possible. Rewarming of deep frostbite (frozen tissue) should not begin until professional medical care can be provided. The person should be kept warm, vital signs should be monitored, and alcohol should *never* be given.

PROGNOSIS

Prognosis varies and depends on length of exposure and depth of the insult. Additional variables

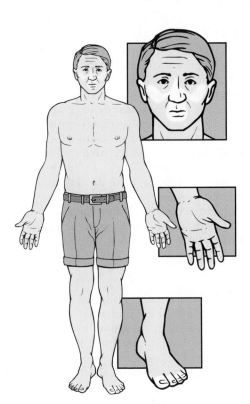

FIGURE 15–15 Usual sites of frostbite.

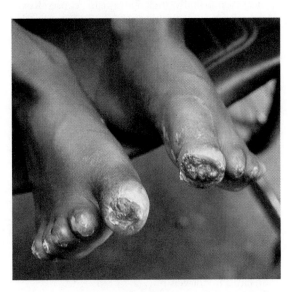

FIGURE 15–16 Frostbite of the toes. Similar changes also may occur in the fingers. (From Stevens A, Lowe J: *Pathology—illustrated review in color*, ed 2, London, 2000, Mosby.)

Bites

are the age of the patient and general health status, as well as underlying pathology.

PREVENTION

Encourage patients to wear gloves, hats, scarves, and heavy socks when the possibility of prolonged exposure to cold is anticipated. Advise them to replace any wet clothing with dry clothing to prevent additional exacerbation from the cold temperature.

PATIENT TEACHING

Provide patients with written information concerning prevention of frostbite. Advise parents to attire children in adequate gloves, hats and scarves during outside winter activities.

Bites

Bites can occur at any time and on any part of the body. They range from the annoying insect bite to bites by domestic animals, reptiles, or even other humans. Insect bites may be insignificant or may be life threatening. Mosquito bites can cause merely itching or can cause *encephalitis,* resulting from infection with, for example, West Nile virus, which is contracted through a bite from an infected mosquito. Additionally, tick bites can cause Rocky Mountain spotted fever, malaria, or Lyme disease. Animal bites range in severity from mere nips that do not break the skin and cause no serious disease to life-threatening bites that carry the risk of rabies and infection.

Insect Bites

DESCRIPTION

An insect bite is puncture of the skin by the bite or sting of any insect or arthropod; that may involve the injection of venom into the tissue of the individual. Examples of insects that commonly bite humans include fleas, mosquitoes, lice, horseflies, fire ants, and mites. Bees, wasps, and hornets can sting an individual and inject venom, thereby causing localized pain and swelling. Spiders also have a tendency to bite or sting humans and inject venom.

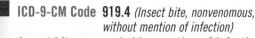

ICD-9-CM Code 919.4 *(Insect bite, nonvenomous, without mention of infection)*
Insect bites are coded by mention of infection. Once the diagnosis has been confirmed, refer to the current edition of the ICD-9-CM coding manual for the appropriate code and modifier.

SYMPTOMS AND SIGNS

The symptoms and signs of an insect bite or sting vary with the type of insect that has bitten or stung the individual (Figs. 15–17 and 15–18). Usually, a sharp, stinging pain is felt, which may be followed by itching, redness, or swelling at the site. If the patient experiences a systemic reaction to the bite, he or she will have itching on the palms of the hands or soles of the feet, the neck, or the groin, or generalized itching, which may include a rash over the entire body. As an allergic reaction develops, the patient experiences generalized edema, *dyspnea,* weakness, nausea, shock, and unconsciousness.

PATIENT SCREENING

Individuals reporting insect stings or bites require prompt assessment. Some bites or stings may precipitate an allergic reaction, often a very rapid and life-threatening reaction. Those with known severe allergic response to certain types of bites or stings usually will require emergency intervention as a life-saving measure. Many such individuals and their families are aware of the potential danger and carry a "bee-sting" kit containing an "Epi-pen" with them at all times for emergency injection of epinephrine to reverse the allergic response. Follow-up appointments will be scheduled to consult with the patient and the family about the dangers of insect stings and preventive measures.

ETIOLOGY

The injury occurs when the insect either bites or stings the patient. *Venom* is injected into the tissue, resulting in the body's response to a foreign protein. Some of the more common types of bites or stings are those of mosquitoes, bees, wasps, hornets, spiders, fire ants, ticks, and fleas. Occurring less often are bites by black widow spiders, brown recluse spiders, and scorpions.

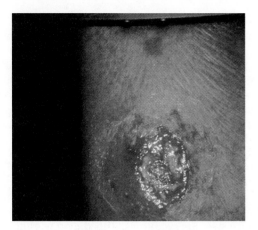

FIGURE 15–17 Brown recluse spider bite after 48 hours of treatment. (From Hill MJ: *Skin disorders—Mosby's clinical nursing series,* St. Louis, 1994, Mosby. Courtesy Dr. William N. New, Dallas, Tex.)

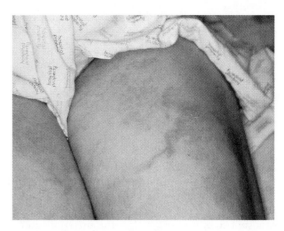

FIGURE 15–18 Multiple bites of imported fire ants. (From Hill MJ: *Skin disorders—Mosby's clinical nursing series,* St. Louis, 1994, Mosby. Courtesy Dermatology Department, University of Texas Southwestern Medical School, Dallas, Tex.)

DIAGNOSIS

Diagnosis is made by visual examination and history. It is hoped that the patient can identify or give a description of the offending insect. Some insect bites or stings leave characteristic signs.

TREATMENT

The first step in treating an insect sting is to determine whether the stinger is still present. If it is present, it must be removed to prevent further damage. The best method of removal is scraping across the site of the sting with a plastic card or a fingernail. (The use of forceps or tweezers squeezes more venom into the site.) The area is then cleansed with soap and water. Application of a dry dressing, cold pack, or *anesthetic* sprays affords some comfort. The person should be observed for any signs of allergic reaction to the sting or bite. Lyme disease, the result of a tick bite, and encephalitis, the result of a mosquito bite, are discussed in Chapters 7 and 13, respectively.

People with black widow spider, brown recluse spider, or scorpion bites should be transported to an emergency facility. Aggressive treatment includes cleansing of the wound, the administration of medication for pain relief, cold applications, the administration of antivenin, and monitoring of vital signs.

PROGNOSIS

Prognosis varies depending on the degree to which the person is sensitized to the offending foreign protein injected during the bite or sting. Many bites or stings resolve without treatment and no sensitization occurs. Recovery for those with moderate to severe reaction may be speedy or slow depending on any underlying pathology. Refer to Chapters 7 and 13 for additional information about Lyme disease and encephalitis.

PREVENTION

Prevention includes avoiding situations where exposure to the offending insect may occur. Use of insect repellant may be helpful. Education of family members and co-workers concerning any possible severe reaction and what actions are necessary to counteract a potentially life-threatening allergic response is beneficial.

PATIENT TEACHING

Provide the patient with information pertaining to prevention of insect bites and stings. Instruct the family about procedures to follow in case of an emergency situation involving severe reaction.

Bites

Bites

Rocky Mountain Spotted Fever

DESCRIPTION

Rocky Mountain spotted fever, a tick-borne disease, is a severe systemic infection. It is the most commonly reported rickettsial disease in the United States.

■ **ICD-9-CM Code 082.0**

SYMPTOMS AND SIGNS

The patient may recall being bitten by a tick, typically during outdoor activity such as camping and hiking. Several days to 2 weeks later, a sudden onset of fever, severe headache, vomiting, *malaise,* and *myalgia* occur. Four days after the onset of fever, a characteristic *maculopapular* rash is noted, which spreads over the body. Small hemorrhages appear under the skin, the characteristic sign that gives the disease its name. Inflammation of blood vessels (vasculitis) affects the skin and other organs, leading to systemic manifestations in the heart, lungs, kidney, and nervous system. After 2 to 3 weeks, the skin begins to peel (Fig. 15–19).

PATIENT SCREENING

Individuals reporting symptoms of fever, severe headache, vomiting, malaise, and myalgia require prompt assessment.

ETIOLOGY

The causative agent, *Rickettsia rickettsii,* is transmitted by the wood tick and is carried in the feces of infected ticks. It is introduced into the bloodstream of a person during a prolonged tick bite (duration of 4 to 6 hours). Once it is in the bloodstream, the organism, an intracellular parasite, reproduces in certain cells and destroys them. The disease cannot be transmitted from person to person.

DIAGNOSIS

Although Rocky Mountain spotted fever is difficult to diagnose, a history of a tick bite or recent outdoor activity in tick-infested areas and the onset of severe systemic symptoms, with the appearance of the characteristic rash, suggest the disease (Fig. 15–20). Laboratory findings include a positive complement fixation reaction, which measures the antigen–antibody reaction occurring in the body, and thereby the severity of infection. Changes in blood-clotting components in the blood may be noted. Isolation of the organism in a blood culture confirms the diagnosis.

TREATMENT

The treatment of choice for Rocky Mountain spotted fever is antibiotic therapy with tetracycline and symptomatic relief with the administration of analgesics. Infection confers lifetime immunity.

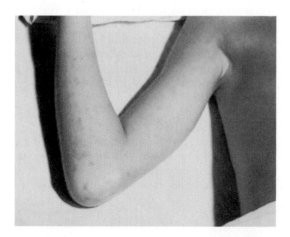

FIGURE 15–19 Rocky Mountain spotted fever rash on wrist. (From Grimes D: *Infectious diseases—Mosby's clinical nursing series,* St. Louis, 1994, Mosby.)

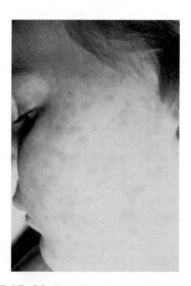

FIGURE 15–20 Rocky Mountain spotted fever rash on side of face 9 days after onset. (From Grimes D: *Infectious diseases—Mosby's clinical nursing series,* St. Louis, 1994, Mosby.)

PROGNOSIS

Prognosis is good with rapid diagnosis and treatment with antibiotic regimen. Underlying pathology or concurrent health problems may complicate the outcome.

PREVENTION

Preventive measures include wearing protective clothing and applying insect repellent to clothing and exposed skin. Visual inspection of the skin for the presence of ticks should be made every few hours during and after outdoor activity in infested areas. If a tick is found, it should be removed carefully with tweezers, avoiding handling of the tick.

PATIENT TEACHING

Encourage individuals to wear proper protective clothing when in environments where ticks may reside. Also, instruct them to make a visual inspection of the skin for ticks or apparent tick bites every few hours.

Malaria
DESCRIPTION

Malaria is a severe generalized infection caused by the bite of an *Anopheles* mosquito that is infected with a *Plasmodium*-type protozoa.

■ **ICD-9-CM Code 084.6**

ENRICHMENT
ALTITUDE SICKNESS

ALTITUDE SICKNESS OR ACUTE MOUNTAIN sickness is a disorder associated with the low oxygen content of the atmosphere at high altitudes. It occurs when individuals make a rapid ascent into altitudes usually above 8000 feet. Symptoms include nausea and vomiting, headache, dizziness, difficulty sleeping, and air hunger. Mild symptoms that mimic jet lag or the flu can subside as the body adjusts to the higher altitude. More severe and even life-threatening altitude sickness can cause prostration, cardiac disturbances, and cerebral edema with possible seizures and death. Pulmonary edema is another severe state of altitude sickness. It is possible for those with heart problems to experience angina and subsequent myocardial infarction triggered by the high altitude (Fig. 15–21).

In addition to the high elevation, dehydration is a contributing factor. Those who experience symptoms should descend to a lower altitude and drink plentiful amounts of water. Rest and curtailing stressful activities helps in relieving symptoms and is a necessary intervention for shortness of breath and increased heart rate.

Prevention includes acclimating one's self to the higher altitudes slowly over a period of a few days, drinking extra fluids, and avoiding alcohol and smoking. It is best not to climb more than 3000 feet a day when at elevations greater than 8000 feet.

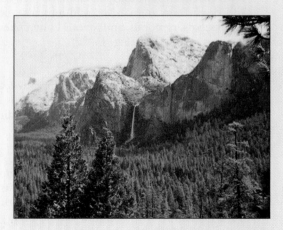

FIGURE 15–21 Typical site for onset of altitude sickness. (Courtesy David L. Frazier, 1999.)

SYMPTOMS AND SIGNS

Malaria is an acute, sometimes chronic, serious, infectious illness. It is characterized by a classic cycle of chills, fever, and sweats, in that order. The patient also may have headache, nausea, fatigue, and myalgia. Although the course and severity of the disease can vary, bouts of malaria usually last from 1 to 4 weeks. Signs include an enlarged spleen, an enlarged liver, and anemia. The symptoms have a tendency to recur and may persist for years.

PATIENT SCREENING

An individual reporting symptoms of chills, fever, and sweats, possibly combined with headache, nausea, fatigue, and myalgia, requires prompt assessment.

ETIOLOGY

Malaria is caused by four species of the protozoan genus *Plasmodium*, which is transmitted from infected human to human by the bite of mosquito **vectors** or, less commonly, by blood transfusion or intravenous drug use. After they are introduced into the body, the protozoan parasites feed on hemoglobin and reproduce within red blood cells (RBCs). Malaria is endemic in tropical and subtropical areas such as South and Central America, Asia, and Africa and usually is brought to the United States by travelers returning from these areas.

DIAGNOSIS

Laboratory testing of infected individuals reveals decreased hemoglobin level, decreased platelet count, prolonged *prothrombin time (PT),* and a positive serum antibody test result. Diagnosis is confirmed by identifying the *Plasmodium* organism in a blood smear.

TREATMENT

Malaria is treated with chloroquine, an antimalarial drug, given orally. **Antipyretics** are given for fever. Infusion of packed RBCs may be required for anemia. Each new case of malaria must be reported to the local board of health.

PROGNOSIS

Prognosis varies depending on the response to treatment and any underlying pathology.

PREVENTION

A prophylactic course of chloroquine may be given before a person embarks on travel to known endemic areas.

PATIENT TEACHING

Provide the patient who may be traveling to endemic areas with information on prophylactic medications. Also, instruct them regarding possible symptoms of malaria and encourage them to seek medical treatment at the onset of any such symptoms.

Animal Bites

DESCRIPTION

An animal bite is any bite inflicted on an individual by another animal. The source may be another human, a domestic pet, or any wild animal.

> **ICD-9-CM Code 879.8** *(Open wound[s] [multiple] of unspecified site[s], without mention of complications)*
> The ICD-9-CM coding manual applies this code to any animal bites. Refer to the current edition of the ICD-9-CM coding manual for additional information and appropriate codes according to site.

SYMPTOMS AND SIGNS

Broken skin with evidence of teeth marks is the usual clinical finding related to an animal bite. Puncture wounds are present, with possible tearing of the skin. Bleeding is usually evident, and the flesh actually may be bitten away. A discoloration of the surrounding skin occurs, indicating bruising to the area. The patient usually reports pain at the site.

ETIOLOGY

Typically the bite occurs when the offending animal is agitated, frightened, threatened, or angry. Bites can be from domestic animals, such as cats and dogs; farm animals; or wild animals, such as skunks, bats, raccoons, and foxes. Human bites also have been recorded (Fig. 15–22).

DIAGNOSIS

Diagnosis is made by a history and by physical examination. The pattern of the teeth marks is helpful in determining the type of animal that did the biting if not immediately known.

TREATMENT

Treatment begins with cleansing of the wound. If bleeding cannot be controlled, *hemostasis* is achieved by **cautery** or suture. Depending on the site and severity of the wound, plastic surgery may be indicated for optimal repair.

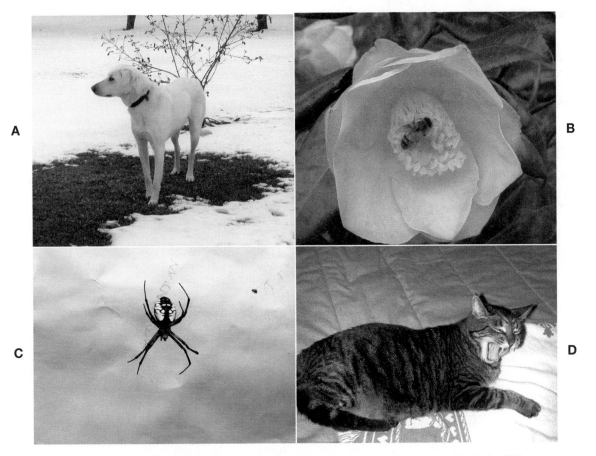

FIGURE 15–22 Insects and animals possibly capable of inflicting bites. (**A-C** courtesy David L. Frazier, 2003; **D** courtesy Mark Boswell, 2003.)

Rabies is transmitted through the saliva of infected animals. If the offending animal is a domestic pet, it usually is not too difficult to confirm the most recent date of rabies inoculation or to quarantine the animal for the time necessary to rule out rabies infection. Most communities require reporting animal bites to the local animal control agency or a local law enforcement agency who will follow through on determining the rabies inoculation status of the animal. If it is not possible to determine whether the animal is rabid, the injured person probably will have to undergo a series of injections to confer immunity to rabies.

As with most invasive trauma, a sterile dressing should be applied. Tetanus prophylaxis is confirmed or administered if necessary, and antibiotics may be prescribed as an additional prophylactic measure.

PROGNOSIS

Prognosis varies depending on the extent of the damage to tissue as well on any existing personal pathology. If the animal is rabid, prognosis becomes guarded.

PREVENTION

Prevention often is difficult, especially when the bite is not knowingly provoked by the actions of the victim.

PATIENT TEACHING

Encourage children not to approach or touch animals, even those who are in a restrained environment. Advise individuals with pets to keep the animal's inoculations, especially for rabies, current. Instruct the patient or family member on wound care and also on the importance of completing any antibiotic therapy that has been prescribed.

Snakebites

DESCRIPTION

A penetrating tissue wound made by the fangs or teeth of a snake is a snakebite.

■ **ICD-9-CM Code** **989.5** *(Bites of venomous snakes, lizards, and spiders)*
Bites of nonvenomous snakes are coded as open wounds. Refer to the current edition of the ICD-

9-CM coding manual for additional information and appropriate codes according to site.

SYMPTOMS AND SIGNS

The patient may have actually seen the snake that gave the bite or may not have been aware of the snake at the time the bite happened. In either event, the patient will have a noticeable bite to the skin or possibly only a slight skin discoloration at the site of injury. Burning pain is present, and swelling begins around the bite; however, this reaction may be delayed, developing slowly over time. The pulse rate becomes rapid, and the patient begins to experience weakness, visual difficulties, and nausea and vomiting. Signs and symptoms of the poisoning may take 30 minutes to several hours to develop. Coral snakes are extremely poisonous and leave small chew-type teeth marks rather than the two distinct fang marks of other poisonous snakes (Fig. 15–23).

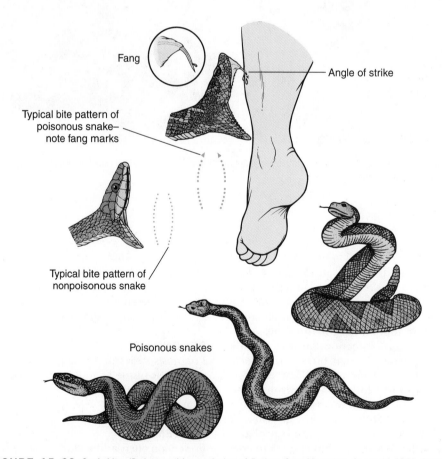

FIGURE 15–23 Snakebite. (Redrawn with permission of Patient Care Magazine. Copyright 1976, Patient Care Publications, Inc., Montvale, NJ.)

PATIENT SCREENING

Complaints reporting a possible snake bite require prompt assessment and intervention. The Emergency Medical System should be activated for transportation of the victim to the nearest emergency care facility.

ETIOLOGY

The poisoning from the snakebite usually takes 1 to 2 days to develop unless the person is allergic to the foreign protein of the venom, which will speed up the reaction time. Four kinds of poisonous snakes are known to inhabit the United States: rattlesnakes, copperheads, water moccasins, and coral snakes. Rattlesnakes account for the greatest number of poisonous snake bites. Some bites are the work of nonpoisonous snakes, but all snakebites should be treated as poisonous by the first aid provider.

DIAGNOSIS

Diagnosis is made by history and visual examination of the affected area. Typically, two fang marks in the skin are indicative of poisonous snakebites the exception is the bite of a coral snake, which appears as a chew-type bite that leaves teeth marks (see Fig. 15–23).

TREATMENT

First aid and intervention at the scene consists of removing the person from the injury site to avoid further risk and keeping her or him calm and quiet. The EMS system should be activated. Cleanse the bitten area with soap and water. Any jewelry, including rings, or other constricting objects should be removed from the affected limb. The extremity should be immobilized and, if possible, kept below the level of the heart. Transportation to the nearest emergency facility should be initiated as soon as possible so that aggressive treatment can begin immediately. If it is not possible to reach emergency care within 30 minutes, consideration should be given to suctioning the bite with equipment from a snakebite kit. Antivenin may be given to the patient and vital functions are supported as needed. The protocol for snakebite treatment indicates that cold should *not* be applied, the wound should *not* be cut, tourniquets should *not* be applied, and electrical shock should *not* be applied.

PROGNOSIS

Prognosis varies depending on the poisonous state of the snake. Bites from nonpoisonous snakes usually resolve and heal with few complications. Recovery from bites of poisonous snakes depends on the availability of anitvenin, the promptness of the treatment, and the location of the bite on the body. Preexisting underlying pathology of the patient may dictate the outcome.

PREVENTION

Using caution in areas known to be inhabited by snakes is prudent (Fig. 15–24). When in an area where snakes are likely to be present, wear heavy "snake" boots to prevent possible bites from penetrating tissue. Avoid grassy wet areas if possible.

PATIENT TEACHING

Encourage individuals to regard all snakebites as being potentially poisonous. Provide information about areas in the community that snakes are likely to inhabit and recommend avoidance of these areas. If travel within or occupation of these areas is necessary, encourage the wearing of heavy boots to prevent bites around feet and lower legs.

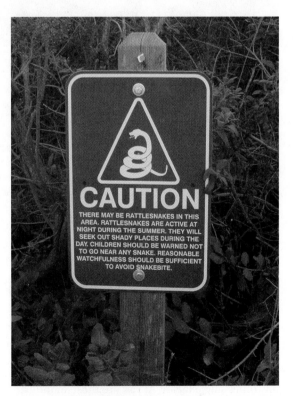

FIGURE 15–24 Warning sign concerning presence of rattlesnakes. (Courtesy David L. Frazier, 2003.)

ENRICHMENT

POISONING

POISONS ARE ANY SUBSTANCES that, when introduced into the body, cause illness or injury; many cause death. Poisoning can be accidental or intentional. Poisons can be introduced into the body by absorption through the skin, ingestion through the gastrointestinal (GI) tract, inhalation through the respiratory system, and injection through a sting, bite, or hypodermic needle. The signs and symptoms vary according to the poison and the method of introduction into the body. Many poisons are found in the domestic setting and often are the cause of exposure. Refer to Table 15–1 for a list of common chemicals found in the domestic setting.

Ingested or swallowed poisons can include foods, alcohol, chemicals, medications, and plants. Inhaled poisons include gases such as carbon monoxide, carbon dioxide, nitrous oxide, chlorine, and fumes from chemicals or drugs. Absorbed poisons include chemicals or oils from certain plants. Injected poisons include venom injected by bites from insects, spiders, ticks, or snakes or drugs given via a hypodermic needle.

Because of the vast number of poisons and methods of introduction into the body, it is impossible to identify symptoms, etiology, diagnosis, and treatment for each toxic substance. General guidelines to follow are (1) identify the toxic substance and (2) contact a poison control center or emergency facility for assistance. Of utmost importance is that the rescuer or care provider not compromise his or her own safety, especially when inhalation of toxic fumes could be involved.

TABLE 15–1
Common Chemical Toxins Available in Domestic Settings

AGENT	EFFECTS
Methyl alcohol	Metabolic acidosis, neurologic damage
Ethylene glycol	Metabolic acidosis, oxalate deposition in kidneys, acute tubular necrosis
Carbon tetrachloride	Centrilobular necrosis in liver, tubular necrosis in kidneys
Carbon monoxide	Tissue hypoxia by forming carboxyhemoglobin
	Headache, dizziness, and confusion (early features)
	Delayed damage to basal ganglia and white matter
	Coma and death with high saturation
Strong alkalis	Ulceration of oropharynx and esophagus

From Stevens A, Lowe J: *Pathology: illustrated review in color*, ed 2, London, 2000, Mosby.

Cumulative Trauma (Repetitive Motion Trauma, Overuse Syndrome)

Cumulative trauma disorders, or repetitive motion injuries, are common to numerous occupations. They account for more time lost from work than any other single factor. At risk are those in industry who perform repetitive tasks, including those who keyboard on a regular and continuous basis, cashiers who scan products across conveyor belts and those who target practice and those engaging in certain sports.

Soft tissue injuries that develop over time as a result of repetitive activities cause continuing stress on specific muscles or nerves. These injuries can result from improper posture of the wrist, arm, back, shoulder, or legs. Many occur because of pressure

ENRICHMENT
DeQuervain Disease

D E QUERVAIN DISEASE is an inflammation of the tendons of the thumb. It is caused by irritation of the long abductor and short extensor tendons. Repetitive motion causes edema and tenderness in the thumb and at its base. Pain is experienced on the radial aspect of the thumb at the base as the thumb is moved away from the hand. Treatment involves splinting the thumb and wrist to restrict movement and hopefully resolve the inflammatory process. Antiinflammatory agents may be prescribed. Steroid injections may be necessary for relief of symptoms. Although most conditions respond to medical management, surgery to split the tendon sheath encasing the tendon is also a treatment option. Prevention involves the avoidance of the repetitive motion, forceful gripping, and excessive movements of the thumb.

centered on the hand or wrist with frequent repetitive motion for an extended time. In the industrial setting, improper use of hand-held tools, especially with excessive or improper grip, can cause cumulative trauma disorders. Additionally, continuous vibration contributes to increased occurrence of trauma. These disorders include but are not limited to white finger *(Raynaud phenomenon),* trigger finger, carpal tunnel syndrome, tennis elbow, thoracic outlet syndrome, de Quervain disease, synovitis, tenosynovitis, and nonspecific **tendinitis.** Cumulative trauma develops over an extended time period, so the onset of symptoms is *insidious.* Much investigation may be necessary to pinpoint the repetitive task that has caused the trauma.

Carpal Tunnel Syndrome

DESCRIPTION
Entrapment and compression of the median nerve in the carpal tunnel causes pain and numbness in the wrist, hands, and fingers.

■ **ICD-9-CM Code 354.0**

SYMPTOMS AND SIGNS
The patient experiences a numbness of hands and fingers, with pain occurring in these areas at night. Swelling of the wrist or hand and "fluttering" of the fingers are additional symptoms. The patient often is observed cradling the arm or rubbing the hand or arm.

PATIENT SCREENING
Although not an emergency, assessment of this painful condition should be accomplished at the earliest available and convenient time.

ETIOLOGY
Tendons, blood vessels, and the median nerve pass through a narrow tunnel that extends from the wrist to the hand (Fig. 15–25). Carpal tunnel syndrome results when the tendons within the tunnel become inflamed from repetitive overuse of the hand, wrist, or fingers, thereby causing entrapment of the median nerve as it passes through the wrist, which results in the pinching of the median nerve (Fig. 15–26).

DIAGNOSIS
The clinical findings, along with the history of the repetitive motion activities, suggests carpal tunnel syndrome. Two specific minor tests aid in the confirmation of the diagnosis. One is the median nerve percussion test (Fig. 15–27), in which the examiner taps his or her fingers along the inside of the affected wrist, eliciting a pins-and-needles sensation in the hand and fingers. The other is the Phalen wrist flexor test, in which the patient presses the backs of the hands together to bend the wrists as far downward as possible, without applying force, and holds them together for 60 seconds. The fingers should be kept pointing toward the floor. In a positive test result, the patient experiences numbness and tingling of the hand or fingers.

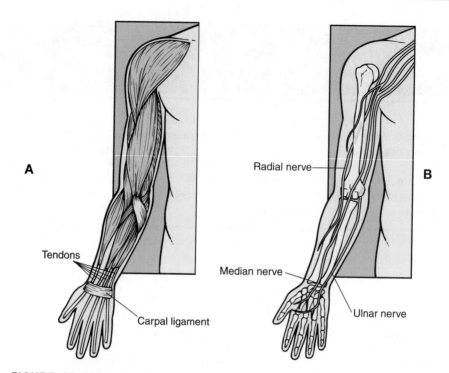

FIGURE 15–25 Anatomy of arm, wrist, and hand. **A,** Muscles, tendons, and carpal ligament. **B,** Nerves. (Redrawn from "Lesson Plan for Ergonomic Seminar Slides," Farmington Hills, Mich, 1994, Ergonomics, Aro, ARO Tool Products/Ingersoll-Rand Professional Tools.)

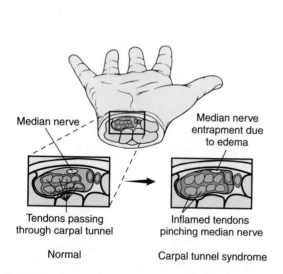

FIGURE 15–26 Entrapment of the median nerve in the carpal tunnel space. (Redrawn from "Lesson Plan for Ergonomic Seminar Slides," Farmington Hills, Mich, 1994, Ergonomics, Aro, ARO Tool Products/Ingersoll-Rand Professional Tools.)

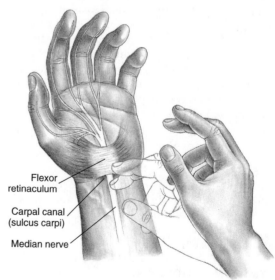

FIGURE 15–27 Elicitation of Tinel sign. (From Seidel HM et al: *Mosby's guide to physical examination,* ed 5, St. Louis, 2003, Mosby.)

TREATMENT

Treatment consists of physical therapy and identification and cessation of the repetitive motion to rest the wrist and hand. Antiinflammatory drugs are prescribed, and a splint may be applied to maintain the wrist in a neutral position. As a final resort, surgery to divide the carpal ligament is performed in an attempt to relieve pressure on the nerve.

PROGNOSIS

Prognosis is usually favorable after surgical intervention. Compliance with suggested or prescribed therapy is helpful for a positive outcome.

PREVENTION

Prevention is important, so **ergonomic** studies and correction of improper repetitive activities should be implemented.

Prevention involves using ergonomically correct devices and positions when engaging in activities that tend to cause the repetitive motion injury.

PATIENT TEACHING

Encourage patients to avoid repetitive motion that places the arm, hand, and wrist in compromised positions. Work with employers to eliminate or modify tasks that require repetitive motion that places the median nerve at risk.

Tennis Elbow

DESCRIPTION

Tennis elbow, technically known as lateral humeral epicondylitis, is the result of repetitive movement involving flexion of the wrist against resistance. The result of this repetitive action is an inflammatory condition of the tissue at the distal portion of the humerus.

 ICD-9-CM Code 726.32

SYMPTOMS AND SIGNS

The patient has pain in the outer (lateral) aspect of the elbow and lower arm. Weakness is exhibited in the affected extremity.

PATIENT SCREENING

Tennis elbow is not an emergency but can be quite painful. Schedule the patient to be seen at the next available appointment.

ETIOLOGY

The extensor attachment to the lateral humeral condyle becomes inflamed. Repetitive motion in the elbow, usually with accompanying stress to the joint, causes this inflammatory condition.

DIAGNOSIS

Diagnosis is made by evaluating the clinical findings and by physical examination.

TREATMENT

Treatment consists of stopping the repetitive task and resting the affected arm. An elastic brace can be placed distal to the elbow to alter the fulcrum of the activity. Nonsteroidal antiinflammatory drugs (NSAIDs) are also helpful in decreasing the inflammation. Steroid injections into the joint space may afford relief.

PROGNOSIS

Prognosis is good when the repetitive motion is alleviated. Resting the affected limb usually affords pain relief and the condition may resolve by itself. When steroid injections are provided, the condition usually improves.

PREVENTION

Use of proper body mechanics when engaging in activities involving the shoulder and arm is helpful as a preventative measure. Recognition of stressful activities and modification of the activity also may be helpful in prevention. If the condition is the result of an occupational task, explore ergonomically correct methods for performing the task.

PATIENT TEACHING

Provide the patient with information and suggestions regarding ergonomically correct methods of performing activities that place stress on the elbow joint. When physical therapy is prescribed, encourage compliance with the recommended exercises.

Trigger Finger

DESCRIPTION

The index finger has a lump or knot that appears on the flexor tendon. Flexion or extension of the finger may be interrupted and then begin again in a jerking type motion.

ICD-9-CM Code 727.03

Cumulative Trauma (Repetitive Motion Trauma, Overuse Syndrome)

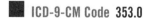

SYMPTOMS AND SIGNS

A lump or knot appears on the flexor tendon of the affected index finger. Movement of the finger may be temporarily interrupted and then continues on with a jerking-type motion.

PATIENT SCREENING

The patient should be scheduled for the next available appointment.

ETIOLOGY

The cause of trigger finger is excessive use of the index finger resulting from difficult repetitive finger movement or trauma to the tendon sheath.

DIAGNOSIS

Diagnosis is made by evaluating the clinical findings, history, and physical examination.

TREATMENT

As with other cumulative trauma, cessation of the repetitive activity and rest of the affected part is the prescribed course of treatment.

PROGNOSIS

Prognosis is good when the repetitive motion is halted.

PREVENTION

No method of prevention other than avoiding the repetitive activity is known.

PATIENT TEACHING

Encourage the patient to allow the finger to rest.

Thoracic Outlet Syndrome (Brachial Plexus Injury)

DESCRIPTION

Thoracic outlet syndrome (TOS) is the compression of the brachial plexus nerves.

■ ICD-9-CM Code 353.0

SYMPTOMS AND SIGNS

Thoracic outlet syndrome causes the patient to experience pain in the arm of the affected side. *Paresthesia* of the fingers also is experienced, along with weakness and diminished grasp capability in the fingers and thumb. The small muscles of the hand may even begin to waste away.

PATIENT SCREENING

Although not an emergency, the condition will cause the patient pain and possibly apprehension because of the numbness in the fingers and the continual dropping of items. Schedule the patient for the next available appointment.

ETIOLOGY

The performance of repetitive tasks that cause continual **hyperabduction** of the arm is one of the causative factors of this condition. Other causes include a continual dropping of the shoulder girdle, a cervical rib, or a fibrous band that develops around the nerve plexus.

DIAGNOSIS

Diagnosis is made by evaluating the clinical findings, history, and physical examination. *Electromyography (EMG)* aids in confirmation of the diagnosis.

TREATMENT

The cessation of any continued hyperabduction of the arm helps to relieve symptoms. When a cervical rib is the cause, it may be surgically removed. Entrapment of the brachial plexus nerves by the anterior scalene muscle usually necessitates a surgical release of any fibrous band or entrapping tissue.

PROGNOSIS

When the condition is the result of hyperabduction of the arm, cessation of the movement is helpful in resolution of the pain. When the condition is caused by a cervical rib or entrapped nerve, prognosis is good with surgical intervention to release the entrapped nerve or remove the cervical rib.

PREVENTION

Cessation of the offending movement of the arm may prevent the continuation of the condition. For a structural cause, there is no prevention.

PATIENT TEACHING

Discuss causative factors with the patient. Provide instructions for care of the incision if surgery is the treatment option.

Tendinitis

DESCRIPTION

Tendinitis (tendonitis) is an inflammation of a tendon that is usually caused by insult or injury to the tendon.

■ ICD-9-CM Code 726.90

SYMPTOMS AND SIGNS

The patient experiences nonspecific pain anywhere along the route of the tendon or its attachments. The most common symptom is acute pain.

PATIENT SCREENING

The patient experiencing severe pain requires prompt assessment. Schedule an appointment as soon as possible.

ETIOLOGY

Tendinitis is an inflammation of a tendon. It is caused by an insult to the tendon resulting from prolonged or improper activity of the affected part. Calcium deposits often are associated with tendinitis, and the bursa around the tendon also may be involved.

DIAGNOSIS

Nonspecific tendinitis is difficult to diagnose. A careful history indicates the event or events that caused the stress to the involved area. If the shoulder is involved, a 50- to 130-degree abduction of the affected arm causes pain.

TREATMENT

Treatment is aimed at reducing pain, decreasing inflammation, and preserving the integrity of the joint involved. Resting the involved area is important, as is administering oral antiinflammatory drugs and applying ice. Steroids may be injected into the joint space. If the joint (e.g., the shoulder) becomes fixed (frozen shoulder), the adhesions that have formed may need to be released surgically to allow full range of motion (ROM) of the joint.

PROGNOSIS

Prognosis is unpredictable because of the tendon being involved and the uncertain response to treatment and rest.

PREVENTION

Prevention involves avoiding the strenuous activity that initiates and subsequently aggravates the condition. With calcium deposit involvement, prevention is unlikely.

PATIENT TEACHING

Encourage patients to be compliant with prescribed drug therapy, physical therapy, and rest of the affected part.

Physical and Psychological Assault Trauma

Violence inflicted on a victim by others takes many forms, including child abuse, spouse abuse, abuse against elders, psychological abuse, sexual abuse, and rape. Victimization of individuals has become so prevalent that health-care providers are now trained to identify people who have been victimized, to treat their physical and emotional trauma, and to report incidents or suspicion of abuse as required by law.

Violence occurs in all areas of society, affecting both sexes, occurring at all socioeconomic levels, and including the entire age spectrum. The number of occurrences continues to increase, even though societal and cultural values typically expressed in the United States do not condone such behavior. Health-care providers are encouraged to provide unconditional support for victims.

Violence has taken on a new dimension in the past few years in the form of terrorist attacks and bioterrorism. (Refer to the Alert box on Bioterrorism for additional information.)

Child Abuse

DESCRIPTION

Physical, psychological, or sexual injury to a child is considered child abuse. The most commonly observed form is physical abuse because the resulting injuries are usually apparent. Signs of psychological abuse may be evidenced in the actions of the child. Sexual abuse may be discovered collaterally when complaints by the child of discomfort in the genital region are investigated or the

ALERT

BIOTERRORISM

Bioterrorism is a source of great public concern. Anthrax, small-pox, plague, botulism, and radiation exposure are possible sources of danger. Government agencies and health-care providers are re-searching these conditions and exploring treatment options. Silent and deliberate attacks can seriously threaten life and cause social disruption. Awareness of the likelihood of the threats and knowl-edge of these conditions and possible intervention measures may prevent a potentially catastrophic final outcome. Updates about these conditions will be provided by the health care communities and government agencies.

The following are thumbnail sketches of bioterrorism agents that a terrorist group would be likely to choose:

Anthrax—Anthrax, a bacterial infection is caused by *Bacillus anthracis,* and can affect the skin, intestinal tract, or respiratory system. Anthrax traditionally has affected mainly agricultural animals and their handlers. Recently pulmonary anthrax has occurred in the United States, and the outbreak has been suspected of being the result of terrorist activity. Pulmonary anthrax begins when a sufficient amount of spores suspended in the air are inhaled into the lungs. Once infected, the person complains of fever, fatigue, muscle aches, chest pain, cough, and severe respiratory distress. Without very early medical intervention, most will die. As soon as exposure to the disease is confirmed, administration of vaccine and antibiotic therapy is begun. Diagnosis is confirmed by examination of blood, skin lesions, or respiratory secretions. Presence of the anthrax bacterium or elevated antibodies causes increased amounts of the protein produced directly as a response to the infection. Every effort is made to find the source of infection. This form of anthrax is not considered contagious.

Skin anthrax starts as a raised, itching lesion; in 1 or 2 days the lesion resembles a blister that ulcerates and develops a coal black center. Caregivers must wear gloves because the skin lesions may be infectious with direct skin contact. This dis-ease is usually not fatal if treated promptly with antibiotics.

Plague—A bioterrorism outbreak of plague is most likely to be brought about by the inhalation of the causative bacteria,

causing a severe life-threatening lung disease within a few days of exposure. The onset is sudden and includes very severe respi-ratory symptoms. Prompt antibiotic treatment is required to save the life of the infected person. Precautions are necessary to prevent the spread of the disease by face-to-face contact.

Smallpox—Smallpox, a highly contagious viral infection caused by the variola virus (a member of the poxvirus family), can be spread in aerosol form as a biologic weapon. It was once eradicated worldwide through vaccination, but now there is con-cern because people under the age of 30 have never been vac-cinated, and some adults vaccinated as children may no longer be immune. Early symptoms resemble a mild viral infection. After a variable incubation (7 to 17 days), symptoms worsen to include high fever, malaise, headache, delirium, and a rash that begins over the face and spreads to the extremities. The rash turns into pustules that leave pitted scars. Treatment is sup-portive only because no treatment or cure has been developed for smallpox. Immediate isolation of the infected individual is required, and every case must be reported to health authorities. Vaccine is once again available and is or has been given to the military, certain public safety providers, and some health care providers. Provisions are in progress to accomplish mass citizen vaccination if an endemic occurrence should come about.

Botulism—Botulism toxin, a powerful poison, is easy to make and store, and can be easily aerosolized. Although other forms of botulism do exist, it is the inhalation form that could possibly be used in a bioterrorist attack. Within a day or two af-ter exposure to the toxin, the infected person experiences a cluster of flu-like symptoms. Shortly thereafter, rapid progres-sion of neurologic symptoms begins that can result in complete respiratory failure. Early intervention with an antitoxin may be helpful in cases in which the toxin is attached to nerve endings. Additionally, treatment with human botulism immune globulin may be used. No other drugs are available to treat botulism toxin or poisoning at this time. Respiratory support is also in-volved in treatment.

child reports the abuse. Neglect also may be con-sidered a form of child abuse.

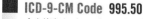
ICD-9-CM Code 995.50

Additional codes may be required to identify any injury, the nature of the abuser or

perpetrator, or the type of abuse.
Once the diagnosis has been confirmed, refer to the current edition of the ICD-9-CM coding manual for additional appropriate codes and modifiers.

SYMPTOMS AND SIGNS

Often children who are victims of child abuse are identified as such by teachers, day-care providers, or health-care providers. The injuries to the child encompass many forms, including bruises, fractures, burns, bites, and welts, and can even be fatal (Fig. 15–28).

Bruising can exhibit many telltale appearances, such as finger marks, which wrap around the child's limb and may show evidence of rings worn by the perpetrator; imprints of electrical cords or hangers; and horizontal wraparound marks left by belts or straps, and possibly buckle marks. These bruises appear on soft tissue and not over bony prominences where normal falls would have caused them to be. The bruising often is in areas normally covered by clothing and the bruises are in various stages of healing.

Burns from cigarettes appear as small circles (the diameter of a cigarette), often on hands, feet, buttocks, or genitals. These are at various stages of healing. Another form of burn is the scald burn with the pattern of "dipping," straight lines with no splash marks, a result of the child's being held in scalding water (Fig. 15–29, *A* and *B*).

Other observable injuries include teeth marks, with bruising caused by human bites, and raised areas or welts caused by spankings with sticks, paddles, or belts on the buttocks or legs. A fracture, usually greenstick in nature, of a long bone may be noted.

Often the child is withdrawn, avoids eye contact, and does not respond appropriately to painful stimuli. When asked how the injury happened, the child denies any abuse and protects the abuser. In other cases, the child exhibits unusually aggressive behavior and has a neglected appearance.

Neglect often is also considered to be a form of child abuse. When children are not provided with food or shelter, the caretaker is considered to be neglectful. Leaving young children unattended, thus endangering their well-being, is also a form of neglect.

PATIENT SCREENING

Any reports of child abuse require immediate investigation. An appointment should be scheduled as soon as possible and if none is immediately available, referral to an emergency facility is made. Follow-up to verify treatment is necessary.

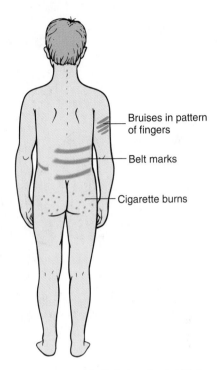

Bruises in pattern of fingers

Belt marks

Cigarette burns

FIGURE 15–28 Typical marks of child abuse.

ETIOLOGY

Child abuse has many causes. These include emotional immaturity of the abuser; stress caused by economic, social, or employment difficulties; poor parenting skills; drug or alcohol abuse; history of the abuser being an abused child; unrealistic expectations of the child; and the limitations of a physically or mentally challenged child.

DIAGNOSIS

Diagnosis is made by history and the clinical findings. Child abuse is not easy to diagnose; nevertheless, health-care providers, teachers, and daycare providers are required by law in most states in the United States to report suspected child abuse to the local or state law enforcement agency or child protective agency.

TREATMENT

Any injuries must be treated in an appropriate manner. Documentation of the injuries is necessary, and the health-care provider must remain alert for patterns of injuries. Radiographic studies of long bones and of the skull of infants and toddlers should be taken to investigate the extent of

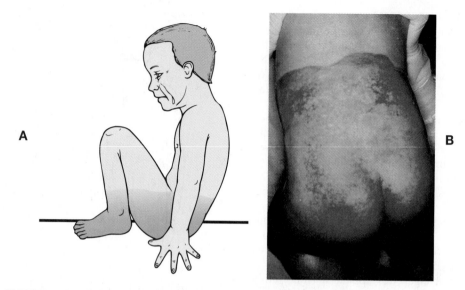

FIGURE 15–29 A, Typical pattern of scald dip burn. **B,** Scalded child. (**B** from Slide Set, Behrman RE, Kliegman RM, Arvin AM, eds: *Nelson textbook of pediatrics,* ed 15, Philadelphia, 1996, Saunders.)

abuse. Emotional support for the child should be given unconditionally. Abusive parents and other perpetrators need help from the appropriate agencies.

PROGNOSIS
Prognosis varies depending on the duration and extent of the abuse and the identity of the perpetrator of the abuse, whether the abuser has custody of or easy access to the child. Removal of the child by appropriate social services agencies from the abusive environment usually is helpful. Emotional attachment of the child to the abuser may play a role in the resolution of this action. This is a difficult and sensitive issue that requires professional interaction.

PREVENTION
Prevention is the best treatment. Parents need to be taught good parenting skills and made aware of resources for crisis intervention. They need to be taught alternatives to striking a child and methods of controlling their abusive reactions to the child's behavior (e.g., counting to 10).

PATIENT TEACHING
Provide written information about prevention of child abuse. Assist the family in locating and contacting community resources. Encourage family and community awareness of signs of child abuse and appropriate interventions.

Shaken Infant (Baby) Syndrome
DESCRIPTION
Shaken infant syndrome or shaken baby syndrome (SBS) refers to the injuries incurred by the infant or toddler who has been shaken forcibly enough to cause intracerebral bleeding with resulting closed head injury.

ICD-9-CM Code 995.55
Additional ICD-9-CM coding for injuries is required. Once diagnosis of the injuries has been confirmed, referral to the current edition of the ICD-9-CM coding manual for appropriate codes and modifiers is recommended.

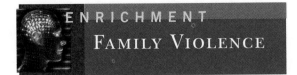

ENRICHMENT

FAMILY VIOLENCE

THE OCCURRENCE OF FAMILY VIOLENCE is increasing. All members of the family, regardless of age, sex, or place in the family line, are at risk for violence or abuse. The elderly and children are often targets of the aggressive behavior of the stronger member of the family. Many members of dysfunctional families do not realize that abusive and violent behavior is not acceptable in today's society.

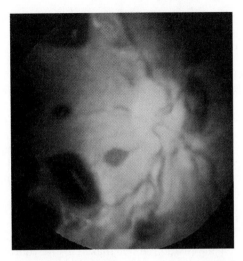

FIGURE 15–30 Shaken baby syndrome: retinal hemorrhages. (From Zitelli BJ, Davis HW: *Atlas of pediatric physical diagnosis,* ed 4, St. Louis, 2002, Mosby. Courtesy Dr. Stephen Ludwig, Children's Hospital of Philadelphia.)

SYMPTOMS AND SIGNS

The shaken baby may experience altered levels of consciousness to complete loss of consciousness. Irritability, changes in skin color to paleness or cyanosis, vomiting, lethargy, and convulsions are additional symptoms. Most of the time, there is no outward indication of physical trauma. Fractured or dislocated bones and neck or spinal injuries may be found. Examination of the eyes may reveal retinal hemorrhages (Fig. 15–30).

PATIENT SCREENING

Shaken baby syndrome is a life-threatening emergency. These children require prompt medical intervention. Contacting Emergency Medical Services for immediate transport to an emergency care facility is a prudent action. A parent calling for an appointment to speak with the physician following diagnosis and treatment of their child should be scheduled so the parent can talk with the physician as soon as possible.

ETIOLOGY

The repeated rapid shaking of an infant results in the brain continually striking the inside of the cranial vault and then recoiling against the other side of the skull. As a result, tiny vessels rupture causing minor or even major bleeds in and around the brain. The swelling and hemorrhage may lead to permanent severe cerebral (brain) damage or even death.

Being a form of child abuse, SBS usually occurs when the caregiver becomes irritated or upset and loses control, shaking the baby violently. Incidents of SBS resulting from tossing the baby into the air and catching it or even jostling the baby in a back pack as the caregiver jogs or runs, causing the baby to bounce up and down, have been documented. Young children have large heads and weak neck muscles and therefore are prone to intracerebral injury.

DIAGNOSIS

The manifestation of three symptoms—subdural hematoma, cerebral edema, and retinal hemorrhage—leads to the diagnosis of SBS. However, it is not necessary for all three conditions to be present.

TREATMENT

Immediate and aggressive intervention, including life-sustaining measures, is necessary. Bleeding and cerebral edema must be controlled and intracranial pressure reduced. Nevertheless, damage may be permanent, even fatal. If the child survives, he or she may have visual deficits from retinal insults, including blindness, mental retardation, or cerebral palsy.

PROGNOSIS

Prognosis varies depending on the extent of the injury. Often the injuries to the brain are nonreversible or even fatal. Those children who do survive may be left with blindness, neurologic insults, and mental retardation.

PREVENTION

SBS may be prevented by educating caregivers about the dangers of shaking a baby in anger and about methods of controlling their outrage. Parents should be made aware of the importance of providing their children with competent caregivers. All caregivers, including parents, should develop a safe plan for dealing with and comforting a crying baby.

PATIENT TEACHING

Provide all parents with infants or young children written information about shaken baby syndrome. Encourage all parents to have competent childcare for their children. Assist parents of shaken babies to locate and contact support groups in the community.

Elder Abuse

DESCRIPTION

Physical, psychological, or sexual injury to an elder is considered elder abuse. The most commonly observed form is physical because the injuries are visually apparent. Psychological abuse may never be uncovered. Sexual abuse may be discovered collaterally with complaints of discomfort in the genital region or by report of the elder.

■ **ICD-9-CM Code** **995.80** *(Adult maltreatment, unspecified)*
Additional ICD-9-CM coding for injuries is required. Once diagnosis of the injuries has been confirmed, referral to the current edition of the ICD-9-CM coding manual for appropriate codes and modifiers is recommended. Additional ICD-9-CM codes are available for various forms of adult abuse. Referral to the current edition of the ICD-9-CM coding manual for other diagnoses, codes, and modifiers is recommended once a diagnosis has been confirmed.

SYMPTOMS AND SIGNS

It is rare for the elderly abuse victim to complain of the abuse. The evidence of the abuse usually is discovered as the result of examination for another purpose. Signs are similar to those of other forms of abuse, are varied, and often are hidden by clothing. Signs include bruising, fractures, malnutrition, poor hygiene, and poor general health status.

Neglect often is also considered a form of elder abuse. When these individuals are not provided with food or shelter, the caretaker is considered to be neglectful. Leaving the disabled elder unattended, especially for long periods of time, thus endangering their well-being, is also a form of neglect.

PATIENT SCREENING

Reports of signs of elder abuse require prompt attention. Schedule the patient to be seen as soon as possible. Often times, the abuse is discovered during a routine examination and follow-up appointments then will be scheduled.

ETIOLOGY

As with other forms of abuse, abuse of the elderly is a complex situation. Often, the elderly are dependent on their children for survival, including financial support and physical care. Society presumes that this group of people are protected by love, gentleness, and caring. Some of the elderly requiring care have diminished mental capacity and are confused. The care of the elderly can be a source of stress to the care provider, not only because of the physical care demands but also because of the financial and emotional pressures. With the breakdown of the nuclear family structure and the stresses of being a single parent, the additional task of caring for an elderly person can become an overwhelming burden. Additionally, current society puts emphasis on youth. Often, the "sandwiched" generation no longer can cope, and abuse takes place. Other cases of elder abuse have a financial basis, either in the caretaker being unable to afford the necessities that the elderly person requires or in taking control of the elderly person's finances for the abuser's personal gain.

DIAGNOSIS

Diagnosis is made by an evaluation of the situation and physical examination. Psychological abuse is difficult to diagnose. Many of the victims believe that revealing their child's abusive behavior toward them will suggest that they have failed as parents or will jeopardize the living arrangements.

TREATMENT

Treatment consists of treating any trauma with the appropriate care. Counseling should be made available to all parties involved. If necessary, the victim should be removed from the abusive environment. Prevention is the best treatment; however, that is not always possible.

PROGNOSIS

Prognosis varies depending on the extent and duration of the abuse and the perpetrator of the abuse. Removal of the elderly individual from the abusive environment usually is helpful.

PREVENTION

Prevention is not always possible. Close monitoring of situations where an elder is dependent on others for care may be helpful. Suggestions of respite care may be helpful. Recognition of signs of extreme stress of the caregiver and suggestions of assistance in the care provision may be helpful.

PATIENT TEACHING

Assist family members in locating and contacting community resources available to them.

Psychological or Emotional Abuse

DESCRIPTION

Psychological or emotional abuse is the intentional and systematic diminishment of another's self-worth or self-esteem.

 ICD-9-CM Code 995.82 *(Adult)*
995.51 *(Child emotional/ psychological abuse)*

SYMPTOMS AND SIGNS

Symptoms of psychological or emotional abuse, the systematic diminishment of another, take on many forms. Often, the abused person offers no complaints. Although emotional battering transcends age groups, children are the most frequent victims. The guilt that these victims carry often leads to self-destructive behavior, including anorexia, bulimia, obesity, alcoholism, self-mutilation, drug addiction, depression, and suicide. Others manifest the guilt by emotional guarding and turn the anger and rage inward against themselves. These persons display a lack of self-esteem and self-worth and often are unable to bond with others.

PATIENT SCREENING

Psychologically or emotionally abused individuals usually do not have enough mental strength to seek out help. Many of these individuals are unaware of the abusive actions directed towards them and feel they deserve any abusive psychological behavior directed at them. Many are often referred from emergency care facilities and require an immediate appointment. The situations often are discovered on a visit to the physician for another reason.

ETIOLOGY

The cause of this form of abuse is unknown. Often, the parent is the abuser, denying the child love and protection. The abuse can be active, with the parent telling the child, "You're stupid," "I'm ashamed of you," or "You'll never amount to anything." It can be passive in the form of intentional neglect. Often, it is a combination of the two. The abuse can take on the verbal form, or it may be shown by the abuser's actions. The response to the abuse often is buried so deeply that it does not surface until later in life.

DIAGNOSIS

Emotional abuse is difficult to diagnose because no physical contact is required. The comments usually are made to the child in private or in the home environment. The abusive behavior takes place over time, making it difficult to identify at a given time. The victim believes that he or she is responsible for the behavior and does not realize that it is a form of abuse. The victims often defend the abusive behavior, believing that they deserved it.

TREATMENT

The best treatment is prevention. Education of the population as to what constitutes emotional abuse and ways to prevent the many forms is important. A building of self-esteem and self-worth is necessary to begin the healing process. Because of the varied forms of emotional abuse, each individual must believe in himself or herself and address his or her specific guilt, possibly with the help of a therapist.

PROGNOSIS

Prognosis varies depending on the duration of the abusive relationship. Psychological therapy may be helpful; however, many of these abused individuals are unable to accept the abusive diagnosis and will be resistant to treatment.

PREVENTION

Prevention relies on education of society as to what constitutes psychological or emotional abuse and how society can be helpful.

PATIENT TEACHING

Patient teaching involves helping the victim to build self-esteem and realize his or her own self-worth. Assist them to locate and contact community resources.

Battered Spouse Syndrome

DESCRIPTION

Battered spouse syndrome is the result of a pattern of behavior in which one spouse is repeatedly physically assaulted by her or his spouse.

 ICD-9-CM Code 995.81

SYMPTOMS AND SIGNS

The victim, most often female, has evidence of bruising in various stages of healing, usually in an area of the body that is concealed by clothing. She or he has a tendency to avoid eye contact with the examiner.

PATIENT SCREENING

An individual reporting physical assault by a spouse or partner requires prompt attention.

ETIOLOGY

Battering of spouses is a complex issue; no one specific cause is known. Stress is suggested as an important factor, along with alcohol ingestion and possible intoxication. Cultural and societal values that made wives their husbands' "property" and the mindset that women are expected to be submissive to their mates have contributed to spouse abuse. Some women are victimized because they do not have the physical or emotional strength that their spouses do. Many of these victims have low self-esteem that adds to their inability to escape the victimization. Women can be the abusers also, and some women abuse their spouses even to the point of dismemberment or setting the spouse on fire. It is believed that many of these cases are retaliation for battering that has been received.

DIAGNOSIS

Diagnosis is made from information provided by the victim or others. Physical examination indicates physical injuries. As with child abuse and sexual abuse, the injuries are varied and often occur on areas of the body that normally are covered by clothing. Assessment of the emotional state is difficult but necessary. Often, intervention results from law enforcement involvement; other times, the abusive trauma is discovered by the physician and staff when the victim is seen for another reason in the office or healthcare facility.

TREATMENT

Treatment involves normal protocol for treating physical injuries. Discussing the situation in a nonjudgmental way is imperative. Referral to appropriate agencies for counseling is indicated; nevertheless, the health-care provider must recognize that the victim may not want or seek counseling and may elect to stay in the abusive situation. Listening is of the utmost importance; however, it is inappropriate to impose one's opinion of the situation on the victim.

PROGNOSIS

Prognosis varies according to the duration and extent of the battering. Additionally, the circumstances of the relationship in which the battering has taken place will affect the long-term outcome of any intervention. Moreover, the willingness of the battered individual to leave the situation and to report the battering to law enforcementalso will affect the outcome.

PREVENTION

Prevention is difficult because many spouses feel that they deserve the battering and that it is accepted behavior in society as they know it. Raising awareness of the issue in the community and in the educational system and teaching that battering is not acceptable behavior may prevent battering and acceptance of battering in future generations.

PATIENT TEACHING

Reinforcing to the victim that no one deserves to be treated in such a manner may be helpful. Acceptance of the victim as an individual with inherent self-worth is a valuable tool in establishing rapport and in building trust between the caregiver and the individual. Provide the victim with local telephone contact numbers to be used in an emergency situation to obtain help. Additionally, assist them in locating and contacting community resources if they desire to do so.

Sexual Abuse

DESCRIPTION

Any form of nonconsensual sexual contact or activity is considered to be sexual abuse. Sexual abuse may involve either sex and may be perpetrated by either sex.

 ICD-9-CM Code 995.83 *(Adult)*
995.53 *(Child sexual abuse)*

SYMPTOMS AND SIGNS

Sexual abuse takes on many forms, thus symptoms and signs can be numerous and different from one patient to the next. Any form of nonconsensual sexual activity can be considered sexual abuse. Some examples of sexual abuse are fondling of the genitals or breasts, penetration of the vagina or rectum with fingers or other objects, and forcing the victim to touch the perpetrator on or around the sex organs. The victim often does not report unwanted advances or activity and usually appears subdued. If the victim is a young female, she may have itching or burning in the urethral and vaginal areas and exhibit symptoms of a urinary tract infection. Sexually abused children have an unusual obsession with the genital region and frequently touch themselves abnormally. They often exhibit aggressive behavior.

PATIENT SCREENING

Any individual reporting sexual abuse requires prompt attention. If no immediate appointments are available, refer the patient to a sexual abuse or emergency facility for immediate intervention. Some victims may be resistant to this option; if so, schedule an appointment as soon as possible.

ETIOLOGY

As with other forms of abuse, the cause of sexual abuse is a complicated matter. Domination, control, and power issues can be reasons for this unacceptable form of behavior. Many of the perpetrators were sexually abused as children, and they do not regard what they are doing as wrong. Some just have a sociopathic approach to society and its norms. It is important to consider that victimization of both sexes occurs and that the abuser can be of either sex. Cases of females sexually assaulting males, of any age, have been reported.

DIAGNOSIS

Diagnosis is made from a history given by the victim and is confirmed by a physical examination. Often the sexual abuse is combined with physical abuse, and the treatment of that abuse may lead to the victim confiding in the caregiver regarding the unwanted sexual activity. Many times, the removal of the victim from a physically abusive environment allows the victim to feel safe enough to discuss the sexual abuse. Perpetrators of sexual abuse of children have been babysitters, relatives, or even a parent.

TREATMENT

Any trauma is treated according to the protocol of the facility. Law enforcement agencies should be notified, with the victim's consent, or according to local or state policy. If possible, the victim is removed from the abusive situation. Emotional support is provided, and reinforcement is given to the victim that he or she is not responsible for the sexual abuse. If the victim is receptive to counseling, arrangements are made to assist the victim in dealing with the abuse. If the victim is a child, child protective services are usually involved, and when the situation warrants, the child is removed from the environment. The social services agencies involved usually determine when a child is to be removed from this type of environment.

PROGNOSIS

Prognosis varies depending on the form and extent of the sexual abuse. The physical wounds may heal quickly, but the emotional wounds often leave permanent scarring. A resulting pregnancy or sexually transmitted disease will require additional intervention.

PREVENTION

Prevention is difficult. It is not often possible to predict who may be a sexual abuser; nor is it possible to predict where or when sexual abuse may take place.

PATIENT TEACHING

Assist the victim in locating and contacting community resource agencies that can provide support and assistance. Reinforce that sexual abuse is not accepted behavior; however, it is important to maintain a nonjudgmental attitude toward the victim.

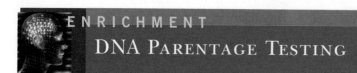

ENRICHMENT

DNA PARENTAGE TESTING

DNA PARENTAGE TESTING is the most reliable and accurate method of determining parentage for legal and medical reasons. It conclusively answers difficult questions, resolves disputes, and helps streamline court proceedings.

Testing is based on a highly accurate analysis of the genetic profiles of the mother, child, and alleged father. Deoxyribonucleic acid (DNA), the unique genetic blueprint within each nucleated cell of a person's body, determines the genetic pattern and individual characteristics. A child inherits half of this DNA pattern from the mother and half from the father. If the mother's and child's patterns are known, the father's can be deduced with virtual certainty.

Age restrictions for DNA testing do not apply because DNA makeup is set at conception. Testing can be performed before a child is born, and newborns can be tested safely at delivery using umbilical cord blood. In fact, samples can be taken from persons of any age, even postmortem. Only ½ teaspoon of blood is required.

DNA technology is so powerful that the genetic patterns of a deceased father can be reconstructed from grandparents, siblings, or other children to determine paternity.

From DNA Diagnostics Center, Fairfield, Ohio, 1999.

Rape

DESCRIPTION
Intercourse forced on the victim against her or his will is termed rape.

 ICD-9-CM Code 959.9 *(Injury by site)*
Refer to the current edition of the ICD-9-CM coding manual for additional codes and/or modifiers for additional diagnosed injuries.

SYMPTOMS AND SIGNS
The symptoms and signs of rape vary with the degree of violence incurred by the victim. Many present to an emergency care facility, physician's office, or clinic, or a law enforcement agency stating, "I've been raped." Some report having pain in the pelvic and perineal regions or being choked or restrained in some manner. Others relate the threat of death. Bruising may be noted in any area of the body, not just the pelvic area. Signs of rape include torn clothing, dirt and debris ground into clothing or hair, disheveled appearance, withdrawal, anxiousness, avoidance of eye contact, and bruising, tears, or lacerations around or on the genitals, rectum, or mouth. Pelvic and rectal examination often reveals tenderness in those areas and evidence of trauma. If the victim has not bathed or douched, evidence of semen may be present on the inner aspects of the thighs, genital areas, mouth, nares, or pubic region. Any part of the body, including the breasts, may be traumatized. If the victim is male, bruising or lacerations in the anal region are indicative of sodomy. Bruises and lacerations also may be discovered in the anal region of the female when she has been sodomized.

PATIENT SCREENING
Many rape victims will go to or be transported to an emergency facility for a sexual assault examination, which includes the gathering of any evidence. However, some victims will resist reporting the attack to authorities and request an appointment to see the physician. Other victims may seek anonymity and seek out a physician with whom they have had no previous contact. Therefore any individual reporting rape or sexual assault and requesting an appointment should be scheduled as soon as possible, and should be treated with complete discretion.

ETIOLOGY
Rape is a crime of violence and domination, not a sexual act. It occurs when mutual consent has not been given by both parties involved in the sexual act, and it is a forceful act. Rape can happen to either female or male victims; most often the victims are females. Rape can be date rape, acquaintance

rape, rape by the victim's spouse, or a violent act perpetrated by an unknown assailant.

DIAGNOSIS

Diagnosis is made by evaluating the history, clinical findings, and physical examination, including pelvic examination and sex crime evidence gathering. Samples of debris, clothing, saliva, hair, pubic hair, fingernails, and scrapings from under the nails are collected. A urinalysis is obtained, along with blood tests for sexually transmitted diseases, AIDS, and possible pregnancy. Photographs may be taken for documentation of injury. It is recommended that this type of complete examination take place in a facility with staff professionally trained in treating sexual assault victims.

TREATMENT

Any patient who has suffered trauma is treated in an appropriate manner. Counseling at a rape crisis center should be offered. Information concerning the risks of possible pregnancy, sexually transmitted diseases, and AIDS is given, along with an explanation of the follow-up testing protocol. If the patient has no religious objection, prophylaxis for pregnancy may be considered.

Reinforcement that the victim is a survivor of a violent crime and is not responsible for the incident is necessary. The victim needs to believe that she or he just happened to be in the wrong place at the wrong time. Everyone dealing with the victim and her or his family must be nonjudgmental and supportive.

PROGNOSIS

Prognosis for victims of rape varies. Physical healing may take place without any complications. However a resulting pregnancy or sexually transmitted diseases will present a complication that needs to be addressed. Psychological counseling may be ongoing and may be required for lengthy periods. Undoubtedly, the physical and psychological effect on victims will be longstanding if not lifelong.

PREVENTION

It is difficult to prevent rape because it is difficult to predict who might be a perpetrator or what place might be a potential location of a rape.

PATIENT TEACHING

Rape victims require a nonjudgmental approach by the caregiver. They should be assisted in seeking counseling. Assist them in contacting the local Rape Crisis Center and encourage them to follow through with the contact.

REVIEW CHALLENGE

Answer the following questions:

1. What are the major types of trauma?
2. What are some ways in which environmental factors can result in trauma?
3. What is the difference between an abrasion and an avulsion?
4. When is it appropriate to use tetanus toxoid in prophylactic treatment?
5. When is debridement of a wound necessary?
6. How are the depth and extent of burns assessed?
7. What are the possible effects of an electrical shock?
8. What are the types of lightning strikes? Which treatments may be required?
9. How are the signs and symptoms of heat stroke and heat exhaustion different?
10. What is the treatment for heat stroke? For heat exhaustion?
11. What are some precautions in the treatment of frostbite?
12. Which spider bites require emergency care?
13. What is Rocky Mountain spotted fever, and how is it transmitted?
14. Why is an animal quarantined after biting a human?
15. What are the signs and symptoms of a poisonous snakebite?
16. What is the relationship between repetitive activities and carpal tunnel syndrome?
17. Which physical patterns may be observed in child abuse?
18. How may elder abuse, child abuse, sexual abuse, or battered spouse syndrome be noted during the history and physical examination?
19. What testing is available for the rape victim?
20. How can parentage be determined in the laboratory?

REAL-LIFE CHALLENGE

Heat Exhaustion

The mother of a 14-year-old girl called the office about her daughter, who had just come home from marching band practice, where she had been for approximately the past 3 hours. The girl was complaining of nausea, weakness, and headache. On questioning, the mother revealed that her daughter's skin appeared pale, cool, and moist. The weather had been hot and humid, and the girl told her mother that she had been practicing the marching routines for about 2½ hours before she felt ill. The mother took the girl's temperature, which was 98.2° F, and said her pulse was faint and fast.

The mother was advised to have her daughter lie down with feet slightly elevated in a cool environment, to loosen her clothing, and to place cool compresses on the girl's face, forehead, neck, chest, abdomen, arms, back, and legs. She also was instructed to give her daughter 4 oz of cool water to drink every 15 minutes. The office advised that they would call back in 1 hour to get a progress report.

The diagnosis was heat exhaustion.

QUESTIONS

1. What is the significance of the cool, moist skin?
2. What measures could have been taken to prevent the onset of heat exhaustion?
3. Compare the moist, cool skin and sweating of heat exhaustion with the skin condition of heat stroke.
4. What could be the anticipated outcome of treatment, as suggested to the mother?
5. If the girl's condition did not improve in an hour, what would you expect the next step in treatment to be?
6. What is the significance of loosening clothing and applying cool compresses?
7. Why would the mother be instructed to use cool compresses and not ice?
8. Why would the patient with heat stroke require treatment in an emergency facility versus the heat exhaustion victim being treated at home?

REAL-LIFE CHALLENGE

Spousal Abuse

A 36-year-old woman is in the office being treated for pain and reduced hearing in the left ear. She is very vague about any history, saying only that her left ear is painful; she has noted some blood coming out of the canal, and she has reduced hearing in her left ear. Bruising is noted around the ear on the left cheek, on the left side of the neck, and behind the left ear on the skull. These areas are tender to touch. The patient is very quiet, at times is tearful, and is wearing a long-sleeved turtleneck shirt and long pants. She is hesitant to remove her shirt for the taking of her blood pressure or for any other examination.

Examination reveals recent trauma to the left ear, blood is visualized in the canal, and otoscopic examination confirms a ruptured tympanic membrane. Audiometry confirms reduced hearing capability in the left ear. Bruises in various stages of healing are noted on arms, neck, and chest. Further examination discloses similar bruising to legs. The patient denies any abusive trauma and says she incurred the injuries in a fall. She avoids eye contact, tending to keep her eyes downward. Her demeanor is subdued, and her posture also appears subdued with slumping shoulders.

Gentle questioning eventually brings out that her husband, a man of large stature, recently lost his job as a result of drinking and aggressive or near-violent behavior. She also admits that in the past 2 weeks since the loss of his job, her husband has been "slapping her around" and that last night he struck her on the left side of her face and across the ear with his open hand. The patient does not want to file a police report and says she cannot leave the situation.

She is referred to an ear, nose, and throat specialist for treatment of the ruptured tympanic membrane. An appointment for follow-up is made for 2 days later, at which time additional support for the psychosocial situation will be supplied. She is instructed to call immediately at any recurrence of the abusive behavior. She also is advised to see whether she can get her husband to make an appointment for an examination.

QUESTIONS

1. What is typical behavior for a "battered" spouse?
2. What is the significance of the alcohol consumption and the loss of employment in the onset of abuse?
3. Why didn't the victim want the abuse reported?
4. What are the legal responsibilities of your office in this situation?
5. What might be the reasons the victim feels she cannot leave the abusive situation?
6. Explain the mechanics of how the impact of the slapping causes the rupture of the tympanic membrane.
7. Discuss the implications of both the abusive husband and the battered wife being patients of the practice.

INTERNET ASSIGNMENTS

1. Research the support available to families of major trauma victims at the American Trauma Society. This same website offers suggested preventive measures.

2. Research suggested measures available to the victim of domestic violence at the National Coalition Against Domestic Violence.

Common Laboratory and Diagnostic Tests

Values may vary according to laboratory reference values. These values are for reference only. Results of one test alone usually are not conclusive and should be considered with results of other diagnostic procedures, the symptoms and signs, and the physical examination to arrive at a diagnosis.

Blood Analysis

Complete Blood Count (CBC)

Evaluation of cellular components of the blood. Includes red blood cell count, red blood cell indices, white blood cell count, white blood cell differential, hemoglobin, hematocrit, and platelet count. Sometimes referred to as hemogram. Often the differential must be ordered specifically as CBC with differential.

Red Blood Count (RBC)

Count of erythrocytes in a specimen of whole blood.

NORMAL RBC:
Adult male: 4.5.7-6.1 million/μl
Adult female: 4.0-5.5 million/μl
Infants and children: 3.8-5.5 million/μl
Newborns: 4.8-7.1 million/μl

An elevated RBC is indicative of many disorders, including but not limited to erythremia, polycythemia, erythrocytosis, dehydration, burns, anoxia, diarrhea, cardiovascular disease, poisoning, and pulmonary disease. A reduced RBC also is indicative of many disorders, including but not limited to anemias, bone marrow suppression, hemorrhage, liver diseases, thyroid disorders, cardiovascular disease,

vitamin deficiency, and ingestion of certain drugs. When the RBC is abnormal, cell morphology should be examined. As with most blood tests, results should be evaluated with other tests, along with symptoms and signs, to determine a diagnosis.

Hemoglobin (Hgb)

Measurement of the oxygen-carrying pigment of the red blood cells.

NORMAL:
Adult male: 14.0-18.0
Adult female: 12.0-16.0
Infants and children: 11.5-15.5
Newborns: 14.5-22.5

An elevated Hgb is indicative of many disorders, including but not limited to CHF, COPD, dehydration, burns, diarrhea, erythrocytosis, high altitudes, and thrombotic thrombocytopenia. A reduced Hgb also is indicative of many disorders, including but not limited to iron-deficiency anemia, hemorrhage, hemolytic reaction to drugs or chemicals, liver diseases, SLE, and pregnancy.

Hematocrit (HCT)

Measurement of the percentage of red blood cells in a volume of whole blood.

NORMAL:
Adult male: 37%-52%
Adult female: 36%-48%
Infants and children: 28%-45%
Newborns: 48%-69%

An elevated HCT is indicative of many disorders, including but not limited to dehydration, burns, diarrhea, eclampsia, pancreatitis, shock, and polycythemia. A reduced HCT also is indicative of many disorders, including but not limited to anemia, bone marrow hyperplasia, CHF, fluid overload, burns, thyroid disorders, pancreatitis, pregnancy, pneumonia, and ingestion of certain drugs.

White Blood Count (WBC)

Count of white blood cells in a whole blood specimen.

NORMAL:

Adult male: 4500-11,000/μl
Adult female: 4500-11,000/μl
Infants and children: 6000-17,500/μl
Newborns: 9000-30,000/μl

An elevated WBC is indicative of many disorders, including but not limited to acquired hemolytic anemia, anorexia, abscess, appendicitis, bacterial infections, bronchitis, burns, biliary disorders, respiratory disorders, disorders of the GI tract, renal disorders, blood disorders, lactic acidosis, poisoning, pregnancy, sepsis, shock, tonsillitis, trauma, uremia, and ingestion of certain drugs. Similar to an abnormal RBC, a differential should be evaluated, and, as with most blood tests, results should be evaluated with other tests, along with symptoms and signs, to determine a diagnosis. A decreased WBC is indicative of many disorders, including but not limited to AIDS, anemias, chemical toxicity, Hodgkin disease, influenza, legionnaire's disease, radiation therapy, shock, septicemia, vitamin B_{12} deficiency, cirrhosis, hepatitis, hypothermia, leukopenia, tuberculosis, and ingestion of certain drugs.

Differential White Blood Cells (Differential Leukocyte Count)

An assessment by percentage of leukocyte distribution in a specimen of 100 white cells.

GRANULOCYTES
NORMAL:

Segmented neutrophils (SEGs) adult: 50%-62%
Band neutrophils (bands) adult: 3%-6%
Eosinophils (EOS) adult: 0%-3%
Basophils (BASOS) adult: 0%-0.75%
Monocytes (MONOS) adult: 3%-7%
Lymphocytes (LYMPHS) adult: 25%-40%

Increased neutrophils are indicative of many disorders, including but not limited to allergies, asthma, acute infections, appendicitis, burns, dia-

betic acidosis, cardiovascular disorders, disorders of the GI tract, leukemia, respiratory disorders, poisoning, pyelonephritis, septicemia, tonsillitis, and ingestion of certain drugs. A decrease in neutrophils is indicative of many disorders, including but not limited to endocrine disorders, anaphylactic shock, carcinoma, chemotherapy, anemias, pneumonia, septicemia, radiation therapy, and ingestion of certain drugs.

Increased bands are indicative primarily of pharyngitis.

Increased SEGs are indicative primarily of pernicious anemia.

Increased eosinophils are indicative of many disorders, including but not limited to allergies, asthma, cancer, dermatitis, diverticulitis, eczema, Hodgkin disease, leukemia, parasitic infection, pernicious anemia, radiation therapy, sickle cell anemia, tuberculosis, and ingestion of certain drugs. Reduced eosinophils also are indicative of many disorders, including but not limited to aplastic anemia, CHF, eclampsia, infections, stress, and ingestion of certain drugs.

Increased basophils are indicative of many disorders, including but not limited to allergic reactions, Hodgkin disease, hypothyroidism, radiation therapy, sinusitis, urticaria, and ingestion of certain drugs. Decreased basophils also are indicative of many disorders, including but not limited to acute infections, anaphylactic shock, endocrine disorders, pregnancy, radiation therapy, stress, and ingestion of certain drugs.

Increased lymphocytes are indicative of many disorders, including but not limited to endocarditis, infectious mononucleosis, leukocytosis, lymphocytic leukemia, syphilis, toxoplasmosis, and ingestion of certain drugs. Decreased lymphocytes also are indicative of many disorders, including but not limited to aplastic anemia, Hodgkin disease, immunoglobulin deficiencies, leukemia, renal failure, SLE, uremia, and ingestion of certain drugs.

Increased monocytes are indicative of many disorders, including but not limited to Epstein-Barr virus, Hodgkin disease, leukemia, rheumatoid arthritis, syphilis, SLE, tuberculosis, and ingestion of certain drugs. Decreased monocytes are primarily indicative of aplastic anemia and hairy-cell leukemia.

Platelet Count (Thrombocyte Count)

Count of platelets in a whole blood specimen.

NORMAL ADULT:

150,000-400,000/µl

Increased platelet count is indicative of many disorders, including but not limited to anemias, carcinoma, fractures, liver disorders, heart disease, hemorrhage, acute infection, inflammation, leukemia, pancreatitis, pregnancy, rheumatoid arthritis, surgery, and ingestion of certain drugs. A decreased platelet count is indicative of many disorders, including but not limited to anemias, bone marrow disorders, autoimmune disorders, severe burns, carcinoma, liver disorders, DIC, hemolytic disease of the newborn, infections, radiation therapy, leukemias, and ingestion of certain drugs.

Blood Chemistries

Chemistries

Normal chemistry profile may contain blood serum levels for albumin, alkaline phosphatase, aspartate aminotransferase, bilirubin, calcium, creatinine, lactate dehydrogenase, phosphorus, total protein, urea nitrogen, and uric acid.

Albumin

Measurement of one of two major protein factions of blood.

NORMAL ADULT:

3.5-5.0 g/dl

Increased levels of serum albumin are indicative of many disorders, including but not limited to dehydration, diarrhea, meningitis, carcinoma, myeloma, nephrosis, nephrotic syndrome, peptic ulcers, pneumonia, rheumatic fever, SLE, uremia, vomiting, and ingestion of certain drugs. Below-normal levels of serum albumin are indicative of many disorders, including but not limited to ascites, alcoholism, burns, CHF, Crohn disease, diabetes mellitus, edema, hypertension, kidney disorders, GI disorders, trauma, stress, and ingestion of certain drugs.

Alkaline Phosphatase

Measurement of enzyme found in bone, liver, intestine, and placenta.

NORMAL ADULT:

2-4 U/dl

Elevated alkaline phosphatase levels are indicative of many disorders, including but not limited to alcoholism, liver disorders, diabetes mellitus, fractures, GI disorders, endocrine disorders, hepatitis, Hodgkin disease, leukemia, neoplasms, myocardial infarction, bone disorders, disorders of the pancreas, kidney disorders, and ingestion of certain drugs. Below-normal levels of alkaline phosphatase are indicative of many disorders, including but not limited to pernicious anemia, cretinism, hypothyroidism, malnutrition, nephritis, and ingestion of certain drugs.

Aspartate Aminotransferase (AST)

Measurement of enzyme found primarily in heart, liver, and muscle.

Normal adult female: 8-20 U/L
Normal adult male: 8-26 U/L

Elevated AST levels are indicative of many disorders, including but not limited to acute myocardial infarction (MI), alcoholism, liver disorders, insult and injury to tissue including trauma, cerebral and pulmonary infarctions, and ingestion of certain drugs. Reduced AST levels are indicative of many disorders, including but not limited to diabetic ketoacidosis, liver disease, uremia, and ingestion of certain drugs.

Bilirubin

A byproduct of hemoglobin breakdown, bilirubin is produced in the liver, spleen, and bone marrow.

Total: Normal adult: <1.5 mg/dl
Direct: Normal adult: 0.0-0.3 mg/dl
Indirect: Normal adult: 0.1-1.0 mg/dl

Total bilirubin is divided into direct bilirubin, primarily secreted by the intestinal tract, and indirect bilirubin, primarily circulating in the bloodstream. Obstructive or hepatic jaundice results in an increased amount of direct bilirubin entering the bloodstream rather than entering the GI tract and being filtered and eliminated by the kidneys. Conditions that cause an increase in direct bilirubin include but are not limited to biliary obstruction, pancreatic cancer (head of pancreas), cirrhosis, hepatitis, and ingestion of certain drugs. Hemolytic jaundice causes the indirect bilirubin to accumulate in the blood because of the increased breakdown of

Hgb. Conditions that cause an increase in direct bilirubin levels include but are not limited to pernicious and sickle cell anemia, autoimmune hemolysis, cirrhosis, hepatitis, intracavity and soft-tissue hemorrhage, MI, septicemia, hemolytic transfusion reaction, and ingestion of certain drugs.

Calcium

Measurement of blood serum calcium levels.

NORMAL ADULT:
8.2-10.2 mg/dl

Calcium acts in bone formation, impulse conduction, myocardial and skeletal muscle contractions, and the blood-clotting process. Elevated serum calcium levels are indicative of many disorders, including but not limited to endocrine disorders, hepatic disease, respiratory acidosis, leukemia, neoplasms, blood disorders, respiratory disorders, and ingestion of certain drugs. Reduced serum calcium levels are indicative of many disorders, including but not limited to alkalosis, bacteremia, burns, chronic renal disease and other renal disorders, endocrine disorders, osteomalacia, rickets, vitamin D deficiency, and ingestion of certain drugs.

Creatinine

Measurement of an indicator of renal function.

Normal adult female: 0.5-1.1 mg/dl
Normal adult male: 0.6-1.2 mg/dl

Serum creatinine is excreted continually by the renal system, and elevated levels are indicative of a slowing of glomerular filtration. Other conditions that may contribute to elevation of serum creatinine include but are not limited to CHF, diabetes mellitus, kidney disorders, hypovolemia, metal poisoning, endocrine disorders, subacute bacterial endocarditis, SLE, and ingestion of certain drugs. Decreased serum creatinine levels are indicative of diabetic ketoacidosis and muscular dystrophy.

Lactate Dehydrogenase

Measurement of body tissue intracellular enzyme released after tissue damage.

NORMAL ADULT:
45-102 U/L

Elevated lactate dehydrogenase levels are indicative of many disorders, including but not limited to alcoholism, anoxia, burns, cardiomyopathy,

CVA, cirrhosis, CHF and myocardial infarction, neoplasms, anemias and leukemia, renal disorders, muscle and bone pain, respiratory disorders, shock, trauma, and ingestion of certain drugs. Decreased levels of lactate dehydrogenase develop after radiation and after the ingestion of oxalates.

Total Protein

A reflection of the total amounts of albumin and globulins in blood serum.

NORMAL ADULT:
6.0-8.0 g/dl

Increased total protein is indicative of many disorders, including but not limited to Addison disease, Crohn disease, dehydration, diarrhea, renal disease, vomiting, protozoal diseases, and ingestion of certain drugs. Decreased total protein is indicative of many disorders, including but not limited to burns, cholecystitis, cirrhosis, CHF, diarrhea, hyperthyroidism, edema, leukemia, peptic ulcer, nephrosis, malnutrition, ulcerative colitis, and ingestion of certain drugs.

Urea Nitrogen/Blood Urea Nitrogen (BUN)

An assessment of the urea content in the blood that gives an indication of the functioning of the renal glomeruli.

NORMAL ADULT:
5-20 mg/dl

An elevated urea nitrogen level can be caused by prerenal (inadequate renal circulation or abnormally high levels of blood protein), renal (impaired renal filtration and excretion), or postrenal (lower urinary tract obstruction) etiologies.

Uric Acid

An end-product of the metabolism of purines.

Normal adult female: 2.4-6.0 mg/dl
Normal adult male: 3.4-7.0 mg/dl

Elevated uric acid levels are indicative of many disorders, including but not limited to gout; hyperuricemia; hemolytic, pernicious, and sickle cell anemias; arteriosclerosis; arthritis; CHF; dehydration; diabetes mellitus; fasting; exercise; hypothyroidism; intestinal obstruction; acute infections; lead poisoning; leukemia; neoplasms; nephritis; polycystic kidney; renal failure; starvation; stress; uremia; urinary obstruction; and ingestion of certain drugs. Reduced uric acid levels are indicative of many disorders, including but not limited to acromegaly, carcinomas, Hodgkin disease, pernicious anemia, and ingestion of certain drugs.

Thyroid Function Tests

An evaluation of all three thyroid levels is important in diagnosing thyroid disorders.

Thyroid Thyroxine (T_4)

The hormone thyroxine is produced in the thyroid gland from iodide and thyroglobulin in response to stimulation by thyroid-stimulating hormone (TSH) produced by the pituitary gland. T_4 stimulates T_3 to be produced. It also stimulates the basal metabolism. In the process of negative feedback, circulating levels of T_4 influence the levels of TSH.

NORMAL ADULT:
   5.0-12.0 μg/dl

Increased levels of T_4 usually indicate the presence of hyperfunctioning thyroid disorders, including Graves' disease, hyperthyroidism, thyrotoxicosis, and ingestion of certain drugs. Decreased levels of T_4 are indicative of hypothyroid disorders, including acromegaly, cretinism, and goiter, as well as hypothyroidism, liver disease, endocrine disorders, GI tract disorders, pituitary tumor, and ingestion of certain drugs.

Triiodothyronine (T_3)

T_3 stimulates the basal metabolic rate for metabolism of carbohydrates and lipids, protein synthesis, vitamin metabolism, and bone calcium release.

NORMAL ADULT:
   80-230 ng/dl

An increase in T_3 levels is indicative of but not limited to Graves' disease, hyperthyroidism, thyrotoxicosis, and ingestion of certain drugs. Decreased levels of T_3 are indicative of but not limited to iodine and thyroid deficiency disorders, including goiter and myxedema, renal failure, starvation, thyroidectomy, and ingestion of certain drugs.

Thyroid-Stimulating Hormone (TSH)

TSH, produced in the anterior lobe of the pituitary gland, stimulates the production and release of T_3 and T_4 by the thyroid gland.

NORMAL ADULT:
   <10 μU/ml

An increase in TSH levels may be indicative of but not limited to Addison disease, goiter, hyperpituitarism, hypothyroidism, thyroiditis, and ingestion of certain drugs. A decrease in TSH may be indicative of but not limited to Hashimoto thyroiditis, hyperthyroidism, and hypothyroidism.

Lipid Profile

A lipid profile consists of comparison of results of four serum lipids, total cholesterol, triglycerides, high-density lipoproteins (HDLs), and low-density lipoproteins (LDLs). One consideration is the ratio of HDL:LDL; the recommended ratio is 3.4:5.0.

Total Cholesterol

A widely distributed sterol that facilitates the absorption and transport of fatty acids. Found in foods of animal origin, cholesterol is synthesized continuously in the body.

NORMAL ADULT:
   <29 years <200 mg/dl
   30-39 years <225 mg/dl
   40-49 years <245 mg/dl
   >50 years <265 mg/dl

Elevated serum cholesterol levels are indicative of many disorders, including but not limited to atherosclerosis, CHD, CHF, biliary disorders, kidney disorders, lipid disorders, and ingestion of certain drugs. Decreased levels of serum cholesterol are indicative of many disorders, including but not limited to anemias, carcinoma, cirrhosis, liver disease, hepatitis, endocrine disorders, GI tract disorders, and ingestion of certain drugs.

Triglycerides

Triglycerides, the principal lipids in blood, are simple fat compounds of three molecules of fatty acid, oleic, palmitic, or stearic.

NORMAL ADULT FEMALE:
   20-29 years 10-100 mg/dl
   30-39 years 10-110 mg/dl
   40-49 years 10-122 mg/dl
   50-59 years 10-134 mg/dl
   >59 years 10-147 mg/dl

Blood Chemistries

NORMAL ADULT MALE:
20-29 years 10-157 mg/dl
30-39 years 10-182 mg/dl
40-49 years 10-193 mg/dl
50-59 years 10-197 mg/dl
>59 years 10-199 mg/dl

Elevated triglyceride levels are indicative of many disorders, including but not limited to arteriosclerosis, MI, aortic aneurysm, hypercholesterolemia, hyperlipoproteinemia, alcoholism, diabetes mellitus, gout, renal disease, starvation, and malnutrition. Decreased triglyceride levels are indicative of many disorders, including but not limited to cirrhosis, malabsorption, hyperalimentation, and ingestion of certain drugs.

HDL Cholesterol
High-density lipoprotein transports cholesterol and other lipids to the liver for excretion. HDL is believed to reduce the risk of coronary artery disease.

Normal adult female: 30-85 mg/dl
Normal adult male: 30-70 mg/dl

Increased levels of HDL are indicative of but not limited to alcoholism, hepatic disorders, cirrhosis, and ingestion of certain drugs. Reduced levels of HDL are indicative of many disorders, including but not limited to arteriosclerosis, hypercholesterolemia, hyperlipoproteinemia, CHD, diabetes mellitus, liver disease, kidney disease, bacterial infections, and ingestion of certain drugs.

LDL Cholesterol
Low-density lipoprotein has a high cholesterol content, and it delivers lipids to body tissues.

NORMAL ADULT:
80-190 mg/dl

Elevated levels of LDL are indicative of many disorders, including but not limited to diabetes mellitus, anorexia nervosa, renal failure, hepatic disease, and ingestion of certain drugs. Decreased levels of LDL are indicative of but not limited to hyperlipoproteinemia, arteriosclerosis, pulmonary disease, stress, and the ingestion of certain drugs.

Electrolytes (lytes)

Blood serum test for chloride, potassium, sodium, and carbon dioxide.

Chloride
An anion found predominately in extracellular spaces.

NORMAL ADULT:
97-106 mEq/L

Increased blood serum levels of chloride may be the result of several disorders, including but not limited to metabolic disorders, dehydration, diabetes insipidus, hyperventilation, hyperparathyroidism, acidosis, respiratory alkalosis, CHF, Cushing disease, nephritis, renal failure, and ingestion of certain drugs. Reduced blood serum levels of chloride may be the result of several disorders, including but not limited to metabolic alkalosis, diabetes, severe vomiting, burns, overhydration, salt-losing diseases, some diuretic therapies, CNS disorders, diaphoresis, fasting, fever, heat exhaustion, acute infections, gastric obstructions, uremia, and ingestion of certain drugs.

Potassium
Potassium is the main cation of intracellular fluid. Potassium is important in nerve conduction, muscle function, osmotic pressure, acid–base balance, and myocardial activity.

NORMAL ADULT:
3.5-5.3 mEq/L

Increased blood serum levels of potassium may be the result of several disorders, including but not limited to renal failure, dehydration, burns, trauma, chemotherapy, metabolic acidosis, Addison disease, uncontrolled diabetes, dialysis, hemolysis, intestinal obstruction, sepsis, shock, pneumonia, uremia, and ingestion of certain drugs. Reduced blood serum levels of potassium may be the result of several disorders, including but not limited to alkalosis, anorexia, vomiting, diarrhea, malabsorption, starvation, diuresis, excessive sweating, draining wounds, severe burns, endocrine disorders, pancreatitis, GI stress, and ingestion of certain drugs.

Sodium
Sodium is the major cation of extracellular fluid and the main base in the blood. Its functions include chemical maintenance of osmotic pressure, acid–base balance, and nerve transmission.

NORMAL ADULT:
135-145 mEq/L

Increased blood serum levels of sodium may be the result of several disorders, including but not limited to severe burns, CHF, excessive fluid loss caused by vomiting, diarrhea, sweating, Addison disease, nephrotic syndrome, pyloric obstruction, diabetes insipidus, hypertension, hypovolemia, toxemia, malabsorption syndrome, diuresis, edema, hypothyroidism, and ingestion of certain drugs. Decreased blood serum levels of sodium may be the result of several disorders, including but not limited to bowel obstruction, dehydration, coma, Cushing disease, diabetes mellitus, glomerulonephritis, hyperthermia, myxedema, certain renal conditions, and ingestion of certain drugs.

Carbon Dioxide

Carbon dioxide in normal blood plasma comes from bicarbonate.

NORMAL ADULT:
    20-30 mEq/L

Increased blood serum levels of carbon dioxide may be the result of several disorders, including but not limited to emphysema, aldosteronism, mercurial diuretics, severe vomiting, airway obstruction, bradycardia, cardiac disorders, renal disorders, and ingestion of certain drugs. Decreased blood serum levels of carbon dioxide may be the result of several disorders, including but not limited to severe diarrhea, diabetic acidosis, salicylate toxicity, starvation, acute renal failure, alcoholic ketosis, dehydration, high fever, head trauma, malabsorption syndrome, uremia, and ingestion of certain drugs.

Clotting and Coagulation Studies

Partial Thromboplastin Time (PTT)

PTT is an evaluation of the functioning of the coagulation sequence. PTT is a screening process used for coagulation disorders and to monitor the effectiveness of heparin therapy.

Normal values or standardized times must be checked with the laboratory because various processes may be used.

Increased standardized times may be indicative of many disorders, including but not limited to cardiac surgery, DIC, abruptio placentae, factor defects, hemodialysis, obstructive jaundice, vitamin K deficiency, presence of circulating anticoagulants, and ingestion of certain drugs. Decreased standardized times are indicative of acute early hemorrhage and extensive cancer.

Prothrombin Time (PT)

Prothrombin time is a measurement of the time taken for clot formation after the addition of reagent tissue thromboplastin and calcium to citrated plasma. In the clotting process, prothrombin converts to thrombin. Adequate vitamin K is necessary for adequate prothrombin production. This test helps in the evaluation of the clotting mechanism and in monitoring oral anticoagulant therapy.

NORMAL VALUES:
    11.0-13.0 sec; may vary according to laboratory

An increase in prothrombin time may be indicative of several disorders, including but not limited to vitamin K deficiency, liver disorders, anticoagulant therapy, prothrombin deficiency, salicylate intoxication, DIC, SLE, clotting disorders, biliary obstruction, CHF, pancreatitis, snakebite, vomiting, toxic shock syndrome, and ingestion of certain drugs. A reduced prothrombin time may be indicative of certain disorders, including but not limited to deep vein thrombosis, MI, peripheral vascular disease, spinal cord injury, pulmonary embolism, and ingestion of certain drugs.

Platelet Count (Thrombocyte Count)

Count of platelets in a whole blood specimen.

NORMAL ADULT:
    150,000-400,000/μl

Increased platelet count is indicative of many disorders, including but not limited to anemias, carcinoma, fractures, liver disorders, heart disease, hemorrhage, acute infection, inflammation, leukemia, pancreatitis, pregnancy, rheumatoid arthritis, surgery, and ingestion of certain drugs. A decreased platelet count is indicative of many disorders, including but not limited to anemias, bone marrow disorders, autoimmune disorders, severe burns, carcinoma, liver disorders, DIC, hemolytic disease of the newborn, infections, radiation therapy, leukemias, and ingestion of certain drugs.

Bleeding Times

Bleeding time is a screening test for coagulation disorders, a measurement of the time required for the platelet clot to form.

Normal time at most laboratories is 3-10 minutes.

Increased bleeding times are indicative of several disorders, including but not limited to thrombocytopenia, DIC, aplastic anemia, platelet dysfunction, vascular disease, leukemias, liver disorders, aspirin ingestion, and ingestion of certain drugs. Decreased bleeding time is clinically insignificant.

Erythrocyte Sedimentation Rate (ESR)

The rate at which red blood cells (erythrocytes) fall out of well-mixed whole blood to the bottom of the test tube. An alteration in blood proteins occurs during inflammatory and necrotic processes, causing an aggregation of red cells, thereby making them heavier and thus causing them to fall rapidly when placed in a special vertical test tube. A higher ESR is the result of faster settling of the cells. Although not diagnostic of any particular disease process, an elevated ESR gives an indication of an ongoing disease process.

NORMAL VALUES BY WESTERGREN METHOD:
Adult male: 0-15 mm/hr
Adult female: 0-20 mm/hr
Children: 0-10 mm/hr

NORMAL VALUES BY WINTROBE METHOD:
Adult male: 0.41-0.51 mm/hr
Adult female: 0.36-0.45 mm/hr

Increased ESRs may be indicative of many disease processes, including but not necessarily limited to collagen diseases, infectious processes, inflammatory disorders, cancer, heavy metal poisoning, toxemia, PID, anemia, pain, pregnancy, pulmonary embolism, renal disorders, arthritis, subacute bacterial endocarditis, and ingestion of certain drugs. Decreased levels may be found in CHF and ingestion of certain drugs.

Glucose Monitoring

Glucose Tolerance Test (GTT)

GTT is a test that evaluates patients who have symptoms of diabetes mellitus or diabetic complications as well as screening for gestational diabetes. The test measures blood glucose levels at the following intervals: fasting, 30 minutes, 1 hour, 2 hours, and 3 hours after ingestion of a dose of glucose. Urine samples also are taken at these intervals.

NORMAL ADULT LEVELS:
Fasting: 70-110 mg/dl
30 min: 110-170 mg/dl
1 hr: 120-170 mg/dl
2 hr: 70-120 mg/dl
3 hr: 70-120 mg/dl

All urine samples should test negative for glucose.

Increased glucose values or decreased glucose tolerance are indicative of certain disorders, including but not limited to diabetes mellitus, excessive glucose ingestion, certain endocrine disorders, hepatic damage, postgastrectomy, CNS lesions, pancreatitis, pheochromocytoma, and ingestion of certain drugs. Decreased glucose values or increased glucose tolerance may be indicative of certain disorders, including but not limited to Addison disease, hypoglycemia, malabsorption, pancreatic disease, liver disease, hypoparathyroidism, hypopituitarism, and ingestion of certain drugs.

Fasting Blood Glucose (FBS) Levels

The amount of glucose found in the blood after 8 hours of fasting.

NORMAL ADULT LEVELS:
Serum: 70-110 mg/dl

Increased levels of blood glucose are indicative of several disorders, including but not limited to diabetes mellitus, excessive glucose ingestion, certain endocrine disorders, hepatic damage, postgastrectomy, CNS lesions, pancreatitis, pheochromocytoma, and ingestion of certain drugs. Decreased glucose values may be indicative of certain disorders, including but not limited to Addison disease, hypoglycemia, malabsorption, pancreatic disease, liver disease, hypoparathyroidism, hypopituitarism, and ingestion of certain drugs.

2-Hour Postprandial

Blood glucose levels 2 hours after ingestion of a normal meal, usually the noon meal.

NORMAL ADULT LEVELS:
65-139 mg/dl

Increased postprandial levels of blood glucose are indicative of several disorders, including but not limited to diabetes mellitus, excessive glucose ingestion, certain endocrine disorders, hepatic damage, postgastrectomy, CNS lesions, pancreatitis, pheochromocytoma, and ingestion of certain drugs. Decreased postprandial glucose values may be indicative of certain disorders, including but not limited to Addison disease, hypoglycemia, malabsorption, pancreatic disease, liver disease, hypoparathyroidism, hypopituitarism, and ingestion of certain drugs.

Glycosylated Hemoglobin/Glycohemoglobin

Glycohemoglobin is a measurement of the blood glucose bound to hemoglobin and gives an overall view of the past 120 days of glucose saturation.

NORMAL ADULT LEVELS:
5.5%-8.5%

Increased glycohemoglobin levels are indicative of several disorders, including but not limited to poorly controlled diabetes mellitus, iron deficiency anemia, splenectomy, alcohol or lead toxicity, and hyperglycemia. Decreased levels of glycohemoglobin may be indicative of certain diseases, including but not limited to hemolytic anemia, chronic blood loss, chronic renal failure, and pregnancy.

Toxicology Studies and Drug Screens

Toxicology studies are conducted on blood, primarily serum, and on urine. Blood levels of various medications are checked by toxicology levels to determine whether the medications are at therapeutic level or approaching or at a toxic level. Blood alcohol levels are the preferred method of screening for blood alcohol content to provide the desired qualitative information. Urine drug screens are used to detect the presence of various drug substances, primarily drugs of common abuse and/or illegal origin as well as blood alcohol. Drugs detected by urine screening include depressants, hallucinogens, sedatives, and stimulants.

Blood Screening Tests

Drug Levels

Common blood serum testing for therapeutic drugs includes, but is not limited to, digoxin, digitoxin, theophylline, lidocaine, lithium, and various drugs for therapeutic or toxic levels.

Digoxin

Digoxin is a cardiac glycoside used to treat CHF and cardiac arrhythmias. Blood level studies produce information about the therapeutic or toxic levels.

NORMAL THERAPEUTIC LEVEL:
0.8-2 ng/ml

Levels above 2 ng/ml indicate a toxicity of the drug. Medical intervention is necessary to return levels to therapeutic. Levels below 0.8 ng/ml indicate that more digoxin is necessary to achieve the expected therapy.

Digitoxin

Digitoxin is a cardiac glycoside used to treat CHF and cardiac arrhythmias. Blood level studies provide information about the therapeutic or toxic levels.

NORMAL THERAPEUTIC LEVEL:
20-35 ng/ml

Levels above 35 ng/ml indicate a toxicity of the drug. Medical intervention is necessary to return levels to therapeutic. Levels below 20 ng/ml indicate that more digitoxin is necessary to achieve the expected therapy.

Theophylline

Theophylline, a bronchodilator, is used to treat asthma and obstructive respiratory disorders. Blood level studies give information about the therapeutic or toxic levels.

NORMAL THERAPEUTIC LEVEL:

8-20 µg/ml

Levels above 20 µ/ml indicate a toxicity of the drug. Medical intervention is necessary to return levels to therapeutic. Levels below 8 µg/ml indicate that more theophylline is necessary to achieve the expected therapy.

Lidocaine

Lidocaine is used to treat ventricular arrhythmias. Blood level studies give information about the therapeutic or toxic levels.

NORMAL THERAPEUTIC LEVEL:

1.5-6 µg/ml

Levels above 6 µg/ml indicate a toxicity of the drug. Medical intervention is necessary to return levels to therapeutic. Levels below 1.5 µg/ml indicate that more lidocaine is necessary to achieve the expected therapy.

Lithium

Lithium is used to treat bipolar disorders.

NORMAL THERAPEUTIC LEVEL:

0.6-1.2 mEq/L

Levels above 1.2 mEq/L indicate a toxicity of the drug. Medical intervention is necessary to return levels to therapeutic. Levels below 0.6 mEq/L indicate that more lithium is necessary to achieve the expected therapy.

Alcohol Levels

NORMAL:

0%

States have established blood levels or content of alcohol that are considered "legally drunk or intoxicated." Refer to state guidelines for these levels.

Cardiac Enzymes/Cardiac Isoenzymes

Cardiac enzymes and isoenzymes are released by the myocardium as a result of an MI. Monitoring the levels of these enzymes helps evaluate the extent of the insult to the myocardium and the progress of the healing process.

C-Reactive Protein

The tissues of the body release a protein, C-reactive protein, that can be detected, helping to evaluate the status of atheromatous plaques. An elevation in the level of this protein often acts as a potential marker of unstable atheromatous plaque. In addition, it is used as an indicator of CAD. Baseline studies are recommended as a reference for future measurement of arterial condition.

NORMAL:

None

An elevation may be indicative of myocardial infarction, rheumatic fever, rheumatoid arthritis, tuberculosis, cancer, pneumococcal pneumonia, SLE, or use of oral contraceptives. This protein is normally elevated in the last half of pregnancy. An inflammation in the body's tissues also must be considered as a source of the elevation.

Creatine Kinase (CK)

Creatine kinase, an enzyme found in certain body tissues, becomes elevated with damage to cardiac and skeletal muscles.

NORMAL ADULT LEVELS:

Female: 96-140 U/L
Male: 38-174 U/L

Values may vary according to laboratory.
In MI, levels begin to rise in 2-6 hours, peak at 18-36 hours, and return to baseline 3-6 days after the onset of the MI. The increased levels should be part of the total evaluation to confirm an MI.

CK Isoenzymes

Isoenzymes increase during an MI and are more specific in the diagnosis of an MI.

NORMAL VALUES:
MM CK3 (muscle): 90%-100%
MB CK2 (heart): 0%-4%
BB CK1 (brain): 0%

MB CK2 begins to rise within 6-24 hours after the myocardial insult; it usually peaks at 24 hours and then returns to normal within 72 hours.

Lactate Dehydrogenase (LDH)

LDH, an enzyme found in kidney, heart, skeletal muscle, brain, liver, and lung tissue, is released from the cell, increasing serum levels and indicating cellular necrosis.

NORMAL VALUES:
150-450 U

Values may vary according to laboratory.
Levels of LDH begin to rise at 12 hours postinsult, reach a peak at 24 hours, and return to normal later than CK.

Lactate Dehydrogenase Isoenzymes

Lactate dehydrogenase isoenzymes are found in many body tissues and are released when tissue necrosis occurs. There are five different LDH isoenzymes, and elevation of LDH1 and LDH2 usually point to cardiac involvement and subsequent necrosis of myocardial tissue.

NORMAL VALUES: % OF TOTAL
LDH1: 17%-27%
LDH2: 29%-39%
LDH3: 19%-27%
LDH4: 8%-16%
LDH5: 6%-16%

LDH1 and LDH2 usually are increased in myocardial insult and necrosis. LDH1 will peak first, and then in 48 hours the ratio between LDH1 and LDH2 reverses.

Aspartate Aminotransferase (AST, SGOT)

Measurement of enzyme found primarily in heart, liver, and muscle.

Normal adult female: 8-20 U/L
Normal adult male: 8-26 U/L

Elevated AST levels are indicative of many disorders, including but not limited to acute MI, alcoholism, liver disorders, insult and injury to tissue including trauma, cerebral and pulmonary infarctions, and ingestion of certain drugs. Decreased AST levels are indicative of many disorders, including but not limited to diabetic ketoacidosis, liver disease, uremia, and ingestion of certain drugs.

Alanine Aminotransferase (ALT, SGPT)

ALT evaluates liver insult and is a measurement of an enzyme product found in the liver, certain body fluids, and in the liver, heart, kidneys, pancreas, and musculoskeletal tissue.

NORMAL ADULT LEVELS:
7-56 μ/L

Elevated ALT levels are indicative of certain disorders, including but not limited to liver insult and liver disease, CHF, muscle injury, MI, pancreatitis, pulmonary embolism, severe burns, trauma, shock, and ingestion of certain drugs. Decreased levels of ALT are not found.

Urine Studies

Urinalysis (UA)

A screening test, using a urine specimen, that gives a picture of the patient's overall state of health and the state of the urinary tract. Measurements include pH and specific gravity of the urine and presence of ketones, protein, sugars, bilirubin, and urobilinogen. Color and odor are noted, as is the presence of abnormal blood cells, casts, bacteria, other cells, and crystals.

Routine urinalysis—Normal
Characteristics
Color and clarity—Pale to darker yellow and clear
Odor—Aromatic
Chemical nature—pH is generally slightly acidic, 6.5
Specific gravity—1.003-1.030, reflects amount of waste, minerals, and solids in urine
Constituent Compounds

Protein—None, or small amount
Glucose—None
Ketone bodies—None
Bile and bilirubin—None
Casts—None, or small amount of hyaline casts
Nitrogenous wastes—Ammonia, creatinine, urea, and uric acid
Crystals—None to trace
Fat droplets—None

Refer to Table 11–1 for abnormal findings and related pathology.

Culture and Sensitivity (C & S) of Urine

Culture

Sample of urine specimen is placed in/on culture medium to see whether microbial growth occurs. If growth occurs, the pathogenic microbe is identified.

Sensitivity

A portion of the specimen is placed on a sensitivity disk (that has been impregnated with specific antibiotics) to determine the antibiotic to which the pathogen is resistant or to which it will be responsive.

NORMAL:
No growth

Growth will indicate pathogens residing in urinary tract. Sensitivity will identify antimicrobials to which pathogens are sensitive.

Cardiology Tests

Electrocardiogram (ECG) (12 lead)

A recording of electrical activity of the myocardium used to diagnose ischemia, arrhythmias, conduction difficulties, and activity of cardiac medications.

Normal—no dysrhythmias/arrhythmias. A 12-lead electrocardiogram (ECG) consists of three limb leads—I, II, III; three augmented limb leads—AVR, AVL, AVF; and six precordial chest leads—V1, V2, V3, V4, V5, and V6. The conduction of the impulse through the myocardium is traced by three specific areas of the systolic and diastolic complex. The P wave represents atrial depolarization, the conduction of the stimulus from the SA node through the atrium to the AV node. The QRS complex represents ventricular depolarization, that is, the conduction of the stimulus from the upper portion of the ventricle and below the AV node through the bundle of His, through the right and left bundle branches, and through the Purkinje fibers, followed by its relay throughout the ventricular myocardium. The T wave represents the repolarization of the ventricular myocardium. The 12-lead ECG is used to detect conduction abnormalities, dysrhythmias, myocardial ischemia, and myocardial damage; to monitor recovery from an MI; and to assist in evaluation of the effectiveness of cardiac medications. Lead II normally is used to evaluate cardiac rhythm. Refer to Table 10–1—Arrhythmias for explanation of cardiac arrhythmias/dysrhythmias.

Echocardiogram

An ultrasound (acoustic imaging) examination of the cardiac structure to define the size, shape, thickness, position, and movements of the cardiac structures, including valves, walls, and chambers.

NORMAL:
Shows no abnormalities

This noninvasive procedure assists in diagnosing cardiac diseases and disorders, including structural abnormalities, congenital defects, myocardial damage, and blood flow through all structures of the heart.

Holter Monitor

A miniature electrocardiograph that records the electrical activity of the heart for an extended period of time, usually 24 to 48 hours. The patient records all activities during the time period to allow the examiner to correlate activity with cardiac abnormalities.

NORMAL:
No dysrhythmias. Refer to ECG.

Thallium Scan

A scan to indicate myocardial profusion and the location and extent of myocardial ischemia or infarction and predict the possible prognosis of the condition.

NORMAL:

No evidence of myocardial ischemia or infarction.

Normal tissue absorbs the isotope on injection, whereas the ischemic area will not immediately absorb the isotope. As the scan is repeated in 5 minutes, ischemic tissue will absorb the isotope, differentiating it from the infarcted areas, which will never absorb the isotope. This test may be done either under stress or without the stress factor.

MUGA Scan (Multigated Blood Pool Study)

A scan that assesses the function of the left ventricle and identifies abnormalities of the myocardial walls.

Normal: 55%-65% ejection fraction, symmetrical contraction of the left ventricle.

A radioactive isotope is injected to show all four chambers and the great vessels simultaneously. A series of images is taken during both systole and diastole, then either shown as a movie or superimposed to relate ventricular function and to allow the ejection fraction to be calculated. This test may be performed either under stress or without the stress factor.

Stress Testing, Treadmill, Exercise Tolerance Testing

An assessment of cardiac function during moderate exercise on a treadmill or stationary bicycle after a 12-lead electrocardiogram.

NORMAL:

Negative

The stress test measures the effects of exercise on myocardial output and oxygen consumption by the concurrent evaluation of the monitored electrocardiogram and oxygen consumption. This test is performed in a safe environment to identify individuals who are prone to myocardial ischemia during activity.

Pulse Oximeter

An instrument (spectrophotometer) that provides a noninvasive measurement of the O_2 saturation of the arterial blood.

NORMAL:

Arterial blood oxygen saturation 95% or greater

Cardiac Catheterization

Fluoroscopic visualization of right or left side of heart by the passing of a catheter into right or left chambers and injection of dye. In angiograms, the catheter is passed into the coronary vessels, where the dye is injected and fluoroscopic images are recorded.

Normal varies with the area being assessed. Normal would indicate normal anatomy and physiology, normal chamber volumes and pressures, normal wall and valve motion, and patent coronary arteries. Normal value for cardiac output is 5-8 L/min.

Imaging Studies

Radiographs

Visualization of internal organs and structures by electromagnetic radiation. Radiographs of bone; the abdomen; the chest; paranasal sinuses; kidneys, ureters, and bladder (KUB); and mammograms do not require contrast medium. Contrast medium is used to distinguish soft tissue and some organs such as the gallbladder, esophagus, stomach, and small and large intestines. Normal results vary with the area being studied by the imaging process. The imaging is interpreted by the radiologist, with a report then dictated and transcribed for the ordering physician. The ordering physician often visually inspects the films or images to evaluate the area himself or herself.

Magnetic Resonance Imaging (MRI)

Uses a magnetic field instead of radiation to visualize internal tissues. It is possible to view tissue and organs in three dimensions with MRI. It helps in determining blood flow to tissues and organs, in studying the condition of blood vessels, to detect tumors, to differentiate healthy and diseased tissues, and to detect sites of infection. The patient is not exposed to ionizing radiation during MRI.

Normal results vary with the area being studied during the MRI. The MRI is interpreted by the radiologist, with a report then dictated and transcribed for the ordering physician. The ordering physician often visually inspects the films or images of the MRI to evaluate the area himself or herself.

Computerized Tomography (CT) Scans

A radiographic technique using a scanner system that can provide images of the internal structure of tissue and organs both geographically and characteristically.

Normal results vary with the area being studied during the CT scan. The scan is interpreted by the radiologist, with a report then dictated and transcribed for the ordering physician. The ordering physician often visually inspects the films or images of the CT scan to evaluate the area himself or herself.

Fluoroscopy

A real-time imaging process that provides continuous visualization of the area being imaged. Films are made of the process for more extensive examination. Used in procedures and to study the functioning of tissues and organs.

Normal results vary with the area being studied during fluoroscopy. The procedure is interpreted by the radiologist, with a report then dictated and transcribed for the ordering physician. The ordering physician often performs a procedure using fluoroscopy as a diagnostic tool and also as a guide for the procedure.

Sonograms, Ultrasound, Echogram

An imaging system that projects a beam of sound waves into target tissues or organs and receives the waves as they bounce back off the target structure. An outline of the structure is produced and recorded on film for examination. Tissue, organs, and systems that may be studied by ultrasound include but are not limited to abdominal aorta, brain, breast, eye and orbit, gallbladder, pelvis for gynecologic structures, heart, kidney, liver, lymph nodes, pancreas, prostate, spleen, thyroid, urinary bladder, upper GI tract, and pregnant pelvis for obstetric diagnostic examination.

Normal examinations vary with the area being examined. The ultrasound scan is interpreted by the radiologist, with a report then dictated and transcribed for the ordering physician. The ordering physician often visually inspects the films or images of the ultrasound to evaluate the area himself or herself.

Myelogram

An imaging examination of the spinal cord and spinal nerve roots. Contrast medium (dye) or air is injected into the subarachnoid space and recorded on radiographic film. Fluoroscopy generally is used in this procedure.

Normal will reveal no lesions or abnormalities.

It is used to diagnose ruptured or bulging disks, spinal cord lesions and tumors, spinal cord and spinal nerve trauma and edema, and other conditions involving the spinal cord and spinal nerves.

Stool Analysis

Guaiac Tests

For occult blood. A qualitative detection of red blood cells in the stool.

NORMAL:
Negative

Presence of blood in the stool specimen is indicative of trauma, lesion, or other insult to the GI mucosa, producing blood.

Ova, Larva, and Parasite Tests

A microscopic examination of stool to detect the presence of parasites at various stages of development.

NORMAL:
None detected

A positive examination result indicates parasitic infection of the GI tract.

Endoscopy Tests

Endoscopy

Visual inspection of internal organs or cavities of the body through the use of a fiberoptic instrument with the appropriate scope. In addition, pathology may be removed and insult to the tissue may be repaired during the diagnostic procedure.

Gastroscopy

Visualization of the stomach by a gastroscope.

Normal: Appearance of upper GI tract is within normal limits.

Hemorrhagic areas or erosion of a vessel may be revealed. Additional abnormal findings may include neoplasm, gastric ulcers, hiatal hernia, gastritis, and esophagitis.

Colonoscopy

Visualization of colon with a colonoscope.

Normal: Appearance of large intestinal mucosa is normal.

Inflammation, areas of ulceration, bleeding areas, strictures, polyps, colitis, diverticula, benign or malignant tumors, or foreign bodies may be observed in abnormal findings.

Sigmoidoscopy

Visualization of the sigmoid portion of the colon and the rectum with a sigmoidoscope.

Normal: Normal appearance of mucosa of sigmoid colon

Inflammatory bowel disease, polyps, benign and cancerous tumors, and foreign bodies may be some of the abnormal findings during a sigmoidoscope examination.

Proctoscopy

Visualization of the rectum with a proctoscope.

Normal: Normal appearance to rectal mucosa and to anal canal

Rectal prolapse, hemorrhoids, rectal strictures, fissures, abscesses, and fistulas are some of the abnormal findings during a proctoscopic examination of the rectum.

Cystoscopy

Visualization of the structures of the urinary tract with a cystoscope.

Normal: The urethra, urethral orifices, urinary bladder interior, and male prostatic urethra appear normal.

Cancer of the bladder, BPH, bladder calculi, prostatitis, ureteral strictures, urinary fistulas, vesicle neck stenosis, ureterocele, polyps, and abnormal bladder capacity are some of the abnormal findings during a cystoscopic examination of the urinary bladder.

Ureteroscopy

Visualization of the ureters and pelvis of the kidney.

Normal: Normal appearance of the ureters and pelvis of the kidney and its structures

Renal or ureteral stones, inflammation or bleeding of the urethral mucosa, and lesions or abnormal structures of the renal pelvis are some of the abnormal findings in a ureteroscopic examination.

Bronchoscopy

Visualization of the trachea and bronchi with a bronchoscope.

Normal: Nasopharynx, larynx, trachea, and bronchi are normal in appearance.

Abnormalities revealed in a bronchoscopic examination include but are not limited to bronchitis, carcinoma and other tumors, inflammatory processes, tuberculosis, abnormal structure and disorders of the larynx and trachea, foreign bodies, and various pulmonary infections.

Arthroscopy

Visualization or inspection of the inner aspect of a joint with an endoscope called an arthroscope. Biopsy specimens may be obtained.

Normal: Normal appearance of the inner aspect of the joint

Abnormal findings in the knee may include tears of meniscus, bone or cartilage fragments, and damage to other structures within the joint. Surgical repair may be attempted. Refer to Chapter 7 for additional information on arthroscopy.

Arterial Blood Gases

Arterial Blood Gas (ABG) Analysis

A measurement of dissolved oxygen and carbon dioxide in arterial blood. Also a measurement of pH and O_2 saturation of the arterial blood. ABGs are used to assess oxygenation and ventilation, along with acid–base balance. In addition, they produce information about the effectiveness of therapy and the status of critical patients and are used in conjunction with pulmonary function studies.

Normal values are listed; however, these studies are complex and require interpretation by a physician along with other diagnostic studies and consideration of symptoms and signs to produce a diagnosis or an evaluation.

Pulmonary Function Studies

NORMAL ADULT VALUES:

pH: 7.35-7.45

$PaCO_2$: 35-45 mm Hg

PaO_2: 75-100 mm Hg

HCO_3: 22-26 mEq/L

O_2 saturation: 96%-100%

Increased pH is indicative of several disorders, including but not limited to alkali ingestion, diarrhea, vomiting, hyperventilation, high-altitude sickness, metabolic acidosis, fever, and ingestion of certain drugs. Decreased pH is indicative of several disorders, including but not limited to asthma, cardiac disease, MI, renal disorders, Addison disease, pulmonary disorders, respiratory acidosis, sepsis, shock, and malignant hyperthermia.

Increased $PaCO_2$ is indicative of several disorders, including but not limited to late-stage asthma, brain death, CHF, respiratory disorders, hypoventilation, renal disorders, poisoning, pneumothorax, respiratory acidosis, near drowning, and ingestion of certain drugs. Decreased $PaCO_2$ is indicative of several disorders, including but not limited to early-stage asthma, hyperventilation, dysrhythmias, respiratory alkalosis, metabolic acidosis, and ingestion of certain drugs.

Increased PaO_2 is indicative of but not limited to hyperventilation and hyperbaric oxygen exposure. Decreased PaO_2 is indicative of several disorders, including but not limited to ARDS, asthma, cardiac disorders, head injury, anoxia, hypoventilation, respiratory disorders, pneumothorax, respiratory failure, shock, smoke inhalation, and CVA.

Increased O_2 saturation is indicative of hyperbaric oxygenation. Decreased O_2 saturation is indicative of several disorders, including but not limited to anoxia, cardiac anomalies and disorders, carbon monoxide poisoning, ARDS, CVA, hypoventilation, respiratory disorders, pneumothorax, shock, smoke inhalation, and near drowning.

Pulmonary Function Studies

Pulmonary function studies are complex and include evaluation of several tests' results. Most tests are performed by respiratory therapists, and results usually are reported to a pulmonologist for evaluation and correlation with symptoms and signs. Normal values are reported here; however, the significance of these values is incomplete without the review and opinion of the pulmonologist, often assisted by the respiratory therapist.

Pulse Oximeter

An instrument (spectrophotometer) that produces a noninvasive measurement of the O_2 saturation of the arterial blood

Normal: Arterial blood oxygen saturation 95% or greater.

Peak Flow

A measurement of inspiratory effort.

Normal: Approximately 300 L/min and is based on sex, height, and age.

Spirometry

A measurement of lung capacity, volume, and flow rates used in the evaluation of asthma, bronchitis, COPD, and emphysema

Methacholine Challenge

A measurement of lung volumes before and after inhalation of methacholine chloride used for diagnosis of asthma

Normal: Negative

Sputum Studies

Sputum studies are analyses and cultures of sputum (material expelled from the respiratory tract) to detect the presence of pathogens. Common studies ordered on sputum include cytology testing, gram stain, and culture and sensitivity.

NORMAL:

Negative

Positive results might include respiratory disorders such as fungal infections, mycobacteria, tuberculosis, or carcinoma.

Pulmonary Function

Normal findings are reported in percentages of observed values and by expected values calculated to include allowances for age, sex, weight, and height. Abnormal results are considered to be less than

80% of calculated values. Consult a respiratory therapist for interpretation of values.

Tidal volume—Normal: 500 ml
Expiratory reserve volume—Normal: 1500 ml
Residual volume—Normal: 1500 ml
Inspiratory reserve volume—Normal: 2000 ml

Miscellaneous Tests

Culture and Sensitivity Studies (C & S)

Specimens are obtained from various tissues and fluids of the body, placed on or in a medium to grow, and then studied for microbes present. The specimens are also placed on a disk impregnated with various antibiotics to determine which antibiotic will be effective in destroying or curbing the reproduction of the microbe.

Tissues and fluids include blood, sputum, CSF, urine, exudates from lesions, nasal secretions, stool, wound drainage, and any excised tissue.

NORMAL:
No growth

The growth of any microbes will require microscopic identification. The antibiotic-impregnated disk will require inspection and identification of antibiotics showing effectiveness against the microbes.

Bone Marrow Studies

Aspiration of bone marrow by needle from the sternum, posterior superior iliac spine, or the anterior iliac crest for diagnosis of neoplasms, metastasis, and blood disorders. Produces a basis for evaluation of hematologic disorders and infectious diseases.

Immune and Immunoglobulin Studies

Studies of the functioning or nonfunctioning of the patient's immune system

NORMAL ADULT:
IgA: 60-400 mg/dl
IgG: 700-1500 mg/dl
IgM: 60-300 mg/dl
IgD: 0-8.0 mg/dl
IgE: 3-42 IU/ml

Increased levels of immunoglobulins are indicative of many disorders and need to be evaluated by a physician. Some disorders include arthritis, cancer, chronic infections, sinusitis, asthma, food and drug allergies, liver disease, SLE, and ingestion of certain drugs. Decreased levels of immunoglobulins are indicative of many disorders, including but not limited to AIDS, bacterial infection, advanced cancer, hypogammaglobulinemia, and ingestion of certain drugs.

Biopsies

The excision of tissue from the living body, followed by microscopic examination, for purpose of exact diagnosis.

Normal: No abnormal cells seen.

Abnormal findings depend on cell structure discovered during microscopic examination.

Lumbar Puncture

A surgical procedure to withdraw spinal fluid for analysis. A measurement and analysis of the chemical components of the cerebrospinal fluid used in diagnosis of CNS diseases and disorders.

NORMAL ADULT:
Appearance: Clear, colorless
Specific gravity: 1.006-1.008
Pressure: 90-150 mm H_2O
AST: 0-19 U
Bicarbonate: 22.9 mEq/L
WBC: 5 cells
Glucose: 40-70 mg/dl
Total protein: 15-60 mg/dl
Lactic acid: 10-24 mg/dl
VDRL: Negative
Bacteria or viruses: None present

Pressure depends on height and whether patient is positioned in a sitting or horizontal position.

Abnormal findings are indicative of disorders or insults to the CNS.

Electroencephalogram

A recording of the electrical activity of the cerebral cortex of the brain, it helps to identify the locale of insult to cerebral tissue.

Normal: Shows symmetric patterns of electrical brain activity.

Abnormal findings include information indicative of CNS or brain insults, hematomas, CVAs, epilepsy, brain tumors, and seizure activity. Lack of any activity is an indication of brain death.

Electromyelogram

An electrodiagnostic assessment and recording of the activity of the skeletal muscles; a nerve conduction study assessing the state of the muscle at rest and during contraction to produce an average picture of local electrical activity of the muscle

Normal: Nerve conduction normal and muscle action potential is normal.

Abnormal findings help to identify the site and cause of muscle disorders and neuronal lesions, particularly of involvement of the anterior horn of the spinal cord.

Gastric Analysis

Used in the diagnosis of pernicious anemia and peptic ulcers. The contents of the stomach are analyzed for acidity, appearance, and volume.

NORMAL ADULT:
Bile: 0 or minimal
Mucus: Evenly mixed
Blood: 0 or scant
Fasting acidity: 2.5 mEq/L
Quantity: 62 ml/hr
PH: 1.0-2.5

Increased levels of gastric acid are indicative of certain disorders, including but not limited to post–massive small-intestinal resection, gastric or duodenal ulcer, hyperplasia, and hyperfunction of gastric cells. Reduced gastric acid levels are indicative of several disorders, including but not limited to pernicious anemia, postvagotomy, renal failure, rheumatoid arthritis, gastric cancer, atrophic gastritis, and vitiligo.

Pregnancy Tests (Human Chorionic Gonadotropin [hCG/UCG])

Used in diagnosis of pregnancy, abortion, ectopic pregnancy, and uterine pathology.

NORMAL:
Negative

A positive result is indicative of pregnancy, either intrauterine or ectopic.

Screening

Tuberculosis (TB) Screening (Mantoux)

An intradermal injection of tuberculin is given, usually on the inner aspect of the lower arm. Results are read in 48 and 72 hours.

NORMAL:
Negative

Positive—Localized thickening of the skin in the area, along with a redness, indicates the presence of active or dormant tuberculosis.

Positive reaction requires further investigation, usually including a chest radiograph.

Cancer or Tumor Markers as Screening Tools

Certain substances are produced by some tumors or cancer, including enzymes, antigens, and hormones. These substances may be present in the blood in higher-than-normal levels and may be an indication of the presence of a tumor. Cancer or tumor markers cannot be used alone to diagnose the presence of cancer or a tumor. Some benign tumors may stimulate the production of these markers. In addition, elevated cancer markers are not always present, especially in the early stages of the disease process. Some physicians will track the progress of tumor growth as well as using them to measure the effectiveness of treatment and for possible recurrence of the tumor. There are several markers, and many are specific in nature. The most widely used screening tool of this nature is the PSA. Other markers include CA 125, carcinoembryonic antigen, alpha-fetoprotein, CA 19-9, CA 15-3, and the Pap smear.

Prostate-Specific Antigen (PSA)

A serum blood test to determine the level of the prostate-specific antigen. This is a screening test that should be followed by a digital rectal examination (DRE) of the prostate gland to identify any abnormalities. Additional diagnostic studies often are indicated.

PSA blood tests are reported as nanograms per milliliter.

PSA is considered a marker in the screening for prostatic cancer. Zero to 4 ng/ml usually are considered to be in the normal range; 4 to 10 ng/ml are considered borderline; values greater than 10 ng/ml are considered high. Increasing age makes slightly higher values acceptable.

ACCEPTABLE LEVELS FOR UP TO AGE 40 YEARS: 0-2 ng/ml
    40-50 years: 0-4 ng/ml
    50-60 years: 0-5 ng/ml
    60-70 years: 0-6 ng/ml

Any increase of 20% or more in the PSA value in 1 year's time is suspicious and requires further investigation. Above-acceptable levels may be indicative of cancer. Additional investigation, including biopsy, is recommended.

The PSA screening should be completed before the DRE. A constant increase in the PSA leads to suspicion of prostate cancer. PSA levels that fluctuate up and down usually are not indicative of cancer but of an inflammatory process in the prostate or of BPH. PSA is a screening tool and must be combined with a DRE for a more accurate screen. Men older than 50 years of age are encouraged to have prostate screening on an annual basis; men older than 70 years of age may or may not be subjected to screening because of the high incidence of prostatic cancer in this group and the treatment protocol of watchful waiting without significant intervention.

CA 125

CA 125 may reflect an increase in production of a marker that may be indicative of cancer of the ovaries.

NORMAL:
    <35 U/ml (conventional units)

Abnormal: An elevation above normal may be indicative of cancer of the ovaries, pelvic organs (including the uterus and cervix), pancreas, liver, breasts, colon, lung, and digestive tract.

CA 19-9

CA 19-9 may reflect an increase in marker levels in the presence of colorectal cancer.

NORMAL:
    <37 U/ml (conventional units)

An elevation may be indicative of the presence of colorectal, pancreatic, stomach, and bile-duct cancer.

CA 15-3

CA 15-3 may reflect an increase in marker levels in the presence of breast cancer.

NORMAL:
    <35 U/ml (conventional units)

An elevation may be indicative of the presence of breast cancer, benign conditions of breast and ovarian disease, pelvic inflammatory disease (PID), endometriosis, pregnancy, lactation, and hepatitis.

Carcinoembryonic Antigen

Carcinoembryonic antigen may be elevated in some people without any form of cancer. This test is used to monitor the spread or metastasis of colorectal cancer and other cancers.

Reference value varies with the health of the individual as well as the smoking history and the presence of existing intestinal or other disease processes. A baseline should be established and monitored for effectiveness of treatment or exacerbation of the condition.

Alpha-Fetoprotein (AFP)

Under normal circumstances, alpha-fetoprotein is produced by the developing fetus with maternal levels decreasing after birth. However, certain conditions involving the fetus may cause an abnormal elevation of this protein as pregnancy progresses, suggesting a possible neural tube deficit or other anomaly in the developing fetus. A maternal AFP level that does not return to normal after parturition is an indication of possible liver or germ cell cancer that demands additional testing.

Normals for amniotic fluid levels as well as blood serum AFP levels: Check with reference laboratory for their normal levels.

Elevations in maternal serum levels as well as amniotic fluid may be indicative of neural tube deficits, including in the non-pregnant female and the male population.

Pap Smear (Papanicolaou test)

A cytologic examination of cells that have been scraped or aspirated from the cervix and cervical os. A screening test done annually, especially before any female hormones are prescribed.

Results of Pap smears are now reported in two different formats. The two methods of reporting results to the physician are a system based on classes, and the Bethesda system, a system using descriptive diagnostic terms.

CLASS SYSTEM:

Class I: Negative with no abnormal or unusual cells seen.

Class II: Negative smear but with some reservation based on the presence of inflammatory cells or evidence of infection. Additional causes may be regeneration of cervical cells or changes related to trauma, infections, or childbirth. A repeat Pap smear and treatment of the underlying cause may be indicated.

Class III: Presence of some abnormal cells that may be considered premalignant. Changes may vary from mild dysplasia to severe dysplasia. Further evaluation, possibly including colposcopy, is indicated.

Class IV: Indicative of a high degree of suspicion for malignancy. Prompt and complete evaluation is indicated.

Class V: Indication of high probability of more extensive malignancy. Prompt and complete evaluation to determine the extent of disease is indicated.

BETHESDA SYSTEM:

Bethesda system: The physician may relate the results as normal or abnormal because surface cervical cells may appear abnormal but are not always malignant.

Dysplasia: Although not cancer, dysplasia may develop into very early cancer of the cervix. The cells in dysplasia undergo a series of changes in their appearance, appear abnormal in microscopic examination, and have not invaded nearby healthy tissue. The cells are described as mild, moderate, or severe according to their appearance under the microscope.

Squamous intraepithelial lesion (SIL) describes the appearance of abnormal changes on the surface of the cervix. SIL cells are classified further as low grade, having early changes in size, shape, and number, or high grade, containing a large number of precancerous cells with an appearance very different from normal cells.

Cervical intraepithelial neoplasia (CIN) is a description of a new abnormal growth of surface layers of cells. Additional information is provided by using the term CIN and the numbers 1, 2, and 3 to describe how much of the cervix contains abnormal cells.

Carcinoma in situ refers to a preinvasive cancer that has not invaded deeper tissues and contains only surface cells.

Atypical glandular cells of undetermined significance (AGCUS) describes slightly abnormal glandular cells of the cervix.

Atypical squamous cells of undetermined significance (ASCUS) describes slightly abnormal squamous cells of the cervix, possibly caused by a vaginal infection or by HPV (human papillomavirus).

Inflammation: Inflammation is present in the cervical cells, and white blood cells also are seen.

Hyperkeratosis: Hyperkeratosis describes dried skin cells on the cervix, often resulting from cervical cap or diaphragm usage or a cervical infection.

Abnormal results range from insignificant to precancerous to invasive cancer of the cervix. Repeat Pap smears in 6 months are often all that is indicated for mild dysplasia and class II Pap smears. Colposcopy and further investigation may be indicated in other abnormal findings. The physician discusses abnormal findings with the patient, and a course of treatment or follow-up is determined.

Mammogram

A radiographic examination of the soft tissues of the breast. A screening test performed on an annual basis for women older than 40 years of age to detect the presence of breast disease. This screening should be accompanied by a manual examination of the breast tissue by a physician. Monthly breast self-examinations are recommended.

NORMAL:

Negative for disease

Identification of abnormal conditions may indicate further investigation. Various benign disorders, including fibrocystic disease of the breast, may be responsible for a positive interpretation. Malignant neoplasms of the breast tissue may be detected, and further investigation, including ultrasound or biopsy of any suspicious area found on the mammogram, is indicated.

Pharmacology

Side effects are listed by various groups of medications and are not specific to any one drug in that group. Referral to the current edition of the *Physician's Desk Reference* (PDR) or other pharmacology reference is recommended to confirm side effects for a specific drug.

This table gives the major drug groups, organized by the action of the medication. The exam-ples are just that—examples—to represent the multiple medications found in each group. The examples are commonly prescribed and may be familiar in some way. Once again, refer to the current edition of the PDR or other pharmacology reference to locate additional drugs in the group.

BODY SYSTEM	DRUG CATEGORY	DRUG ACTION	EXAMPLES	SIDE EFFECTS	COMMENTS
CHAPTERS 1 AND 2					
Drugs for pain and fever	Analgesics Opioids (Narcotics)	Relieve pain	codeine, meperidine (Demerol)	May cause drowsiness; constipation can occur	May become addictive. Patients should not drive or operate machinery while taking.
	Nonopioid		acetaminophen (Tylenol) acetylsalicylic acid (aspirin)	Aspirin may cause stomach upset and tinnitus	Aspirin also has anti-coagulant, antiprosta-glandin effects. Both are antipyretic medications
	Anesthetics General	Produce loss of sensation by interfering with nerve impulses	thiopental Na (Pentothal) midazolam (Versed)	Versed: amnesia, hypotension, headache	Versed is used for conscious sedation.
	Local		lidocaine (Xylocaine) procaine (Novocain)		Xylocaine may be topical form, also is used system-ically as cardiac drug.
Drugs for infectious diseases	Antibiotics	Destroy or inhibit the growth of bacterial strains of microorganisms but have not been found to be effective for viral infections	penicillin v potassium (Pen-V-K) tetracycline (Sumycin) amoxicillin (Amoxil) cephalosporins (Keflex, Ceclor) ciprofloxacin (Cipro)	Common side effects of any are nausea, GI upset, urticaria	Caution must be used when administering penicillin IM regarding observation after injection for potential of anaphylaxis. Cipro: acute infections and prophylactic postanthrax exposure
	Antifungals	Inhibit and kill fungal growth	griseofulvin (Grisactin) ketoconazole (Nizoral) clotrimazole (Lotrimin)	Nausea, vomiting, abdominal pain, itching, urticaria	Some are available in oral form for systemic treatment, others are available in topical form
	Antivirals	Inhibit viral growth	acyclovir (Zovirax) zidovudine (Retrovir) amantadine (Symmetrel)	GI disturbances, headache, malaise, insomnia, dizziness	Should be taken at first sign of onset of viral attack for best relief of symptoms.
	Antiprotozoals	Inhibit protozoal infections	chloroquine HCl	Headache, pruritus, GI	Also known as antimalarials.

Category	Classification	Use	Drugs	Side effects/adverse reactions	Special considerations
	Antipyretics	Reduce fever	acetaminophen (Tylenol) acetylsalicylic acid (aspirin) ibuprofen (Motrin)	Toxic doses of acetaminophen may cause irreversible and fatal liver damage	Caution must be exercised when administering Tylenol drops or syrup to infants and children. Check dosage for either before administering. These drugs usually are given in combination.
Drugs used to treat cancer	Antitubercular	Suppress mycobacterium causing tuberculosis	Isoniazid (INH) ethambutol (Myambutol)	GI disturbances and hepatic disturbances	Historically used in combination to treat cancer. Cytoxan is considered an alkylating agent.
	Antineoplastics	Used as chemotherapy to inhibit the growth of neoplasms. May be used in conjunction with radiation or surgery.	cyclophosphamide (Cytoxan) methotrexate (Mexate, Folex) fluorouracil (5-FU)	Nausea, vomiting, hair loss and interference with blood cell production resulting in anemia and suppression of the immune system.	Fluorouracil is used topically to treat actinic keratosis and basal cell carcinoma.
	Antimetabolites	Treat carcinomas and sarcomas	methotrexate (Tolex) mercaptopurine (Purinethol)	Bone marrow depression, stomatitis, mouth ulcers, GI upset, loss of hair, fever and chills	Side effects are relatively mild. Blood counts and liver studies are recommended.
	Estrogen receptor blocker	Used to treat breast cancer	tamoxifen (Nolvadex)	Reduces platelet count; may cause hot flashes night sweats, and insomnia	
Drugs used as nutritional supplements and alternative medicines	Electrolytes	Replace electrolytes	KCl (K-Tab) 0.9% sodium chloride (normal saline) Na polystyrene (Kayexalate)	Rapid heart rate when levels are abnormally high	Potassium replacement therapy in use of diuretics. Potassium levels should be monitored.
	Vitamin/mineral supplements	Supplement or replace essential vitamins and minerals	vitamin B_{12} (cyanocobalamin), multiple vitamins (One-A-Day), vitamins with minerals (One-A-Day with Minerals), ferrous sulfate (Feosol)	Oral iron supplements may cause constipation Excessive oral iron intake may cause GI bleeding	Vitamin B_{12} for treatment of pernicious anemia is by injection. Caution must be used to avoid excessive ingestion of fat-soluble vitamins and iron to prevent toxicity. Folic acid supplements are encouraged for females of childbearing capability to reduce incidence of neural tube deficits in developing fetus.

Continued

BODY SYSTEM	DRUG CATEGORY	DRUG ACTION	EXAMPLES	SIDE EFFECTS	COMMENTS
CHAPTER 3 Drugs used to treat disorders of the immune system, immunizations	Immunizations	Provide artificially acquired active immunity to diseases; produce an antigen–antibody reaction	diphtheria-tetanus-pertussis vaccine (DPT), measles-rubella-mumps vaccine, polio vaccine, oral (Sabin) and injectable (Salk)	Redness may develop at injection site, generalized malaise and fever	Follow American Academy of Pediatrics schedule recommendation
	Immune globulins and antitoxins	Provide artificially acquired passive immunity	Rho (D) immune globulin (Rho GAM), immune globulin (Gamastan), tetanus antitoxin	Local inflammation at the injection site, slight fever	RhoGAM is given prenatally and postnatally to Rh neg mothers to prevent Rh incompatibility in the infant and in subsequent pregnancies.
	Immunosuppressants	Reduce the body's autoimmune response to its own tissues	methotrexate (Rheumatrex), cyclosporine (Neoral), azathioprine (Imuran)	Imuran: lower white cell count, upper GI symptoms, fatigue, alopecia, diarrhea, joint pain	Used to prevent rejection in transplant patients and to treat rheumatoid arthritis. Increases risk of cancer in long term use
CHAPTER 4 Drugs for the endocrine system	Hypoglycemics A. Insulin	Replacement for insulin needed in diabetes mellitus	isophane suspension insulin (NPH-Humulin-N; Novolin-N; Lantus) regular insulin (Iletin R; Humulin R)	Side effects of insulin include hypoglycemia or insulin shock	Glucophage reduces absorption of glucose from the intestine, helps to prevent gluconeogenesis, and increases insulin utilization.
	B. Oral Hypoglycemics	Stimulates insulin release	glipizide (Glucotrol) metformin (Glucophage) glyburide (Glynase) ploglitazone (Actos)	Sulfonylureas also may cause hypoglycemia	Patients taking Glucophage should be warned about the danger of iodine-media–based contrast imaging studies and the importance of advising any imaging technicians that they are taking Glucophage.

Insulin antagonists or hyperglycemics	Elevate blood sugars	Glucagons	Increase in blood glucose	Glucose tablets and gels are effective in emergency situations of low blood glucose.
Corticosteroids	Regulation of immune response system and control of artificial immune response	hydrocortisone (Cortef) dexamethasone (Decadron) prednisone (Deltasone) methylprednisolone (Medrol)	Nervousness; sleepiness; hypertension; muscle weakness; dry, itching, burning skin; depression	Must be "weaned" off by reducing dosages. Long-term use may cause severe effects.
Thyroid replacements	Treat hypothyroidism	thyroid extract levothyroxine (Synthroid)	Increased or irregular heart beat, SOB, headache, nervousness, irritability, sleeplessness, tremors, heat intolerance, weight changes, vomiting or diarrhea	Take 30 minutes before breakfast on empty stomach. Once diagnosed as hypothyroid, patient must take replacement therapy for life.
Antithyroid preparations	Inhibit the production of thyroid hormone	methimazole (Tapazole) propylthiouracil (PTU)	Blood dyscrasias	Medication should be taken around the clock. Used to treat Graves' disease.

CHAPTER 5
Drugs for the sensory system

A. Eyes				
Mydriatics	Dilate the pupil of the eye	epinephrine (Epifrin, Glaucon) phenylephrine (Isopto Frin, Prefrin Liquifilm)	Systemically will cause increased heart rate, increased BP	Adrenergic drugs.
Miotics	Constriction of pupil of the eye	pilocarpine (Isopto Carpine, Ocusert Pilo) carbachol (Isopto carbachol) timolol maleate (Timoptic)	May slow heart rate and cause drop in BP	In the beta-blocker class.
B. Ears				
Cerumenolytics	Soften and emulsify ear wax	carbamide peroxide (Debrox)	None noted, do not use if tympanic membrane is ruptured or there is a discharge from ear	Must not be used when ruptured tympanic membrane is present.

Continued

BODY SYSTEM	DRUG CATEGORY	DRUG ACTION	EXAMPLES	SIDE EFFECTS	COMMENTS
Drugs for the sensory system B. Ears—cont'd	Antiinfectives	Inhibit the growth of bacteria, as in swimmer's ear	boric acid solution (swimmer's ear) hydrogen peroxide/ ethyl alcohol	Rash	Used routinely after swimming.
CHAPTER 6 Drugs for the integumentary system	Anesthetics	Produce a lack of sensation to pain or abolishes the sensation to pain	Topical: ethyl chloride dibucaine (Nupercaine) Local: lidocaine (Xylocaine) bupivacaine (Marcaine)	Neurotoxicity, local reaction	May be mixed with epinephrine, causing vasoconstriction and extending duration of anesthesia.
	Antiparasitics	Rid body of parasites (e.g., lice)	lindane (Kwell) pyrethrin (RID)	Possibly carcinogenic	May be a blood toxin, must be used with care; follow all directions completely.
	Antipruritics	Stop itching	calamine lotion diphenhydramine HCl cream (Benadryl cream) corticosteroid creams and ointments	Unlikely. Skin rash may rarely occur.	Provides topical relief for dermatitis-type irritation.
	Antiseptics	Retard bacterial growth, usually used on living tissue	Hexachlorophene (pHisoHex) silver sulfadiazine (Silvadene)	pHisoHex: dermatitis, may be toxic when absorbed systemically.	Used as preoperative scrubs and cleansing. Silvadene is used on burn patients.

Category	Purpose	Drugs	Side effects	Comments
Disinfectants	Kill or inhibit bacterial growth; usually used on inanimate objects	hydrogen peroxide povidone iodine (Betadine) isopropyl alcohol	[...Silva]dene has a solid base and may cause reactions in those allergic to sulfa-based products. Betadine may cause skin rash when applied to those who have allergic reactions to topical iodine.	
		Formaldehyde glutaraldehyde (Cidex) phenol (Lysol)	Not for use on humans. May cause skin rash.	Effective as disinfectant on inanimate objects
Emollients	Soothe irritated tissue	A+D Cream	None likely	Frequently used to treat diaper rash or other localized skin irritation
Demulcent (emollients and demulcents often are classified together)	Protects tissues	A+D Ointment Diaparene, vitamin E ointment Desitin, Sween Cream	None likely	Frequently used to treat diaper rash or other localized skin irritation
Keratolytics	Control abnormal skin scaling or promote peeling of overgrowths/neoplasms of skin	coal tar (Tegrin Shampoo) salicylic acid benzoyl peroxide (Clearasil) fluorouracil (Efudex) tretinoin (Retin A)	Retin A: erythema, crusting lesions on skin; itching, burning, and dryness of skin	Efudex is used to treat actinic keratosis and basal cell carcinoma.

CHAPTER 7 Drugs for the musculoskeletal system

Category	Purpose	Drugs	Side effects	Comments
Antiarthritics	Treat arthritic symptoms, especially rheumatoid arthritis	auranofin (Ridaura) gold sodium thiomalate (Myochrysine) celecoxib (Celebrex)	Bone marrow depression, hematuria, GI upset, ulcerative colitis	Celebrex is a cox-2 inhibitor reported to have fewer gastric side effects.
Antigouts	Treat chronic gout	colchicine allopurinol (Zyloprim) probenecid (Benemid)	Rash, headache, GI disorders, blood dyscrasias	Helpful in reducing excessive amounts of uric acid produced by body
Antiinflammatories	Reduce inflammation in joints and muscles			
A. Steroidal (See endocrine system)		prednisone, etc.	GI upsets and bleeds, renal disturbances. Steroids may mask infections.	Patients usually are instructed to follow instructions carefully and report any side effects ASAP.
B. NSAIDs (nonsteroidal antiinflammatory drugs)		ibuprofen (Motrin, Advil) naproxen (Naprosyn) indomethacin (Indocin)	GI symptoms, bleeding tendencies, changes in liver enzymes	

Continued

BODY SYSTEM	DRUG CATEGORY	DRUG ACTION	EXAMPLES	SIDE EFFECTS	COMMENTS
Drugs for the musculoskeletal system—cont'd	Bone replacement therapeutics	Treatment and prevention of osteoporosis	alendronate (Fosamax) calcitonin (salmon) (Miacalcin nasal spray)	Abdominal pain, muscle pain, constipation or diarrhea, nausea, flatulence	Instruct patients to take Fosamax on an empty stomach with a glass of water and not to eat for at least 30 minutes. Vitamin D is necessary for calcium absorption.
	Muscle relaxants	Relax skeletal muscles	methocarbamol (Robaxin) cyclobenzaprine HCl (Flexeril)	GI upset, miosis, increased bronchial secretions, muscle cramps, tachycardia, elevated liver enzymes	May make patients drowsy; advise against driving or operating machinery
CHAPTER 8 Drugs used for the gastrointestinal system	Antacids	Neutralize stomach acid	calcium carbonate (Tums) magaldrate (Riopan) magnesium–aluminum hydroxide (Maalox)	Constipation or diarrhea	Chronic use of antacids may cause acid rebound effect.
	Antidiarrheals	Control diarrhea	bismuth subsalicylate (Pepto-Bismol) loperamide (Imodium) diphenoxylate HCl/atropine (Lomotil)	Constipation, abdominal cramping	Prolonged uncontrolled diarrhea should be reported to a physician.
	Antidotes	Neutralize toxins and poisons	syrup of ipecac activated charcoal	Syrup of ipecac is never given if the ingested substance is corrosive (e.g., lye, Drano), is petroleum based, or patient is lethargic or unconscious. Charcoal will cause stool to be black.	Syrup of ipecac: administration is followed by drinking a minimum of 4-6 glasses of water (adults). Be prepared for vomiting. The activated charcoal is given after the vomiting has ceased; protect clothing; give with a straw to get medication to back of mouth and prevent charcoal color on teeth.

Classification	Action/Use	Examples	Adverse Reactions	Comments
Antiemetics	Prevention and treatment of nausea and vomiting	Prochlorperazine (Compazine) metoclopramide HCl (Reglan) dimenhydrinate (Dramamine) ondansetron (Zofran)	Drowsiness, dizziness, blurred vision, anticholinergic effects, hypotension, skin reactions	Slow peristalsis, may cause abdominal cramping and related constipation. Zofran may be given to cancer patients on chemotherapy to aid in nausea and vomiting. Also used to treat infant colic.
Antiflatulents	Symptomatic relief of gastric bloating and intestinal gas	simethicone (Mylicon, Phazyme)	None noted	
Anthelmintics	Eradication of helminths (worms)	mebendazole (Vermox) pyrantel pamoate (Antiminth)	Abdominal pain, diarrhea	Treatment of entire family is recommended.
Antispasmodics	Relieve smooth-muscle spasms of the stomach and intestines	hyoscyamine sulfate (Levsin) belladonna hyoscyamine (Donnatal) dicyclomine HCl (Bentyl)	Decreased peristalsis, dry mouth, headache, dizziness, palpitations, fatigue	Used to treat irritable bowel syndrome and similar intestinal disorders.
Antiulcer	Reduce gastric acid secretions by acting as histamine 2 receptor antagonists	cimetidine (Tagamet) ranitidine (Zantac) nizatidine (Axid)	Headache, fatigue, myalgia, alopecia, diarrhea, rash, dizziness	Helpful in treatment of GERD
Digestants	Assist with digestion of food by replacing pancreatic enzymes	pancrelipase (Ultrase, Pancrease) pancreatin (Creon)	GI upset, rashes	Instruct patient not to chew or crush capsules.
Emetics	Cause vomiting	Syrup of ipecac	Syrup of ipecac is never given if the ingested substance is corrosive (e.g., lye, Drano), is petroleum based, or patient is lethargic or unconscious.	Syrup of ipecac administration is followed by drinking a minimum of 4-6 glasses of water (adults). Be prepared for vomiting.
Laxatives/cathartics	Induces defecation and relieves constipation	bisacodyl (Dulcolax) mineral oil psyllium (Metamucil)	Cramping, diarrhea	Caution patients about excessive continued use that may have reverse reaction.
Stool softeners	Soften feces	docusate sodium (Colace) docusate calcium (Surfak)	Leakage of oil-like substances from rectum, increased peristalsis, cramping	Used to ease evacuation of bowel contents.

Continued

CHAPTER 9
Drugs used for the respiratory system

BODY SYSTEM	DRUG CATEGORY	DRUG ACTION	EXAMPLES	SIDE EFFECTS	COMMENTS
Drugs used for the respiratory system	Asthma prophylactics	Prevention of exercise-induced asthma	cromolyn sodium (Intal)	Bronchospasm, cough, wheezing, nasal congestion	An antiallergic agent that has best action when used before exposure.
	Antihistamines	Inhibit histamine to relieve allergy symptoms	diphenhydramine (Benadryl) clemastine (Tavist) chlorpheniramine (Chlor-Trimeton) fexofenadine (Allegra) cetirizine (Zyrtec) loratidine (Claritin)	Drowsiness, dry eyes, dry mouth, hypotension constipation, anorexia, palpitations	May cause drowsiness. Advise patient not to drive or operate machinery while taking medication. Contraindicated in patients with glaucoma.
	Antitussives	Cough suppressants	dextromethorphan (Benylin) hydrocodone bitartrate (Triaminic)	CNS stimulation, blurred vision, palpitations, anxiety, weakness, insomnia	Instruct patients to follow directions.
	Bronchodilators	Relax smooth muscle of bronchial tree; relieve bronchospasm	albuterol sulfate (Proventil) epinephrine (Primatene) theophylline (Theo-Dur)	Hyperactivity, excitement, tremor, nervousness, insomnia, tachycardia	Routine theophylline blood level studies are recommended.
	Decongestants	Shrink nasal mucous membranes	oxymetazoline (Afrin) pseudoephedrine HCl (Sudafed) phenylephrine (Neo-Synephrine)	Nasal sprays may cause irritation to nasal membrane. Constricts vessels; hypertension	Prolonged use of sprays may cause rebound effects. Should not be used by pregnant females as possible constriction of vessels may occur.
	Expectorants	Increase respiratory secretions and reduce viscosity to allow for the expulsion of sputum	guaifenesin (Robitussin) iodinated glycerol (Organidin)	Excitability, constipation, nausea, vomiting, drowsiness	May cause drowsiness. Advise patient not to drive or operate machinery while taking medication.

Mucolytics	Liquefy respiratory secretions	acetylcysteine (Mucomyst)	Runny nose, throat irritation, nausea	Used to treat asthma and cystic fibrosis. Also used as antidote in acetaminophen overdose.
Smoking cessation aids	Reduce nicotine levels while assisting with smoking-cessation programs	nicotine (Nicorette, Nicoderm) bupropion (Zyban)	Tobacco withdrawal symptoms, local effects from patches or sprays, dry mouth, insomnia	Patient may require emotional support while using these products.
CHAPTER 10 Drugs used for the cardiovascular system and for hematology				
Antianginals	Prophylactic treatment of angina; dilate coronary arteries	nitroglycerin (Nitrostat, Transderm-Nitro)	Lightheadedness, headache	Nitrostat sublingual tablets should be placed under the tongue to treat angina. May be repeated every 5 minutes three times to relieve angina. If no relief, entry into the emergency medical system is advised.
Antiarrhythmics	Suppress cardiac arrhythmias	propranolol (Inderal) verapamil (Isoptin) procainamide (Pronestyl)	Hypotension, GI upset, headache, fatigue	Regular monitoring of arrhythmias is recommended.
Anticoagulants	Prevent formation of clots	warfarin sodium (Coumadin) heparin sodium	Tissue or organ hemorrhage, rash, abdominal pain, headache	Blood coagulation studies are performed on a regular basis.
Antihypertensives	Treatment and management of hypertension	metoprolol (Lopressor) atenolol (Tenormin) clonidine (Catapres) methyldopa (Aldoril)	Hypotension, lethargy, GI symptoms, slow heart rate, dizziness	Atenolol is a beta-blocker. These medications should not be stopped abruptly.
Antihyperlipidemics	Reduce serum cholesterol and low-density lipoproteins	gemfibrozil (Lopid) cholestyramine (Questran) simvastatin (Zocor) atorvastatin (Lipitor) ezetimibe (Zetia)	Myalgia, GI upset, headache, rash, dizziness, elevated liver enzymes. Zetia: stomach pain, tiredness	Statin drugs are reported to reduce existing arterial plaque. Zetia is a cholesterol-lowering drug with less reported myalgia.

Continued

BODY SYSTEM	DRUG CATEGORY	DRUG ACTION	EXAMPLES	SIDE EFFECTS	COMMENTS
Drugs used for the cardiovascular system and for hematology—cont'd	Cardiotonics/cardiac glycosides	Strengthen heart beats	digoxin (Lanoxin) digitoxin (Crystodigin)	Irregular heartbeat, palpitations, loss of appetite, nausea, vomiting, diarrhea, visual changes	Instruct patient to take in morning, record daily weights, and take apical pulse before taking medication. If pulse is below 60 BPM, hold dose and recount pulse in 1 hour. If still below 60 BPM, hold medication and contact physician. Patient may be digitalis toxic.
	Coagulants/hemostatics	Control or stop bleeding by promoting coagulation	phytonadione (Aquamephyton) menadiol sodium (Synkayvite)		Administered to newborns to prevent hemorrhagic disease of newborns.
	Platelet Inhibitors	Inhibit platelet clumping	aspirin dipyridamole (Persantine)	Normal aspirin side effects, Persantin, dizziness, headache, rash, GI upset	Work best in combination.
	Thrombolytics	Dissolve blood clots	streptokinase (Streptase) alteplase (Activase)	GI bleeds, bleeding in other sites	Best if administration begins within 2-3 hours after onset of MI chest pain.
	Vasoconstrictors	Constrict blood vessels	metaraminol (Aramine) norepinephrine (Levophed) epinephrine (Adrenalin)	Nausea and vomiting, cardiac arrhythmias, decreased urine output	Used to treat shock.
	Vasodilators	Dilate blood vessels	nitroglycerin isosorbide dinitrate (Isordil) isoxsuprine HCl (Vasodilan) isosorbide mononitrate (ISMO)	Lightheadedness, headache	Nitrostat sublingual tablets should be placed under the tongue to treat angina. May be repeated every 5 minutes three times to relieve angina. If no relief, entry into the emergency medical system is advised.

CHAPTER 11
Drugs used for the urinary system

Classification	Action	Drug	Side Effects	Nursing Considerations
Urinary analgesics	Lessen pain and burning of urinary tract infection	phenazopyridine HCl (Pyridium)	Produces orange to red-colored urine that may stain clothing.	Advise patients about possibility of stains to clothing from the orange or red-colored urine.
Urinary antiseptics	Specific antibacterials for urinary tract	nitrofurantoin (Furadantin) nitrofurantoin monohydrate/ macrocrystals (Macrobid)	GI disturbances, may turn urine orange	Inform patients about possibility of urine turning orange and suggest sanitary napkin protection for underwear.
Urinary antispasmodics	Relief of urgency, frequency, and incontinence	oxybutynin HCl (Ditropan) flavoxate (Urispas)	Dry mouth, constipation, somnolence, tachycardia	Relaxes bladder muscles and helps to reduce incontinence.
Diuretics	Remove excessive fluid from body tissues; increase urinary output	furosemide (Lasix) hydrochlorothiazide (HydroDiuril) bumetanide (Bumex)	Hypokalemia, excessive diuresis, GI upset, dizziness, vertigo	Characterized by site of action. Many require monitoring of potassium levels and require daily potassium replacement. Instruct patients to take medication in AM so they can have restful nights. Encourage recorded daily weights.
Enuretic agents	Control enuresis	desmopressin acetate (DDAVP nasal spray) tolterodine tartrate (Detrol)	Dry mouth, constipation, somnolence, tachycardia	Relax bladder muscles and help to reduce incontinence.

CHAPTER 12
Drugs used for the reproductive system

Classification	Action	Drug	Side Effects	Nursing Considerations
Contraceptives	Prevent conception or pregnancy	estrogen/progestin (Ovral, Triphasil, Ortho-Novum)	Thromboembolism associated with MI and CVA. Elevated blood pressure and blood glucose levels, acne, hair loss, gall bladder disease, hirsutism	A missed pill may lead to pregnancy. Antibiotic therapy may render contraceptive ineffective. Now available in an intradermal patch form.
Fertility enhancers	Induce ovulation	clomiphene citrate (Clomid)	GI symptoms, CNS symptoms, acne, ovarian enlargement, ectopic pregnancies	Occurrence of multiple pregnancies

Continued

BODY SYSTEM	DRUG CATEGORY	DRUG ACTION	EXAMPLES	SIDE EFFECTS	COMMENTS
Drugs used for the reproductive system—cont'd	Hormone Replacements	Replace reproductive hormones			
	A. Androgens	Stimulate the development of male characteristics	testosterone (Depo-Testosterone) methyltestosterone (Testred)	Urinary urgency, breast tenderness, priapism	Supplement low levels of testosterone
	B. Estrogens	Stimulate the development of female characteristics	estradiol (Estrace) conjugated estrogens (Premarin)	Anorexia, nausea, headaches, edema of lower extremities, hypercalcemia, thrombophlebitis	Used to treat symptoms of menopause, increases risk of breast and cervical cancer. Caution must be used in females that smoke; may cause DVT
	C. Progestins	Treat amenorrhea and abnormal uterine bleeding	progestins (Depo-Provera, Provera) medroxyprogesterone (Provera)	Weight gain, stomach disturbances, edema, headaches, breakthrough bleeding	May be used for contraception, used in combination with estrogen for postmenopausal HRT.
	Drugs used to treat prostatic conditions	Treats BPH and urinary retention	doxazosin (Cardura) tamsulosin (Flomax) terazosin (Hytrin) finasteride (Proscar)	Hypotension, fatigue, edema, dyspnea	Used to relieve urinary retention and nocturia caused by enlarged prostate.
	Drugs used to treat erectile dysfunction		sildenafil citrate (Viagra) tadalafil (Cialis)	Nasal congestion, blurred vision, hypertension, dizziness, rash	Alert patients who have cardiac disease not to take Viagra. Drug should be taken on an empty stomach an hour before eating.
CHAPTER 13 Drugs used for the neurologic system	Adrenergics	Mimic sympathetic nervous system	epinephrine (Adrenalin) dopamine (Intropin)	Increased blood pressure and rapid heart rate	Initiate "fight or flight" system
	Adrenergic blockers	Block the action of sympathetic nervous system	propranolol (Inderal) methyldopa (Aldomet)	Hypotension, bradycardia, constricted bronchioles	Used to treat hypertension; Inderal also used for migraine headaches

Classification	Action	Drugs	Side Effects	Comments
Analgesics				
A. Opioids (Narcotics)	Relieve pain	codeine, meperidine (Demerol)	May cause drowsiness; constipation can occur.	May become addictive. Patients should not drive or operate machinery while taking.
B. Nonopioids		acetaminophen (Tylenol) acetylsalicylic acid (aspirin)	Aspirin may cause stomach upset and tinnitus.	Aspirin also has anti-coagulant, antiprostaglandin effects. Both are antipyretic medications.
Anesthetics	Produce loss of sensation by interfering with nerve impulses			
A. General		thiopental sodium (Pentothal) midazolam (Versed)	Versed: amnesia, hypotension, headache	Versed is used for conscious sedation.
B. Local		lidocaine (Xylocaine) procaine (Novocaine)		Xylocaine may be topical form, also is used systemically as cardiac drug.
Anticholinergics	Block parasympathetic nervous system	atropine scopolamine	Dry mouth, increased heart rate, constipation, urinary retention. Dilate pupils.	May be used in treatment of Parkinson disease.
Antiepileptics	Reduce the number and/or the severity of seizures due to epilepsy	phenytoin (Dilantin) clonazepam (Klonopin) gabapentin (Neurontin)	Reduced coordination, involuntary eye movement, slurred speech	Encourage good mouth care as Dilantin may cause gingival hyperplasia. Neurontin may be prescribed to treat post-therapeutic neuralgia. Do not stop these medications abruptly.
Antiparkinsonism medications	Relieve symptoms and increase mobility of patients with Parkinson disease	levodopa (L-dopa) amantadine (Symmetrel)	Dystonia, GI symptoms, dry mouth, increased hand tremors	Used to increase levels of dopamine in the brain.
Cholinergics	Mimic parasympathetic nervous system by liberating acetylcholine	neostigmine (Prostigmin) pilocarpine (Isopto Carpine)	Increased peristalsis	

Continued

BODY SYSTEM	DRUG CATEGORY	DRUG ACTION	EXAMPLES	SIDE EFFECTS	COMMENTS
Drugs used for the neurologic system—cont'd	Hypnotics/Sedatives A. Barbiturates	Produce sedation or sleep	amobarbital (Amytal) secobarbital (Seconal)	Increased excitability, hostility, confusion, hallucinations	May cause drowsiness, do not drive or operate machinery. Do not consume alcohol while using.
	B. Nonbarbiturates		choral hydrate (Noctec) flurazepam (Dalmane)		
	Stimulants	Increase the activity of brain/spinal cord	caffeine methylphenidate HCl (Ritalin) amphetamines	Anorexia, euphoria, sleeplessness, dry mouth, GI disturbances	May be addictive. Ritalin is used to treat hyperactivity in children.
	Drugs used in the treatment of Alzheimer disease	Enhance transmissions of cholinergic neurons to improve thought processes	tacrine (Cognex) donepezil (Aricept)	GI disturbances, insomnia, vomiting, anorexia	Help with memory and thinking processes, improve everyday activities, improve behavior.
CHAPTER 14 Drugs used for mental disorders	Antianxiety/Anxiolytics/ Minor Tranquilizers	Short-term treatment of anxiety disorders, some psychosomatic disorders, and nausea and vomiting	diazepam (Valium) lorazepam (Ativan) clorazepate (Tranxene) alprazolam (Xanax)	CCNS symptoms, GI disturbances, skin rash, nasal congestion	May cause drowsiness; use caution when driving or operating machinery. Patient should not stop medication abruptly but be "weaned" off by reducing dosages.

Category	Use	Drugs	Side effects	Comments
Antidepressants/mood elevators	Treat patients with depression	amitriptyline (Elavil) phenelzine (Nardil) sertraline (Zoloft)	CNS symptoms, GI disturbances, weight gain, somnolence. SSRIs have a lower incidence of side effects.	May take 2–4 weeks for effects to be realized. Consumption of alcohol should be avoided.
Antimanics	Treat manic disorders	lithium (Lithobid)	Dry mouth, excessive thirst, weight gain, GI disturbances, tremors, cardiac arrhythmias, visual impairment, and unsteady gait	Used to treat bipolar disorders. Blood level should be monitored on a regular basis.
Antipsychotics/ Neuroleptics/ Major Tranquilizers	Relieve symptoms of psychosis and severe neurosis	haloperidol (Haldol) fluphenazine HCl (Prolixin) chlorpromazine (Thorazine) imipramine (Tofranil)	Tachycardia or bradycardia, vertigo, postural hypotension, dry mouth, constipation, urinary retention, anorexia, blurred vision, fever, CNS system reactions	May cause drowsiness; use caution when driving or operating machinery.

CHAPTER 15
Drugs used for first aid, emergency situations

Category	Use	Drugs	Side effects	Comments
Sulfonamides used for burns	Topical burn treatment	silver sulfadiazine (Silvadene) mafenide acetate (Sulfamylon)	Rash and redness	Helpful in treating infections; broad spectrum effective against both Gram-positive and Gram-negative organisms.
Antivenoms	Counteract toxins such as those from snake bites, spider bites	crotaline Fab antivenom (FAB) (rattlesnake) Black widow spider antivenom	Made from sheep serum so less likely to produce severe reaction than antivenom from horse serum. Compartment syndrome may occur in affected limb.	Often preceded by administration of antihistamine to lessen any allergic effects. Observation of individual for a minimum of 24 hours usual protocol.

Resource Agencies

Chapter 1

Cancer Information Service
National Cancer Institute
NCI Public Inquiries Office, Suite 3036A
6116 Executive Blvd., MSC8322
Bethesda, MD 20892-8322
(800) 4-CANCER
www.nci.nih.gov

Centers for Disease Control and Prevention
1600 Clifton Rd.
Atlanta, GA 30333
(800) 311-3435
www.cdc.gov

American Academy of Allergy, Asthma and
  Immunology
611 E. Wells St.
Milwaukee, WI 53202
(800) 822-2762
www.aaaai.org

National Council on Aging
300 D Street, SW, Suite 801
Washington, DC 20024
(202) 479-1200
www.ncoa.org

Genetic Alliance, Inc.
4301 Connecticut Ave. NW, Suite 404
Washington, DC 20008-2369
(202) 966-5557
www.geneticalliance.org

Chapter 2

American Academy of Pediatrics
National Headquarters
141 Northwest Point Blvd.
Elk Grove Village, IL 60007-1098
(847) 434-4000
www.aap.org

Cystic Fibrosis Foundation
6931 Arlington Rd.
Bethesda, MD 20814
(800) FIGHT-CF, (800) 344-4823
www.cff.org

United Cerebral Palsy Association
1660 L Street, NW, Suite 700
Washington, DC 20036
(800) 872-5827
www.ucpa.org

Muscular Dystrophy Association – USA
National Headquarters
3300 E. Sunrise Dr.
Tucson, AZ 85718
(800) 572-1717
www.mdausa.org

Shriner's Hospitals for Children
2900 Rocky Point Dr.
Tampa, FL 33607-1460
(800) 237-5055
www.shrinershq.org

Cleft Palate Foundation
104 S. Estes Dr., Suite 204
Chapel Hill, NC 27514
(800) 24-CLEFT
(919) 933-9044
www.cleftline.org

Asthma and Allergy Foundation of America
  (AAFA)
1233 20th Street, NW, Suite 402
Washington, DC 20036
(800) 7-ASTHMA
(202) 466-7643
www.aafa.org

National Immunization Hotline (English)
(800) 232-2522
National Immunization Hotline (Spanish)
(800) 232-0233

Chapter 3
National Institute of Allergy and Infectious
  Diseases (NIAID)
Building 31, Room 7A-50
31 Center Dr., MSC 2520
Bethesda, MD 20892-2520
www.niaid.nih.gov

National HIV/AIDS Hotline
(800) 342-2437
(800) 344-7432 (Spanish)
STD Hotline (800) 227-8922
www.ashastd.org/nah

Arthritis Foundation
P.O. Box 7669
Atlanta, GA 30357-0669
(800) 283-7800
www.arthritis.org

Lupus Foundation of America
2000 L St., NW, Suite 710
Washington, DC 20036
(800) 558-0121
(202) 349-1155
www.lupus.org

National Multiple Sclerosis Society
733 Third Ave.
New York, NY 10017
(800) Fight-MS (344-4867)
www.nmss.org

Chapter 4
National Institute of Diabetes and Digestive and
  Kidney Diseases
Building 31, Room 9A04, 31 Center Drive, MSC 2560
Bethesda, MD 20892-2560
(301) 496-4000
www.niddk.nih.gov

American Diabetes Association
Attention: National Call Center
1701 N. Beauregard St.
Alexandria, VA 22311
(800) 342-2383
www.diabetes.org

Endocrine Society
8401 Connecticut Ave., Suite 900
Chevy Chase, MD 20815-5817
(301) 941-0200
www.endo-society.org

American Thyroid Association
6066 Leesburg Pike, Suite 650
Falls Church, VA 22041
(800) THYROID
www.thyroid.org

Chapter 5
American Foundation for the Blind (AFB)
AFB Headquarters
11 Penn Plaza, Suite 300
New York, NY 10001
(800) 232-5463
(212) 502-7600
www.afb.org

National Institute on Deafness and Other
  Communication Disorders
National Institutes of Health
31 Center Dr., MSC 2320
Bethesda, MD 20892-2320
www.nidcd.nih.gov

American Academy of Ophthalmology
P.O. Box 7424
San Francisco, CA 94109
(415) 561-8500
www.aao.org

Glaucoma Research Foundation
4900 Post St., Suite 1427
San Francisco, CA 94102
(800) 826-6693
www.glaucoma.org

Chapter 6
American Academy of Dermatology
P.O. Box 4014
Schaumburg, IL 60168-4014
(888) 462-DERM (3376)
(847) 330-0230
www.aad.org

Chapter 6–cont'd

American Academy of Dermatology (Washington office)
1350 I Street, NW, Suite 880
Washington, DC 20005-4355
(202) 842-3555
www.aad.org

The Melanoma Research Foundation
23704-5 El Toro Rd., #206
Lake Forest, CA 92630
(800) MRF-1290
www.melanoma.org

Chapter 7

American Lyme Disease Foundation
Mill Pond Offices
293 Route 100
Somers, NY 10589
(914) 277-6970
www.aldf.com

Amyotrophic Lateral Sclerosis Association
27001 Agoura Rd., Suite 150
Calabasas Hills, CA 91301
(800) 782-4747
www.alsa.org

National Osteoporosis Foundation
1232 22nd St. NW
Washington, DC 20037-1292
(202) 223-2226
www.nof.org

National Eating Disorders Association
603 Stewart St., Suite 803
Seattle, WA 98101
(206) 382-3587
www.nationaleatingdisorders.org

American Liver Foundation
75 Maiden Ln., Suite 603
New York, NY 10038
(800) GO-Liver (465-4837)
www.liverfoundation.org

Chapter 8

Traveler's Hotline
Centers for Disease Control
(877) 394-8747

American Dental Association
211 E. Chicago Ave.
Chicago, IL 60611-2678
(312) 440-2500
www.ADA.org

American Society for Gastrointestinal Endoscopy
1520 Kensington Rd., Suite 202
Oakbrook, IL 60523
(630) 573-0600
www.asge.org

National Eating Disorders Association
603 Stewart St., Suite 803
Seattle, WA 98101
(206) 382-3587
www.nationaleatingdisorders.org

American Liver Foundation
75 Maiden Ln., Suite 603
New York, NY 10038
(800) GO-Liver (465-4837)
www.liverfoundation.org

Chapter 9

American Lung Association
61 Broadway, Sixth Floor
New York, NY 10006
(800) 586-4872
(212) 315-8700
www.lungusa.org

National Institute of Allergy and Infectious Diseases (NIAID)
Building 31, Room 7A-50
31 Center Dr., MSC 2520
Bethesda, MD 20892-2520
www.niaid.nih.gov

Chapter 10

American Heart Association (AHA)
7272 Greenville Ave.
Dallas, TX 75231
(800) AHA-USA1 or (800) 242-8721
www.americanheart.org

American Red Cross
National Headquarters
2025 E St., NW
Washington, DC 20006
(202) 303-4498
www.redcross.org

Leukemia & Lymphoma Society
Home Office
1311 Mamaroneck Ave.
White Plains, NY 10605
(800) 955-4572
(914) 949-5213

Chapter 11

National Kidney Foundation
30 East 33rd St., Suite 1100
New York, NY 10016
(800) 622-9010
www.kidney.org

American Urological Association
1000 Corporate Blvd.
Linthicum, MD 21090
(866) RING-AUA or (866) 746-4282
www.auanet.org

American Foundation for Urologic Disease
1000 Corporate Blvd., Suite 410
Linthicum, MD 21090
(800) 828-7866
www.afud.org

The Organ Procurement and Transplantation
  Network
P.O. Box 2484
Richmond, VA 23218
(888) TX-INFO-1
www.optn.org

Chapter 12

Women's National Health Resource Center
157 Broad St., Suite 315
Red Bank, NJ 07701
(877) 986-9472
www.healthywomen.org

American Social Health Association
P.O. Box 13827
Research Triangle Park, NC 27709
(919) 361-8400
www.ashastd.org

American Society for Reproductive Medicine
1209 Montgomery Highway
Birmingham, AL 35216-2809
(205) 978-5000
www.asrm.org

Endometriosis Association
8585 North 76th Place
Milwaukee, WI 53223
(414) 355-2200
www.endometriosisassn.org

North American Menopause Society
P.O. Box 94527
Cleveland, OH 44101
(800) 774-5342
(440) 442-7550
www.menopause.org

Chapter 13

National Spinal Cord Injury Association
6701 Democracy Blvd.
Suite 300-9
Bethesda, MD 20817
(800) 962-9629
www.spinalcord.org

National Parkinson Foundation
Bob Hope Parkinson Research Center
1501 N.W. Ninth Ave.
Bob Hope Rd.
Miami, FL 33136-1494
(800) 327-4545
www.parkinson.org

American Association of Neurological Surgeons
5550 Meadowbrook Drive
Rolling Meadows, IL 60008
(888) 566-2267
www.aans.org

National Multiple Sclerosis Society
733 Third Ave.
New York, NY 10017
(800) 344-4867
www.nationalmssociety.org

Brain Trauma Foundation
5841 Cedar Lake Road, Suite 204
Minneapolis, MN 55416
(952) 545-6204
www.aneuroa.org

Chapter 14

Alzheimer's Association
225 N. Michigan Ave., Suite 1700
Chicago, IL 60601-7633
(800) 272-3900
www.alz.org

National Center for Post-Traumatic Stress
  Disorder
VA Medical Center
215 N. Main St.
White River Junction, VT 05009
(802) 296-5132
www.ncptsd.org

National Institute of Mental Health (NIMH)
Office of Communications
6001 Executive Blvd., Room 8184 MSC 9663
Bethesda, MD 20892-9663
(866) 615-6464
www.nimh.nih.gov

Alcoholics Anonymous
475 Riverside Drive, 11th floor
New York, NY 10115
(212) 870-3003
www.alcoholics-anonymous.org

American Academy of Sleep Medicine
One Westbrook Corporate Center 0930, Suite 920
Westchester, IL 60154
(708) 492-0930
www.aasmnet.org

Chapter 15

American Trauma Society (ATS)
8903 Presidential Parkway, Suite 512
Upper Marlboro, MD 20772
(800) 556-7890
www.amtrauma.org

National Center for Missing and Exploited
  Children
Charles B. Wang International Children's
  Building
699 Prince St.
Alexandria, VA 22314-3175
(866) 411-5437 (toll-free)
www.missingkids.org

Girls and Boys Town
14100 Crawford St.
Boys Town, NE 68010
(800) 448-3000
www.girlsandboystown.org

National Coalition Against Domestic Violence
P.O. Box 18749
Denver, CO 80218
(800) 799-SAFE (7233) (National Hotline)
(303) 839-1852
www.ncadv.org

FaithTrust Institute (Formerly Center for
  Prevention of Sexual and Domestic Violence)
Faith Trust Institute
2400 N 45th St. #10
Seattle, WA 98103
(206) 634-1903
www.cpsdv.org

Rape, Abuse, and Incest National Network
635-B Pennsylvania Ave., SE
Washington, DC 20003
(800) 656-4673, extension 3
www.rainn.org

American Burn Association
ABA Central Office—Chicago
625 N. Michigan Ave., Suite 1530
Chicago, IL 60611
(800) 548-2876
(312) 642-9260
www.ameriburn.org

Abduct (*Sp. Abducción, separar*): move an arm or leg away from the body

Abruptio placentae (*Sp. Desprendimiento de la placenta*): detachment of the placenta from the uterus before birth; often results in severe bleeding

Abscess (*Sp. Absceso*): a localized collection of pus surrounded by swollen tissue

Acidemia (*Sp. Acidemia*): a decreased pH of the blood (increased hydrogen ion concentration)

Acidosis (*Sp. Acidosis*): a pathologic condition resulting from an abnormal increase in the level of hydrogen ion in the body (decrease in pH) resulting from the accumulation of acid or loss of the alkaline reserve

Acute abdomen (*Sp. Abdomen agudo*): an abdominal condition of sudden onset, accompanied by pain resulting from intraabdominal inflammation or infection

Adenocarcinoma (*Sp. Adenocarcinoma, carcinoma glandular*): a cancerous tumor arising from glandular tissue

Adenoma (*Sp. Adenoma*): a benign neoplasm in which cells are derived from glandular epithelium

Adenosarcoma (*Sp. Adenosarcoma*): a cancerous gland-like tumor, such as Wilms' tumor

Adnexal (*Sp. De los anexos*): pertaining to accessory organs or tissues; an appendage(s)

Agglutination (*Sp. Aglutinación*): the clumping of antigens with antibodies, or of the red blood cells from one type of blood with the red blood cells of another type

Aggregation (*Sp. Agregación*): the coming together of entities such as platelets, blood cells, or diseases

Agranulocytosis (*Sp. Agranulocitosis*): a condition of the blood marked by a sudden decrease in the number of granulocytes (a type of white blood cell); occurs in lesions of the throat or other mucous membranes or as a side effect of the administration of certain drugs or radiation

Alkalosis (*Sp. Alcalosis*): excessive alkalinity of body fluids

Allergen (*Sp. Alérgeno*): an antigenic substance capable of producing an allergic response in the body

Allograft (*Sp. Injerto alogénico*): a graft of tissue between genetically different individuals of the same species

Amblyopia (*Sp. Ambioplía*): reduced vision in an eye without a detectable organic lesion

Amnesia (*Sp. Amnesia*): a loss of memory; inability to recall past experiences

Amniography (*Sp. Amniografía*): radiography (after injection of radiopaque contrast medium into the amniotic fluid) of the pregnant uterus to detect placement of the placenta, the amniotic cavity, and the fetus

Amniotic fluid (*Sp. Líquido amniótico*): a transparent albuminous liquid made by the amnion and the fetus; surrounds and protects the fetus during pregnancy

Amyloid (*Sp. Amiloide*): a waxy, starch-like protein that tends to build up in tissues and organs in certain pathologic conditions

Analgesia, analgesic (*Sp. Analgesia, analgésico*): relief of pain

Anaphylaxis (*Sp. Anafilaxia*): a severe systemic allergic response characterized by redness, itching, swelling, and water buildup (angioedema); in severe cases, life-threatening respiratory distress occurs and the blood pressure drops rapidly (anaphylactic shock)

Anaplastic (*Sp. Anaplástico*): a change in the orientation and structure of cells; a loss of differentiation that is characteristic of malignancy

Anastomosis (anastomoses) (*Sp. Anastomosis*): the surgical or pathologic connection between two vessels or tubular structures

Anesthesia, anesthetic (*Sp. Anestesia, anestésico*): partial or complete loss of sensation caused by injury, diseases, or the administration of an anesthetic agent

Angina pectoris (*Sp. Angina de pecho*): paroxysmal chest pain, which often radiates to the arms and may be accompanied by a feeling of suffocation and impending death; the most common cause is a shortage of oxygen to the cardiac muscle linked with coronary artery disease

Angioplasty (*Sp. Angioplastia*): repair of a narrowed blood vessel through surgery or other angiographic procedures

---

The Glossary contains all chapter Key Terms plus important terms italicized in the text.

Angiotensin-converting enzyme (ACE) (*Sp. Enzima de conversión de la angiotensina—ECA*): an enzyme found on the surface of blood vessels in the lungs and other tissues with vasopressive action

Angiotensin-converting enzyme inhibitors (*Sp. Inhibidores de la enzima de conversión de la angiotensina*): agents that inhibit angiotensin-converting enzyme (a potent vasoconstrictor) and promote relaxation of blood vessels

Ankylosis (*Sp. Anquilosis*): immobility of a joint

Anorexia, anorectic (*Sp. Anorexia, anoréxico*): loss of appetite for food

Antibody (antibodies) (*Sp. Anticuerpo*): an immunoglobulin that may combine with a specific antigen to destroy or control it

Anticholinergic (*Sp. Anticolinérgico*): a drug used to block the transmission of parasympathetic nerve impulses

Anticholinesterase (*Sp. Anticolina esterasa*): any enzyme that counteracts the action of the choline esters

Anticoagulant (*Sp. Anticoagulante*): any substance that delays or prevents blood clotting

Antiemetic (*Sp. Antiemético*): a medication that prevents or relieves nausea and vomiting

Antigen (*Sp. Antígeno*): any substance that stimulates the immune system to produce antibodies

Antimicrobial (*Sp. Antimicrobiano*): a substance that kills microorganisms or suppresses their growth

Antipyretic (*Sp. Antipirético*): a drug or treatment that reduces or relieves fever

Antitrypsin (*Sp. Antitripsina*): a substance that inhibits trypsin, an enzyme that hastens the hydrolysis of protein

Anxiolytic (*Sp. Ansiolítico*): a substance that diminishes anxiety

Aphasia (*Sp. Afasia*): a nerve defect that results in loss of speech

Aphonia (*Sp. Afonía*): inability to produce normal speech sounds or loss of voice

Aphthous ulcers (*Sp. Úlceras aftosas*): recurrent painful canker sores in the mouth

Apnea, apneic (*Sp. Apnea, apneico*): the temporary cessation of breathing

Apoptosis (*Sp. Apoptosis*): a pattern of cell death affecting single cells; refers to *programmed cell death*

Arrhythmia (*Sp. Arritmia*): variation or loss of normal rhythm of the heartbeat

Arthrodesis (*Sp. Artrodesis*): the immobilization of a joint accomplished surgically

Arthroplasty (*Sp. Artroplastia*): surgical reconstruction or replacement of a diseased joint

Ascites (*Sp. Ascitis*): abnormal intraperitoneal accumulation of serous fluid

Asymptomatic (*Sp. Asintomático*): without symptoms

Asystole (*Sp. Asístole*): the absence of contractions of the heart; cardiac standstill

Ataxia (*Sp. Ataxia*): an uncoordinated gate associated with pathology of the central nervous system

Atrophy (*Sp. Atrofia*): a wasting away; a degeneration of a cell, tissue, organ, or muscle because of disease or other influences

Audiogram (*Sp. Audiograma*): the record of a hearing test

Aura (*Sp. Aura*): a sensation or phenomenon that signals the onset of an epileptic seizure or a migraine

Auscultation (*Sp. Auscultación*): a diagnostic technique of listening for sounds within the body, particularly the lungs, heart, or abdominal viscera

Autoantibody (*Sp. Autoanticuerpo*): an antibody that attacks and destroys the body's own cells

Autoimmunity, autoimmune (*Sp. Autoinmunidad, autoinmune*): an immune response resulting in the presence of self-antigens or autoantigens on the surface of certain body cells; may result in allergy or autoimmune disease

Autosome, autosomal (*Sp. Autosoma, autosómico*): any of the 22 ordinary paired chromosomes in humans, distinguished from the sex (X and Y) chromosomes

Azoospermia (*Sp. Azoospermia*): an absence of spermatozoa in the semen

Azotemia (*Sp. Azotemia*): an excess of urea or other nitrogenous bodies in the blood

Barium (*Sp. Bario*): a pale, soft, alkaline metallic element; a radiopaque barium (barium sulfate) compound commonly used in radiographic studies of the gastrointestinal tract

Battle's sign (*Sp. Signo de Battle*): bogginess of the temporal region of the head that may indicate fracture at the base of the skull

Bicornate uterus (*Sp. Útero bicorne*): a uterus having two horns or horn-shaped branches

Bifurcate (*Sp. Bifurcado*): split into two branches

Bilirubinemia (*Sp. Bilirrubinemia*): the presence of bilirubin in the blood

Bilirubinuria (*Sp. Bilirrubinuria*): the presence of bilirubin (a yellow- or orange-tinged pigment in the bile) in the urine

Biopsy (*Sp. Biopsia*): the excision of tissue from the living body, followed by microscopic examination, for the purpose of exact diagnosis

Blood gases (*Sp. Gases sanguíneos*): the gases present in the blood that are a result of utilization of oxygen and production of carbon dioxide during metabolism; the blood is analyzed for evidence of deviations (acidosis or alkalosis) from normal levels

Blood urea nitrogen (BUN) (*Sp. Nitrógeno ureico en sangre—BUN*): a measurement of urea nitrogen (a substance formed during protein breakdown) in the serum or plasma; an elevated BUN level may indicate impaired renal function

Breech (*Sp. Nalgas*): buttocks

Bronchoscopy (*Sp. Broncoscopía*): examination of the bronchial tree with a bronchoscope to obtain a biopsy, remove an obstruction, or diagnose a disease

Bruit (*Sp. Ruido*): an abnormal sound heard in auscultation

Cachexia (*Sp. Caquexia*): a profound and marked wasting disorder, usually associated with malnutrition and such diseases as cancer and tuberculosis

Calculus (calculi) (*Sp. Cálculo*): a stone usually composed of mineral salts (e.g., kidney stones and gallstones); or calcified deposits on the teeth

Carcinogen, carcinogenic (*Sp. Carcinógeno*): a substance that produces cancer or that causes transformation of a normal cell to a cancerous one

Cardiac sphincter (*Sp. Esfínter cardiaco*): the circular muscle at the opening of the esophagus into the stomach

Cardiomegaly (*Sp. Cardiomegalia*): enlargement of the heart

Cast (*Sp. Impresión*): a negative mold or copy formed in a hollow organ or part (e.g., kidney or bronchi); a urinary cast is a small structure formed within the urinary system from mineral or protein matter and extruded from the body in the urine

Cataract (*Sp. Cataratas*): a progressive disease in which the lens of the eye becomes cloudy, impairing vision or causing blindness

Catatonic posturing (*Sp. Estado catatónico*): a state of not being able to move, with the assumption of a rigid, often bizarre posture

Cautery (*Sp. Cauterio*): an instrument or chemical that destroys tissue, as a therapeutic measure

Cephalgia, cephalalgia (*Sp. Cefalea*): pain in the head; headache

Cephalic (*Sp. Cefálico*): referring to the head; cranial

Cerclage (*Sp. Cerclaje*): encircling of the cervix with a metal ring or suture ring to treat cervical incompetence during pregnancy to help prevent spontaneous abortion

Cheilectomy (*Sp. Queilotomía*): surgical removal of abnormal bone around a joint; also refers to surgical removal of a lip

Cholangiogram (*Sp. Colangiograma*): a diagnostic radiographic study of the gallbladder and bile ducts

Cholecystogram (*Sp. Colecistografía*): a diagnostic radiographic study of the gallbladder

Cholinergic (*Sp. Colinérgico*): an agent that produces the effect of acetylcholine at the connections of muscles and nerves

Chorea (*Sp. Corea*): the ceaseless occurrence of involuntary muscular movements of the limbs or facial muscles

Circadian rhythm (*Sp. Ritmo circadiano*): the biologic clock in humans; the rhythmic repetition of certain phenomena, such as hunger, fatigue, and changes in blood pressure, that tend to fluctuate within a 24-hour period

Circumoral cyanosis (*Sp. Cianosis circumoral*): a bluish discoloration around the mouth

Clean-catch urine specimen (*Sp. Espécimen de orina limpia*): a urine specimen obtained by cleaning the genitalia and then capturing a midstream urine sample for laboratory analysis

Closed reduction (*Sp. Reducción cerrada*): the nonsurgical manipulative reduction of a dislocation or fracture

Coagulation (*Sp. Coagulación*): the process of clot formation

Cognitive (*Sp. Cognitivo*): pertaining to the mental processes of thinking, knowing, remembering, and perceiving

Collateral (*Sp. Colateral*): a small side branch of a blood vessel or nerve

Colporrhaphy (*Sp. Colporrafia*): suturing of the vagina

Colposcopy (*Sp. Colcospia*): examination of the vagina and cervix with an optical magnifying instrument

Comedo (comedones) (*Sp. Comedón*): a blackhead, as seen in acne

Commissurotomy (*Sp. Comisurotomía*): surgical incision of component parts at the sites of junction between adjacent cusps of the heart valves to increase the size of the opening

Comorbid (*Sp. Comórbido*): two or more existing medical conditions

Computed tomography (CT) (*Sp. Tomografía asistida por computadora—TAC*): a diagnostic technique using ionizing x-rays passed through a patient around specific sections of the body at multiple angles; useful in the detection of tumors

Continuous positive airway pressure (CPAP) (*Sp. Presión positiva continua de las vías respiratorias—CPAP*): a form of respiratory therapy in which ventilation is assisted by a flow of oxygen delivered at a constant pressure throughout the respiratory cycle

Contracture (*Sp. Contractura*): immobility of muscles or a joint caused by shortening or wasting of tissue or muscle fibers

Controlled drug (*Sp. Drogas controladas*): a drug regulated by the Federal Controlled Substance Act

Corneal ulcer (*Sp. Úlcera de la córnea*): ulcerative keratitis

Corticotropin, or adrenocorticotropic hormone (ACTH) (*Sp. Corticotropina u hormona adrenocorticotrópica—ACTH*): a hormone secreted by the anterior lobe of the pituitary

Craniotomy (*Sp. Craneotomía*): incision into the skull, usually to relieve pressure, to remove a lesion, or to control bleeding

Creatinine (*Sp. Creatinina*): an important nitrogen compound that is a normal constituent of urine and blood; increased levels may indicate renal damage

Crede maneuver (method) (*Sp. Maniobra—método de Crede*): manual external compression of the bladder to aid in expulsion of urine.

Cryoablation (*Sp. Crioablación*): the removal of tissue by destroying it with extreme cold

Cryotherapy (*Sp. Crioterapia*): the therapeutic use of cold

Cryptorchidism (*Sp. Criptorquidismo*): failure of one or both testicles to descend into the scrotum

Cul-de-sac (*Sp. Fondo de saco*): an area at the end of the abdominal cavity that is midway between the rectum and the uterus

Cyanosis, cyanotic (*Sp. Cianosis, cianótico*): bluish appearance of the skin and mucous membrane that usually indicates reduced hemoglobin levels in the blood

Cytology, cytologic (*Sp. Citología, citológico*): the scientific study of cells

Cytoreduction (*Sp. Citorreducción*): a decrease in the number of cells (such as in a tumor)

Debride (*Sp. Desbridar*): remove foreign material or dead tissue in a wound

Demise (*Sp. Fallecimiento*): destruction or death

Demyelination (*Sp. Desmielinización*): loss of the myelin sheath of a nerve

Dermatomes (*Sp. Dermatoma*): a configured zone of skin innervated by a spinal cord segment

Dialysate (*Sp. Dializado*): the fluid that passes through a semi-permeable membrane during dialysis

Dialysis (dialyses) (*Sp. Diálisis*): a procedure that filters out unwanted substances from the blood, usually in cases of renal failure

Diaphoresis, diaphoretic (*Sp. Diaforesis, diaforético*): profuse perspiration

Diplopia (*Sp. Diplopía*): double vision

Discoid (*Sp. Discoide*): shaped like a disk

Diuresis, diuretic (*Sp. Diuresis, diurético*): increased formation and excretion of urine

Doppler (*Sp. Doppler*): ultrasonographic technique used to evaluate blood flow velocity

Dorsiflexion (*Sp. Dorsiflexión*): to bend a joint toward the posterior aspect of the body; for example, the hand is dorsiflexed when it is extended or bent backward at the wrist

Dyspareunia (*Sp. Dispareunia*): pain or discomfort in the pelvis or vagina during or after sexual intercourse

Dysphagia (*Sp. Disfagia*): difficulty in swallowing

Dysphasia (*Sp. Disfasia*): difficulty in speaking, usually caused by a lesion in the central nervous system

Dysphonia (*Sp. Disfonía*): hoarseness; difficulty in speaking

Dysplastic (*Sp. Displástico*): marked by abnormal adult cells

Dyspnea (*Sp. Dispnea*): labored or difficult breathing

Dysrhythmia (*Sp. Disritmia*): an abnormal cardiac rhythm

Echocardiogram, echocardiography, echocardiographic (*Sp. Ecocardiograma, ecocardiografía, ecocardiográfico*): an ultrasonographic study of the motion of the walls or structures of the heart

Ectopic (*Sp. Ectópico*): out of normal position

Effacement (*Sp. Borramiento*): the thinning or obliteration of the cervix during labor

Electrocardiogram, electrocardiography, electrocardiographic (*Sp. Electrocardiograma, electrocardiografía, electrocardiográfico*): a record of the electrical activity of the heart

Electromyogram, electromyography, electromyographic (*Sp. Electromiograma, electromiografía, electromiográfico*): an electrodiagnostic assessment of the activity of skeletal muscles

Embolus (emboli) (*Sp. Émbolo*): a mass (e.g., foreign body, blood clot, or a piece of tumor) that breaks off and causes occlusion of an artery

Emergency medical service (EMS) (*Sp. Servicios médicos de urgencia—EMS*): trained services provided on the scene

Encephalitis (*Sp. Encefalitis*): inflammation of the brain

Endarterectomy (*Sp. Endarterectomía*): the surgical excision of the innermost lining of an artery to remove blockage

Endemic (*Sp. Endémico*): condition in which a disease is prevalent in a particular geographic area or in a population

Endometriosis (*Sp. Endometriosis*): a growth of endometrial tissue at various sites outside the uterus

Endometrium (*Sp. Endometrio*): the lining of the uterus that changes with the menstrual cycle; if the ovum is fertilized, the endometrium serves as the place where implantation occurs

Endoscopy (*Sp. Endoscopia*): examination of any cavity of the body with an endoscope

Enzyme-linked immunosorbent assay (ELISA) (*Sp. prueba de inmunoabsorción enzimática—prueba ELISA*): a test used to detect antibodies to the acquired immunodeficiency syndrome (AIDS) virus in blood serum

Epigastric (*Sp. Epigástrico*): refers to the upper middle region of the abdomen

Epiphysis (epiphyses), epiphyseal (*Sp. Epífisis, epifiseal*): the long end of a bone where bone growth occurs

Epistaxis (*Sp. Epistaxis*): bleeding from the nose

Ergonomics (*Sp. Ergonomía*): the science concerned with people and their work; it explores mechanical principles enhancing efficiency and well-being in the work environment

Ergot (*Sp. Cornezuelo*): a drug obtained from a fungus that grows on rye plants

Erythrocyte sedimentation rate (ESR) (*Sp. Tasa de sedimentación eritrocítica*): a measurable reflection of the acute-phase reaction in inflammation and infection

Esophagoscopy (*Sp. Esofagoscopia*): examination of the esophagus with an esophagoscope

Exacerbation (*Sp. Exacerbación*): an increase in the severity of a disease or aggravation of its symptoms

Exotoxin (*Sp. Exotoxina*): bacterial toxins excreted outside of the bacterial cell

Exsanguination (*Sp. Desangramiento*): excessive loss of blood from a part

Exudate (*Sp. Exudado*): fluid, cells, or cellular debris that has oozed into tissue because of injury or swelling

Fascia (*Sp. Fascia*): a fibrous membrane that covers, separates, and supports the muscles

Fasciculation (*Sp. Fasciculación*): involuntary contraction or twitching of muscles

Fibrin (*Sp. Fibrina*): a protein material produced by the action of thrombin on fibrinogen

Fibrosis, fibrotic (*Sp. Fibrosis, fibrótico*): the abnormal formation of fibrous tissue

Fissure (*Sp. Fisura*): a crack or groove on a surface

Fistula (*Sp. Fístula*): an abnormal tube-like passageway

Fluorescein angiography (*Sp. Angiografía fluoresceínica*): a procedure in which light-sensitive material is injected into a blood vessel

Foramen (foramina) (*Sp. Foramen*): an opening or hole in a bone, allowing the passage of nerves or blood vessels

Fowler's position (*Sp. Posición de Fowler*): a semisitting position, usually at 45 degrees, used to facilitate breathing and drainage

Fulguration (*Sp. Fulguración*): tissue destruction with high-frequency electrical sparks

Fulminant (*Sp. Fulminante*): occuring with great intensity; refers to severe pain with sudden onset

Gamete (*Sp. Gameto*): male or female sex cell

Gangrene (*Sp. Gangrena*): death of tissue caused by a decrease or absence of blood supply

Gastrectomy (*Sp. Gastrectomía*): surgical removal of the stomach

Gastroscopy (*Sp. Gastroscopía*): visual examination of the stomach using a gastroscope

Giemsa stain (*Sp. Tinción de Giemsa*): a process of staining bacteria for identification

Glenoid (*Sp. Glenoideo*): having the semblance of a socket

Glomerulosclerosis (*Sp. Glomeruloesclerosis*): hardening of the renal glomerulus

Glomerulus (glomeruli) (*Sp. Glomérulo*): a tiny ball of microscopic blood vessels on the end of the renal tubules

Goitrogenic (*Sp. Bociógeno*): pertaining to substances causing goiters

Gram stain (*Sp. Coloración de Gram*): a process of staining bacteria for identification

Guthrie test (*Sp. Prueba de Guthrie*): a test to detect phenylketonuria

Gynecomastia (*Sp. Ginecomastia*): abnormal enlargement of breast tissue in men

H_2-receptor antagonist (*Sp. Antagonista del receptor H_2*): chemical agent that blocks the interaction of histamine or acetylcholine with receptors in stomach cells; drugs that inhibit secretion of gastric acid

Hallucination (*Sp. Alucinación*): a false perception of reality; may be visual, auditory, or olfactory

Hallux (*Sp. Hallux*): the great toe

Hematemesis (*Sp. Hematemesis*): vomiting of blood

Hematocrit (*Sp. Hematocrito*): the percentage of the total blood volume consisting of erythrocytes

Hematopoiesis, hematopoietic (*Sp. Hematopoyesis, hematopoyético*): pertaining to the production and the development of blood cells or a substance that stimulates their production

Hematuria (*Sp. Hematuria*): blood in the urine

Hemiparesis (*Sp. Hemiparesia*): paralysis affecting one side of the body

Hemoccult (*Sp. Hemoccult*): trademark for a guaiac reagent strip test for occult blood

Hemodynamic (*Sp. Hemodinámica*): refers to forces involved in the circulation of blood within the body

Hemolysis, hemolytic (*Sp. Hemólisis, hemolítico*): the destruction of red blood cells with the release of hemoglobin

Hemoptysis (*Sp. Hemoptisis*): spitting up blood

Hemostasis (*Sp. Hemostasis*): the condition of controlled bleeding

Hepatomegaly (*Sp. Hepatomegalia*): enlargement of the liver

Histoplasmosis (*Sp. Histoplasmosis*): a systemic respiratory disease caused by a fungus

Homeostasis (*Sp. Homeostasis*): a state of equilibrium within the body

Human chorionic gonadotropin (hCG) (*Sp. Gonadotropina coriónica humana—GCH*): hormones produced by the placenta and detected in the urine and blood of a pregnant woman

Humoral (*Sp. Humoral*): refers to body fluids or substances found in them

Hyaline membrane (*Sp. Membrana hialina*): a membrane that forms in the lung sacs of a developing fetus; a respiratory distress syndrome of the newborn

Hydronephrosis (*Sp. Hidronefrosis*): accumulation of urine in the renal pelvis caused by obstruction, forming a cyst

Hymen (*Sp. Himen*): the membrane partially covering the entrance to the vagina

Hyperalimentation (*Sp. Hiperalimentación*): infusion of life-sustaining fluids, electrolytes, and elements of nutrition intravenously or via the gastrointestinal tract

Hypercapnia (*Sp. Hipercapnia*): increased carbon dioxide levels in the blood

Hypercoagulable (*Sp. Hipercoagulable*): refers to the increased ability of any substance to coagulate, especially blood

Hyperemic (*Sp. Hiperémico*): refers to an excessive amount of blood in a part or area

Hyperesthesia (*Sp. Hiperestesia*): increased sensitivity to pain

Hyperglycemia (*Sp. Hiperglicemia*): an increase in the normal blood glucose level

Hyperlipidemia (*Sp. Hiperlipemia*): an increase of fat levels in the blood

Hyperparathyroidism (*Sp. Hiperparatiroidismo*): a condition caused by overactive parathyroid glands

Hyperplasia (*Sp. Hiperplasia*): abnormal multiplication of the number of cells resulting from an increased rate of cellular division

Hypertrophy, hypertrophic (*Sp. Hipertrofia, hipertrófico*): enlargement of an organ or structure

Hyperuricemia (*Sp. Hiperuricemia*): excessive uric acid levels in the blood

Hypoalbuminemia (*Sp. Hipoalbuminemia*): low albumin levels in the blood

Hypocalcemia (*Sp. Hipocalcemia*): low calcium levels in the blood

Hypokalemia (*Sp. Hipocalemia*): low potassium levels in the blood

Hypoparathyroidism (*Sp. Hipoparatiroidismo*): a condition caused by greatly reduced function of the parathyroid glands

Hypovolemic shock (*Sp. Choque hipovolémico*): a condition that occurs when blood in the circulatory system is decreased (e.g., as a result of hemorrhage)

Hypoxia (*Sp. Hipoxia*): low oxygen levels in the tissues

Idiopathic (*Sp. Idiopático*): refers to a disease without a known or recognizable cause

Immunocompetence (*Sp. Inmunocompetencia*): the ability of the immune system to defend the body against disease

Immunocompromised (*Sp. Con inmunidad comprometida*): refers to an immune system incapable of fighting disease

Immunodeficiency (*Sp. Inmunodeficiencia*): the diminished ability of the immune system to react with appropriate cellular immunity response; often the result of loss of immunoglobulins or aberrance of B or T cell lymphocytes

Immunogen (*Sp. Inmunógeno*): an antigen (i.e., a substance capable of stimulating an immune response)

Immunoglobulin (*Sp. Inmunoglobulina*): a protein that can act as an antibody

Immunoincompetence (*Sp. Inmunoincompetencia*): immunodeficiency

Immunosuppressive (*Sp. Inmunosupresor*): having the property of suppressing the body's immune response to antigens

Incompetent cervix (*Sp. Cervix incompetente*): premature painless dilation of the cervical os during pregnancy

Infarct, infarction (*Sp. Infarto, infartado*): an area of dead tissue caused by lack of blood supply

Insidious (*Sp. Insidioso*): refers to the onset of a disease without symptoms

Intractable (*Sp. Incurable*): incurable or resistant to treatment

Intravenous pyelogram, intravenous pyelography (*Sp. Pielograma intravenoso, pielografía intravenosa*): radiographic study of the renal pelvis and ureter using injected dye

Intravenous urogram, intravenous urography (*Sp. Urograma intravenso, urografía intravenosa*): radiographic study of the urinary tract using injected dye

Intrinsic (*Sp. Intrínseco*): refers to the essential nature of a substance or structure

Intrinsic factor (*Sp. Factor intrínseco*): a substance normally found in gastric juices; essential for the absorption of vitamin B_{12}

Iontophoresis (*Sp. Iontoforesis*): the therapeutic introduction of ions into the body tissues by direct current

Ischemia, ischemic (*Sp. Isquemia, isquémico*): holding back or obstructing the flow of blood

Ischemic necrosis (*Sp. Necrosis isquémica*): the death or sloughing off of small areas of tissue or bone, caused by insufficient circulation or lack of blood supply

Jaundice (*Sp. Ictericia*): yellowing of the skin

Karyotype (*Sp. Cariotipo*): a picture of chromosomes in the nucleus of a cell

Kegel exercises (*Sp. Ejercicios de Kegel*): isometric pelvic exercises used by women to strengthen pelvic muscles and/or to improve retention of urine

Keratin (*Sp. Queratina*): a hard protein substance found in hair, nails, and skin

Keratoconjunctivitis sicca (*Sp. Queratoconjuntivitis seca*): dryness of the conjunctiva resulting from a decrease in lacrimal function

Keratolytic (*Sp. Queratolítico*): a substance that causes shedding of the skin

Kernicterus (*Sp. Kernicterus*): a form of icterus (bile pigmentation of tissues and membranes) occurring in infants

Laparoscopy (*Sp. Laparoscopia*): a surgical procedure to examine the abdomen using an endoscope called a laparoscope

Laryngoscopy (*Sp. Laringoscopia*): visual examination of the larynx using a laryngoscope

Laser ablation (*Sp. Ablación por láser*): separation, detachment, destruction, or removal of a part using laser surgery

Laser photocoagulation (*Sp. Fotocoagulación por láser*): coagulation of the blood vessels in the eye using a laser

Lavage (*Sp. Lavado*): the cleaning out of a cavity with liquid

Leukocytosis (*Sp. Leucocitosis*): a slight increase in the numbers of white blood cells

Leukopenia (*Sp. Leucopenia*): a decrease in the number of white blood cells

Leukorrhea (*Sp. Leucorrea*): a white or yellow mucous discharge from the vagina

Lipase (*Sp. Lipasa*): a fat-splitting enzyme produced by the pancreas

Liposome (*Sp. Liposoma*): a small spherical particle in an aqueous solution, formed by a bi-layer of phospholipid molecules

Lithotripsy (*Sp. Litotripsia*): crushing of stones (e.g., kidney stones and gallstones)

Lumbar puncture (*Sp. Punción lumbar*): a surgical procedure to withdraw spinal fluid for analysis or the injection of an anesthetic solution

Lumpectomy (*Sp. Tumorectomia*): removal of just the tumor from the breast

Lymph (*Sp. Linfa*): a mostly clear, colorless, transparent, alkaline fluid found within the lymphatic vessels; formed in tissues throughout the body

Lymphadenitis (*Sp. Linfadenitis*): inflammation of the lymph nodes

Lymphadenopathy (*Sp. Linfadenopatía*): disease of the lymph nodes

Lymphocyte (*Sp. Linfocito*): one of two types (B cells and T cells) of leukocytes (white blood cells) found in blood, lymph, and lymphoid tissue

Lymphocytosis (*Sp. Linfocitosis*): an excessive number of lymph cells

Macrophage (*Sp. Macrófago*): a monocyte blood cell

Macula (*Sp. Mácula*): a small spot or a colored area

Maculopapular (*Sp. Maculopapular*): pertaining to or consisting of macules and papules

Magnetic resonance imaging (MRI) (*Sp. Formación de imágenes por resonancia magnética—MRI*): a procedure similar to computed tomography that does not require radiographs; a large magnetic field is applied and creates an image; useful in visualizing the cardiovascular system, brain, and soft tissues

Malaise (*Sp. Malestar*): a feeling of discomfort, illness, or uneasiness

Malocclusion (*Sp. Maloclusión*): improper positioning and faulty contact of the teeth

Mastectomy (*Sp. Mastectomía*): surgical removal of breast tissue; can be partial or radical

McBurney's point (*Sp. Punto de McBurney*): the point of special tenderness in acute appendicitis; corresponds with the normal position of the base of the appendix

Meconium (*Sp. Meconio*): the first stool of a newborn, greenish black and with a tarry consistency

Mediastinal shift (*Sp. Desplazamiento mediastinal*): abnormal movement of the structures within the mediastinum to one side of the chest cavity

Mediastinum (*Sp. Mediastino*): the area in the chest between the lungs

Megakaryocyte (*Sp. Megacariocito*): a large bone marrow cell having large or many nuclei

Megaloblastic (*Sp. Megaloblástico*): pertaining to abnormally large red blood cells found in pernicious anemia

Melanin (*Sp. Melanina*): the black pigment found in the basal layer of the epidermis

Melena (*Sp. Melena*): the passage of very dark, tarry stools stained with digested blood

Meningitis (*Sp. Meningitis*): inflammation of the coverings around the brain and spinal cord

Menorrhagia (*Sp. Menorragia*): painful menstruation

Metabolic acidosis (*Sp. Acidosis metabólica*): excessive acid in the body fluids caused by dehydration, diarrhea, vomiting, renal disease, or hepatic impairment

Metaplastic (*Sp. Metaplástico*): characterized by metaplasia (a reversible change of cells usually caused by stress or injury); cancer formation can occur with chronic inducing stimulus by injury or irritation

Metastasis (metastases), metastatic, metastasize (*Sp. Metástasis, metastásico, metastatizar*): spreading of a malignant disease or pathogenic microorganisms from one organ or part to another not directly connected with it

Metatarsophalangeal (*Sp. Metatarsofalángico*): pertaining to the metatarsus and phalanges of the toes

Monoclonal antibodies (MAB) (*Sp. Anticuerpos monoclonales—MAB*): antibody produced from a single clone of B lymphocytes

Monocyte (*Sp. Monocito*): a phagocytic white blood cell that engulfs and destroys cellular debris

Murmur (*Sp. Murmullo*): a blowing sound heard when listening to the heart or vessels with a stethoscope

Mutation (*Sp. Mutación*): a variation or change in genetic structure

Mutism (*Sp. Mutismo*): a condition of being unable to speak

Myalgia (*Sp. Mialgia*): muscle pain

Mycoplasma (*Sp. Micoplasma*): microscopic organisms that lack a rigid cell wall; some species cause infections in humans

Myelin (*Sp. Mielina*): the protective fat and protein covering around the axons of many nerves

Myelogram, myelography (*Sp. Mielograma, mielografía*): radiographic study of the spinal cord after the injection of a dye

Necrosis, necrotic (*Sp. Necrosis, necrótico*): death of tissue

Neoplasm, neoplasia, neoplastic (*Sp. Neoplasma, neoplasia, neoplástico*): abnormal formation of new tissue; can be benign or malignant

Neovascularization (*Sp. Neurovascularización*): the formation of new blood vessels

Nephron (*Sp. Nefrona*): the functioning unit of the kidney or renal tubule

Neurotransmitter (*Sp. Neurotransmisor*): a chemical released by the terminal end fibers of an axon

Nociceptors (*Sp. Nociceptor*): nerves that receive and transmit painful stimuli

Normal flora (*Sp. Flora normal*): the presence of normal bacteria and fungi adapted for living in, and characteristic of, the area considered (e.g., skin, intestine, or vagina)

Nuchal rigidity (*Sp. Rigidez en la nuca*): neck stiffness

Nullipara (*Sp. Nulípara*): a woman who has never produced viable offspring

Odynophagia (*Sp. Odinofagia*): painful swallowing

Oligospermia (*Sp. Oligospermia*): insufficient number of spermatozoa in the semen

Oliguria (*Sp. Oliguria*): scanty urination

Oncogene (*Sp. Oncógeno*): a gene in a virus that can prompt a cell to turn malignant

Oophorectomy (*Sp. Ovariotomía*): the surgical removal of one or both ovaries

Opacity (*Sp. Opacidad*): the state of being opaque or not transparent

Open reduction (*Sp. Reducción abierta*): exposure of a fractured or dislocated bone through a surgical incision to realign the bone ends

Ophthalmoscopy, ophthalmoscopic (*Sp. Oftalmoscopia, oftalmoscópico*): an examination of the interior of the eye

Opportunistic infection (*Sp. Infección oportunista*): infection resulting from a defective immune system

Orchiectomy (*Sp. Orquiectomía*): the surgical removal of one or both testes; also called orchidectomy

Orchitis (*Sp. Orquitis*): inflammation of the testes

Orthodontics (*Sp. Ortodoncia*): branch of dentistry concerned with correction of dentofacial structures (e.g., teeth)

Orthopnea (*Sp. Ortopnea*): a condition in which breathing becomes easier in an upright standing or sitting position

Orthoptic training (*Sp. Entrenamiento ortóptico*): eye muscle exercises

Ortolani's sign (*Sp. Prueba de Ortolani*): an assessment maneuver designed to detect a hip dislocation

Osteophyte (*Sp. Osteofito*): a bony outgrowth, usually branch-shaped

Ostomy (*Sp. Ostomía*): a surgical opening of the bowel to the outside of the body

Otitis media (*Sp. Otitis media*): middle ear infection

Otoscopy (*Sp. Otoscopia*): visual examination of the ear using an otoscope

Oxygen saturation (*Sp. Saturación de oxígeno*): refers to the oxygen content in blood, divided by oxygen capacity and expressed in volume percent

Palliative (*Sp. Paliativo*): alleviating symptoms without curing the underlying cause

Panhypopituitarism (*Sp. Panhipopituitarismo*): a condition in which the entire pituitary gland ceases to function and is not producing any pituitary hormones

Papule (*Sp. Pápula*): a circular area on the skin that is reddened and elevated

Paresis (*Sp. Paresia*): partial paralysis

Paresthesia (*Sp. Parestesia*): abnormal, usually increased, sensations

Parietal (cells) (*Sp. Células parietales*): the cells on the wall of a cavity; pertaining to or located near the parietal bone (as the parietal lobe)

Paronychia (*Sp. Paroniquia*): inflammation of soft tissue surrounding the nail

Partial thromboplastin time (PTT) (*Sp. Tiempo parcial de tromboplastina—TPT*): a measure of the coagulation sequence of plasma and screen for platelet abnormalities

Patch test (*Sp. Prueba del parche*): a screening test in which a small piece of material containing the allergy-causing substance is placed on the skin; redness or edema indicates a positive reaction

Pathogenesis (*Sp. Patogénesis*): the development of disease; pathologic mechanisms

Pathologist (*Sp. Patologista*): one who specializes in the study of disease

Peau d'orange (*Sp. Piel de naranja*): condition in which the skin is dimpled, resembling the skin of an orange

Pelvic inflammatory disease (PID) (*Sp. Enfermedad inflamatoria pélvica—EIP*): inflammation of the female pelvic organs, usually caused by bacteria

Perfusion (*Sp. Perfusión*): delivery of oxygen and other nutrients to the tissue by the blood

Pericoronitis (*Sp. Pericoronitis*): inflammation of the gum around the crown of a tooth

Periosteum (*Sp. Periostio*): the fibrous covering of long bones

Peritonitis (*Sp. Peritonitis*): inflammation of the membrane that lines the abdominal cavity and covers the viscera

Pessary (*Sp. Pesario*): an object placed in the vagina to support the uterus

Petechia (petechiae) (*Sp. Petequia*): a tiny spider-like hemorrhage under the skin

Phagocyte, phagocytic, phagocytosis (*Sp. Fagocito, fagocítico, fagocitosis*): the process by which cells surround and digest certain particles (e.g., bacteria, protozoa, and debris)

Phlebotomy (*Sp. Flebotomía*): surgical puncture of a vein to withdraw blood

Phonological (*Sp. Fonológico*): refers to oral communication or vocal sounds

Photophobia (*Sp. Fotofobia*): unusual sensitivity to light

Phototherapy (*Sp. Fototerapia*): treatment of disease by exposure to light

Plaque (*Sp. Placa*): a deposit of hardened material lining the blood vessel; or a gummy accumulation of microorganisms that clings to teeth and is considered the forerunner of caries and periodontal disease

Plasmapheresis (*Sp. Plasmaféresis*): the process of separating blood into its components by centrifuging

Polyposis (*Sp. Poliposis*): a condition of multiple polyps

Positive end-expiratory pressure (PEEP) (*Sp. Presión positiva al final de la expiración—PEEP*): mechanical ventilation with pressure maintained, thereby increasing the volume of gas remaining in the lungs at the end of expiration

Positron emission tomography (PET) (*Sp. Tomografía por emisión de positrones—PET*): a noninvasive radiographic study of the blood flow in specific organs and body tissues

Postprandial (*Sp. Posprandial*): after meals

Primipara (*Sp. Primípara*): a woman who has delivered one child of at least 20 weeks' gestational age

Proctoscopy (*Sp. Proctoscopia*): visual examination of the rectum with a proctoscope

Prodromal (*Sp. Prodrómico*): refers to the initial stage of a disease before the onset of actual symptoms

Prophylaxis, prophylactic (*Sp. Profilaxis, profiláctico*): the prevention of disease

Prostate-specific antigen (PSA) (*Sp. Antígeno específico de la próstata—PSA*): an enzyme that is measured in a blood test to detect cancer of the prostate

Proteinuria (*Sp. Proteinuria*): the presence of protein in the urine

Prothrombin time (PT) (*Sp. Tiempo de protrombina—TP*): a measure of the time taken for clot formation

Proton pump inhibitor (*Sp. Inhibidor de la bomba de protones*): a drug that blocks gastric acid secretion; used to treat ulcers of the gastrointestinal tract and gastroesophageal reflux disease (GERD)

Pruritus (*Sp. Prurito*): itching

Pseudoneurologic (*Sp. Pseudoneurológico*): refers to a neurologic symptom that is without clinical basis

Pseudopregnancy (*Sp. Pseudoembarazo*): false pregnancy, also known as pseudocyesis

Psychotropic drugs (*Sp. Drogas psicotrópicas*): drugs that have an effect on the mind, or that alter the state of mind

Purpura (*Sp. Púrpura*): a red-purple discoloration of the skin caused by multiple minute hemorrhages in the skin or mucous membrane

Purulent (*Sp. Purulento*): containing pus

Pustule (*Sp. Pústula*): a small elevation of the skin containing pus

Putrefaction (*Sp. Putrefacción*): decomposition of organic matter

Pyelonephritis (*Sp. Pielonefritis*): a purulent infection of the kidney tissue and renal pelvis

Pyuria (*Sp. Piuria*): pus in the urine

Raccoon eyes (*Sp. Ojos de mapache*): dark discoloration (bruising) around the eyes; a sign of possible basilar skull fracture

Radioimmunoassay (*Sp. Radioinmunoanálisis*): a test that measures minute amounts of antibodies or antigens by the use of radioactive substances

Rale (*Sp. Estertor*): an abnormal crackling sound made by the lungs during inspiration; indicative of fluid in a bronchus

Raynaud's phenomenon (*Sp. Fenómeno de Raynaud*): a temporary constriction of arterioles in the skin causing short episodes of numbness and color changes in the fingers and toes. This condition is usually idiopathic

Reflux (*Sp. Reflujo*): a backward flow

Renal calculi (*Sp. Cálculo renal*): kidney stones

Reticuloendothelial (*Sp. Reticuloendotelial*): refers to the system responsible for phagocytosis of cellular debris, pathogens, and foreign substances and for removing them from the circulation

Retrovirus (*Sp. Retrovirus*): a family of viruses that contains RNA (ribonucleic acid) and reverse transcriptase; some retroviruses are oncogenic and can induce tumors

Rheumatoid factor (*Sp. Factor reumatoide*): a macroglobulin type of antibody; increased levels are found in the blood of persons with rheumatoid arthritis

Rhonchus (*Sp. Ronquido*): dry rattling in the throat or bronchus caused by partial obstruction

RNA (*Sp. ARN*): ribonucleic acid; controls protein synthesis in cells and takes the place of DNA in some viruses

Salpingo-oophorectomy (*Sp. Anexectomía*): the surgical removal of a fallopian tube and an ovary

Schick test (*Sp. Prueba de Schick*): an intradermal skin test to detect immunity to diphtheria; a positive result indicates lack of immunity or negative immunity

Sclerosis, sclerosing (*Sp. Esclerosis*): hardening of a body part

Sclerotherapy (*Sp. Escleroterapia*): a form of treatment for varices in which a sclerosing solution is injected into a vein

Seborrhea (*Sp. Seborrea*): the excessive secretion of sebum from sebaceous glands

Sebum (*Sp. Sebo*): oily secretion of sebaceous glands

Semi-Fowler position (*Sp.* ***Posición semi-Fowler***): position of lying on the back with the head elevated 8 to 10 inches and the knees flexed

Senile (*Sp.* ***Senil***): refers to growing old with decreased physical and mental capacity

Senile plaque (*Sp.* ***Placa senil***): microscopic patch of fragmented nerve around amyloid deposits found in the cerebral cortex of normal elderly people; found in larger amounts in people with Alzheimer disease

Septicemia (*Sp.* ***Septicemia***): a disease in which pathogenic microorganisms or toxins are present in the blood

Sequestrum (*Sp.* ***Secuestro***): a segment of dead bone; the result of an abscess from a bacterial infection in a bone and bone marrow

Serology, serologic (*Sp.* ***Serología, serológico***): a study of blood serum to measure antibody titers

Sigmoidoscopy (*Sp.* ***Sigmoidoscopia***): visual examination of the sigmoid colon with a sigmoidoscope

Sinopulmonary (*Sp.* ***Sinopulmonar***): pertaining to the paranasal sinuses and lungs

Skeletal traction (*Sp.* ***Tracción ósea***): a method of immobilization and reduction of a long-bone fracture in which traction is applied by means of pins and wires

Somatoform (*Sp.* ***Forma somática***): psychogenic symptoms without an underlying disease process

Splenomegaly (*Sp.* ***Esplenomegalia***): enlarged spleen

Squamous cell (*Sp.* ***Células escamosas***): flat and scaly epithelial cell

Status asthmaticus (*Sp.* ***Estado asmático***): severe asthmatic episode that does not respond to normal treatment

Steatorrhea (*Sp.* ***Esteatorrea***): the presence of malabsorbed fat in the feces

Stenosis, stenosed (*Sp.* ***Estenosis, estenosado***): narrowing of an opening

Stent (*Sp.* ***Stent***): a device used to hold tissue in place or provide support

Steri-Strips (*Sp.* ***Steri-Strips***): trademark for sterile adhesive strips used to approximate and hold together the edges of a wound

Stomatitis (*Sp.* ***Estomatitis***): an inflammatory condition of the mouth

Stress incontinence (*Sp.* ***Incontinencia por presión***): leakage of urine when stress is placed on the perineum

Stridor (*Sp.* ***Estridor***): a high-pitched respiratory sound caused by obstruction of air passageway

Subluxation (*Sp.* ***Subluxación***): partial dislocation

Substernal retraction (*Sp.* ***Retracción del esternón***): condition in which the chest wall under the sternum sinks in with each respiration

Sulfonylurea (*Sp.* ***Sulfonilurea***): oral hypoglycemic agent that stimulates the pancreas to produce insulin

Supine (*Sp.* ***Supino***): lying on the back

Surfactant (*Sp.* ***Agente de superficie***): an agent (normally present in the lungs as a phospholipid) that lowers surface tension; abnormal in the lungs of premature infants or in hyaline membrane disease

Symptomatic (*Sp.* ***Sintomático***): concerning the nature of a symptom indicative of a disease

Syncope (*Sp.* ***Síncope***): fainting, lightheadedness

Synovial (*Sp.* ***Sinovial***): pertaining to fluid around a joint

Synthesize (*Sp.* ***Sintetizar***): to produce a substance by combining two or more elements or chemicals

Tachycardia, tachycardic (*Sp.* ***Taquicardia, taquicárdico***): rapid heartbeat; more than 100 beats per minute

Tachypnea (*Sp.* ***Taquipnea***): rapid and shallow respirations

Tamponade (*Sp.* ***Tamponar***): compression of a part by pressure or a collection of fluid

Tendinitis (*Sp.* ***Tendinitis***): inflammation of a tendon

Tetany (*Sp.* ***Tetania***): hyperexcitability of nerves and muscles resulting from low serum calcium levels; a syndrome characterized by intermittent tonic spasms of the extremities, cramps, and convulsions

Tetralogy of Fallot (*Sp.* ***Tetralogía de Fallot***): a congenital cardiac condition

Thallium scan (*Sp.* ***Escáner con talio***): a cardiac stress test using intravenous thallium injection to diagnose ischemia and coronary artery disease

Thoracentesis (*Sp.* ***Toracentesis***): surgical puncture into the thoracic cavity to remove accumulated air or fluid

Thrill (*Sp.* ***Estremecimiento***): vibration felt on palpation, especially over the heart

Thrombocytopenia (*Sp.* ***Trombopenia***): reduced number of thrombocytes (platelets)

Thyroidectomy (*Sp.* ***Tiroidectomía***): surgical removal of the thyroid gland

Thyrotoxicosis (*Sp.* ***Thyrotoxicosis***): a toxic condition caused by hyperactivity of the thyroid gland

Tinnitus (*Sp. Tinnitus*): ringing in the ears

Tonometry (*Sp. Tonometría*): measurement of intraocular pressure

Toxin, toxic (*Sp. Toxina, tóxico*): poisonous substance

Toxoplasmosis (*Sp. Toxoplasmosis*): a disease caused by infection with protozoa found in many mammals and birds

Transcutaneous electrical nerve stimulation (TENS) (*Sp. Estimulación nerviosa eléctrica transcutánea*): electrical stimulation of nerves for relief of pain

Transferrin (*Sp. Transferrina*): globulin in blood serum that transports iron

Trousseau's phenomenon (*Sp. Fenómeno de Trousseau*): sign in which pressure applied to the upper arm produces muscular spasms, indicating latent tetany

Truss (*Sp. Braguero*): a device that holds a reduced hernia in place

Turgor (*Sp. Turgor*): normal tension in a cell that results in normal strength and tension of the skin

Tympanic membrane (*Sp. Membrana del tímpano*): eardrum

Tzanck test (*Sp. Análisis de Tzanck*): diagnostic test that examines the tissue of a lesion to determine the type of cell present

Ulcer, ulceration (*Sp. Úlcera, ulceración*): a crater-like sore on the skin or mucous membrane

Ultrasound diathermy (*Sp. Diatermia por ultrasonidos*): medical diathermy (heating of body tissue) using ultrasound

Uremia (*Sp. Uremia*): toxic condition of excessive waste products, protein, and nitrogen in the blood caused by renal insufficiency

Urodynamics (*Sp. Urodinámica*): study of the mechanics of urinary bladder, filling and emptying liquid

Urothelium (*Sp. Urotelio*): transitional epithelium in the wall of the bladder

Vaginismus (*Sp. Vaginismo*): a spasm of the muscles surrounding the vagina, causing painful contractions of the vagina

Valsalva maneuver (*Sp. Maniobra de Valsalva*): forced exhalation with the mouth and nose closed, causing increased intrathoracic pressure, slowing of the heart rate, increased venous pressure, and a reduced amount of return blood flow to the heart

Varicocele (*Sp. Varicocele*): a condition in which the veins in the scrotum near the testicles are swollen and enlarged

Vector (*Sp. Vector*): carrier of infectious agent of disease from one person to another (usually insects)

Venom (*Sp. Veneno*): poison secreted by an animal

Ventricular shift (*Sp. Desplazamiento ventricular*): lateral movement of one of the ventricles of the brain to one side caused by pressure on the other side

Vertex (*Sp. Vertex*): top of the head

Vesicle (*Sp. Vesícula*): a small blister-like elevation of the skin containing clear fluid

Vitrectomy (*Sp. Vitrectomía*): a surgical procedure that removes the contents of the vitreous chamber of the eye

Western blot test (*Sp. Prueba Western blot*): a laboratory blood test to identify and analyze specific protein antigens; sometimes used to confirm the validity of the ELISA test

Wheal (*Sp. Ampolla*): a smooth, round, elevated area of the skin with red edges and a white center, usually accompanied by itching; hives

White blood cell, white blood cell count (WBC) (*Sp. Glóbulos blancos, conteo de glóbulos blancos*): See Appendix 1, Common Laboratory and Diagnostic Tests, under Blood Analysis

Xerostomia (*Sp. Xerostomía*): dry mouth; reduced amount of saliva

Zygote (*Sp. Zigoto*): fertilized ovum

f, Figure; t table; b box.